I0882334

Carbon-Based Nanomaterials for Sustainable and Technological Applications

Carbon-Based Nanomaterials for Sustainable and Technological Applications covers the fundamentals of carbon-based nanomaterials (CNMs) and their potential for technological and industrial applications. Addressing recent advancements in technology and improvement in material synthesis, the book outlines how functionalized CNMs are used in nanobiotechnology, for active sorbent materials, and in pharmaceutical applications. Chapters cover macro-scale applications, biosensors and drug delivery, and treatment in cancer and coronavirus diseases.

Key features:

- Through up-to-date references, this book demonstrates that carbon-based nanomaterials are one of the most promising nanomaterials in medical applications, such as drug and gene delivery carriers, as well as nonmedical, environmental applications.
- Discusses the synthesis methods of processing (CQDs), (GQDs), (CPDs), and (g-C3N4) materials-based nanocomposites for biotechnological applications.
- Chapters address various classes of carbon nanomaterials and their innovative technologies.
- Opens up further exploration of environmental nanotechnology, bionanotechnology, and biomedical applications of novel carbon nanomaterials.
- Full references can be found via the Support Material: www.routledge.com/9781032635934.

Written by a leading expert, this volume provides the reader with thorough coverage of bionanotechnology and biomedical applications of novel carbon nanomaterials.

Carbon-Based Nanomaterials for Sustainable and Technological Applications

Loutfy H. Madkour
Professor, Tanta University, Egypt

CRC Press
Taylor & Francis Group
Boca Raton London New York

CRC Press is an imprint of the
Taylor & Francis Group, an **informa** business

Designed cover image: Shutterstock

First edition published 2025
by CRC Press
2385 Executive Center Drive, Suite 320, Boca Raton, FL 33431

and by CRC Press
4 Park Square, Milton Park, Abingdon, Oxon, OX14 4RN

CRC Press is an imprint of Taylor & Francis Group, LLC

ISBN: 978-1-032-63593-4 (hbk)
ISBN: 978-1-032-63596-5 (pbk)
ISBN: 978-1-032-63598-9 (ebk)

DOI: 10.1201/9781032635989

Typeset in Times
by Apex CoVantage, LLC

Access the Support Material: www.routledge.com/9781032635934

Contents

Preface

Carbon is a versatile element; there are three naturally occurring allotropes of carbon (diamond, amorphous carbon, and graphite). Specifically, researchers' attention exponentially increased after exploring new multidimensional fullerenes, carbon nanotubes (CNTs), and finally the synthesis of graphene (GR), because of their potential and technological applications. Carbon nanotubes (CNTs) are nanotechnology's utmost distinctive inventions. Carbon nanomaterials (CNMs) have attracted significant scientific and technological interest due to their unique structural characteristics and their excellent electronic, mechanical, and thermal properties. Based on these properties, they have been used in a wide range of applications, including fillers in composite materials, sensors, drug delivery systems, antibacterial agents, and others. Carbon is one of the most abundant elements on Earth. The ultimate goal of any technology is to improve the lifestyle of humans and their well-being. In today's 21st century, carbon nanomaterials (CNMs) are the most researched material, with worldwide investigation of the growing industry, due to their various properties for use in many applications, either in the medical field or in other potential applications. The applications of CNTs include various disciplines, like nanotechnology, transistors, nanomedicine, biosensors, bioimaging, actuators, and condensers. Carbon, which is the source of our lives, apart from our metabolic activities, attracts attention with its extraordinary structures created in nature. These structures are materials that are formed and discovered over time in the environment of high temperature and pressure. The chemical properties of these materials are very different from those of inert carbon. Conductivity, strength, and catalytic properties are only a few of the properties of carbon nanomaterials. This type of structure is also known as a fullerene. Nanomaterials are at the leading edge of the rapidly developing field of nanotechnology. Their unique size-dependent properties make these materials superior and indispensable in many areas of human activity. By taking advantage of these features, today's technology will have the ability to further develop products or make R&D increases. This, together with costs, can facilitate the development of technology. Depending on the purpose of use, carbon nanomaterials increase sensitivity by increasing surface area and conductivity, especially in diagnostic systems. A promising sub-branch of diagnostic systems has made great progress in recent years, creating an important area in the development of point-of-care diagnostic tests. This area is especially developed on the fundamentals of sensors, biosensors, and drug delivery nanotechnologies. The technology consists of a recognition agent placed on a physicochemical transducer.

Key Features

Some specific distinguishing features of the book that express what the reader will gain from the book (benefits) and how the book will deliver it (features):

- Provides insight into, with emphasis on, future trends to vision for life sciences regarding the synthesis processing and novel applications of carbon nanomaterials and nanodevices in industries, nanoscience, biomedical, and research laboratory.
- Addresses sustainable, cutting-edge, innovative technologies, studying, explaining, and discussing in detail the bright technologies of future-based carbon nanomaterial (CNMs) classes: CNTs, fullerene, and graphene derivatives.
- Describes the status of fundamentals and technical approaches in processing and behavior of carbon nanostructured materials to provide the readers systematic, comprehensive, and brief information in the challenging field of carbon nanomaterials (CNMs) with nanotechnology.
- Reviews recent advances of clear vision for the different allotropes of carbon related to device type, classification, new modification in synthesis, functionalization processing, properties, and novel promising applications of CNMs among the researchers.
- Describes the role and the biointerfaces behavior between biology systems and carbon nanoelectronics systems, with some examples of essential applications.
- Focuses on the novel applications of various forms of allotropic elemental carbon nanomaterials (fullerene, nanodiamond, graphite, carbon nanotubes [CNT], graphene) and two-dimensional transition metal dichalcogenides (2D TMDCs), discussed in detail, with examples of the different morphologies and corresponding applications for CNMs.
- Emphasizes the most promising systems of significant modification for the specific immobilization of enzymes attachment on carbon nanotubes without affecting their activity, which will give a solution to the problems and allows reusability by easing the process of separation, with respect to the techniques and innovative support materials employed for immobilization of biocatalysts that have potential implication with improved stability to various environmental factors on future enzyme market.
- Presents answers about the many scientific essentials and important questions throughout its chapters for all the various classes of carbon nanomaterials and their innovative daily applications in technologies.
- Generally, the book gives emphasis to current and future trends to vision for life sciences of synthesis processing and the novel applications of carbon nanomaterials and nanodevices in industries and research laboratory. Thus, the book is considered actually as

an essential academic and scientific updated reference book for sustainable and technological applications–based carbon nanomaterials (CNMs).

The book, titled *Carbon-Based Nanomaterials for Sustainable and Technological Applications*, is a compilation of eight chapters written by author Loutfy H. Madkour.

These chapters will cover the fundamentals of technical and cutting-edge, innovative advances in the nanobiotechnology of carbon-based nanomaterials (CBNMs):

1. Comprehensive Study of Carbon Nanomaterials-Based Nanostructured Materials: Potential for Technological and Industrial Applications
2. Progression in Synthesis Processing and Growth Mechanism of Carbon Nanomaterials for Advanced Macro-Scale Applications
3. Bionanotechnological Applications of Fullerene (C60)-Based Modified Development Imaging and Biosensing Devices
4. Computational Simulation Optimization and Pharmaceutical Role of CNTs-Based Development of New Target Drug Delivery Systems (DDSs) for Enhanced Efficacy in Anticancer Therapy
5. Cutting-Edge Nanobiotechnology in Advanced Drug Delivery Nanosystems for CNTs, Fullerenes, NDs, and Graphene-Based Materials
6. Bright Future of Carbon Nanomaterials for Cancer Nanomedicine-Based Enzyme Immobilization Conjugates
7. CNMs-Based Develped Biosensors for Rapid Technologies Detection of Antiviral Infection and the Management Coronavirus Markers
8. Insights on Carbon-Based Nanomaterials as Smart Nanosystems Platform for Cancer Theranostics Sustainable Technology

Carbon nanomaterials (CNMs) are widely used in the aerospace, automotive, and electronics industries because of their stability and enhanced metallic and electrical properties. CNTs are also being investigated for biomedical applications, such as in drug delivery systems and in biosensors. The application of CNTs to improve the performance of many products, especially in healthcare, has led to an occupational and public exposure to these nanomaterials. The production and applications of carbon-based nanomaterials (CBNMs) have gained speed in recent years. Carbon nanomaterials that can be found in different conformations with sp^2 hybridization can be extremely useful. These nanomaterials include nanotubes, graphene, carbon nanoparticles, carbon fibers, and fullerenes. Among these materials, fullerenes are nanomaterials that have gained speed in recent years due to their structure and unique properties. It is well acknowledged that CBNMs are a potential new class of nanomaterials for technological advancement. With the advancement in technology and improvement in material synthesis, functionalized CNMs are used in nanobiotechnology, for active sorbent materials, for environment sensing, and in renewable energy. In the past few decades, there has been an increasing amount of studies reported in carbon-based nanomaterials (CBNMs) (Figure FM.1) in the

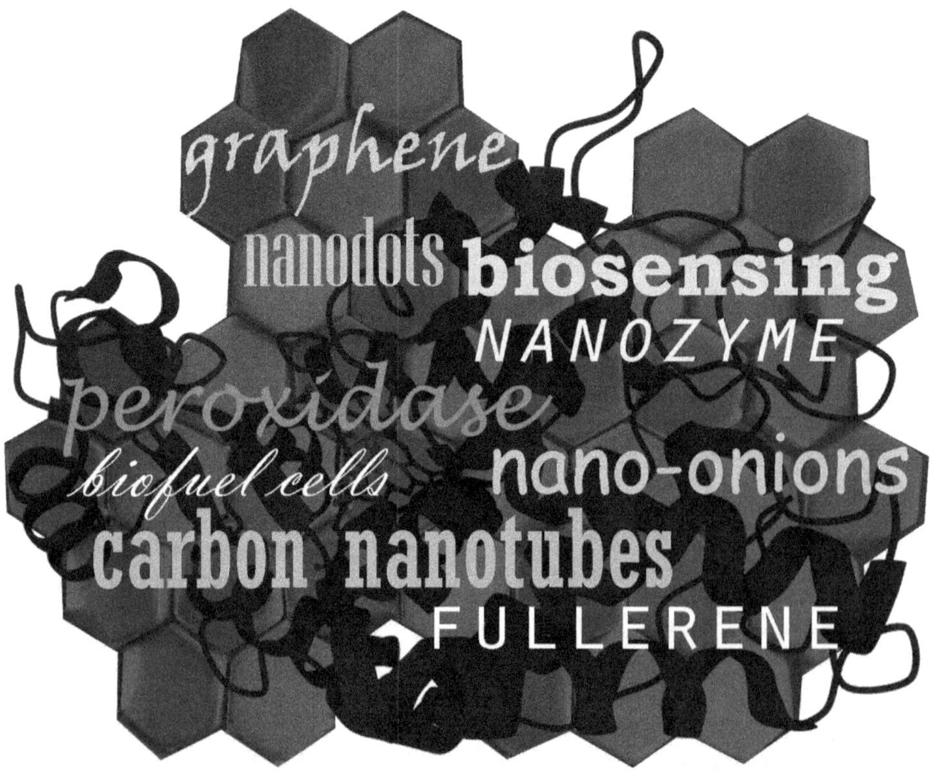

FIGURE FM.1

engineering of various interfaces to enhance the performance of current state-of-the-art devices.

CBNMs up to now are the most researched materials of the 21st century, with an international intention of growing industrial quantities due to their superior properties for use in many applications, either in medical or other potential industrial and environmental applications. Carbon-based nanomaterials are emerging as a new class of technological materials with numerous novel and useful properties. Different types of CNT delivery have been explored in various biomedical applications. The contents of the book are well-organized, where this book presents the current understanding about the roles and mechanisms of the fundamentals and technical approaches in processing and behavior of carbon nanostructured materials, to provide the readers systematic, comprehensive, and brief information in the challenging field of carbon nanomaterials (CNMs) with nanotechnology. CBNMs have attracted substantial research interest in bionanotechnology, rendered from its unique structure, electronic, mechanical, and optical properties. As CNTs have attracted the fancy of many scientists worldwide, the work beyond our expectations and their simple mechanism with long-lasting life makes it more reliable to use. The unique and unusual properties of these structures make them a unique material with a whole range of promising applications. CBNMs become increasingly popular in various fields simply because of their small size and amazing optical, electric, and magnetic properties when used alone or with the addition of metals. Carbon nanotubes (CNTs) are described as a cylindrical rolled graphene sheet. They are capped, with the end containing the pentagonal ring, and also cylindrical graphene with a diameter of 12 nm. The use of carbon nanostructures dates back to 1985, when the first carbon nanotube was discovered. Since this time, the field has undergone rapid development and will play an important role in the future of material and medical technology.

Carbon nanomaterials (CNMs) are engineered nanomaterials (ENMs) made with carbon. They show vast diversity in their structures and size, for example, fullerenes, graphene, carbon nanotubes (CNTs), nanocones, carbon dots, nanobeads, nanofibers, etc. These materials possess a high surface area and an enormous absorption potential. The properties of these materials can be further modified by introducing organic functional groups in the CNMs via covalent and non-covalent functionalization. The introduction of organic molecules changes the physical and chemical properties of the material. CNTs are allotropes of carbon with a nanostructure which is cylindrical in its shape. There are single-walled as well as double-walled nanotubes. They have many biological and biomedical applications not because of its small size alone but due to their remarkable optical, electric, and magnetic properties. They are promising candidates for targeted drug delivery as they can detect and deliver drugs to neoplastic cells. They are a new alternative and efficient tool for transport and translocation of therapeutic molecules as they have easy access to cytoplasm and nucleus without immunogenic response or toxicity. CNTs even serve as a very simple, rapid, sensitive, and electrical sensor.

CNMs are emerging as a new class of technological materials with numerous novel and useful properties. Different types of CNMs delivery have been explored in various biomedical applications. CNTs and their structured materials are likely to become important biomaterials in the near future due to their superior and unique characteristics over conventional biomaterials. Their electrical, optical, thermal, and spectroscopic properties make them unique for the detection of biomolecules, such as DNA, antigen–antibody, cells, and other biomolecules, thereby leading to great advancement in therapy. CNTs will find numerous applications as biomaterials and have important roles in the development of emerging technologies. It also acts as lubricant or glidants in the pharmaceutical industry for the manufacture of tablets. Carbon nanotubes (CNTs) have recently garnered interest in today's world of medicine and are being highly researched in the fields of efficient drug delivery and biosensing methods for disease treatment and health monitoring.

Nanotubes are categorized as single-walled carbon nanotubes (SWCNTs) and multiple-walled carbon nanotubes (MWCNTs). Various techniques have been developed to produce carbon nanotubes in sizeable quantities, including arc discharge, laser ablation, chemical vapor deposition, silane solution method, and flame synthesis method. Research on the properties and characteristics of CNTs has barely begun to tap into the potential of these structures.

The recent discovery of diverse kinds of carbon nanostructures has sparked interest in the potential applications of these materials in a variety of disciplines. Numerous distinct carbon nanotube (CNT) production methods have been developed, and their characterization, separation, and manipulation of individual CNTs are now possible. Structure, surface area, surface charge, size distribution, surface chemistry, aggregation state, and purity of the samples all have a significant impact on the reactivity of carbon nanotubes, as does the purity of the samples. Our book discusses the different types, structures, and properties of CNMs, as well as their synthesis and purification methods, how to functionalize CNTs, and their application in medicinal, pharmaceutical, and biomedical fields, toxicological properties and their assessment, as well as *in vivo* pharmacology and biodegradation pathways.

Despite the diverse potential applications, the integration of CNMs in biomedical research is one of the most challenging areas, where nanotubes fall under much scrutiny. Pristine nanotubes are highly hydrophobic and non-dispersible in most of the common aqueous and organic solvents, and to render nanotubes biocompatible, functionalization is one of the key prerequisites. In this regard, covalent and non-covalent functionalizations are the two widely adopted approaches for cotethering biologically active molecules on the CNTs. Likewise, the hollow cavity of the nanotube facilitates the endohedral encapsulation of biomolecules, peptides, DNA oligonucleotides, and proteins, thereby retaining the physiological attributes of the biological molecules.

Carbon nanomaterials have potential therapeutic applications in various fields, like drug delivery for API, diagnostics, and biosensing. Functionalized carbon nanotubes can also act as vaccine delivery systems. With the increasing interest shown by the nanotechnology research community in this field, it is expected that a lot of applications of carbon nanotubes are going to be explored in the future for medical as well as other file. These compounds have become increasingly popular in various fields simply because of their small size and amazing optical, electric, and magnetic properties when used alone or with the addition of metals. Carbon nanotubes have potential therapeutic applications in the field of drug delivery, diagnostics, and biosensing. In addition to the well-known crystallographic modifications, such as graphite and diamond, other allotropic carbon modifications, such as graphene-based nanomaterials and carbon nanotubes, have recently come to the fore. These carbon nanomaterials can be designed to help deliver or target drugs more efficiently and to innovate therapeutic approaches, especially for cancer treatment, but also for the development of new diagnostic agents for malignancies, and they are expected to help combine molecular imaging for diagnosis with therapies. The basic concept is to link the antigen to carbon nanotubes while retaining its conformation, thereby inducing antibody response with the right specificity. With the increasing interest shown by the nanotechnology research community in this field, it is expected that plenty of applications of CNTs will be explored in the future.

Over the last two decades, widespread research efforts have been conducted on CBNs as one of the most widely used classes of nanomaterials. Having their inherent mechanical, optical, electrochemical, and electrical properties, CBNs have been extensively used in multiple areas. In addition, owing to their versatile surface properties, sizes, and shapes, over the past decade, CBNs have drawn great attention in biomedical engineering. Interestingly, CBNs are becoming promising materials due to the existence of both inorganic semiconducting properties and organic π–π stacking characteristics. Hence, it could effectively interact with biomolecules and respond to light simultaneously, by taking advantage of such aspects in a single entity. The nanotubes of carbon are a widely considered allotropic carbon which has many unique properties. Carbon nanotubes and their related materials have many characteristic properties and applications, making them a suitable choice in the biomedical field, such as in tissue engineering, drug release, biosensors, and gene therapy. However, CNT toxicity has played an important role in various biomedical applications, which makes them difficult to use. There are many such aspects that lead to CNTs toxicity, such as agglomeration, size, impurities, and length.

This book concludes the different aspects and operations that influence the toxicity of carbon nanotubes. In this book, we have also covered the various applications of carbon nanotubes that are related to the biomedical field, biodistribution effects, and potential health-related deleterious effects that nanotubes may have during interactions with cultured cells and living organisms. Advances in the synthesis and scalable manufacturing of carbon-based nanomaterials (CBNMs) remain critical to realizing many important commercial applications.

Summary

Carbon nanomaterials (CNMs) are allotropes of carbon, made of graphite, and constructed in cylindrical tubes with nanometer in diameter and several millimeters in length. Their impressive structural, mechanical, and electronic properties are due to their small size and mass, their strong mechanical potency, and their high electrical and thermal conductivity. Among the various nanomaterials, carbon nanomaterials offer wide advantages due to their outstanding electrical, thermal, chemical, and mechanical properties. Carbon nanomaterials (CNMs) are found to have unique and promising substances due to their nanoscale diameter and high aspect ratio. Composite materials derived from carbon nanomaterials are used in energy storage and conversion, sensors, drug delivery, field emission, and nanoscale electronic components. Carbon nanotubes (CNTs) are cylindrical nano-sized structures made entirely out of carbon atoms. Each carbon atom is covalently bonded to three other carbon atoms, forming strong hexagonal structures from which the tube is made. Carbon nanotubes become increasingly popular in various fields simply because of their small size and amazing optical, electric, and magnetic properties when used alone or with the addition of metals. The electrical, optical, mechanical, and thermal properties of CNTs make them a very attractive material for the detection and therapy of cancers and other diseases. The unique properties of CNTs also enable them to efficiently deliver pDNA, siRNA, and miRNA. Even though these substances show anomalous properties, their commercialization is still limited due to their bundle- and layer-forming behavior, and hence, there is a need of functionalization in suitable position. The functionalized carbon nanomaterials (*f*-CNMs) have outstanding mechanical, electrical, dispersion, solubilization, and biological functions.

This book, in which a wide range of research studies, especially from the last years till now, is discussed, is an update on the previous work regarding advanced nanobiotechnology of carbon-based nanomaterials (CBNMs). A *CNT* is considered as a cylinder formed by rolling up a graphene sheet with caps which are similar to parts of the fullerenes and exhibits extraordinary strength and unique electrical properties and is an efficient conductor of heat [1]. The diameters of single-walled carbon nanotubes (SWNTs) and multi-walled carbon nanotubes (MWNTs) are typically 0.8–2 nm and 5–20 nm, respectively, although MWNT diameters can exceed 100 nm. Individual CNT walls can be metallic or semiconducting, depending on the orientation of the lattice with respect to the tube axis, which is called chirality. Fullerenes (also called buckyballs) are molecules of varying sizes composed entirely of carbon that take on the form of hollow spheres or ellipsoids. Fullerenes were the subject of intense research in the 1990s, both because of their unique chemistry and for their technological applications, especially in materials science, electronics, and nanotechnology. Graphyne is a one-atom-thick planar sheet of sp- and sp^2-bonded carbon atoms arranged in a crystal lattice. It can be seen as a lattice of benzene rings connected by acetylene bonds. Graphyne has been a theorized allotrope of carbon for a long time and attracted great attention after the discovery of graphene [2]. CFs are a long thin strand of materials about 5–10 μm in diameter and composed mostly of carbon atoms that are bonded together in microscopic crystals aligned parallel to the long axis of the fiber [3]. The crystal alignment makes the fiber incredibly strong for its size. Several thousand CFs are twisted together to form a yarn, which may be used by itself or woven into a fabric. The yarn or fabric is combined with epoxy and wound or molded into shape to form various composite materials. CFs-reinforced composite materials are used in many areas, including spacecraft parts, racing car bodies, golf club shafts, bicycle frames, fishing rods, automobile springs, sailboat masts, and other components where light weight and high strength are needed. Other carbon-based materials include glassy (or vitreous) carbon, a class of carbon widely used as an electrode material in electrochemistry as well as in prosthetic devices and high-temperature crucibles; pure atomic and diatomic carbon; and linear acetylenic carbon, a one-dimensional carbon polymer with the structure single bond $(C{=}C)_n$ [4].

This book reviews the emerging synthesis, characterization, and growth properties for new macro-scale applications of CNTs and discusses the perspectives and obstacles of these promising nanomedicinal approaches. The book focuses on carbon nanomaterials (CNMs) synthesis, functionalization, characteristics, pharmacokinetics, toxicity, biosafety, and applications (Figure FM.2) [5]. The book reviews the emerging synthesis, characterization, and growth properties of new macro-scale applications of carbon nanomaterials (CNMs) and discusses the perspectives and obstacles of these promising industrial and nanomedicinal approaches.

In general, the book will be satisfying the following criteria:

1. A comprehensive classification and characterization study of carbon nanomaterials (CNMs)–based nanostructured materials
2. Production and main processing synthesis methods for tuning the technological strategies on carbon nanomaterials (CNMs)
3. Applications of fullerenes for the development of biosensors-based modified biosensing devices in bionanotechnology
4. Quantum and computational molecular dynamics simulation optimization studies of CNMs-based development of new targeted strategies for drug delivery systems (DDSs)
5. Applications of CNTs, fullerenes, NDs, and graphene for the development of nanobiotechnology in advanced drug delivery nanosystems

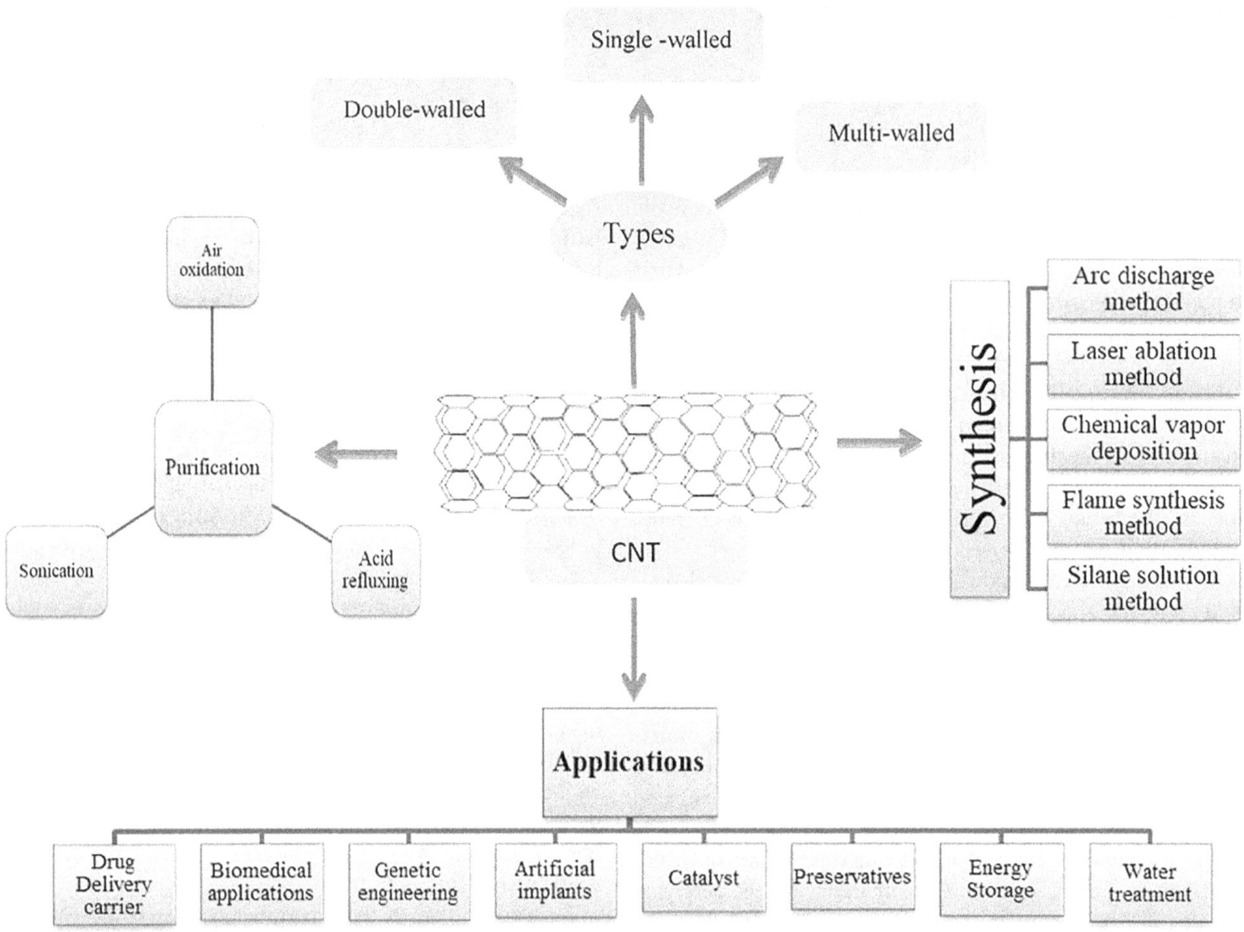

FIGURE FM.2

6. Enzyme immobilization conjugates studies-based CNMs aiming for bright future therapy and theranostic approach in cancer treatment
7. Developing new technologies for the treatment of antiviral infection and the management of coronavirus diseases
8. Applications studies of carbon-based nanomaterials (CBNMs) as smart nanostructured materials for sustainable technological approach in cancer theranostics platform

In conclusion, this book is very important and essential for all areas of study within nanotechnology and advanced nanoelectronics materials in public health, industry, nanotoxicology, environmental chemistry, and pollution. The book is an essential and very important topic for research, the environmental industry, and/or in teaching. The book answers many essential and important questions throughout its chapters for all various classes of carbon nanomaterials and their daily innovative industrial applications and research technologies. The book gives emphasis to the present and future novel applications of carbon nanomaterials and nanodevices in industries and research laboratory technological applications.

In general, more research is needed on the field of "sustainable innovative technologies–based carbon nanomaterials (CNMs)."

Finally, we would like to thank the editor, all reviewers, and all the CRC publishing editorial board members' team for their invaluable contributions and for the professional assistance and support.

BIBLIOGRAPHY

[1] Baughman, R.H., A.A. Zakhidov, W.A. de Heer, Carbon nanotubes—the route toward applications, *Science* 297 (5582) (2002) 787–792.
[2] Enyashin, A.N., A.L. Ivanovskii, Graphene allotropes, *Phys. Status Solidi B* 248 (8) (2011) 1879–1883.
[3] Hiremath, N., J. Mays, G. Bhat, Recent developments in carbon fibers and carbon nanotube-based fibers: A review, *Polym. Rev.* 57 (2) (2017) 339–368.
[4] Hoffmann, R., A.A. Kabanov, A.A. Golov, D.M. Proserpio, Homo citans and carbon allotropes: For an ethics of citation, *Angew. Chem.* 55 (37) (2016) 10962–10976.
[5] Jha, Roopali, Amit Singh, P.K. Sharma, Neeraj Kumar Fuloria, Smart carbon nanotubes for drug delivery system: A comprehensive study, *J. Drug Deliv. Sci. Technol.* 58 (August 2020) 101811.

Author

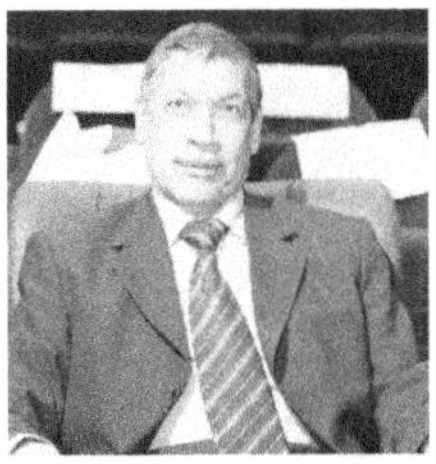

Loutfy H. Madkour is a professor of physical chemistry and nanoscience at Tanta University, Egypt. He received his BSc, MSc, and PhD in physical chemistry from the Cairo, Minia, and Tanta Universities in Egypt, respectively. He has published 200 peer-reviewed original research articles, 26 review articles, 12 books, and 5 book chapters. His name has been listed in the top 2% of the most distinguished and influential scientists globally according to the ranking and database of Stanford American University of Scientists. He is an editorial board member of several international journals, including the *International Journal of Industrial Chemistry* (IJIC-Springer), *International Journal of Ground Sediment & Water, Global Drugs and Therapeutics, Chronicles of Pharmaceutical Science, Journal of Targeted Drug Delivery, UPI Journal of Pharmaceutical, Medical and Health Sciences, Global Journal of Nanomedicine, Clinical Pharmacology and Toxicology Research, Journal of Pharmacology & Pharmaceutical Research, LOJ Pharmacology & Clinical Research, CPQ Medicine, Pharmaceutical Sciences & Analytical Research Journal, Japan Journal of Research, Organic & Medicinal Chemistry International Journal, Nanotechnology & Applications, Materials Science Journal, Journal of Chemical Science and Chemical Engineering, United Journal of Nanotechnology and Medicine, Clinical Practice (Therapy), Journal of Materials New Horizons, Journal of Radiology and Medical Imaging* (MedDocs Publishers), *World Journal of Pharmacy and Pharmaceutical Sciences, Journal of Material Science and Technology Research, Ecronicon: EC Clinical & Medical Case Reports (ECCMC), Medical Research and Health Sciences*, and *Acta Scientific Women's Health Journal, PHARMACOGNOSY Journal, Journal of Community Medicine and Health Care Management, Environmental Degradation of Materials of Frontiers in Materials, Journal of Cancer Therapy and Research, Journal of Materials and Polymer Science, Journal of Clinical and Biomedical Investigation, Radiology & Imaging Journal, International Journal in Pharmaceutical Sciences (IJPS), EC Clinical and Medical Case Reports, BOHR International Journal of Pharmaceutical Studies (BIJOPS), General medicine and Clinical Practice, Journal of Gastroenterology Hepatology and Digestive Disorders, International Journal of Organic and Inorganic Chemistry, ACTA SCIENTIFIC PHARMACEUTICAL SCIENCES, Medvix Publications LLC, International Journal of Cardiology Research & Reviews, International Journal of Nursing Care and Research, International Journal of Medical Science and Clinical Invention (IJMSCI) and Universal Library of Chemistry* (https://ulopenaccess.com/ulpages/editorialboardUlche).

1

Comprehensive Study of Carbon Nanomaterials-Based Nanostructured Materials: Potential for Technological and Industrial Applications

1.1 Background of Carbon-Based Nanostructured Materials

Carbon-based nanomaterials (CBNMs) are considered as one of the ideal materials, due to their high surface area, high aspect ratio, and impressive material properties, such as mechanical strength, and thermal and electrical conductivity, for the manufacture of next-generation composite materials. In spite of the mentioned attractive features, however, they tend to agglomerate due to their inherent chemical structure, which limits their application. CNMs are a subject of interest for several researchers and industrialists for their remarkably unprecedented and versatile functionalities.

This chapter seeks to provide a comprehensive review on the structure, characterization, synthesis, properties, functionalization, classification, and promising technological applications of carbon-based nanomaterials (CBNMs). Carbon nanotubes are discussed in this chapter in terms of characters, history, structures, properties, synthesis, purification, characterization methods, toxicity, and applications. The purification of nanotubes includes many techniques: acid treatment, oxidation, annealing, ultrasonication, cutting, magnetic purification, chromatography techniques. Further functionalization enhanced the water solubility of CBNMs and completely transformed their biocompatibility profile. Predictive analysis of the behavior is difficult without detailed knowledge of the differences between various carbon nanomaterials and their surface functionalization, thus leaving the selection process to traditional trial-and-error work. The present characterization fills this knowledge gap for carbon nanomaterial surface properties with respect to chemical states and functionalization. In fact, 1 nm (nanometer) is a billionth of a meter, that is, 1 nm = 10^{-9} m = 10 Å (Scheme 1.1).

The most commonly adopted method of classification is based on their dimension, as shown in Scheme 1.2 (https://doi.org/10.1016/B978–0–12–821713–9.00011–1).

Carbon nanotubes (CNTs) have recently garnered interest in today's world for biomedical applications and are being highly researched in the fields of efficient drug or gene delivery system in therapeutics and biosensing methods for disease treatment and health monitoring.

1.1.1 Structure of Carbon Nanotubes (CNTs)

An understanding of SWNT structure requires familiarity with the concept of nanotube chirality, since the chirality of an SWNT dictates many of its properties. The chirality map, illustrated in Scheme 1.3, has been developed as a tool for understanding chirality and its implications.

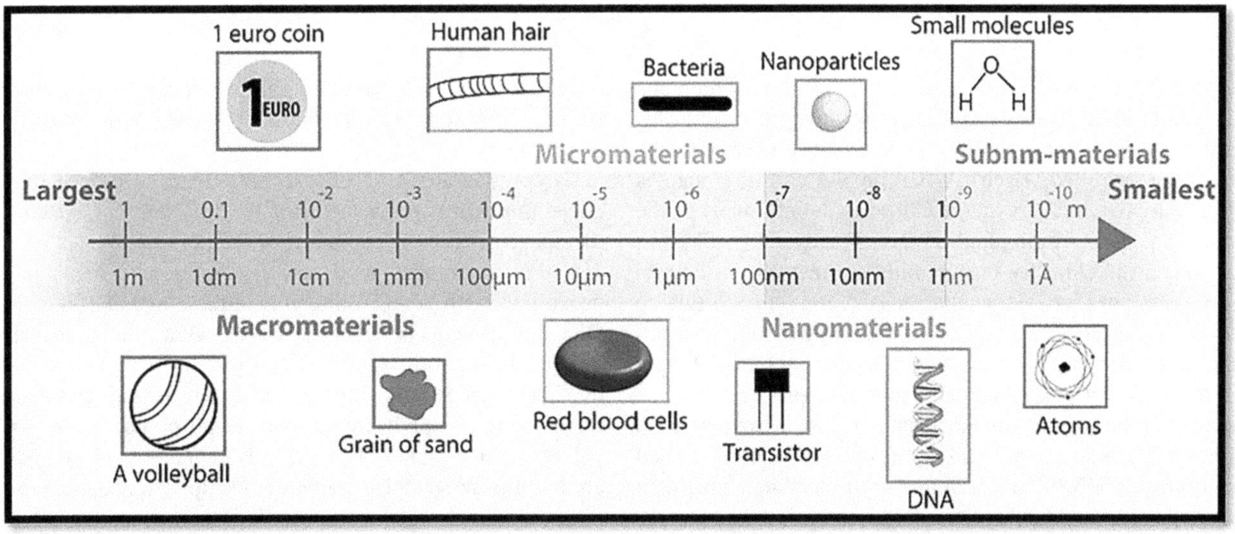

SCHEME 1.1 Nanomaterials range.

DOI: 10.1201/9781032635989-1

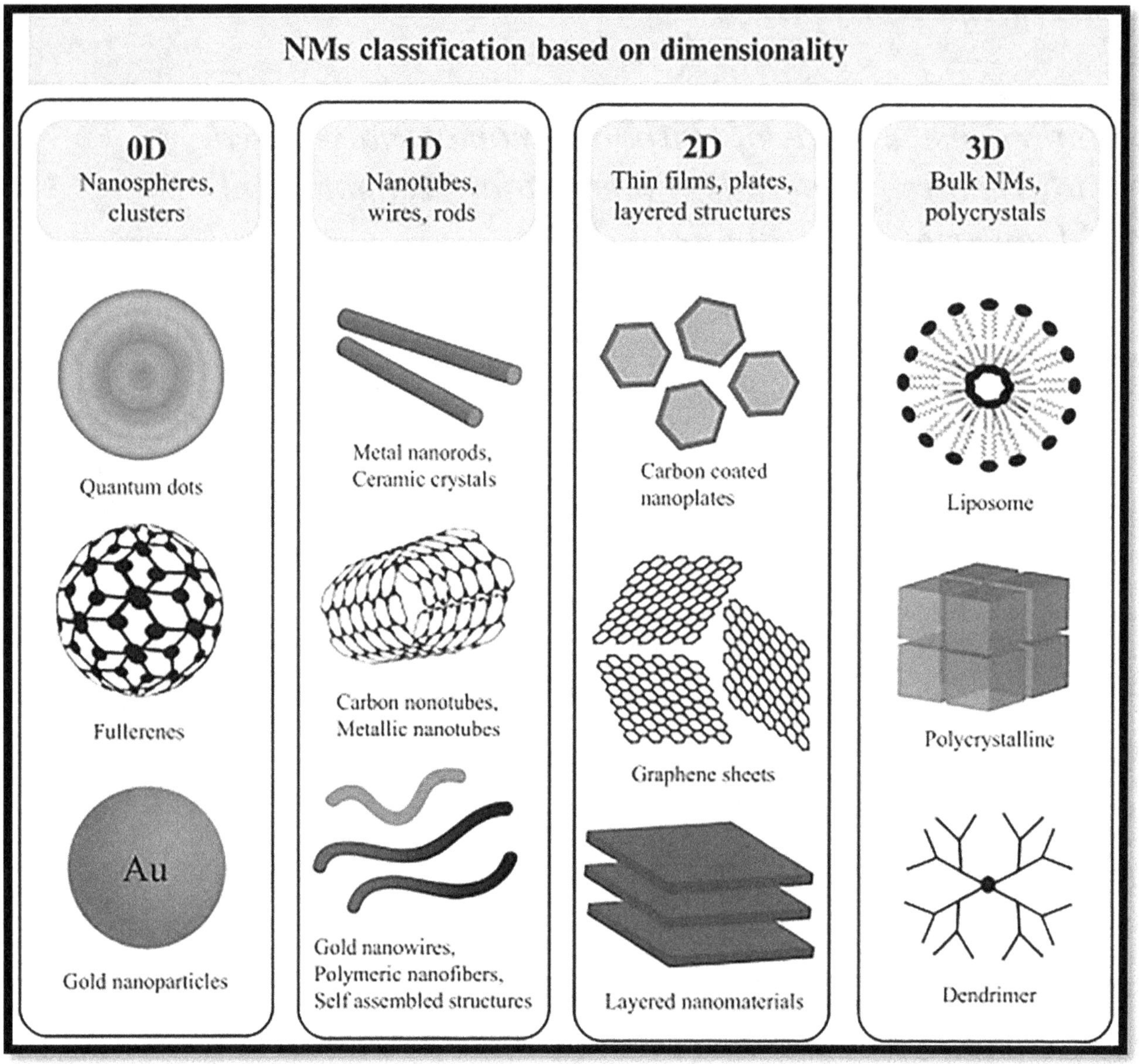

SCHEME 1.2 Classifications of nanomaterials.

An SWNT can be envisioned as a sheet of graphene one atom thick rolled into a tube (inset in Scheme 1.3). The chirality describes both the orientation and diameter to which the sheet is rolled. Each SWNT on the chirality map is defined by two integers (n, m). Chirality defines many of the properties of the individual SWNT. For example, SWNTs shown on the chirality map in blue are metallic in nature. These are tubes where $n = m$ (armchair) or $n - m = 3i$ (where i is any integer). Those depicted in yellow are semiconducting, displaying different bandgaps depending on the length of the chiral vector. Another significant property of carbon nanotube is carrying electricity so that it carries 1,000 times more than copper and silver do. Most single-walled nanotubes (SWNT) have a diameter of close to 1 nm, with a tube length that can be many millions of times longer [1]. Chemical functionalization is a new, promising approach that enlarges the application field of CNTs by developing novel nanomaterials based on value added by several materials to CNT armature that can be realized by the means of multiple strategies.

Carbon nanotubes (CNTs), in particular, have been introduced in pharmacy and medicine for drug delivery system in therapeutics since the beginning of the 21st century.

Carbon nanotubes tend to have impressive mechanical properties, with Young's modulus in the range of 100–1,000 GPa and strengths between 2.5 and 3.5 GPa. Nanotubes have a diameter ranging from 1 to 100 nm and lengths of up to millimeters. Their densities can be as low as ~1.3 g/cm^3, and their Young's moduli are superior to all carbon fibers with valves greater than 1 TPa [2]. CNTs have received much attention from scientific communities up to this date mainly because of their superior properties, such as having a wide bandgap, high melting point, high tensile strength, and high thermal conductivity.

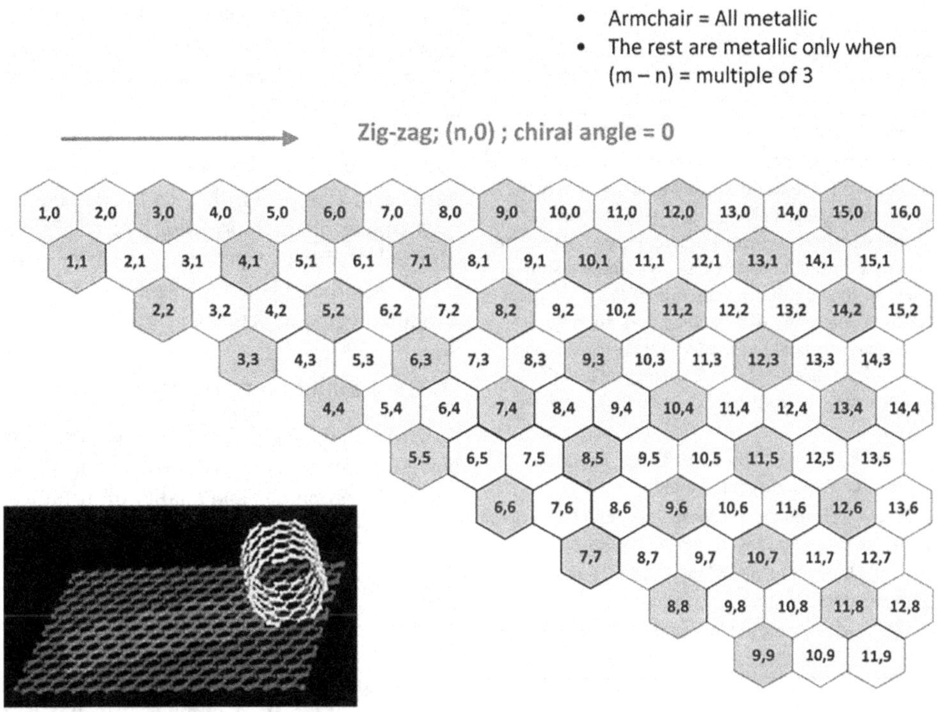

SCHEME 1.3 A graphic displaying chirality map which shows the various types of SWNTs that can be formed. The properties are governed by the way in which they are rolled, as shown in the inset. The SWNT will be metallic in the armchair configuration or when m-n is a multiple of 3.

CNTs have extremely high tensile strength (≈150 GPa, more than 100 times that of stainless steel), high modulus (≈1 TPa), large aspect ratio, low density (1,100–1,300 kg/m^3, one-sixth of that of stainless steel), good chemical and environmental stability, high thermal conductivity (3,000 W/m/K, comparable to diamond), and high electrical conductivity (comparable to copper) [3]. Carbon nanotubes have various applications, like electrodes for electrochemical double-layer capacitors, field emitters, nanoelectronic devices, hydrogen storage, functional polymers, etc.

Recently, strong and stretchable CNT fibers were spun from 0.65 mm long CNT forests which have the strength and Young's modulus of 1.91 GPa and 330 GPa, respectively. SWCNT/PVA composite fibers are tougher than any natural or synthetic organic fiber described so far. Carbon nanotubes bulk production in an economical way is the route for the feasibility of these applications. For large-scale production of carbon nanotubes, contrast chemical vapor deposition (CVD) has been proven to be a preferred route [4].

1.2 History of Carbon Nanotube Composites

CNTs can be assumed to have a history of approximately 30 years, as you can see in Table 1.1.

1.2.1 History of Fullerenes (C_{60})

Fullerene consists of curved pentagons and hexagons that form a fused structure. Pioneering studies (Table 1.2) on fullerene discovery were carried out between 1983 and 1990.

TABLE 1.1
Historical Progress of CNTs

Date	Event
1952	Carbon nanofilaments were observed.
1958	Dense bamboo structure of carbon nanofilaments was reported.
1960	The graphite layer was synthesized.
1976	The production of carbon nanofibers (CNF) was carried out via chemical vapor deposition.
1991	MWCNTs were reported and explained.
1993	SWCNTs were synthesized.

1.3 Characterization of CNTs

The following are the methods that are currently used for the characterization of CNTs:

- RAMAN spectroscopy—suitable for the quick and reliable screening of the presence of SWCNT.
- Transmission electron microscopy (TEM)—assessment of detailed structures.
- Scanning electron microscopy (SEM)—provides an overview of sample structures and is less sensitive to sample preparation and homogeneity than TEM.
- Thermogravimetric analysis—gives information about the relative abundance of catalyst particles, nanotubes, and other carbonaceous structures.
- Electron energy loss spectroscopy.
- High-resolution transmission electron microscopy.

TABLE 1.2
Historical Progress of Fullerene

Date	Event
1966	D. E. H. Jones thought of the structure of a giant fullerene.
1970	Osawa proposed the spherical Ih-symmetric (the construction of *Ih* symmetrical fullerenes from pentagons) soccer ball structure for the first C_{60} molecule. Twelve pentagons are sufficient and necessary to form a fullerene cage. According to this structural feature of fullerenes, we propose a simple and efficient method for the construction of *Ih* symmetrical fullerenes from pentagons. This method does not require complicated mathematical knowledge; yet it provides an excellent paradigm for students to learn the construction of molecular structures manually and develop their spatial visualization.
1984	It was observed that large carbon clusters (Cn) could be obtained via laser evaporation of graphite.
1985	Kroto and Smalley proved the existence of C_{60} and C_{70}, which can be produced under specific clustering conditions.
1990	Krätschmer and Huffman identified the C_{60}'s absorption line in laboratory analogs of interstellar powders.
2010	Fullerenes (C_{60}) were discovered in a cloud of cosmic dust at 6,500 light-years away.

Thermogravimetric analysis, scanning electron microscopy, transmission electron microscopy, atomic force microscopy, Raman spectroscopy, infrared spectroscopy, and nuclear magnetic resonance have been used. While TEM, SEM, and AFM have been used for the majority part to qualitatively ascertain the widespread structural studies of carbon nanotubes, infrared spectroscopy, Raman spectroscopy, and nuclear magnetic resonance spectroscopy have been used to authenticate the presence of useful moiety on carbon nanotubes. All procedures have advantages when used in combination with other techniques.

1.3.1 Transmission Electron Microscopy (TEM)

The internal microstructure and crystal structure of samples, which are thin enough to transmit electrons, can be analyzed with TEM. It is used to measure outer and inner radius and linear absorption coefficient for CNT studies [5], the effects of nitrogen doping in MWNTs, and SWNT peapod structures, to name a few, which can be investigated by TEM. It also identifies various layers of MWCNTs and separates SWNTs from the bundles. Electron diffraction and electron energy loss spectroscopy (EELS), along with TEM, have the advantage that the average helicity and local variation of helicity in individual SWNT and ropes of SWNTs can be determined on the nanoscale.

1.3.2 Scanning Electron Microscopy (SEM)

This is one of the main surface analysis instruments. It is used in the preliminary evaluation of CNT morphology. It can measure the diameter of CNT, not precisely, but roughly. In its conventional situation, the technique is controlled by its incapacity to set apart catalyst and carboniferous impurities from CNTs. However, the metallic content of CNT samples is customarily quantifiable by SEM tied with an energy-dispersive X-ray analysis detector (SEM-EDX).

Despite the consequences, SEM is perhaps the only technique that will give data on each CNT structural information and also the metal impurity content was shown in Abdulkareem and Afolabi (2007).

It provides a summary of sample constituents though not as much of susceptible to preparation of sample and its homogeneity than TEM. This is often being used in the prior assessment of the morphology of CNT. SEM is presumably the only method capable of providing information on both CNT metallic impurity content and morphology as shown in Abdulkareem and Afolabi (2007).

1.3.3 Raman Spectroscopy

For the characterization of carbon-based materials, Raman spectroscopy is an equally valuable method and is applied to study the properties and quality of metallic, superconducting, and pristine phases of graphite intercalation compound and solids based on fullerene [5]. Inelastic light scattering from nanotubes causes an increase or decrease in an incident light energy because of the emission or absorption of the photon, thereby resulting in scattering, known as Raman scattering [5]. This technique gives information with details about the configuration of CNTs. A number of walls, the presence of crystalline and amorphous carbon, and the diameter of SWNTs can be determined with Raman spectroscopy.

1.3.4 Proton Nuclear Magnetic Resonance (Proton NMR)

H1-NMR is used to analyze the synthesis of and as well as attaching the functional group to CNTs. The H1-NMR of functionalized CNTs is portrayed by wide peaks for protons close to the CNT, fitting sharper with separation. H1-NMR has been accustomed to analyze the synthesis and attachment of functional moiety to CNTs.

1.3.5 Absorption Spectroscopy (UV, Vis, and IR)

IR spectroscopy is often used to determine impurities remaining from synthesis or molecules capped on the CNT surface. Numerous works are performed on organic molecules and CNTs: IR spectroscopy exhibits all the modification of the CNTs structure and reveals the nature of compounds added to the CNTs. The difference is in the catalytic activity performance between CNTs activated carbon and graphite samples in the oxidative dehydrogenation of ethylbenzene. The highest catalytic activity is obtained with MWCNTs which are oxidized before the catalytic experiments. The possibilities of the use of CNTs for catalytic removal of NOx (NO, NO_2, NO_3) were also investigated by FT-IR [5]. For a correct characterization of CNTs, all these techniques described herein cannot be used individually but must be used in complementary ways.

1.3.6 Thermal Analysis (TGA/DTG)

Thermal analysis methods are useful for identifying relative changes due to processing. It is used to study the degree of CNTs purification [5]. Thermal gravimetric analysis (TGA) and derivative thermal gravimetric (DTG) analysis methods control the oxidation process, which gives quantitative data on the weight fractions of carbon and metal catalysts in the sample, and the temperatures of bulk oxidation events [5]. It is fundamentally a subjective instrument acclimated set up useful gatherings and furthermore the idea of their connection to CNT sidewalls. Very surprising functional moieties retain characteristic frequencies of IR radiation, offering prompt fingerprint recognition of bonds. It is a harmonizing technique for magnetic resonance to substantiate the presence of bonds between CNTs and coupled moieties.

The high sensitivity of the TGA, which is in the order of 0.1 mg/min, acceptable weight loss determinations at a given heating rate, within a short time, without overwhelming too much material. The oxidation rates of carbon nanotubes measured in air at atmospheric pressure within the TGA are exceptional for each CNT sample of diverse wall thicknesses. This analysis is being implemented to quantitatively ascertain the concentration of carbonaceous and non-carbonaceous materials present in bulk samples of CNT, the homogeneity, and thermal stability of CNT. It also provides data on the comparative abundance of nanotubes, catalytic constituent part, and additional carbonaceous structures.

1.3.7 Atomic Force Microscopy (AFM)

Among the current microscopy methods, AFM is the most widely employed method of characterization. The comprehensive use of AFM is attributed to the short time in three-dimensional sample topography by means of atomic resolution, for a relatively low price. This method also provides us with information on the nanotube's length and an estimated assessment on the diameter of bundles.

1.3.8 Elemental Analysis

The elemental analysis of raw purified MWCNTs depicted carbon and hydrogen content in nanotubes. The purification of raw MWCNTs allowed the elimination of some catalyst impurities in oxidized form, and also, raw MWCNTs could be functionalized with some oxygen-containing groups, like –COOH groups and –OH groups, which would be later confirmed by elemental analysis [5].

1.3.9 X-Ray Diffraction (XRD)

This technique is used to obtain some information on the interlayer spacing, the structural strain, the impurities, the SWNT bundles, and several layers of MWNTs and allows morphological information for an unlimited number of crystals [5]. In an X-ray diffraction system, electrons emitted from the filament (cathode) are accelerated to target (anode), and X-ray characteristics of atoms in the irradiated area are emitted. By analyzing their energy, the atoms can be identified, and by counting the emitted X-ray number, the atom concentration in the specimen can be determined. X-ray diffraction (XRD) is mostly used for bulk structure analysis. However, if the concentration of the active component is large enough, it can be appropriate for size determination. Quantitatively, a number average size is obtained from the following equation [5].

$$d = \frac{0.85\lambda}{(B^2 - b^2)^{1/2=\cos\theta}}$$

Where b = value for a well-crystallized specimen, and λ = wavelength.

1.4 Classification of the Categories of Carbon Nanotube Types and Their Properties

Elemental carbon displays a complex allotropy, depending on the nature of hybridization: diamond (sp^3 hybridized), graphite, graphene, fullerenes, and carbon nanotubes (sp^2 hybridized). Graphite is the most common allotrope of carbon, and the word *graphite* in Greek means "to write." *Graphene*, an acronym for the 2D-layered graphite, is the mother of all carbon materials as shown in Geim and Novoselov (2007), as a graphene sheet can be wrapped to form 0D fullerenes, rolled to form 1D nanotubes, or stacked to form 3D graphite, as depicted in Figure 1.1. The unearthing of "ground-breaking experiments regarding the two-dimensional material graphene" by Geim and Novoselov in 2010 heralded graphene as the next-generation carbon material was shown in Novoselov, Geim, Morozov (2004).

1. *Zigzag.* Named after the pattern of the hexagon as one moves circumferentially around the body of the tubule.
2. *Chiral.* Most commonly occurring SWNT. *Chiral* means "handedness" and indicates that the tubes may twist in either direction.
3. *Armchair.* Describes one of the two conformers of cyclohexane, a hexagon of carbon atoms, and describes the shape of the hexagons as one moves around the body of the tubules.

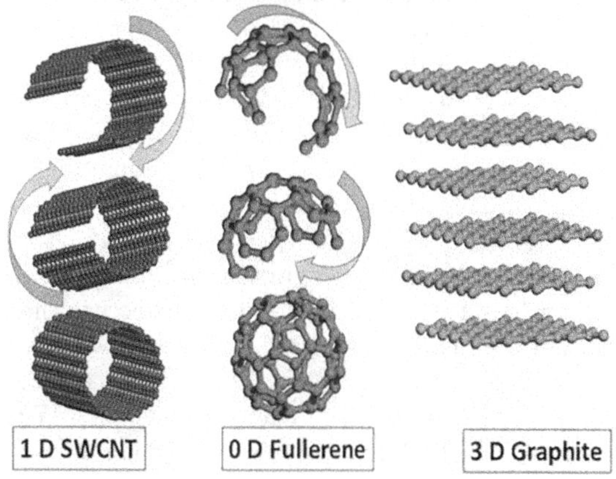

FIGURE 1.1 Formation of SWCNT, fullerene, and graphite from a single graphene monolayer.

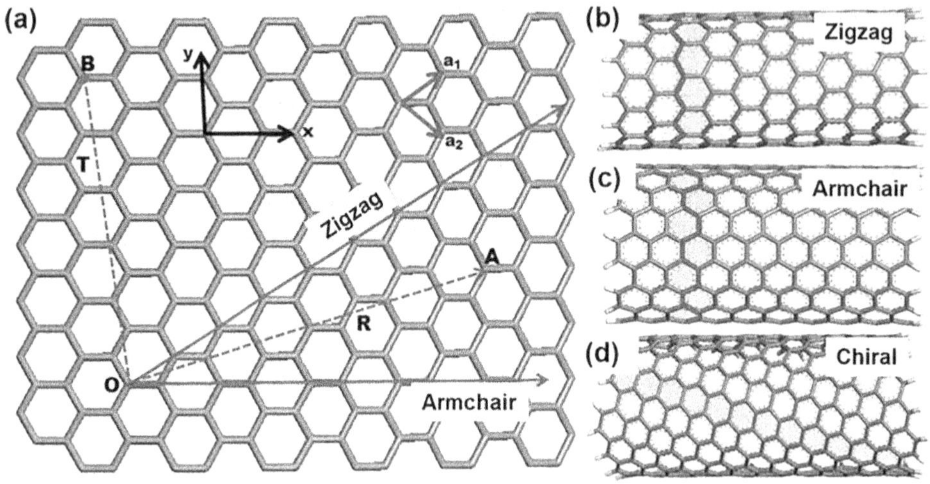

FIGURE 1.2 (a) A graphene sheet depicting (b) zigzag, (c) armchair, and (d) chiral CNT based on the rolling of carbon atoms along chiral vectors through the circumference (OA) of a nanotube.

CNTs are hexagonally arranged, honeycombed lattice of carbon atoms formed by the rolling of graphene into seamless cylindrical structures (see Figure 1.2a). Nanotubes like graphene have a high diameter-to-length ratio (aspect ratio) and demonstrate high electrical, mechanical, and thermal conductivity along with structural stability. CNTs are broadly classified as single-wall CNTs (SWCNTs) and multi-wall CNTs (MWCNTs). SWCNTs comprise of a single graphene sheet with diameter ~0.5–1.5 nm and length of ~100 µm, while MWCNTs are formed from the coaxial stacking of SWCNTs with diameter ~1.4–100 nm, length between 1 nm and 1 µm, and internuclear distance of 0.3–0.4 nm between the coaxial tubes. The representation of a zigzag ($m = 0$), armchair ($n = $ m), and chiral ($n \neq$ m) nanotube is depicted in Figure 1.2b-d. The (n, m) indices render remarkable electronic properties to the CNTs, and the sp^2 hybridization along the tubular axis makes it chemically inert by nature.

The unique electronic properties exhibited by CNT are governed by the quantum confinement of electrons, where the periodic boundary conditions come into play. Hence, a detailed *in vivo* and *in vitro* toxicity analysis is mandatory in understanding CNT-based therapeutic regimes for sustained drug delivery applications.

Based on the structure of the wall, carbon nanotubes (CNTs) are of following two types. These are single-walled carbon nanotubes (SWNTs) and multi-walled carbon nanotubes (MWNTs). The classifications of CNTs are described in Figure 1.3 [6].

The various features of SWNTs and MWNTs are described in Figure 1.4.

SWCNTs consist of a single graphene cylinder with diameter varying between 0.4 and 2 nm and usually occur as hexagonal close-packed bundles. MWCNTs consist of two to several coaxial cylinders, each made of a single graphene sheet surrounding a hollow core. The outer diameter of MWCNTs ranges from 2 to 100 nm, while the inner diameter is in the range of 1–3 nm, and their length is 0.2 to several μm.

The differences between the two classes are highlighted in Figure 1.5, and they affect their solubility and dispersion both in surfactants and in other common solvents. Ideally, chiral vector C with indices (n, m) is employed to categorize SWCNTs into zigzag, armchair, and chiral. Zigzag and armchair structures are obtained when (n, 0) or $m = 0$ and $n = m$, respectively, while chiral nature exists when $n > m > 0$ [7]. Given that SWCNTs are combined to form MWCNTs, their individual optical, chemical, mechanical, and thermal properties dictate the potential applications of MWCNTs.

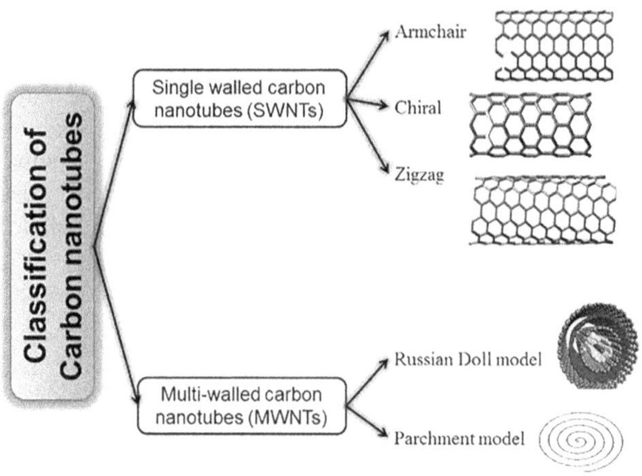

FIGURE 1.3 Classifications of CNTs.

Nanotubes may indeed be alienated into various classifications based upon the number of sheets of graphene existent in the CNTs. Carbon nanotubes are classified into the following three types:

- Single-walled carbon nanotubes (SWCNTs)
- Double-walled CNTs
- Multiple-walled carbon nanotubes (MWCNTs)

We discuss some details for the three types.

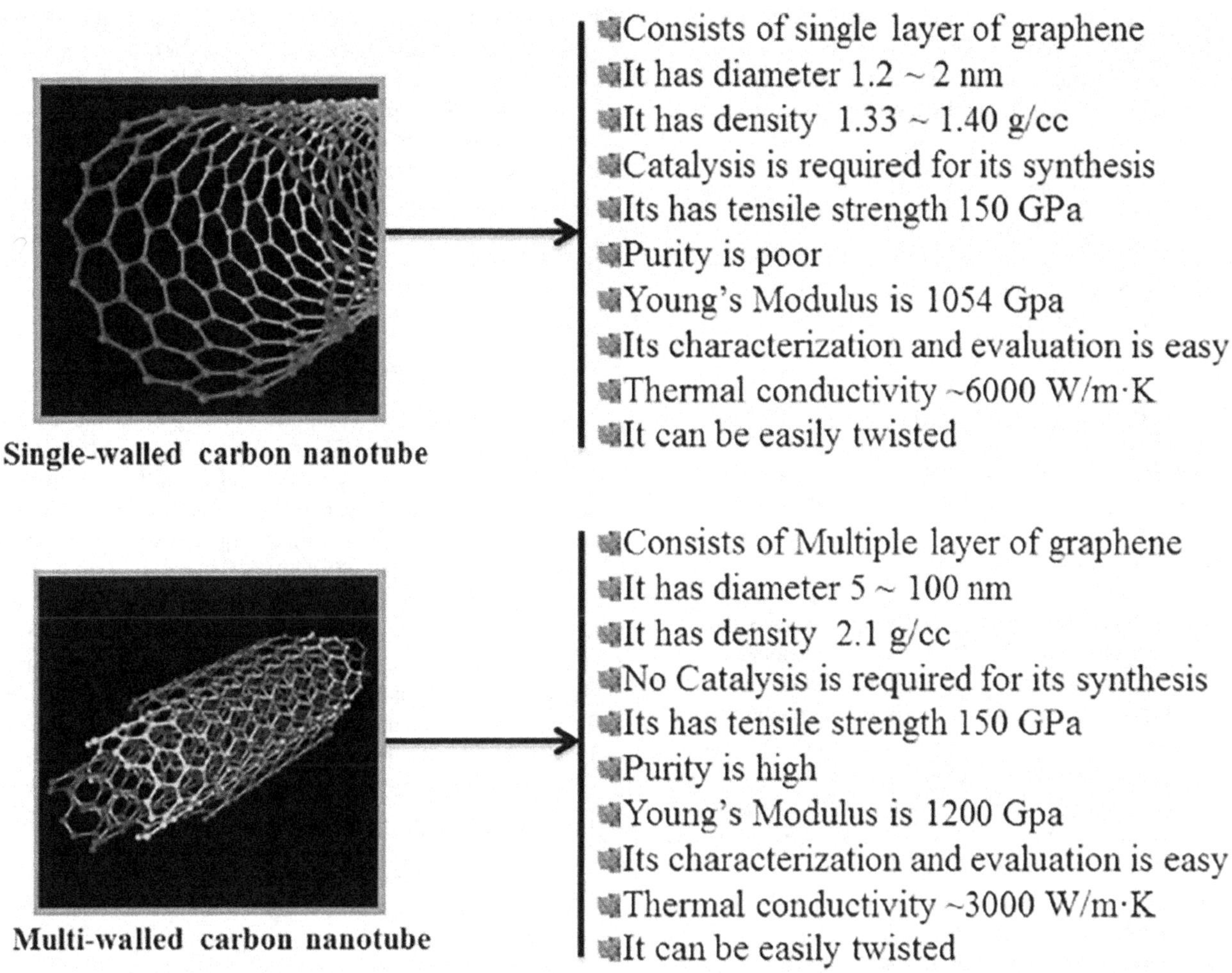

FIGURE 1.4 Various features of single-walled carbon nanotubes (SWNTs) and multi-walled carbon nanotubes (MWNTs).

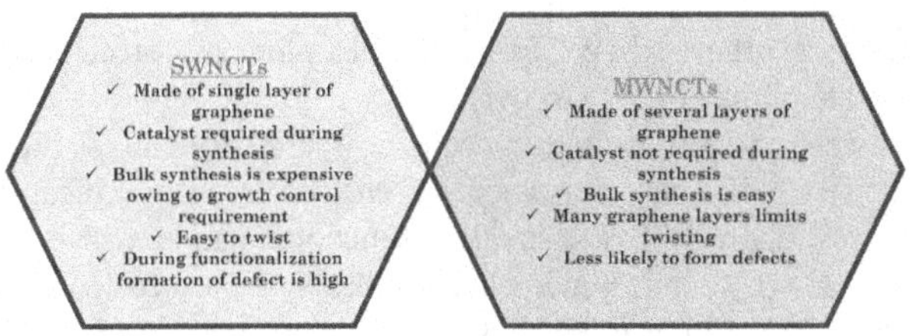

FIGURE 1.5 Differences between SWCNTs and MWCNTs.

1.4.1 Unique Properties of Single-Walled Carbon Nanotubes (SWCNTs)

Diameter: Ranging from 1 to 10 nm.

Length: 20–1,000 nm.

Properties: Consist of one layer of cylinder graphene sheet.

Mechanical: Individual SWNTs are significantly stronger than steel. Calculated values for tensile strength of SWNT are ~100 times greater than steel at 1/16th the weight. The highest measured value is approximately half of the predicted theoretical strength, the difference possibly being due to defects in the structure.

Electrical: Individual SWNTs have current-carrying capacities of 10^9 amp.cm^{-2}, higher than those of copper or gold, and semiconducting species exhibit higher electron mobility than silicon.

Optical: SWNTs have a distinct optical absorption and fluorescence response, with each chirality demonstrating its own characteristic absorption and fluorescence spectrum.

Thermal: Room-temperature thermal conductivity of a single nanotube may be comparable to that of diamond or in-plane graphite, which is generally thought to display the highest measured thermal conductivity of any known material at moderate temperatures.

The structural features of SWNTs are generally illustrated by means of an (n, m) vector that describes the chirality and diameter [5]. There are three SWNTs: (a) armchair (10, 10), (b) chiral (13, 6), and (c) zigzag (14, 0). The number of unit vectors along the two directions is represented by the integers n and m in the honeycomb crystal lattice of graphene. The nanotubes are called zigzag when m = 0. The nanotubes are called armchair when n = m. Otherwise, they are called chiral. From the following equation, the diameter of a nanotube can be calculated using its (n, m) indices, where $a = 0.246$ nm.

$$d = \frac{a}{\pi}\sqrt{(n^2 + nm + m^2)}.$$

SWCNTs have shown a marked drop in price recently, from around \$1,500 per gram as of year 2000 to retail prices of around \$50 per gram of as-produced 40–60% by weight SWCNTs as of March 2010.

1.4.1.1 Challenges of SWNTS

Technical hurdles in the areas of purity, selectivity, and dispersibility have so far limited the widespread application of SWNTs. However, much recent progress has been made to address each of these obstacles.

Purity: The various manufacturing processes used in the production of SWNTs lead to products which are contaminated to varying degrees with residual catalyst and other forms of carbon. For many applications, further purification processes are necessary to remove these contaminants to provide a product of sufficient purity. More recently, methods of synthesis that minimize the "synthesized" impurities have become commercially available.

Selectivity: As described earlier, SWNTs are a mixture of tubes of different chiralities, some of which are electrically conducting and some are semiconducting. Laboratory-scale methods to achieve a very high degree of selectivity have been reported, and efforts to develop scalable separation processes are bearing fruit. Manufacturing processes such as the CoMoCAT® catalytic CVD process have been shown to provide a high degree of selectivity toward certain chiralities in SWNTs as synthesized, making the yield of secondary purification processes substantially higher or even unnecessary.

Dispersibility: SWNTs can be difficult to disperse, partly because of their well-known tendency to form ropes or bundles due to van der Waals attraction between the tubes.

Additionally, dispersion of SWNTs in resins and thermoplastics is limited by a dramatic buildup in viscosity caused by the entanglement of the SWNTs bundles.

1.4.1.2 Synthesis of SWNTS

Various methods have been used in the manufacture of SWNTs. These include laser ablation, carbon arc, and CVD processes, either involving a gaseous catalyst, as in the HIPCO® process, or using a supported catalyst, as in the CoMoCAT® process. The laser ablation process is used primarily for research materials. The carbon arc process produces long tubes with diameters in the range 1.4 to 2.0 nm, but the carbon arc material has a large amount of impurities and, for most applications, will require extensive purification. The CVD processes offer the best approach to the manufacture of larger SWNT quantities, with perhaps the most scalable being the CoMoCAT® process, which uses a fluidized bed reactor similar to those used in petroleum refining, albeit currently on a much smaller scale. The supported catalyst approach also offers the unique ability to provide a substantial degree of chirality control during synthesis.

1.4.1.3 Characterization of SWNTS and Quality Assurance Parameters

As discussed earlier, the properties of carbon nanotubes vary with the individual SWNT chirality. Since at this time all SWNTs are produced as a mixture of chiralities, the properties of the material will depend on the proportions of chiralities present. Many analytical techniques have been deployed to determine the structure of SWNT materials. These range from observational techniques, such as SEM, TEM, AFM, and STM, to spectroscopic techniques, such as UV-Vis-NIR, photoluminescence (PL), and Raman. In addition to these methods, X-ray diffraction has been used by Miyata et al. to confirm the chirality assignments in the optical spectrum of SWNTs. TEM and SEM have been widely used to assess SWNT purity.

1.4.2 Double-Walled CNTs (DWCNTs)

Apart from these, there is another type of CNTs that resembles SWCNTs, that is, they are structurally similar. These nanotubes constitute of two concentric layers encasing its inner cylindrical tube inside its outer tube. They are of significant concern in the pharmaceutical sector.

Since the name is given, this CNT is comprised of two concentric CNTs, where an external layer of the carbon chamber is completely encased inside the internal chamber (outside cylinder is encased in inside cylinder) [8]. No catalyst is needed for its synthesis. MWCTs are highly pure and structurally complex. It is not easy to twist.

Their properties and morphology are similar to those of SWCNTs, but resistance to chemicals is significantly improved. In SWCNT, covalent functionalization will break some C = C double bond, leaving holes in the structure on the nanotube and thus modifying both its mechanical and electrical properties, while in case of DWCNTs, only the outer wall is modified. Structure and TEM are described.

1.4.3 Multi-Walled CNTs (MWCNTs)

Multi-walled carbon nanotubes (MWCNTs) are a special form of carbon nanotubes in which multiple single-walled carbon nanotubes are nested inside one another. Although MWCNTs are still classed as a one-dimensional form of carbon, the unique properties that are seen within single-walled and double-walled carbon nanotubes are not as prominent. The reason for this is the higher probability of defects occurring. These disadvantages are offset by the increased dispersibility of MWCNTs and the reduced cost in synthesis and purification of these materials.

What Are Multi-Walled Carbon Nanotubes?

Diameter: Approximately 5–30 nm
Length: 1 to several μm
Properties: Contain several concentric graphene sheets

MWCNTs consist of multiple carbon nanotubes nested within one another. The number of nanotubes that are within an MWCNT can vary—from as little as 3 to over 20.

MWCNTs have an inner diameter ranging from 0.4 nm to 3 nm, whereas the outer diameter ranges from 2 nm to 100 nm, and their length is from 0.2 to a few micrometers. MWCNTs have closed tips with dome-shaped half-fullerene molecules (pentagonal defects) and range in axial size from 1 m to a few centimeters. Half-fullerene molecules (pentagonal ring defect) help close the tube at both ends.

MWCNTs have a multilayer of graphene and move upon one another, having a width of 2–50 nm, which depends upon the quantity of graphene cylinder present, and the separation between this graphene cylinders is 0.34 nm. In the amalgamation of MWCNTs, they do not require any impetus and can be delivered by the mass union, having greater virtue than SWCNTs.

MWCNTs consist of multiple rolled layers (concentric tubes) of graphite. The SEM image of the MWCNT is illustrated in the two models which can be used to describe the structures:

1. **Russian Doll Model:** Graphite sheets are arranged in concentric cylinders, for example, a (0, 8) single-walled nanotube (SWCNT) within a larger (0, 17) single-walled nanotube.
2. **Parchment Model:** A single graphite sheet is rolled in around itself like a scroll of parchment or a rolled newspaper, and the interlayer distance is approximately 3.4 Å.

1.4.4 Differences in SWNTs and MWNTs

Carbon nanotubes are mainly classified into two types: SWCNTs (single-walled carbon nanotubes) and MWCNTs (multiple-walled carbon nanotubes). The comparison between SWCNT and MWCNT is presented in Table 1.3.

Detailed explanations of CNT structures can be found in several recent review articles cited herein [9]. The structures and characterizations of SWCNTs and MWCNTs are summarized in Table 1.3, according to Singh et al. [9].

TABLE 1.3
Comparative Characteristics of SWCNTs and MWCNTs

SWCNTs	MWCNTs
Single layer of graphene.	Multiple layer of graphene.
Catalyst is required for synthesis.	Can be produced without catalyst.
Bulk synthesis is difficult as it requires proper control over growth and atmospheric condition.	Bulk synthesis is easy.
Not fully dispersed, and form bundled structures.	Homogeneously dispersed, with no apparent bundled formation.
Resistivity usually in the range of 10^{-4}–10^{-3} Ω·m.	Resistivity usually in the range of 1.8×10^{-5}–6.1×10^{-5} Ω·m
Purity is poor. Typical SWCNT content in as-prepared samples by chemical vapor deposition (CVD) method is about 30–50 wt%. However, high purity up to 80% has been reported by using arc discharge synthesis method.	Purity is high. Typical MWCNT content in as-prepared samples by CVD method is about 35–90 wt%.
A chance of defect is more during functionalization.	A chance of defect is less, especially when synthesized by arc discharged method.
Characterization and evaluation is easy.	It has very complex structure.
It can be easily twisted and is more pliable.	It cannot be easily twisted.
Less accumulation in body.	More accumulation in body.

1.4.5 Types of CNTs Justified on the Basis of Chirality

In determining the electrical characteristics of CNTs, chirality is a very significant variable. There is around three varieties of CNTs based on chirality, namely, armchair, zigzag, and also chiral. All the aforementioned three forms are illustrated in Figure 1.6 [10]. In armchair, the bonds are arranged where the chiral vector has chairs perpendicular to the axis of the tube. In zigzag, bonds are organized where the tube has a V shape perpendicular to the axis of the tube, and likewise in chiral or helical configuration, unlike the preceding two arrangement types.

Other related structures of carbon nanotubes are as follows:

1. Torus
2. Nanobud
3. Cup-stacked carbon nanotubes
4. Extreme carbon nanotubes

1.4.5.1 Torus

Nanotorus is a carbon nanotube bent into a torus (doughnut) shape. Nanotori are predicted to have many unique properties, such as magnetic moments 1,000 times larger than previously expected for certain specific radii. Depending on radius of the torus and radius of the nanotube, the magnetic moment, thermal stability, and other properties vary widely.

1.4.5.2 Nanobud

Nanobuds are the newly synthesized combination of carbon nanotubes and fullerenes that possess useful properties of both. The fullerene-like buds are covalently bonded to the outer sidewalls of the underlying carbon nanotube. Nanobuds are exceptionally good field emitters and improve the mechanical properties of composite material (the attached fullerene molecules may function as molecular anchors, preventing slipping of the nanotubes).

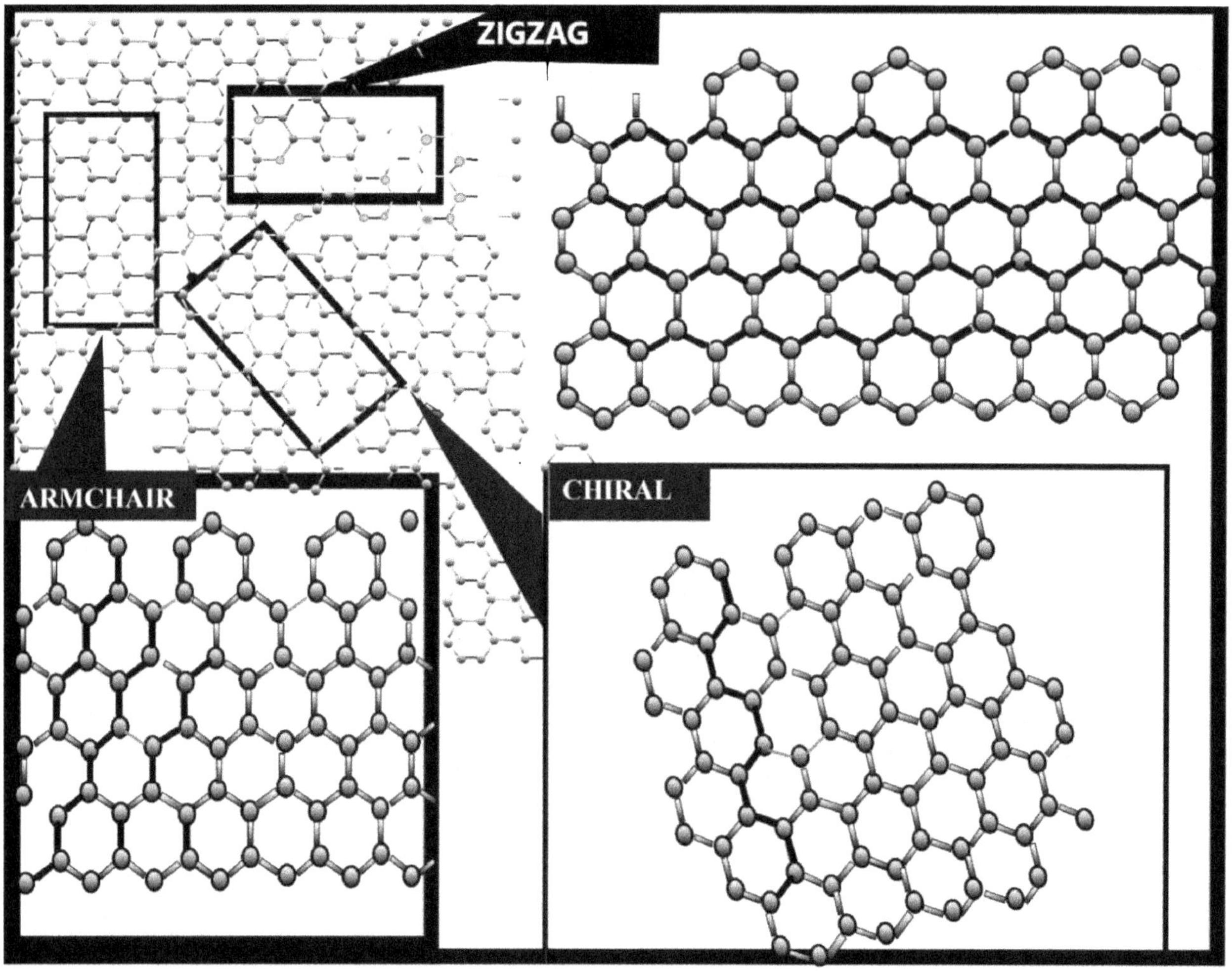

FIGURE 1.6 Type of CNTs based on chirality.

1.4.5.3 Cup-Stacked Carbon Nanotubes (CSCNTs)

CSCNTs exhibit semiconducting behaviors due to the stacking microstructure of graphene layers and thus differ from other quasi-1D carbon structures that behave as a metallic conductor of electrons.

1.4.5.4 Extreme Carbon Nanotubes

The longest carbon nanotubes (18.5 cm long) were reported in 2009, which were grown on Si substrates using an improved chemical vapor deposition (CVD) method and represent electrically uniform arrays of single-walled carbon nanotubes. The shortest carbon nanotube synthesized is that of cycloparaphenylene, in the early 2009. The thinnest carbon nanotube is armchair (2, 2) CNT, with a diameter of 3 Å, grown inside a multi-walled carbon nanotube. The characterization of carbon nanotube type was done by a combination of high-resolution transmission electron microscopy (HRTEM), Raman spectroscopy, and density functional theory (DFT) calculations.

The thinnest freestanding single-walled carbon nanotube is about 4.3 Å in diameter, with questionable indices, but the suggested indices can be either (5, 1) or (4, 2) SWCNT. (3, 3), (4, 3), and (5, 1) carbon nanotubes (all about 4 Å in diameter) were unambiguously identified using more precise aberration-corrected HRTEM. However, they were found inside double-walled carbon nanotubes (Figure 1.7).

1.5 Different Allotropes of Carbon Related to Devices

Initially, 3D materials such as diamond and graphite were used for device applications. The research on carbon-based nanomaterial has caught the attention of scientists and technologists after the discovery of fullerene, a 0D carbon allotrope. Furthermore, the discovery of carbon nanotubes (CNT), a 1D carbon allotrope, by Iijima [11] in 1991 provided a major boost in the field of carbon-based nanomaterials for device applications. Moreover, the demonstration of graphene as the basal structure for all allotropes can be understood from Figure 1.7.

With different hybridizations, carbon atoms can be arranged into materials with different structures, such as diamond, graphite, fullerene, and CNTs. Diamond and graphite are two of the most common forms in the carbon family.

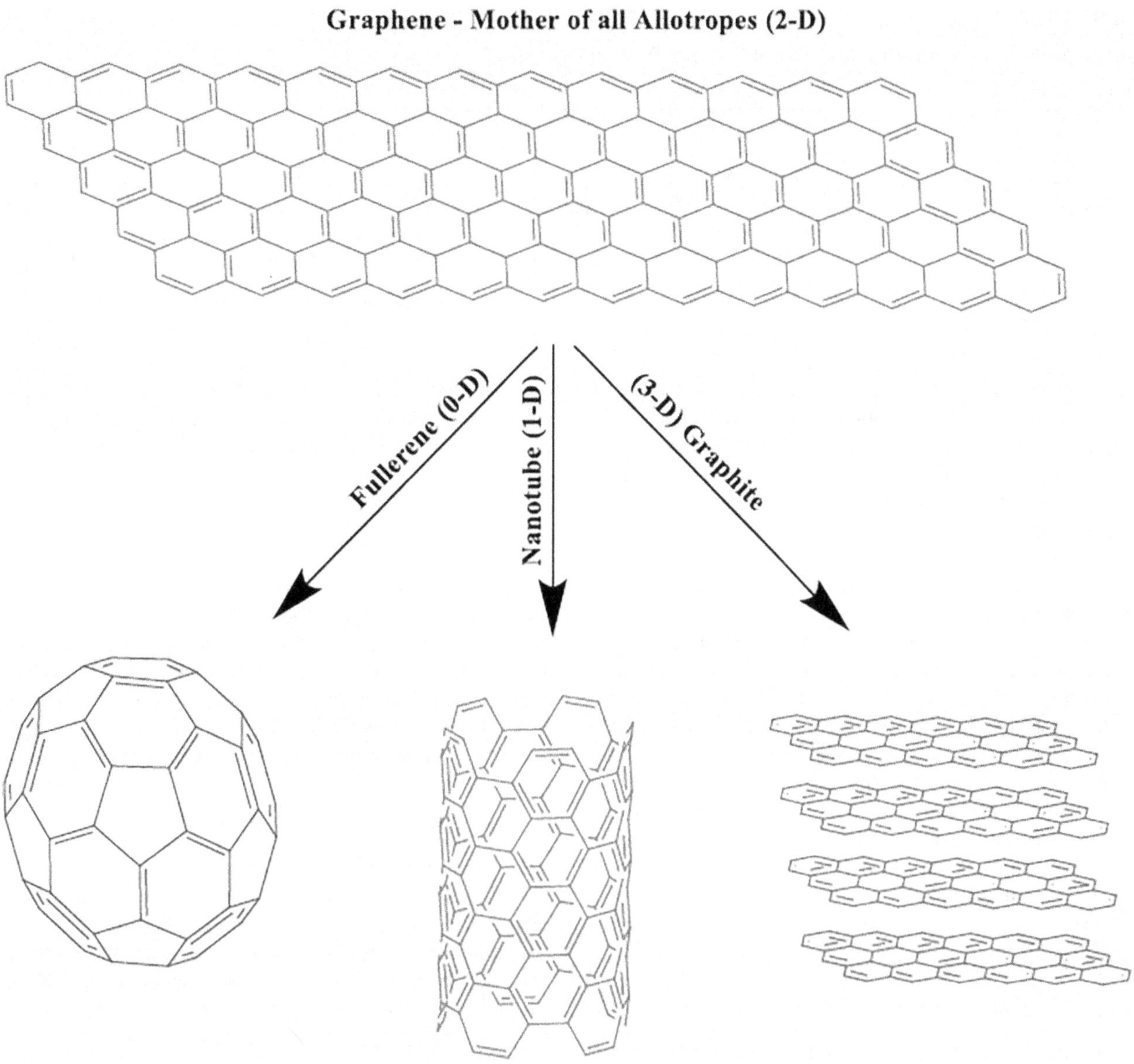

FIGURE 1.7 Graphene represented as the origin of all carbon allotropes. Materials when enveloped, rolled, and stacked form 0D buckyball, 1D nanotube, and 3D graphite, respectively (redrawn).

Various carbon allotropes, including diamond (the carbon atoms are bonded together in a tetrahedral lattice arrangement, 3D), graphite (the carbon atoms are bonded together in sheets of a hexagonal lattice, 3D), graphene (2D), carbon nanotubes (single-walled carbon nanotubes (SWCNT), multi-walled carbon nanotubes (MWCNT, 1D), and fullerenes (the carbon atoms are bonded together in spherical, tubular, or ellipsoidal formations, 0D), have very different physical and electrochemical properties from each other (see Table 1.4).

1.5.1 Zero-Dimensional Allotropes

1.5.1.1 Fullerene

Buckyball, or fullerene, is named after the American architect Richard Buckminster Fuller for his inspiring design of geodesic domes, which is a closed caged structure made by the periodic arrangement of graphene layers having the chemical formula C_{60}. It is made up of truncated icosahedral symmetry with 32 faces, 60 corners, and 90 edges composed of 20 hexagons and 12 pentagons where the 6:6 ring bonds (between two hexagons) are regarded to be double bonds with shorter bond lengths than the 6:5 bonds (between a hexagon and a pentagon), with an average bond length of 1.4 Å. Fullerenes are also known to have other isomers, C_{70}, C_{76}, C_{78}, and C_{84}. The electronic structure of C_{60} is represented by a fivefold degenerate HOMO (hu) and a threefold degenerate LUMO (t1u) having a bandgap of 1.8 eV (or 2 eV in certain literature), thus showing semiconductor behavior.

1.5.1.2 Graphene Quantum Dots (GQDs)

Carbon quantum dots (CQDs), widely regarded as carbon dots (CDs), are a 0D allotrope composed of carbon having

TABLE 1.4
Important Parameters of Carbon Materials of Different Dimensionalities [12]

Dimension	0D	1D	2D	3D
Isomer	Fullerene	Nanotube	Graphene	Diamond
Hybridization	sp^2	sp^2	sp^2	sp^3
Density (g/cm^3)	1.72	1.2–2.0	2.26	3.515
Bond length (Å)	1.40 (C = C) 1.46 (C–C)	1.44 (C = C)	1.42 (C = C)	1.54 (C–C)
Electronic properties	Semiconductor E_g = 1.9 eV	Meta/semiconductor E_g = ~0.3–1.1 eV	Zero-gap semiconductor	Insulator

size <10 nm. Its attractive photoluminescent and photophysical properties, such as exceptional photostability and photocatalytic activity, along with appreciable conductivity and extensive optical absorption, make it an appropriate material for viable photoelectrical devices. However, most of the luminescent CQDs exhibit fluorescence only on excitation arising from surface defects by trapping excitons, thus posing a hindrance in the performance of carrier injection for optoelectronic applications [13].

The modification of 2D graphene sheets into 0D GQDs with a radius smaller than exciton Bohr's radius [14] generates modification in electron distribution, thus demonstrating new phenomena by means of quantum confinement and edge effects, as observed in CDs leading to fluorescent properties, along with different chemical and physical functionalities in contrast to other allotropes. Furthermore, GQDs are superior against organic dyes and semiconductive QDs in terms of their excellent photostability, low toxicity, and biocompatibility [15], along with suitable surface grafting.

1.5.2 One-Dimensional Allotropes

1.5.2.1 Carbon Nanotubes (CNTs)

In 1991, a Japanese physicist, Iijima [11], revolutionized the field of carbon-based nanomaterials with his discovery of the carbon nanotubes (CNTs). It received great recognition by researchers all over the world for its unique set of characteristics. The CNTs are further classified into single-walled carbon nanotubes (SWCNTs), which are just a layer of graphene rolled up into hollow cylindrical product, and multi-walled carbon nanotubes (MWCNTs) can be thought of as several layers of graphene rolled up, forming a similar structure. These elongated tubes comprise of carbon hexagons orchestrated in a concentric fashion, with the two closures typically topped by fullerene-like structures containing pentagons [14]. Further, CNTs can be structurally classified as zigzag, armchair, and chiral.

1.5.2.2 Carbon Nanofibers (CNFs)

Carbon nanofibers are cylindrical fibrous structures with various stacking conformations of graphene sheets, like stacked platelet, ribbon, or herringbone. CNFs have lengths measured up to a few micrometers, while its diameter ranges from a couple of tens of nanometers to several hundreds of nanometers. Additionally, CNFs exhibit a unique set of physical and chemical properties, for instance, excellent electrical conductivity, large surface area, biocompatibility, characteristic chemical functionalities, and convenience in fabrication, thus making it an ideal candidate for device applications.

1.5.2.3 Carbon Nanohorns (CNHs)

Carbon nanohorns (otherwise called nanocones) are conical carbon nanostructures developed from an sp^2 carbon sheet. They give a practical and valuable option in contrast to CNTs, in a wide scope of utilizations. CNHs are known to comprise of a funnel-shaped upper area and, subsequently, a short round and hollow nanotube area. CNH is also well-known for its porosity, enabling it to be reliable for adsorption and storage activities.

1.5.2.4 Graphene Nanoribbons (GNRs)

Graphene nanoribbons, a quasi-1D derivative of graphene, are shown to have two possible edge geometries, namely, armchair and zigzag, having nomenclatures AGNRs and ZGNRs, respectively, with absolutely contrasting electronic properties as a result to their dissimilar boundary conditions. AGNRs can be determined into three categories, in the order of N_a = {3p}, {3p + 1}, and {3p + 2} where *p* is a positive integer with widely varying electronic properties and N_a is the number of dimer lines along the ribbon. The periodic AGNRs with Na = {3p + 2} show metallic behavior, whereas the other two show semiconducting behavior within the tight binding (TB) formalism. Relating to its novel edge symmetry, ZGNRs express a wide variety of electronic properties by means of its width and edge shape, tunability in terms of electronic configuration, and bandgap through structural or chemical adjustments, as well as doping and external perturbations [16]. The magnetism in ZGNRs is known to rise from π-orbitals of carbon confined at the edge. These properties, along with the ballistic electronic transport and quantum Hall effect, make GNRs regarded to be a versatile material for forthcoming nanoelectronic and spintronic devices.

1.5.3 Two-Dimensional Carbon Allotropes

1.5.3.1 Graphene (GR)

Although its discovery is late, GR is widely regarded as the mother of all carbon allotropes. It is considered as the base structure of graphite, large fullerenes, nanotubes, and others. It has a phenomenal intrinsic carrier mobility of 200,000 $cm^2/V^{-1}\ s^{-1}$

and exhibits excellent thermal as well as electrical conductivity. GR has a wide surface area of 2,630 m^2g^{-1} [17], which is greater than that of SWCNTs, while possessing remarkable mechanical properties, elastic properties, and so on. From the four valence states of GR (s, p_x, p_y, p_z), three atomic orbitals (s, p_x, p_y) form strong covalent bonds, with three neighboring carbon atoms forming sp^2 hybridization, thus conforming into a chicken wire-like structure, while one "p_z" orbital is found to overlap with three neighboring atoms of its own to relate *p* and *p** orbitals, resulting in HOMO and LUMO states, respectively.

1.5.4 Three-Dimensional Carbon Allotropes

1.5.4.1 Graphite

Graphite is a 3D carbon allotrope of sp^2 hybridization having each carbon atom bonded with three other atoms, thus forming a planar array of fused hexagons. It is further pigeonholed as a progression of GR layers along the XY plane, stacked in Z-direction. Within a layer of GR, the carbon atoms are located at the corners of hexagons. Further, each atom of carbon displays three σ bonds along its edges. Graphite with only three out of four valence electrons contributing implies that pz orbital does not have a role in the hybridization. Hence, they create a π-cloud, which is delocalized across the layer of GR. Graphite, owing to its layered structure and van der Waals force acting between the layers, hence allows the layers to glide past each other, which can be exploited for its appreciable thermal as well as electrical conductivity besides its well-known lubricative property.

1.5.4.2 Diamond

Diamond is another 3D allotrope of carbon in which the atoms are organized in a detailed type of cubic lattice called diamond cubic. Diamond is the hardest natural material as a result of its conformation, in which individual carbon atoms have four neighboring atoms joined to it by covalent bonds, exhibiting sp^3 hybridization state. Diamond as a semiconductor has a wide bandgap of 5.45 eV, which is a factor for its larger breakdown field strength in contrast to narrow bandgap semiconductors. A serendipitous creation is the diamond-like carbon (DLC), consisting of a combination of sp^2 and sp^3 hybridization energy states [18]. DLC exhibits remarkable properties, such as great hardness, low coefficient of friction, excellent wear and corrosion resistance, good chemical stability and biocompatibility, large electrical resistivity, infrared transparency, high refractive index, and excellent smoothness [18].While most SWNTs are chiral ($m \neq n$), some of them present armchair ($m = n$) or zigzag ($m = 0$) configurations (Figure 1.8A).

In the most general case, a CNT is composed of a concentric arrangement of several cylinders (Figure 1.8C). Such MWNTs can reach diameters of up to 100 nm, and the distance between two walls is very close to the distance between two graphene layers in graphite (~3.5 Å). Double-walled carbon nanotubes (DWNTs) are a special case of MWNTs composed of just two concentric cylinders (Figure 1.8B). DWNTs bridge the gap between SWNTs and MWNTs, thereby cumulating properties of both kinds of CNTs. More specifically, DWNTs resemble SWNTs with respect to their small diameter, length, and ability to form bundles, but their mechanical stability is much greater than that of the SWNTs, especially when covalently functionalized. Moreover, the outer wall of DWNTs can be functionalized without affecting the mechanical and electrochemical properties of the inner tube, just like MWNTs.

Besides, CNTs have a large specific surface area (SSA), which enables immobilization of a large number of functional units at the carbon nanotube surface, such as receptor moieties for biosensing applications.

The most important feature in the Raman spectrum of CNTs is the radial breathing mode (RBM), which is often located between 100 and 250 cm^{-1}, providing information about CNT diameters. The increase of the RBM frequency indicates that the CNTs agglomerate in bundles.

All the possible ways the graphene sheet can be rolled up to a cylinder can be represented by a pair of integer numbers or chiral indices *n* and *m* that predefine the chiral vector (c_h→). Chiral angle (θ) and chiral vector (c_h→) can be classified into three categories, namely, zigzag, armchair, and chiral, in terms of the chiral vector c_h→, as shown in Figure 1.9 [19].

MWCNTs and SWCNTs have similar properties. The sp^2 bonds between the individual carbon atoms in CNTs give the carbon nanotube intrinsic mechanical properties. This bond is even stronger than the sp^3 bond found in diamond; for this reason, carbon nanotubes are considered the strongest materials. CNTs have remarkable flexibility and resilience due to the high anisotropy of graphite. Their Young's modulus is superior to all carbon fibers, greater than 1 TPa; compared to steel, it is approximately five times higher. This specific characteristic gives carbon nanotubes a possible use in composite materials with improved mechanical properties [20].

CNTs have high thermal conductivity: SWCNTs up to 3,500 W/m.k, and MWCNTs more than 3,000 W/m.k [21]. Their densities can be drawn up or below 1.3 g/cm^3. CNTs also have extraordinary electronic properties comparable to copper. They have high electrical conductivity because of the chirality (the chiral angle between hexagons and the tube axis). CNT can be metallic or semiconducting; in another way, the energy gap decreases with increasing tube diameter [21].

In general, SWCNT is a single molecular nanomaterial which is formed of only a layer that rolls a single sheet of graphite (graphene) into a seamless molecular cylinder. Its diameter distribution and length are at the range of 0.75–3 nm and 1–50 m, respectively. While MWCNT is composed of more than two layers of curly graphite sheet and its diameter is at the range of 2–30 nm—and some even more than 100 nm—the distance between each layer is approximately 0.42 nm. The armchair CNTs have a metallic attribute with the most stable structure.

1.6 Basic Structure and Morphology Features of CNTs

There are three types of SWCNTs: armchair, chiral, and zigzag. The chiral vector (n, m) describes the SWCNT structure and directly affects the electrical characteristics of nanotubes.

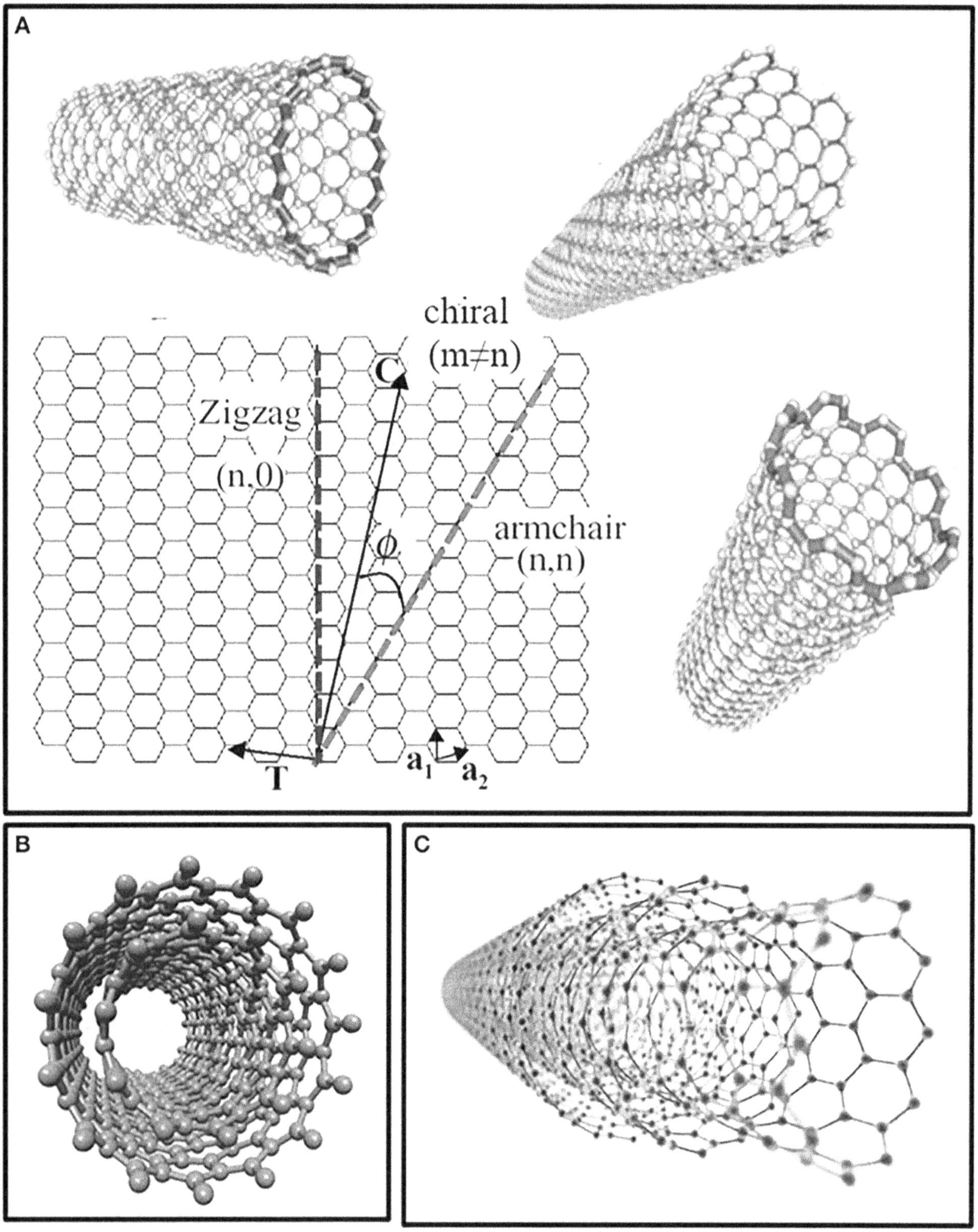

FIGURE 1.8 Structure and models of carbon nanotubes in function of their number of walls: (a) single-walled carbon nanotube (SWNT) structures in function of their chirality (zigzag, armchair, and chiral); (b) model of double-walled carbon nanotubes (DWNTs); (c) structure of multi-walled carbon nanotubes (MWNTs) made up of several concentric shells.

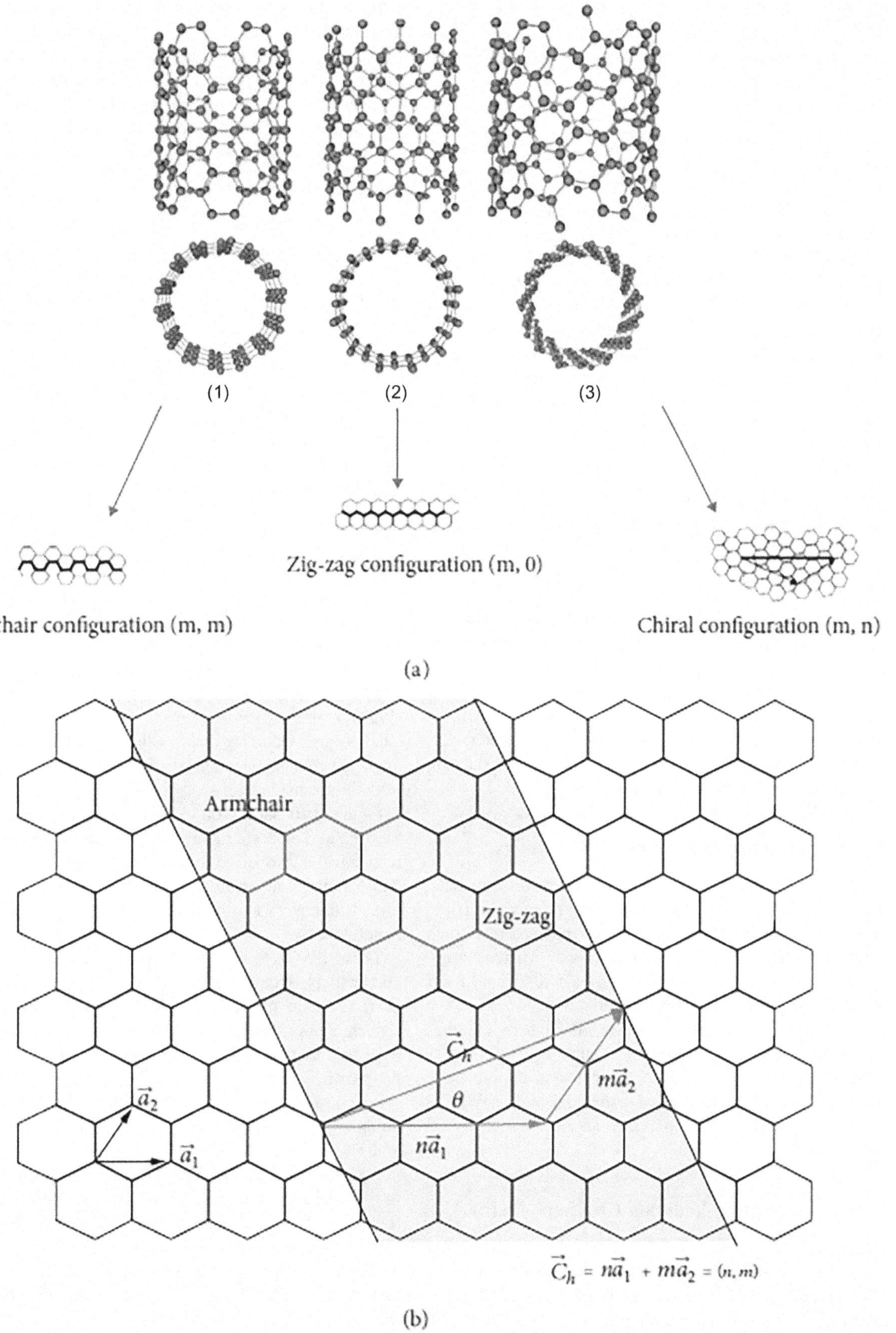

FIGURE 1.9 (a) Configuration of nanotubes (1) armchair, (2) zigzag, and (3) chiral. (b) Representation of the schematic diagram of the chiral vector $c_h \rightarrow$ and the chiral angle (θ). This vector can be decomposed in two components $a_1 \rightarrow$ and $a_2 \rightarrow$, $c_h \rightarrow = na_1 \rightarrow + ma_2 \rightarrow$, where the integration pair (n, m) is the indices of translation which decide the winding of tube.

The integers *n* and *m* determine the number of unit vectors in the honeycomb crystal lattice of graphene.

Accordingly, the diameter of a carbon tube may be estimated using the formula

$$d = \frac{a\sqrt{m^2 + mn + n^2}}{\pi}$$

where a = 1.4223, and $\sqrt{Å}$ is the graphite sheet lattice constant. Nanotubes are metallic or highly conducting when their n–m ratio is 3. If not, they are semimetallic or semiconducting. Other forms can turn the nanotube into a semiconductor, but the armchair form will always remain metallic. Two structural models of multi-walled carbon nanotubes exist: Russian doll and parchment. The *Russian doll* model is when a carbon nanotube contains another nanotube with a larger diameter than the inner nanotube. The *parchment* model refers to a single graphene sheet wrapped around itself like a scroll of parchment. MWCNTs and SWCNTs are comparable (Table 1.3). Because MWCNTs are multilayer, their outer walls not only protect the inner carbon nanotubes from external chemicals but also have exceptional tensile strength compared to SWCNTs.

1.6.1 Structure of SWCNT and MWCNT

Based on wrapping mechanism, three different forms of SWCNTs include chiral, armchair, and zigzag patterns. The single-walled structure is primarily characterized by a set of indices (*n* and *m*) which describe the vector mechanism of chiral, and it absolutely impinges (impacts) on the electrical tendency of both nanotubes. As a general prediction, when n = m, these nanotubes are known as armchair ones; if m = 0, they are said to be zigzag; and for other range as chiral.

1.6.2 Formation of Multi-Walled Nanotubes

Such MWCNTs can be developed via two distinct models, namely, the Russian doll and parchment-type models. If the diameter of the outer CNT exceeds that of the inner tube, such a model is described as a Russian-type model, whereas wrapping of a single graphite sheet to many a fold around itself constitutes the simple parchment model.

Owing to the presence of sp^2 bonds available betwixt indigenous carbon atoms, CNTs possess higher tensile property compared to steel as well as Kevlar. Such a bond exhibits more strength rather than sp^3 bonding of diamond. Hence, SWCNTs possess maximum tensile property, which may be nearly 100 times as that of steel.

1.6.3 Graphene and Reduced Graphene Oxide

Graphene consists of a single sheet of carbon atoms that bind with each other in a honeycomb lattice. Graphene sheets are one-atom thick and 2D layers of sp^2-bonded carbon. It is the basic building block for graphitic materials of all other dimensionalities. Graphene can be wrapped up into a spherical shape to form 0D fullerenes (buckyballs), rolled into a cylindrical shape to form 1D nanotube, or stacked in layers to form 3D graphite [12]. This revolutionary discovery has added a new dimension of research in the fields of physics, chemistry, biotechnology, and materials science [12]. Technologists and materials scientists have rapidly grabbed some of the assets of graphene and are already exploring the ways of incorporating graphene into applied devices and materials.

1.6.4 Carbon Dots (CDs)

Carbon dots (CDs) are zero-dimensional carbon nanomaterials that have been polymerized. CDs have been extensively used as biosensors. CDs are a subclass of nanoparticles, defined by a quasi-spherical morphology with a single unit with a characteristic size <10 nm. They show low toxicity, stability, and biocompatibility for their application as electrochemical biosensors. CDs can also be classified as carbon quantum dots (CQDs) and graphene quantum dots (GQDs); we mention these alternative acronyms here as they are widely used in the literature. CQDs and GQDs have a diameter ranging from 1 to 10 nm. GQDs consist of graphene layers of size less than 10 nm [22].

1.6.5 Structure Morphologies of SWCNTs

Single-walled carbon nanotubes (SWCNTs), which can be considered as seamless cylinders of graphene, have been at the forefront of nanotechnology research for the past two decades [23]. They possess a range of exceptional properties, including high strength (~37 GPa), thermal conductivity (~3,500 W/m/K), and ballistic electronic transport. Importantly, they can be semiconducting or metallic, depending on their helical angle (χ), that is, the angle between the tube axis and the edge of the graphene lattice.

Figure 1.10 shows the SWCNT application space (with existing and emerging applications in square and oval boxes, respectively) in relation to their physical properties (diameter and helicity) and organizational architecture. At one end lie mixed diameters and helicities as well as randomly aligned nanotubes.

These SWCNTs are mostly processed in powdered form and available from a number of suppliers (c.f. Table 1.5 in ref [24]). Over the past decade, global CNT production, primarily centered on low-cost multi-walled CNTs (MWCNTs), has increased tenfold and is predicted to rise to over 15 kilotons per year by 2020.

As can be seen in Figure 1.10, most of the existing technologies, such as reinforced composites, Li-ion batteries, and electromagnetic (EM) shielding, use randomly aligned, mixed helicity/diameter SWCNTs. An emerging application in this space is conductive SWCNT-based inks and thin-film transistors for flexible electronic applications. Transitioning from applications that are independent of alignment properties to more organized structures (along the horizontal axis in Figure 1.10) motivates the synthesis and processing of architectures like horizontally and vertically aligned SWCNTs and fibers and yarns. These materials can be used in semiconductor electronics, advanced composites, filtration membranes, and multifunctional fabrics [24]. Some of

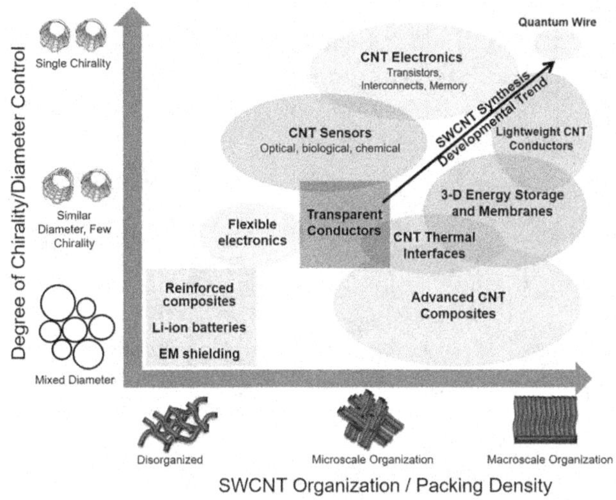

FIGURE 1.10 Structure–property relationship diagram showing the application space of SWCNTs with respect to tube diameter/helicity and architecture. The horizontal axis shows the organization of the SWCNTs from a random network to highly aligned architectures (vertically aligned fibers, etc.), while the vertical axis shows the degree of diameter/helicity control from mixed to single helicity. Existing and emerging SWCNT applications are shown in the square and oval boxes, respectively. The diagonal arrow in the graph shows the general direction of developments in synthesis over time.

these applications (along the vertical axis in Figure 1.10) will also benefit from SWCNTs with a narrower diameter range or fewer helicities, for example, SWCNT fiber-based conductive cables that possess a higher fraction of metallic tubes, and horizontally aligned semiconducting SWCNTs for next-generation semiconductor devices.

1.6.6 Helicity Control of SWCNTs

Helicity control remains the most significant challenge for the synthesis of SWCNTs. Often referred to as the holy grail of nanotube synthesis, control over the structure of SWCNTs (Figure 1.11a) is desirable for electronics applications that require semiconducting SWCNTs, for conducting cables where metallic SWCNTs are highly desirable, and for single SWCNT devices.

These concerns have prompted researchers to look toward other catalyst systems for helicity-controlled growth.

1.6.7 Catalyst Design for Selective SWCNTs Growth

One way to ensure that the catalyst remains solid at growth temperature is to use a high-melting-point catalyst which does not undergo significant surface reconstruction due to carbon adsorption. A recent example is the successful demonstration of selective growth of (12, 6), (16, 0), and (14, 4) SWCNTs from W-Co intermetallic compound nanoparticles (Figure 1.11b). The atomic arrangements of the W_6Co_7 nanocrystals are believed to play key roles in the selective growth. SWCNTs grow epitaxially from the solid-state catalysts, and thus, their helicities are defined. Under optimized carbon feeding conditions, SWCNT specific helicities can be synthesized.

TABLE 1.5

Producers of CNT powders and dispersions

Company	Country	URL
Arkema	France/USA	http://www.arkema-inc.com/ http://www.graphistrength.com
Bayer MaterialScience AG	Germany	www.bayer.com http://www.baytubes.com/
BlueNano	USA	www.bluenanoinc.com
Catalytic Materials	USA	http://www.catalyticmaterials.com
Chengdu Organic Chemical Co. Ltd.	China	www.timesnano.com
Cnano	China/USA	http://www.cnanotechnology.com
Eden Energy	Australia/India	http://www.edenenergy.com.au/
Eikos	USA	www.eikos.com
Hanwha Nanotech Corporation	South Korea	www.hanwhananotech.com
Hodogaya	Japan	http://www.hodogaya.co.jp
Hyperion Catalysis	USA	www.hyperioncatalysis.com
Hythane Co.	USA	http://hythane.net/
Idaho Space Materials	USA	www.idahospace.com
KleanCarbon	Canada	http://www.kleancarbon.com/
Meijo-Nano Carbon	Japan	www.meijo-nano.com
Mitsubishi Rayon Co.	Japan	http://www.mrc.co.jp
Mitsui	Japan	www.mitsui.com
Nanocyl S. A.	Belgium	www.mitsui.com
Nanointegris	USA	www.nanointegris.com
Nanolab	USA	http://www.nano-lab.com/
Nanothinx	Greece	http://www.nanothinx.com
Nano-C	USA	http://www.nano-c.com
Raymor Industries Inc.	Canada	www.raymor.com
Rosseter Holdings Ltd.	Cyprus/USA	www.e-nanoscience.com
Shenzhen Nanotech Port Co. Ltd.	China	www.nanotubes.com.cn
Showa Denko K. K.	Japan	www.sdk.co.jp
South West Nano Technologies Inc.	USA	www.swentnano.com
Sun Nanotech Co. Ltd.	China	www.sunnano.com
Thomas Swan and Co. Ltd.	England	www.thomas-swan.co.uk
Toray	Japan	www.toray.com
Ube Industries	Japan	www.ube-ind.co.jp
Unidym Inc.	USA	www.unidym.com
Zyvex	USA	www.zyvex.com

Source: [24].

Note: This information is gathered from online sources and through personal communications. It is not meant to be a comprehensive list of all activities in this area.

1.6.8 Structure and Features of Fullerenes (C_{60})

Fullerene offers a high symmetrical lattice in different sizes (C60, C76, and so on), with its unusual structure containing sp^2 carbons. The most abundant types of fullerene synthesized are C_{60} and C_{70}. Each fullerene has 2n + 20 carbon atoms

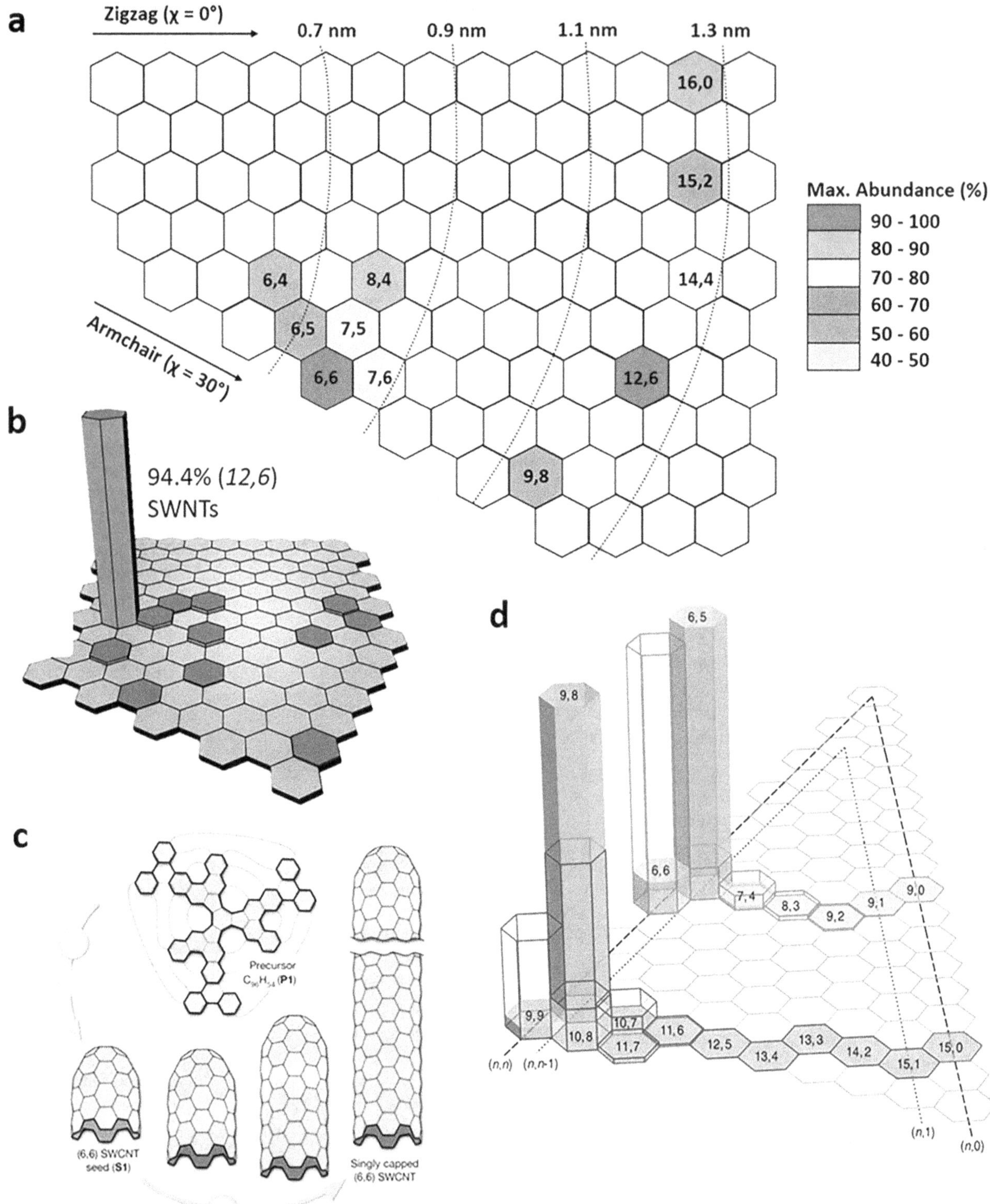

FIGURE 1.11 Recent advances toward helicity-controlled SWCNT growth. (a) Chiral index map showing the (n, m) indices of all the SWCNTs that have been grown with high purity. The color scale indicates the maximum reported abundance for that particular SWCNT. (b) Relative abundances of various helicities of SWCNTs grown from W-Co alloy catalyst particles. The inset shows a schematic illustration of a SWCNT growing from a W-Co alloy particle. (c) Schematic illustration of bottom-up synthesis of helicity-controlled SWCNTs using molecular end-cap precursors. (d) (n, m) distributions calculated based on atomistic computations for two CNT sets (d ≈ 0.8 and 1.2 nm). The solid and empty bars correspond to solid and liquid catalysts.

Source: Reproduced with permission. Copyright 2014 Nature Publication Group.

consisting of n hexagon. The C_{60} contains 60 carbon atoms, and in terms of shape, the fullerene C60 is as a soccer ball; it comprises 12 pentagons with 60 vertices and a polygon with 32 faces, 20 of which are hexagons.

1.7 Production and Workplace Exposure to CNTs

Different techniques have been developed to produce nanotubes in appropriate amounts, including arc discharge, laser ablation, high-pressure carbon monoxide disproportionation, and chemical vapor deposition (CVD). The laser ablation method yields around 70% and produces primarily SWCNTs with a controlled size determined by the reaction temperature. However, it is more expensive than both arc discharge and CVD. In plasma torch method, a gas mixture composed of argon, ethylene, and ferrocene is introduced into a microwave plasma torch, where it is atomized by the atmospheric pressure plasma, which has the form of an intense "flame." We present in details recent chemical approaches according to Figure 1.12 with the functionalization of CNTs including practical uses of functionalized CNTs in many fields of applications. In light of this fact, we have an intention to do a thorough study reviewing exclusively the recent advances in CNT functionalization, which will provide researchers a global insight of the main functionalization strategies of carbon nanotube nanostructures [25].

1.8 Synthesis of Carbon Nanotubes (CNTs)

CNT is generally produced by three main techniques:

Arc discharge: Two electrodes of carbon in the presence or absence of a catalyst are taken, and an arc is discharged between them. Resulting vapors of carbon get self-assembled and give rise to nanotubes.

Laser ablation: Collision occurs between the high-power laser pulse and volume of carbon, which contains the methane or carbon monoxide as a feedstock gas and produce nanotubes in small quantity.

Chemical vapor deposition (CVD): Produce MWNTs or SWNTs of poor quality and range of large diameter. The CVD process is scaled up easily and favors the viable manufacture.

From the preceding three main methods, CVD shows the most prospect for commercial CNT production. In addition to enabling higher atomic quality and percent yield than the other methods, CVD provides manufacturers with control over nanotube orientation, length, diameter, and other parameters. CVD is capable of making bulk quantities of multi-walled nanotubes for composites or individual-aligned SWNTs on substrates to utilize in electronics. A brief description of methods contributing to mass production with their effectiveness is given in Scheme 1.4 [5].

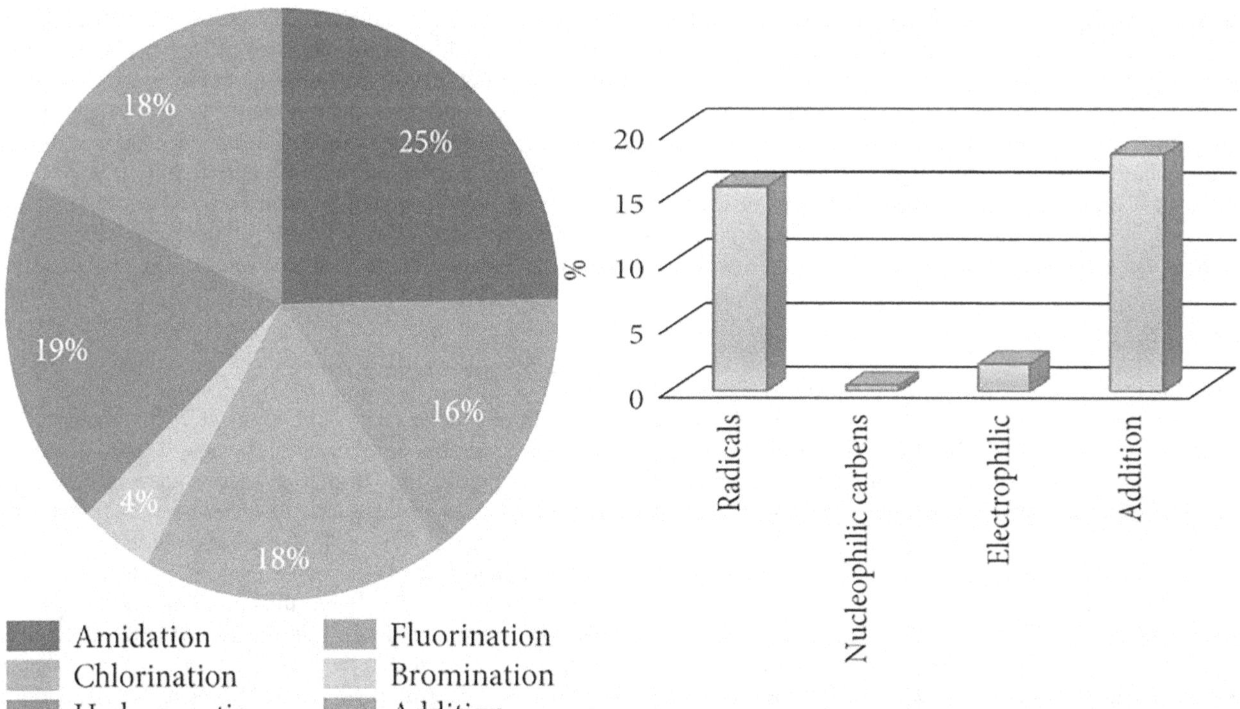

FIGURE 1.12 (a) Statistical published papers on CNT functionalization using new approaches. (b) Different types of CNT addition approach in 2020.

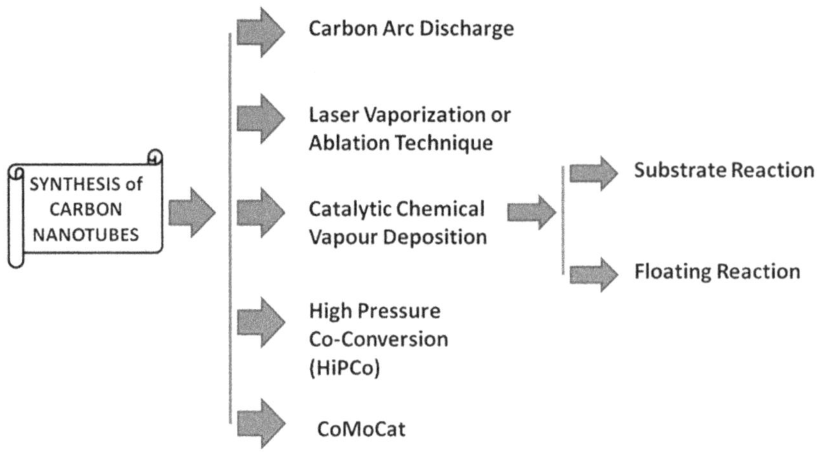

SCHEME 1.4 Methods of synthesis for carbon nanotubes.

Techniques have been developed to produce nanotubes in sizeable quantities, including arc discharge, laser ablation, and chemical vapor deposition. A numbers of different procedures have been established for the production of CNTs. Gas-phase methods such as chemical vapor deposition (CVD), laser ablation, and arc discharge are the most well-established methodologies for achieving effective growth in a controlled environment. Electrolysis and sonochemical techniques are two other options. CVD is the most cost-effective, most controlled, and most productive of these techniques, allowing for the most precise control over nanotube diameter, length, alignment, and purity. CVD is also the most environmentally friendly technology.

Three main techniques generally used for SWCNTs and MWCNTs production are the arc discharge method (using arc vaporization of two carbon rods), laser ablation method (using graphite), and chemical vapor deposition (using hydrocarbon sources: CO, methane, ethylene, acetylene).

There are various methods of production of carbon nanotubes, such as by arc discharge, chemical vapor deposition, laser ablation, flame synthesis, high-pressure carbon monoxide (HiPco), electrolysis, pyrolysis, etc. But they can be mainly classified into the following groups: (1) physical processes, (2) chemical processes, and (3) miscellaneous processes.

1.8.1 Physical Processes

These are the processes which make use of physical principles of carbon conversion into nanotubes. These include popular processes of carbon nanotube production, such as arc discharge and laser ablation. Due to their widespread popularity, they are by far the most widely used processes for nanotube production for experimental purposes.

1.8.1.1 Arc Discharge

It is possible to synthesize carbon nanotubes using the electric arc discharge process, also known as the plasma arcing method. It is used in this approach to apply a voltage between pure graphite electrodes that are separated by 1 mm and to keep the pressure of flowing helium gas within the quartz chamber constant at 500 torr (see Figure 1.13), while the electrodes are separated by 1 mm. This method is used to manufacture multi-walled carbon nanotubes, and it is also used to synthesize single-walled carbon nanotubes. To synthesize multi-walled carbon nanotubes, catalyst nanoparticles of iron, cobalt, and nickel are inserted into the middle region of the positive electrode. [5, 26].

This is one of the oldest methods of carbon nanotube production, first utilized by Iijima [11] in 1991 at NEC's Fundamental Research Laboratory to produce a new type of finite carbon structures consisting of needle-like tubes. The tubes were produced using an arc discharge evaporation method similar to that used for fullerene synthesis. The carbon needles, ranging from 4 to 30 nm in diameter and up to 1 mm in length, were grown on the negative end of the carbon electrode used for the direct current (DC) arc discharge evaporation of carbon. During the process, Iijima used a pressurized chamber filled with a gas mixture of 10 torr methane and 40 torr argon. Two vertical thin electrodes were installed in the center of the chamber (Figure 1.13). The lower electrode (cathode) contained a small piece of iron in a shallow dip made purposefully to hold iron.

The arc was generated by running a DC current of 20 V between the electrodes. The use of the three components, namely, argon, iron, and methane, was critical for the synthesis of SWNT.

1.8.1.2 Laser Ablation

In the laser ablation process, a graphite target is vaporized by a laser source, similar to the physical vapor deposition method shown in Figure 1.14. In this procedure, the graphite target is put in the center of a quartz chamber filled with argon gas and maintained at 1,200°C for the duration of the experiment. Either a continuous laser source or a pulsed laser source is used to melt the graphite target material. The flow of argon gas sweeps the vaporized target atoms (carbon) toward a cooled copper collector, where they are collected. This approach is used to manufacture multi-walled carbon nanotubes, and it is also used to synthesize single-walled carbon nanotubes, with the catalyst nanoparticles of Fe, Co, and Ni being employed in both cases [26].

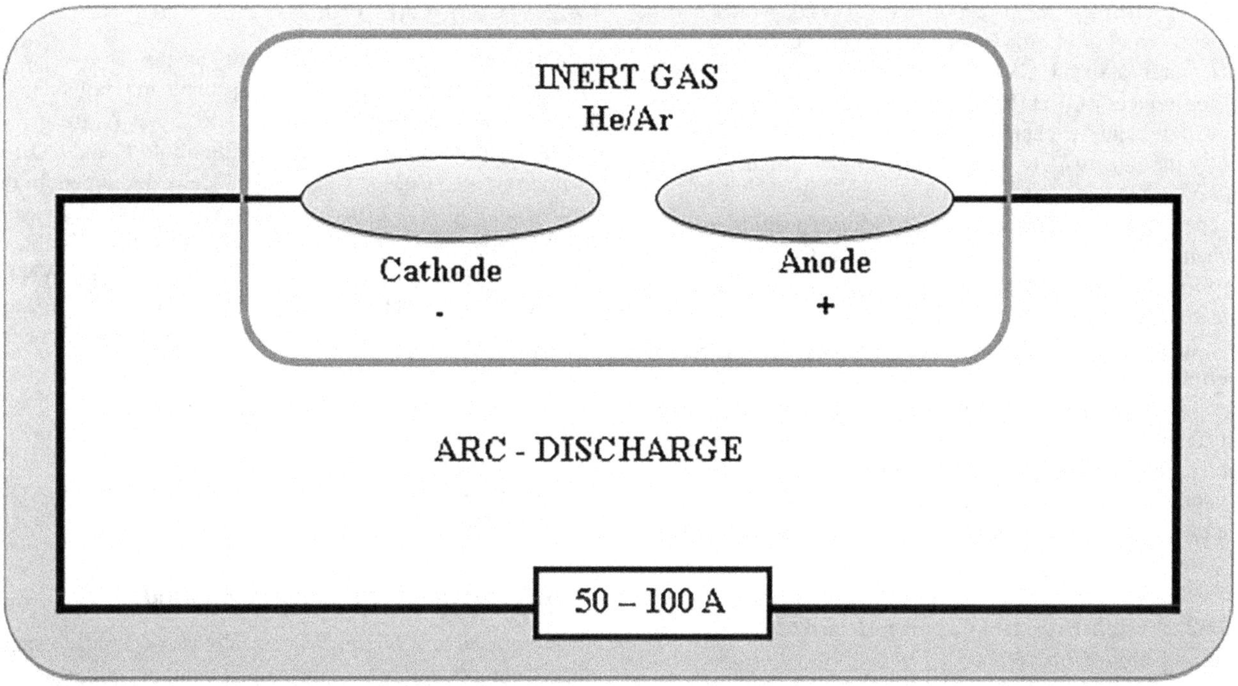

FIGURE 1.13 Diagrammatic representation of arc discharge setup for synthesis and growth of the nanotube.

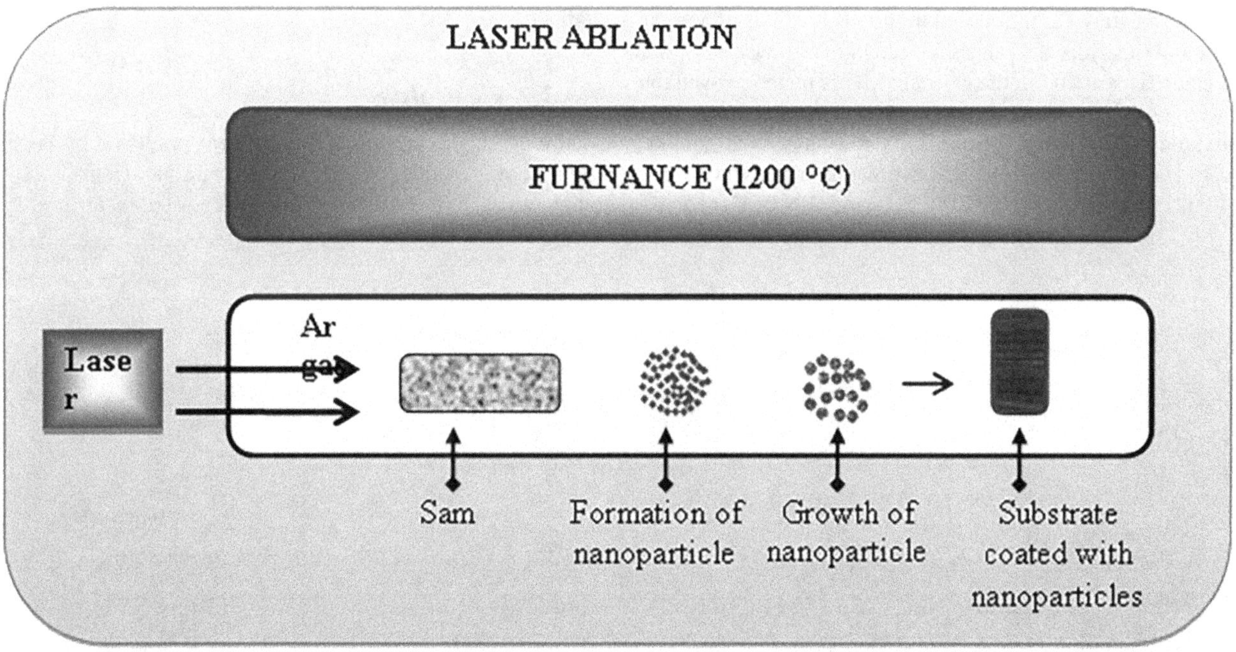

FIGURE 1.14 Diagrammatical representation of laser ablation setup for nanotube synthesis and growth.

In the laser ablation process, a pulsed laser is made to strike at a graphite target in a high-temperature reactor in the presence of inert gas, such as helium, which vaporizes a graphite target. The nanotubes develop on the cooler surfaces of the reactor as the vaporized carbon condenses. A water-cooled surface is also included in the most practical systems to collect the nanotubes (Figure 1.14).

1.8.2 Chemical Processes

1.8.2.1 Chemical Vapor Deposition (CVD)

Chemical vapor deposition, sometimes known as CVD, is one of the most widely used processes for producing carbon nanotubes. The term "chemical vapor deposition" (CVD) encompasses many different types of processes, including catalytic chemical vapor deposition (CCVD), which can be either thermal or plasma enhanced (PE) oxygen assisted CVD [11] water assisted CVD, microwave plasma (MPECVD), radio frequency CVD (RF-CVD), and hot-filament (HFCVD). However, catalytic chemical vapor deposition (CCVD) is currently the most widely used approach for the manufacture of carbon nanotubes in industry.

Chemical vapor deposition is a type of deposition in which a chemical vapor is deposited on a surface. CVD is a technology in which the vaporized reactants react chemically with one another to generate a nanomaterial product that is placed on a substrate during the deposition process (Figure 1.15). The thermal CVD process is used to synthesize CNTs, with hydrocarbon gas serving as the carbon source. It is necessary to use this technology in order to keep the temperature of the quartz tube high (500–900°C), which is maintained by an RF heater + catalyst nanoparticles of iron, cobalt, and nickel utilized in the production of single-walled carbon nanotubes. [26]

1.8.2.2 High-Pressure Carbon Monoxide Reaction (HiPco®)

This is a unique method developed at Rice University in 1999 for the production of carbon nanotubes. Unlike other methods in which the metal catalysts are deposited or embedded on the substrate before the deposition of the carbon begins, in this method, a catalyst is introduced in the gas phase. Both the catalyst and the hydrocarbon gas are fed into a furnace, followed by catalytic reaction in the gas phase. This method is suitable for large-scale synthesis because the nanotubes are free from catalytic supports and the reaction can be operated continuously. Usually, CO gas is used as hydrocarbon gas which reacts with iron pentacarbonyl $Fe(CO)_5$ to form SWNT.

1.8.2.3 CoMoCAT® Process

Recently, an effort has been made at the University of Oklahoma to develop a process using cobalt and molybdenum catalysts and CO gases. In this method, SWNTs are grown by CO disproportionation (decomposition into C and CO_2) in the presence of a CoMo catalyst (specifically developed for the purpose) at 700–950°C in flow of pure CO at a total pressure that typically ranges from 1 to 10 atm. This process is able to grow a significant amount of SWNTs (about 0.25 g SWNT/g catalyst) in a couple of hours, keeping selectivity toward SWNT better than 80%. The secret of the process is in the synergistic effect of Co and Mo.

1.8.3 Miscellaneous Processes

Some miscellaneous and relatively less used processes of carbon nanotube production are given in the following.

1.8.3.1 Helium Arc Discharge Method

It was reported in 2006 by scientists of NASA's Goddard Space Flight Center that they have developed a simple, safe, and very economical process of single-walled carbon nanotube production. In this method, scientists used a helium arc welding process to vaporize an amorphous carbon rod and then form nanotubes by depositing the vapor onto a water-cooled carbon cathode.

1.8.3.2 Electrolysis

In this method, carbon nanotubes were produced by depositing alkali metals on a graphite cathode from a high-temperature molten salt system. The deposited metallic atoms

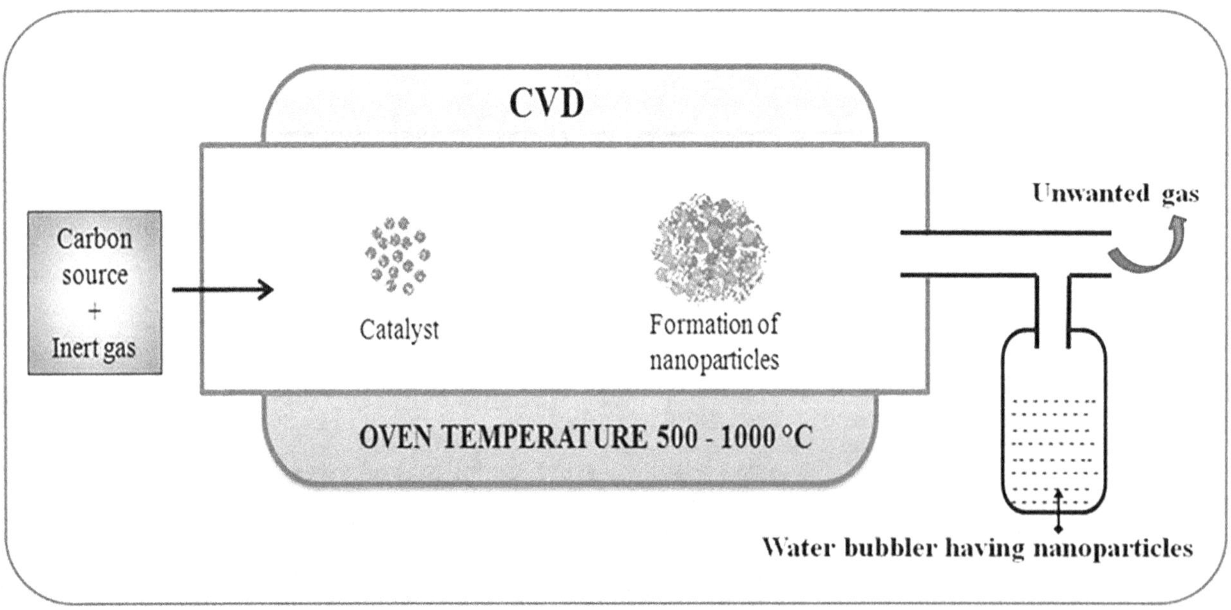

FIGURE 1.15 Diagrammatical representation of chemical vapor deposition (CVD) setup for nanotube synthesis and growth.

intercalate into the space between the graphitic sheets and diffuse towards the bulk of the graphite cathode, causing some mechanical stress inside the graphite. This stress induces the ablation of separate graphitic sheets, which will turn into carbon nanotubes due to interfacial forces, trying to recombine broken carbon–carbon bonds. Though this method has been reported to yield a good quality of carbon nanotubes, it is not scalable to a large-scale production method to produce carbon nanotubes.

1.8.3.3 Flame Synthesis

This method is based on the synthesis of SWNT in a controlled flame environment, which produces the temperature, forms the carbon atoms from the inexpensive hydrocarbon fuels, and forms small aerosol metal catalyst islands. SWNTs are grown on these metal islands in the same manner as in laser ablation and arc discharge. These metal catalyst islands can be made in three ways. The metal catalyst (cobalt) can either be coated on a mesh, on which metal islands resembling droplets are formed by physical vapor deposition. These small islands become aerosol after exposure to flame.

1.9 Growth Mechanism of Carbon Nanotubes (CNTs)

The techniques are not known exactly for the formation of the nanotube, and more than one method of growth mechanism might be effective for the construction of carbon nanotubes, which is still a conflict. The mechanism comprises the steps shown in Scheme 1.5, and the simple diagrams of growth mechanism are shown in Scheme 1.6. Firstly, C_2 acts as a precursor for the construction of nanotubes and fullerenes on the surface of the metal catalyst particle.

A rod-like carbon is produced quickly from a metastable carbide particle. Secondly, the CNT's wall contributes to slow graphitization. For all nanotube techniques, the actual growth mechanism seems similar. On a growth mechanism of nanotubes, there are several theories, one of which is described in Scheme 1.5. For supported metals, filaments can form either by "extrusion/root/base growth" or by "tip growth." Catalyst size plays a role in the type of nanotube obtained, whether SWNTs or MWNTs.

1. Particles of metal catalyst are supported or float on graphite or on a different substrate, which anticipates the spherical or pear shape of the catalyst particles.
2. The deposition will occur only on one-half of the surface, and the carbon diffuses along the concentration gradient and is precipitated on the opposite half, around and below the bisecting diameter; it does not take part from the tip of the hemisphere, which accounts for the vacant core that is distinctive of these filaments.
3. Extrusion or root growth: nanotube grows upward from the metal particles that remain attached to the substrate. Tip growth: the particles detach and move at the head of the growing nanotube.

The formation of single- or multi-walled CNT is governed by the size of the catalyst nanoparticle. Generally speaking, when the particle size is a few nanometers, SWCNTs form, whereas if the particles are a few tens of nanometers wide, it favors MWCNT growth (Figure 1.16).

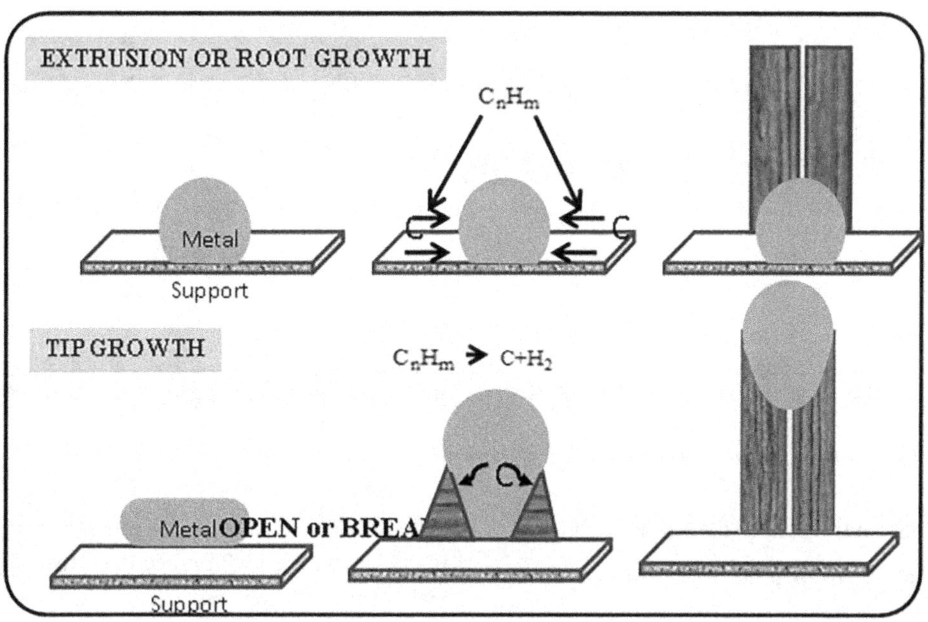

SCHEME 1.5 The visual image of a possible carbon nanotube growth mechanism.

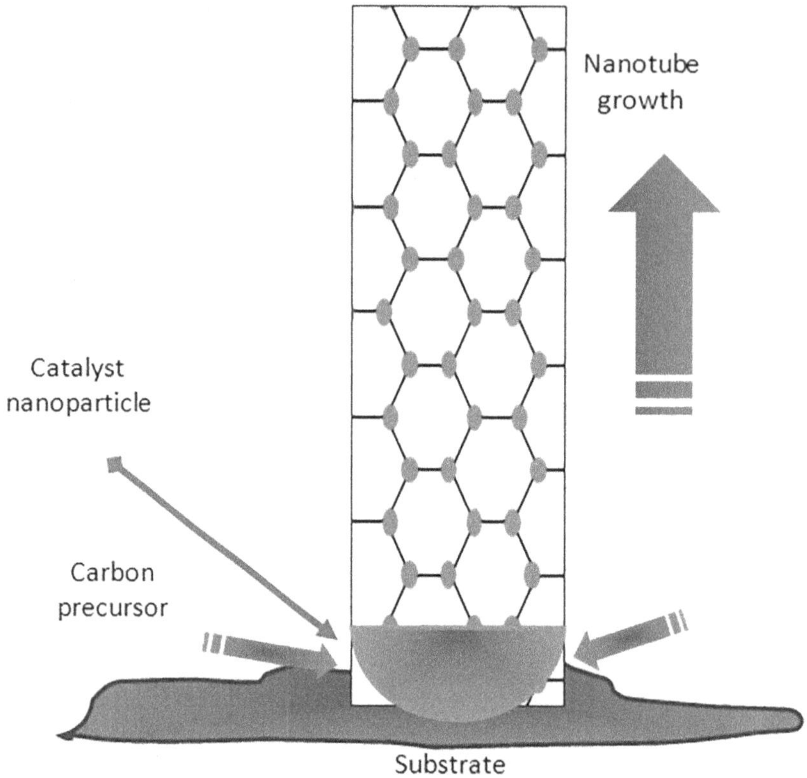

SCHEME 1.6 Growth mechanisms of nanotubes: gas based on carbon breaks apart on the surface of the catalyst by CVD, and nanotube grows outward from the surface.

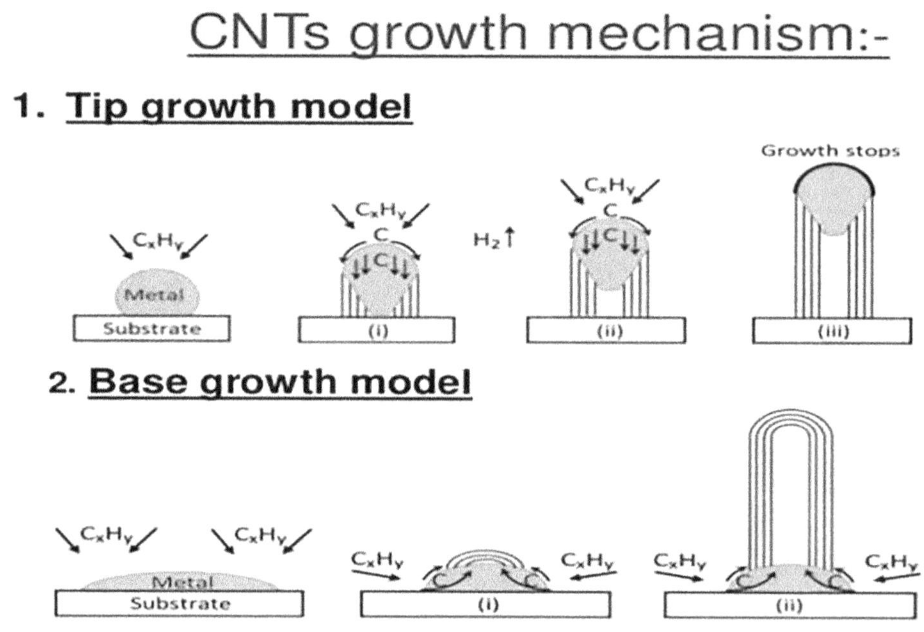

FIGURE 1.16 Schematic diagram of growth mechanisms of carbon nanotubes.

1.9.1 SWCNT Growth from Molecular Seeds

With this approach, seeds of three SWCNTs with different helicity—(7, 6), (6, 5), and (7, 7)—have been elongated significantly from a few hundred nanometers to tens of micrometers using methane or ethanol as the carbon source, and the helicity of the nanotube seeds was successfully inherited during this metal-free VPE process. Further improvement in the yield of the VPE process was demonstrated by introducing a small amount of ethylene along with methane, resulting in the successful cloning of several nanotubes spanning the whole range of chiral angles: (9, 1), (10, 2), (8, 3), (6, 5), (7, 6), (6, 6), and (7, 7) SWCNTs. Considering that carbon nanotube seeds could be highly pure and metal-free, SWCNTs synthesized by VPE could be directly utilized without any post-synthesis purification.

1.9.2 Computational Modeling of SWCNT Growth

Computational modeling studies targeting various aspects of SWCNT growth mechanisms pertinent to catalytic CVD have since grown considerably in number and complexity, and recent reviews present an ample account of theoretical efforts. This kinetic route of chiral selectivity, controlled by the R factor, may produce preferentially the fastest-growing (2 m, m) tubes, corresponding to $\chi \simeq 19°$, where the number of kinks reaches maximum (Figure 1.11d).

The preceding model not only explains the sometimes-contrasting experimental observations but also suggests a route toward structure-controlled growth. For example, realizing nucleation on a solid catalyst and then transitioning to steady-state growth on a liquid catalyst may provide access to achiral SWCNTs. However, very recently, based on large-scale first-principles calculations combined with kinetic Monte Carlo simulations, it was shown that such selectivity in the case of Co_7W_6 instead can be a result of complex growth kinetics [27]. Computational studies have also revealed the formation of a Ni-C core inside the Ni nanocatalyst that persists throughout the nucleation and growth of SWCNTs, although this may perturb and alter the steady growth of the SWCNT.

1.9.3 Related Advances in Graphene and Other 2D Material Growth

Indeed, well-defined single crystalline planar substrates serve as simplified model systems for fundamental studies of SWCNT catalysis (Figure 1.17) that can be readily probed with powerful surface science techniques while avoiding some of the complexities of SWCNT growth, such as diverse nanoparticle populations, nanosizing effects, and support interactions.

1.9.4 Graphene Growth Mechanisms

Growth models incorporating kinetic effects have been developed, highlighting in particular that graphene nucleation simply requires a local carbon supersaturation to be developed at the catalyst surface, while the concentration in the bulk of the catalyst can remain much lower. Graphene growth thus depends on the balance between precursor dissociation

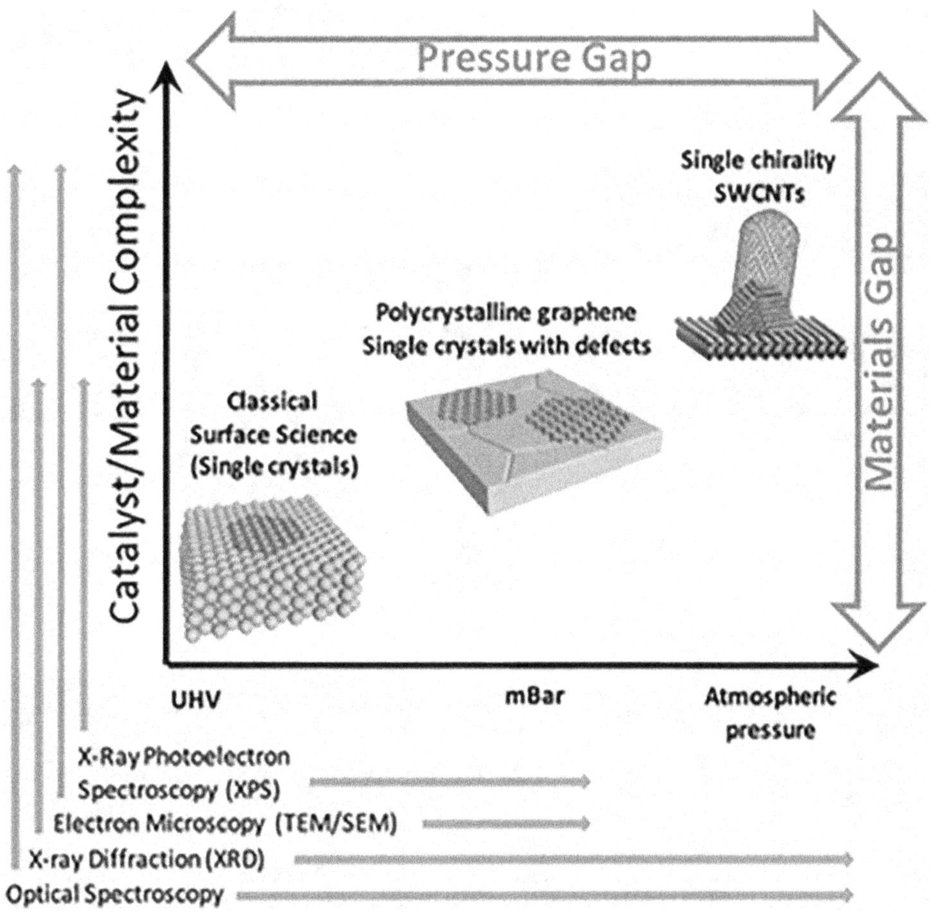

FIGURE 1.17 Pressure and materials gap for catalytic growth of SWCNTs and graphene. Overlaid on the chart are various in situ methods that have been used to characterize SWCNT and graphene growth, and their operating ranges in terms of pressure and characterization capabilities.

and diffusion into the catalyst bulk as well as the transport of carbon across the catalyst surface and attachment to the graphene edges. Centimeter- and even meter-sized domains can be achieved on appropriately treated Cu–Ni alloy foils (Figure 1.18f) or single-crystal Cu foils (Figure 1.18g), while wafer-scale growth of epitaxially aligned domains has been demonstrated on Ge (110).

1.9.5 In Situ Transmission Electron Microscopy

Early pioneering work focused on the direct observation of SWCNT growth within an ETEM. The in situ ETEM experiments have enabled the observation of catalyst surface and shape reconstruction and step-flow dynamics during SWCNT nucleation, as well as catalyst particle dewetting and glimpses into the early stages of organized growth. In the case of graphene growth, scanning electron and optical microscopy has been used to directly image isothermal growth on polycrystalline metal foils. Meanwhile, low-energy electron microscopy (LEEM) has been used to study graphene growth on a variety of single-crystal substrates. However, the optimum imaging conditions within an ETEM impose restrictions on the SWCNT growth conditions, such as lower pressures and temperatures, which limit its use. The ultrahigh vacuum

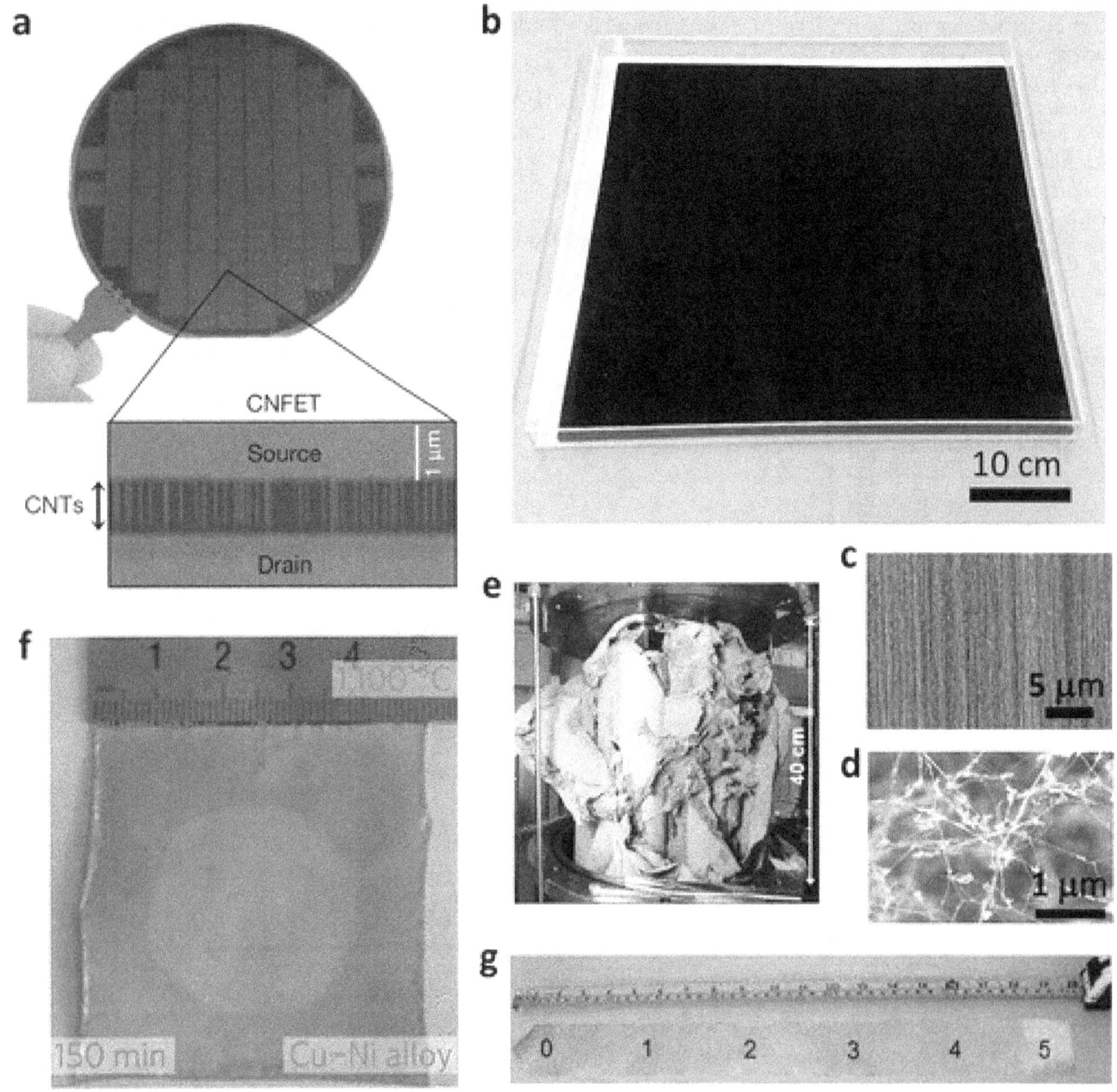

FIGURE 1.18 Recent advances in large-area growth and applications of SWCNTs, BNNTs, and graphene. (a) Top: Optical image of a 4 in wafer after fabrication of SWCNT field-effect transistors (FET) for logic operations. Bottom: SEM image of an SWCNT FET showing horizontally aligned semiconducting SWCNTs between the source and drain electrodes. (b) Optical image of a 50 × 50 cm^2 SWCNT forest grown by water-assisted CVD. (c) SEM image showing the alignment of SWCNTs in an array. (d, e) SEM and optical image of BNNTs produced by RF thermal plasma. (f) Synthesis of large-area single-crystal graphene on a 2 × 2 in^2 $Cu_{85}Ni_{15}$ alloy substrate from a single nucleus. (g) Graphene grown on a 2 × 50 cm^2 single-crystal Cu (111).

conditions and consequent slower kinetics in these studies can reveal the behavior close to thermodynamic equilibrium but are usually far from the realistic conditions used for large-scale graphene or CNT growth (Figure 1.17).

1.9.6 In Situ Spectroscopy

In addition to microscopy, in situ spectroscopic measurements during synthesis have furthered our understanding of SWCNT and graphene growth mechanisms. X-ray-based techniques such as X-ray photoelectron spectroscopy (XPS) and X-ray scattering/diffraction have been particularly effective. On the one hand, XPS can probe the chemical state of the catalyst, and ambient pressure XPS (AP-XPS) studies using synchrotron radiation allow high temporal and energy resolution to be achieved and have shown that the catalyst should be in a reduced state prior to SWCNT nucleation.

1.9.7 Growth Challenges

Although impressive progress has been made over the past decade, to achieve the level of growth control demanded by many of the proposed high-value applications of graphene and other 2D materials, a number of key challenges still remain. The integration of graphene with other materials is also critical to applications, for example, as a passivating coating, functional device layer, or in lateral and vertical heterostructures with other 2D materials. Continuing to build on the progress to date in graphene CVD will be critical to addressing these challenges and realizing many of the envisioned applications of graphene.

1.10 Methods of Purification and Dispersion of Carbon Nanotubes

Purification is the primary step and is always needed before any further use of CNTs. Prepared CNTs contain an assortment of impurities that are essential to be removed prior to their utilization in drug, gene, or vaccine delivery. These vanish by post-manufacturing treatments, and three fundamental methods have been reported for purification:

1. Gas phase
2. Liquid phase
3. Intercalation techniques

Depending on the method of carbon nanotube synthesis used, there are numerous distinct purification methods and procedures to choose from. All purification procedures consist of the following major steps: filtration to remove large graphite particles and aggregations, dissolution in appropriate solvents to eliminate catalyst particles (concentrated acids as solvents) and fullerenes (use of organic solvents), microfiltration and chromatography to size-separate and remove amorphous carbon clusters. Purification of MWNTs produced by arc discharge procedures can be accomplished by the use of oxidation processes that can separate MWNTs from polyhedral graphite-like particles. Most of the techniques used are combined with other techniques. The various steps used in the purification of nanotubes are as follows.

1.10.1 Air Oxidation

Air oxidation treatment of the CNTs is a useful way to eliminate carbon impurities (defect carbon) and metal catalyst. The main disadvantage of this process is that not only the impurities but also the CNTs are oxidized. The reason that impurity oxidation is preferred is that these impurities are most commonly attached to the metal catalyst, which also acts as an oxidizing catalyst. The optimum yield of this process is highly dependent on a lot of factors, such as metal content, oxidation time, oxidizing agent, and temperature.

1.10.2 Acid Refluxing Treatment

Acid treatment—it removes the metal catalyst by exposing the metal surface to oxidation or sonication. Then the metal catalyst is exposed to acid and solvated so that the nanotubes remain in the suspended form. When HNO_3 is used for the treatment, it only affects the metal catalyst, but not the nanotubes or other particles of carbonaceous nature [5]. With HCl, less effect on single-walled carbon nanotubes and other carbon particles was observed during reflux, but unlike HNO_3, metal should be exposed to acid for the lysis of graphitic carbon and short fullerenes. The metal will be melted and can be removed by using vacuum having high temperature [5].

This is among the most expedient techniques for reducing the load of contaminants from nanotubes. Various acids which are employed could be sulfuric acid (H_2SO_4), hydrochloric acid (HCl), and nitric acid (HNO_3).

1.10.3 Surfactant-Aided Ultrasonication, Filtration, and Annealing Purification Methods

Annealing. High temperature between 873 and 1,873 K will result in the rearrangement of nanotubes, with the consumption of defects resulting in the pyrolysis of graphitic carbon and short fullerenes. The metal will be melted and can be removed by using vacuum with high temperature [5].

1.10.4 Ultrasonication

Sonication is well-known as one of the effectual processes to get rid of the amorphous impurities adhering or binding to the walls of CNTs using suitable solvents [5]. During sonication, the solvent molecules are able to interact with CNTs and hence lead to solubilization, which can improve purification efficiency [5]. In ultrasonication, vibration caused by sonic waves result in separation of particles and dispersion of nanoparticles agglomerates. This process demands that nanoparticles be isolated utilizing ultrasonic vibrations.

1.10.5 Magnetic Purification

In this process, ferromagnetic nanoparticles are mechanically separated from their graphitic lattice. Magnetic purification—the removal of ferromagnetic (catalytic) particles occurs mechanically from their graphitic shells. To get rid of these ferromagnetic particles in an ultrasonic bath, the SWNTs suspension and inorganic nanoparticles (ZrO_2 or $CaCO_3$) are mixed together, followed by the trapping of particles by stable magnetic poles. Since SWNT of high purity will be obtained by chemical treatment, a large equipment is not required, and the production of laboratory-sized quantities of SWNTs containing no magnetic impurities has been observed [5].

1.10.6 Microfiltration

This method is employed to remove carbon nanoparticles by microfiltration, which is completely based on size or particle separation. The other nanoparticles, such as catalyst metal and fullerenes, also pass through the filter. One way of separating fullerenes from CNTs by microfiltration is to immerse the as-synthesized CNTs first in a carbon disulfide solution. The contents that are insoluble in carbon disulfide (as-synthesized CNTs) are then trapped in a filter. The fullerenes that are solvated in the carbon disulfide pass through the filter.

1.10.7 Cutting

The nanotubes can be shortened or cut by three steps: chemically, mechanically, and the combination of both.

1. **Chemically:** Chemicals are used for cutting CNTs. After partially functionalizing the CNTs, followed by pyrolization in the form of CF_4 or COF_2, fluorinated carbon will be driven off the sidewall, which leaves behind the nanotubes; those are chemically cut [5].
2. **Mechanically:** Due to high friction between the nanoparticles and the nanotubes, the bonds will break and disordered, and the cutting is caused by ball milling [5].
3. **The combination of both (chemically and mechanically):** In an acid solution, cutting of the nanotubes is ultrasonically induced; thus, the ultrasonic vibration will provide the sufficient energy for the nanotubes to leave the catalyst surface [5].

1.10.8 Functionalization of Carbon Nanotubes

Functionalization depends on making carbon nanotubes more hydrophilic in nature than the contaminations by appending different groups to the tubes. Presently, it is anything but difficult to isolate them from insoluble contaminations, for example, metal particles, by filtration. An added functionalization procedure also leaves the carbon nanotubes' structure unblemished and makes them solvent for chromatographic size division. For recovery of the purified carbon nanotubes, the helpful functional moieties can be evidently cleared by heat treatment process, such as annealing.

1.10.9 Chromatography

This system is primarily used to isolate little amounts of CNTs into fractions with little length and diameter dispersion. The CNTs overflow into a column comprised of permeable materials, through which the CNTs will run. The columns utilized are gel permeation chromatography and high-performance liquid chromatography size-exclusion chromatography columns. The number of pores the CNTs will move through relies upon their size. This implies that the littler the particle, the more drawn out the pathway as far as possible of the section will be, and that the bigger atoms will succeed first.

To separate the CNTs in relation to small length and diameters, chromatography is mainly used. Carbon nanotubes with a porous material are run through a column, through which CNTs will pass. The GPC (gel permeation chromatography)

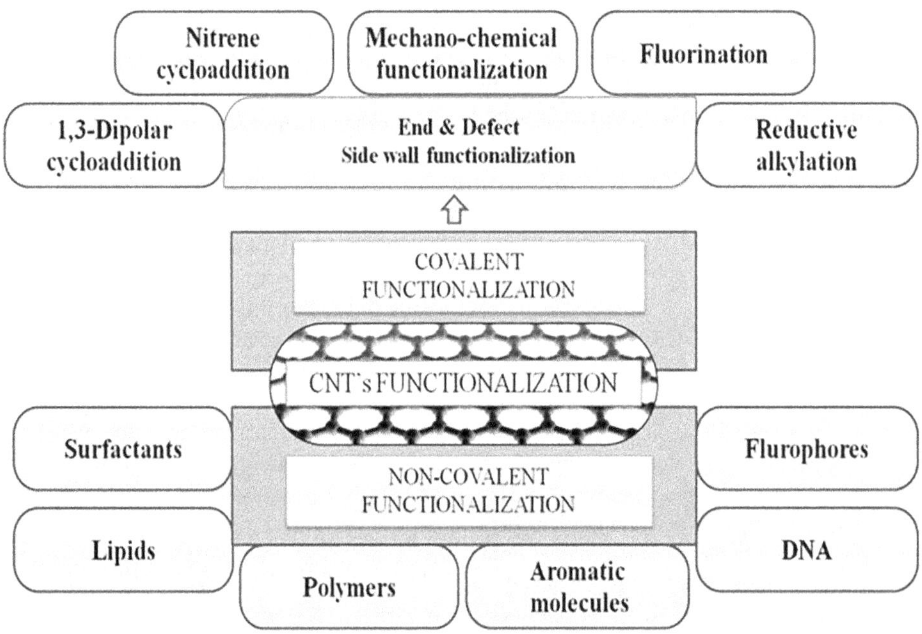

SCHEME 1.7 Approaches for CNT functionalization.

and HPLC-SEC (high-performance liquid chromatography size-exclusion chromatography) columns are some examples which are used in the technique of separation.

1.11 Limitations and Modification (Functionalization)

Carbon nanotubes are poorly soluble in aqueous media and need to be functionalized or modified before use as drug delivery vehicles. The limitation in the applications of CNTs can be defeated, to some extent, by a process named functionalization [5]. Functionalization of CNTs can be achieved in two ways, as shown in Scheme 1.7.

1. **Non-covalent functionalization:** Various non-covalent interactions, for example, π-stacking, hydrophobic, and van der Waals interactions, have allowed for the functionalization of CNTs with a wide range of molecules.
2. **Covalent functionalization:** May is described as a chemical grafting of molecules onto the sp^2 carbon atoms of the π-conjugated skeleton of the CNTs. The basic reaction for CNT functionalization is oxidation [5], performed under strongly acidic conditions. There are two main strategies for covalently functionalizing nanotubes:
    a. End and defect modification
    b. Sidewall modification

Due to its stable structure and the large absorption capacity of the inner tube, CNTs are not soluble in most solvents. To overcome this problem, which significantly restricts the use of CNTs in biosensor applications, CNT functionalization is required [28]. Since its discovery, numerous studies have been carried out to dissolve in solvents and functionalize. The pioneering works in the functionalization of CNTs have developed three main approaches, as follows:

1. Covalently linking chemical groups to the skeleton of CNTs
2. Adsorption of various functional molecules to CNTs
3. Endohedral filling of the internal cavity of CNTs

It is also vital to stabilize the dispersion to prevent the re-agglomeration of CNTs. Thus, a wide range of surface functions can be created on CNTs [28, 29].

Covalent functionalization, non-covalent functionalization, external decoration with inorganic materials, and endohedral functionalization are the four basic techniques accessible for the functionalization of carbon nanotubes. Figure 1.19 illustrates the basic techniques accessible for the functionalization of carbon nanotubes.

1.11.1 Oxidation

The primary method of functionalizing carbon nanotubes includes oxidation by strong acids, resulting in a reduction

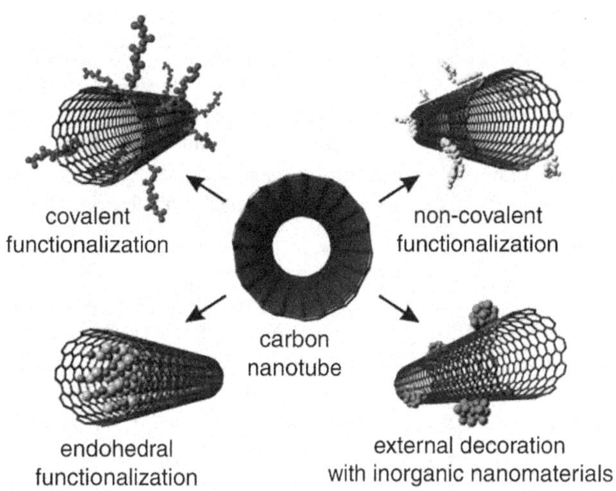

FIGURE 1.19 Basic techniques accessible for the functionalization of carbon nanotubes.

in their length while generating exposed carboxylic groups, improving dispersibility in aqueous solutions.

1.11.2 Addition Reactions

A second method is based on addition reactions to the external wall of the carbon nanotube, based on the 1,3-dipolar cycloaddition of azomethine ylides and heating in DMF in the presence of α-amino acids and an aldehyde.

1.11.3 Other Methods

Other functionalization methods include attaching one or more drugs intended to function as and constituting a single powerful payload that can be triggered to release in the target location. Also recognition units able to encourage the uptake of the carbon nanotube by the target cells, and imaging agents, such as a fluorescent probe, to allow the carbon nanotube to be tracked within the body.

1.11.4 Covalent Functionalization

To improve dispersion, purification, conjugation with biomolecules, anchoring to polymeric composites, and other properties of CNTs, covalent functionalization has been widely used. A covalent bond is much more stable than other methods, like surface adsorption. Direct sidewall functionalization and defect group functionalization are the two main covalent functionalization strategies for CNTs. Both strategies have been used to integrate CNTs into diverse applications, such as tuning electronic properties with active moieties, introducing them into polymeric composites, and fabricating biosensors, drug delivery systems, and tissue engineering scaffolds.

1.11.5 Non-Covalent Functionalization

Non-covalent functionalization of carbon nanotubes entails the adsorption or wrapping of various functional molecules onto the CNTs' tubular surface. This kind of functionalization is particularly fascinating since it is based on p–p stacking, van der Waals interactions, or charge transfer interactions, which retain the tubes' extensive network. The majority of research on non-covalent functionalization has focused on increasing the dispersibility of carbon nanotubes through bundle exfoliation to create individual carbon nanotubes, which are notoriously difficult to distribute homogeneously in solution.

1.11.6 Endohedral Functionalization

The interest of using inorganic chemicals to decorate carbon nanotubes is twofold. On the one hand, it is rapidly developing into a highly effective technology for identifying and detecting faults and functions on external sidewalls. A detailed examination of carbon nanotubes labelled with inorganic elements enables the precise location, distribution, and density of defects or functions on the carbon nanotube backbone to be determined down to the atomic scale. Atomic force microscopy (AFM), scanning tunnelling microscopy (STM), high-resolution transmission electron microscopy (HRTEM), and scanning transmission electron microscopy are the most frequently utilized techniques for characterizing these tagged carbon nanotubes (STEM). On the other hand—and this is the area in which the most interest is being generated—the production of hybrid materials such as CNT-inorganic composites frequently results in increased performance in terms of the quality of the separate components for a given application.

1.11.7 Ends and Defects

The ends of the CNTs are more reactive than the sidewalls. Treating the CNTs with oxidative agents results in introducing oxygenated groups, for instance, carboxylic acid, ketone, alcohol, and ester, at the nanotube ends and defect sites [5] (Scheme 1.5), thus leaving the ends open and possibly cutting and shortening CNTs [5]. Such treatments eliminate amorphous carbon and metal catalyst particles and can remove smaller-diameter (more reactive) tubes. Techniques have been developed to probe the degree of oxidation and the type of oxygenated groups formed [5]. Oxidation also results in hole-doping of the CNTs, causing disruption of its electronic structure [5], though the disruption is less pronounced than those produced in the case of sidewall modification. Other modifications of oxidized CNTs by non-covalent interactions have also been performed through zwitterionic interactions and nonspecific protein binding, which have coupled CNTs to crown ether [5].

1.11.8 Sidewall Functionalization

To introduce higher concentrations of covalently attached functional groups onto the surface of CNTs with the substitution of significant disruption in the electronic structure or the method used to break down the bonds present on the wall of CNTs, which help attach the different functional groups.

1.11.9 External Decoration with Inorganic Materials

A novel method for functionalizing carbon nanotubes is to fill their interior holes with host materials. Filled carbon nanotubes may be used in a variety of applications, from nanoelectronic devices to drug delivery systems that pass through functional ceramics. Carbon nanotubes exhibit bandgap modulation when encapsulated in various materials, making them excellent candidates for molecular electronics.

Thus, functionalization heightens the scope of CNTs as raising nanovectors for the delivery of therapeutics [5].

1.12 Drug Loading Mechanism and Cellular Uptake of CNTs

Functionalized carbon nanotubes are easily internalized by cells through passive and endocytosis-independent mechanisms. Nanotubes conform to a perpendicular position with the cell membrane during uptake, perforating and diffusing through the lipid bilayer to enter the cytoplasm. Other methods of cell penetration are under experimentation, including the use of magnetic carbon nanotubes that "spear" a target cell by the use of an external rotating magnetic field. Molecules containing aromatic groups can be easily bound to CNTs non-covalently by strong π–π interactions. Thus, CNTs possess unique and excellent structural, optical, and electrical properties for the development of advanced drug delivery systems [5] (Figure 1.20).

1.13 Uptake *of* CNTs *by* Cell

CNTs have been aimed and actively explored as multipurpose, innovative nanocarriers for drug delivery systems. Thanks to their very high aspect ratio, CNTs can penetrate the cell membrane and be taken up by cells. After entering the cell, CNTs are mainly located inside cell endosomes and lysosomes. Individualized CNTs are able to travel through various cellular barriers and even enter the nucleus [5]. The applicable cell-internalization mechanisms for CNTs are the endocytosis–phagocytosis pathway. Endocytosis represents the engulfing of an extracellular particle by the cell (for example, viruses ~100 nm in size) through the formation of a vesicle that is then integrated into the cell. Endocytosis is an energy-using process in which cells absorb molecules (proteins) by engulfing them. Endocytosis is mediated by the formation of vesicles, so-called endosomes, containing cell-bound materials that segregate from the plasma membrane and get internalized.

Passive diffusion–phagocytosis is similar to endocytosis but usually involves an uptake of larger particles, such as bacteria (~1 μm). In the passive diffusion pathway, CNTs cross the lipid bilayer in a needle-like manner [5]. The uptake mechanism of SWCNTs through phagocytosis can be enhanced by functionalization through conjugation with phospholipids. Raffa et al. reported the cellular uptake of nanotubes within lysosomes and phagosomes of healthy and normal cells [5].

These two processes are energy-dependent and are hindered at low temperatures (Figure 1.21). Energy-dependent endocytosis was reported as the main internalization mechanism of SWCNTs bound to various types of proteins [5]. In addition, the imaging of SWCNTs within the phagosomes and lysosomes of healthy cells also suggests uptake by phagocytosis [5]. Uptake by diffusion was reported for MWCNTs [5]. The

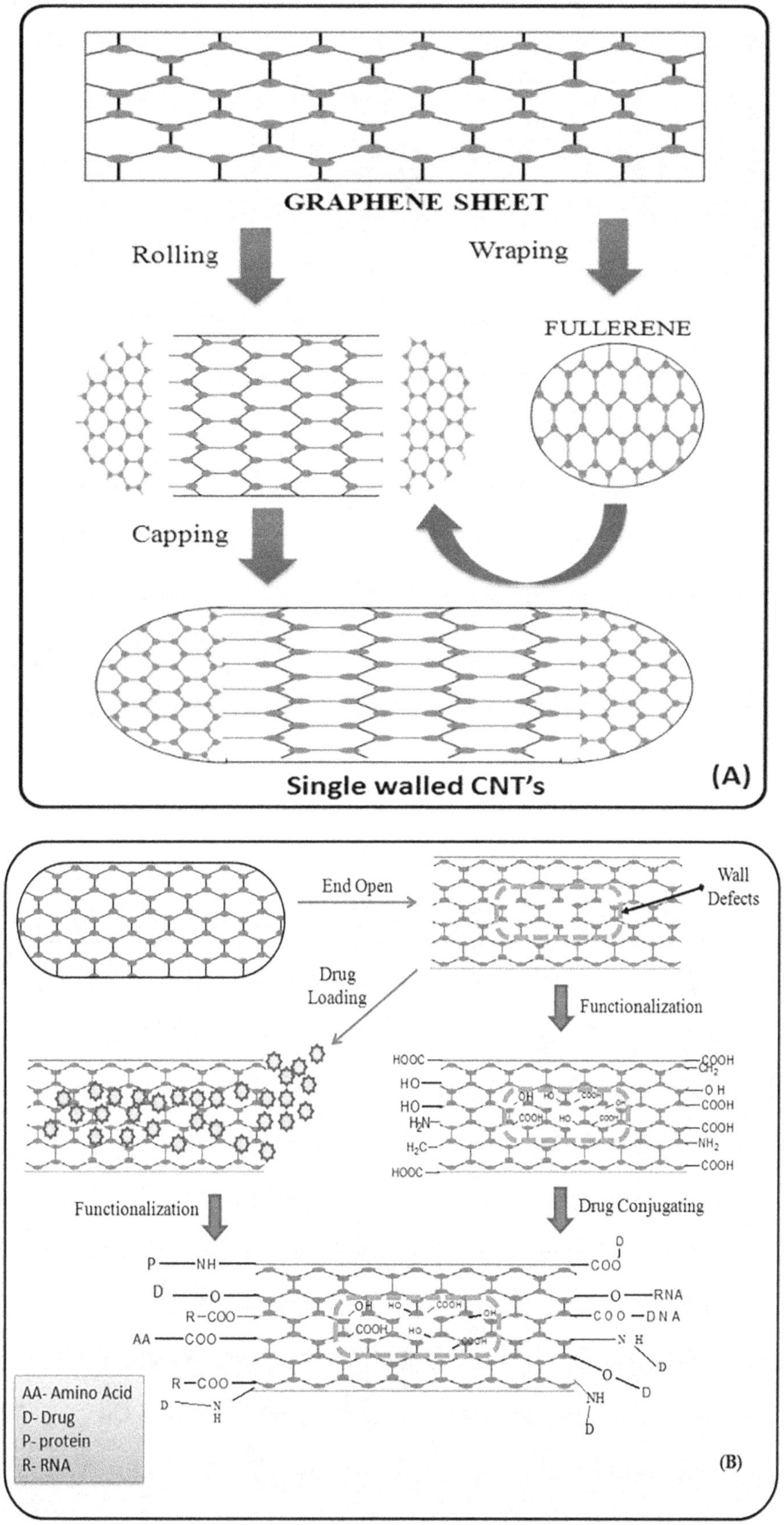

FIGURE 1.20 Building of SWCNTs/MWCNTs and its physical and chemical treatment for use as drug carriers. (A) Demonstration of the structure formation of SWCNTs with the two ends closed. (B) The diagram of the strategy for the preparation of CNT-based drug delivery systems. (C) Schematic representation of receptor-mediated endocytosis of CNTs: (a) receptor association of ligand-conjugated drug-loaded CNTs, (b) endosomal uptake of conjugates, (c) release of drug at the targeted site, (d) formation of recycling vesicles, and (e) receptor regeneration.

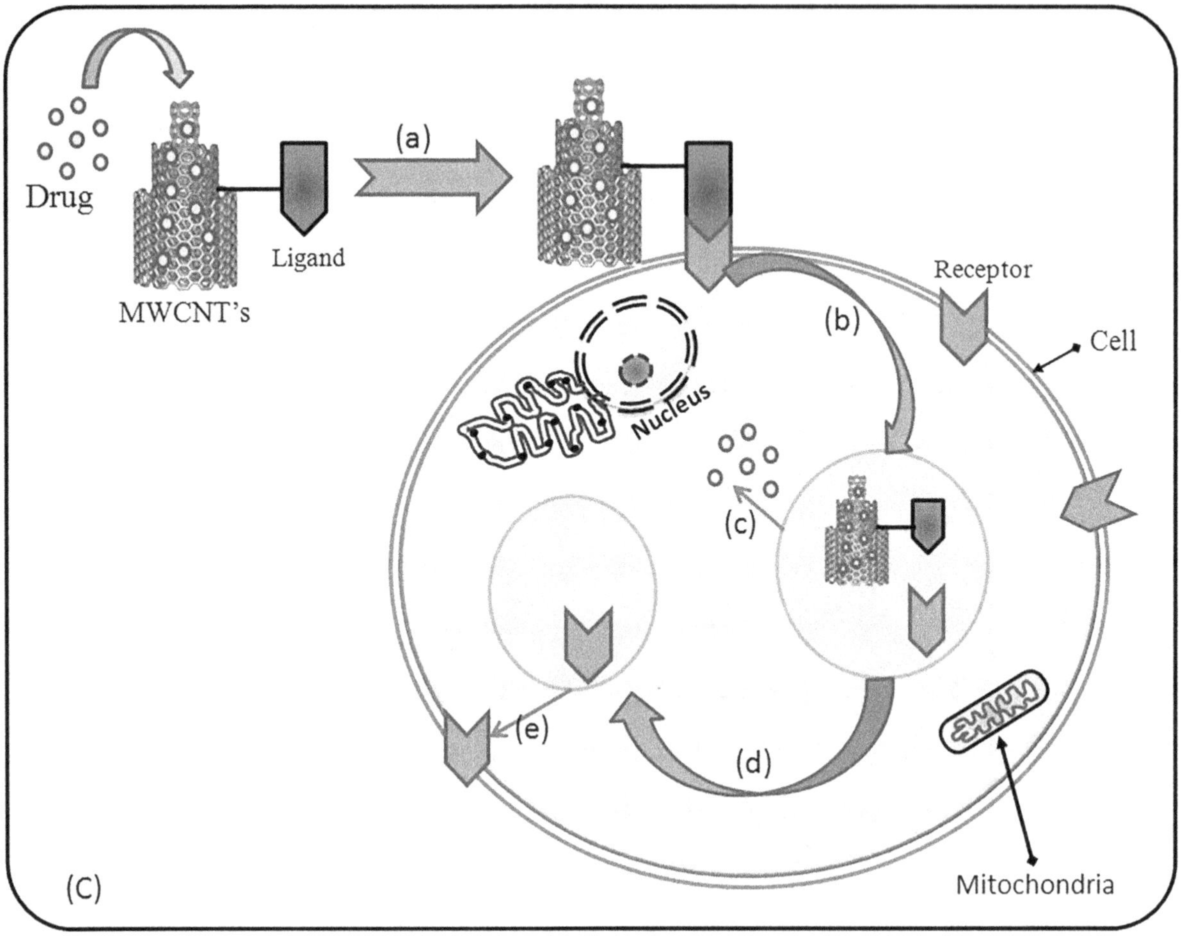

FIGURE 1.20 (Continued)

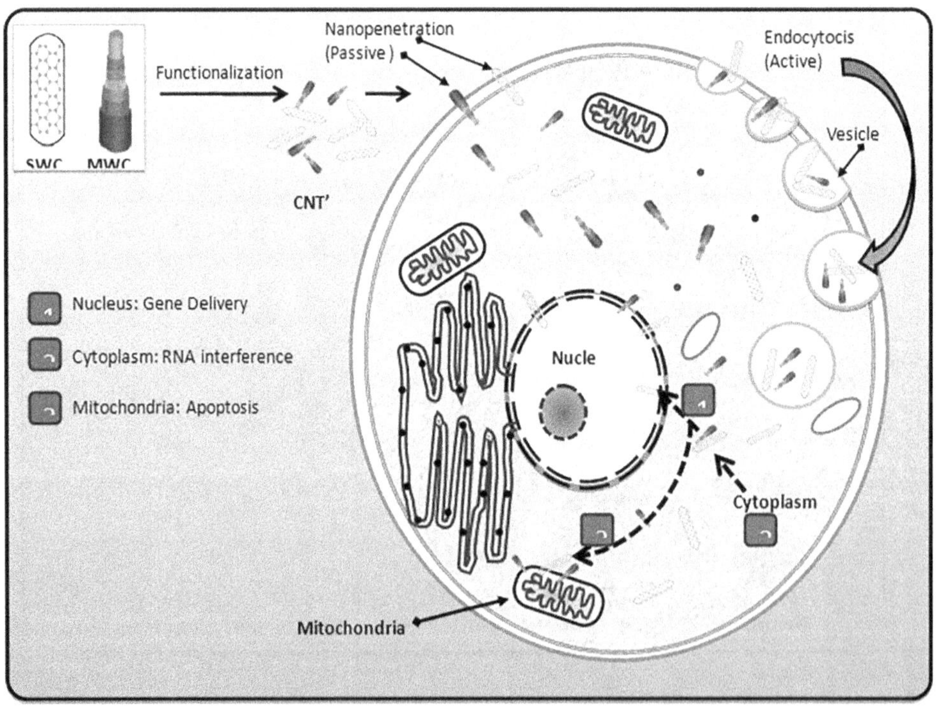

FIGURE 1.21 Possible mechanisms of CNT and cell interactions showing receptor-mediated endocytosis or nanopenetration, which is functionalization-dependent.

f-CNTs penetrate inside cells at 4°C. They may also penetrate into cells in the presence of inhibitors of endocytosis, that is, sodium azide, 2, 4-dinitrophenol (DNP).

1.14 Breakdown Mechanism of CNTs in the Body

A group of Swedish and American scientists has shown for the first time that carbon nanotubes can be broken down by a lysosomal enzyme, myeloperoxidase (MPO), an abundant enzyme of neutrophils granulocytes found in white blood cells and, to a lesser extent, also in certain macrophages [5], since it clearly shows that endogenous MPO neutralizes harmful bacteria and that the enzyme also works on carbon nanotubes, breaking them down into water and carbon dioxide. Shvedova et al. (2012) [30] reported that, in simple biochemical model systems, MPO turned out to be effective in oxidative biodegradation of SWCNT via a plethora of intermediate aliphatic and aromatic products to ultimately yield carbon dioxide (CO_2) and water (H_2O) by a combination of two pathways associated with the following:

1. Hypochlorite generated by the enzyme in the presence of chloride
2. Reactive intermediates of the enzyme [5]

The researchers also showed that carbon nanotubes that have been broken down by MPO no longer give rise to inflammation in mice [5].

1.15 Toxicity *of* CNTs

In cases where CNTs have a toxic interaction by cells, the mechanisms of toxicity are coming into focus. Results suggest that CNTs may cause harm to cells by activating many pathways at once, mostly involving DNA damage [5]. In one study, most cells incubated with CNTs halt at the G1 phase of the cell cycle [5]. Another study showed that mesothelial cells exposed to SWCNTs at concentrations ~25 μg/cm^2 activated DNA recovery along with changes in the cell cycle and generation of apoptotic signals. It was also observed that CNT/DNA interaction was the preferred route of toxicity in a 3 h incubation study with 96 μg SWCNT/cm^2, which induced DNA damage (through micronucleus generation) in lung fibroblasts [5]. It should be possible, through the observation of specific toxic events that result from incubations with different types of f-CNTs, to test for functional groups that reduce the severity of such events.

The harmful effect of nanoparticles arises because of high surface area and intrinsic toxicity of the surface [5]. CNT, in the context of toxicology, can be classified as "nanoparticles" due to their nanoscale dimensions; therefore, unexpected toxicological effects upon contact with biological systems may be induced.

The study of the adverse effects of nano-sized particles and fibers and their interaction in the living organism has been termed as "nanotoxicology." A nano-sized particle could have the potential to cause the toxicity.

Certain properties determine the toxicity of nano-sized particles:

- The surface area/mass ratio of the particles. If the particle has a larger surface area, it provides greater contact with the cellular membrane and as well as provides greater capacity for adsorption and transport of toxic substance.
- Retention of particles within a physiological environment. Retention time determines the cellular contact and therefore causes greater chances for damage. Retention time also determines its mobility either through clearance or migration to nearby tissue.
- Inherent toxicity of contaminants present in nanomaterials.

SWCNT elicited cytotoxicity in a concentration-dependent manner, while SWCNT-PEG was less cytotoxic. ROSs were generated after exposure to both nanomaterials. Gene expression analysis using a real-time PCR array showed that the genes involved in oxidoreductases and antioxidant activity, nucleic acid or lipid metabolism, and mitochondria dysfunction were highly represented (Scheme 1.8) [30]. The alterations of genes were surface coating-dependent. The findings suggest that surface functionalization of SWCNT decreases the oxidative stress–associated response. It has been found in [30] that the exposure of primary human immune-competent cells to cytotoxic ZnO nanoparticles results in upregulation of genes encoding metallothioneins, low-molecular-weight proteins with metal-binding capacity, and antioxidant properties (unpublished observations). The results are not unexpected in light of the fact that ZnO nanoparticles undergo dissolution when immersed in cell culture.

The basic idea of nanomaterials' toxicity can be revealed by its lung deposition. The lung deposition of a nano-sized material depends upon its surface area/mass ratio. C_{60} fullerenes do not prove significant toxicity; it shows the speedy distribution in rates and deposition in many tissues like brain, liver, and spleen [5]. Studies showing the toxicity profile of CNTs are summarized in references [5, 30].

1.16 Different Impressive Properties of Carbon Nanotubes

The properties of CNTs depend on atomic regulation (the shape of rolling graphite layers), the diameter and length of the tubes, and the morphology or nanostructure. CNTs are found as single-walled or multi-walled structures, and MWCNTs are simply composed of concentric SWCNTs. Besides, MWCNTs offer superior opportunities than SWCNTs, as they are easier to produce due to lower product cost per unit, advanced thermal and chemical stability, and easier control of the growth process [49].

All the extraordinary features of the CNTs, especially the superior electrical features, such as electron mobility

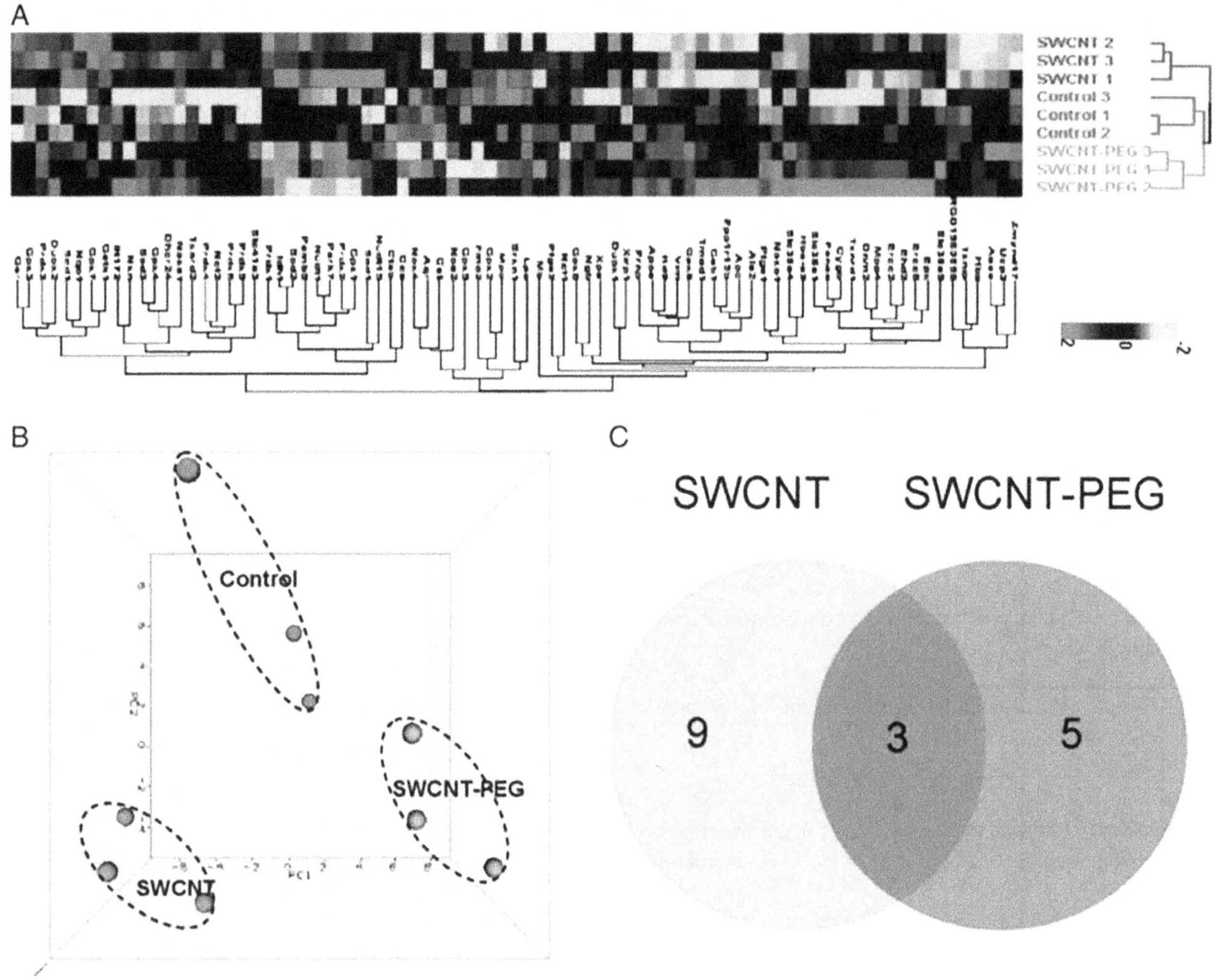

SCHEME 1.8 Transcriptomic assessment of cytotoxic effects of SWCNT. The effect of surface modification of SWCNT on oxidative stress genes was determined using real-time PCR array to evaluate 84 genes related to oxidative stress. (a) Hierarchical cluster analysis (HCA) and (b) principal component analysis (PCA) of nine array data from neuronal PC12 cells treated with SWCNT (blue dots), SWCNT-PEG (green dots), and vehicle (red dots). (c) Venn diagram of the genes significantly changed by SWCNT or SWCNT-PEG treatment.

(100,000 cm^2/Vs), field-effect mobility (79,000 cm^2/Vs), and electrical conductivity (10^4 S/cm), have made CNTs the perfect candidate for improving biosensing tools.

The important properties of carbon nanotubes are the following:

1. Carbon nanotubes are cylindrical tubes of nanoscopic dimensions. There are two types of nanotubes: CNT-SW (single-walled nanotubes) and CNT-MW (multi-walled nanotubes).
2. Typical diameters range from a few nanometers (approx. 5–30 nm, and even <1 nm for single-walled nanotubes); typical lengths are in the range of a few millimeters [31].
3. The substructure of carbon nanotubes ("armchair," "zigzag") is derived from the type of process used during synthesis and affects features, such as the existence of semiconductor properties. The electric and thermal properties of the raw materials are greatly superior to those of conventional materials. In particular, the correct insertion of the carbon nanotubes into a material matrix will cause a significant shift of the percolation curve toward reduced material concentrations [32].
4. Another interesting property of carbon nanotube is that their electrical resistance changes significantly when other molecules attach themselves to the carbon atoms.
5. Another property of nanotubes is that they can easily penetrate membranes, such as cell walls. In fact, nanotubes' long, narrow shape makes them look like miniature needles, so it makes sense that they can function as a needle at the cellular level. Medical researchers are using this property by attaching molecules that are attracted to cancer cells to nanotubes to deliver drugs directly to diseased cells.

6. These promising properties are based on the emergence of a network that takes advantage of the high aspect ratio between the length and the diameter. The formation of networks also supports the improvement of mechanical properties within the matrices, particularly as the basic material has a tensile strength (11–63 GPa) 20 times that of steel.

Carbon nanotubes' elasticity is another outstanding attribute. Nanotubes are flexible to shape and will recover their original shape when exposed to high axial compressive forces, but their elasticity is limited and can be momentarily deformed by very strong force presses. Atomic vacancies or a rearrangement of carbon bonds might impair the nanotube's strength. A nanotube's elasticity is measured by its elastic modulus. Transmission electron microscopes (TEM) measure the elasticity modulus of multi-wall nanotubes (MWNTs) (TEM). TEM scientists analyze heat vibrations at both ends of tubes. They can tolerate high temperatures and also act as excellent heat conductors due to the strength of the atomic bonds in carbon nanotubes. They can endure temperatures up to 750°C and 2,800°C in a vacuum. The thermal conductivity of carbon nanotubes is affected by tube and ambient temperature. Table 1.6 summarizes some significant carbon nanotube physical properties.

A number of properties result from the regular formation of carbon atoms in graphene cylinders. Carbon nanotubes are a huge cylindrical large molecule consisting of a hexagonal arrangement of sp^2-hybridized carbon atoms (C–C distance is about 1.4 Å). The wall of CNTs consists of single or multiple layers of graphene sheets, of which those formed by rolling up of single sheet are called single-walled carbon nanotubes (SWCNTs) and those formed by rolling up of more than one sheet are called multi-walled CNTs (MWCNTs). Both SWCNTs and MWCNTs are capped at both ends of the tubes in a hemispherical arrangement of carbon networks called fullerenes wrapped up by the graphene sheet (Figure 1.20). The interlayer separation of the graphene layers of MWCNTs measures approximately 0.34 nm on average, each forming an individual tube, with all the tubes having a larger outer diameter (2.5 to 100 nm) than SWCNTs (0.6 to 2.4 nm). SWCNTs have a better-defined wall, whereas MWCNTs are more likely to have structural defects, resulting in a less-stable nanostructure. In the medical field, three main attributes of CNTs have been exploited:

- Their small size.
- Their high surface-area-to-volume ratio.
- Their ability to contain chemicals.

TABLE 1.6

The Physical Properties of Carbon Nanotubes

Physical Properties		Values
Equilibrium structure	Average diameter of SWNTs	1.2 to 1.4 nm
	Distance from opposite carbon atoms (line 1)	2.83 Å
	Analogous carbon atom separation (line 2)	2.456 Å
	Parallel carbon bond separation (line 3)	2.45 Å
	Carbon bond length (line 4)	1.42 Å
	C–C tight bonding overlap energy	Approximately 2.5 eV
	Group symmetry (10, 10)	C5V
	Lattice: bundles of ropes of nanotubes	Triangular lattice (2D)
Lattice constant		17 Å
Lattice parameter	(10, 10) Armchair	16.78 Å
	(17, 0) Zigzag	16.52 Å
	(12, 6) Chiral	16.52 Å
Density	(10, 10) Armchair	1.33 g/cm^3
	(17, 0) Zigzag	1.34 g/cm^3
	(12, 6) Chiral	1.40 g/cm^3
Interlayer Spacing	(n, n) Armchair	3.38 Å
	(n, 0) Zigzag	3.41 Å
	(2n, n) Chiral	3.39 Å
Fundamental gap (optical properties)	For (n, m); n–m is divisible by 3 [metallic]	0 eV
	For (n, m); n–m is not divisible by 3 [semiconducting]	Approximately 0.5 eV
Electrical transport	Conductance quantization	(12.9 k O)-1
	Resistivity	10–4 O -cm
	Maximum current density	1,013 A/m2
Thermal transport	Thermal conductivity	Approximately 2,000 W/m/K
	Phonon mean free path	Approximately 100 nm
	Relaxation time	Approximately 10 to 11 s
Elastic behavior	Young's modulus (SWNT)	Approximately 1 TPa
	Young's modulus (MWNT)	1.28 TPa
	Maximum tensile strength	Approximately 100 GPa

Carbon nanotubes can be produced small enough to pass through holes in tumors or to transport DNA. The large surface-area-to-volume ratio provides a good platform for efficient transportation of chemicals and for the reactions needed for ultrasensitive glucose detection. The carbon nanotube is among the most robust as well as rigid materials, respectively, in aspects of elastic modulus and tensile strength.

1.16.1 Electrical Conductivity Properties of CNTs

The unique electrical properties of CNTs are derived from their 1D characteristics and the peculiar electronic structure of graphite. These unique electrical properties are utilized for fabricating field emission displays (FEDs) as well as constructing electronic computer circuits entirely out of carbon nanotubes.

In chiral forms, CNTs exhibit electrical characteristics. Investigators have shown that CNTs have distinctive conductive characteristics. According to the type of chirality, CNTs could perhaps be conducting or semiconducting, accordingly. Semiconducting SWCNTs are generally p-type semiconductors, but MWCNTs comprise of many SWCNT pipes and therefore may not be strictly one-directional conductors. The varying conducting characteristics stay induced by means of the molecular structure, which consequences in some other band structure, then consequently a varying bandgap.

CNTs can be very conducting and, henceforth, can be said to be metallic. Their conductivity has been demonstrated to be a function of their chirality, the level of bend, just as their width. CNTs can be either metallic or semidirecting in their electrical conduct. The conduct of the ropes of semiconducting single-walled nanotubes is unique, in that the transport current changes unexpectedly at different situations on the CNTs.

CNTs have chiral-shaped electrical characteristics. SWCNTs are resistivity-type metals ranging from 0.34×10^{-4} to 1.0×10^{-4} ohm-cm from carbon atom bonding within. With CNTs prearranged in a hexagonal pattern, every carbon atom is covalently linked by sp^2 molecular hybridization to three distinct neighboring carbons. Thus, in all parts, the fourth valence e- leftovers are free, and these free e- are arranged in an irregular pattern across all atoms, giving the electrical behavior of CNTs. CNTs can be applied in sophisticated electronics in transistors and further switching applications. The significant aspect of CNT emitters is that, at a reduced voltage, the discharge can be achieved.

1.16.2 Strength and Elasticity Property

The elasticity property for both single-walled and multi-walled CNTs is examined by the term known as *modulus of elasticity*, or *elastic modulus*. Such property of multi-walled CNTs can be analyzed using transmission electron microscopy (TEM). Using such an apparatus, the researchers examine and investigate the molecular vibrations owing to thermal forces created at both edges of the tubes.

As the atomic bond strength is high, CNTs not only withstand elevated temperature levels but also act as excellent thermal conductors. Hence, under vacuum atmospheric pressure ranges, they are able to withstand 2,900°C and nearly 800°C at normal pressure conditions. But the prevailing tube temperature and ambient environment may have an impact on thermal conductivity of carbon nanotubes. The prescribed physical properties are outlined in Table 1.7.

Various types of indigenous single-walled CNTs obtained using chemical vapor deposition technique onto a supporting chemical agent are mostly of semiconducting nature (I type). Such nanotube type depicts the impact of field transistor (FET) nature at atmospheric conditions, and these have recently attained greater interest and also achieved extensive exploration toward their application as nanoelectronic materials, indulging logic circuit devices and electronic transistors. Such growing CNTs seem to be p-type, containing doped holes

TABLE 1.7
Physical Properties of CNTs

Physical Properties	Parameter	Range	References
Structure during equilibrium	Mean diameter	1.3–1.5 nm	[33]
Density	Zigzag (16, 0)	1.33 g/cm^3	[34]
	Armchair (10, 9)	1.32 g/cm^3	[34]
	Chiral (12, 5)	1.41 g/cm^3	[35]
Lattice parameter	Zigzag (16, 0)	16.53 nm	[35]
	Chiral (12, 5)	16.53 nm	[36]
	Armchair (10, 9)	16.55 nm	[35]
Interlayer distance	Zigzag	3.40 Å	[36]
	Chiral	3.38 Å	[36]
	Armchair	3.37 Å	[37]
Elastic nature	Young's modulus	1.0–1.27 TPa	[38]
	Tensile strength	About 100 GPa	[38]
Thermal property	Mean free path	Around 100 nm	[39]
	Thermal conductivity	Around 2,000 W/m-K	[40]
Electrical behavior	Current density	1,015 A/m^2	[41]
	Conductance	13.0 (K.Ohms)−1	[41]

with absolute hole depletion and reduced conductance values (100 kΩ to 1 MΩ) in specific to positive logic gate voltages. In the present context, it has been demonstrated that adsorption of molecular oxygen onto the CNTs is a contributing factor to drive the hole doping effect of SWCNTs. Oxygen removal can even lead to the mere existence of a semiconducting nature. Instead, day by day, investigations on CNTs reveal that the electrical properties of such carbon nanotubes are much sensitive to chemical doping impacts and charge transfer mechanism in spite of exhibiting extreme robustness [39].

The type-II CNTs developed by CVD technique appear to be quasi-metallic, consisting of smaller bandgaps in the order of 10 meV. Such CNTs are not sensitive compared to the semiconducting type, due to their electrostatic doping mechanism through gate potentials, but exhibit a mere conductance dip occluded with that of smaller bandgap. These CNTs' origin is a class of non-armchair single-walled CNTs, and band origin may be due to shift of sp^2 to sp^3 orbital hybridization, which occurs prominently by the existence of non-flat hexagonal nature of tube walls. Quasi-metallic types exhibit enhanced electrical conductivity at low-temperature levels when subjected to temperature-dependent experimental studies [40].

1.16.3 Mechanical and Electromechanical Characteristics of CNTs

CNTs possess high stiffness and axial strength as a result of carbon–carbon sp^2 bonding. They are the stiffest known fiber, with a measured Young's modulus of 1.4 TPa. Their elongation to failure is 20–30%, which, combined with the stiffness, projects a tensile strength above 100 GPa, the highest known so far. For example, the Young's modulus of high-strength steel is around 200 GPa, and its tensile strength is 1–2 GPa.

As of now, CNTs are the most grounded issue in disposition. The audit of the writing says CNTs are well-manufactured materials, especially inside the pivotal course. The Young's modulus esteems fewer than 270 to 950 GPA, having highly pliable power between 11 and 63 GPA. Because of one of the unbelievably solid holdings in nature, the carbon–carbon bonding found inside graphite, CNTs have amazingly brilliant power, as they are the hardest game plan still delivered by any analyst. Table 1.8 represents the comparison of the mechanical properties of CNTs with other string materials [42].

TABLE 1.8

Comparison of Mechanical Properties of CNTs with Other String Materials

Material	Young's Modulus (GPa)	Tensile Strength (GPa)	Density (g/cm³)
Single-wall nanotube	1,054	150	N/A
Multi-wall nanotube	1,200	150	2.6
Steel	208	0.4	7.8
Epoxy	3.5	0.005	1.25
Wood	16	0.008	0.6

Source: [42].

A schematic pattern of growth has been extensively used to obtain suspended CNTs in a single wall across certain trenches, along with normal nanotubes, which may be electrically wired up with relative easiness. Operated NEM switches and accessible memory devices have also been envisioned in the nearby future. A powerful control and deterministic mode of synthesis of CNT will further explore exciting opportunities and greater possibilities of finding novel nanomaterials and other devices [41].

1.16.4 Optical Properties of CNTs

Speculative researches have shown that the chiral nanotube's optical activity disappears when CNTs grow larger. Consequently, these parameters also influence other physical characteristics. The optical activity could lead to optical devices where CNTs play a major role.

Carbon nanotubes are novel "one-dimensional frameworks" which can be imagined as moved single sheets of graphite (or all the more accurately, graphene). This rolling should be possible at various points and ebbs and flows, bringing about various nanotube properties. The width normally fluctuates in the range of 0.4–40 nm (i.e., "just" ~100 times), yet the length can shift ~100,000,000,000 times, from 0.14 nm to 55.5 cm. The nanotube perspective proportion, or the length-to-breadth proportion, can be as high as 132,000,000:1, which is unmatched by some other material. Thusly, all the properties of the carbon nanotubes comparative with those of common semiconductors are incredibly anisotropic (directionally reliant) and tunable.

1.16.5 Thermal Conductivity and Expansion Properties of CNTs

CNTs are of high significance not only because of their mechanical and electronic characteristics but also because of their thermal characteristics. Entirely, nanotubes are anticipated to be there as a very exceptional thermal conductor besides the tube, illustrating a feature called "ballistic conduction."

CNTs have been shown to display superconductivity underneath 20°K (roughly at 253°C). Investigations propose that these intriguing strands, as of now, proclaimed for their unparalleled strength and unique capacity to promote the electrical properties of either semiconductors or perfect metals, may sometime in the not-so-distant future, too, discover applications as smaller-than-expected warm conduits in gadgets and materials. It is anticipated, hence, that nanotube reinforcement in polymeric materials may also appreciably progress the thermal and thermomechanical properties of the composites.

1.16.5.1 Field Emission

Field emission comes about from the tunneling of electrons from a metal tip into a vacuum, underneath the utilization of a strong electric field. The little breadth and high aspect ratio of carbon nanotubes is extraordinarily ideal for field discharge. Undeniably for direct voltages, a strong electric field is made at the free conclusion of backed carbon nanotubes because of their sharpness.

1.16.5.2 High Aspect Ratio

Carbon nanotubes address an extremely minimal high aspect ratio conductive-added substance for plastics of numerous types. Their high aspect ratio suggests that a lower stacking of carbon nanotubes is required, contrasted with other conductive-added substances to perceive the equivalent electrical conductivity. This low loading protects more of the polymer resins' robustness, mostly at low temperatures, as well as keeping up other key performance properties of the matrix resin. Carbon nanotubes have shown to be an astounding added substance to give electrical conductivity in plastics. Their high angle proportion, around 1000:1, gives electrical conductivity at lower loadings, contrasted with standard included substance materials, for example, carbon dark, cleaved carbon fiber, or stainless steel fiber.

1.16.6 Dimensional and Small Size

Due to their nanoscale dimensions, electron transport in carbon nanotubes will take place through quantum effects and will only propagate along the axis of the tube. These electrical and structural properties best serve CNTs as far as biosensing is concerned, because current changes in the CNTs can signify the specific biological entities they are designed to detect. The fact that CNTs are small (nanometer scale) allows them to deliver smaller doses of drugs to specific disease cells in the body, thus reducing the side effects and harm to healthy cells, unlike conventional drugs, whilst improving disease cell–targeting efficiency.

The biggest advantage of CNTs is their small diameter, due to which they have been attached onto normal AFM tips in order to improve their resolving capability. The small size of SWCNTs makes it easier to study chemical bindings between only one pair of receptor/target. Another application utilizing the small size of SWCNTs is as electron emitters. This kind of emitter can be used to extract electrons to generate light, either visible (TV) or X-ray (portable and high-resolution X-ray machine).

1.16.7 Chemical Properties and Species Interaction

SWCNTs are mostly inert in nature. The covalent attachment that agglomerated the molecular species with fully bonded sp^2 hybridization onto sidewalls of CNT proves to be complex. The adsorbed molecules onto CNTs through the development of non-covalent forces have evidently turned to be facile and consequently lead to possible effects on their physical properties and also with their potential applications.

Similarly, illumination of UV light at low photon intensity forces a drastic molecular desorption rate from SWCNTs at even ambient conditions, whereas wavelength-governing measurements predict that the photo-desorption process may occur due to the sudden excitation of electrons occluded in the nanotubes, and perhaps it is a non-thermal process.

1.16.7.1 Solubility

Though SWCNTs have attracted considerable interest owing to their novel, structure-dependent mechanical and electronic properties, research on the applications of SWCNTs has been hampered by difficulties associated with processing and manipulation [43]. Considerable efforts [44] have thus been devoted to the modification of SWCNTs to improve their solubility in solvents and to enhance their compatibility in composite materials. Among various modification methods, sidewall functionalization of SWCNTs has been studied extensively as a route to their separation [45,46], solubilization, and subsequent reactivity. Most of these efforts have involved the use of conventional chemical techniques, such as refluxing and sonication. Many research initiatives have been carried out on carbon nanotubes using such mechanochemistry method, especially with high-speed vibration mill (HSVM) technique. Konya introduced functional groups like thiol, amine, amide, carbonyl, chlorine, etc. onto carbon nanotubes by ball milling in reactive atmospheres.

1.16.7.2 Highly Absorbent

The huge surface area and high absorbency of CNTs make them perfect contender to utilize in air, various gases, and water purification. A lot of investigation is being done in substituting activated charcoal with CNTs in certain ultrahigh purification purposes.

1.16.8 Outline Information

While mechanical, electrical, and electrochemical (supercapacitor) properties of carbon nanotubes are entrenched and have quick applications, the down-to-earth utilization of optical properties is yet muddled. The previously mentioned tunability of properties is conceivably helpful in optics and photonics. Specifically, light-discharging diodes (LEDs) and photograph detectors dependent on a solitary nanotube have been created in the lab. Their exceptional element is not the effectiveness, which is yet moderately low, but the limited selectivity in the frequency of discharge and recognition of light and the chance of its adjusting through the nanotube structure.

1.17 Advantage and Disadvantage of Carbon Nanotubes (CNTs)

1.17.1 Advantage of CNTs

Carbon nanotubes (CNTs) are considered as one of the ideal materials due to their high surface area, high aspect ratio, and impressive material properties, such as mechanical strength and thermal and electrical conductivity, for the manufacture of next-generation composite materials. In spite of the mentioned attractive features, they tend to agglomerate due to their inherent chemical structure, which limits their application.

1. High electrical along with warm conductivity
2. Very high elasticity
3. Highly adaptable and flexible (~18% lengthening before disappointment)
4. High perspective proportions
5. Good field emanation

1.17.2 Disadvantage of CNTs [47, 48]

In spite of their excellent properties and widespread applications, the lack of solubility in aqueous and organic media has been a major technological barrier for CNTs. This is due to their stable structure having a pure carbon element. In addition, they have very high long-range van der Waals forces of attraction, due to which they have a tendency to aggregate together, and it becomes very difficult to disperse them. Thus, the poor processability due to their insoluble and intractable nature has hindered their use in many applications. To overcome this problem of poor processability, and in order to take full advantage of the properties of CNTs, functionalization and solubilization of CNTs have received much recent attention. This helps to extend their application areas immensely.

1. More current innovation, so not as much testing has been completed
2. Lower lifetime (1,750 hours contrasted with 6,000 hours for silicon tips)

The most notable disadvantage of CNTs is the lack of aqueous solubility when exposed to any media, and in order to eradicate such a problem, surface modification is introduced on the carbon nanotubes, that is, stable fictionalization of surface with suitable hydrophilic substituents and reaction chemistries, which can improve both aqueous solubility as well as biocompatibility of CNT.

1.18 Administration of Carbon Nanotubes

Carbon nanotubes have so far been delivered to patients by subcutaneous, abdominal, and intravenous routes. Shorter carbon nanotubes are absorbed into the body more easily through oral routes, passing through columnar cells of the intestines. Carbon nanotubes delivered subcutaneously tend to linger in the area of injection before slowly diffusing away from the region and passing through the lymph system. This is potentially useful for targeting metastatic cancer cells that migrate in this manner.

The pharmacological and toxicological profile of carbon nanotubes requires further investigation before they can be used in clinical settings.

1.19 Examples of Medical and Therapeutic Applications for Carbon Nanotubes

Since the beginning of the 21st century, CNTs have been introduced in pharmacy and medicine for drug delivery system in therapeutics. A number of biomedical applications of CNTs are proposed, including drug vectors, biomolecule, gene delivery to cells or organs, tissue regeneration, and biosensor diagnostics and analysis. In fact, due to their high surface area, excellent chemical stability, and rich electronic polyaromatic structure, CNTs are able to adsorb or conjugate with a wide variety of therapeutic molecules (drugs, proteins, antibodies, DNA, enzymes, etc.) and to carry them near the targeted cell.

CNTs bound to an antibody, which is developed by chickens, have been shown to be useful in laboratory tests to demolish breast cancer tumors. The antibody-containing nanotubes are attracted to proteins produced by one type of breast cancer cell. Then the nanotubes absorb light from an infrared laser, incinerating the nanotube and attaching to the tumor. Using nanotubes as a cellular-scale needle to convey quantum dots and proteins in cancer cells improves the healing process for broken bones by putting up a carbon nanotube scaffold for new bone material to grow on [5].

An additional application of CNTs in medicine is for sensing molecules or species. Many studies on the electrochemical reactivity of carbon nanotubes showed that carbon nanotubes can enhance biomolecules and promote the transfer of electron in proteins (heme-containing proteins). In heme-containing proteins, carbon nanotubes are able to access the heme center of biomolecules that is generally not sensed by glass electrodes. CNTs can also be utilized as blood vessels in order to deliver drugs to their target site. When the drug delivery is done that way, the drug dosage can be lowered (and it is cheaper for pharmaceutical companies). There are two methods, both equally effective:

1. The drug can be attached to the side or behind.
2. The drug can actually be placed inside the nanotube.

For synthetic muscles—due to their high contraction/extension ratio given an electric current—CNTs are ideal.

In artificial muscles, CNTs have enough contractility to make them candidates to replace muscle tissue [5].

Nanotubes function like a needle at the cellular level. This property is used in attaching molecules that are attracted to cancer cells to nanotubes to deliver drugs directly to diseased cells. The attachment of ethylene glycol molecules to nanoparticles of nanotubes stops WBCs from recognizing the nanoparticles as foreign materials, allowing them to circulate in the bloodstream long enough to attach to cells in cancer tumor therapy. Magnetic fields drive drug-loaded nanoparticles to reduce blood vessel blockages in an animal study. Functionalized CNTs are used as emerging nanovectors for the delivery of therapeutics. Functionalization of SWCNTs enhances solubility and allows for efficient tumor-targeting drug delivery. It prevents SWCNTs from being cytotoxic and altering the function of immune cells [5].

The applications of CNTs encompass major fields and various disciplines, which include nanotechnology, medicine, construction, manufacturing, electronics, peripheral hardware, software, and so on (Scheme 1.9). The mentioned applications can be considered: actuators, composites with maximum strength, energy storage as well as energy-conversion equipment, media for H_2 storage, nanosensors and probes, electronic instruments, and process catalysis. Anyway, the forthcoming sections will highlight the detailed applications of CNTs in the biomedical field. There are three parameters which may act as barriers before using CNTs in the fields of biotechnology and biomedical-based industry. These barriers have to be overcome: toxicity, pharmacology, and functionalization perspectives of CNTs.

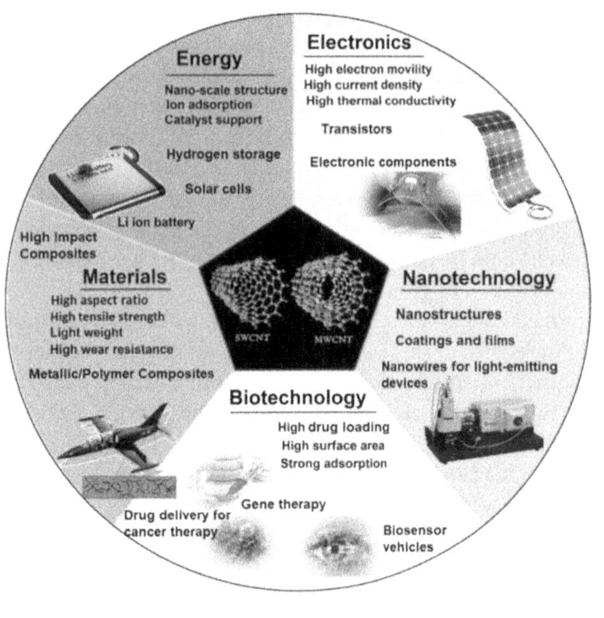

SCHEME 1.9 Applications of enzyme-linked functionalized CNTs.

The most prominent barrier is the toxic nature of CNTs. In general, the coexistence of maximum surface area rendered by CNT, along with the intrinsic toxic nature of nanosurface, can become the most important for the harmful impacts of aggregated nanoparticles. The toxic nature of CNTs can be influenced by the particle size of designed nanotubes. If the particles are less than a size of 100 nm, they are able to exhibit definite harmful effects, such as enhanced potential hazard to the liver and lungs, protein structure modification, escape from usual phagocytic powerful attacks, activation of immunological and inflammatory responses, and explicit redistribution strategy from their spot of tube deposition. Previously made studies have demonstrated that CNTs of water-soluble nature are much more biocompatible with the inbuilt human body fluids and also do not show any toxic ill-effects or abnormal mortality.

1.19.1 Artificial Implant Scopes

Nanomaterials portray their chosen probability and trusted promise in the field of regenerative medicine due to their extraneous physical/chemical properties. In general, in order to avoid rejection of implant materials, which may be the cause of post-administration implant pain, nanotubes were attached to amino acids and to proteins, thereby achieving a promising development. Both the single- and multi-walled forms can be effectively utilized as implants, which may be either artificial joints or other implant materials without any kind of host rejection output response. Perhaps due to its unique material properties, such as maximum tensile strength, these can effectively act as implant materials for bone substitutes, and if suitably filled with calcium, such implants can be shaped or arranged within the bone structure [49, 50].

It has also been shown that proliferation and cellular adhesion can increase with the availability of SW and MW carbon nanotube composites; hence, these can be essentially integrated into natural nanomaterials and synthetic-type materials to fabricate suitable nanocomposites. The specific type of CNT accustomed to artificial implants is represented in Table 1.9.

1.19.2 Tissue Engineering

The scope of tissue engineering lies in the substitution of damaged tissues using biological alternatives that can possibly replace/repair original and normal function. The recent advances in the emerging fields of material science have been promisingly supported in the growth of tissue engineering and regenerative medicine.

CNTs can be recommended for use in the field of tissue engineering under four different perspectives. They are cell tracking/labeling, sensing cellular nature and mechanism, augmenting the mechanism, and enhancing the tissue matrices. Cell tracking/labeling is the specific capacity to identify implanted cell structures and to record the noteworthy improvement of tissue growth *in vivo* as well as non-invasively [51]. Hence, CNTs can be more feasible as contrast imaging agents for optical resolution, for magnetic resonance behavior, and also for radio tracer simulating models.

Novel nanosensors will be effectively utilized in such a way as to determine continuous monitoring associated with the working performance of engineered tissues.

1.19.3 Cancer Cells Tracing

Nanodevices have been investigated that have the effective potential to generate new techniques in cancer treatment, diagnosis, as well as detection. The geometric structures of these nanomaterials may be very small (<100 nm), such that the body will evacuate it rapidly so as to become more efficient, either through detection or by imaging, and thereby enter the damaged cells and organelles inside the body to

TABLE 1.9

Nature of CNT in Artificial Implants Application

Type of CNT	Background Materials	Properties	References
SWCNT impregnated	Chitosan type	Enhancement in cell morphology and growth	[49]
SWCNT (pore type)	Membrane of polycarbonates	Increase in cytoskeletal extensions	[50]
SWCNT	Sodium alginate	Elevated proliferation	[50]
MWCNT	Collagen type	Enhancement in cellular adhesion	[51]
MWCNT	Polyacrylic acid type	Improves cellular discrimination	[52]

have interaction with DNA or protein molecules. The possible detection of cervical cancer–causing cells among human beings can be improved by carrying out modification on the graphene electrode using the peptide form of nanotube folic acid.

Special categories of tumor biomarkers have been tremendously applied and also conceivably utilized in the diagnosis and treatment of hepatocellular carcinoma, pancreatic cancer, colorectal cancer, prostate cancer, and ovarian tumor on epithelial cells, which include CA19–9 (carbohydrate antigen), carcinoembryonic antigen (CEA), alpha-fetoprotein (AFP), human chorionic gonadotropin (hCG), carcinoma antigen 125 (CA125), and specific antigen to prostate (PSA).

1.19.4 Gene and Drug Delivery Applications (CNTs in the Delivery of Bioactives)

Bioactives are chemicals or chemical molecules that have some biological effect on our bodies. For example, hydroxyapatite is a form of calcium phosphate that has a chemical resemblance with the mineral component of bones and teeth tissues. Tissue adhesion and bone growth get promoted and form a bone-like apatite layer which is biologically active. Thus, hydroxyapatite is classified as a biocompatible and bioactive material that has biological applications, such as skeletal implants or dental and bone repair scaffolds [5]. Amphotericin B–loaded MWCNT is employed as an efficient nanocarrier for antileishmanial therapy [5], and gemcitabine-loaded smart CNTs for effective targeting of cancer cells.

As shown in Table 1.10, CNTs possess specific features, such as ultrapure/maximum surface distribution, which essentially provoke them to act as a promising tool for drug delivery, nucleic acids, and peptides.

The releases of drugs using CNTs ae highlighted in Table 1.10.

TABLE 1.10

Release of Drugs from CNTs

Nucleic Acid/ Drug–CNT Type	Cell/Tissue	Properties
Doxorubicin–SWCNT	Colon cancer	Efficient take-up of cancer-causing cells and then transfer to nucleus
Radionuclide–SWCNT	Burkitt lymphocytes	Targeted tumor both in vitro and in vivo
siRNA–SWCNT	Human neuro cells	Improves the working of siRNA-assisted gastrin peptide receptor
Toxic siRNA–MWCNT	Human lung system	Inhibits discrete tumor growth
Cisplatin–SWCNT	Neurocarcinoma	Tumor development—drastic recession
Paclitaxel–SWCNT	Breast cancer	Improved efficacy in treatment with minimal effects

1.19.5 Sensor-Based Biomedical Applications

In the cardiology field, CNTs are used for artificial valves to heart blocks, pacemakers, etc. These CNTs may be involved either individual or in combined form to synthesize smart sensors and various multi-functional materials. They possess maximum aspect ratios that make the CNT to be extremely ideal for operating longer durations and of course continuous sensing. Their greater surface distribution shall be definitely exploited for providing material deposition in order to generate hybrid variety of functional materials or better functionalized to formulate different electrodes for certain applications.

CNTs are much prone to promote its ballistic conductivity, which may occur owing to minimum scattering of electrons in their one-dimensional solid structure containing mean free paths in the measurable range of tens to microns. The exerted mechanical stress/strain can even aid few reproducible changes acquainted with the electrical properties involved in CNT fibers, thereby felicitating it extremely viable to act as electro mechanical sensor devices. The occluded changes are noted as capacitance, inductance, and electric resistance, which can be directly correlated to the impact of strain. Moreover, such CNTs are hugely responsive to compressive, flexural, tensile/torsional strain.

The working mechanism of sensors derived from a simple CNT macroscopic assembly inculcates the change of their electrical resistance or resistivity resulting from mechanical strain is said to be piezo-resistivity, change of its inductance/capacitance via mechanical strain, variation of its electrical resistivity with a plausible variation with temperature is said to be thermoresistivity and a magnetoresistance may result due to variation in electrical resistance, which may be due to varying magnetic field is known as magnetoresistance was shown in Kahng, Gates, Jefferson (2008), In: NASA Technical Report. SAMPE "08 Fall Technical Conference, Memphis, TN, United States; 2008.

Even electrical resistance change can occur owing to variation in mechanical resonance frequency thereby resulting changes in temperature, mass, pressure, and strain. In contrast, the simultaneous change in electrical conductance/resistance is most predominant than any other mild variation accustomed in electrical properties. This happens partially due to selective and simple separation of charge carriers under the influence of temporary/permanent deformation which may lead to certain elevation in resistance. For every minute strain effects, the deformation is shown to be extremely elastic and the electrically conductive mechanism can be completely withdrawn due to its associated strain removal, and thereby leads to a deduction in resistance. However, plastic deformation has been proved to be much different. Though the resistance approaches zero due to strain removal, and hence hysteresis curve has been fully observed. The various sensors involved with such CNT fiber yawns were strain type, pressure sensor devices, chemical sensors, and even mass sensors.

Drug delivery, biomolecule distribution, gene transfer to cells or organs, tissue regeneration, and biosensor diagnostics and analysis are the major applications of carbon nanotubes in the medicinal field. The drug can either be loaded into the CNT structure or be attached to the CNT surface. Two different systems of drug delivery conjugate with CNT have been described either without internalization of the CNT carrier or both the drug and the CNT carrier entering the cells either via the endocytosis pathway or via the insertion-and-diffusion pathway. The internalization method is more effective than surface attachment. In fact, in the former method, after entering the cells, the intracellular environment degrades the conjugated drug releasing pharmacological agents inside the cells, while in the surface attachment method the drug can be degraded in the physiological fluids prior to being internalized by the cells. These novel approaches in drug delivery were first used to bind antineoplastic and antibiotic drugs to CNTs for cancer and infection treatment, respectively.

1.19.6 Drug Delivery and Gene Delivery

The following is a brief recap of the overall procedure of employing CNTs for drug delivery in general. The drug is adhered to the surface or the inside of functionalized CNTs, depending on the application. The conjugate obtained is subsequently administered into the animal's body using traditional methods (oral administration, injection) or directly to the target spot through the use of a magnetic conjugate, which is guided to the target organ, such as lymphatic nodes, by an external magnet, for example. The drug CNT capsule is ingested by the cell, and eventually, the nanotube spills its contents into the cell, resulting in the delivery of the drug. Figure 1.22 depicts a diagrammatic illustration of the drug delivery method in action.

As previously stated, carbon nanotubes (CNTs) have unique features, such as an extremely high surface area, that make them a viable delivery vehicle for medicines, peptides, and nucleic acids, among other things (Table 1.11). Specific drugs or genes can be integrated into the walls and tips of CNTs, which can then recognize cancer-specific receptors on the cell surface. As a result, CNTs can cross the mammalian cell membrane by endocytosis or other mechanisms, allowing them to transport therapeutic drugs or genes more safely and efficiently into cells that were previously inaccessible. If this system comes into contact with cancer cells, it has the potential to activate receptor-mediated endocytosis by recognizing cancer-specific receptors on the surface of cancer cells, resulting in the efficient and targeted release of chemotherapeutic drugs from cancer cells.

1.19.7 Identification of Cancerous Cells (CNTs in Cancer Therapies)

Cancer is a disease characterized by out-of-control cell growth. Cancer harms the body when damaged cells divide uncontrollably to form lumps or masses of tissue, called tumors. CNTs are hopeful drug carriers in the target drug delivery systems for cancer therapies.

It has been demonstrated that the combination of radioisotope-labeled SWCNTs and radionuclide-based imaging modalities (PET and SPECT) can improve tissue penetration, sensitivity, and medium resolution. The presence of numerous characteristic protein biomarkers, which are frequently overexpressed in cancer cells, provides an opening gate for early diagnosis and prognosis, maintaining surveillance after curative surgery, monitoring therapy in advanced disease, and predicting therapeutic response in cancer patients. Many important tumor markers, such as carbohydrate antigen 19–9 (CA19–9), alpha-fetoprotein (AFP), carcinoembryonic antigen (CEA), carcinoma antigen 125 (CA125), human chorionic gonadotropin (hCG), and prostate-specific antigen (PSA), have been widely applied and used in the diagnosis of hepatocellular carcinoma, colorectal cancer, pancreatic cancer, prostate cancers, and epithelial ovarian cancer (PSA). Several cancer biomarkers that can be detected by CNT-based detection devices are listed in Table 1.12 and discussed more later.

TABLE 1.11
Examples of Drugs and Nucleic Acids Released by Carbon Nanotubes

Drug/Nucleic Acid	CNT Type	Cell or Tissue	Properties
Taxoid	SWNTs	Leukemia	High potency toward specific cancer cell lines
Doxorubicin	SWNTs	Colon cancer	Efficiently taken up by cancer cells, then translocates to the nucleus while the nanotubes remain in the cytoplasm
Cisplatin	SWNTs	Squamous carcinoma	Rapid regression of tumor growth
Cisplatin	SWNTs	Nasopharyngeal epidermoid carcinoma, etc.	High and specific binding to the folate receptor (FR) for theSWNT-1 conjugate
Doxorubicin	SWNTs	Breast cancer Glioblastoma	Show large surface areas on single-walled carbon nanotubes (SWNTs)
Doxorubicin	SWNTs	Cervical carcinoma	Increase nuclear DNA damage and inhibit the cell proliferation
Radionuclide	SWNTs	Burkitt lymphoma	The selective targeting of tumor *in vitro* and *in vivo*
Paclitaxel	SWNTs	Breast cancer	High treatment efficacy, minimum side effects
siRNA	SWNTs	Tumor cells both in *in vitro* and *in vivo* mouse models	Increase suppression of tumor growth
Toxic siRNA sequence (siTOX)	Functionalized MWNTs	Human lung xenograft model	Significant tumor growth inhibition
siRNA	SWNT	Human neuroblastoma	Enhance the efficiency of siRNA-mediated gastrin-releasing peptide receptor (GRP-R) gene silencing
SOCS1 siRNA	sWNT	Dendritic cells (DCs)	Reduced SOCS1 expression and retarded growth of established B16 tumor in mice

TABLE 1.12

An Example of How Carbon Nanotubes Are Used to Identify a Cancer Biomarker

Carbon Nanotube	Biomarker	Cancer Type
P-type carbon nanotubes	Prostate-specific antigen (PSA)	Prostate cancer
Multilabel secondary antibody–nanotube bioconjugates	Prostate-specific antigen (PSA)	Prostate cancer
Microelectrode arrays modified with single-walled carbon nanotubes (SWNTs)	Total prostate-specific antigen (T-PSA)	Prostate cancer
Multi-walled carbon nanotubes–thionine chitosan (MWCNTs-THICHIT) nanocomposite film	Chlorpyrifos residues	Many forms
Carbon nanomaterial	Carcinoma antigen-125 (CA125)	Carcinoma
MWCNT–platinum nanoparticle-doped chitosan (CHIT)	AFP	Many forms
Poly-lysine/hydroxyapatite/carbo n nanotube (PLL/HA/CNT) hybrid nanoparticles	Carbohydrate antigen 19–9 (CA19–9)	Many forms
MWCN–polysulfone (PSf) polymer	Human chorionic gonadotropin (hCG)	Many forms
Multi-walled carbon nanotube–chitosan matrix	Human chorionic gonadotropin (hCG)	Many forms
MWCNT–glassy carbon electrode (GCE)	Prostate-specific antigen (PSA)	Prostate cancer
Nanoparticle (NP) label/immunochromatographic electrochemical biosensor	Prostate-specific antigen (PSA)	Prostate cancer
SWNT–horseradish peroxidase (HRP)	Prostate-specific antigen (PSA)	Prostate cancer
Carbon nanotube field effect transistor (CNT-FET)	Prostate-specific antigen (PSA)	Prostate cancer
Carbon nanoparticle (CNP)/poly(ethylene imine) (PEI)–modified screen-printed graphite electrode (CNP-PEI/SPGE)	Carcinoembryonic antigen (CEA)	Urothelial carcinoma
Tris(2,2′-bipyridyl)cobalt(III) (Co(bpy)33+)- MWNTs-Nafion composite film	Carcinoma antigen-125 (CA125)	Carcinoma
Gold nanoparticles and carbon nanotubes–doped chitosan (GNP/CNT/Ch) film	Alpha-fetoprotein (AFP)	Many forms
Multiple enzyme layers–assembled multi-wall carbon nanotubes (MWCNTs)	Alpha-fetoprotein (AFP)	Many forms

Source: [53].

1.19.8 Uses in Anticancer Treatment (CNTs in Cancer Therapies)

Many anticancer drugs, such as epirubicin, doxorubicin, cisplatin, methotrexate, quercetin, and paclitaxel, have been conjugated with functionalized CNTs and successfully assessed both *in vitro* and *in vivo*. The chemotherapy agents can be bound to a complex formed by CNT and antibody against antigen overexpressed on the cancerous cell surface. In this way, it is possible to carry the drug mostly at the level of the tumor cells. Drugs can be linked with a magnetic CNT complex, obtained by fixing a layer of magnetite (Fe_3O_4) nanoparticle on the surface of the nanotubes. In this case, the system CNT drugs can be guided by an externally placed magnet to target a desired organ interested by the cancer cell localization sparing normal counterparts [16]. Moreover, due to their tiny size and accessible external modifications, CNTs are able to cross the blood–brain barrier (BBB) by various mechanisms targeting for acting as effective delivery carriers to treat brain tumors.

CNTs showed some peculiarity in targeting the drug in different tumor types. Molecular and ionic migration takes place by carbon nanotubes, thus offering novel opportunities designed for molecular sensors and electronic nucleic acid sequencing. The variation of a carbon nanotube on a molecular level via biological molecules is effectively an example of the "bottom-up" fabrication principle of bionanotechnology.

1.19.9 Tissue Regeneration

Cell and organ transplantation research, as well as improvements in CNT chemistry, have all made significant contributions to the sustained development of CNT-based tissue engineering and regenerative medicine in the last few years. Carbon nanotubes, among numerous other materials, such as natural and synthetic polymers for tissue scaffolds, may be the most promising tissue engineering candidate because this nanomaterial is biocompatible, resistant to biodegradation, and can be functionalized with biomolecules to enhance organ regeneration. CNTs can be employed as additions to tissue scaffolding to increase the mechanical strength and conductivity of the scaffolding by integrating with the host's body.

1.19.10 Artificial Implant

Because of their appealing chemical and physical features, nanomaterials have the potential and promise to be used in regenerative medicine. Implants are generally rejected because of the post-administration pain, and the attachment of nanotubes to proteins and amino acids has shown promise in preventing this rejection in some cases. In the form of artificial joints and other implants, carbon nanotubes, both single- and multi-walled, can be used as implants without causing a host rejection response. Furthermore, because of their unique qualities, such as high tensile strength, carbon nanotubes (CNTs) can be used as bone substitutes and implants if they are filled with calcium and shaped/arranged into the bone structure.

SWCNT and MWCNT composites have been researched for their ability to improve cellular adhesion and proliferation, and as a result, these nanotubes have been incorporated into a variety of natural and synthetic materials to create nanocomposites. Table 1.13 lists some of the applications of nanotubes as artificial implants, with a brief description of each.

1.19.11 CNTs as Biosensor

Although the use of carbon nanotubes in biosensor nanotechnology is relatively new, it represents an extremely promising application area for therapeutic monitoring as well as *in vitro* and *in vivo* diagnostics. CNTs and glucose-oxidase biosensors, for example, have been combined by numerous researchers to improve the accuracy and ease of manipulation of blood sugar control in diabetic patients, compared to using biosensors alone. Other CNT–enzyme biosensors, such as CNT-based dehydrogenase biosensors, peroxidase, and catalase biosensors, have also been created for a variety of therapeutic monitoring and diagnostic applications. CNTs as biosensor vehicles are highly recommended for the development of sensitive procedures for diagnostics and analyses from the laboratory to the clinic, owing to their length scale and unique structure.

1.19.12 Stimuli-Responsive CNT-Based Drug Delivery Systems

Environmentally sensitive drug delivery systems, also known as smart structures, were developed to deliver therapeutic cargo to diseased tissues by leveraging certain elements that are present in the unhealthy tissue. Later, it was discovered that this notion may also be used to regulate the release behavior of single or several payloads in the context of a cocktail therapy regimen. A number of CNT-based smart systems have been developed to initiate and manipulate cargo release in response to irregularities in physiological/environmental conditions, such as pH, enzymatic, redox gradients, and temperature.

1.19.13 CNTs as Antioxidants

Recent research has revealed that CNTs, namely, carboxylated SWCNTs, are natural antioxidants that may have important medicinal applications in the prevention of chronic illnesses, the slowing of ageing, and the preservation of food. Several anti-aging cosmetics and sunscreen creams have benefited from their antioxidant properties, which have been employed to protect skin against free radicals produced by the body or by ultraviolet light. It will be necessary to do additional research into different CNT forms over the next few years in order to further enhance their valuable free radical scavenger action for biomedical and environmental applications, as free radicals are widely recognized to be extremely harmful species.

1.19.14 CNTs for Infectious Therapy

The use of carbon nanotubes (CNTs) has been investigated as a means of resolving infectious agent resistance to a wide range of antiviral and antibacterial medications, as well as vaccination inefficacy in the body. CNTs that have been functionalized

TABLE 1.13

Application of Carbon Nanotubes as Artificial Implants

CNT Type	Natural or Synthetic Materials Type	Cell or Tissue Type	Properties
Porous SWCNT	Polycarbonate membrane	Osteoblast-like cells	Increase lamellipodia (cytoskeletal) extensions, and lamellipodia extensions
SWCNT-incorporated	Chitosan scaffolds	C2C12 cells/C2 Myogenic cell line	Cell growth improvement
MWCNT	Collagen sponge Honeycomb scaffold	MC3T3-E1 cells, a mouse osteoblast-like cell line	Increase cellular adhesion and proliferation
MWCNT	Polyurethane	Fibroblast cells	Enhance interactions between the cells and the polyurethane surface
SWCNT	Alginate	Rat heart endothelial cell	Enhance cellular adhesion and proliferation
MWCNT	Poly(acrylic) acid	Human embryonic stem cells	Increase cellular differentiation toward neurons
SWCNT	Propylene fumarate	Rabbit tibia	Support cell attachment and proliferation

Source: [53].

have been shown to be capable of acting as antimicrobial agents, including the antifungal amphotericin B. CNTs have the ability to bind covalently to amphotericin B and transport it into mammalian cells, as demonstrated in the earlier study. When compared to the free medication, this combination has been shown to minimize antifungal toxicity by around 40%. Using the antibacterial drug pazufloxacin mesilate in conjunction with amino-MWCNT with high adsorption, our lab has effectively coupled the two compounds. The combination will be used in experimental testing for infection treatment.

1.19.15 CNT for Vaccine Delivery

It has also been demonstrated that functionalized CNTs can be used as vaccine delivery methods. The association of a bacterial or viral antigen with carbon nanotubes (CNTs) allows for the preservation of the antigen structure, resulting in the induction of an antibody response with the appropriate specificity. It has been shown that the attachment of functionalized CNTs with B and T cell epitopes can result in a multivalent system capable of inducing a powerful immunological response, making it a promising candidate for vaccine administration. CNTs that have been functionalized may be a good carrier system for the delivery of vaccine antigens that are in the development stage. Furthermore, because germs can be adsorbed onto the surfaces of CNTs, as in the case of *E. coli*, it is possible that CNTs themselves have antibacterial properties. The antibacterial activity of carbon nanotubes has been related to the oxidation of the intracellular antioxidant glutathione caused by the carbon nanotubes, which results in increased oxidative stress on the bacterial cells and, ultimately, cell death.

1.19.16 Antimicrobial Application

Functionalized CNTs can be used in vaccination procedures. CNTs were shown to activate cells deriving from the innate immune system, such as monocytes, macrophages, and dendritic cells. Microarray profiling of a monocytic cell line, THP-1, showed that CNTs, both functionalized and non-functionalized, activate several genes involved in monocyte response to infection or vaccination, such as nuclear factor kappa-light-chain-enhancer of activated B cells (NF-κB), interleukin-1β (IL-1β), IL-6, tumor necrosis factor-α (TNF-α), among others.

CNTs activate the class II major immuno-compatibility complex (MHC) in antigen-presenting cells, which can, in turn, promote an antibody-based response. The linkage of either a bacterial or viral antigen to CNTs allows the maintenance of antigen conformation integrity, thereby inducing antibody response, increasing both the specificity and the sensitivity.

It has also been suggested that SWNT conjugated with unmethylated CpG DNA motifs can be used as an adjuvant in vaccines. Functionalized CNTs have been demonstrated to be able to act as carriers for antimicrobial agents, such as the antifungal amphotericin B. CNTs covalently attached to amphotericin B reduced the undesired toxicity by about 40% as compared to the free drug.

Moreover, CNTs themselves might have antimicrobial activity through oxidation of the intracellular antioxidant glutathione, resulting in increased oxidative stress on the bacterial cells and eventual pathogen death.

1.19.17 Treatment of Central Nervous System Disorders

Central nervous system (CNS) disorders consist of neurodegenerative diseases and brain tumors. It is more difficult to diagnose and treat CNS disorders than any other diseases because of the unique and complex environment and the restricted anatomical access (blood–brain barrier) of the CNS. Both pristine and chemically functionalized CNTs have positive effects on neuronal growth, charge on the nanotubes could be manipulated to control neurite outgrowth [5], and CNTs functionalized with nerve growth factor or brain-derived neurotrophic factor could stimulate growth of neurons on the nanotube scaffold [5], proving that conventional tungsten and stainless steel wire electrodes coated with CNTs could enhance both recording and electrical stimulation of neurons in culture, rats, and monkeys. CNT-coated electrodes are expected to improve current electrophysiological techniques and to promote the development of long-lasting brain–machine interfacing devices, both of which will aid the diagnosis and treatment of CNS disorders. The nanoparticle-based formulations of some chemotherapeutic agents (e.g., doxorubicin) [5] have the potential for systemic chemotherapy of brain tumors with higher efficacy than the free agents. MWCNTs (p-MWCNTs or MWCNTs functionalized with DNA and siRNA) were found to be internalized by brain microglia (macrophage derived from migratory monocytes in the brain that are believed to be an effective target for brain cancer treatment) *in vitro* and *in vivo* without inducing proliferative and cytokine changes [5]. It indicated that MWCNTs may possibly act as a safe nanovector delivery system for immune therapies of brain cancers (e.g., gliomas) [5].

1.20 Applications of Graphene

Due to the exemplary properties of graphene, such as light weight, electrical conductivity, strong mechanical and thermal strength, graphene is widely involved in different applications, such as electrochemiluminescence (ECL) sensor [54], transistors, water filtration, energy storage, biosensors, and solar cells.

1.20.1 Energy Storage

Graphene is applied in energy storage devices, such as batteries and supercapacitors, because of its high surface area. In Li-ion batteries, graphene is widely used as anode and has a capacity of about 1000 mAh g^{-1}, which is three times higher than that of graphite electrode. Graphene also offers longer-lasting batteries and faster recharge time in seconds. Also, due to its flexibility, graphene is used as a solid-state supercapacitor printed device in textiles for wearable electronics (Figure 1.22a). The theoretical specific energy density increases with increase in graphene content in the supercapacitor, as illustrated in Figure 1.22b.

1.20.2 Water Filtration Technology

Graphene nanoporous membranes can ideally be used for water desalination and filtration with an efficiency of 33% to 100%, depending on the pore size and the applied pressure. Tanugi and Grossman first studied the classical molecular dynamics and reported that water could flow through graphene membranes at a range of up to 100 L cm^{-2} day^{-1}, which is higher in magnitude than RO-diffusive membranes. The desalination capacity of salt water depends on the pore size of the membrane, the quantity of chemical composition, and the applied pressure. Graphene membranes have the capacity to reject 97% of NaCl from seawater.

1.20.3 Transistors

At room temperature, the carrier mobility of graphene is very high; this property makes graphene able to be applied in transistors. The top gate modulates the drain current, and one-layer graphene has better field-effect characteristics compared to silicon transistors. Graphene transistors have been used in antenna-coupled field-effect to detect radiation of terahertz, and from then, field-effect graphene transistors have been applied in sensing proteins, biomolecules, cells, gas, and DNA.

1.20.4 Solar Cells

Recently, solar cells have played a vital role in the production of electrical power. Solar cells efficiency is an important factor in converting light energy into electricity. Graphene, because of their exemplary optical, mechanical, and electrical properties, has been incorporated in dye-sensitized solar cells (DSSC) and used as electrodes to boost the efficiency of photovoltaic cells. They were, for the first time, used as transparent electrodes in 2008 to replace fluorine-doped tin oxide (FTO) at the photo anode. CdS/graphene nanocomposites exhibit superior photocatalytic activities. The introduction of graphene in CdS semiconductor improves photostability, increases the number of reaction sites, and enhances light-absorption capacity in solar cells.

1.20.5 Other Applications

The linkages of other biomolecules, such as genes, proteins, DNA, and biosensors, to CNTs have also been assessed for gene therapy and tissue regeneration. CNTs can effectively transport the genes inside mammalian cells, maintaining their integrity. In fact, when bound to SWCNTs, DNA probes are protected from enzymatic cleavage and interference from nucleic acid–binding proteins; consequently, the DNA–SWCNT complex exhibits superior biostability and increased self-delivery capability of DNA in comparison to DNA used as free moieties. CNTs can interact directly with DNA through van der Waals and hydrophobic forces.

SWCNTs appear to be an excellent platform for biomedical molecular imaging. Scheme 1.10 represents the applications of enzyme-linked functionalized CNTs.

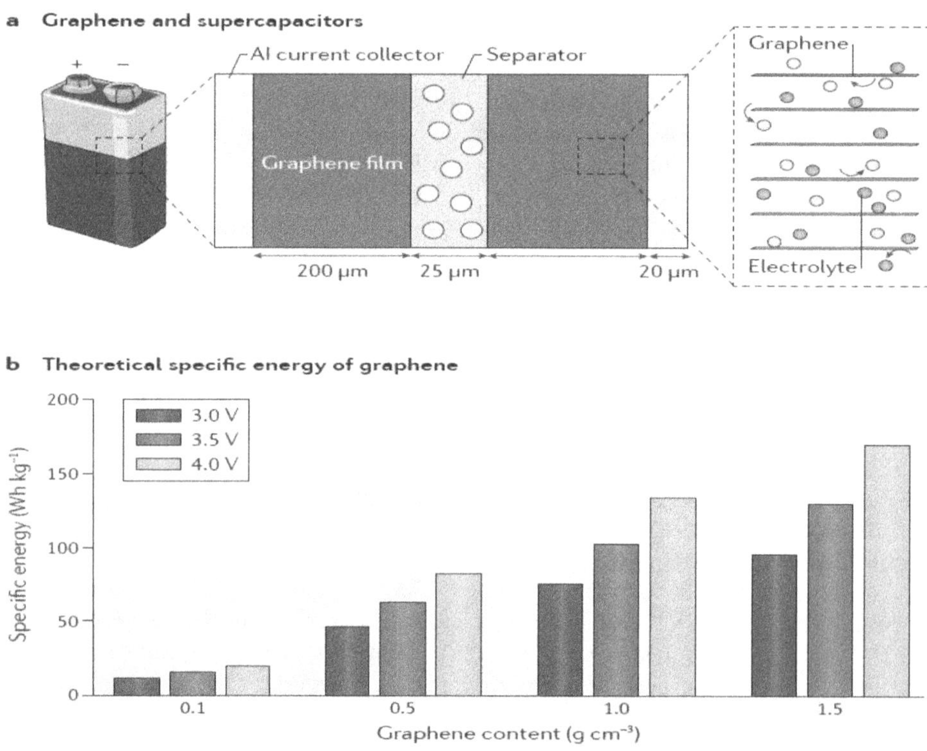

FIGURE 1.22 Schematic diagram of (a) magnified view of the graphene supercapacitor structure. (b) theoretical specific energy density of graphene supercapacitor at different graphene density content.

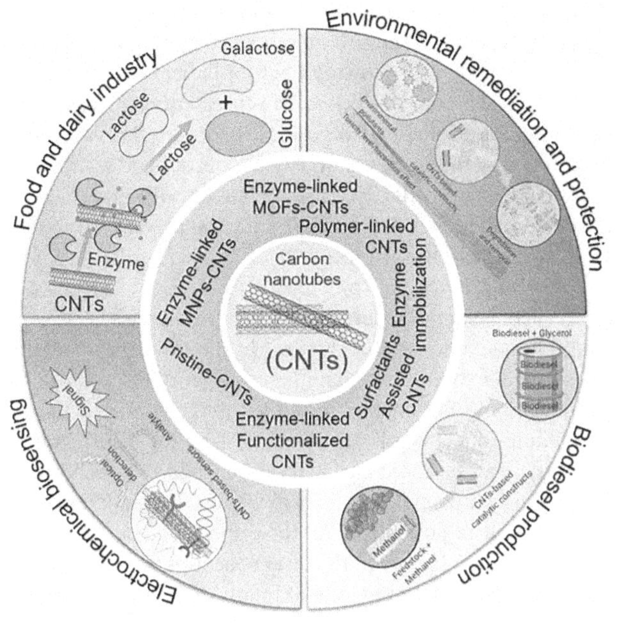

SCHEME 1.10 Sustainable and technological applications of carbon-based nanomaterials.

Polymethyl methacrylate denture base material modified with multi-walled carbon nanotubes showed better results in terms of fatigue resistance, flexural strength, and resilience compared to conventional materials used in dentistry. Besides these main applications of CNTs, they have been shown as a powerful tool for enantiomer separation of chiral drugs and chemicals in the pharmaceutical industry.

1.21 Conclusions

This chapter provides a concise, comprehensive review on recent advances in carbon nanomaterials and their potential applications. We aimed to describe in detail the different types, structures, and properties of CNTs; synthesis and purification methods of CNTs; how to functionalize CNTs; its application in the medicinal field; its toxicological properties and its assessment; *in vivo* pharmacology; and biodegradation pathways of CNTs. A brief history, the structure, properties, growth mechanisms, characterizations, and sustainable and technological applications of carbon-based nanomaterials are discussed (Figure 1.23 and Scheme 1.9). Graphene is considered as one of the most attractive functional nanomaterials in the world due to its excellent unique properties, such as high tensile strength, high electrical conductivity, high carrier mobility, high elasticity, high thermal conductivity, and optical transparency of about 97%. Since its discovery in 2004, graphene has enticed a wide array of applications in different fields like transistors, solar cells, water purification technologies, sensors, batteries, and supercapacitors, which have incredibly attracted a lot of attention among scientists and engineers around the globe.

Nanomaterials provide an enriched knowledge on distinct probability and also definitely sound well in biomedical regenerative therapy for its uniqueness, owing to its excellent physical as well as chemical properties. Thus, CNMs, both in modified and purified type, have a definite potential of establishing promising applications in wide sectors of scientific fields. Perhaps the prompt impregnation of other substituents in carbon nanoforms would confirm its strong perspective for their enhancing biomedical applications and in general

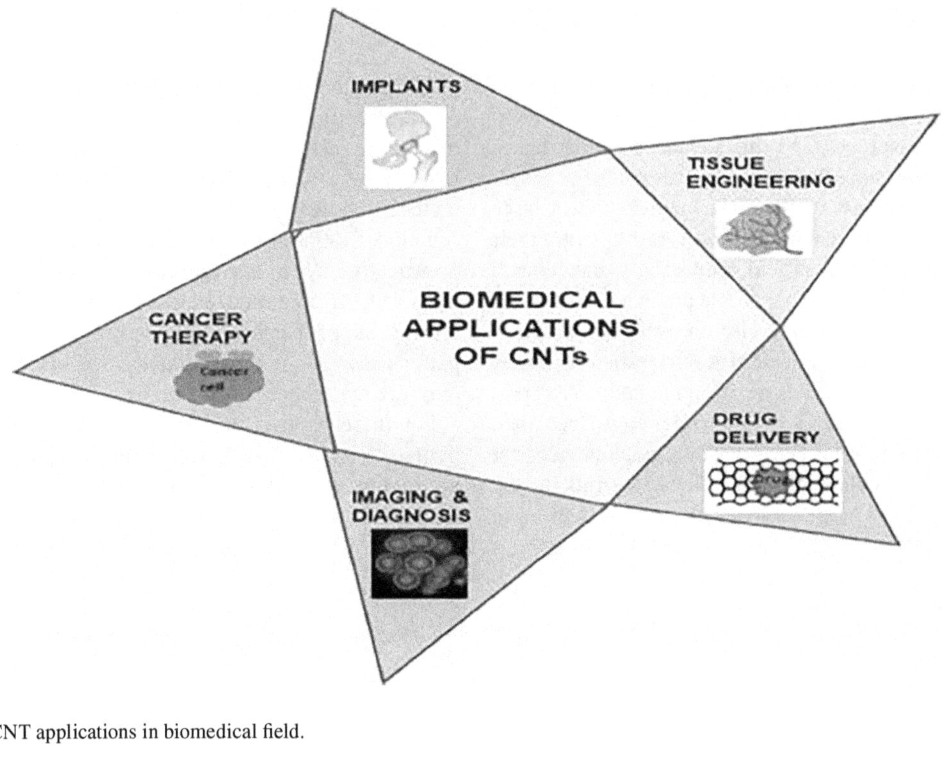

FIGURE 1.23 CNT applications in biomedical field.

medicine. Still then, there exist questions on unsolved issues, whereas proximate homogeneity of the selected nanomaterial contains extensive distribution of nanotubes radius, unlike its geometric structures, classification of nanotubes, trace inclusion of residual elements, and a marked sensitivity to different species and other toxic gases.

CNMs are discussed and described in this chapter from their discovery to the present day in the requisites of historical background, structure, properties, growth mechanism, synthesis, purification, characterization methods, cellular uptake of CNTs, breakdown mechanism, toxicity, and its biomedical applications. Carbon nanotubes may have only recently caught the attention of the world, but many modernizations have been made since their discovery. They are unique nanostructures that display the desirable properties of any other known material. Production methods include many approaches, which change types, yields, and structural surfaces of CNMs, which results in the change in the electrical and mechanical properties, and the actual structure of CNTs. Useful techniques for CNM characterization that are used are electron microscope, XRD, etc. But the most powerful technique to characterize CNMs remains Raman spectroscopy, in which, without sample preparation, a fast and nondestructive analysis is possible. Significant advances have been made in the delivery of anticancer and anti-inflammatory drugs and bioactive molecules, namely, DNA, RNA, and proteins. Drugs and biomolecules can be loaded in CNTs, which can then be utilized as targeted molecules. The toxicity of pristine CNTs is still a major concern based on the highly conflicting results obtained by various researchers. However, functionalized CNMs have been considered biocompatible and safe for drug and biomolecule delivery applications, as they are soluble in physiological media and non-toxic. They have shown no accumulation in the tissues; conversely, once functionalized, they can be readily excreted through the renal route by means of degradation through the myeloperoxidase (MOP) enzyme. However, CNT-based delivery systems are undoubtedly very promising in terms of their numerous advantages over existing technologies.

In this chapter, we have summarized various synthesis techniques of carbon nanotubes, and this advanced carbon nanomaterial has emerged since their discovery about 25 years ago. The broad scope of these applications suggests that a large number of CNT-based technologies will result from their unique properties of high electrical conductivity, mechanical strength, high aspect ratio, and nanoscale diameter. This chapter on carbon nanotubes revealed also an overview on structure, morphology, purification, and characterization methods. The distinct structural properties of carbon nanotubes, in particular, their high aspect ratio, strength, and high surface area, have the added advantage of being potential nanodevices for various medical and industrial applications. Overall, recent studies regarding CNTs have shown a very promising glimpse of what lies ahead in the future of science. In this work, we also reported a variety of familiar methods to synthesize carbon.

Nanomedicine is a growing field for patient care (treatment and diagnosis), especially for life-threatening diseases like cancer. Theranostic and regenerative approaches are being explored vigilantly and vigorously. Properties and characteristics of CNMs are still being researched heavily, and scientists have barely begun to tap into the potential of these structures. However, research has proved that CNTs are safer and more effective alternatives to previous drug delivery methods. In brief, current studies regarding CNTs have shown a very promising glimpse into what lies ahead in the future of medicine. Like single-walled carbon nanotubes, MWCNTs are insoluble. For dispersing in aqueous solutions, we recommend the use of sodium dodecylbenzene sulfonate if an ionic surfactant is suitable; if a non-ionic surfactant is needed, we recommend surfactants with high molecular weights. For functionalized nanotubes, it is possible to disperse them without the use of any surfactants. However, the total concentration of dispersed nanotubes will be lower. A maximum of 0.1 mg/mL can be achieved for COOH and OH.

The use of nanotechnology in medicine is expected to spread rapidly. In recent years, the pharmaceutical industry has used nanoparticles to reduce toxicity and the side effects of drugs. Until now, it was not realized that NPs as CNT systems themselves could impose risks to both patients and exposed workers. In fact, as clearly described by Kostarelos and colleagues:

> The use of CNTs in medicine is now at the crossroads between a proof-of-principle concept and an established preclinical candidate for a variety of therapeutic and diagnostic applications. Progress towards clinical trials will depend on the outcomes of efficacy and toxicology studies, which will provide the necessary risk-to-benefit assessments for carbon nanotube, based materials.
>
> [55–58]

CNMs are not completely inert materials and can be endowed with intrinsic cytotoxicity that can cause potential deleterious effects in normal tissues. Experimental studies have given evidence that factors determining CNT toxicity include size, length, diameter, purity, production method, and functionalization. However, these studies have been conducted prevalently *in vitro* and in animals, and it is difficult to translate results from animal studies to humans, because exposure doses in experiments are frequently higher than those of occupational and living environments, and also the exposure systems are not the real ones.

For these reasons, more toxicological investigations, particularly *in vivo*, of different forms of functionalized CNMs are highly recommended before they can be effectively used in clinical study and then marketed worldwide.

2

Progression in Synthesis Processing and Growth Mechanism of Carbon Nanomaterials for Advanced Macro-Scale Applications

2.1 Production and Main Processing Synthesis Methods of Carbon Nanotubes

This is the first comprehensive chapter to discuss the effect of nanostructured energy materials on the electrochemical properties of carbon nanotube–based fibers, which covers the various compositions, spinning, and fabrication conditions on the performance of wearable energy storage.

A few key applications that capitalize on the properties of SWCNTs are also reviewed with respect to the recent synthesis breakthroughs and ways in which synthesis science can enable advances in these applications.

There are various methods of production of carbon nanotubes, such as production of nanotubes by arc discharge, chemical vapor deposition, laser ablation, flame synthesis, high-pressure carbon monoxide (HiPco), electrolysis, pyrolysis, etc. But they can be mainly classified into the following groups: (1) physical processes, (2) chemical processes, and (3) miscellaneous processes.

Various generation methods for carbon nanotubes (CNTs) involve chemical deposition of vapor, discharge using electric arc, and laser ablation mechanism, which are driven by functionalization, chemical addition, doping, and filing, such that in-depth characterization and manipulation of CNTs are possible. The inbuilt elasticity, electromechanical, chemical, and optical properties of CNTs have a notable impact on its stability and reactivity. Perhaps the flexibility, along with its determined strength, makes them validate their potential application in diverse fields, which enables these CNTs to definitely procure a prominent role in nanotechnology.

Although there are many methods to synthesize CNTs, there are three methods that are the most important and commonly used: (1) electric arc discharge method, (2) laser ablation method, and (3) chemical vapor deposition method.

The arc discharge method uses high temperature (i.e., >3,000°C) necessary for evaporating carbon atoms into a plasma, forming both multi- and single-walled CNTs. The existence of a catalytic agent is not mandatory for MWNT, whereas during the preparation of individual SWNT, a catalytic agent is required, such as cobalt, yttrium, nickel, iron, etc. The chemical vapor deposition method involves hydrocarbon sources, such as cobalt, methane, ethylene, etc. The laser ablation method involves the vaporization of graphite in an electrical furnace heated at 1,200°C. The graphite purity ensures a high-level purity for the resulting products and a high converting ratio.

Carbon materials can be grouped into three classifications based on their period of advancement: classical carbons, nano ones, and new carbons [1]. Cracking carbons incorporate engineered graphite squares principally utilized as anodes, carbon blacks, and enacted carbons, for which creation systems were created before the 1960s. During the 1960s, carbon materials not quite the same as these great carbons were designed: carbon filaments from different forerunners, including fume-developed carbon filaments; pyrolytic carbons delivered by means of concoction fume testimony forms; glasslike carbons with high hardness and gas impermeability; high-thickness isotropic carbons created by isostatic squeezing; intercalation mixes with various functionalities, for example, high electrical conductivity; and precious stone like carbons as straightforward carbon sheets. These recently evolved carbon materials are grouped as new carbons. Since the 1990s, different fullerenes with shut-shell structure, carbon nanotubes with nanometer distances across, and graphene pieces of just a couple molecules' thickness have stood out from nanotechnology; these are ordered as nanocarbons.

On the off chance that these carbon materials are considered from the perspective of their surface, be that as it may, they might be ordered into two gatherings: nano-textured and nano-sized carbons. Most carbon materials in the new carbon classification are delegated nano-textured carbon, in light of the fact that their nano texture is controlled by means of various procedures in their creation, notwithstanding the basic control. Then again, fullerenes, carbon nanotubes, and graphene can be delegated nano-sized carbon—the shell size of fullerenes, breadth of carbon nanotubes, and thickness of graphene drops are on the nanometer scale. Carbon blacks in great carbon are made out of nano-sized particles, yet they are not typically named nanocarbons, since they have different applications as a mass, not as individual nano-sized particles.

CNTs have outstanding mechanical, thermal, electrical, and optical properties that are used exclusively or in mix to deliver keen sensors or, on the other hand, multifunctional materials. They have high angle proportions that are perfect for long and persistent detecting. Their high surface region, for example, can be misused for storing materials to make half-breed useful materials or functionalized to make cathodes for an assortment of uses. CNTs are additionally known to display ballistic conductivity because of insignificant electron dispersing in their 1D structure with mean freeways of the request of several microns.

Mechanical strain may cause reproducible changes in the electrical properties of CNT filaments, making it conceivable

DOI: 10.1201/9781032635989-2

to misuse them as electromechanical sensors. The partner changes incorporate inductance, capacitance, and obstruction, which can be associated to the strain. Of incredible significance is that CNT filaments are receptive to elastic, compressive, flexural, and torsional strain.

Thus, the presented chapter highlights the synthesis details, associated properties, and current applications of carbon nanotubes.

Several methods have been reported for the synthesis of CNTs, but the most common methods are arc discharge, [2] laser ablation, [3] and chemical vapor deposition (CVD) [4–7].

CNT synthesis has been known to occur in a wide range of environments. The prerequisites required for its synthesis are an active catalyst, a carbon source, and an adequate energy source. Commonly used techniques for the production of SWNTs and MWNTs involve (1) arc discharge synthesis, (2) laser ablation, and (3) chemical vapor deposition (CVD). High-temperature techniques like arc discharge and laser ablation methods are now being replaced with low-temperature preparative methods, such as CVD (<800°C), for CNT synthesis, wherein a great degree in the control of purity of synthesized CNTs, nanotube orientation, length, diameter, and density can be achieved. The arc discharge method (Scheme 2.1A) [6], the first recognized preparative method, utilizes a high-purity graphite anode and cathode under a helium atmosphere, where a stable arc is achieved at a voltage of 12–25 V. An arc is produced across a 1 mm gap; between these two graphite electrodes, the nanotubes deposit on the cathode as the anode is consumed during the process. Using this process, both MWNTs and SWNTs can be synthesized, where doping the graphite electrodes with metallic catalysts yields SWNTs; on the contrary, using unmodified electrodes yields MWNTs. In laser ablation method (Scheme 2.1B), the graphite target is vaporized using a laser generally in a quartz tube furnace in an inert atmosphere of ~500 torr of Ar or He. The growing nanotubes, as a result of the plume of vaporized graphite, are collected on a water-cooled copper target.

Both of these techniques (arc discharge and laser ablation) are limited by the amount of samples (CNTs) produced with respect to the carbon source being used for synthesis, and they are also plagued by undesirable by-products that require laborious purification steps post-synthesis. These drawbacks are overcome in the CVD technique, where a bulk quantity of CNTs in grams can be obtained with even aligned SWNTs on silica substrates for electronic applications can be attained easily. Additionally, CNTs produced through this method have a higher atom quality owing to the lower operating temperatures used in CVD technique. This technique (Scheme 2.1C) involves the use of gaseous carbon feedstock such as ethanol, methane, benzene, naphthalene, camphor, alcohol, carbon monoxide, hexane, cyclohexane, and anthracene which is passed through transition metal (Fe, Ni, and Co) nanoparticles, which act as catalysts at temperatures between 550–800°C in a furnace. CVD offers a greater feasibility of forming CNTs. For instance, MWNTs are formed at lower temperatures (300–800°C), whereas SWNTs require higher temperatures (600–1,000°C).

A comparative description of these three methods is given in Table 2.1. In addition to these, a few less frequently used approaches for synthesizing nanotubes are the gas-phase catalytic process (HiPCO), flame synthesis, core shell polymer microsphere method, aerosol precursor method, arc water process, low-temperature route, plasma method, fluidized bed method, and nebulized spray process.

Among the many ways CNTs can be fabricated, the three primarily used techniques include chemical vapor deposition (CVD), laser ablation, and arc discharge. Another set of techniques, called top-down or bottom-up approaches, is sometimes used by researchers to form CNTs. However, among the three primary techniques, CVD is the standardized technique suitable for industries due to its simple methodology, low cost of fabrication, and the ability to be produced on a large scale. These three methods are explained through examples in the following sections. The main differences between the three methods in terms of yield, defects, and characteristics of the produced SWCNTs and MWCNTs are shown in Table 2.2 [10]. Both SWCNTs and MWCNTs can be produced with high yield using all three methods, but their physical characteristics, length, and diameter vary according to the processes involved. Additionally, all three methods have effects on the CNTs that require further processing prior to their use as electrodes in sensing systems. These processing steps mostly include the use of nanotubes to form the electrodes of the prototypes. Apart from these techniques, scientists have also used laser torching and liquid electrolysis [11]. These two techniques have not been used as much as the others due to some disadvantages, like non-uniform temperature distribution over the heated spot, which is still a primary concern for laser torches. For liquid electrolysis, one of the limitations is the requirement of high pressure and electric power.

Although high-quality CNTs could be produced in enormous quantities using arc discharge and laser ablation method, these are applicable for research purposes only. CVD is the most conjoint method used for the production of CNTs on large commercial scale and is comparatively cheaper than others. Because of the increasing concern of researchers and inventors, the demand for CNTs has progressively increased. CVD is perhaps the most extensively used technique for the production of CNTs, which typically utilizes the fluidized bed reactor to permit both undeviating diffusion of gas and transfer of heat to the metal catalyst for production of CNT. This method offers a mean large-scale production of nanotubes, and also advantages of being economical, a high yield, less consumption of energy, and lesser production of waste by-products. Nonetheless, CNTs formed using this technique are often not pure enough, or even the contaminants could vary the characteristics of CNT, and these often require purification to get rid of contaminants using chemical treatment and/or thermal annealing, which is costly. Pure single-walled nanotubes could indeed be produced by density gradient centrifugation that could be used in conjunction with a specific surfactant or using gel chromatography. Using CVD, the production of SWCNTs need much more stringent quality control than MWCNT production; therefore, the cost of SWCNTs is still far superior to that of MWCNTs.

The prevalence of the biosensor applications of CNTs has led to an increased need for CNTs in the sector. Therefore, several different methods have been proposed to synthesize

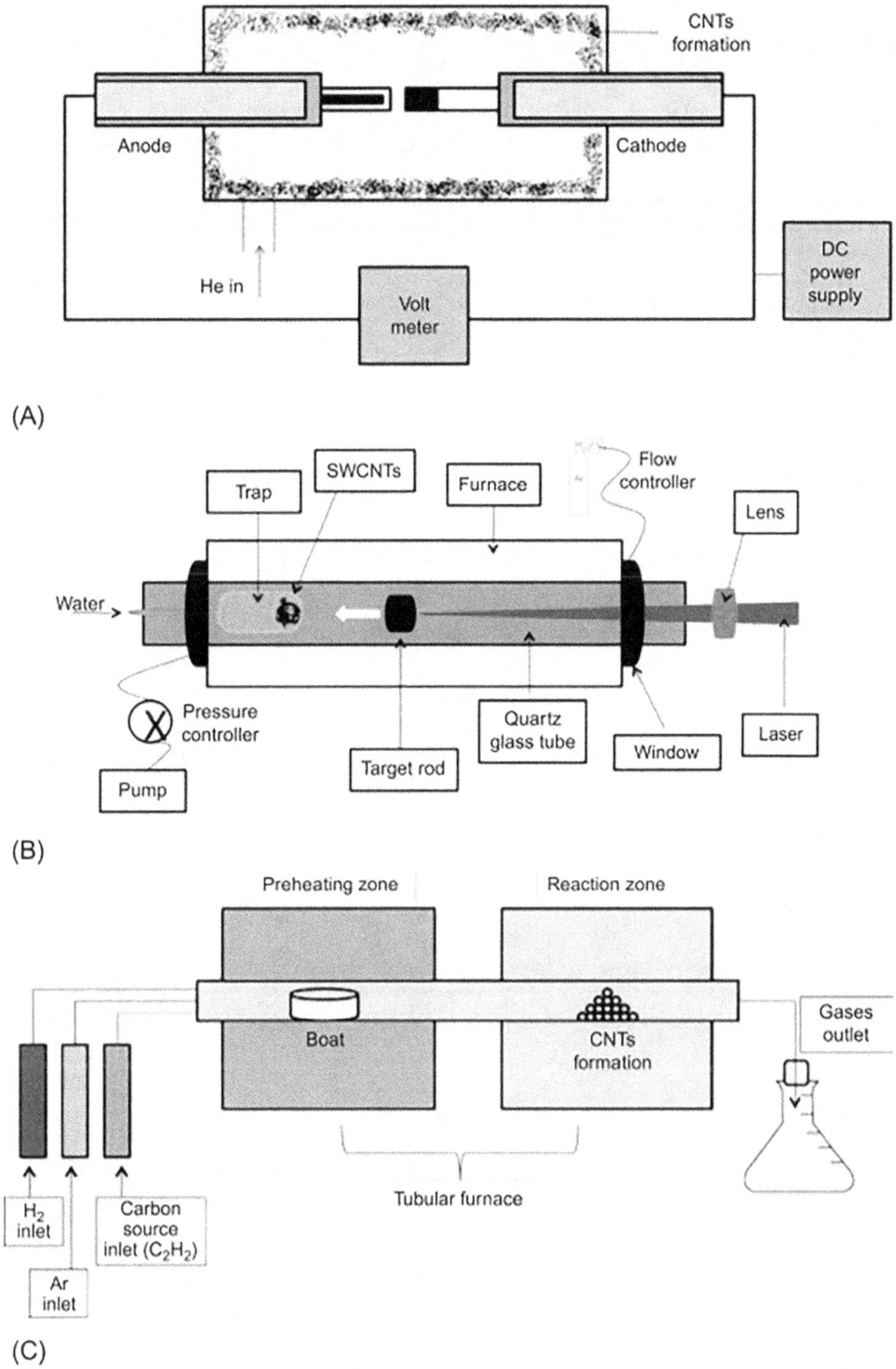

SCHEME 2.1 Different approaches for CNT synthesis: (a) arc discharge synthesis, (b) laser ablation, and (c) chemical vapor deposition.

CNTs in recent years. However, there are three main synthesis techniques (arc discharge, laser ablation, and chemical vapor deposition [CVD]) for CNT production. Compared to arc discharge and laser ablation methods, CVD is a simple and economical method for the synthesis of CNTs at low temperature and ambient pressure. Additionally, it allows serial CNT production with higher efficiency and purity. Moreover, CVD is the most efficient technique for control of the structure or CNT architecture [12]. In the CVD method, a catalyst material is heated to high temperatures in a tube furnace, while the precursor hydrocarbon gas flows through the tube for a while. In the process, the method is also versatile because the versatile hydrocarbons can be used in any state (solid, liquid, or gas). Furthermore, since various substrates are used, it allows the production of a wide range of different structures.

TABLE 2.1
Comparison of Main Synthesis Methods of Carbon Nanotubes

Method/ Requirements	CVD	Laser Ablation	Arc Discharge
Raw materials and availability	Fossil-based and botanical hydrocarbon, abundantly available	Graphite, difficult to get.	Pure graphite, difficult to get.
Nature of process and description	Continuous, substrate placed in an oven, and heated to high temperature, followed by slow addition of carbon-bearing gas, such as methane; gas decomposes to liberate carbon atoms, which combine to form nanotubes	Batch intense laser pulse used to blast graphite to generate carbon gas to form CNTs, and different conditions were tried to get optimum, which produces a sufficient amount of SWCNTs	Batch 2 graphite rods placed a few millimeters apart and connected to a power supply; at 100 amps, carbon vaporizes and forms hot plasma
Process condition	High temperatures within 500 to 1,000°C at atmospheric pressure	Argon or nitrogen gas at 500 torr	Low-pressure inert gas (helium)
Production cost	Low	High	High
Post-treatment	Not required	Required	Required
Yield	High, 20–100%	Moderate, 70% max	Good, 30–90% max
SWCNT	Long tubes with diameters ranging from 0.6 to 4 nm	Long bundles of tubes with length 5–20 μm, and individual diameter 1–2 nm	Short tubes having diameters in range 0.6–1.4 nm
MWCNT	Long tubes with the diameter in the range of 10–240 nm	MWNT synthesis possible but too expensive	Short tubes with inner diameter 1–3 nm and the outer diameter approximately 10 nm
Purity	High	High	High
Production rate	High	Low	Low
Energy requirement	Moderate	High	High
Reactor design	Easy	Difficult	Difficult
Advantages	Easy to scale up, simple process, long-length SWCNTs with a controllable diameter and good purity	Good-quality SWNTs with high yield and narrow distribution compared to arc discharge	Less expensive, with open-air synthesis; can easily produce SWNT and MWNTs—SWNT with few structural defects and MWNTs even without a catalyst
Disadvantages	Synthesized CNTs usually with defects	Costly technique since it requires expensive lasers and high power, limited to lab scale	Extensive purification required since nanotubes are short, tangled, with random sizes and directions
References	[4–7]	[3 and 8]	[2,9]

TABLE 2.2
Effect of the Three Production Methodologies on the Physiochemical Properties of CNTs

Parameters	Chemical Vapor Deposition	Arc Discharge	Laser Ablation
Yield (%)	20–100	30–90	≤70
SWCNTs	Long tubes with a diameter of 0.6–4 nm	Short tubes with a diameter of 0.6–1.4 nm	Long bundles of tubes with individual diameters of 1–2 nm
MWCNTs	Long tubes with a diameter of 10–240 nm	Short tubes with an inner diameter of 1–3 nm and an outer diameter of approximately 10 nm	Synthesis possible, but because of its cost, used less often
Defects	Often riddled with defects	Need a lot of purification	Fewer defects, but technique expensive
Advantages	Easy scaling up	Inexpensive	Good diameter of the CNTs
	Simple process	Few structural defects, particularly on SWCNTs	Few defects
	High purity		
Disadvantages	Many defects	Nanotubes short and randomly oriented	Very expensive
		Requirement of post-processing steps	High power requirement

Source: [10].

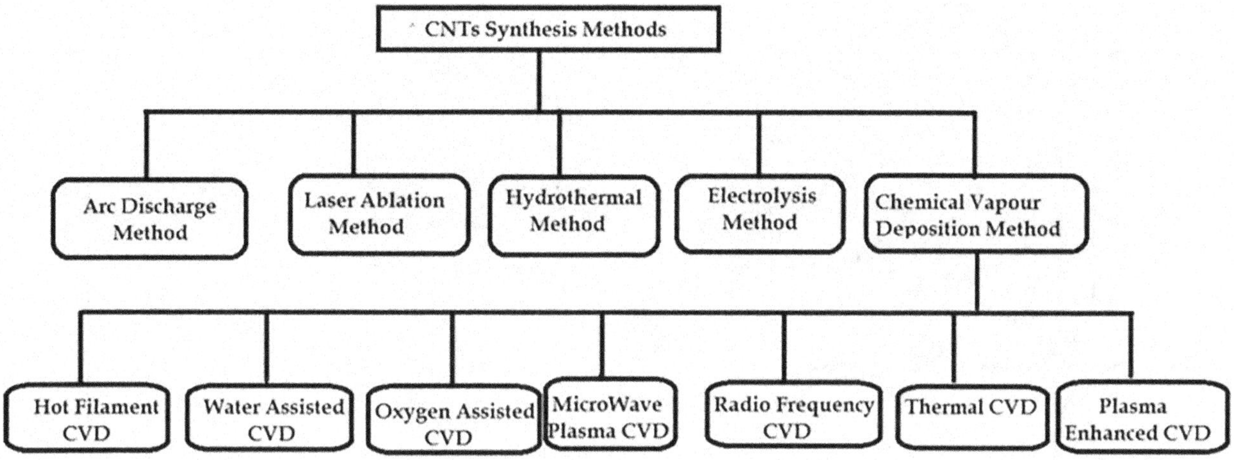

FIGURE 2.1 Schematic diagram of different synthesis methods of CNTs.

The development of carbon nanotubes during synthesis expected to commence from the recombination of carbon molecules came apart by warmth from its precursor. In spite of the fact that a number of more up-to-date fabrication procedures are being designed, three fundamental strategies are laser ablation, electric arc discharge, and chemical vapor deposition. Chemical vapor deposition is getting to be exceptionally well-known because of its potential for scale-up generation (Figure 2.1).

The fact that carbon atoms can combine with each other, resulting in the formation of unique and diverse structures, presents the carbon element as the most intriguing element worldwide. Through hybridization of the form sp, sp^2, and sp^3, novel and specialized nanostructures like NPs, NN diamonds, NN onions, peapods, NN fibers, NN rings, fullerenes, and NN tubes have been realized. Their broad range of structures comprises zero-dimensional (0D) (fullerenes and diamond clusters), 1D (NN tubes–NTs), 2D (graphene [Gr]), and 3D structures (NN crystalline diamond and fullerite) [13], which have gained considerable attention. Particularly, CNT, which was discovered by Iijima in 1991 [14], is considered a milestone in NM production, as can be attested by the steady growth in volumes of existing/available articles and researches connected to the topic. CNTs have attracted substantial attention due to the combination of excellent chemical and physical (outstanding elastic module, high electrical conductivity, and great fracture strength) properties [13].

Conceivably, the CNT structure consists of one or more rolled-up sheets of graphene, as shown in Figure 2.2 (diagram schematically showing synthesis techniques and formation of SWCNTs and MWCNTs from graphene layer). Here, an sp^2 hybridized meshwork of carbon atoms is arranged hexagonally to obtain cylindrical geometry of one-dimensional CNT NN structure with a high aspect ratio. Based on the number of sheets involved, two configurations are generally used to classify CNTs. When one layer of graphene is rolled up, single-walled CNTs (SWCNTs) are designed, with typical diameters of nearly 1 nm. The formation of multi-walled CNTs (MWCNTs) involves several layers to form concentric cylinders enclosed in each other with a spacing of layers of between 0.3 and 0.4 nm [13].

CNTs can be synthesized by diverse means, like laser ablation, chemical vapor deposition techniques (CVD) (such as hot filament, water-aided, oxygen-aided, microwave plasma, radio frequency, thermal and plasma-improved), electrolysis, arc discharge, and sonochemical hydrothermal methods. The pristine CNTs synthesized have remarkable properties, which have catapulted them to high levels of advanced technological applications. Through re-engineering, chemical modification, and functionalization, the properties can even be improved. These outstanding properties have seen CNTs being used in the field of solar cells, energy storage, sensing, flexible displays, electronics (e.g., computer chips), biological field (cancer treatment, drug delivery, tissue reengineering, etc.), and water splitting [13].

Concerning the mechanical possessions of CNTs, these constituents have been found to be stiff and extremely strong. They are endowed with remarkable tensile strength (11–62 GPa) and Young's modulus (E = 0.27–3.6) [15]. Their density normalized is approximately 56.0 times higher when compared to steel wire, as well as around 1.70 times more when compared to that of silicon NN rods [16]. Now, in comparison with raw/pristine CNTs, CNT-based composites have even higher electrical conductivity and mechanical properties, which are vital ingredients for the electrochemical sensing technology aimed at tracing, detecting, and mitigating pollutants, pathogens, and wastewater matrices [17].

High-quality nanotube materials are desired for both fundamental and technological applications. *High quality* refers to the absence of structural and chemical defects over a significant length scale (e.g., 1–10 μm) along the tube axes. The number of patents and publications on the synthesis of carbon nanotube is increasing rapidly. However, there are many challenges remaining that must be resolved regarding the synthesis of CNT. Currently, there are four main challenges in the field of nanotube synthesis: (1) mass production, that is, the development of low-cost, large-scale processes for the synthesis of high-quality nanotubes, including SWCNTs; (2) selective

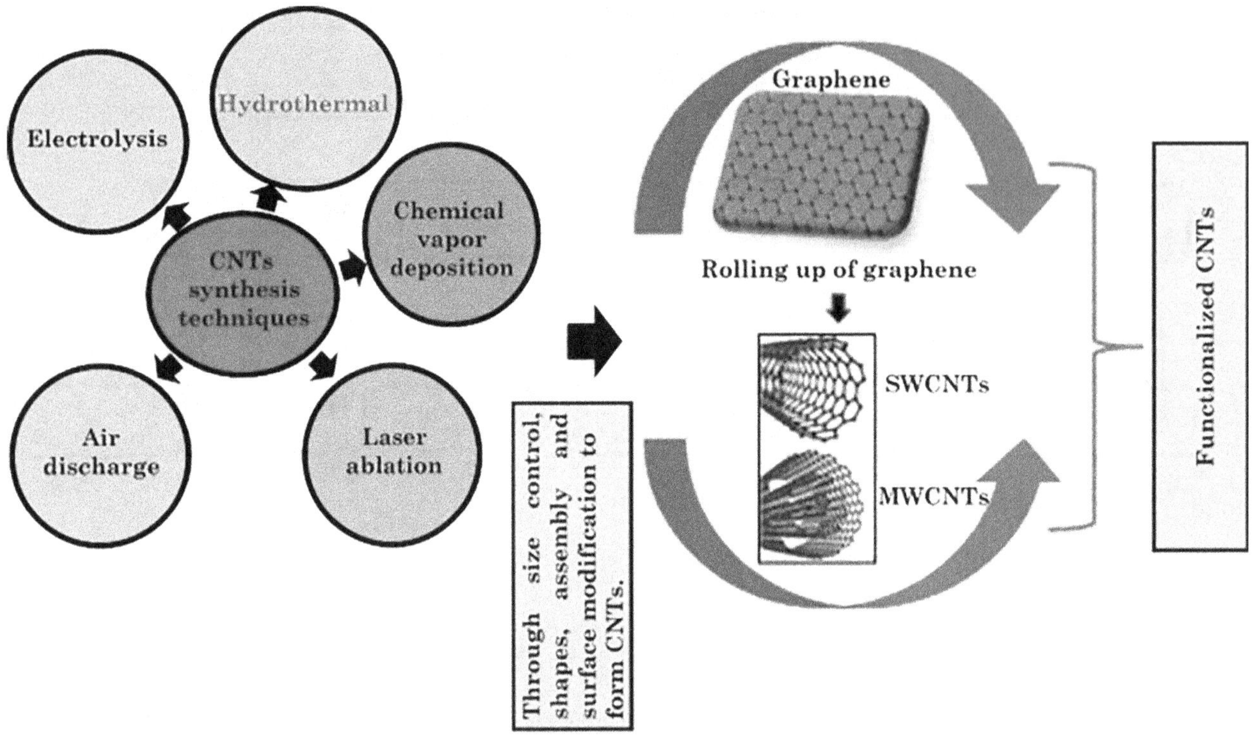

FIGURE 2.2 Representation of CNT synthesis methods and formation of SWCNTs and MWCNTs from rolling up graphene sheet.

production, that is, control over the structure and electronic properties of the produced nanotubes; (3) organization, that is, control over the location and orientation of the produced nanotubes on a flat substrate; (4) mechanism, that is, the development of a thorough understanding of the processes of nanotube growth. The growth mechanism is still a subject of controversy, and more than one mechanism might be operative during the formation of CNTs.

The increase in momentum in research on CNTs has resulted in the high demand of CNTs in industry, and recently, it is becoming increasingly urgent in demand. There are three basic methods for synthesis of SWCNTs and MWCNTs: electrical arc discharge, laser ablation (laser vaporization), and chemical vapor deposition (CVD) (or catalytic decomposition of hydrocarbons). Research on CNTs is more and more extensively pursued, and the synthetic methods of CNTs have been improved. In arc discharge, the current through two graphite electrodes creates a deposit of CNTs on the cathode. By altering conditions, either SWCNTs or MWCNTs can be synthesized. Laser vaporization of graphite in a lined silica tube with high-temperature furnace generally results in MWCNTs, but with the use of catalytic metal nanoparticles, SWCNTs can be synthesized. MWCNTs are produced by CVD during the pyrolysis of hydrocarbon gases at high temperatures. Table 2.3 shows a list of various methods for preparing various kinds of CNTs in recent years.

We will discuss in detail the following synthesis methods generally used to synthesize CNTs:

- Arc discharge production method
- Laser ablation production method
- Chemical steam deposition or vapor deposition
- Vapor-phase growth
- Flame synthesis method
- Hydrothermal process
- Electrolysis process
- Spray pyrolysis
- Silane solution method

2.2 Electric Arc Discharge Method

Carbon nanotubes are synthesized by electric arc discharge method [22–25], which is also called plasma arcing method. This method is applicable for the preparation of a large amount of CNTs. This method is used for producing C_{60} fullerene; it is the most common and the easiest way to produce carbon nanotubes. The arc discharge strategy produces a number of carbon nanostructures, such as fullerenes, whisker, carbon soot, and profoundly graphitized carbon nanotubes, from high-temperature plasma that approaches 3,700°C.

Description

Electrodes: Pure graphite rods (both positive and negative electrode). The positive electrode is adjustable from outside to maintain the gap between the two electrodes.

Diameter of electrodes: 5–20 μm.

Gap between electrodes: 1 mm.

TABLE 2.3
The Synthetic Methods of CNTs

Method	Progress	Consequence	Refs.
Arc discharge	Synthesized between two graphite rods in water bath at different voltage	Good-quality and high-yield CNTs obtained	[19]
	Two graphite electrodes submerged in different liquid media	Yielding various dimensional nanocarbon structures	
	Using strong oxidizing agent, HNO_3/H_2O_2, instead of metal catalyst and vacuum devices	Improving purity of MWCNTs	
	Discharge maintained in a magnetic field	High-quality MWCNTs obtained	
	Using physical forces both during synthesis	Relatively straight and defect-free MWCNTs obtained	
Laser ablation	Dynamic light scattering, micro-Raman and high-resolution transmission electron microscopy used	Controlling their nanostructures	
	Using binary catalysts combining the transition metals Fe, Co, and Ni	Different carbon nanostructures can be obtained	
	Direct synthesis using pulsed laser ablation	SWCNTs show fast and strong photo-response (as high as 1,350% at 405 nm)	
	Irradiating of a CO_2 laser in continuous wave mode onto a boron-containing graphite target at room temperature	Fine crystalline structure of MWCNTs can be obtained	
	Ablating a nickel/carbon composite target in ethanol or ambient air	MWCNTs	
CVD	Growing on iron catalyst film using plasma-enhanced chemical vapor deposition (PECVD) system	Vertically aligned single-walled carbon nanotubes of diameter 0.8–1.5 nm can be obtained	[20]
	Co used as catalysts, at 700°C, using hydrogen-to-acetylene-gas ratio at 25:25 Sccm	High yield of MWCNTs	
	Using NiO powder as catalysts and LPG as carbon source	Yield of CNTs increased	
	$AlPO_4$ used as catalysts	Y-shaped CNTs	
	Taking iron nanoparticles as catalyst	SWCNTs	
	Taking Co-Mo as catalyst and using CH_4 at 900°C	SWCNTs	
	Metal catalyst-free mist flow	SWCNTs synthesized without any treatment	[21]
	Ni over Cr layer as a catalyst at 600°C	CNTs	
	Taking Ni/MgO as catalyst and using CH_4 in micro-fluidized bed	CNTs exhibiting relatively small and mean outer diameter, less defect, and high purity	[21]
	Photochemical deposition	MWCNTs	
Low-temperature plasma	Plasma causes dissociation of carbon resource	CNTs with highly distributed active species and catalyst activation	
Low-temperature plasma reduction	Facile glow discharge plasma reduction operated at room temperature	CNTs	
Solvothermal	At the low temperature of 180°C	MWCNT bundles	
Low-temperature solvothermal	Dichlorobenzene as a carbon source catalyzed by a solvothermal approach at 200°C	Well-aggregated carbon nanotubes achieved	
Solvothermal	At temperature of 200°C and a reaction for 10 h	Magnetic MMWCNTs with alterable structure	
Sol-gel	Mixed solution evaporated at 80°C for 8 h	MWCNT-$LiMn_2O_4$	
Hydrothermal	Solution transferred into a 100 mL autoclave and kept at 160°C for 8 h	CNTs with well-dispersed Fe_3O_4	[22]
Hydrothermal	Solution transferred into a 30 mL autoclave and kept at 150°C for 4 h	CNT core/porous MnO_2	[23]
Flame	Diffusion flames acted as reaction environments, using catalysts as aerosols and supported upon substrates	CNTs	[24]
Flame	CNT growth occurs the decomposition of flame-generated carbon precursors	CNTs with higher physical properties	[25]
Flame	Using rotating opposed-flow ethylene diffusion flames and a catalytic Ni substrate	Controlling the synthesis of CNTs	[26]
Flame	Taking $Fe/Mo/Al_2O_3$ as catalyst	Self-oriented CNTs	[27]

Source: [18].

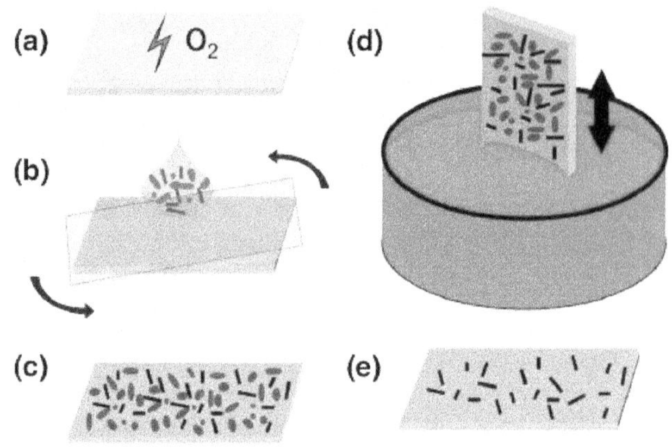

FIGURE 2.3 Schematic diagram of the fabrication steps that were used for the purification of the CNTs: (a) is the silicon chip after being made hydrophilic with reactive ion etching, (b) and (c) represent spin coating of the CNTs synthesized by arc discharge performed on the hydrophilic silicon chips, (d) shows the silicon chip containing the CNTs and debris immersed, and (e) shows the obtained purified form.

Current: 50–120 A.

Voltage: 20–25 V.

Inert gas pressure: 100–500 torr (no CNT formed below 100 torr). Inert gas is used for cooling and condensation of atoms to form the CNTs. Inert gas determines the structure of carbons to be present in CNTs. Commonly used inert gas is helium.

Temperature: 3,000–3,500°C.

Reactor: It contains a quartz chamber which is connected to a vacuum pump and a diffusion pump to inert gas supply. Initially, the chamber is made vacuum by the vacuum pump, and then the chamber is filled with helium gas by the diffusion pump.

Although researchers have obtained CNTs with more optimized characteristics using CVD compared to the arc discharge method, the latter has been the most primitive and well-accepted technique to form the CNTs, as these were the first techniques used by Iijima to form MWCNTs. Some of the advantages of this technique are its simplicity, low-cost process, and no requirement for multistep purification [28]. Another major advantage that sets this technique apart from the others is its ability to form CNT hybrids. Both alternating current (AC) and direct current (DC) are used as input for the evaporation of carbon sources to form the CNTs.

Apart from the formation of CNTs using the arc discharge method, another study demonstrates the purification of CNTs [29]. Figure 2.3 [29] shows a schematic diagram of the purification steps of CNTs. The CNTs synthesized by the arc discharge method, along with the amorphous carbon debris, were initially dispersed in 1,2-dichloroethane to form relatively high concentrations of 0.25 ppm. Clean silicon substrates were taken and made hydrophilic through reactive ion etching. The CNT-based dispersions were then spin-coated on the silicon substrates. The purification was carried out carefully to avoid any damage to the synthesized CNTs. Surface tension between the liquid and the contact line of the substrate selectively swept away larger amorphous carbon debris while leaving behind clean CNTs on the substrate. Patterns were formed in the shape of etched trench-like grooves where CNTs were deposited. The entire process was carried out in a non-invasive manner, that is, without causing any mechanical damage or chemical modification to the CNTs.

This technique produces a mixture of components and requires separating nanotubes from the soot and the catalytic metals present in the crude product. This is regarding arc vaporization of two carbon rods placed end to end on the site, separated by about a 1 mm, in an enclosure filled with inert gas (helium or argon) at low pressures, that is, between 50 and 700 mbar.

The arc discharge technique has already been proposed, intended for the development of CNTs. It is plausible to use this method for the highest-quality nanotubes. The arc discharge concerning two electrodes of carbon by means of or shorn of a catalyst creates a vapor. The consequential of carbon self-assembled to form nanotubes, as shown in Figure 2.4. A 50 A current is conceded amid two graphite electrodes involved in the manifestation of helium.

This method is for the preparation of large amounts. This method is used for producing C_{60} fullerene; it is the most common and the easiest way to produce carbon nanotubes. This technique produces a mixture of components and requires separating nanotubes from the soot and the catalytic metals present in the crude product. This is arc vaporization of two carbon rods placed end to end, separated by approximately 1 mm, in an enclosure filled with inert gas (helium of argon) at low pressures, that is, between 50 and 700 mbar.

Arc evaporation production technique is known as the best technique to produce the greatest quality of CNTs. It involves the passage of the current into two separate graphite electrodes having helium environment, and the current passing between this electrodes is 50 amps. This substance is accumulated on cathode known as CNTs. SWCNTs are obtained after the addition of copper (Co), nickel (Ni), and additional metal on anode electrode.

Arc discharge is the oldest and most common technique to produce CNTs. It also produces carbon soot material, which is

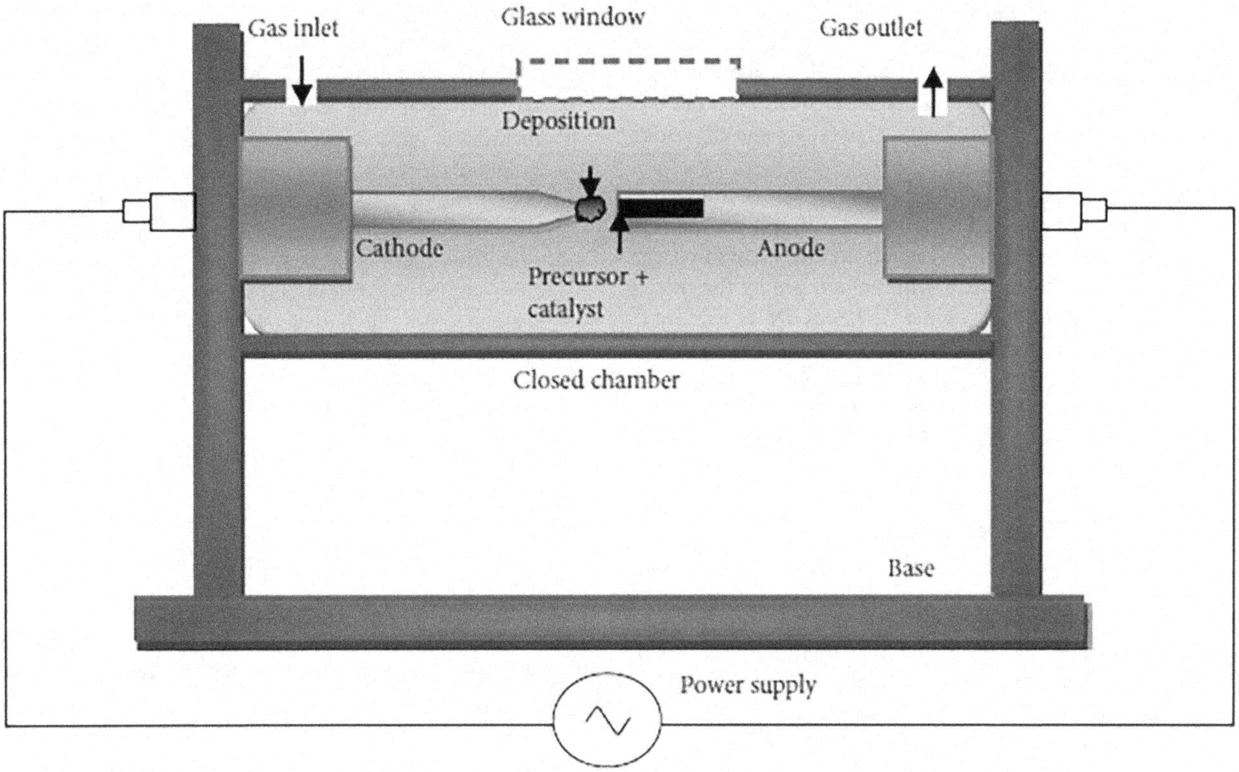

FIGURE 2.4 Schematic of an arc discharge chamber.

formed of fullerene molecules. This method relies on the electrical breakdown of a gas to generate plasma. It uses higher temperatures (above 1,700°C) to evaporate carbon atoms in plasma, providing the growth of CNTs with minimum structural defects in comparison with other techniques. A schematic of an arc discharge chamber is shown in Figure 2.4. The chamber consists of two electrodes, one of which is an anode, and the other is cathode. The anode is filled with a mixture of graphite powder and catalyst. The catalyst favors the growth of SWNTs rather than MWNTs [30]. The cathode consists of a pure graphite rod. Initially, electrodes are kept independent under a gaseous atmosphere (typically argon/hydrogen mixture), then distance between the electrodes is reduced, and an electric arc of 60–100 A or 50–150 A intensity is applied, associated to a potential drop of 25 V. The inert gas flow is maintained at 50–600 torr; the temperature in the interelectrode zone is above 1,700–4,000°C. The electrodes become red hot, and a plasma is formed, so carbon sublimes from the positive anode that is consumed and condenses as filamentous carbon product on the cathode due to the temperature gradient. The reaction takes up from 30–60 s to 2–10 min. At the final stage of the reaction, the machine is left for cooling. Later, CNTs and soot deposited on the walls of the chamber are collected, then purified, and finally observed under an electron microscope to investigate their morphology. Flow rate, inert gas pressure, and metal concentration are the fundamental process parameters to obtain a high yield of CNTs.

The synthesis of CNTs using arc discharge with fewer defects has better thermal conductive performance and greater mechanical strength. But there are also some problems, for example, the synthesis of CNTs is required under the vacuum environment, but the vacuum environment is hard to maintain, and it is also very expensive. In addition, low-current arc is conducive to the formation of CNTs, but this will make the arc unstable. However, if the arc current is higher, the generated impurities, such as amorphous carbon and graphite of CNTs, will be increased. Moreover, because the electrodes need continuous change, it will result in discontinuity of the process. Therefore, the yield of CNTs via arc discharge is lower.

Arc discharge is one of the most mature synthetic methods for SWCNTs, and it is also used more extensively. Research has shown that different catalysts for the synthesis of SWCNTs would cause different diameter distribution. Ferrocene was found to be a better catalyst precursor, and it can form SWCNT products with very high purity and an overview and high-resolution TEM images (inset) of the CNT product.

2.2.1 Procedure for Synthesis of CNTs by Electric Arc Discharge Method

In this method, a potential of 20–25 V is applied across the pure graphite electrodes separated by 1 mm distance and maintained at 500 torr pressure of flowing helium gas filled inside the quartz chamber. When the electrodes are made to strike each other under these conditions, it produces an electric arc. The energy produced in the arc is transferred to the anode, which ionizes the carbon atoms of pure graphite anode and produces C+ ions and forms plasma (plasma is composed of atoms or molecules in vapor state at high temperature). These positively charged carbon ions move toward the cathode, get reduced and deposited, and grow as CNTs on the cathode. As the CNTs grow, the length of the anode decreases, but the electrodes are adjusted and always maintain a gap of 1 mm between the two electrodes.

Reactor: It contains a quartz chamber which is connected to a vacuum pump and a diffusion pump to inert gas supply. Initially, the chamber is made vacuum by the vacuum pump, and then the chamber is filled with helium gas by the diffusion pump [31]. If proper cooling of electrodes is achieved, uniform deposition of CNTs is formed on the cathode, which is achieved by inert gas maintained at proper pressure. By this method, multi-walled carbon nanotubes are synthesized, and to synthesize single-walled carbon nanotubes, catalyst nanoparticles of Fe, Co, and Ni are incorporated in the central portion of the positive electrode. The obtained CNTs are further purified to get the pure form of CNTs.

The preparation of SWNTs by arc discharge method usually requires a transition metal catalyst, and the anode generally is made of a composite material, such as graphite composited with a commercial metal, like Ni, Fe, Co, Ag, Pt, or a composite of two metals, such as Co-Ni, Fe-Ni, Fe-No, Co-Cu, Ni-Cu, etc. In order to ensure the high efficiency of production, it is necessary to guarantee a stable current density and anode consumption rate during the reaction process so that a constant spacing between the electrodes should be maintained. Although the production of carbon nanotubes by arc discharge method has gradually become more and more mature by adjusting the preparation conditions in terms of catalyst, electrode size, electrode spacing, and types of raw materials, the yield of carbon nanotubes produced by such method is relatively low due to the difficulties in arc control and high cost of fabrication.

2.2.1.1 Production of SWCNTs

An anode is used which is dipped by means of a metal catalyst, for instance Y, Co, Fe, Ni, or Mo. The SWCNTs produced are of diameter 1.2–1.4 nm. The efficiency of CNTs developed using arc discharge method can be enhanced by (1) the choice of inert gas used for synthesis, (2) the optimum pressure of inert gases for the production of nanotubes of appropriate diameters, (3) selection of catalyst, (4) Synthesis in open air using soldering arc torch, etc.

In the production of SWCNTs, an anode is dipped with a metal catalyst, such as Fe, Co, Ni, Y, or Mo. It produces SWCNTs with a diameter of 1.2 to 1.4nm. The efficiency of SWCNTs production by arc discharge method is improved with:

1. Inert gas: Argon with a lower diffusion coefficient and thermal conductivity has given nanotube a smaller diameter (1.2 nm) and a 0.2 nm diameter decrease, with 10% increase in argon–helium ratio, when nickel and yttrium are used as a catalyst (4.2:1).
2. **Optical plasma control:** As the distance between anode and cathode increases, anode vaporization increases, due to which strong visible vortices around the cathode occur.
3. **Catalyst:** By changing metal catalysts, nanotubes with a diameter of 0.6 to 1.2 nm are produced. Catalysts used are Co and Mo.
4. Open-air synthesis with welding arc torch: This method is specifically used for SWCNTs with a graphite rod containing a metal catalyst. The arch is operated at 100 amps current, and a shielding Ar gas flows through the torch to enhance arc jet formation. This method is very convenient and inexpensive, with Ni:Y (3.6:0.8). Nanotubes produced by this method are of the diameter 1.32 nm.

2.2.1.2 Production of MWCNTs

Pure graphite arc by means of an innermost diameter of 1–3 nm and an external diameter 10 nm approximately can be produced using this method. There is no prerequisite for heavy acid purification, as the catalyst is not used in this method. MWCNTs can, therefore, be produced with fewer defects. The manifestation of hydrogen gas into the growth region has been proven toward providing an optimal synthesis of MWCNTs of high crystallinity and few intrinsically intertwined CNTs. Various approaches for synthesizing MWCNTs have been utilized likewise: (1) synthesis of nanotubes in liquid nitrogen, (2) magnetic field synthesis, (3) arc discharge via plasma rotation, etc.

MWCNTs are produced with the use of pure graphite arc with an inner diameter of 1–3 nm and outer diameter of 10 nm (approx.). Since a catalyst is not used in this process, there is no need for a heavy acidic purification. So MWCNTs can be formed with a fewer number of defects. Different methods used to synthesize are:

1. **Synthesis in liquid nitrogen:** MWCNTs are formed by generating arc discharge in liquid nitrogen, for which low pressure and expensive inert gas are not needed. Yield is about 70% of reaction product.
2. **Magnetic field synthesis:** MWCNTs formed by this method are defect-free and have high purity. In this, arc discharge is controlled by a magnetic field around the arc plasma. Extremely pure graphite rods (purity >99.999%) are used as electrodes. Highly pure MWCNTs (purity >95%) are obtained without further purification, which disorder walls of MWCNTs.
3. **Plasma rotating arc discharge:** The centrifugal force caused by the rotation generates turbulence and accelerates the carbon vapor perpendicular to the anode, and the rotation distributes the micro discharges uniformly and generates stable plasma. Consequently, it increases the plasma volume and raises the plasma temperature. At the rotation speed of 5,000 rpm, a yield of 60% was found at a temperature of 1,025°C without the use of a catalyst. The yield can be increased up to 90% after purification if the rotation speed is increased and the temperature is enlarged.

2.3 Laser Ablation Method

The third most popular technique for processing carbon-based precursors of CNTs is laser ablation. This technique has been carried out using several different types of lasers. The quality of the CNT has been examined with reference to certain parameters, like laser power, pulse per index, frequency, and speed. Generally, a carbon source like graphite is vaporized using a laser system under controlled temperature, pressure, and gas environment conditions. The fabrication of CNTs with fine crystallinity was accomplished using a CO_2-based laser ablation technique. The target for laser ablation was formed using carbon and boron. Boron-containing graphite was laser-ablated using CO_2 lasers in a continuous wave (CW) mode. The entire process was carried out at room temperature in the presence of Ar gas. The pressure of the gas was varied at 50, 150, 400, or 760 torr. The ablation process was carried out with a power, time duration, and speed of 3.5 kW, 10 s, and 6 rpm, respectively. The gas flow was fixed at 10 L/min, while the power density of the laser was around 50 kW/cm^2. The synthesized CNTs had a fine crystal structure with diameters ranging between 5 and 40 nm. The quantity and the intensity of graphitization of the developed CNTs were directly proportional to the pressure exerted by Ar gas. The optimal pressure was 760 torr when highly oxidative and stable CNTs were formed. The CNT-based cathode of the sensors had a reliable response and a β value of 3.6×10^4 cm^{-1}.

The use of laser ablation to form CNT-based composites is also demonstrated in ref. [32], where the execution is carried out in pulsed liquid media to develop CNTs decorated with cadmium oxide (CdO) nanoparticles. Cadmium sheets immersed in precursor solutions were laser-ablated to form subsequent metal oxide nanoparticles decorated on the CNTs. Figure 2.5 [32] shows a schematic diagram of the fabrication steps depicting the functionalization of the CNTs with CdO nanoparticles via pulsed laser ablation in liquid media. Initially, the functionalization process was carried out using hydrochloric acid (HCl) and nitric acid (HNO_3) solutions, followed by overnight drying at 90°C. Then, the target was placed at the bottom of a glass vessel to synthesize the nanocomposites.

2.3.1 Procedure for Synthesis of CNTs by Laser Ablation Method

The laser ablation method is a physical vapor deposition method in which graphite target is vaporized by a laser source. In this method, the graphite target is placed at the center of a quartz chamber filled with argon gas and maintained at 1,200°C.

2.3.2 Procedure for Pulsed Laser Deposition Method

Pulsed laser deposition is a thin-film deposition technique in which the target material is vaporized by pulsed laser beam, and vaporized target atoms are made to deposit on substrates (Figure 2.6). The furnace contains a target at the bottom and a substrate mounted on the top. A pulsed laser beam from an Nd:YAG laser source is made to strike the target to produce vaporized target atoms, called the plume (*plume* is vaporized atoms at high temperature).

This synthesis was first reported in 1995 by Smalley's group at Rice University. A periodic or continuous laser is employed to vaporize a graphite target in an oven at 1,200°C. The main distinction between continuous and periodic laser is that periodic laser demands a way higher intensity (100 KW/cm^2 compared with 12 KW/cm^2). The oven is stuffed with helium or argon gas to keep the pressure at 500 torr.

A very highly powered beam of laser or continuous pulse intends a bulk of carbon-containing feedstock gas (CO, CH_4), as shown in Figure 2.7 [33]. It consists of graphitic rods and the catalytic blend of Ni and Co (50:50) at around 1,200°C argon gas streaming through it. The carbon source used is graphite, and this technique is very expensive. For the graphite target to

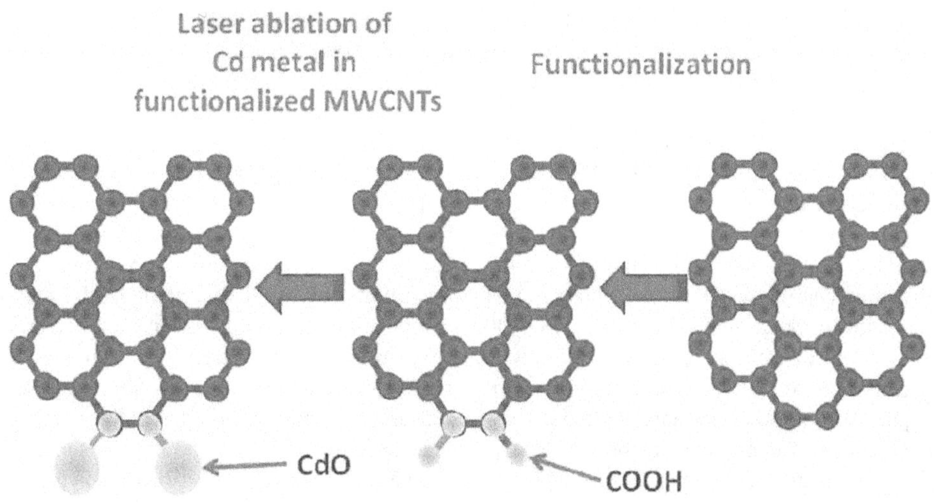

FIGURE 2.5 Schematic diagram of the fabrication steps depicting the functionalization of CNTs using pulsed laser ablation in liquid media.

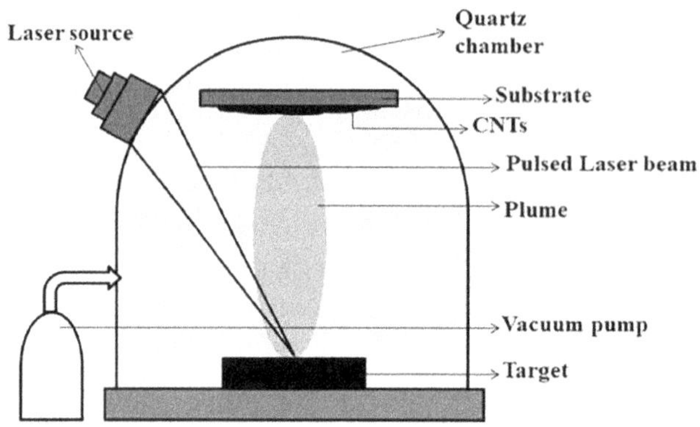

FIGURE 2.6 Pulsed laser ablation method—schematic representation.

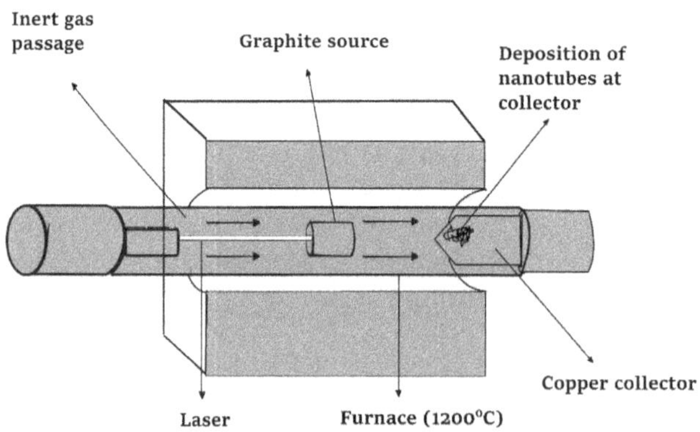

FIGURE 2.7 Diagram illustrating laser ablation method.

turn to vapor at 1,200°C into an oven, a constant laser has been used. Helium and argon gases are used to retain the pressure at about 500 torr. The method is much comparable to the arc discharge technique. It has generally been used for the production of SWCNTs, as this method is very expensive. It results in a high yield of SWCNTs [34]. Different methods used for the synthesis include thus: (1) A method called free electron laser method (FEL) using a pulse width of ~400, a preheated argon gas jet dissipating the carbon soot commencing the anterior of the carbon source. (2) The other technique, called laser powder technique, has CO_2 laser in a stream of argon. Laser ablation of a blend of carbon source and powder of catalyst is employed, resulting in a substantial decline in thermal conductivity losses. The catalyst used in this method is Ni:Co (1:1), and the yield is around 5 gm/hr.

Laser ablation strategy incorporates the use of laser bar to vaporize an object of a mix of graphite and metal impetus; the main difference between continuous and pulsed laser is that the pulsed laser demands a much higher light intensity (100 KW/cm^2 compared with 12 KW/cm^2). The oven is filled with helium or argon gas in order to keep the pressure at 500 torr. A very hot vapor plume forms, then expands and cools rapidly. As the vaporized species cool, small carbon molecules and atoms quickly condense to form larger clusters, possibly including fullerenes. The catalysts also begin to condense and attach to carbon clusters and prevent their closing into cage structure.

Laser ablation is a simple and effective new method developed from the arc discharge by Smalley and his coworkers. The principle of this method can be described thus: Firstly, a piece of graphite is placed in a vacuum furnace which is filled with some inert gas (e.g., helium) under the condition of high temperature. After that, using high-energy laser beam to irradiate the metal catalyst and carbon atoms of targeted graphite, a high temperature will be produced instantly to prompt them to evaporate, and then the carrier gas will bring these carbon molecules and catalyst particles to the high-temperature zone.

With a similar principle and mechanism of the arc discharge method, carbon nanotubes produced by laser ablation method exhibit a relatively high crystallinity and straightness.

The performance of CNTs prepared by laser ablation is mainly affected by the following parameters: laser parameters (energy fluence, peak power, continuous wave and pulse wave, repetition rate, oscillation wavelength), pressure and material composition of the combustion chamber, structure and chemical composition of the target material, flow and pressure of the buffer gas, spacing between target material and matrix, and the temperature of matrix and ambient.

Laser ablation (LA) is one of the superior methods to produce SWNTs; however, this method is not very much interesting for the synthesis of MWNTs because of its expensive cost.

Laser irradiation focuses on targeting through the window and under high temperature (800–1,400°C), or mostly

1,200°C, and an inert gas flow or mixed gas composition inside the quartz tube (Ar, N_2). The pressure is between 200 and 400 torr, allowing for the evaporation of the target rod swept by inert gas and depositing the soot on a water-cooled collector located at the exit of the furnace which filters them to deposit CNTs.

The properties of CNTs prepared by the LA process are strongly dependent on different parameters: the laser properties, the composition of the target material, the chamber temperature, pressure, the chemical composition, and flowing buffer gas [35]. Chrzanowska et al. have studied the effect of laser wavelength on SWCNT synthesis yield and properties by using a double pulse Nd:YAG laser, working at a wavelength of 355 or 1,064 nm. They have found that properties of synthesized CNTs depend much more on the laser fluence, and the SWCNT synthesis is favored at narrower UV laser radiation fluence.

Arc discharge and laser ablation were the first methods that allowed the synthesis of SWCNTs in relatively large (gram) amounts. Both methods involve the condensation of hot gaseous carbon atoms generated from the evaporation of solid carbon. For the growth of single-wall tubes, a metal catalyst is needed in the arc discharge system. The growth of high-quality SWCNTs at the 1–10 g scale was also produced using a laser ablation (laser oven) method. Besides the laser oven method, there are reports regarding the usage of a typical industrial continuous wave CO_2 laser system for the production of SWCNTs. Nevertheless, the equipment requirements and the large amount of energy consumed by these methods make them less favorable for nanotube production. With the arc and laser methods, only powdered samples with nanotubes tangled into bundles can be produced. The common feature of arc discharge and laser ablation methods is the need for a high amount of energy to induce the reorganization of carbon atoms into CNTs. The temperature used is even higher than 3,000ºC, which is beneficial for good crystallization of the CNTs; thus, the products are always produced with good graphite alignment. However, the basic requirements of these systems, including vacuum conditions and continuous graphite target replacement, pose difficulties to the large-scale production of CNTs.

2.4 Purification of CNTs

The synthesized CNTs can be separated from the amorphous carbon, carbon nanoparticles, residual catalyst, and other impurities by various methods. The conventional methods of purification are not very successful, but methods like gas-phase, liquid-phase, and intercalation methods show good results.

2.4.1 Gas-Phase Purification of CNTs

In this method, the CNTs are subjected to a high-temperature oxidation, followed by repeated extractions with nitric acid and hydrochloric acid. This procedure makes the synthesized CNTs purer and highly stable, with fewer amounts of residual catalyst and other non-CNTs formed.

2.4.2 Liquid-Phase Purification of CNTs

A series of steps is followed in the liquid-phase purification of synthesized CNTs. They are:

- Preliminary filtration to remove bulk graphite particles
- Dissolution in both organic solvents and concentrated acids to remove the fullerenes and catalyst, respectively
- Centrifugal separation of CNTs (solid part) from the solution (containing impurities).
- Microfiltration
- Chromatography to isolate multi-walled carbon nanotubes, single-walled carbon nanotubes, etc.

2.4.3 Intercalation Purification of CNTs

In this method, the nanoparticle impurities present are oxidized by metallic copper, which acts as an oxidation catalyst formed from the reduction of copper chloride added during the process. This process introduces intercalate residues and damages CNTs during the oxidation process.

2.5 Chemical Vapor-Phase Growth Production Deposition Method (CVD)

Sources for CVD used. Based on the heating source, the CVD can be:

- Thermal-activated CVD, which is heated by IR radiation, RF heater, etc.
- Photo-assisted CVD, which is heated by arc lamps, CO_2 laser, argon ion laser, Nd–YAG laser, etc.
- Plasma-assisted CVD, which is heated by microwave radiation, etc.

Conditions maintained: The following conditions are maintained inside the furnace.

- Temperature: 500–900°C
- Inert gas atmosphere: Argon gas

In CVD, the deposition of carbon molecules and CNT formation occur on the surface of the catalyst particles. This is the best technique for CNT preparation and has been described by several researchers for the large-scale production of CNTs. In this method, the CNT growth is directional and controlled. There are two types of CVD methods: thermal CVD and plasma-enhanced CVD. The most common sources of carbon include carbon monoxide (CO), methane (CH_4), and acetylene (C_2H_2). However, for the large-scale production of SWCNTs and DWCNTs, a mixture of hydrocarbons, such as ethylene (C_2H_4), CH_4, or C_2H_2, and a process gas, such as ammonia (NH_3), nitrogen (N_2), or hydrogen (H_2), is used to react in a closed vessel under 700–900°C. This is also a

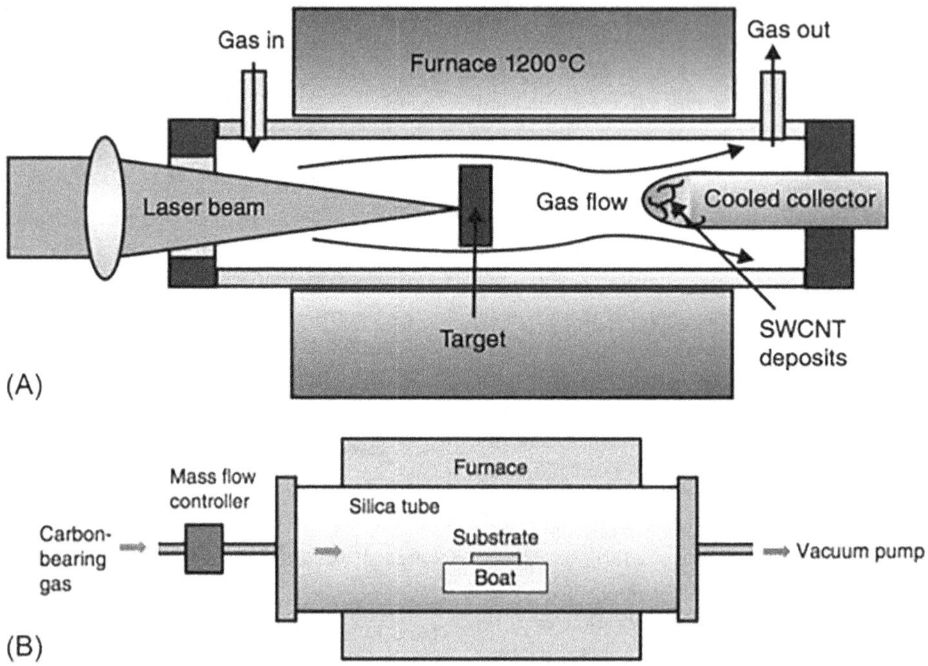

SCHEME 2.2 (a) Laser ablation method of CNT perpetration. (b) Chemical vapor deposition technique for CNT preparation.

Source: (a) Henley, S., Anguita, J., Silva, S., 2012. Synthesis of Carbon Nanotubes. Springer, The Netherlands. Copyright permission from Springer Nature, The Netherlands. (b) Homma, Y., 2015. Carbon Nanotube Synthesis and the Role of Catalyst. Springer, Japan, pp. 125–129. Copyright permission from Springer Nature, Japan.

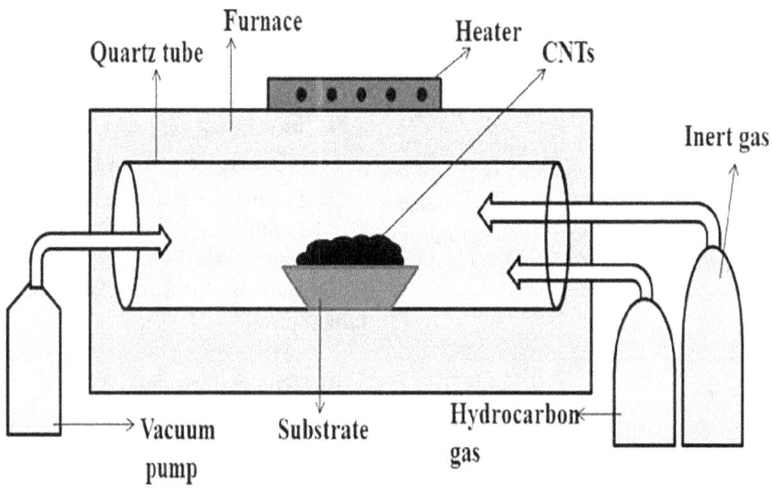

FIGURE 2.8 Schematic representation of chemical vapor deposition (CVD).

Sources for carbon: The precursors for carbon nanotubes are hydrocarbon gases, such as acetylene, ethylene, methane, etc.

Substrate used: Substrates are materials on which the CNTs are grown. The commonly used substrates in CVD method are zeolite, silica, silicon plate coated with iron particles, etc.

Catalyst used: To produce single-walled carbon nanotubes, metal catalyst nanoparticles such as iron, cobalt, nickel, molybdenum, iron–molybdenum alloys, etc. are used.

two-step synthesis, including a catalyst preparation step and the temperature-dependent reaction step following heating of about 500–1,000°C (Scheme 2.2). Plasma-induced CVD is a process in which plasma is emitted during the synthesis of CNTs. Cumings and coworkers from the University of California, Berkeley, first reported the synthesis of DWCNTs by using the plasma CVD method.

Chemical vapor deposition (CVD): CVD is a technique in which the vaporized reactants react chemically and form a nanomaterial product that is deposited on the substrate (Figure 2.8).

2.5.1 Procedure for Synthesis of CNTs by Thermal CVD Method

CNTs are synthesized by thermal CVD method by using hydrocarbon gas as carbon source. In this method, a quartz tube is placed inside a furnace maintained at high temperature (500–900°C) heated by RF heater. A crucible containing the substrate coated with catalyst nanoparticles is placed inside a quartz tube filled with an inert gas such as argon gas. The hydrocarbon gas (carbon source) is pumped into the quartz tube, which undergoes pyrolysis reaction and forms vapor carbon atoms. These carbon atoms bind to the substrate and join to each other by van der Waals force of attraction and grow as multi-walled carbon nanotubes (MWCNTs) on the substrate. To synthesize single-walled carbon nanotubes, catalyst nanoparticles of Fe, Co, and Ni are used. The obtained CNTs are further purified to get the pure form of CNTs.

It is achieved by putting a carbon supply (methane, carbon monoxide, and acetylene) in the gas phase and using an energy source, such as plasma or a resistively heated coil, to transfer energy to a gaseous carbon molecule. Nanotubes could be developed upon a diversity of constituents utilizing the approaches of CVD, which enables them to participate more effectively in ongoing processes of electronics manufacturing. The mentioned process could also be additionally divided into the following categories comprising microwave plasma (MPECVD), CCVD (catalytic CVD), plasma-enhanced CVD (PE-CVD), and oxygen-assisted CVD [36]. The CVD method includes volatile or otherwise gaseous compound decomposition catalyzed using metallic nanoparticles that correspondingly function as the nucleation site intended for the induction of progression of CNTs. In comparison to the two previously mentioned methods, CVD is a preferred way of large-scale production of CNTs and is economical as well. CNTs can be developed at a comparatively low temperature and by altering the particle size of the catalyst; their size could moreover be supervised. The commonly used source of carbon in this method is carbon monoxide (CO), methane (CH_4), acetylene, etc. Catalysts with a small particle size are challenging to synthesize, although with the small particle size of the catalyst, a range of catalyst sizes is acquired, which results in the development of nanotubes with a range of diameters [37]. If appropriate considerations have been retained, it results in the development of CNTs.

It is a two-step process: (1) nucleation and deposition of catalyst by thermal annealing or chemical engraving; (2) growth of nanotubes over a substrate at 500–1,000°C temperature. The tube length depends upon the time of reaction, and tubes up to 60 mm in length could be produced.

CVD is one of the most widely used and the most in-depth investigated method for the synthesis of CNTs; actually, it is essentially a thermal dehydrogenation reaction which needs a transition metal catalyst. The principle of CVD is, firstly, the carbon source gas enters into the reaction chamber together with carrier gas under the temperature of 600–1,000ºC, and the gas will be decomposed to produce the carbon atoms on a coated catalyst substrate under high temperature. And finally, CNTs are generated. The often-used transition metal catalysts are Co, Fe, Ni, Cu, Cr, and Mo, and sometimes their alloy. The carbon source generally uses carbon gases, such as methane, ethanol, ethylene, acetylene, benzene, and so on. This can help in reducing the required temperature for the decomposition of gaseous hydrocarbon into carbon and hydrogen. The key process parameters of CVD are carbon source, gas flux, carrier gas flux, and growth temperature and catalyst concentration. According to the loading and dispersion methods of catalyst, CVD is divided into matrix method and floating catalyst method. The advantages of CVD are that CNTs can grow on the substrate directly and the equipment is simple and low-cost. It is worth noting that this method can be operated continuously for mass production.

There are different CVD techniques, such as plasma-enhanced (PECVD), microwave plasma (MPECVD), or radio frequency (RF-CVD), hot filament (HFCVD) [35], oxygen-assisted and water-assisted, and floating catalyst (FCCVD) method [38]. Recently, CVD has been considered as an uncomplicated and flexible technology used in the synthesis of CNTs compared to arc discharge and laser ablation. The main advantages of CVD are easy control of the reaction, high yield, low impurity production, low cost of CNT, and relatively low operating temperature—lower than 1,200°C.

CVD process parameters (deposition time, temperature, and gas flow rate) can be independently utilized to produce CNTs with similar or different dimensions and characteristics with distinctive advantages. The increase in reaction temperature and flow rate of the precursor gas increases the mean diameter of MWCNTs, while increasing processing time decreases the diameter. Additionally, the diameter distribution and quality of MWCNTs are strongly influenced by the diameter of the catalyst particles [39]. High hydrogen content can induce catalytic hydrogenation of carbon and lead to surface modification of CNTs—as a result, the mean and core diameters. The crystallinity of the graphene walls and the length of CNTs are greatly influenced by hydrogen flow. Recently, it has been reported that hydrocarbons are not the only source for synthesis of CNTs. Bhongade et al. reported the synthesis of MWCNTs using waste toner powder as carbon source by CVD method, then confirmed that waste toner is a good source of carbon for the synthesis of CNTs [40].

The difference between these conventional methods is in the quality and purity of the obtained CNTs, although scientists are searching for other possibilities, namely, more economic ways to grow nanotubes, but they have had less success. The main causes can be summed up in the reaction in the devices, the reaction conditions (pressure, temperatures of liquid nitrogen), and the cost of the catalyst material. Thus, the CVD technique is carried out in a two-step process:

1. Catalyst is deposited on the substrate, and then nucleation of the catalyst is carried out via chemical etching or thermal annealing. Ammonia is used as an etchant. Metal catalysts used are Ni, Fe, or Co.
2. The carbon source is then placed in its gas phase in the reaction chamber. Then carbon molecule is converted to atomic level by using an energy source like plasma or heated coil. This carbon will get diffused toward the substrate, which is coated with a catalyst, and the nanotubes grow over this metal catalyst. Carbon source used is methane, carbon monoxide, or acetylene. Temperature used for synthesis of nanotube is in the 650–9,000°C range. The typical yield is 30%.

The CVD method has attracted significant interest by researchers. This method mainly uses a hydrocarbon substance as a carbon source to be cleaved into carbon clusters on the surface of the catalyst particles and then regrouped when the carbon source gas is in contact with the catalyst in the quartz tube at a suitable temperature. A transition metal, such as iron, cobalt, nickel, molybdenum, niobium, and tantalum, is generally used as a catalyst. The experimental results show that the size of the metal catalyst particles predominantly determines the inner and outer diameter of the carbon nanotubes. Therefore, carbon nanotubes with higher purity and uniform size distribution can be grown by selectively controlling the type and particle size of the catalyst.

Compared with other methods, the CVD method has the advantage of easy control of the reaction process, simple and convenient preparation apparatus, relatively low growth temperature, and high purity, low cost, strong adaptability, and large-scale production. The method also has the ability to align carbon nanotube arrays by controlling the application of catalysts and increasing the density of the array by the liquid-induced process, which has been widely used in the preparation of carbon nanotubes.

The CVD method involves the decomposition of a gaseous or volatile compound of carbon, catalyzed by metallic nanoparticles, which also serve as nucleation sites for the initiation of carbon nanotube growth. In contrast to the previous two methods, CVD has been proven to be a preferred route for large-scale production of carbon nanotubes. Thus, the CVD method has the advantages of mild operation, low cost, and controllable process. Over the last 12 years, several methods have been developed that have the potential for industrial-scale preparation of nanotubes. All of them are based on CVD methods. Among these methods, five different approaches have been shown to be the most promising:

1. Methane CVD. It was first reported in 1998, where a bulk amount of SWCNTs was synthesized by CVD from methane at 900°C. The yield of this method has been significantly improved using Al_2O_3 aerogels impregnated with Fe/Mo nanoparticles as a catalyst.
2. HiPCO, which stands for high-pressure catalytic decomposition of carbon monoxide, uses high-pressure CO as the carbon source for the preparation of SWCNTs. The catalysts used in a HiPCO process are in the gas phase, produced from a volatile organometallic catalyst precursor.
3. CO CVD uses CO as a feed gas. Compared with samples made using the same catalyst and methane, the amount of amorphous carbon can be reduced. An important advance in the CO CVD method is the development of the Co-Mo catalyst. In that process, Co-Mo bimetallic catalysts and a fluidized bed CVD reactor were used to produce a large quantity of SWCNTs. The most important advantage of fluidized bed reactors is that they permit continuous addition and removal of solid particles from the reactor, without stopping the operation.
4. Alcohol CVD was reported in 2002, which produced high-purity SWCNTs without any amorphous carbon coating using alcohols such as methanol and ethanol as a carbon source. It was proposed that the OH radical formed at high temperature from alcohols can remove amorphous carbon efficiently during nanotube growth, leaving only pure SWCNTs as a product.
5. Plasma-enhanced CVD (PECVD) methods have also been widely used for making carbon materials, including MWCNTs and SWCNTs, recently. The reactive species in the plasma system could affect the growth of very small diameter tubes, with implications to both diameter control and selective etching of metallic SWCNTs.

At present, the production of MWCNTs accounted for more than 90% of the output. Therefore, how to synthesize MWCNTs effectively with more yields has become a particularly important issue. As the MWCNTs can be grown effectively, CVD has become the main synthetic method of MWCNTs. Camilli et al. developed a new method for synthesizing MWCNTs by CVD using a stainless steel as catalyst. It is worth noting that a continuous production of CNTs from the same substrate is achievable, and the stainless steel substrate can be reused after carefully removing the synthesized CNTs. The presence of native nanoscale substrate structures, which look like hills, still persists after the substrate has been used for the synthesis of CNT.

CVD is the most popular technique used to form CNTs due to its distinct advantages over other techniques. Some primary advantages include an inexpensive fabrication process, the requirement of temperatures less than 1,000°C, and high purity of obtained CNTs [41]. CVD was first used by Endo et al. in 1993 to synthesize CNTs. This was carried out by using carbon feedstock in the form of hydrocarbons with metallic catalysts at a defined temperature in the fabrication chamber. CVD has been largely used to form CNTs due to the diversified characteristics of the resultant products [42]. The CVD process can be optimized by changing the experimental parameters, like pressure, catalyst, type and rate of gas flow, grain size, types of CVD, and others. The effect of some of these parameters has been shown by significant research, which will be expanded upon in the following subsections.

2.5.2 Effect of Catalyst

The nature of the catalyst used by different research groups to obtain different products in the fabrication process has been varied. Pure and metallic alloys are mostly used to carry out the synthesis process. It was seen that each of the parameters, such as the reaction temperature, flow of precursor gas, and the process, changed the mean diameter of the CNTs. CNTs were selectively grown on an NiO catalyst supported by Al_2O_3 nanoparticles. This process also included C_2H_2 as the carbon precursor gas and argon (Ar) as the carrier gas. The synthesis was performed with reaction temperatures below 700°C and above 1,000°C, which led to the formation of disoriented CNTs. CNT alignment was improved by increasing the precursor rate of the gas flow, which correspondingly led to an increase in the number of tubular CNTs.

Catalysts play a crucial role in the CVD synthesis of CNTs; therefore, improving the desired characteristics of catalyst will enhance the obtained CNTs' quality as well as the process yield. Carbon nanostructures are commonly synthesized using transition metal nanoparticles as catalysts. Transition metals in the form of nanoparticles are considered as the most effective catalysts. The peculiar ability of transition metals to promote CNT growth is strongly related to these factors: (1) catalytic activity for decomposition of volatile carbon compounds, (2) ability of metastable carbides formation, and (3) diffusion of carbon through and over the metallic particles. The catalytic CVD process for CNT growth utilizes heterogeneous catalysts, which are the catalytically active metal particles, typically with a diameter of 1–10 nm, anchored on a high-surface inert area. The transition metals used to date as catalysts include Fe, Ni, Co, and Mo. More recent studies, however, have shown that other metals, such as In, Cu, Ag, Pd, Mn, Mo, Cr, Al, and Au, can also be used for SWCNT formation.

So far, the published results concerning catalysts have mainly focused on the synthesis of monodispersed CNTs, but there have been very few detailed experimental studies of the reaction pathways. Furthermore, the interaction between catalysts and the surface of substrates need to be further investigated and characterized. Efforts in the future will be geared toward finding optimal CVD conditions to discover the detailed mechanism of catalysis, and facilitating control over the growth of CNTs for future fabrication of nanotube-based devices.

2.5.3 Types of CVD

CVD is also varied to develop CNTs and obtain optimized characteristics. Each category simultaneously varies in terms of intrinsic parameters, such as current, atmospheric pressure, and temperature. Most of these eight categories are used in industrial sectors to form high-quality SWCNTs and MWCNTs. The type of CVD used for the fabrication process invariably changes the physicochemical properties of the CNTs. The optimized version of the two layers allows the effective growth of CNTs with patterned and non-patterned substrates. The underlayer increases the surface roughness, which subsequently increases the active nucleation sites.

2.5.4 Carbon Sources

One of the major barriers to the industrial application of CNTs lies on the cost of their carbonaceous precursors.

There are two main carbon sources for the synthesis of CNTs using CVD method: fossil-based hydrocarbon and plant-based hydrocarbon. Hydrocarbon has long been widely used as the conventional carbon source in the field of CNT research. Natural gas becomes the most preferable carbon source to many researchers. Because of its stability at high temperature against self-decomposition, methane catalytic decomposition by transition metal catalyst particles is the dominant process in carbon nanotubes growth. Besides methane, several other carbon species, such as acetylene, benzene, xylene, toluene, and so forth, have been used as a carbon feedstock to synthesize CNTs. These carbons precursors are related to fossil fuels, and in view of the insufficient available source in the near future and its environmental effects, it is necessary to consider developing carbonaceous materials from natural sources. Efforts are now directed to the use of nonpetroleum products. Syntheses of CNTs from natural precursors are rare; however, over the past several years, natural renewable resources have become more attractive because of their environmental benefits and lower cost. One such appreciable effort is the use of nondegradable polymers for synthesis of CNTs. There have been reports on the use of natural precursors, such as camphor ($C_{10}H_{16}O$), turpentine oil ($C_{10}H_{16}$), eucalyptus oil ($C_{10}H_{18}O$), castor oil ($C_{54}H_{100}O_7$), coconut oil ($C_{39}H_{74}O_6$), and palm oil ($C_{67}H_{127}O_8$), for synthesis of CNTs. Published data show that some researchers have used waste cooking palm oil as the biocarbon precursor in their studies. Waste cooking oil, which is much less expensive than virgin vegetable oil, is a promising alternative to vegetable oil for CNT production. Suriani and coworkers reported the use of waste cooking palm oil for the synthesis of vertically aligned carbon nanotubes (VACNT). The result showed that the complex composition of the waste oil (leaching of fats and other hydrocarbons from the fried objects) did not affect the synthesis process.

2.5.5 Gas Flow

One of the most significant parameters that affect the length and diameter of CNTs is the type of gas used during the experimental process. The presence of different types of gases as carrier flow simultaneously varies the amount of deposition and the electrical characteristics of CNTs. One such example shows the use of multiple gases (Ar and H_2). Their analysis was done in terms of Young's modulus (E) by using a vibrating reed technique. The experiments were conducted using three different precursors that resulted in differing densities of defects in the tube walls. The developed CNTs were electrostatically driven in the air over a dark-field light microscope for study.

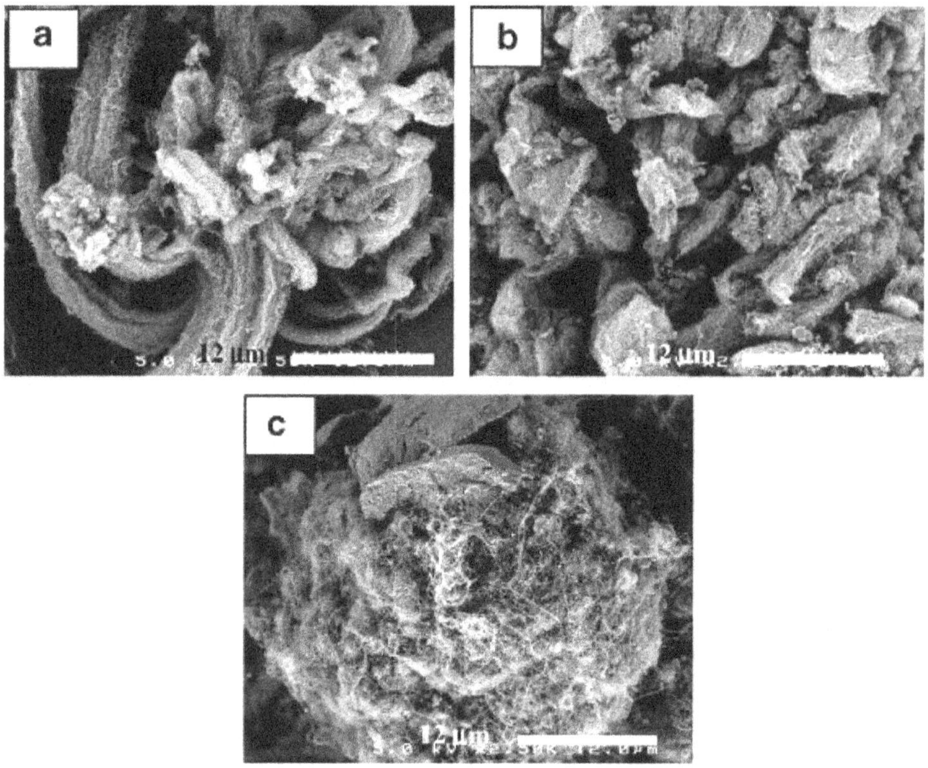

FIGURE 2.9 SEM micrographs of the synthesized CNTs at (1) 550°C, (b) 650°C, and (3) 750°C.

Source: [43].

2.5.6 Grain Size

Consideration of the grain size of substrates and catalyst metals is very effective to optimize the physiochemical properties of the CNTs. The selective growth of CNTs on the multi-gram scale was done using CVD from ethylene. With the formation of CNTs in the macropores of the catalyst, an explosion of catalyst grains was induced. Figure 2.9 [43] shows the scanning electron microscopy (SEM) images of the CNTs formed at temperatures of 550°C, 650°C, and 750°C.

With the constant growth of industrial companies working on the mass production of CNTs, it is essential for each working unit to fabricate these nanotubes with low-cost experimental setups while maintaining a production of high-quality CNTs. Although both SWCNTs and MWCNTs are being fabricated and utilized equally in the academic sector, the optimization of the experimental parameters affects SWCNTs comparatively more than MWCNTs. This is due to the high chirality of the simple structure. Also, the proportion of semiconducting tubes is higher in SWCNTs than in MWCNTs; thus, their properties are found to be more influenced by the temperature and atmospheric conditions. Apart from the mentioned parameters, other variables like reaction time, carbon precursors, and supporting materials were also studied to increase the yield and to purify the synthesized CNTs.

2.6 Vapor-Phase Growth Production Method

Physical vapor deposition (PVD): PVD is a technique by which a material can be vaporized into gaseous form and then deposited on the surface of a substrate.

Target source: The most common carbon source target used is solid graphite, which is irradiated by laser source and vaporized into vapor carbon atoms.

Laser source: The laser source used for the vaporization of target material into target vapor atoms can be a continuous laser source, such as CO_2 laser, or a pulsed laser source, such as Nd:YAG laser (neodymium-doped yttrium aluminum garnet, Nd:Y3A15O12).

Substrate used: The substrate used in this method is water-cooled copper collector, on which the vaporized carbon atoms deposit and grow as CNTs.

Inert gas atmosphere: Argon gas is commonly used as inert gas which flows at a constant flow rate toward the water-cooled copper collector.

It is a new method also known as the converted type of CVD technique. The central dissimilarity in this technique is that CNTs are produced straight from the reaction gas plus catalytic metal within the slab, not including any substrate. Two heating systems are located within the reaction slab. Catalyst used inside this process is ferrocene. Carbon catalytic vaporization maintains a small temperature in the initial furnace. Fine catalytic atoms are produced now, and after they arrive at the subsequent furnace, at that time, fresh carbons are absorbed within this medium through diffusion, where they are transformed into CNTs.

2.7 Other Emerging Methods

Except the preceding three main synthetic methods, there are some other emerging methods for the preparation of CNTs, such as low-temperature plasma/solvothermal process hydrothermal, flame, and the microwave. But the yield of these methods is relatively lower, and the process conditions are very difficult to control.

2.7.1 Flame Synthesis Method

SWCNTs are formed from hydrocarbon fuels and tiny aerosol metal catalysts in a controlled flame environment. Flames are considerably less expensive than existing methods for the fabrication of nanotubes in large quantities. Three crucial components for the development of CNTs are necessary: these are a carbon source, metal catalyst particles, and a heat source. Catalytic precursors have been usually incorporated through the flame system in this method and, in addition, are nucleated and finally condensed into solid metal spherical nanoparticles. The composition of even the final synthesized product might also be swayed by both the catalytic properties and the alteration of the flame parameters. As a repercussion, various flame patterns inclusive of inverse diffusion are shown; partially mixed and premixed flames would have also been employed for the manufacturing of nanotubes as well as nanofibers. By utilizing the vapor of pentacarbonyl and iron as a source of a metal catalyst, nanotubes with single walls could have perhaps been identified in the post-flame area of the premixed argon/oxygen/acetylene flame, conducted at about 50 torr (6.7 kPa). Nanotubes are detected to form and amalgamate into bunches amid 40 and 70 nm height directly above the burner (within ~30 ms).

The flame synthesis technique is another method where CNTs are able to be produced. During this technique, hydrocarbon blazes are re-used. These blazes give out beginning growths of nanotubes. Gases such as carbon monoxide, methane, C_2H_4, ethane, and C_2H_6 are present inside the after-flame portion and are a great source of carbon.

2.7.2 Hydrothermal Process

In a typical synthesis, ferrocene and sulfur in 1:2 proportions are dissolved in a mixed solution of water, and ethanol and NaOH pellets are added to the solution under a stirring condition for 30 min in a magnetic stirrer. The resulting homogeneous mixture is transferred to the reactor. The autoclave is heated to 200°C and maintained at this temperature for 20 h, and then it is cooled to room temperature naturally; the resulting black precipitate is filtered, washed, and dried at 60°C in air.

2.7.3 Electrolysis Process

Soluble base and alkaline earth chloride salts are generally hygroscopic. Thermally drying (250°C) the salt in air is typically acceptable for CNT production. (For CNT production, on account of the utilization of graphite crucible, melting the salt ought to be directed under inert climate.) This procedure is called pre-electrolysis. After pre-electrolysis, a graphite bar of 1.4 cm^2 diameter with 5 cm^2 height is embedded into the melt as cathode. The cathode is embedded into the melt up to 4 cm^2 deepness in the graphite crucible as anode just as holding vessel for electrolyte. The control of DC power supply additionally needs to give an adequately wide range of currents and voltages. This procedure is completed at the steady current of 3 A and voltage of 4.6 V. The current, voltage, and temperature of the bath are recorded all throughout the procedure.

2.7.4 Spray Pyrolysis

Progress metal nanoparticles ware directly put in a quartz boat and kept at the center of a quartz tube, which is put inside a tubular heater. The inert gas nitrogen is presented at a rate of 100 mL/min into the quartz tube to expel any oxygen from that point and to make an inert environment (Figures 2.10). The temperature is raised from room temperature to the preferred growth temperature. In this way, the carbon precursor is brought into the quartz tube through a spray nozzle, and the stream is kept up at a rate of 0.5 mL/min at a temperature of 650°C. This process is carried out for 45 min, and thereafter, the furnace is cooled to room temperature. Nitrogen atmosphere is maintained throughout the experiment.

2.7.5 Silane Solution Method

Nanotubes are produced by means of the silane solution technique by immersing the substrate into a silane solution along with a metallic catalyst, if possible Co–Ni, in or around a proportion of 1:1, along with a carbon source, such as ethylene containing feedstock gas, fed over the substrate, and the deposition of the catalyst thereon as heating is provided to the substrate by utilizing an electric current. Carbon nanotubes are produced using a silane solution method, in which a substrate such as carbon paper or stainless steel mesh is immersed in a silane solution of a metal catalyst, preferably Co–Ni in a 1:1 ratio, and a feedstock gas containing a carbon source such as ethylene is fed through the substrate and the catalyst deposited thereon while the substrate is heated by applying an electrical current thereto. Thus, a reaction occurs between the catalyst and the gas to yield CNTs supported on the conductive substrate.

2.8 Experimental Reproducibility

A crucial aspect of CVD synthesis is the inherent variability in the day-to-day experimental process parameters (ambient humidity, furnace cleanliness, substrate placement, etc.), which can severely impact reproducibility. One solution is to automate processes involved in SWCNT growth, which can

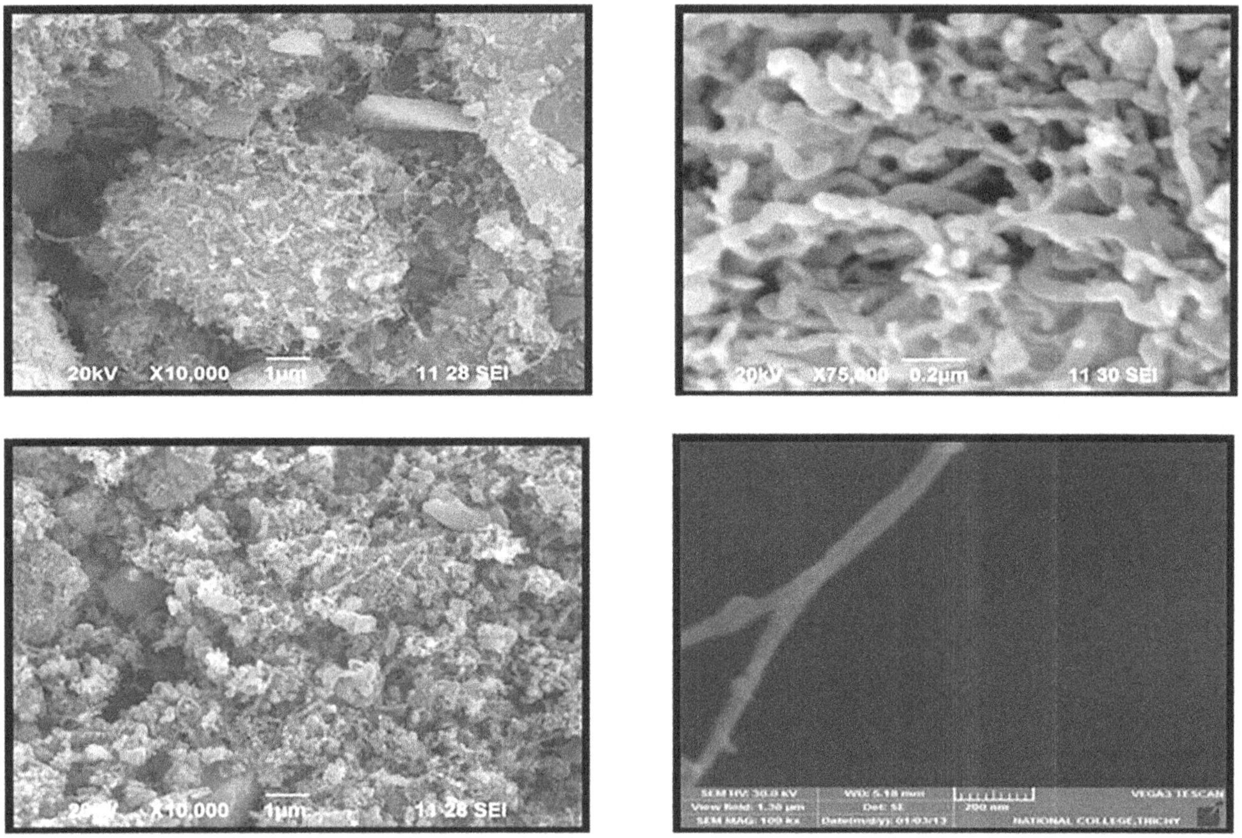

FIGURE 2.10 SEM images of carbon nanotubes from different carbon sources.

mitigate reproducibility issues. Another problem with CVD synthesis is the huge experimental parameter space (catalyst, hydrocarbon, substrate, temperature, pressure, flow rates, etc.), which makes progress prohibitively slow. This presents a drawback for most in situ techniques that study nonideal growth scenarios (for example, low pressures and temperatures) using a small number of controlled growth parameters while providing little statistics to account for variations between experiments. To that end, the recently developed autonomous research system (ARES) uses robotics and machine learning (ML) to execute, evaluate, and plan subsequent growth experiments by handling the multidimensional parameter space through computations. ARES is a fully autonomous, closed-loop research robot for materials development. It relies on a variety of ML planners, such as random forest and knowledge gradient, and has shown that it can learn to grow SWCNTs at a desired growth rate. Future advance with operando and in situ techniques will greatly benefit from implementation of automation and autonomous feedback control to increase reliability.

2.9 In Situ Growth Deposition of CNTs and 2D Material Synthesis on Fibers

Another alternative for coating micron-sized fibers with CNTs is by growing them in situ—that is, by using the fiber surface as a substrate for CNT synthesis. The biggest advantages of in situ growth are the high control of the growth, uniformity, thickness, and density of CNTs, by means of the control of the process parameters. For this approach, chemical vapor deposition (CVD) has been established as the most effective and practical route. The main drawbacks of the CVD technique are related to the usage of high temperatures, which induce thermal damage on the fibers, decreasing their mechanical properties [44]. Among the first efforts on this area are those reported by Downs and Baker, where a novel concept involving the generation of vapor-grown carbon filaments on the surface of CFs was proposed. The carbon filaments were grown on the fiber by impregnation with copper-nickel catalyst precursors as a product of the decomposition of selected hydrocarbons and carbon monoxide. During this reaction, the hydrocarbons are adsorbed and decomposed at the catalyst particles, followed by the diffusion of carbon species through the catalyst particles, producing the filament structure. Since this early study, many research efforts have been devoted to CVD growth of nanostructures on micron-sized fibers.

A schematic of the general process for in situ growth is shown in Scheme 2.3. Unsized fibers are typically used as substrates for CNT growth, with GFs and CFs the most commonly reported ones. To remove the fiber surface coating (sizing) usually present on commercial fibers, preheating treatments (>450°C) under different atmospheres are customarily used [44]. After sizing removal, metallic catalyst

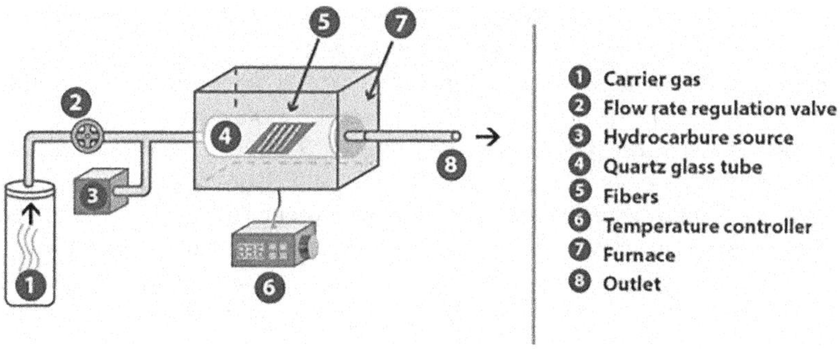

SCHEME 2.3 Schematic of the process of in situ growth of carbon nanotubes on engineering fibers by CVD.

Source: [44].

particles are deposited onto the fiber surface. Different means are reported to deposit the metal catalyst required for thermal CVD reactions, including incipient wetness (solution impregnation) methods, polymer–metal complex deposition, sputtering, electron beam evaporation, thermal evaporation, and electrodeposition.

The ability to directly monitor SWCNTs or other low-dimensional nanostructures during growth can provide valuable insights into their growth mechanisms, and in situ or operando measurements have become increasingly important. Because each in situ method has its own operational parameter space and information delivered about SWCNTs or 2D materials, the choice of characterization tool is significant. This challenge is often expressed in terms of the so-called pressure and materials gaps, where traditional surface science is typically performed in ultrahigh vacuum and on well-defined model surfaces/single crystals, while scalable catalytic growth of SWCNTs and 2D materials is performed at higher pressures and involves complex material architectures (Figure 1.22). It is important to bridge these gaps to fully understand the catalytic process under real working conditions. Also, shown in Figure 1.22 are the selected in situ characterization methods that have been employed to study 1D and 2D material growth, mapped with respect to their operating ranges in terms of pressure and characterization capabilities.

2.10 Substrate-Bound SWCNT Synthesis

When grown on flat substrates, SWCNTs are generally surface-bound, unless the interactions among sufficiently dense SWCNTs force their vertical growth. The formation of these surface-bound SWCNTs requires a dispersed distribution of catalyst particles so that forces exerted by the substrates on the SWCNTs can either horizontally align them in parallel to each other or distribute them in a random network. Horizontally aligned arrays of SWCNTs exceed the performance of traditional crystalline channel materials (e.g., silicon, GaAs) in digital and analog or radio frequency (RF) electronics. As discussed previously, Figure 1.23a shows a recent example of horizontally aligned CNT-based field-effect transistors (FETs) used in a computer. Random networks of SWCNTs, on the other hand, may replace amorphous silicon and organic materials in flexible electronics and flat panel displays. Both arrangements of SWCNTs are also considered for use in applications such as transparent electronics and bio/chemical sensors.

As the substrate-bound SWCNTs require dispersed distributions of catalyst particles, sometimes in the form of parallel stripes for aligned growth, the particles are introduced on the substrate either from solutions of preformed catalysts (by drop-casting or spin-coating) or by lithographic patterning of catalyst films. Such catalyst deposition is always followed by calcination (i.e., high-temperature annealing in air), generally for approximately an hour, at 900–950°C, to remove the solvents or lithographic residues. This process causes catalyst coarsening and reduced catalytic efficiency, resulting in a low density of SWCNTs on the substrate. Interestingly, calcination on sapphire substrates at a higher temperature (1,100°C) and for a longer time (8 h) dissolves catalyst particles into the substrate, mitigating catalyst coarsening and yielding a high density of surface-bound, aligned SWCNTs. These catalysts, which are dissolved within the substrate during calcination, precipitate slowly during the growth phase and have been named Trojan catalysts in reference to the "Trojan horse" of Greek mythology.

Major applications of surface-bound SWCNTs are in electronics and sensors, which require semiconducting SWCNTs (s-SWCNTs) at levels much higher than the 66.67% obtained from standard CVD growth of SWCNTs (digital electronics, for example, require 99.99% s-SWCNTs in aligned arrays). To achieve this goal, SWCNTs are grown using different catalysts, [45] engineered catalyst supports, carbon feedstock, and recently with the application of electric field along the direction of growth [46]. Promising techniques among these revised growth recipes use catalyst supports like ceria that have active oxygen or gases like CH_4 and water vapor.

2.11 Vertically Aligned SWCNTs

Vertically aligned SWCNT arrays (also called forests, carpets, and VANTAs) are formed by a bottom-up, self-organization process, which renders a hierarchical and anisotropic morphology. The multitude of interactions among neighboring CNTs growing in concert causes individual CNTs to self-align. Researchers have been exploiting this paradigm since 1996 to synthesize relatively well-ordered MWCNTs and SWCNTs without requiring post-processing steps, which promises to transform a range of applications. In recent years, CNT forests have been shown to be advantageous for supercapacitor electrodes, electronic interconnects for vertical vias, electron emitters, broadband optical absorbers, terahertz technologies (generators, polarizers, detectors), optical rectennas, thermopower wave guides, thermal interface materials, anisotropic surfaces, gecko-inspired dry adhesives, flexographic printing, mechanical dampers, selective membrane nanochannels, and advanced yarns and sheets. Aside from pure applications, CNT forests are heavily studied because they are model systems for analyzing growth kinetics, wherein the average collective height of the forest is related to the length of individual constituent CNTs.

To make CNT forests competitive in each application space, targeted growth must advance to hone application-specific properties. Researchers have sought to focus control on one or a few critical characteristics, including intrinsic CNT forest properties like crystallinity/defect density, wall number, diameter (and polydispersity), alignment, and areal density. Importantly, there are inherent tradeoffs between these characteristics, which limit the extent of independent control and thus should be considered in the application design. Other growth challenges that remain critical bottlenecks to applications are achieving ultralong CNT forests (>mm scale), large-area forests (>wafer scale), and growth on conductive or flexible substrates, all of which remain nontrivial. Here, we focus on highlighting recent trends in the collective body of forest growth literature aimed at manipulating the support and catalyst layers to control SWCNT diameter, density, and forest height (yield).

The observation that the alumina support's bulk porosity (for subsurface diffusion) and surface roughness (for Ostwald ripening) can be modified to control catalyst migration, and hence diameter, revealed a coarse knob to control aligned CNT growth. For example, recent strategies decreased the amount of Fe loss into the support layer by manipulating the physical density (or oxidation state) of the alumina support via pretreatments (prior to Fe deposition) of either oxygen plasma or thermal annealing. Furthermore, both ion and electron bombardment of a sapphire surface, which is otherwise inactive for CNT growth, was shown to increase surface roughness and enable CNT forest growth [47]. This approach of engineering the topography of the support layer by ion bombardment promoted the growth of small-diameter CNTs, suggesting that smaller particles remained sufficiently stable for nucleation and growth. Such a pretreatment of oxide supports to improve growth has also been extended to other supports, such as sputtered MgO.

While not all the synthesis challenges for SWCNT forests have been resolved, we now have sufficient understanding to address industrial issues, such as continuous production, uniform gas delivery over large areas, and cost. Wafer-scale growth has already been demonstrated in a lab-scale tool. Moreover, Zeon Corp., under the subsidiary company Zeon Nano Technology Co. Ltd., recently established an industrial-scale SWCNT production plant. In collaboration with the National Institute of Advanced Industrial Science and Technology (AIST) in Japan, Zeon Corp. has developed a continuous belt conveyor process to synthesize aligned SWCNTs on flat 50 × 50 cm^2 metal substrates (see Figure 1.23b, c) for ton-scale production of long, pure, and high-surface-area aligned SWCNTs. Vertically aligned CNT growth has been demonstrated on catalyst-supported ceramic spheres in a fixed, monolayer bed of the beads. Fluidized bed CVD using catalyst supported on porous powders has realized commercial production of MWCNTs at hundreds of tons annually, although CNTs are not in aligned arrays but in agglomerates with catalyst powders. However, recent advances, such as using a lamellar catalyst and spherical ceramic beads with sputtered CVD catalyst, have enabled the growth of tens- to hundreds-of-micrometer-long SWCNT and few-wall CNT arrays. These methods provide a high carbon yield of 65–70% in spite of the small residence times (0.2–0.3 s). Moreover, the CNT arrays are easily separated from the ceramic beads by gas flow, yielding carbon purity levels as high as >99.6 wt% without the need for additional purification steps. The submillimeter-long CNT arrays can be easily transformed to sponge-like papers by dispersion filtration, showing excellent performance as 3D current collectors for rechargeable batteries and electrochemical capacitors. Because the materials need to cost less than 100 USD/kg to be used in practical batteries, scale-up of the production of CNT arrays in volume is highly demanded.

2.12 Recent Advances in Synthesis of Boron Nitride Nanotubes (BNNTs) Growth

Besides carbon, other materials with layered crystal structures, such as hexagonal boron nitride (hBN) and metal chalcogenides (e.g., WS_2), are known to form tubular structures at the nanoscale. Among them, boron nitride nanotubes (BNNTs) have been of particular interest due to their properties complementary to those of CNTs. BNNTs are seamless rolled-up cylinders composed of single- or few-layered hBN sheets. Owing to the structural similarity, BNNTs possess exceptional mechanical strength comparable to that of CNTs; however, they are a wide-bandgap semiconductors (~6.0 eV) and transparent in the visible spectrum. They also exhibit a remarkable oxidation resistance up to 900°C, electrical insulation with high thermal conductivity, thermal neutron absorption ability, and piezoelectricity. This makes BNNTs better suited than CNTs for many applications under extreme conditions, such as high-temperature, corrosive, and radioactive environments, where they can be used in thermal management for electronics, transparent nanocomposites, flame retarding/resistance, radiation shielding, and electroactive materials.

Many BNNT synthesis methods have been explored based on CNT synthesis methods; however, it has been challenging to produce high-quality BNNTs at large scale owing to their heteroatomic nature, limited access to boron sources, and necessity of extreme synthesis conditions. High-temperature routes (e.g., arc discharge, laser, plasma) have demonstrated good potential in the scalable manufacturing of highly crystalline, small-diameter BNNTs (<10 nm) directly from pure B or BN sources; however, the major challenge was the relatively slow reaction between B droplets (seeds for BNNT nucleation) and N_2 (renitridation agent) due to the strong triple bond of N_2, which limits the yield below 1 g/h.

Very recently, there has been notable progress that led to successful commercialization of BNNTs. High-pressure environments were found to be effective in driving the B–N_2 reaction toward BN formation by improving their collision frequency. Using a CO_2 laser to evaporate a B target under high N_2 pressures (0.7–1.4 MPa), a high temperature–pressure method was developed by the NASA-Langley team and demonstrated the growth of highly crystalline, small-diameter (<5 nm) BNNTs. This technology was licensed by BNNT LLC (Newport News, USA), and high-quality, small-diameter BNNTs became commercially available in 2014.

A different method based on an induction thermal plasma used hydrogen as a growth enhancer, significantly increasing the yield of small-diameter BNNTs (~20 g/h) at atmospheric pressure (see Figures 1.23d,e) [48]. Optical emission spectroscopy showed that the presence of hydrogen facilitates the formation of B–N–H containing intermediate species (e.g., NH and BH free radicals), while suppressing the recombination of freed N radicals into N_2 [49]. Compared to N_2, such species can provide faster chemical pathways to the BN formation owing to the relatively weak bonds of N–H or B–H. A recent numerical simulation also suggested improved particle heating and quenching rates (~105 K/s) in the presence of hydrogen due to the high thermal conductivity of hydrogen over the temperature range of 3,500–4,000 K. These turned out to be important for the complete decomposition of the hBN feedstock and rapid formation of nano-sized B droplets for the subsequent BNNT growth [49]. As discussed before, Figure 1.23d and e show photos of the as-produced BNNT material (~200 g) in the filtration chamber following an 11 h synthesis experiment, and its SEM image, respectively [48]. In 2015, this technology was licensed by Tekna Systems Inc. (Sherbrooke, Canada), and high-quality BNNTs became accessible in kilogram quantities. Enabled by this technology, the scalable fabrication of macroscopic high-purity assemblies of BNNTs (such as buckypapers, yarns, and thin films) was also successfully demonstrated [48]. A similar induction plasma process (now licensed to BNNT LLC, Newport News, VA) [50] at high pressure (>0.3 MPa) was also reported to produce small-diameter BNNTs at a large scale (~35 g/h) without using hydrogen.

Despite the recent progress, the current production capacity of BNNTs is still far behind that of SWCNTs. For the expedient development of BNNT-based applications, more effort is needed to understand the growth mechanisms through modeling and in situ diagnostics. Suitably engineered BNNTs will have transformative impact by providing a rich variety of geometrical or electronic structures and allow nanomaterial-based products not addressable by SWCNTs. Tuning the structure of BNNTs, such as bucking or faceting, has opened possibilities to control their torsional or shear stiffness, atomic-scale interlayer friction, and chemical reactivity. A systematic study of tunable BCN nanotubes is needed to elucidate how the electronic, optical, and physical properties of BNNTs can be tailored upon altering their composition or the distribution of hybrid domains of B, C, N, or BN. While atomically thin hBN layers have served as an excellent platform for this research, nanotube analogs using coaxial BNNTs and CNTs have received limited attention. The knowledge accumulated over two decades of SWCNT synthesis can provide useful guidance toward identifying critical pathways for the successful exploration of unchartered areas in BNNT science and technology.

2.13 Influence of Precursor Gas Chemistry

While researchers have analyzed the impacts of the catalyst, cocatalyst, and catalyst–substrate interactions on the resultant SWCNT product, less attention has been devoted to the carbon feedstock beyond the hydrocarbon metal solubility and, to some extent, its "cracking" behavior. However, over the past decade, bodies of evidence have emerged demonstrating the multiple critical roles of reactive gas feedstocks. For example, oxygen-containing species can influence lifetime through oxidative polishing, growth temperature by promoting dehydrogenation, and diameter control by influencing catalyst sintering behavior, while the hydrocarbons and their reaction products can influence nucleation efficiency and catalyst reduction as well as CNT alignment, growth rate, and defect density.

A burgeoning area where choice of precursor might have a significant impact is toward scale-up and more environmentally benign production of CNTs. A variety of renewable sources ranging from naturally occurring materials (oils, biodiesel, food-based products) and vegetable and animal waste products has shown their efficacy for producing CNTs. However, these feedstocks are inherently heterogeneous, which could lead to undesirable toxic by-product emissions and reduced product quality. In contrast, recent efforts to employ the by-product of Fischer–Tropsch (FTS) synthesis have been shown to produce SWCNT forests with enhanced growth rates and smaller average tube diameters compared to growth using traditional precursors such as ethylene. In addition, the FTS precursor also enabled MWCNT forest growth at low temperatures (<400°C). While all these precursors are still employed in a typical tube furnace-based thermal CVD process, alternate CNT synthesis routes are possible. In that regard, recent experiments in an open electrochemical system have demonstrated that CO_2 can be captured directly from the air and converted to CNTs, while O_2 evolves as a reaction by-product from the system [51]. These techniques represent an emerging direction for nanomaterials research that brings together the scientific discoveries of yesterday with the scaling and environmental challenges of tomorrow. Moreover, nontraditional chemical precursors may allow us to better understand the chemical pathways involved in SWCNT nucleation, while providing industrially viable routes for large-scale economic and sustainable production of CNTs.

2.14 Recent Trends in the Synthesis of CNTs

The production of MWNTs has also been used with a recent nebulized pyrolysis technique. A unique ultrasonic atomizer generates a nebulized spray, which is the principal variable in this process. MWNTs have been achieved using this method with a relatively even diameter in aligned bundles. This method is the most favorable method among all, and also a modified form of the CVD method. MWCNTs with high purity can be obtained by the use of various aliphatic and aromatic hydrocarbons and ferrocene as a catalytic precursor. By means of an ultrasonic nebulizer, the source of carbon, the catalyst, along with the solvent, is sprayed underneath an argon flow of 1 L/min keen on a tube-like furnace at a constant temperature of around 800°C. In arrears to their nonpolluting nature, being economical, unobtrusive derivatives (i.e., carbon monoxide [CO]), as well as easy management, ethanol is used in this method as a carbon source in addition to a solvent. The major benefit of this method above other CVD techniques is that the catalyst antecedent as well as the liquid hydrocarbon could be unswervingly acquainted with the reaction region; henceforth, the fabrication of MWCNTs becomes more economical in addition to semi-continuous.

Modern nebulizer spray pyrolysis technique has been utilized for the production of MWCNTs. Nebulizer spray is a primary factor in this technique, where it is obtained through the particular ultrasonic atomization method. MWCNTs have been produced through this technique with objectively homogeneous diameters within range bunches with the utilization of an ultrasonic nebulizer, where ferrocene is used as a catalyst, ethanol is used as a solvent, and a carbon supply is sprayed inside the tubular heating system at 8,000°C set temperature underneath argon movement within 1 L/min range. Ethanol is used as a solvent and carbon supplement because of its muddy characterization, less cost, nontoxic by-product, and ease in handling. Elevated development of MWCNTs on the surface is formed. The benefit of using nebulizer spray is its simple production into industrial-level manufacturing, because reactants are continuously fed into the furnace.

2.15 Methods of Carbon Nanotube-Based Fibers Production

Two distinct routes have been developed for manufacturing neat CNT fibers. One route employs a solid-state process wherein CNTs are directly spun into a fiber from either the synthesis reaction zone or from a CNT forest grown on a solid substrate. This approach does not lend itself to the typical easy scale-up of chemical processes, as it combines multiple steps into a single one, limiting the options for process and material optimization. Indeed, solid-state fibers have low packing and poor orientation and include impurities within their structure. Despite these shortcomings, solid-state CNT fibers have delivered the best properties so far. The reason for this relative success is the length of the CNTs that constitute these fibers—1 mm or more. Longer CNTs reduce the number of CNT ends in a fiber, yielding greater strength and reducing CNT junctions, which increase electrical and thermal conductivity. The alternate fiber production route—wet spinning—was the first method for producing CNT fibers. In this process, premade CNTs are dissolved or dispersed in a fluid, extruded out of a spinneret, and coagulated into a solid fiber by extracting the dispersant. Wet spinning is easily scaled to industrial levels and is indeed the route by which high-performance fibers are manufactured (including ballistic fibers, such as Kevlar and Twaron, and structural fibers, such as Toho Tenax and Thornel carbon fibers). Decoupling the synthesis of CNTs from the spinning of the fibers allows the independent optimization of the two steps and enables CNT purification. An important variation of the original wet spinning method was the use of acid as solvent and standard coagulants like water, thereby simplifying the original method by avoiding surfactants in the CNT dispersion and eliminating polymer from the coagulation bath. So far, wet spinning from acid has yielded the most highly ordered and dense CNT fibers. Yet their properties have been disappointing. Inadequate CNT length (~0.5 mm) has been the presumed culprit, and the literature concurs that wet spinning is inappropriate for handling long CNTs. Here we show that exciting properties can be achieved by wet spinning ~5 mm "short" CNTs into high-performance multifunctional fibers. High-quality CNTs were dissolved in chlorosulfonic acid (the only known CNT solvent) at a concentration of 2 to 6 wt% and filtered to remove particles, in order to form a spinnable liquid crystal dope (Figure 2.11A) [52].

The dope was extruded through a spinneret (65–130 mm diameter) into a coagulant (acetone or water) to remove the acid. The forming filament was collected onto a winding drum (Figure 2.11, b to e). The linear velocity of the drum was higher than the dope speed at the spinneret exit, to ensure high CNT alignment, by continuous stretching and tensioning of the filament. The fibers were further washed in water and dried in an oven at 115°C.

High performance is only one of the two requisites for technology adaptation. Ease of manufacturing is key for cost control through process scale-up [52]. Scalability of solution spinning has been demonstrated by using a multihole spinneret under the same conditions, as for the single-hole spinning—same linear extrusion rate (~10 m/min) per hole and spinneret diameter (Figure 2.11E). The only required change was a simple switch of the spinning plate, with no alteration of any other hardware. The produced 19-filament fibers showed properties comparable to those of the monofilament ones.

The production of continuous fibers made purely of carbon nanotubes has paved the way for new macro-scale applications which utilize the superior properties of individual carbon nanotubes. These wire-like macroscopic assemblies of carbon nanotubes were recognized to have the potential to be used in electrical wiring. Carbon nanotube wiring may be extremely light and mechanically stronger and more efficient in transferring high-frequency signals than any conventional conducting material, being cost-effective simultaneously. However, transfer of the unique properties of individual CNTs to the macro-scale proves to be quite challenging. This feature section gives an overview of the potential of using carbon nanotube fibers as next-generation wiring, state-of-the-art developments in this field, and goals to be achieved before carbon nanotubes may be transformed into competitive products.

Commonly, the production processes of CNT fibers are divided into two basic categories, that is, wet and dry spinning. There are also a few reports of spinning of the fibers using electrical methods, which probably should be treated as a separate category.

The wet methods rely on extrusion of a liquid solution of nanotubes into a bath with a coagulant, which is a liquid that can mix with the solvent but cannot disperse nanotubes. The

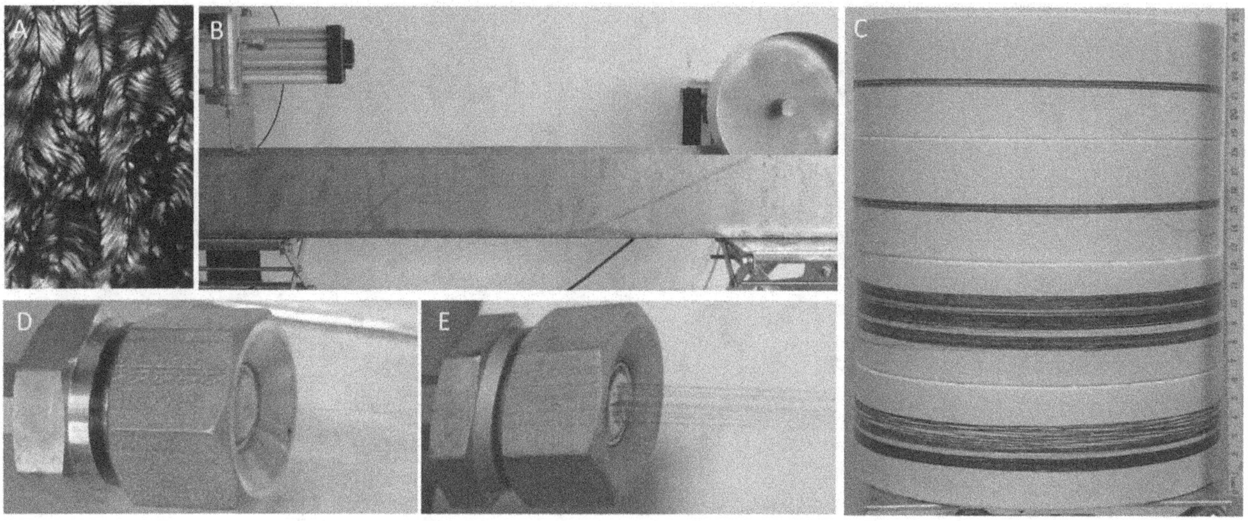

FIGURE 2.11 (a) Light micrograph of a birefringent fiber spinning dope (3 wt% CNT in chlorosulfonic acid). (b) Fiber spinning setup. The fluid is extruded from the spinning chamber (left) through a spinneret immersed in a coagulation bath; the fiber is continuously collected on the winding drum (right). (c) Winding drums with collected fibers (100 to 500 m on each drum). (d and e) Close-up view of a single- and 19-filament spinning.

Source: [52].

CNTs, therefore, get precipitated in the form of long fibers. There are three basic spinning approaches reported, that is, spinning (1) out of liquid crystalline suspensions of SWNTs in superacids or MWNTs in ethylene glycol; (2) out of surfactant-stabilized suspensions, which normally use sodium or lithium dodecyl sulfates as surfactants; and (3) out of dispersions prepared with the aid of biomolecules, for example, DNA or hyaluronic acid. Quite a wide range of substances may be used as coagulants, including water, alcohols, polymeric compounds, acids, and so forth. So as to obtain fibers made purely of CNTs, the post-process annealing has to be applied to remove residual chemicals from the as-made fibers.

The most popular wet spinning process is the method proposed first by Ericson et al., which is the spinning from superacid LC phase. The LC phase is prepared from SWNTs produced via high-pressure decomposition of CO and superacid which protonates the nanotubes and causes their electrostatic repulsion, thus causing the formation of homogenous SWNT solutions. Next, the LC is continuously extruded through a capillary into the coagulation bath and then, depending on the coagulant used, either directly wound on a rotating spindle or washed prior to the collection. Figure 2.12 presents an example of a setup used by Ericson et al. for spinning of the fibers. Similarly to other wet-spun fibers, to obtain pure material, the fibers need to be annealed at very high temperatures; otherwise, they stay severely doped with the superacids used for dispersion.

Dry methods include a one-step process in which the fibers are directly drawn from CVD reactor, and two-step techniques which rely on spinning out of other CNT assemblies: CNT arrays, CNT cotton, and CNT films.

The direct spinning of CNT fibers from a CVD reactor is shown schematically in Figure 2.13. The vertical arrangement of the reactor is shown as an example; however, it may as well be orientated horizontally. In the direct spinning of CNT fibers from a CVD reactor process, the feedstock comprising hydrocarbons, ferrocene, a sulfur compound and hydrogen is introduced into the hot zone of a CVD furnace (temperatures above 1,000°C).

Among the two-step dry methods of CNT fiber production, the most widely applied is that of drawing of the fibers from CNT vertical arrays (forests). In the first step, the forests are prepared using CVD techniques. In order to obtain CNT forests, the catalyst particles are placed on a substrate, which is inserted into a furnace. The hydrocarbons are introduced into the furnace with the flow of carrier gases, such as a mixture of 5 mol% acetylene in helium. The synthesis takes place in the hot zone of the reactor, normally at temperatures above 600°C.

In the second step of fiber spinning, depicted in Figure 2.14, a chosen cluster of CNT is pulled out of the assembly. The following nanotubes get attached at the ends of the previous ones, thus forming a sparse wire-like network of axially aligned CNTs. Most often, the networks are condensed via twisting.

The process taking place during the drawing of the fibers from the arrays is not yet fully understood. However, it is known that not all the arrays are spinnable. Such factors as over-waviness of CNTs, improper length, or the presence of impurities were suggested, which prevent the formation of continuous fibers. The existing theories indicate two potential explanations of the mechanisms of spinning of CNT fibers from CNT arrays. The first one suggests that during drawing, the bigger CNT bundles get joined at the ends by smaller bundles. The small bundles slide along the big bundles during separation. They accumulate at the tips of the big bundles, knotting them together, and thus a continuous chain of nanotubes is formed. The second theory, based on SEM observations of the spinning process, suggests that natural slight entanglement of nanotubes results in the formation of connections between the ends of drawn CNT bundles due to the compression of the entanglements.

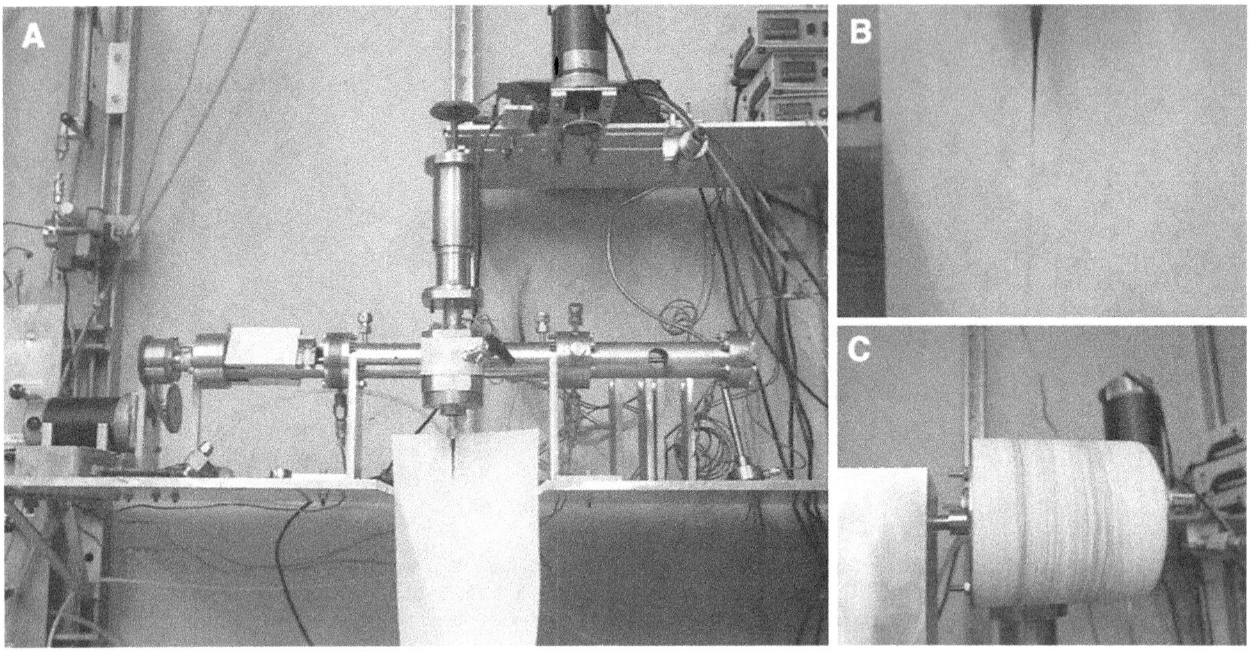

FIGURE 2.12 (a) The system used to spin CNT fibers from liquid crystalline phase. (b) Fiber extruded from capillary tube. (c) CNT fiber wound on a rotating spool.

Source: Reproduced with permission form Ericson et al. Science 2004, 305, 1447. Copyright 2012, American Association for the Advancement of Science.

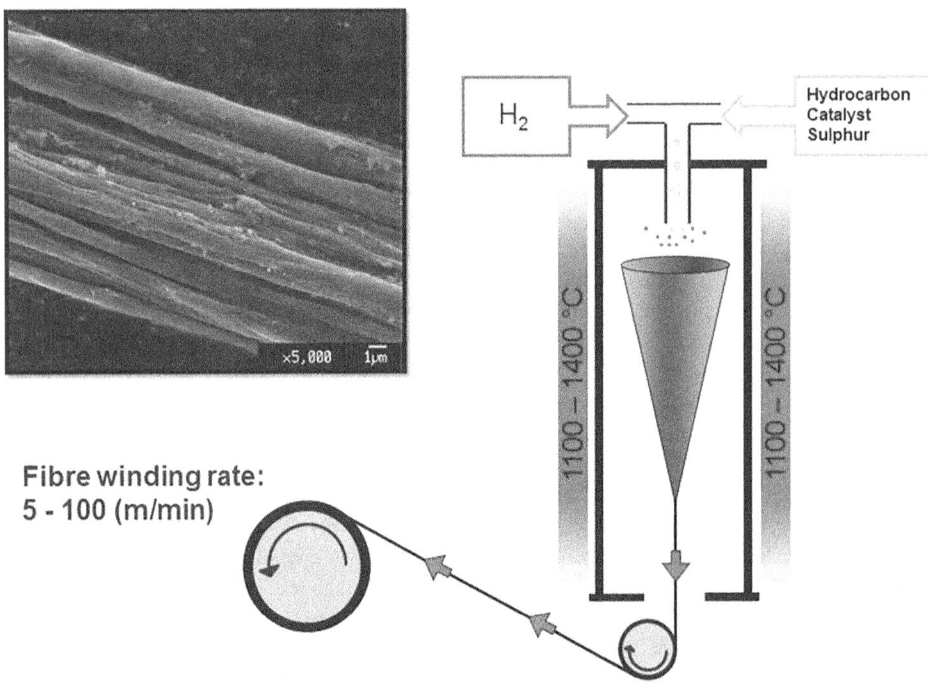

FIGURE 2.13 Top left: scanning electron microscope image of CNT fiber produced directly from CVD reactor presented on the right. Feedstock is introduced at the top of vertical furnace. CNTs are synthesized in the hot zone of the reactor and extracted at the bottom in the form of fiber. The fibers are condensed and wound on a rotating collector.

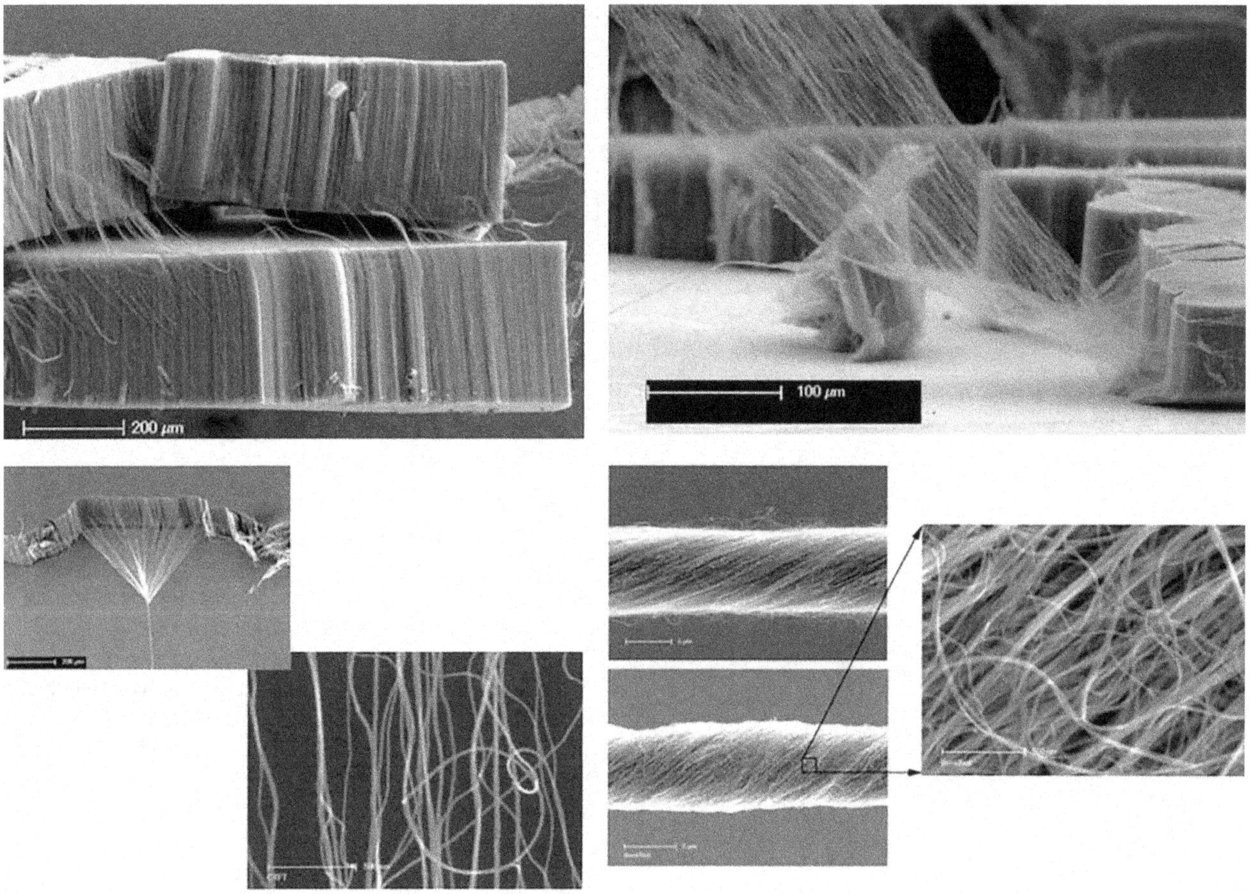

FIGURE 2.14 Top left: An image of spinnable CNT array used by Huynh et al. Top right: Initial part of a spun CNT fiber. Bottom left: Twisting of the fiber. Bottom right: Images of CNT fibers before and after densification with acetone, with an insight into the internal structure of the spun fibers.

Source: Reproduced with permission. Huynh et al. Carbon 2010, 48, 1105. Copyright 2012, Elsevier.

In a similar fashion to the spinning from a vertical array of CNTs, the fibers may be spun from the CNT cotton or film. The cotton is prepared via the CVD method. In this process, catalyst particles are mixed with hydrocarbon, and their solution is introduced into the hot zone of the reactor by a carrier gas. The cotton is grown on substrates analogously to CNT arrays or on the walls of the CVD furnace. Then a cluster of nanotubes is pulled out of the assembly, which drags along further nanotubes.

CNT films for fiber spinning were prepared in a process analogous to the one used for one-step direct spinning of CNT fibers from CVD reactor described earlier. To obtain the CNT films, the partly aligned sparse material extracted directly from the furnace is not condensed but directly wound on a rotating collector. Many layers of material form thick free-standing films of CNTs, which then may be spun like CNT arrays and cottons.

Finally, it was shown that CNT fibers may be spun using electrical methods. Ma et al. demonstrated the spinning out of aqueous solutions of SWNTs. The CNT solution was placed in a vessel, which constituted the first electrode. A second electrode was made of a wire attached to a movable stage, which allowed the withdrawal of the fiber out of the solution. A low voltage (10 V) at high frequency (2 MHz) was applied between the electrodes. To obtain longer fibers, the wire used as the second electrode was replaced by a metal ring with saline solution suspended in it. The fiber was withdrawn through the ring and collected on a rotating rod.

In the process suggested by Imaizumi et al., MWCNTs were dispersed in polyvinyl butyral. A high voltage of 15 kV was applied between the metal nozzle (first electrode) of an infusion pump containing the MWNT/polymer solution and the rotating collector (second electrode). Thus, composite CNT/polymer fibers were spun. Further, the output material was annealed to obtain pure CNT fibers. Figure 2.15 shows the setup used.

Carbon nanotubes have been widely utilized as electrode materials owing to their extraordinary physical and chemical properties, and assemblies of CNTs in fiber format have been shown to be a viable platform to take these properties from the nanoworld to macroscopic scale. As the electrode materials, the conductivity and strength of CNT fibers should be satisfied with the requirement of a supercapacitor. The formation of carbon nanotube-based fiber can be divided into wet-spun method and solid-state spun method.

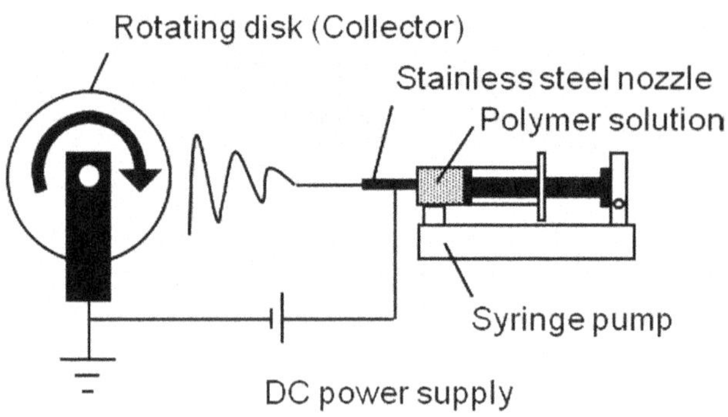

FIGURE 2.15 Schematic drawing of a system used for spinning CNT fibers via electrical method used. The fibers dispersed in polymer are extruded from a nozzle with the aid of DC voltage applied between the nozzle and a rotating winder on which the fibers are collected.

2.15.1 Wet-Spun CNT Fibers

Wet spinning is one of the conventional fiber fabricating methods and can enlarge the yield of fibers. A 60 wt% carbon nanotube (prepared by arc discharged method) that contained fiber was firstly developed by Vigolo and coworkers, in which the fiber was prepared by extruding the surfactant-stabilized single-walled carbon nanotube (SWNT) solution into a polyvinyl alcohol (PVA) coagulation bath. In previous researches, dispersing CNTs with polymers or surfactant could form a stable spinning solution; the composite fibers were prepared by following extrusion into coagulation bath and extension. With the existence of polymers, large-molecule surfactant, the electrical and thermal conductivity of the fiber was extremely poor, although the mechanical properties were reasonable, owing to the enhancement of CNTs. Using this technology, the existing polymer can only be completely removed by thermal annealing that causes pyrolysis of the polymer, which will degrade the mechanical properties of the fibers by decreasing strength and modulus and making them rather brittle. Polymer-free carbon nanotube fibers can alternatively be achieved by utilizing a small-molecule coagulation bath system, pH-adjusting flocculation-based process, and superacid-based wet-spun fabrication. The spinning parameters can also draw an important role in the preparation, including the diameter and shape of the needle or the spinneret, extruding speed, and rotating speed in rotate spinning method, which will affect the morphologies and performances of the obtained fibers.

2.15.2 Solid-State Spun CNT Fibers

CNT fibers prepared by solid-state spinning can be expanded with the following methods: directly spinning from a CVD-grown CNT aerogel, spinning from vertically grown CNT arrays, twisting/rolling from "cotton" like CNT bundles or a CNT film. The carbon nanotubes can be self-assembled into fiber due to the van der Waals interactions, by which CNTs hold together to form aligned bundles.

Floating CVD was initially utilized to grow CNTs, then developed a method to draw a fiber from the CNT aerogel formed in a vertical furnace with a purity of 85–95 wt% of MWNTs inside, as well as a good electrical conductivity of 8.3×10^5 S/m. This direct spinning method can be used to obtain a variety of products, including nanotube fibers, ribbons, and coatings. On this basis, Li and coworkers improved the process and successfully achieved a few kilometers of CNT fiber; meanwhile, the strength reached more than 1 GPa.

The key to directly spinning from carbon nanotube arrays is to prepare arrays that are uniform and enough material for continuous spinning. Firstly, draw an ultralong CNT fiber from a spinnable CNT array with extraordinary electrical property. Twisted CNT sheets have been proved to enhance the strength of fibers; the height of the grown CNT arrays can also influence the mechanical performance of the fiber. It is mainly due to the defects, which are the density of the end points on the grown ultralong carbon nanotubes, which are relatively low, so that the contact area of the adjacent carbon nanotubes is large, to prevent slipping of the bundles. Zhang et al. (2007) reported a strong, stiff, and lightweight CNT fiber which was spun from an ultrahigh (1 mm) individual CNT forest. In addition, the density, diameter, number of walls, and content of amorphous carbon of the carbon nanotubes in the array will affect the forming process of fibers and ultimately determine the properties of the CNT fibers.

By using the ancient spinning approach, a CNT "cotton" was twisted into a fiber, as the CNT assemblies were readily transferred to fiber format. The film-like CNTs similarly can be rolled or twisted into a fiber, which has been demonstrated. As followed by Feng et al. (2010), they developed another method by rolling a synthesized double-layered carbon nanotube (DWNT) film into a fiber, which had a superior electrical conductivity of 8.0×10^4 S/m.

Generally, the length, diameter, defects, and post-treatment of the prepared carbon nanotubes predominately affect the dispersion of CNT in aqueous or super-acid system to form continuous and uniform CNT fibers in the followed procedure. Besides, the strength, stiffness, and flexibility of the formed CNT fibers are also determined by these characteristics of the prepared CNTs by utilizing the wet spinning method. Due to the specific fabrication approach of solid-spun CNT fibers, carbon nanotubes that are grown by CVD have been demonstrated as the major method to obtain the desired fibers. The fibers fabricated by wet spinning technology exhibit a higher electrical conductivity and lower mechanical properties compared to those of solid-state spun fiber, which can be illustrated in reference [53].

2.16 Nanostructured Energy Materials in Fibers

Although the stability and high power density of double-layered capacitance materials like carbon nanotube are demonstrated and well-known, the limitation of the energy density has drawn a wide attention to improve. Combing high-electrochemical-capacitance materials, such as graphene, active carbon, metal oxide, transition sulfide, and conducting polymer, with prepared carbon nanotube–based fibers can extremely enhance the specific capacitance of original fibers and maintain the cyclical properties meanwhile. In this part, we will mainly discuss the nanostructured energy materials used in fiber-based supercapacitors from the perspective of compositing approaches. The different methods used for fiber electrode fabrication have been summarized in [53].

2.16.1 Co-Spinning

With the features of self-stacking and self-assembling during the spinning process of carbon nanotube–based fibers, which has been demonstrated to affect the electron exchange between ions and materials in the electrolyte, nanostructured energy materials can simultaneously incorporate with these carbonaceous materials by bonding or simply sticking. It is found that combining carbon nanotubes with two-dimensional sheet-like materials can prevent effective surface area reduction and capacitance loss caused by stacking of materials.

Peng and coworkers prepared a CNT/graphene hybrid fiber by dip-coating the GO dispersions on the as-grown MWNT arrays and then spinning to form a fiber through the approach described earlier, as shown in Figure 2.16a.

Due to the strong interaction of the π–π bond between the graphene oxide sheet and the carbon nanotube, the transfer efficiency of electrons in the composite fiber is greatly improved, and the graphene oxide sheet can reduce the stacking of the carbon nanotubes and increase the paths of ions. The tensile strength of the chemical-reduced hybrid fiber was reached at ~500 MPa, compared to that of bare CNT fiber (~630 MPa); meanwhile, the electrical conductivity of the hybrid fiber can be achieved as high as 450 ± 20 S/cm. The calculated specific capacitance of the hybrid fiber could be reached at ~31.5 F/g, compared with ~5.83 F/g of the bare CNT fiber. Depending on a similar principle, a novel type of conductive carbon nanotube–graphene composite fiber was explored by electro-spinning a chemical-reduced graphene within and cover the surface of MWNT fibers during the drawing procedure (Figure 2.16B). The electrical conductivity of the prepared hybrid fiber could be reached at 900 ± 50 S/cm, while the tensile strength, modulus, and elongation at break of the fiber were about 140 MPa, 2.58 GPa, and 6%, respectively. The specific capacitance was dramatically improved to 111 F/g at a scan rate of 2 mV/s.

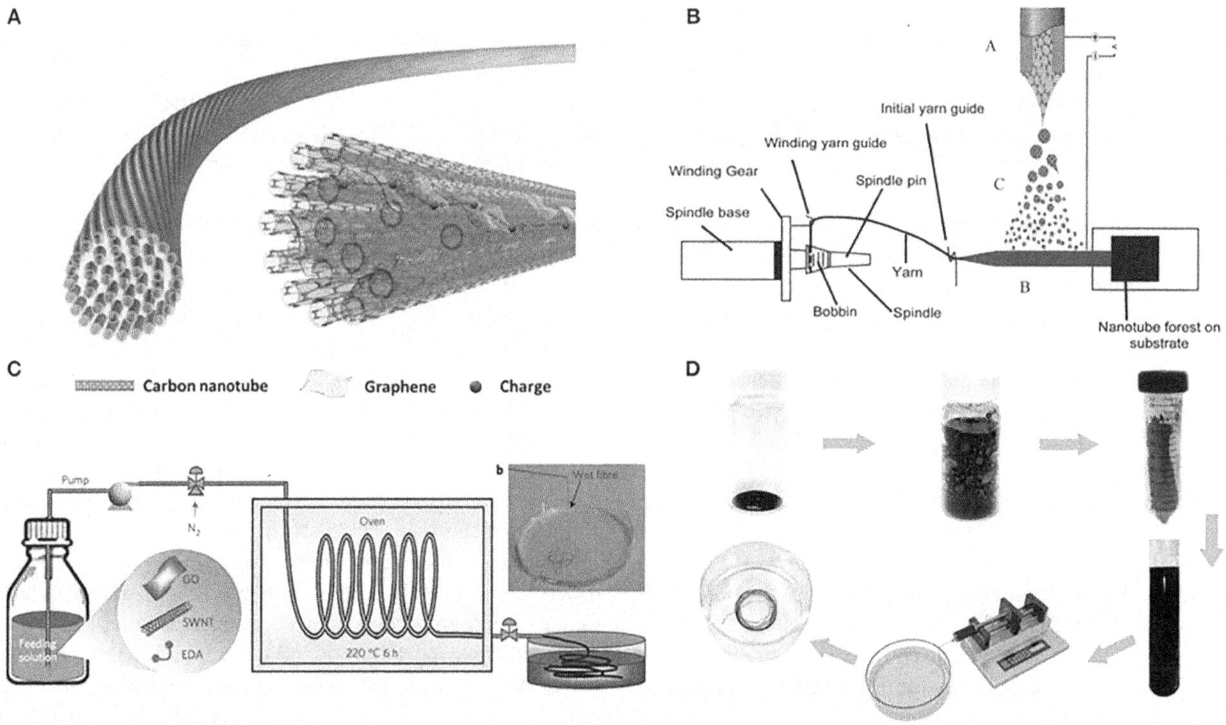

FIGURE 2.16 Schematic illustration of (a) a solid-spun carbon nanotube fiber with internal graphene sheets; (b) co-spinning of CNT/graphene hybrid fiber with solid-spun and electrospinning methods; (c) hydrothermal procedures of rGO/SWNT composite fiber; (d) super-acid exfoliated graphene sheets co-spun with carbon nanotubes.

Source: [54].

A wet-spinning process was proposed by Ma and coworkers to fabricate a CNT-rGO fiber. The pure few-walled carbon nanotubes (FWNTs) with 3–5 walls were first dispersed in water with the assistance of ultrasonication, then mixed with a GO solution that was synthesized from expanded graphite. The mixture was extruded into a chitosan/acetic acid coagulation bath to form a fiber, followed with washing and drying. The interaction of FWNT and rGO sheets can dramatically increase the stress strength from 193.3 to 385.7 MPa, and electrical conductivity from 53.3 to 210.7 S/cm, compared to pristine rGO fiber, by using a similar method, while the fiber-based supercapacitor illustrated a specific capacitance of 38.8 F/cm^3.

As a good surfactant to disperse nitric acid–treated SWNTs, GO dispersion can homogenously be mixed with SWNTs as an aqueous suspension for composite fiber spinning. Such suspension has been proposed to be fed into a homemade silica column and heated in an oven with optimal parameters (Figure 2.16c). The composite SWNT/rGO fiber was self-assembled by hydrothermal method and successively pushed into water by gas flow and further dried in air. The fiber enjoyed a tensile strength of 88 MPa, and the electrical conductivity was ~100 S/cm compared to that of SWNT fiber and rGO fiber, which are 50–150 MPa and ~12.5 S/cm, respectively. The assembled hybrid fiber supercapacitor expressed an ultrahigh volumetric specific capacitance of ~45.0 F/cm^3.

Recently, we used the violent exothermic reaction of chlorosulfonic acid and hydrogen peroxide to exfoliate graphite powder to form graphene with a small number of layers and mixed the prepared graphene and carbon nanotubes with chlorosulfonic acid as a spinning solution. The graphene/carbon nanotube composite fiber was prepared by wet-spun technology with a three-dimensional structure, as shown in Figure 2.16d. It can be shown that electron channels were formed when the two-dimensional graphene sheets were stacked and upheld by the carbon nanotube bundles, leading to a good electrical and ionic conductivity. The specific surface area of the fiber cross section was greatly increased, and the specific capacitance of the composite fiber was thus increased by about 38% compared with the carbon nanotube fibers prepared by us previously [54].

With the assistance of nanoparticles or nanosheets, the co-spun CNT-based fiber can also increase the integral electrochemical performances compared with the bare CNT fiber. A suspension of ordered microporous carbon (OMC) has been creatively painted on ten layers of aligned CNT sheets drawn from a spinnable CNT array, and the combined sheets were rolled into a hybrid fiber as one electrode. The electrochemical performances of the OMC/CNT hybrid fiber were investigated in a three-electrode system, which indicated a rectangular-shaped CV curve even at a scan rate of 200 mV/s. The prepared negative electrode enjoyed a specific volumetric capacitance up to 121.4 F/cm^3 (or 116.3 F/g) at 0.43 A/cm^3, which was controlled by the content of OMC particles in the hybrid fiber (~76 wt%).

Choi and coworkers also developed a novel method that biscrolled CNT sheets with drop-casting of MnO_2 dispersion into a fiber (shown in Figure 2.17; [55]). The strategy of biscrolling can dramatically expand the loading mass of active nanoparticles as high as 99 wt% without any influences on the mechanical properties of fiber. The biscrolled MnO_2/CNT fiber was able to achieve an areal specific capacitance of 889 mF/cm^2 (or 155 F/cm^3) and possessed an energy density of 35.8 μWh/cm^2 (or 5.41 mWh/cm^3).

Sun et al. (2015) [56] pre-coated the MoS_2 nanosheets, which are dispersed in DMF, on the carbon nanotube arrays during the spinning process. The prepared composite fibers had significantly improved the volumetric specific capacitance. Li et al. also illustrated a cathode active material (V_2O_5)–enhanced CNT fiber by wet-spinning method, which showed a maximum energy density of 1.95 mWh/cm^3 at a power density of 7.5 mWR/cm^3, although the PVA-based coagulation bath relatively influenced the conductivity of the fiber. Recently, Chen's group prepared an MnO_2/CNT fiber by mixing the nanosheet structured MnO_2 with SWNT dispersion to form a spinning solution for wet spinning. The fabricated fibers had a content of active substance with more than 75% [57].

The co-spinning method can be appropriate for solid-state spinning and wet spinning of CNT fibers by mixing or casting active materials dispersed solution with intrinsic spinnable suspension or arrays. CNT fibers have the feasibility to be incorporated with the nanostructured materials during the wet spinning, hydrothermal reactions (with graphene), and assembling process. Consequently, such an approach can be considered to apply various functional materials into the CNT-based fibers (Figures 2.17d,e).

2.16.2 Dip-Coating

As we know, the obtained CNT-based fibers have a potential to embrace nanostructured energy materials. Dip-coating, as one of the most utilized methods to compose different substances, has been frequently reported and is relatively more effective than co-spinning. PEDOT, as a conducting polymer with good film-forming properties, high concentration in aqueous solution, and high stability and conductivity, has attracted a lot of interest recently. The salt-doped PEDOT has been proved to be directly spun into a conductive fiber and well film-forming. Commercial PSS-doped PEDOT solution has been used as a doping medium, in which SO_3H groups improved the electroactivity of principal conducting polymers in a neutral electrolyte due to the "doping effect" of PSS, and a gamma-irradiated CNT fiber as a current collector to produce a fiber-based supercapacitor. The easy preparation of fiber electrode could be scaled up, and the existing PEDOT and CNT illustrated a rectangular shape of CV curves, as well as remarkable fast charge–discharge properties during electrochemical measurement. The gravimetric specific capacitance of the supercapacitor was achieved at 18.5 F/g, which was almost twice compared to that of bare irradiated CNT fiber supercapacitor (9.2 F/g).

To enhance the adhesion of the applied electrochemical active materials on the fibers, polymer-assisted dispersions are good medium to be further utilized for dipping and coating. Meanwhile, the format of asymmetric fiber supercapacitor can extend the operating potential window and result in much higher energy and power densities of the whole device. A mass of MnO_2 nanoparticles in PVA solution has been dispersed by vigorous stirring to form a uniform MnO_2-PVA

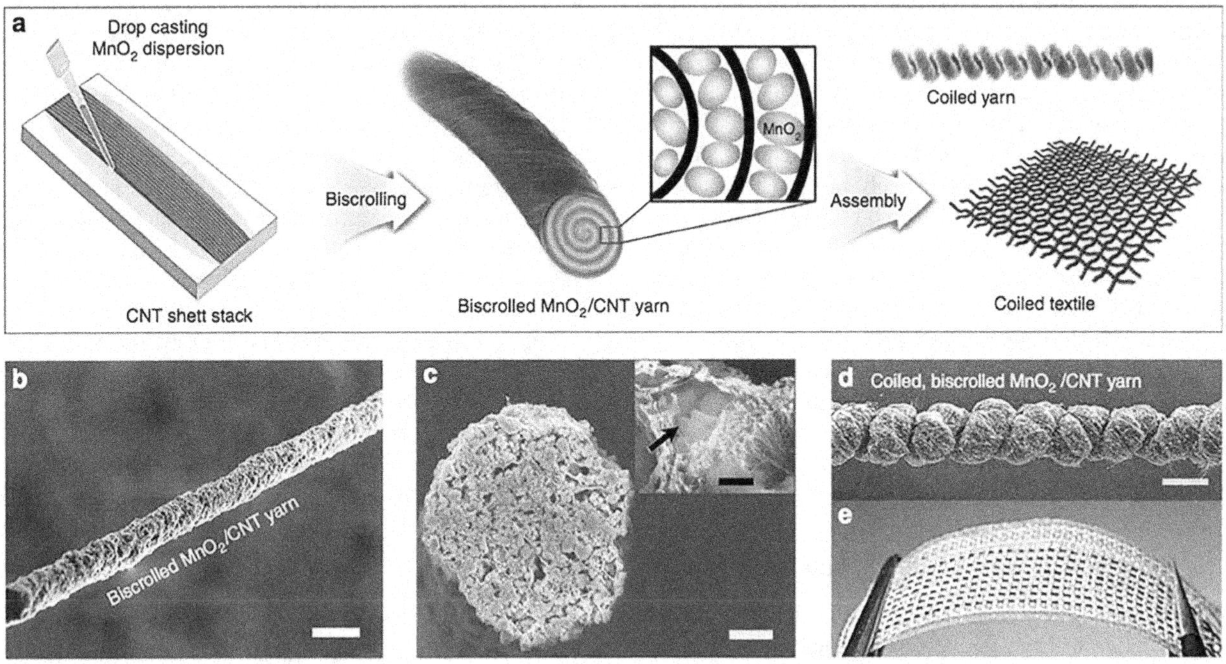

FIGURE 2.17 Schematic showing the (a) preparation and structure of biscrolled CNT/MnO_2 hybrid fiber, SEM morphologies of (b, c) as-spun biscrolled hybrid fiber, and (d, e) two-ply coiled yarn integrated in a fabric.

Source: [55].

paste. The as-spun CNT fibers were then dip-coated with the prepared paste by a self-designed setup, and the obtained CNT/MnO_2/PVA fiber electrode was twisted with a bare CNT fiber by overall casting of a gel electrolyte to form an asymmetric supercapacitor. This type of supercapacitor expressed a wide operating potential window of 2.0 V, and the highest energy and power densities reached were 42.0 Wh/kg and 19,250 W/kg, respectively. With a similar method, they synthesized a PANI nanowire solution before fiber spinning; the obtained irradiated CNT fiber was orderly covered with PANI-PVA and PVA gel electrolyte. The composited fiber revealed a gram-specific capacitance of 78 F/g (or 43 mF/cm^2), which was almost twice compared to that of a bare CNT/PANI fiber-based supercapacitor.

The dip-coating method can not only fill the interspaces in carbon nanotube–based fibers but also enhance the mechanical properties of the original fibers by specifically selecting film-forming solutions. Many active materials are insoluble or reactive in aqueous dispersions by using co-spinning; dip-coating can alternatively be chosen to incorporate such materials with a suitable solvent.

2.16.3 In Situ Compositing

In situ composition is derived from the concepts of in situ crystallization and in situ polymerization. The second phase in the material of the composite is formed during the formation of the material or synthesized on a substrate. The in situ formation may be a phase of metal, ceramic, or polymer, which may be presented in the matrix in the form of microstructures, such as particles, whiskers, crystal plates, or microfibers. For fiber-based electrodes, in situ synthesis and electrochemical deposition have been generally utilized to enhance electrochemical performances.

2.16.3.1 In Situ Synthesis

As-spun all-carbon fibers can be regarded as a scaffold to deposit pseudocapacitive materials, such as metal oxide (i.e., MnO_2, $Ni(OH)_2$, Fe_2O_3, V_2O_5), polypyrrole, and polyaniline, in room temperature or using the hydrothermal procedure [58,59]. The porous CNT- or graphene-based fibers are hydrophilic, which facilitates the diffusion of deposition ions throughout the fibers. Based on the CNT fiber prepared with CNT aerogel, the fiber has been immersed in ethanol, which was added with a $KMnO_4$ aqueous solution. The fiber could reduce aqueous permanganate to obtain MnO_2 by the following reaction:

$$4MnO_4^- + 3C + H_2O \rightarrow 4MnO_2 + 3CO_3^- + 2HCO_3^- \quad (1)$$

The obtained CNT/MnO_2 fibers were designed and applied in a stretchable asymmetric configuration, extending the potential window from 0.8 to 1.5 V with a high linear specific capacitance of ~157.53 μF/cm at 50 mV/s. The calculated energy density was reached from 17.26 to 46.59 nWh/cm when the power density varied from 7.63 to 61.55 μW/cm.

Yao's group has dramatically increased the capacitance of the as-spun CNT fiber electrode by inducing the cathode materials–based active materials in recent years. The dandelion-like molybdenum-nickel-cobalt ternary oxide (MNCO) nanowire arrays were grown on the surface of the as-prepared solid-spun carbon nanotube fiber as the positive electrode and a vanadium nitride (VN)@C coated CNT fiber as negative electrode to form a fiber-shaped asymmetric supercapacitor. The growth of the crystal was controlled by the hydrothermal method and largely increased the surface area of the fiber electrode, which obviously enhanced the specific capacitance of the supercapacitor. They then improved the volumetric capacitance of the supercapacitor by alternating the positive electrode to the three-dimensionally aligned zinc-nickel-cobalt oxide (ZNCO)@$Ni(OH)_2$ nanowire arrays–coated CNT fiber; the capacitance increased from 62.3 to 94.7 F/cm^3. Recently, a $CoNiO_2$@$Ni(OH)_2$-grown CNT fiber electrode was demonstrated by them, and assembled with a TiN@VN-coated CNT fiber, the supercapacitor showed a higher capacitance of 109.4 F/cm^3 [60].

2.16.3.2 Electrochemical Deposition

Electrochemical deposition refers to a technique in which electrons are transferred through anions and cations in an electrolyte solution under an external electric field, and a redox reaction of specific ions occurs on the electrode to form a plating layer. Electrochemical deposition is widely used and can form nanostructure crystals or conductive polymers to greatly improve the capacitive properties of fiber electrodes. Peng's group firstly applied the electrochemically deposited MnO_2 nanoparticles on an MWNT fiber spun from an aligned MWNT forest. They used $Mn(CH_3COO)_2$- and Na_2SO_4-mixed solution as sources for growing MnO_2 particles at a potential range, from 0.2 to 0.8 V. The as-prepared composite fibers showed a mass specific capacitance of 13.31 F/g (or 3.01 mF/cm^2 or 0.015 mF/cm) when they were in a twisted supercapacitor configuration, and the fibers could further be utilized as a linear Li-ion battery. Then the solid-stated spun CNT fiber has been utilized as a substrate to composite with MnO_2 nanoparticles, in which the fiber was immersed in a $MnSO_4$ and Na_2SO_4 contained solution. By using a three-electrode system and applying constant voltage of 1.3 V, the flower-like MnO_2 nanoflakes were uniformly deposited outside and inside the porous CNT fiber (Figure 2.18a). The consequent specific capacitance of the all-solid-state fiber-based supercapacitor was 25.4 F/cm^3, and the average energy density was 3.52 mWh/cm^3 when the average power density was 127 mW/cm^3. Based on this principle, we also pioneered a high-performance flexible fiber supercapacitor by using the super-acid spun CNT fiber (shown in Figure 2.18b). The as-spun fiber was highly conductive, with many micropores, and MnO_2 nanoflakes were deposited by electrodeposition. The characterized specific capacitance of the assembled supercapacitor was over 152 F/g (or 156 F/cm^3), which was about 500% higher than that of Choi's device at the same scan rate. The measured energy density was 14.1 Wh/kg at a power density of 202 W/kg.

The as-spun fiber was first dipped into the electrolyte-containing H_2SO_4 and aniline monomer, and the well-infiltrated fiber was then applied with a potential of 0.75 V. To form an all-solid-state fiber supercapacitor, the gel electrolyte

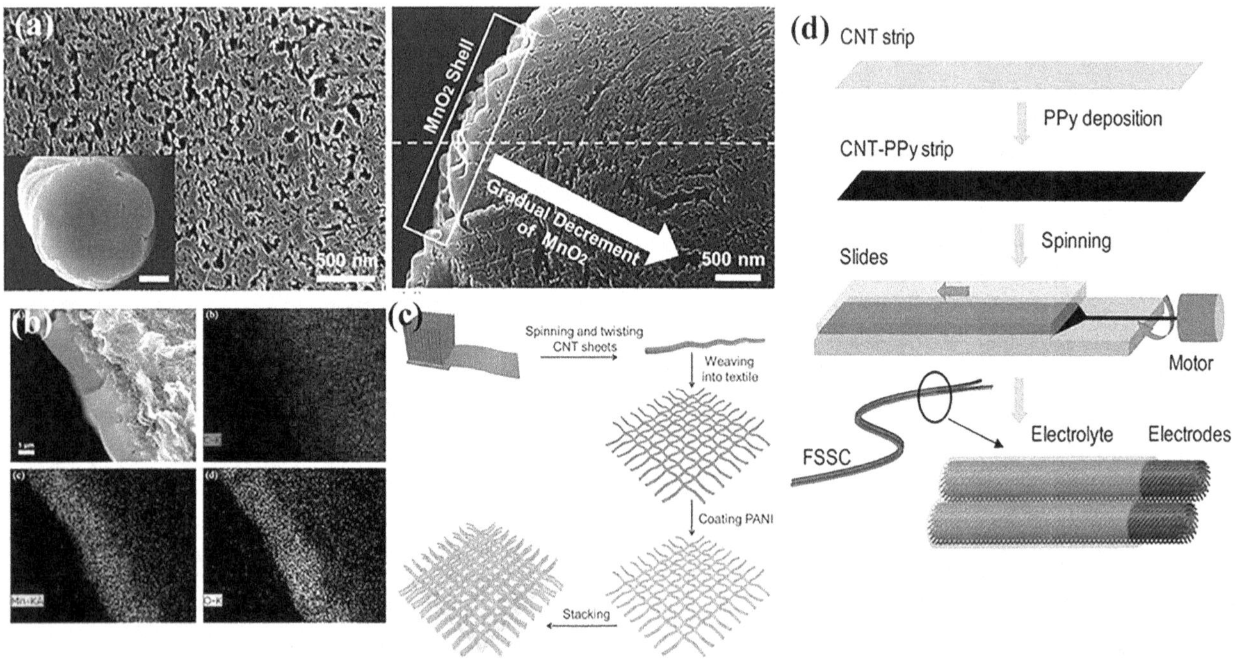

FIGURE 2.18 Cross-section morphologies of (a) the solid-spun CNT fiber with electrodeposited MnO_2 nanoparticles, (b) EDS of each element of the deposited MnO_2 in wet-spun CNT fiber, (c) schematic fabrication procedures of electrodeposited PANI/CNT textile supercapacitor [61], and (d) solid-spun CNT fiber from pre-deposited PPy carbon nanotube film.

Source: Xu et al., RSC Adv. (2015), 5, 22015–22021, doi: 10.1039/C5RA01917F.

was coated on the overall fiber as the separator. The assembled supercapacitor was fabricated by twisting two composite fibers with a corresponding gravimetric specific capacitance of 274 F/g (or 263 mF/cm). Furthermore, in their following improvement, two pieces of CNT/PANI composite fiber–based textiles were attached together with gel electrolyte to form a thin, lightweight, transparent, and flexible supercapacitor (Figure 2.18c; [61]). The as-prepared supercapacitor displayed a high specific capacitance of 272.2 F/g, which could be further integrated in a garment to store the energy that was converted from solar energy. Lu et al. (2018) [54] reported a super-elastic wire-like supercapacitor by springing the polyaniline electrodeposited carbon nanotube/graphene hybrid fiber covered with SEBS rubber. The obtained coil-like supercapacitor presented a superior stretchability of 800%, with a specific capacitance of about 138 F/g at a current density of 1 A/g, which could be further allied in the stretchable textiles to afford the shape deformation of body gesture.

Besides the conducting polyaniline, polypyrrole (PPy) has also been drawn with a superior pseudocapacitive performance. A thin layer of PPy has been electrodeposited on an aligned CNT film by placing the film between two pieces of stainless steel mesh as the working electrode. The deposited films were then coiled into fibers in wet state by two motors with opposite direction (shown in Figure 2.18d). High specific capacitance (350 F/g) and extreme stability were then exhibited by the as-prepared fiber electrode in cyclic testing even under bending and twisting.

It can be seen from [53] that the method of electrochemical deposition facilitates the composition between double-layer capacitive carbon nanotube–based fibers with high capacitive active materials. In some occasion, such an approach can extend to the stretchable fibers which are prepared by wrapping the CNT film on a stretched substrate. The stretchable composite fibers, like CNT/MnO_2, CNT/PANI, CNT/PPy, and CNT/PEDOT fibers, possessed reasonable electrochemical performances even under a large elongation, showing the potential to be applied in large deformation devices.

2.17 Processing and Applications of Novel Functionalized Carbon Nanotubes (CNTs)

Chemical vapor deposition (CVD) is the dominant mode of high-volume CNT production and typically uses fluidized bed reactors that enable uniform gas diffusion and heat transfer to metal catalyst nanoparticles. Scale-up, use of low-cost feedstock, yield increases, and reduction of energy consumption and waste production have substantially decreased MWNT prices. However, large-scale CVD methods yield contaminants that can influence CNT properties and often require costly thermal annealing and/or chemical treatment for their removal. These steps can introduce defects in CNT sidewalls and shorten CNT length. Currently, bulk purified MWNTs are sold for less than \$100 per kilogram, which is one- to tenfold greater than commercially available carbon fibers.

The understanding of CVD process conditions has enabled preferential synthesis of metallic or semiconducting SWNTs with selectivity of 90 to 95%, doping of CNTs with boron or nitrogen, and flow-directed growth of isolated SWNTs up to 18.5 cm long. However, improved knowledge is urgently needed on how CNT chirality, diameter, length, and purity relate to catalyst composition and process conditions. In situ observation of CNT nucleation and molecular modeling of the CNT–catalyst interface will be critical to advance chirality selective synthesis.

Moreover, because SWNT synthesis by CVD requires much tighter process control than MWNT synthesis, and because of legacy costs of research and process development, bulk SWNT prices are still orders of magnitude higher than for MWNTs. Use of MWNTs is therefore favored for applications where CNT diameter or bandgap is not critical, but most emerging applications that require chirality-specific SWNTs need further price reduction for commercial viability.

The synthesis of SWCNTs, graphene, and other nanostructures is a concept intrinsically tied to their processing and applications. In some cases, processing or applications can be directly enabled by synthesis, such as in the case of fiber spinning from solid CNT arrays, where synthesis-controlled properties of the material dictate the feasibility of dry spinning methods. In other cases, processing or applications are passively dependent on synthesis since the parameters controlled in synthesis studies can be related to their performance or processing requirements but do not dictate the feasibility of making a device or application.

In the remainder of this section, we discuss selected important applications that capitalize on the properties of SWCNTs and also highlight ways in which synthesis science can enable advances in the processing or application platform. The synthesis challenges for each application are shown schematically in radar/spider plots in Figure 2.19 with respect to the current status and future needs. While there are numerous parameters that can impact a particular application, for the sake of general discussion, we have chosen length, diameter, alignment, helicity, and density. Moreover, comparison between various applications necessitates vagueness in the units, for example, low and high density. Similar analogies could be made for processing and applications of 2D-layered materials.

2.18 Synthesis of Fullerenes

The recent synthesis of fullerenes and carbon nanotubes and the separation of graphene have generated enormous interest in these carbon materials. Carbon allotropes of this type offer not only a highly exciting and vast area for scientific exploration but also the potential for a wide spectrum of novel engineering applications due to their properties.

Fullerene can be produced by a laser beam on graphite in the helium atmosphere. However, the total yield is insufficient, considering the potential application areas and industrial areas. Therefore, various methods are developed for the synthesis of an effective and efficient fullerene. The second method proposed in the synthesis of fullerene is the laser ablation of graphite. This method permits the production of macroscopic amounts of fullerene from graphite under high-temperature conditions. In this method, materials are removed from the solid surface using a laser beam. When the

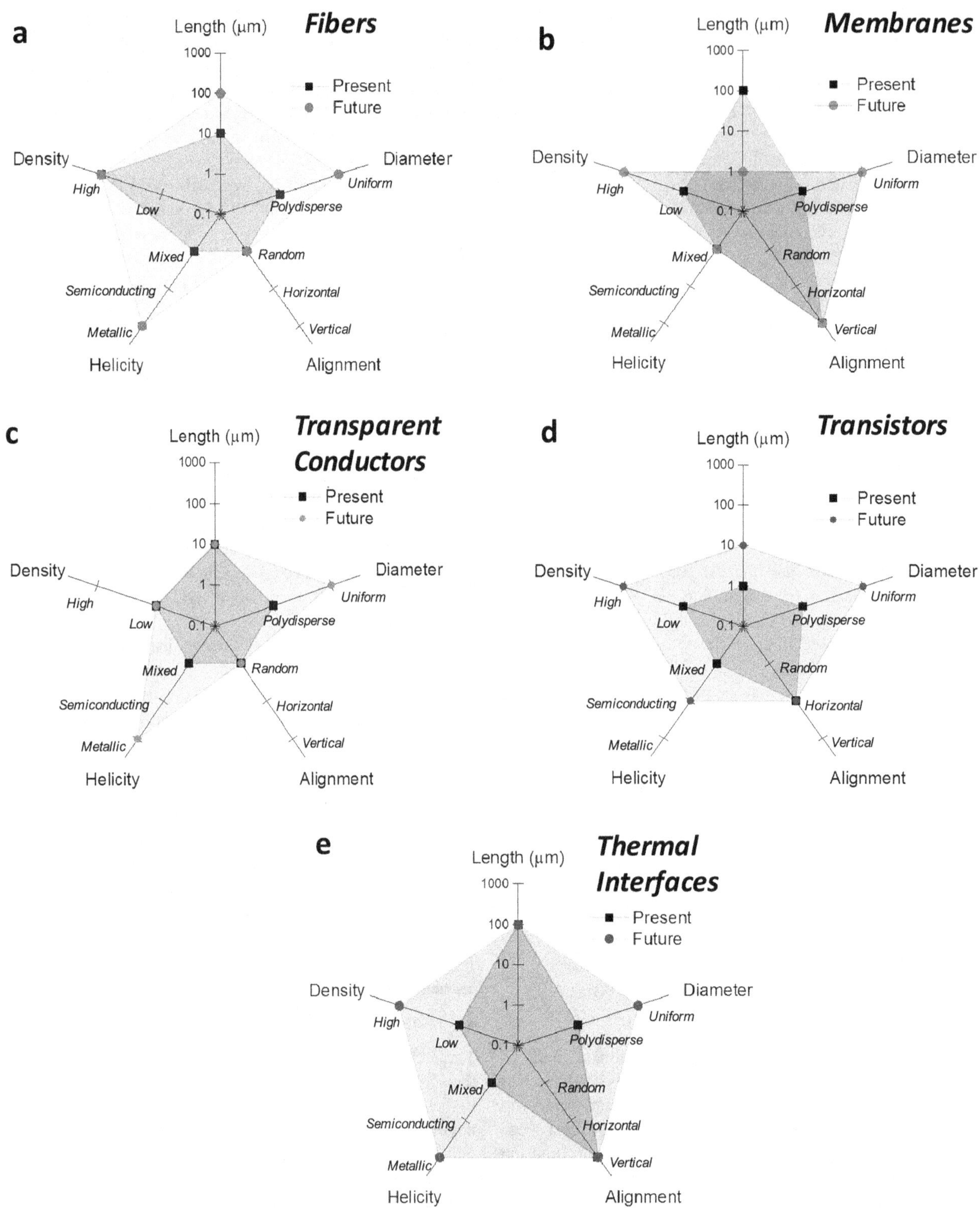

FIGURE 2.19 Radar charts showing the present state of SWCNT synthesis with respect to physical properties, and future requirements for the properties for various applications.

graphite is exposed to the laser beam, the materials removed from the solid surface evaporate and become plasma. By cooling the gas, the vaporized and combined atoms form the fullerene. Another alternative method proposed in the synthesis of fullerene is the arc discharge process. The arc discharge of graphite is one of the most common techniques used in the production of novel fullerenes. In this method, the graphite evaporates with the electric arc formed between the two electrodes. However, the temperature conditions of the carbon arc prevent an existing device from detecting the types that occur during the production. On the other hand, there are also non-equilibrium plasma methods where fullerene is produced without high temperature [62].

2.19 Methods of Graphene Preparation

The rapid adoption of graphene as a material of interest lies in its actual availability by a range of techniques and methods. In 2004, Geim and coworkers first reported graphene sheets prepared by mechanical exfoliation (repeated peeling) of highly oriented pyrolytic graphite. This method, which is called the "scotch-tape" method, is still widely used in many laboratories to obtain pristine, perfect structured graphene layer(s) for basic scientific research and for making proof-of-concept devices. However, this method is not suitable for the large-scale production of graphene necessary to fulfill the requirements in different areas. A large amount of recent effort has been devoted to develop methods to synthesize graphene at large scale for practical electronic applications. These methods include mechanical exfoliation and cleavage of natural graphite, chemical vapor deposition on metals, electric arc discharge, epitaxial growth on electrically insulating surfaces, unzipping of carbon nanotubes, solution-based chemical approaches (chemical or thermal reduction of graphite oxide), and thermal decomposition of SiC wafer under ultrahigh vacuum conditions.

2.19.1 Structure and Properties of Graphene

Graphene is a carbon nanomaterial made of two-dimensional layers of a single-atom-thick planar sheet of sp^2-bonded carbon atoms packed tightly in a honeycomb lattice crystal. Graphene's structure is similar to lots of benzene rings jointed, where hydrogen atoms are replaced by carbon atoms (Figure 2.20a) and considered hydrophobic because of the absence of oxygen groups [63]. Furthermore, it is a carbon allotrope in the structure of a plane of sp^2-bonded atoms with a molecule bond length of 0.142 nm. Layers of graphene are piled together to form graphite, with an inter-planar spacing of 0.335 nm.

This stacking makes a three-dimensional structure of graphite (Figure 2.20b), while graphene is a two-dimensional, one-atom-thick material. Graphene has a hybridized sp^2 bonding. It displays a single π orbital and three σ bonds perpendicular to the plane (Figure 2.20c). The strong in-plane σ bonds act as the hexagonal rigid backbone structure, while the out-of-plane π bonds control the interaction between different graphene layers. In any case, the changes in the structure of graphene are mainly due to the absence of one or more sp^2 carbon atoms or the presence of one or more different atoms with sp^3 hybridization. Over the previous decades, single sp^2-bonded carbon atom allotropes from 0 to 3 dimensionalities, such as nanotube, fullerene, graphene, and graphite, have been integrated into diverse polymer matrices due to their exceptional thermal, mechanical, and electrical properties and light weight [64].

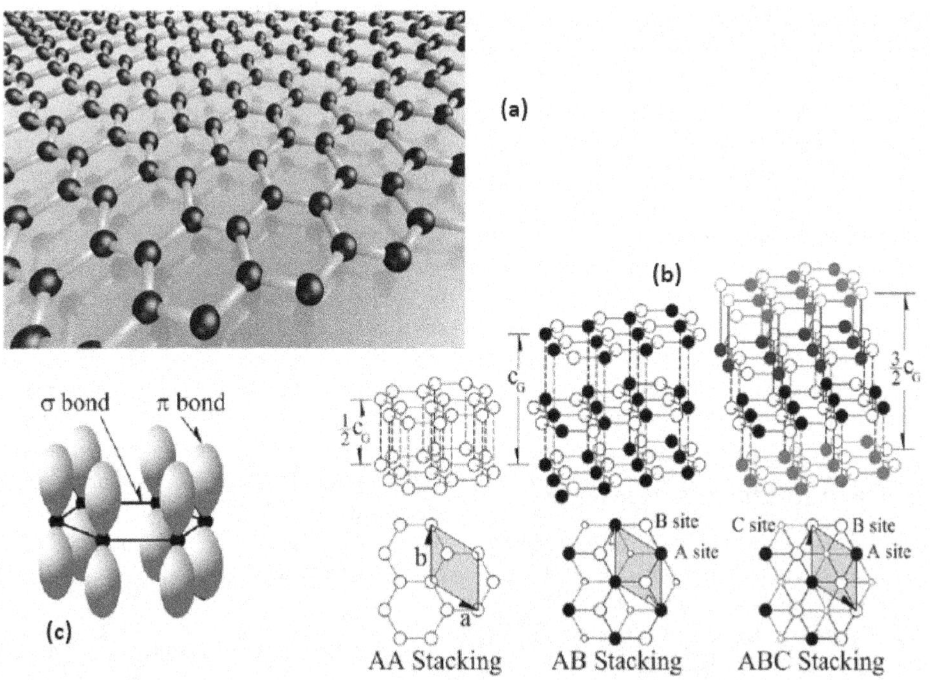

FIGURE 2.20 (a) Schematic presentation of graphene's hexagonal lattice structure [64], (b) three most typical graphite structures and stacking arrangements of graphene, and (c) schematic of the out-plane π orbitals and in-plane σ bonds perpendicular to the plane of the graphene sheets.

With the carbon atoms bonded covalently within the plane, forming σ bonds with three neighboring carbon atoms and one out-of-plane π bond, this network of sp^2 carbon atoms gives graphene its unique properties [65]. Graphene's tensile strength is around 125 GPa, and its elastic modulus is 1.1 TPa; this makes the strength of graphene be 100 times more than that of steel. The thermal conductivity of graphene is around 5×10^3 W/mK, henceforth 10 times higher than that of copper (401 W/mK). Graphene's electron mobility has a conductivity of 106 S/m and resistance of 31 Ω/sq, which account for an ultrahigh mobility of 2 × 105 cm^2/V.s, that is, 140 times more than that of silicon. The reason for this ultrahigh mobility is sp^2 hybridization, which donates an extra electron to the π bond; these pi electrons are delocalized at room temperature, yielding high conductivity.

Besides, graphene is naturally a semimetal, and its benzene ring–like electronic structure comprises six π orbitals with three occupied bonding and three unoccupied antibonding orbitals, separated by a bandgap. Fusing of these benzene rings leads to a little overlap between the valence and conduction bands; thus, the electrons from the top valence band can flow to the bottom conduction band without stimulating any heat [66]. Aggregation of the layers of graphene determines the specific surface area. The modification of pristine graphene with other compounds decreases the aggregation and increases the effective surface area. In recent years, graphene has fascinated much attention of researchers, owing to its extraordinary electronic, optical, magnetic, thermal, and mechanical properties as well as large surface area.

2.19.2 Growth Mechanism of Graphene

Recently, there have been several methods used to synthesize graphene. This synthesis process is known as extracting graphene, depending on the purity and the desired product. After the 2004 discovery of graphene, different techniques have been developed to produce layers and thin films of graphene. As shown in Figure 2.21, chemical vapor deposition (CVD), chemical exfoliation, chemical synthesis, and mechanical cleaving are some of the commonly used methods of graphene synthesis.

Top-down and bottom-up synthesis methods are determined by the number of layers, thickness, nature, and average size of graphene materials. In top-down growth mechanism process, graphene sheets are produced by exfoliation/separation of graphite and its derivatives, including graphite oxide (GO). [67] summarizes both top-down and bottom-up synthesis methods as well as their advantages and disadvantages.

2.19.3 Micromechanical Exfoliation/Cleavage

Mechanical exfoliation is also known as scotch tape or peel-off method. It was the first method to be used by Novoselov and Geim for the production of graphene with the help of an adhesive tape to force the graphene layers apart. In this method, multiple layers of graphene remain on the tape after peeling off, but with recurrent peeling, it splits open into a handful of graphene flakes. For detachment, the tape is attached to a certain substrate (acetone), and a final peeling by using a fresh tape is carried out to obtain flakes different in both size and thickness, which can be observed under a light microscope on SiO_2/Si substrates. This process is slow and imprecise; hence, the material produced is most often used to study the properties of graphene rather than actually using it commercially. This method can also be performed by using different agents, such as electric field, epoxy resin, and by transfer-printing technique.

2.19.4 Electrochemical Exfoliation

Graphite exfoliation by electrochemical techniques has become a simple yet high-yielding method in recent times for the mass production of graphene. This method involves the use of various forms of graphite, such as graphite foils, plates, rods, and graphite powders, as electrodes in an aqueous or non-aqueous electrolyte and electric current to bring about the expansion of electrodes. The electrodes could be of two types based on the power applied, that is, cathodic (negative) and anodic (positive) electrodes [68]. Graphite rods have been accommodated in an electrochemical cell which was filled with the electrolyte. A persistent current of 5 V was applied. Few minutes of electrolysis resulted in the accumulation of a black material at the anode. The exfoliation process was carried on for 4 h to isolate the product from the cell. It was then centrifuged at 1,000 rpm, and then the product was gradually poured out. The dispersion obtained was found to be extremely stable. Powdered dry graphene was achieved by washing the dispersion with deionized water and alcohol, followed by vacuum drying. Then the yield was calculated by weighing the dry powder and sediment.

2.19.5 Pyrolysis

The word *pyrolysis* originated from the Greek-derived element *pyro* and *lysis*. *Pyro* means "fire," and *lysis* stands for "separating." Synthesized carbon atom on a metal surface is a simple procedure used to fabricate few-layer graphene. One of the common techniques of graphene synthesis is the thermal decomposition of silicon carbide (SiC). At high temperature, Si is desorbed, leaving behind C atom, which forms few graphene layers, as shown in Hibino et al. (2010). This technique has received a significant improvement through the continuous production of graphene films in millimeter scale at a temperature of 750°C on a thin film of nickel coated with an SiC substrate. The advantage of this method is the continuous production of graphene films over the entire SiC-coated surface. However, this method cannot be used in the synthesis of graphene in large scale. A similar approach is applied in the thermal decomposition of ethylene at 1,000 K. The advantage of this synthesis method is the production of high-purity graphene monolayer.

2.19.6 Chemical Vapor Deposition (CVD)

Up to date, CVD is the synthesis technique of high-quality graphene on a large-scale basis. However, to explore the full

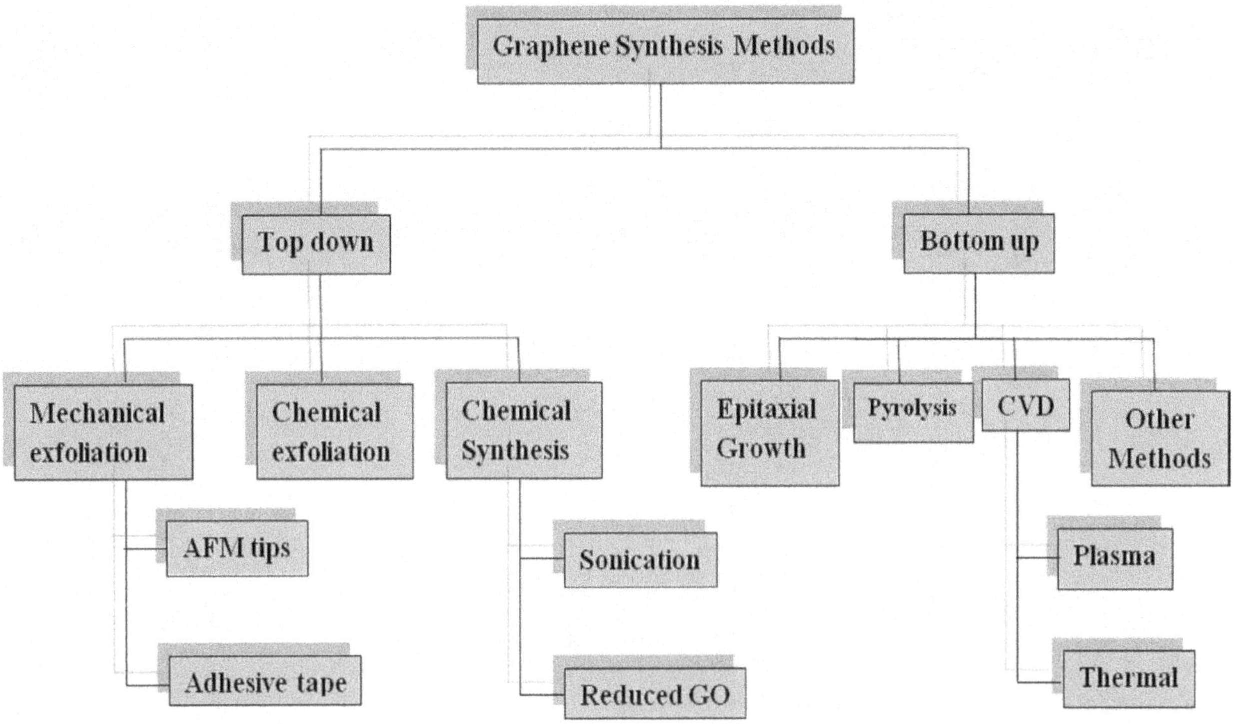

FIGURE 2.21 Schematic representation of different methods of graphene synthesis.

Source: [64]. Copyright 2017 Elsevier Ltd.

potential of graphene economically, some critical points, such as toxicity, long-term stability, and environmental effects, need to be addressed. Chemical vapor deposition (CVD) is a bottom-up synthesis technique used for the production of high-quality graphene on a large-scale basis. This method involves combining a gas molecule with a surface substrate inside a reaction chamber under temperature, pressure, and gas flow rate conditions. A typical CVD instrument includes a quartz reaction chamber, a mass flow controller, a pump, thermocouples for temperature measurement, a gas delivery system, a vacuum system, an energy system, and a computer for auto-control (Figure 2.22) [69,70]. Different substrates are used in CVD for graphene film growth; they include nickel (Ni), copper (Cu), iron (Fe), and stainless steel. Methane (CH_4) and acetylene (C_2H_2) are normally used as a carbon source. Two CVD processes are used to activate the carbon source, including thermal CVD and plasma-enhanced CVD (PECVD).

Thermal CVD consists of a vacuum tube, high-temperature heating furnace, vacuum pump, vacuum gauge to control pressure, and a mass flow controller to regulate carbon and carrier gas used in the synthesis of graphene. In PECVD, plasma leads to the decomposition of the gas source and then reacts with the metal substrate, resulting in the growth of graphene films. Power sources such as direct current (DC), microwave, and radio frequency (RF) have been used as a plasma source. The advantage of PECVD over thermal CVD is that the graphene growth mechanism can occur under low pressure and temperatures. The carbon source decomposes at high temperature into hydrogen and carbon atoms.

$$(i)CH_{4(g)} ----greater\ than\ 2H_{2(g)} + C_{(S)}$$
$$(ii)C_2H_{2(g)} --> H_{2(g)} + 2C_{(s)}$$

In this CVD method, hydrogen and argon gases are used as carrier gases to remove and clean unwanted oxides on the metal catalyst surface.

Transition metal substrates such as Cu and Ni have typically been utilized for the CVD growth of graphene [71]. This growth process follows two main steps: (1) formation of carbon by pyrolysis of the gas precursor and (2) formation of the carbon structure of graphene using the segregated carbon on the surface of the metal catalyst [72]. For instance, the production of graphene by using polycrystalline Ni is achieved by first annealing Ni in an H_2 atmosphere at the desired temperature of 900–1,000°C with grain size. The substrate is exposed to H_2/CH_4 gas mixture; here, CH_4 is used as the source of carbon. The decomposition of hydrocarbon makes the carbon atom dissolve in the Ni film, where the solid solution is formed. Ni has high solubility at high temperature, and the solid solution of Ni is cooled down in argon gas to form Ni–C precipitate, which etches graphene (Figure 2.23) [73]. Although Ni is a good substrate for the production of graphene, the quality of Ni film can affect the percentage and size of the monolayer graphene. The cooling rate affects the thickness and quality

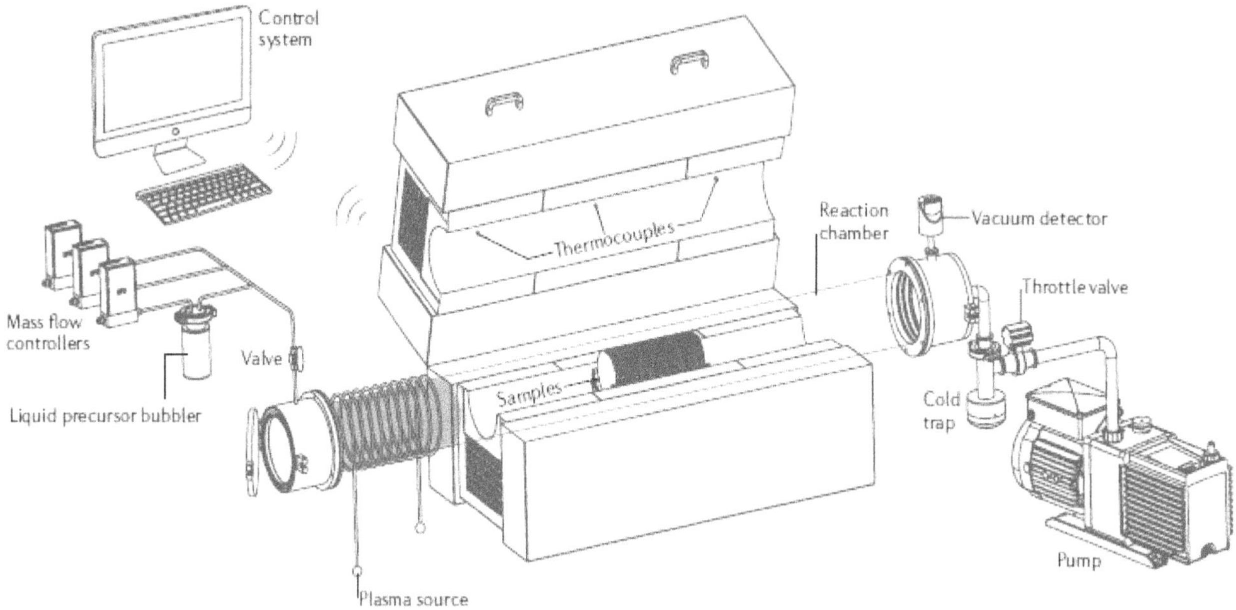

FIGURE 2.22 Schematic diagram of typical CVD equipment.

Source: Excerpted from refs. [69,70]. Copyright 2021 Nature Reviews.

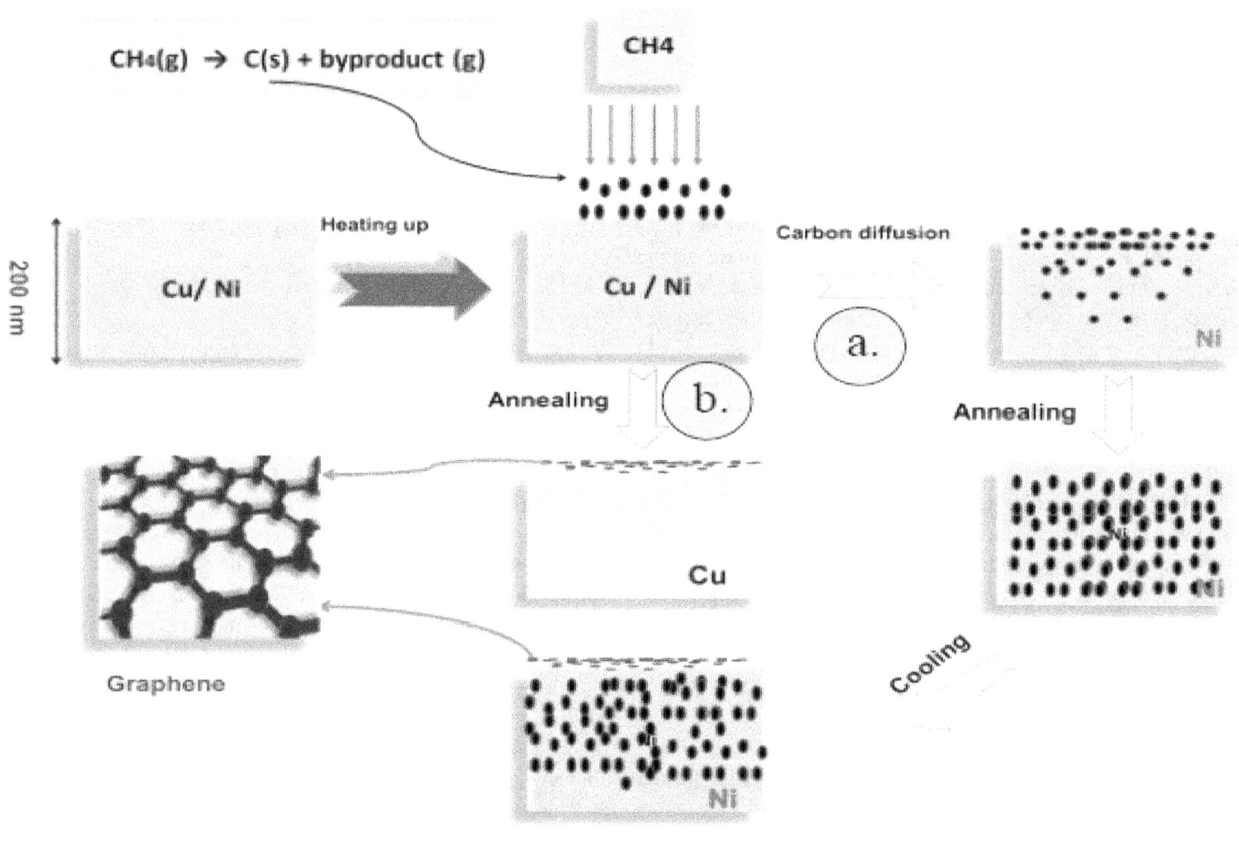

FIGURE 2.23 A schematic diagram showing the growth mechanism for CVD graphene growth on Ni substrate: (a) graphene growth by dissolution–precipitation mechanism and (b) graphene growth direct by deposition mechanism.

Source: [73].

of graphene, and the microstructure of Ni can also affect the formation of graphene morphology.

Chemical vapor deposition (CVD) is a simple, scalable, and cost-efficient method to prepare single- and few-layer graphene on various substrates. It opens a new route to large-area production of high-quality graphene films for practical applications. In general, CVD techniques involve the decomposition of fluid (gas and liquid sprays) at high temperature to form either thin films on substrates or powders through filters. There are many forms of CVD, like hot-wire CVD, thermal CVD, plasma-enhanced CVD, radio frequency CVD, and ultrasonic spray pyrolysis. Evaporated Ni film on SiO_2/Si wafers or copper foils are ideal substrates for graphene synthesis. Synthesis of graphene on Ni supported on Si/SiO_2 wafers facilitated the breakthrough approach for large-scale graphene. This is attributed to the excellent geometrical fit of the ordered graphene/graphite phase of carbon to the crystalline metal surface that is provided by Ni films. Another reason is the convenient interactions that favor bond formation between carbon atoms at specific conditions. Carbon atoms dissolve into the Ni crystalline surface, and they arrange epitaxially on the Ni (111) surface to form graphene at certain temperatures (Figure 2.24). CVD synthesis of graphene can be carried out at ambient pressure or vacuum by systematically varying parameters such as gas composition and flow rate, temperature, and deposition time. The carbon precursor in CVD is methane. By using diluted methane, single- and few-layer graphene (less than five layers) are grown, while using concentrated methane results in multilayer growth. Other carbon precursors can be used in CVD, such as ethanol, isopropanol, ethylene, acetylene, and others.

2.19.7 Unzipping of CNTs into Monolayer Graphene

The method of unzipping single-walled carbon nanotubes to form monolayer graphene has been reported recently, accomplished by harsh acids and the right thermodynamic conditions (Figure 2.25) [74]. Recently, Dai and coworkers have taken a unique approach to fabricating graphene nanoribbons (GNRs) with well-controlled dimensions. Based on the concept that

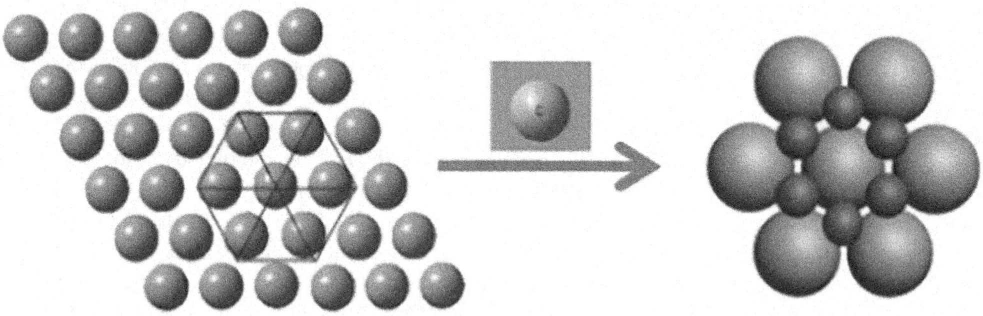

FIGURE 2.24 Schematic representation of the atomic arrangement of the hexagonal lattice of the (111) face of nickel (blue spheres) and how carbon atoms (gray spheres) would arrange on the Ni (111) surface to form graphene.

Source: Arco L et al, Croatia: InTech; 2011. pp. 161–184. DOI:10.5772/1742.ch10.

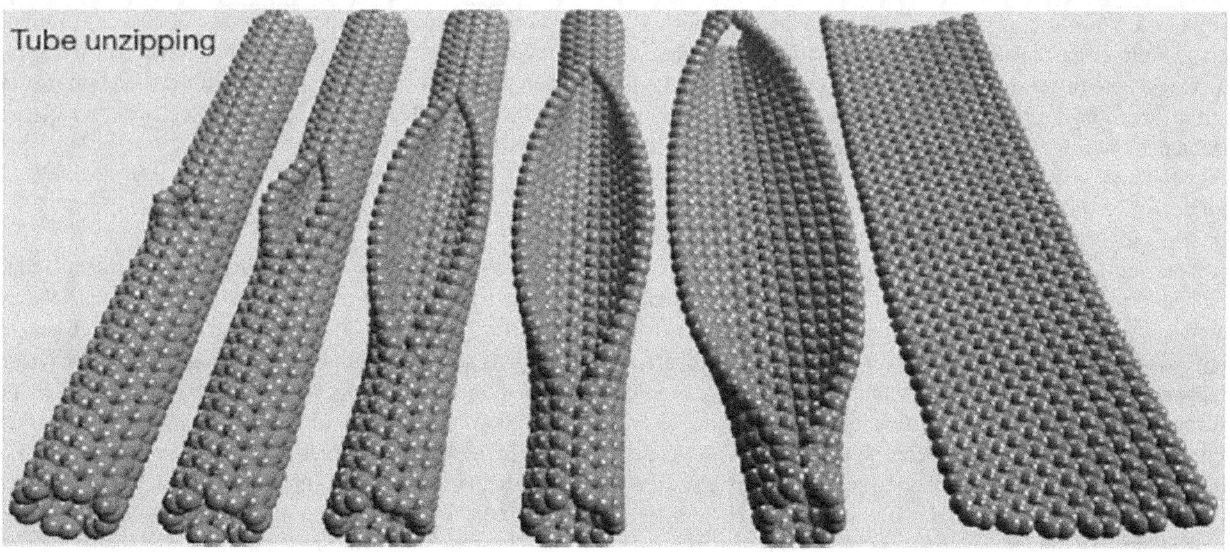

FIGURE 2.25 Modelling illustration of the SWCNT unzipped into monolayer graphene.

Source: [74].

CNTs are considered to be GNRs rolled up into seamless tubes and the fact that the size of CNTs has been well controlled, Dai's group developed a method to produce GNRs through controlled unzipping of CNTs using the Ar plasma etching method. Shimizu and coworkers produced GNRs through the oxidization and longitudinal unzipping of MWCNTs in concentrated sulfuric acid, followed by treatment with $KMnO_4$. Another approach involved the preparation of longitudinal unzipped MWCNTs by controlled oxidation and intercalation through reaction with concentrated H_2SO_4 and HNO_3 at room temperature in order to control the reaction rate. The unzipped MWCNTs are thermally treated up to 1,000°C and 2,500°C in an inert atmosphere to exfoliate and reduce the edge defects. The sonication process is responsible for chemo-mechanical breaking and the separation of multi-layer nanoribbons. Furthermore, graphene nanoribbons were synthesized by the oxidative unzipping of SWCNTs using a mixture of concentrated HNO_3/H_2SO_4 in a 1:3 volume ratio, followed by 8 h of ultrasonic treatment performed at 50 W at 45°C. In addition, catalytic unzipping of single-, double-, and multi-walled carbon nanotubes (SWCNTs, DWCNTs, and MWCNTs) in the presence of Pd nanoparticles and an oxygen-containing liquid medium yielding few-layer graphene sheets was performed under microwave irradiation.

2.19.8 Arc Discharge

Arc discharge is a versatile and low-cost method for producing various kinds of carbon nanomaterials. Compared to other methods, the graphene sheets synthesized by arc discharge method have merits of good dispersibility in organic solvent, few defects, and high thermal stability. In the arc discharge technique, graphite rods (purity: 99.99%) are used as electrodes for high-voltage arcing. At extremely high voltages between the electrodes that are separated by very small distances, very high electric fields can be produced, leading to instantaneous sparks, like in a welding process. The fall-out during the discharge process is the end product that contains the carbon nanostructures. To prepare pure few-layered graphene, a direct current arc discharge of graphite evaporation was carried out in a water-cooled stainless steel chamber filled with different buffer gases after evacuating the chamber by a mechanical pump. When the arc discharge process ended, the generated soot was collected under ambient conditions. The soot deposited on the inner and top walls of the reaction chamber was only collected in order to exclude relatively heavy products (amorphous carbon nanoparticles or multi-layered graphene sheets) dropped to the bottom of the chamber during the arc discharge process. Different discharge atmospheres may induce different chemical bonds that cause the prepared graphene sheets to have different properties. Direct current hydrogen arc discharge evaporation of pure graphite electrodes in various gas mixtures can be used to mass-produce high-crystalline few-layer graphene sheets. Various gas mixtures were reported, such as H_2, He, mixture of H_2 and He, mixture of NH_3 and He, and mixture of CO_2 and He, to synthesize few-layered graphene sheets with high electrical conductivity. On the other hand, a novel method for the large-scale production of graphene flakes in an arc discharge enhanced with a specially shaped magnetic field and a custom-designed catalyst was reported.

2.19.9 Reduction of Graphene Oxide into Graphene

Graphene oxide (GO) was synthesized by the strong oxidation of flake graphite using acid via Hummers' method [75] or modified Hummers' method [76]. GO, an oxidized form of graphene, is decorated by hydroxyl and epoxy functional groups on the hexagonal network of carbon atoms with carbonyl and carboxyl groups at the edges. GO is highly hydrophilic and forms stable aqueous colloids due to the large number of oxygen-containing functional groups as well as the repulsive electrostatic interactions at the edges of the platelets. It was reported that GO can be reduced via thermal, chemical, electrochemical, and laser-scribing methods.

2.19.9.1 Thermal Reduction

The thermal method is believed to be a green method, in which no hazardous reductants are used. This process requires heating up to 1,050°C in an oven under argon gas, up to 800°C under hydrogen gas, or up to 700°C in a quartz tube. The thermal reduction of GO was accompanied by the elimination of epoxy and carboxyl groups in the forms of O_2, CO, CO_2, and H_2O, as predicted from thermogravimetry data. Recently, graphene sheets were prepared by a solvothermal reduction of GO suspension in water, octadecylamine, butanol, or N,N-dimethylacetamide. Wei Huang synthesized high-performance graphene nanosheets by thermal reduction of GO under ethanol atmosphere at 900°C. This method can effectively remove the oxygen-containing functional groups and restore its graphic structure compared to the ones obtained using hydrazine or hydrogen. It can provide a simple, low-cost, and high-yield approach for the preparation of high-performance graphene nanosheets. Furthermore, graphene sheets with different reduction levels were produced through thermal reduction of GO in the temperature range of 200–900°C under N_2 atmosphere for supercapacitor applications. Thermal reduction can produce few layer graphene with less agglomeration, higher specific surface area, and higher electrical conductivity compared to other reduction routes.

2.19.9.2 Chemical Reduction

GO formation was followed by subsequent chemical reduction with a reducing agent such as hydroquinone, sodium borohydride, hydrazine, and hydrazine with NH_3. Hydrazine hydrate was proven to be the best reducing agent for the chemical reduction of GO into graphene, and very thin graphene-like sheets were obtained. Moreover, the hydrazine treatment resulted in the formation of unsaturated and conjugated carbon atoms, which in turn imparts electrical conductivity of the graphene sheets. These reducing agents, particularly hydrazine, are highly toxic and explosive, and their use should be with extreme care and minimized. Chemical reduction may also leave some residual epoxide groups on the reduced GO sheets, leading to some loss in electron mobility. On the basis of these observations, a new approach was employed to develop a "green" synthesis method for the production of graphene, by using environmentally friendly reducing agents, such as vitamin C, reducing sugars, and L-glutathione, under mild conditions.

On the other hand, the chemical reduction methods of exfoliated GO with reducing agents such as hydrazine hydrate provide a promising approach to the efficient large-scale production of chemically converted graphene (CCG) sheets. However, in most cases, heating to nearly 100°C over several hours is required. A novel, facile, convenient, and scalable method for the synthesis of CCG sheets as well as metallic and bimetallic nanoparticles supported on the CCG sheets using a simple household microwave oven was utilized. It was reported that graphene is a good microwave-absorbing material and can reach a high temperature in minutes. Microwave irradiation (MWI) has been demonstrated for the synthesis of a variety of nanomaterials with controlled size and shape without the need for high temperature or high pressure. The main advantages of MWI over other conventional heating methods are (1) rapid reaction velocity, (2) clean and energy efficiency, and (3) uniform heating of the reaction mixture. Due to the difference in the solvent and reactant dielectric constants, selective dielectric heating can provide significant enhancement in the transfer of energy directly to the reactants, causing an instantaneous internal temperature rise. Dried GO was sonicated in deionized water until homogenous dispersion was obtained. After that, it was placed inside a conventional microwave after adding 100 μl of a reducing agent (hydrazine hydrate, ethylenediamine, or ammonium hydroxide) in 30 s cycles for a total reaction time of 60 s. A black color was obtained, indicating the complete chemical reduction to graphene. The graphene sheets were separated by using a centrifuge operated at 5,000 rpm for 15 min and dried overnight under vacuum. Microwave-assisted methods allowed the rapid chemical reduction of GO using a variety of reducing agents in either aqueous or organic media. By using this method, many types of metallic and bimetallic nanoparticles can be dispersed on the graphene sheets via simultaneous reduction of GO and a variety of metal salts to create novel nanocatalysts supported on the large surface area of the thermally stable 2D graphene. Moreover, this method provides a low-cost approach to the facile production of nanoparticles/graphene composites on a large scale for applications.

2.19.9.3 Electrochemical Reduction

As pointed out by Kaner and coworkers, both chemical and thermal reduction techniques have some obvious drawbacks, namely, the highly toxic reductant hydrazine, lack of control of the film thickness, and the incompatibility of the thermal reduction process under some conditions. Thus, the electrochemical method was adopted as an effective and controllable alternative technique for the modification of electronic states. It has drawn great attention due to its fast and green nature. This is done by adjusting the external power source to change the Fermi energy level of the electrode surface that reduces GO in the presence of direct current bias. Typically, the electrochemical synthesis of graphene is carried out via two steps, namely, GO being first assembled on the electrodes by solution deposition methods, then being subjected to electrochemical reduction by scanning the potential (cyclic voltammetry) or by applying constant potential (bulk electrolysis). Another approach was achieved via a one-step technique in which graphene films can be prepared on electrodes directly from GO dispersions by simultaneous electrodeposition and electroreduction. The reduction of GO can be confirmed from the color of GO electrodes that changes from yellow (before reduction) to black (after reduction), involving the reduction of the high number of functional groups present in the GO sheets, such as OH, COOH, and epoxides.

The properties of electrochemically converted graphene (ECG) are quite different from those of other nanostructured carbons (CNTs), and even different from CCG. The morphology of CCG and ECG on glassy carbon sheet was characterized by high field emission scanning electron microscopy (FE-SEM), respectively. The micrographs show that CCG sheets are rippled and crumpled with a dimension of several nanometers to a few micrometers, while ECG sheets are more homogeneous and more compact on the surface than CCG. ECG exhibits greatly enhanced activity for the electrocatalytic reduction of O_2 and H_2O_2, and much higher electrochemical capacitance for potential application in ultracapacitors. Moreover, the ECG coating is very stable as a result of its poor insolubility in common solvents.

2.19.9.4 Laser-Scribing Technology

Compared to chemical and thermal methods, pulsed laser irradiation reduction is simple, rapid (shorten the reaction time from several hours to a few minutes), energy-efficient, and free from poisonous material and high temperature. Also, the pulsed laser reduction of GO in the solution makes it particularly attractive for producing graphene composites by premixing with other materials. Moreover, Feng-Shou Xiao fabricated graphene microcircuits by direct reduction and patterning of GO films using femtosecond laser representing well conductivity for electrical applications. Recently, Kaner and coworkers prepared graphene using standard laser-scribing technology more typically used to etch labels and images onto DVDs. Initially, a thin film of GO dispersed in water was drop-cast onto a flexible substrate (a DVD covered with a layer of plastic). Irradiation of the film with an infrared laser inside an inexpensive commercially available light scribe CD/DVD optical drive reduces the GO to laser-scribed graphene (LSG), as indicated by the change in film color from golden brown to black. Analysis of cross sections of the film with scanning electron microscopy showed that the initially stacked GO sheets were converted into well-exfoliated LSG sheets without any sticking together through laser irradiation.

2.20 Synthesis and Tuning Strategies of GQDs

The synthetic strategies of GQDs can be generally classified into two types, top-down and bottom-up methods [77]. A brief summary of the typical synthetic strategies of GQDs is listed in [78]. The top-down methods cut carbonaceous materials by using physical, chemical, or electrochemical processes, which were widely employed to prepare GQDs due to the simple operation. The precursors of this method could be various materials, such as graphene oxide (GO), multi-walled carbon nanotubes (MWCNTs), glucose, graphite, and so on. However, this method suffers from low yield, accidental damage of graphene structure, and less-uniform GQD morphologies. Bottom-up methods, though chemically more difficult, provide opportunities for producing GQDs with smaller and more uniform morphologies. Solution chemistry routes using precursor pyrolysis, hydrothermal synthesis, electrochemical synthesis, and cage opening have also been successfully applied to synthesize GQDs. Herein we will introduce both the top-down and bottom-up strategies for GQD synthesis in detail.

2.20.1 Top-Down Method

Top-down methods generally produce small amounts of GQDs through cutting large carbon materials, including GO, graphene sheets, MWCNTs, etc., through the use of strong oxidants and acids. GQDs synthesized by top-down method always contain functional groups at the edge, which is adaptable to further functionalization. However, this method suffers from low yield, accidental damage of graphene structure, and less-uniform GQD morphologies.

2.20.1.1 Oxidative Cleavage

Oxidative cleavage is one of the most common methods applied to produce GQDs, which is simple, is cheap, and can produce high-quality GQDs. Dong et al. prepared GQDs by chemically oxidizing a commonly used carbon source of CX-72 carbon black with concentrated nitric acid and separated the as-prepared GQDs by centrifuging in acidic solution. In another study, GQDs were synthesized by cutting GO powder into smaller pieces and then reducing by L-ascorbic acid (l-AA) with a surfactant of sodium polystyrene sulfonate (PSS). GQDs could also be synthesized using acid treatment and chemical exfoliation of MWCNTs, and the as-prepared GQDs have a uniform size distribution, zigzag edge structure, and 2D morphology.

2.20.1.2 Hydrothermal Synthesis

Hydrothermal synthesis is a relatively facile method to synthesize GQDs among various synthetic routes. Pan et al. developed a hydrothermal method for cutting preoxidized graphene sheets into ultrafine GQDs with blue luminescence. The cutting mechanism may involve the complete breakup of mixed epoxy chains composed of epoxy groups and carbonyl groups under hydrothermal condition. Zhao et al. reported a facile and high-efficient (≈35 wt% conversion rate) approach to prepare GQDs using a commonly hydrothermal method with the assistance of KO_2. The as-prepared GQDs exhibited rarely reported yellow emissive PL property and respectable quantum yields (8.9%) in aqueous media. Chen et al. presented a one-pot hydrothermal method for the synthesis of GQDs by using starch as a precursor (Figure 2.26) [79]. The reactants consisted of only starch and water. Post-processing steps are avoided because the products are only GQDs, water, and carbide precipitate. Furthermore, the reaction is rapid, and the entire synthetic process requires only 120 min.

2.20.1.3 Electrochemical Synthesis

Electrochemical synthesis generally obtains GQDs via oxidatively cleaved working electrode which contains graphene, graphite, or carbon nanotubes under high redox potential (±1.5 to ±3 V). GQDs with a uniform size of 3–5 nm and green luminescence were prepared by Li et al. via electrochemical method, which performed in 0.1 M phosphate buffer solution (PBS) with a filtration-formed graphene film as working electrode. The as-prepared GQDs can retain stability in water for several months without any changes. In another study, boron-doped GQDs (B-GQDs) were synthesized by electrochemical exfoliation of graphite in borax electrolyte. The B-GQDs borax ($Na_2B_4O_7{\cdot}10H_2O$) solution showed highly green fluorescence. Upon evaporation, bright-green fluorescent crystals were generated. Red-emission GQDs were prepared by electrochemical exfoliation of graphite in 0.01 M $K_2S_2O_8$ solution. The as-prepared GQDs were demonstrated to be isolated sp^2 domains with a diameter of ≈3 nm generated by the active $SO_4^{\cdot-}$ radicals produced from $S_2O_8^{2-}$ as electrochemical "scissors" to sharply cut the graphene sheets into small intact sp^2 structures.

2.20.1.4 Microwave-Assisted Methods

Microwave-assisted methods dramatically shorten the reaction time compared to other approaches, such as oxidative cleavage and hydrothermal and electrochemical methods. Meanwhile, it can also improve production yields and purities. Therefore, many groups employed microwave-assisted methods for the synthesis of GQDs. With the assistance of microwave irradiation, Li et al. prepared greenish-yellow luminescent GQDs (quantum yield: 11.7%) from GO nanosheets under acid conditions (3.2 M HNO_3 and 0.9 M H_2SO_4) within 3 h. Brightly blue-luminescent GQDs (QY: 22.9%) were also obtained via moderately reducing GQDs with $NaBH_4$ within 2 h. Red-fluorescence GQDs were prepared via microwave-assisted methods using mango leaves as a carbon source. The obtained GQDs were in quantum size, ranging from 2 to 8 nm, and showed selective emission in the near-infrared (NIR) region between 650 and 750 nm. Nair et al. prepared GQDs from GO by a sonochemical method with intermittent microwave heating in half an hour. The synthesized GQDs were of high quality and exhibited good QY (23.8%), high product yield (>75%), and low cytotoxicity (tested up to 1,000 μg mL^{-1}).

2.20.2 Bottom-Up Method

The *bottom-up strategy* refers to a series of reactions in which GQDs are synthesized from small carbon precursors, including glucose, citric acid, and other carbon sources. GQDs produced by the bottom-up method always have a well-defined molecular size, morphology, and stable properties. However, some preparation processes are complicated.

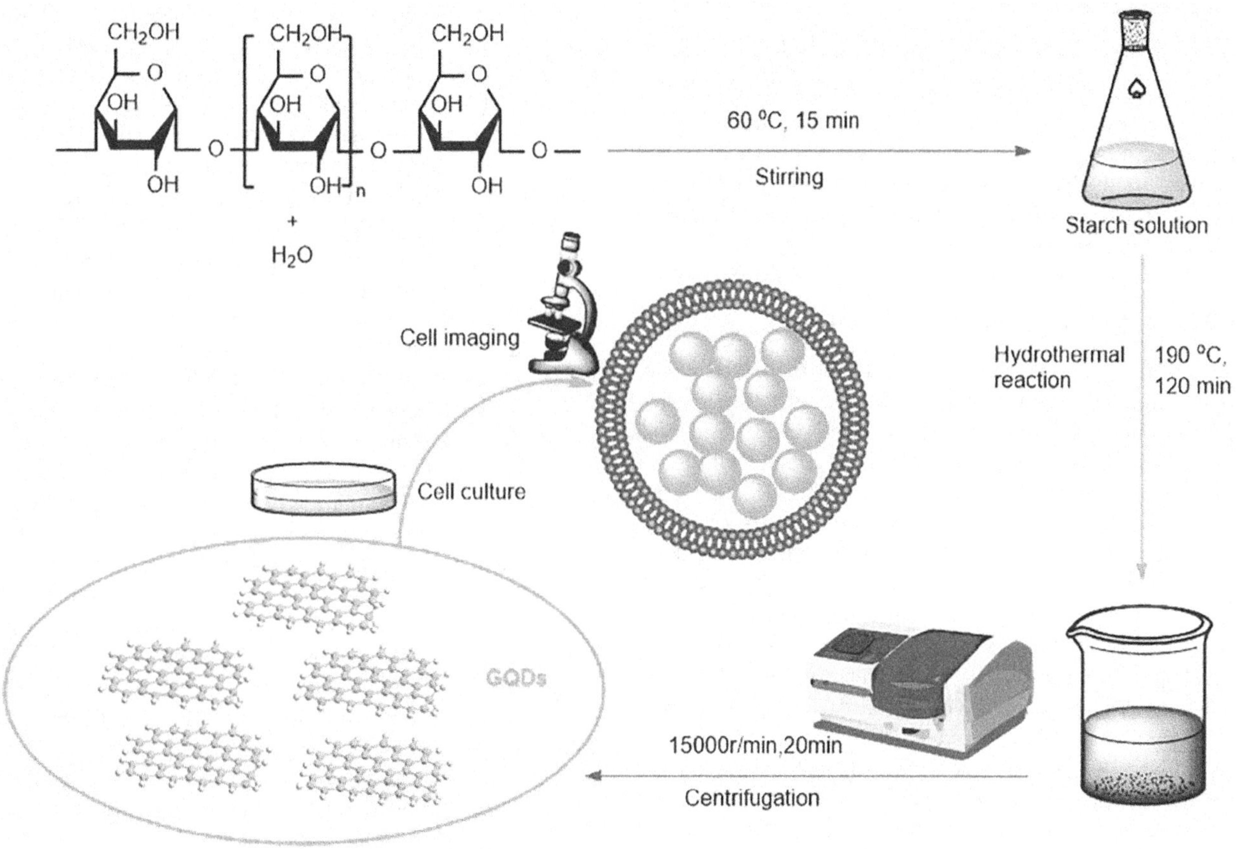

FIGURE 2.26 Schematic illustration of the green route of GQD synthesis.

Source: Reproduced with permission from [79]. Copyright 2018, The Royal Society of Chemistry.

2.20.2.1 Precursor Pyrolysis

Precursor pyrolysis for preparation of GQDs has been reported largely. Citric acid (CA) is a typical nonconjugate organic precursor that can be used in the precursor pyrolysis approach. Qu et al. synthesized N-doped GQDs using CA as a carbon precursor and different amines as the N source. Under basic reaction conditions, the CA molecules self-assembled into sheet structure, followed by condensation reactions through intermolecular dehydroxylation, forming nanocrystalline GQDs. Gevaerd et al. also synthesized GQDs with an average diameter of 7 nm based on citric acid pyrolysis at 200°C. The GQDs were electrodeposited directly at electrode surface under cyclic voltammetric conditions [80]. Besides CA, L-glutamic acid and 1,3,5-triamino-2,4,6-trinitrobenzene (TATB) were also employed as nonconjugate organic precursors. Wu et al. synthesized GQDs for *in vitro*/*in vivo* imaging and sensing applications by using the direct and simple pyrolysis of L-glutamic acid. The GQDs not only showed a stable, strong excitation-dependent photoluminescence with a high QY (54.5%) in the blue to red range but also provided an excitation-dependent NIR fluorescence emission in the range of 800–850 nm. Li et al. synthesized N-GQDs with green fluorescence by using TATB as the only precursor. The synergetic effects of exfoliation caused by the expanding gas and intramolecular carbonization during the pyrolysis process of TATB played dominant roles in the formation of N-GQDs in this process. In addition to nonconjugate organic precursors, conjugated precursors were also used in precursor pyrolysis. For example, Liu et al. prepared multicolor PL GQDs with a uniform size of ≈60 nm diameter and 2–3 nm thickness by using unsubstituted hexa-peri-hexabenzocoronene as the carbon source, [81] and the resultant GQDs possess a high PL efficiency of 3.8%.

2.20.2.2 Cage Opening

Lu et al. synthesized GQDs on a ruthenium surface using C_{60} molecules as a precursor. Results showed that the structures were formed through the ruthenium-catalyzed cage opening of C_{60}. Chua et al. demonstrated that small GQDs (≈2–3 nm) could be prepared by treating fullerene C_{60} with a mixture of strong acid and chemical oxidant. The as-prepared GQDs exhibited strong luminescence properties when excited at 340 nm. Furthermore, the red- and blueshift of the luminescence resulted from the chemical treatments with hydrazine hydrate and hydroxylamine.

2.21 Regulation Properties of GQDs

GQDs have attracted tremendous attention due to their excellent physicochemical properties. To satisfy various application scenarios, it is necessary to regulate the properties of GQDs. Here we briefly discuss three strategies of tuning GQDs' properties, including intrinsic properties control, surface functionalization, and heteroatom doping.

2.21.1 Intrinsic Properties Control

As demonstrated by Peng et al., the PL of the GQDs can be tailored through controlling the reaction temperature to effectively produce GQDs with various sizes [114]. Considerable research work is devoted to controlling the size of GQDs. Until now, many strategies, such as precursor pyrolysis [81], sonication, column chromatography, etc., have been successfully used to control the size of GQDs. Liu et al. synthesized GQDs with uniform size of ≈60 nm in diameter and 2–3 nm in thickness by using unsubstituted hexa-peri-hexabenzocoronene as the carbon source [81]. Yan et al. synthesized large, stable colloidal GQDs with desired sizes and structures through solution chemistry. The as-prepared GQDs consisted of graphene moieties containing 168, 132, and 170 conjugated carbon atoms, respectively. Kim et al. fabricated GQDs with a relatively narrow size distribution by varying the length of the carbon tube attached. GQDs with different core sizes but similar surface chemistry were prepared by solvothermal synthesis [82].

Apart from size regulation, control of some other intrinsic properties, including shape, number of layers, and edge state, was also continuously investigated. For example, Liu et al. reported that the shape of the graphene can be tailored by optimizing the annealing temperature and the density of the carbon clusters. Hassan et al. synthesized activated GQDs (aGQDs) enriched with both free and bound edges though ultrasonic approach with chemical activation using KOH. Unlike their nonactivated counterparts, the aGQDs emitted enhanced intense blue luminescence and exhibited electrochemical double-layer capacitance greater than that of graphene.

2.21.2 Surface Functionalization

Polyethylene glycol (PEG) is one of the most commonly used reagents in surface functionalization of GQDs due to its great biocompatibility and resistance to nonspecific binding by using as short as 12–14 ethylene glycol units. The PEG-functionalized GQDs always showed stronger PL emission. Shen et al. prepared PEG-modified GQDs by a one-pot hydrothermal reaction using small GO sheets and PEG as starting materials. The prepared GQDs showed strong blue emission and green fluorescence under an ultraviolet and an 808 nm laser irradiation, respectively. Wang et al. synthesized PEG surface-passivated GQDs, which possessed PL quantum yields as high as 18.8%.

Amine functionalization is another significant surface modification strategy owing to its unique protonation mechanism. Tetsuka et al. synthesized amino-functionalized graphene quantum dots (af-GQDs) by the ammonia-mediated bond-scission reaction from oxidized graphene sheet. Af-GQDs exhibited clear multiple colors under a single-wavelength UV excitation, and their luminescence quantum yields were over 40%. Jin et al. synthesized GQDs with 1–3 layers thickness and less than 5 nm in diameter that were functionalized with amine group. The amine-functionalized GQDs exhibited a redshift of PL emission compared to the unfunctionalized counterparts. Meanwhile, the PL emissions of the GQDs and the amine-functionalized GQDs were also pH-dependent due to the protonation or deprotonation of the functional groups. Polyethylenimine (PEI) is also proven to be a useful reagent for surface functionalization of GQDs. Wang et al. applied PEI-functionalized GQDs (GQDs-PEI) for the bioimaging of MG-63 cells. The GQDs-PEI showed brighter luminescence and minor cytotoxicity and were clearly rendered in the nucleus region compared to unfunctionalized GQDs. Blue-emitting PEI_{1800} GQDs and red-emitting PEI_{600} GQDs were prepared by coating GQDs with different molecular weights of PEI, which demonstrated to be feasible strategies in U-87 cells bioimaging. GQDs-PEI can also be synthesized from coffee grounds. The GQDs-PEI showed a highly efficient fluorescent property and a low cytotoxicity in favor of bioimaging applications.

Apart from PEG, amine, and PEI, aryl has also been applied as an effective reagent in tuning GQDs' optical properties. Thus, the modification of aryl groups changed the edge structures of GQDs, protected their PL active edge sites, and introduced the interaction of graphene basal planes and aryl grafts. Luo et al. modified GQDs with aryl groups, including phenyl, 4-carboxyphenyl, 4-sulfophenyl, and 5-sulfonaphthyl, via diazonium chemistry method, which tuned the PL bands of GQDs with increased fluorescence QY (Figure 2.27). Feng et al. fabricated alkylated GQDs (AGQDs) via the solvothermal reaction of propagatively alkylated graphene sheets (PAGenes). The synthesized AGQDs possessed a pH-independent character and emitted ultrabright PL with a relative quantum yield up to 65%. Further studies indicated that the synthesized AGQDs were nearly oxygen-defect-free, with alkyl groups decorated on edges and basal plane, which can be attributed to their greatly improved pH tolerance and high quantum efficiency.

2.21.3 Heteroatom Doping

Heteroatom doping is an effective way to tune the PL intensity and emission wavelength of carbon-based quantum dots. Since the first successful nitrogen-doped GQDs reported in 2012, doping GQDs with heteroatoms has received considerable attentions in scientific communities. Several types of dopants, including but not limited to nitrogen, boron, sulfur, phosphorus, fluorine, etc., have been utilized in GQD modification. The introduction of heteroatom into the carbon sheet of GQDs will result in the disturbance of local electronic environment, which can be used to regulate the surface chemistry, elemental composition, as well as bandgap and eventually affect the optical behavior of GQDs [83]. Theoretical and experimental studies have proven that the properties of GQDs vary with the heteroatom types and their bonding configurations. Reference [78] lists the information of partial GQDs doped with various types of heteroatoms.

Among the numerous potential heteroatoms, nitrogen is one of the most extensively used elements in heteroatom doping of

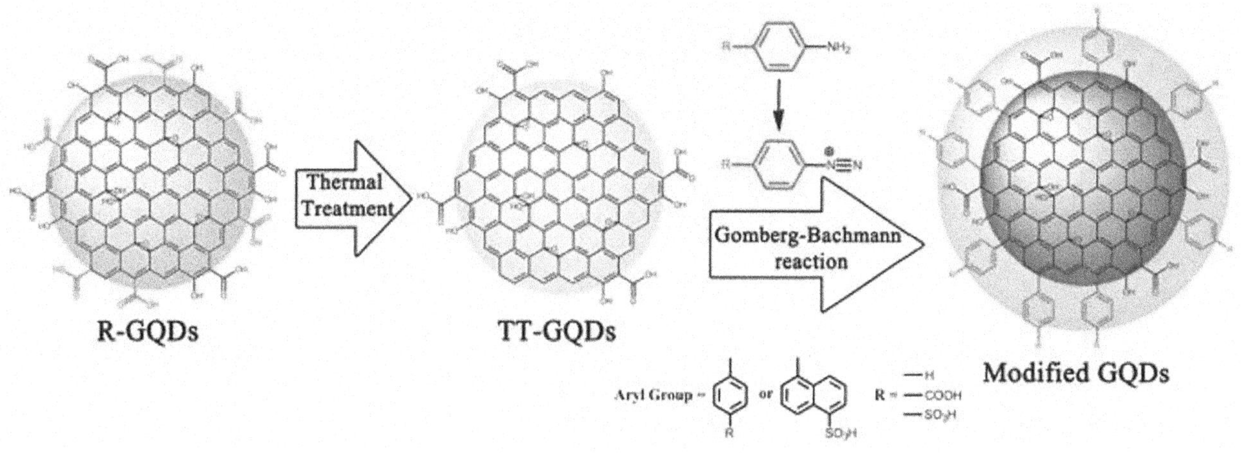

FIGURE 2.27 The scheme of modifying GQDs with aryl groups via Gomberg–Bachmann reaction.

GQDs. In the periodic table, nitrogen ($1s^22s^22p^3$) is adjacent to carbon ($1S^22s^22p^2$), with one more valence electron than carbon. Meanwhile, nitrogen displays a greater electronegativity (χ = 3.04) than carbon (χ = 2.55). Therefore, nitrogen tends to incorporate into carbon network via substitution doping. Numerous methods, including hydrothermal, [84] solvothermal, precursor pyrolysis, electrochemistry, etc., were used to prepare the N-GQDs. The nitrogen-doped multilayer GQDs were prepared by microwave-assisted hydrothermal method using glucose and urea as the starting materials. Li et al. prepared CH_2O-responsive NGQDs encapsulated with switchable "on–off" fluorescence via hydrothermal method using citrate and urea as carbon and nitrogen precursor [85]. N-GQDs were prepared using one-step pyrolysis, where citric acid acted as a carbon source, and tris(hydroxymethyl)amino-methane (Tris-HMA) worked as a surface passivation agent and a dopant. Fu et al. synthesized multicolor fluorescent N-GQDs about 20 nm by electrochemical method, and the as-synthesized N-GQDs emit three primary color fluorescence (blue, green, and red) independently [86].

Boron has also been introduced in graphene because its atomic radius is similar to that of carbon. Boron ($1s^22s^22p^1$) has one less valence electron than carbon ($1s^22s^22p^2$). A boron–carbon bond is 0.5% longer than that of a carbon–carbon bond. Thus, the incorporation of boron into GQDs will lead to the disturbance of the electron network and ultimately regulate the optical properties of GQDs. The graphite powder, or GO, always acts as a carbon source during the boron doping (B-doping), while B source can be varied from H_3BO_3 to B_2O_3, B_4C, and so on [87]. Wang et al. synthesized B-GQDs at 200°C using 4-vinylphenylboronic acid (VPBA) and boric acid as the precursor (Figure 2.28a) [88]. B-doped GQDs were prepared via a microwave approach with GO as the carbon source and borax as the boron source (Figure 2.28b). The as-prepared B-GQDs exhibited excitation-independent PL behaviors, with an excitation/emission maximum at 320/430 nm, and a fluorescence quantum yield of 21.1%. Moreover, the PL was stable over a wide range of pH 3.0–11.0.

Other types of dopants, such as sulfur, [89] phosphorus, [90] fluorine, etc., have also been successfully introduced to synthesize doping GQDs. Ma et al. reported a general method for the synthesis of doped GQDs based on the direct carbonization of organic precursors at a solid state under controlled experimental conditions. GQDs doped with different heteroatoms, including O, N, S, and P, can be successfully synthesized depending on the chemical compositions of precursors. Fluorinated GQDs (F-GQDs) were synthesized with controllable sizes and tunable fluorine contents from bulk fluorinated graphite. The doped fluorine atoms made F-GQDs resistant to pH effects and displayed stable luminescence in both acid and alkali conditions.

Notably, the co-doping may produce GQDs with new properties compared to the single-doping counterparts. Previous studies have demonstrated that co-doping could enhance the coupling effect between heteroatoms and thus improve the PL properties of GQDs. Luo et al. proposed a facile, inexpensive, and environmentally friendly hydrothermal method to synthesize nitrogen and sulfur co-doped graphene quantum dots (NS-GQDs). The NS-GQDs had a high quantum yield of 41% and a diameter of 1–5 nm. The PL emission of the NS-GQDs exhibited an obvious blueshift of 54 nm compared to that of the NGQDs. Nitrogen and phosphorus co-doped GQDs were synthesized using a biomolecule (ATP) as the precursor. The prepared co-doped GQDs showed a high quantum yield (≈27.5%) and strong two-photon excitation with a two-photon absorption cross section (20,000 Göppert–Mayer [GM] unit). Kundu et al. reported N-, F-, and S-co-doped GQDs in customized ionic liquid medium without using any tedious separation technique. The as-prepared GQDs showed a high yield of about 85%, along with a higher quantum yield of 70%. Manganese ion (Mn^{2+})–bonded nitrogen-doped graphene quantum dots (Mn(II)-NGQDs) were prepared by hydrothermal carbonization of glycine and sodium citrate [91]. The as-prepared Mn(II)-NGQDs exhibited advantages of low toxicity, superior brightness, and high photostability for fluorescence live cell.

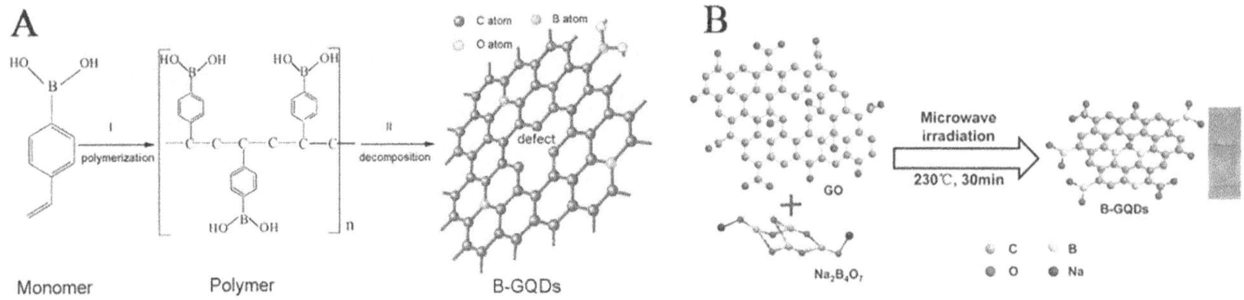

FIGURE 2.28 (a) The schematic representation of the formation of B-GQDs. (b) Preparation scheme for the B-GQDs by using GO and borax as carbon and boron sources.

Source: Reproduced with permission from [88]. Copyright 2017, Wiley-VCH.

2.22 Conclusion

In this chapter, we have summarized various synthesis techniques of carbon nanotubes, and this advanced carbon nanomaterial has emerged since their discovery about 25 years ago. This report on carbon nanotubes reveals also an overview on the structure, morphology, purification, and characterization methods. The distinct structural properties of carbon nanotubes, in particular, their high aspect ratio, strength, and high surface area, have the added advantage of being potential nanodevices for various medical and industrial applications. Overall, recent studies regarding CNTs have shown a very promising glimpse of what lies ahead in the future of science. In this work, we also reported a variety of familiar methods to synthesize carbon nanotubes, such as arc discharge, laser ablation, and spray pyrolysis–assisted chemical vapor deposition, and the types, properties, purifications, characterization, and some notable applications in diverse field. We also covered some recent synthesis of CNTs from a range of hydrocarbons using spray pyrolysis.

As excellent electrode materials, carbon nanotubes can be widely used as compatible electrochemical active materials, as well as the carrier or substrate integrated in wearable energy storage devices. In this chapter, we first summarize the main methods that synthesize the carbon nanotube and briefly describe the development of wet spinning and solid-state spinning methods that are presently utilized to form carbon nanotube fibers, with an extension of approaches to manufacture the composite fibers based on them. We subsequently focus on the potential applications of the fibers in energy storage system and elaborately discuss how to combine the prepared fibers with nanostructured active materials with different compositing approaches to intrinsically enhance their capacitive performances.

Various modified synthesis techniques have been developed in order to produce CNTs in large scale for commercial application. At the moment, the CVD method is the most promising method to produce large quantities of CNTs, since the cost is relatively low compared to other methods. Commercial applications of CNTs have been rather slow to develop, however, primarily because of the high production costs of the best-quality nanotubes. Enormous strides have been made in the chemistry of CNTs, and it is clear that this subject will drive the applications of carbon nanotubes. Functionalization of CNTs, and particularly CNTs of defined length, diameter, and chirality, will lead to a better control of CNT-based materials and devices at the molecular level.

Flexible energy storage technology has been regarded as the key supporting technology for smart wearable electronics. The flexible energy storage device assembled from carbon nanotube fiber-based electrodes has the advantages of being bendable, lightweight, and invisibly encapsulated, which will be the foundation of wearable smart textiles and promotes the rapid development of flexible energy storage devices. The relatively low specific capacitance and yield have been the most significant drawbacks of carbon nanotube–based fibers; these points can be theoretically overcome from the perspective of fiber structure, proper nanostructured active materials, and the improvement of existing fiber fabrication method. The summarization of appropriable nanostructured energy materials equally enriches the paths to synthesize high-performance fibers and provides a reference for the development of other novel fiber-based electrode materials in the future.

3

Bionanotechnological Applications of Fullerene (C_{60})-Based Modified Development Imaging and Biosensing Devices

3.1 Introduction

Fullerene is a compound of carbon. In October 1996, the Nobel Prize for Chemistry was awarded to researchers Harold Kroto, Robert F. Curl, and Richard E. Smalley for the discovery of fullerenes. Fullerene receives its name from the architect Buckminster Fuller, who designed homes in the shape of a geodesic dome based on pentagons and hexagons, sometimes even referred to as "buckyball." There are three important types of fullerenes: C_{60}, C_{70}, and fullerenols.

In the world of nanoscience and nanotechnology, fullerenes have opened a new door of opportunity and fields of science. Before fullerenes were discovered, only diamond and graphite allotropes existed. The first fullerene molecule was discovered in outer space later on and first synthesized in 1985 by Richard Smalley, Robert Curl, James Heath, Sean O'Brien, and Harold Kroto at Rice University [1]. The name comes from Buckminster Fuller, whose geodesic domes it resembles. Since its first discovery, fullerene C_{60} has been the object of extensive research. Its unique and favorable characteristics of easy chemical modification, conductivity, and electrochemical properties have led to its tremendous use in (bio)sensor applications. Fullerenes create such artistic structures that they are found to be intriguing in not only the scientific community but also in the worlds of mathematics, the visual arts, and architecture. The serendipitous discovery of fullerene triggered the research of carbon structures into the world of symmetric nanomaterials. Consequently, in 1996, Robert F. Curl, Harold W. Kroto, and Richard E. Smalley were awarded the Noble Prize in Chemistry for their discovery of the buckminsterfullerene (C_{60}, with a cage-like fused-ring structure). Since its first discovery, fullerene C_{60} has been the object of extensive research. Their unique and favorable characteristics of easy chemical modification, conductivity, and electrochemical properties have led to their tremendous use in (bio)sensor applications. The discovery of them has led to the expansion of other carbon allotropes, with intense research interest in the scientific community in electronics, material science, and nanotechnology. Fullerenes' unique structure and morphology make them sensitive to free radicals, introducing them as potential agents for biomedical applications. Even though fullerenes are originally soluble in non-polar solvents, polar solvent–soluble fullerenes have been developed in order to facilitate their application in aqueous solutions.

Bionanotechnology is a new, emerging field of nanotechnology and combines knowledge from engineering, physics, and molecular engineering with biology, chemistry, and biotechnology, aimed at the development of novel devices, such as biosensors, nanomedicines, and biophotonics.

With the development of biotechnology and interdisciplinary sciences over time, the use of nanoscale materials is increasing in biotechnological process developments. Nanomaterials created new opportunities, especially in biotechnology, with their easy modification advantage, especially in the field of diagnosis, and they offered significant advantages over traditional diagnostic methods in terms of sensitivity and selectivity. Diagnosis is the most important step in terms of developing health technologies. The correct diagnosis brings with it the rightful treatment, the right prognosis, the well-being of the patient, and a decrease in health expenditures. The important parameters in the exact diagnosis are sensitivity and accuracy. These two terms can describe the technological power of the diagnostic systems. In the development of sensitivity and accurate measurement, nanomaterials have an important place in today's technologies [2]. Nanotechnology is becoming increasingly important in the field of (bio)sensors. The performance and sensitivity of biosensors are greatly improved with the integration of nanomaterials into their construction.

Sensor and biosensor technologies have shown rapid progress in recent years. These technologies use nanomaterials that have an important place in immobilization materials for recognition of analyte molecules. Although fullerenes, among these materials, have attracted much attention in recent years, their number of studies is less than that of other carbon-based nanomaterials. However, the present chapter covers all aspects of biosensors based on fullerene C_{60}.

A *biosensor* is an analytical device that consists of a biological recognition element in direct spatial contact with a transduction element, which ensures the rapid and accurate conversion of the biological events to measurable signals. However, the discovery of rich nanomaterials has opened up new opportunities in the field of biosensing research and offers significant advantages over conventional biodiagnostic systems in terms of sensitivity and selectivity.

Among various nanostructure materials, carbon nanomaterials have been receiving great attention, owing to their exceptional electrical, thermal, chemical, and mechanical properties, and have found application in different areas as composite materials, energy storage and conversion devices, sensors, drug delivery systems, field emission devices, and nanoscale electronic components. Moreover, the possibility to customize their synthesis with attached functional groups or to assemble them into three-dimensional arrays has allowed researchers to design high-surface-area catalysts and materials with high photochemical and electrochemical

DOI: 10.1201/9781032635989-3

activity. Their exceptional electrochemical properties lead to their wide application for designing catalysts for hydrogenation, biosensors, and fuel cells. The wide application of carbon nanomaterial for the construction of biosensors is partly motivated by their ability to improve electron-transfer kinetics, high surface-to-volume ratios, and biocompatibility. In addition, the use of nanomaterials can help address some of the key challenges in the development of biosensors, such as sensitive interaction of an analyte with biosensor surface, efficient transduction of the biorecognition event, and reduced response times.

Various kinds of zero-, one-, two-, and three-dimensional carbon nanomaterials have been used. Examples of such materials include carbon nanotubes, nanowires, nanoparticles, nanoclusters, graphene, etc. Fullerenes are a very promising member of the carbon nanostructure family. The closed-cage, nearly spherical C_{60}, and related analogues have attracted great interest in recent years. Multiple redox states, stability in many redox forms, easy functionalization, signal mediation, and light-induced switching are among their exceptional properties. In different applications, fullerenes have been used for the development of superconductors, sensors and biosensors, catalysts, and optical and electronic devices. Their superior electrochemical characteristics, combined with their unique physiochemical properties, enable the wide application of fullerenes in the design of novel biosensor systems. It is the aim of this chapter to present the most recent and relevant contributions in the development of biosensors based on fullerene C_{60}, graphene, and different biological components. A brief introduction and history of fullerene C_{60} are first presented. Available methods for synthesis and functionalization of fullerene C_{60} are mentioned also. We briefly outline the current status and future direction for electrochemical biosensors based on fullerene C_{60}, especially fullerene C_{60} and graphene as immobilizing platform for DNA. Recently, Afreen et al. introduced a review on functionalized fullerene C_{60} as nanomediators for the construction of glucose and urea biosensors [3].

Now, we consider that it is time to review the progress of fullerene-based research from its birth until now. Although the advent of other carbon nanomaterials like carbon nanotubes and two-dimensional graphene put fullerenes in the shadow, this form of carbon, which can be considered as 0D carbon nanostructure, deserves great attention in nanomaterials studies, especially considering that, contrary to the other cited materials, its structure is perfectly defined, the reproducibility of its functionalization is not an issue, and its characterization can take advantage of both classical and innovative techniques. In this chapter, the production method, modification, and use of fullerene, which is a nanomaterial in the development of biosensor and sensor systems developed with biological or non-biological recognition agents, are described. This chapter provides a concise review of the advances in fullerene C_{60} research and its use as a nanomaterial for the development of biosensors. Research work reported in the literature on the synthesis, functionalization, and approaches to nanostructuring electrodes with fullerene has been examined, and some of the exciting applications in the field of (bio)sensing are outlined.

We aim for this to be a comprehensive chapter with a broad interest to the biomedical engineering community, being a substantial overview of the most recent advances on fullerenes in the field of biosensing and bionanotechnology applications that have not been exhaustively and critically reviewed in the past few years.

3.1.1 What Are Fullerenes?

Fullerenes are the allotropic form of carbon and closed convex polyhedra composed of an even number of carbon atoms. The name *fullerene* originated from that of Richard Buckminster Fuller (1895–1983), an American engineer, architect, inventor, and writer known for having discovered the structural principle of tensegrity, the property of a structure that makes it stand through the forces of tension and compression. Fuller is also known for his works on synergetic systems; his participation in the Gaia hypothesis, especially as creator of the architectural concept of the geodesic dome, is of utmost importance. A fullerene material is one of the allotropes of carbon. Any kind of substance that consists of carbon elements only and is formed with a spherical, elliptical, or tubular structure can be called a fullerene. The structure of fullerene is similar to that of graphite; the difference is that five-membered rings exist in fullerene, while there are six-membered rings in graphite. Fullerene is a molecule with a hollow center and is made up of carbon. Many shapes can represent fullerenes, such as spheres, cubes, or tubes. A *fullerene* is the three-dimensional allotrope of carbon shaped like a sphere, tube, or ellipsoid, with the carbon molecules bound to each other through single and double bonds, forming pentagonal and hexagonal fused rings. Due to their π electrons, fullerenes exhibit interesting phenomena that are easily manipulated by chemical methods.

Nowadays, we know fullerenes exist in nature and interstellar space. In the past, fullerene was Molecule of the Year in 1991 and has attracted a majority of research projects compared to other scientific subjects, to the extent that the average rate of publications was every 13 h in the first few years after its discovery.

Nanodiamond, which is a significant member in the carbon nanomaterials family, has been discovered before fullerene in 1963–1982. Indeed, fullerene can be considered as the first discovery among symmetric carbon nanostructures, and its discovery revealed new perspectives in carbon-based materials that resulted in research on carbon nanotubes, cylindrical cousin of buckyball, and rapid developments in advanced materials field.

Although the emergence of 2D carbon nanomaterials, such as graphene, reported in 2004by Geim and Novoselov, who were awarded the Noble Prize in 2010, marginalized fullerenes and moved majority of the studies toward other carbon nanostructures, the incredible properties of fullerene cannot be underestimated.

3.1.2 Drawing Fullerene Graphs

Fullerenes are presented with the empirical formula of Cn to adopt a closed-mesh morphology, with the most famous member called buckminsterfullerene (sometimes buckyball), with the molecular formula of C_{60}, named after the Americana architect and system theorist Buckminster Fuller. The term *buckyball* is used for C_{60} because of its similarity to a soccer ball. Fullerenes resemble the structure of graphite, which is constructed of sheets of carbon molecules in hexagonal shapes. Unlike graphite, fullerenes are typically pentagonal in shape and therefore do not lie in flat sheets. The most common fullerenes are constructed of 60 carbon atoms (C_{60}) and are bound by single and double bonds. These are the most common types of fullerenes and are referred to as **buckminsterfullerenes**, or simply buckyballs. We also must remember that all forms of fullerenes have a hollow core, similar to footballs and soccer balls.

Tubular shapes can also represent the fullerene structure. The tubes are referred to as nanotubes. Sheets of hexagonal carbon form tube shapes and typically have capped ends. They can vary in length but are always hollow. Cube-shaped fullerenes can also be formed. The cube fullerenes contain 540 carbon molecules.

Since geodesic domes designed by Buckminster Fuller in 1960s provided clues to realize fullerene C_{60}'s structure, this molecule, buckminsterfullerene, was named after this American architecture. After this discovery, in 1990, Wolfgang Krätschmer of the Max Planck Institute for Nuclear Physics and Donald Huffman of the University of Arizona, with their students, prospered in producing fullerene in bulk quantities.

In the following sections, we will detail the different formations that fullerenes can take.

3.1.2.1 Buckminster Fullerenes

If $\rightarrow x_0$ is chosen sufficiently close to the face, and if the points of the polyhedron lie on a sphere, the resulting 2D embedding will be planar. While Schlegel only proved that the projection produces a planar layout when the vertices lie on a sphere, it still works in many cases where this is not the case, and the method is widely used to the extent that planar graph embeddings sometimes (incorrectly) are called Schlegel diagrams. However, Schlegel diagrams are specifically the embeddings that result from the Schlegel projection. The Schlegel projection is illustrated in Figure 3.1(a). A problem with the Schlegel projection is that it often fails and produces crossing edges when used with many non-spherical polyhedra or when the parameters are not well chosen. The cone-projection method, shown in Figure 3.1(b), which projects the vertices out on an enveloping cone of the fullerene polyhedron and then down onto a plane, seems to be more robust.

As stated previously, Buckminster fullerenes also go by "buckyballs." Buckyballs were named after the famed architect and designer R. Buckminster Fuller. They are the most common of all the fullerenes, consisting of 60 carbons (C_{60}). Buckminster fullerenes form what resembles a soccer ball and have 32 sides, of which 12 sides are pentagonal, and 20 sides are hexagons. Buckyballs are extremely strong, making them valuable in the construction of different types of materials.

Other spherical fullerenes can consist of as few as 20 carbons and range to being over 100 carbons.

3.1.2.2 Carbon Nanotubes

Carbon nanotubes are exactly as they sound. They are fullerenes that have formed a tube or cylindrical shape from a sheet of carbon molecules in a hexagonal shape. The nanotubes can be of various lengths, and although most are capped at the end, some are open. As they are fullerenes, they are all internally hollow.

The hexagonal layout of the rings and helical orientation of the rows can cause some nanotubes to be metallic. This property makes the nanotubes semiconducting.

Fullerene, namely C_{60}, has a structure similar to that of a soccer ball and is named after architect Richard Buckminster Fuller; it was produced by vaporizing graphite in a laser beam. Fullerenes are soluble in organic solvents and not in water. C_{60} fullerenes are the smallest ones, like the buckyball; meanwhile,

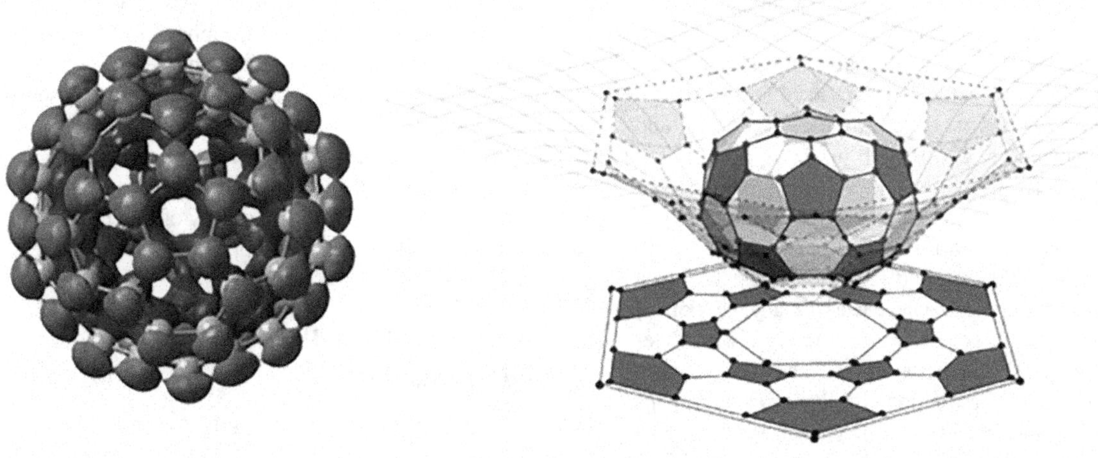

(a) (b)

FIGURE 3.1 (a) Schlegel projection of C_{60}-I_h. (b) Cone projection of disk-shaped C_{72}–D_{6d}.

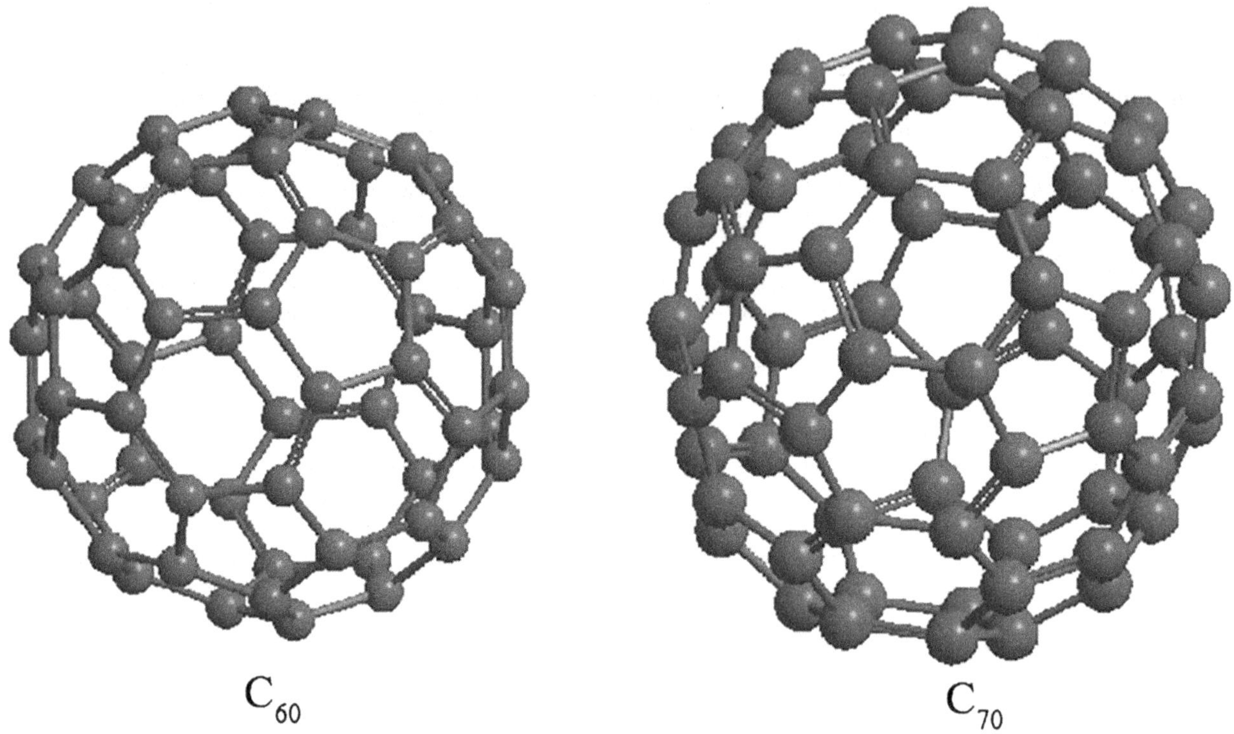

FIGURE 3.2 Schematic of fullerene molecules (C_{60} and C_{70}).

C_{70} has the structure of a rugby ball. Nowadays, most of carbon 60 is manufactured in the laboratory. The remarkable carbon cage structure makes them a potential agent for many therapeutic applications, in biomedicine and diagnostics.

Fullerene, with its unique structure consisting of sp^2 carbons, presents a high symmetric cage with different sizes (C_{60}, C_{76}, and so on). The most abundant fullerene in the as-synthesized composition is C_{60}, the molecular structure of which, together with that of C_{70}, can be observed in Figure 3.2. C_{60} consists of 60 carbon atoms with C_5–C_5 single bonds which form 12 pentagons and C_5–C_6 double bonds which form 20 hexagons [1]. Indeed, each fullerene with 2n + 20 carbon atoms contains "n" hexagons. As shape, fullerene C_{60} is like a soccer balls, and Yadaf et al. have stated that the ratio of fullerene molecule to soccer ball is the same as the ratio of soccer ball to Earth, where the diameters of the Earth, the soccer ball, and the fullerene molecule are 12.75×10^6 m, 2.2×10^{-1} m, and 7.0×10^{-10} m, respectively.

In relation to the crystallographic properties of the fullerene molecule, the presence of symmetric elements, including 30 twofold axes, 20 threefold axes, and 12 fivefold axes, has made fullerene the most symmetrical molecule (as already mentioned) that is controlled by the golden mean rule. C_{60}, with face-centered cubic lattices (FCC) in solid phase, has a stable structure, to the extent that the destruction of fullerene cage happens at temperatures higher than 1,000°C. Divergent spectroscopic methods like Raman spectroscopy, UV-vis, NMR, and FTIR could be deployed to characterize fullerene. Moreover, fullerene results into a compatible nanomaterial with biomolecules specially structured by Fibonacci sequence and possess golden mean properties too. Among the different characteristics of this molecule, C_{60} has the ability to produce oxygen species upon exposure to visible light, which makes it a suitable candidate for photodynamic therapy. The interesting behavior of fullerene in solutions presents a unique solvent–solute interaction in which the rigid molecular structure of fullerene has not undergone conformational and solvent-dependent changes.

As mentioned earlier, different strategies have been exploited in order to promote fullerenes' behavior in solvents, especially aqueous dispersions, which play a crucial role in biological applications.

The divergence of publications and research articles using the Scopus database (date of search: November 21, 2016) regarding the biomedical applications (cancer, photodynamic therapy, antiviral, antibacterial, HIV, DNA, RNA, toxicity, biosensor, antioxidant, imaging, drug deliver, and stem cell) of fullerene is demonstrated in Figure 3.3. The number of papers with the word "toxicity" is more than that of other keywords, demonstrating the great importance placed on the toxicity of fullerenes, which is a prerequisite for the biomedical applications of fullerenes.

3.2 Fullerenes, Their Properties and Production

Fullerenes have several specific properties:

- They bind with single and double covalent bonds.
- Nanotubes make up the strongest/toughest material known.

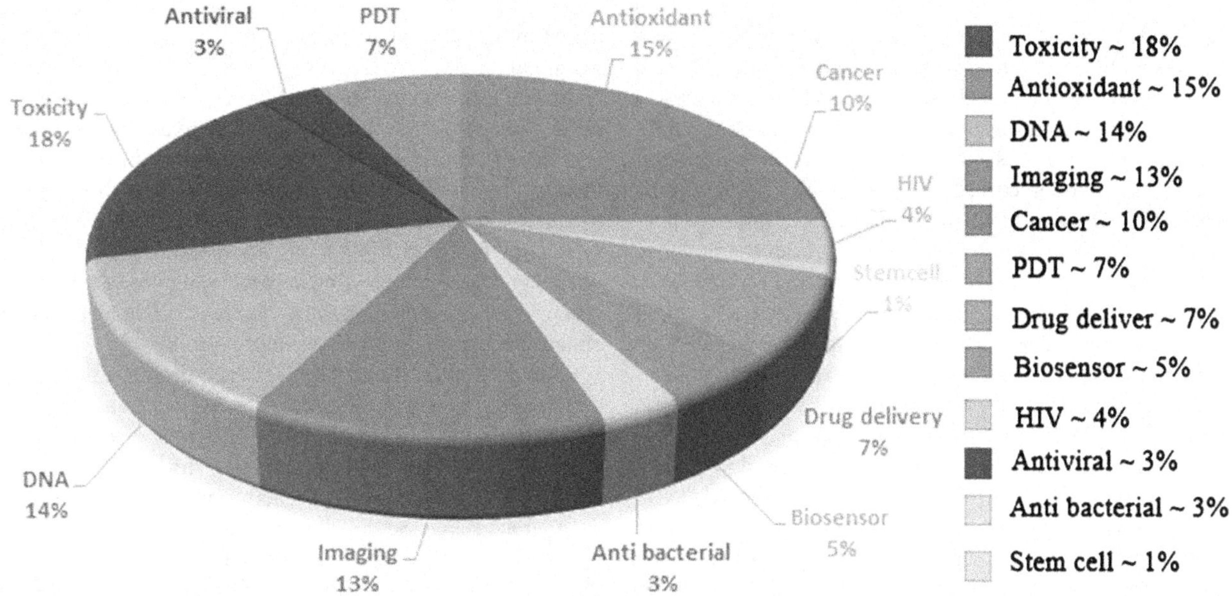

FIGURE 3.3 Distribution of various biomedical applications of fullerene.

- Nanotubes contain strong graphene bonds.
- Due to the negative space, nanotubes are highly compressible, and that compression is easily reversed.
- Buckyballs react differently under different types of temperature and pressure.

Thanks to its completely closed structure and at least 30 double bonds, it can be modified from 30 points, which provides a great advantage. At these points, thanks to the ability to modify amine, thiol, carboxyl, or metallic groups, modification residues can be created for all kinds of immobilization. According to the zero-dimensional nanomaterial class, fullerenes provide an extremely large surface area. Therefore, it provides more biological or non-biological recognition receptors immobilized on this surface area. Moreover, increasing the surface area with more recognition agent also increases sensitivity. This is the most important parameter of sensor technologies, which is provided by fullerenes. In this book chapter, the development of fullerene-modified sensor and biosensor technologies is explained with examples, and fullerene modifications are given in figures as fullerene derivatives. Contribution is made in the method development stage by giving comparison of fullerene type sensor and biosensor systems.

In this simple system, electrodes, optic systems, or piezoelectric systems can be used as physicochemical transducers. Electrodes are physicochemical conductors that can detect electrochemical signals in a solution. On the other hand, optical sensors can detect light–matter interactions, and piezoelectric systems can perform specific and sensitive mass analysis. The recognition layer on these transducers plays a key role for biosensors and sensors. In biosensor systems, this recognition receptor is called a *biorecognition agent*, such as enzymes, antibodies, DNA, RNA, and other proteins that can be used as biorecognition elements. As a result of the interaction of these biomolecules with the target molecule, catalytic or affinity-based biosensor systems can be developed. Otherwise, molecularly imprinted polymers, nanoparticles, and other polymers can be used as recognition agents in sensor systems instead of biological receptors. Increasing the effectiveness of these recognition agents depends entirely upon the properties of the immobilization/modification material used in the modification of the physicochemical transducer. Fortunately, nanomaterials can be used in sensor and biosensor systems in order to increase the power of the measurement system or to use it as a recognition material. These materials increase the surface area to obtain more sensitive signals and increase the possibility of interacting with more target molecules by binding more recognition agents to the surface. Technically, nanomaterial forms of inert metal/organic materials can be used as catalytic agents when they are in nanoform.

3.2.1 Basics and History of Fullerene (C_{60})

The fullerene molecules of carbon atoms are arranged in a regular six tops and pentagons that make up the surface of the sphere or ellipsoid. Fullerenes have multiple types, but the most renowned forms are C_{60}, C_{70}, and fullerenols because of their important uses.

Fullerene is built up of fused pentagons and hexagons forming a curved structure. The smallest stable, and the most abundant, fullerene obtained by the usual preparation method is the Ih-symmetrical (the construction of *Ih* symmetrical fullerenes from pentagons) buckminsterfullerene (C_{60}). The next stable homologue is C_{70}, followed by higher fullerenes, C_{74}, C_{76}, C_{78}, C_{80}, C_{82}, C_{84}, and so on. Since the discovery of fullerenes, buckminsterfullerene (C_{60}) has fascinated a large number of researchers due to its remarkable stability and electrochemical properties. The stability of the C_{60} molecule is due to the geodesic and electronic bonding present in its structure. In 1966, Deadalus (also known as D. E. H. Jones) considered the possibility of making a large hollow carbon cage (giant fullerene). Later on, in 1970, Osawa first proposed the spherical Ih-symmetric (the construction of *Ih* symmetrical fullerenes from pentagons) football structure for the C_{60} molecule. In 1984, it was observed that upon laser vaporization of graphite, large carbon clusters of Cn with n = 30–190 can be produced. The breakthrough in the discovery of fullerene happened in 1985, when Kroto and Smalley proved the presence of C_{60} and C_{70}, which can be produced under specific clustering conditions. The second breakthrough in fullerene research was achieved by Krätschmer and Huffman. They invented the laboratory analogues of interstellar dust by then vaporization of graphite rods in a helium atmosphere and observed that upon choosing the right helium pressure, the IR spectrum shows four sharp, strong absorption lines which were attributed to C_{60}.

In 1985, three scientists produced a fullerene, named C_{60}, in fewer quantities by vaporizing graphite in the arc or the laser beam or with an electric current in a low-pressure argon or helium atmosphere. Since then, they have gained significant attention in different fields. The newly found molecule was named by these scientists after Richard Buckminster Fuller; in 1967, he made a dome shaped like the carbon cluster, whereas in 1970, the possibility of fullerene's existence was predicted. Later, it was observed that fullerenes occur in interstellar dust and also in Earth's geological formations, only in the ppm range. Fullerenes, also known as buckyballs, are carbon's new allotrope, and their appearance also resembles soccer balls. Fullerenes consist of 20 hexagons and 12 pentagons with a carbon atom in each edge of the lattice structure. Fullerenes also exist in different stones, naturally. Earlier, on cave walls, they were deposited as soot. In 1990, fullerenes were produced on a larger scale for the first time. In this chapter, the making of fullerene is explained properly, and the fact that fullerene's unique structure joined with immense derivatization makes them a possible agent for many therapeutic applications, including free radical scavenger, anti-HIV protease activity, antimicrobial action, photodynamic DNA cleavage, and their use as diagnostic agents and in biomedicine.

Each carbon in a fullerene C_{60} atom is bonded to three others and is sp^2-hybridized. The C_{60} molecule has two bond lengths; the 6:6 ring bonds can be considered as double bonds and are shorter than the 6:5 bonds. C_{60} is not "superaromatic," as it tends to avoid double bonds in the pentagonal rings, resulting in poor electron delocalization. Therefore, the C_{60} structure behaves like an electron-deficient alkene and reacts readily with electron-rich species. The estimated values of electron affinity (EA) (2.7 eV) and ionization potential (IP) (7.8 eV) of C_{60} indicate that it can easily contribute to the electron transfer reaction and reveal a very rich electrochemistry, which makes them attractive candidates for electroanalytical applications.

3.2.2 Fullerene Structure

Fullerene is carbon's third allotrope, after graphite and diamond. They are carbon molecules inside a closed cage, produced in the gas phase during graphite's laser desorption. Fullerene has molecules that consist of carbon atoms joined by double and single bonds to make a partially closed or closed mesh, with fused rings of 5 to 7 atoms. Carbon's allotropes were limited to graphite, diamond, etc., but then carbon's third form, called fullerenes, got discovered. C_{60} fullerenes (CFs) constitute a fused-ring structure of carbon atoms comprising of 12 pentagons and 20 hexagons. Fullerenes can be used in lipid-like systems, serving as a reservoir and even crossing membranes of cells and the blood–brain barrier. The behavior of controlling the drug–disease rate, high loading of the drug, substantial biocompatibility, immuno-neutrality, mononuclear phagocytic system bypassing capability, nature of long circulation, and extraction of tissue by virtue of retention effect and enhanced permeability are its major promises.

Fullerenes can serve as stages for the transportation of drugs and imaging agents. Fullerenes, when surface-functionalized, can have direct antioxidant activity. They also serve as drug vectors or scaffolds of drug delivery with covalent or non-covalent linkages between bioactive moiety and fullerene. A fullerene subclass known as endohedral fullerenes offers a robust shell, and in their interior spaces they contain atoms that are supposed to be prevented from contacting the body, for example, in contrast enhancement for MRI and as radionuclides carrier. C_{60} is of soccer ball shape, and it is the archetype fullerene of the family. Higher fullerenes have larger cases, including C_{74}, C_{78}, C_{70}, C_{84}, C_{76}, etc. Cages of fullerenes are comprised of pentagons and hexagons with alternating carbon–carbon bonds of single-bond character (at the pentagon–hexagon junctions) or of double-bond character (at the hexagon–hexagon junctions). Also, the larger the cage of fullerene, the more possible the structural isomers. With the help of their all-carbon surfaces, minimum derivatization is needed to use them for the delivery of drugs. The effectiveness of the drug is increased due to the properties of the nanomaterials, including a specific size, the characteristics of the surface, a rare spherical structure with a strong apolar character, and compositions of material, well recognized to provide potentially valuable advances over traditional drug delivery.

Fullerene is an allotrope of carbon with molecules that consist of carbon atoms joined by double and single bonds to make a partially closed or closed mesh, with fused rings of 5 to 7 atoms. Carbon's allotropes were limited to graphite, diamond, etc., but then carbon's third form, called fullerenes, got discovered. An experiment was done in which laser irradiation vaporized graphite's surface into plasma containing free ions and atoms. Due to the collision with helium atoms, those free atoms and ions were chilled down. Clusters containing numerous amounts of carbon atoms were made because of the collision, ranging in size from 20 carbon molecules to larger ones. It has also been discovered that carbon 60 molecule concentration is increased by permitting the plasma to react longer; a mass spectrometer examined the clusters, and it was seen that clusters having 70 to 60 carbon atoms dominated, making up carbon 60, 40 times more as compared to carbon's other structures. These were the most studied fullerenes. In the beginning, only less than 10–15 g was prepared, but in 1990, new preparation methods for a high yield of fullerenes were developed. Fullerenes got named after an architect, Richard Buckminster Fuller, who made a so-called geodesic dome structure of hexagonal and pentagonal cells in 1967, very similar to the fullerene molecules. Fullerenes exist in nature, particularly where high energy and carbon exist and close to volcano craters. They are even formed when gas burns in the household cooker, in regular lighter's flame, or in places of ancient carbon rock accumulation. In 1999, C_{60} fullerenes were found in schungite.

Fullerenes are constituted by a network formed by 12 pentagons and 20 hexagons, closing the sphere. Each carbon of a fullerene is sp-hybridized in the form of a sigma bond (simple bond) with three other carbon atoms, subtracting one electron from each carbon. The most important property of fullerenes is its high symmetry. In this one, there are 120 symmetry operations, such as axis rotations or reflections in the plane. This makes the C_{60} molecule the most symmetrical molecule, since it has the largest number of symmetry operations. For the C_{60} molecule, there are three types of rotation axes: C2, C3, and C5.

Fullerenes are spherical carbon nanomaterial derivatives. This structure, unlike other carbon structures, consists of a closed form of pentagonal and hexagonal carbon structures fused together.

Graphene nanomaterials are called two-dimensional nanomaterials because they consist of only one layer, while fullerenes are classified as zero-dimensional, closed-cage type of nanomaterial. The spherical form of the fullerene nanomaterial gives this nanomaterial a large surface area [4]. This feature is a sought-after feature for biosensors and sensor systems. The most advantageous feature of the double bonds formed by the carbon structure is that they can be modified, as they can easily respond to chemical reactions. Most of the chemical reactions that occur through nucleophilic attacks can form active sides on the fullerene sphere. With these modifications, fullerenes can be chemically modified. Chemical modification is important for biomolecule immobilization or surface modification. Fullerene in 60 carbons has the capacity to form 30 bonds due to its spherical structure, and 30 double bonds. These bonds can be modified with different chemical agents to form fullerene derivatives.

3.2.3 Fullerenes Properties

One very important property of fullerenes is that they are highly symmetric, with 120 symmetrical operations, including rotation and reflection in a place. Resistance to heat and superconductivity are the properties of fullerenes that have been extensively investigated. Accordingly, fullerenes have been found to be unusually reactant in many organic reactions, namely, Bingel reaction. Through modification and attaching active functional groups, the reactivity of fullerenes has been increased. Normally, fullerenes are electrically insulated; however, in the case of crystallization by alkali metals, they turn out to be superconductors. Some fullerenes are chiral because of their D2 symmetry, which can be used as specific sensors to detect their relevant enantiomers. Fullerenes can be built atom by atom based on the bottom-up synthesis approach or inversely by top-down approach through breaking the larger structure into smaller parts. Taking the advantage of the top-down method, asymmetric but more stable fullerenes can be achieved.

Fullerenes, due to their remarkable properties and structure, attracted many different scientists. Properties like symmetric nature, nanometric size, chemical tailoring opportunities, thermal conductivity, photoconductivity, and capabilities to load drugs are the reason that fullerenes are good in applications of drug delivery. Fullerenes also have neuroprotective, antiviral, MRI contrast, antioxidant, and anti-inflammatory properties. Fullerenes and its derivatives also provide enormous promises in drug delivery, especially to cancerous cells, due to its benefits, therapeutically and chemical modifications. The highly symmetrical C_{60} sphere has elegance and beauty that excites the imagination of scientists, as they cover aesthetic gaps between architecture, the sciences, and the visual arts. Fullerenes have a broad range of properties in both mechanic and electric field and are also great conductors of electricity and heat and have astonishing tensile strength. Due to such properties, they have a great future in the field of medicine, pharmacy, structural materials, and electronics.

1. **Topology:** Schlegel diagrams are usually used for viewing closed-shell fullerenes' 3D structure. A closed fullerene of the sphere-like shell should have some heptagon or pentagon cycles at least. Open fullerenes, for example, graphene and carbon nanotubes, consist entirely of rings of the hexagon. In theory, a long nanotube with joined ends forms a torus-like closed sheet that could also consist entirely of hexagons.
2. **Bonding:** Three neighbors are connected with each carbon atom, so it is usual to label those bonds as a mixture of single and double covalent bonds.
3. **Encapsulation:** Endohedral fullerenes are one of the fullerene derivatives that have small molecules or ions incorporated inside the cage atoms.
4. **Aromaticity:** Scientists have increased the reactivity of the fullerene by assigning active groups to their surfaces. Superaromaticity is not exhibited by fullerenes. C_{60} diameter is 0.7 nm, and it is just like a soccer ball, due to which it is usually called a "soccer ball molecule." Comparing one such molecule's dimensions with the Earth, one finds that the soccer ball–fullerene relation resembles the relation between the Earth and a soccer ball. Fullerenes have a very low density of 1.68 g/cm³, in comparison with graphite having a density of 2.1–2.3 g/cm³, or diamond having a density of 3.51 g/cm³, which is because of their hollow ball shape. C_{60} is the smallest stable fullerene because of the two pentagons that are side by side. C_{60} molecule's important property is high symmetry, because there are 120 symmetrical operations, like rotation around the axis and reflection in a plane, which map the molecule onto itself. Bond lengths are of two types in fullerene: C5–C6 double bonds (hexagons) and C5–C5 single bonds (pentagons). Each C atom bonds via sp^2 hybridization with three other adjacent atoms.

A C_{60} molecule has a diameter of 7 Å. C_{60} molecules form a solid bond of weakly bound molecules together. Fullerites are fullerenes' crystalline state. It looks like a yellow powder, but after dissolving in toluene, it turns pink. The molecule is quite stable chemically. Temperature of over 1,000°C is required to break the balls. In the absence of air, fullerenes can transform into graphite when heated up to 1,500°C. C_{70} looks more like a rugby ball and has 25 hexagons. When hexagons are removed or added from the structure of the soccer ball, fullerene begins to lose its roundness. Giant fullerenes appear in the shape of a pentagon. Smaller fullerenes appear as asteroids. Carbon 60 is the most stable one. A loss of stability comes with the loss of roundness. Other than C_{60} and C_{78}, C_{70}, C_{86}, C_{76}, and C_{84} have been separated and discussed in detail. Carbon disulfide, toluene, and xylene are good solvents.

- Fullerene is harder than diamond.
- The ductility of fullerene is 100 times stronger than that of steel.
- Fullerene conducts electricity and has stronger conductivity than copper.
- Fullerene weighs only one-sixth of a copper material.
- Fullerene is made of carbon so can be extracted from waste.

3.2.4 Fullerene Derivatives and Chemical Reactions

Fullerenes are not self-inflammable and are mostly yellow in color. Under an ignition source's influence, fullerenes are flammable (dust explosion). Fullerenes are the only carbon modifications that are not soluble in water but soluble in organic solvents. Hydrated C_{60} fullerene helps an organism return to its "normal condition" in the case of any negative changes, and it does that for the maintenance and restoration of those structures it has generated as a matrix in the process of life's origin. C_{60} fullerenes are the smallest ones, like the buckyball; C_{70} is the next larger fullerene, having the shape of a rugby ball. Nowadays, most of carbon 60 is synthesized in the laboratory by treating soot with organic solvents to extract carbon 60. The soot is made between two carbon electrodes by using an electric arc. Extracted carbon 60 can be separated and then purified using chromatography, along with other fullerenes. C60 molecules are incorporated into frames and shafts to achieve very thin-walled and lightweight, robust structures of carbon. These are highly used in medical fields and have various applications in biomedicine.

The most isomerically found types of fullerene derivatives are C_{60} and C_{70} fullerenes. These derivatives can only be dissolved in highly non-polar liquids, such as toluene and benzene. Thanks to this hydrophobic property, it can be used as a drug carrier, intercalator, or modification material in hydrophobic layers as lipid layers. In computer studies about fullerene, solubility attempts that were made in 75 different solvents were examined.

Although it is possible to dissolve fullerene in different solvents, surface modification of fullerenes for biosensor and sensor technology is the most effective way to use it. The solubility in water can be achieved by modifying fullerenes with polar groups. In the method developed by Hirsch and colleagues, fullerene is modified by 18 carboxyl groups, gaining solubility in water as 34 mg/mL at pH = 7.4. In these studies, a nucleophilic cyclopropanation procedure was performed; protection was removed with the help of bis-(polyamide)-malonate dendrimer, and 18 carboxyl groups were created. With this modification, a material which can be used as an advantage in water solubility for modification of the carboxyl group, especially for sensor and biosensor technology, is obtained. With the activation of EDC/NHS, 18 carboxyl groups can be made to bind the amino group, or a fullerene nanomaterial containing carboxyl groups can be modified on an amino group–modified transducer.

In another study, Cusan and his colleagues synthesized three ethylene glycol and three ammonium groups in polycharged fullerene–pyrrolidone derivatives. In that study, which was carried out on two strategies, 2,2′-(ethylenedioxy) diethylamine was reacted by amino esterification with benzyl bromoacetate. Subsequently, the substance was interacted with carboxylate groups on fullerene to obtain fulleropyrrolidine in toluene. In this method, the authors have shown that purification is difficult and yield is low. For fullerene-PEG, in terms of biosensor and sensor technology, the fullerene derivative has two different arms, with an amino group that can be used for modification by activating amino groups with glutaraldehyde as cross-linker.

Fullerene modifications can be carried out entirely through the modification of the C = C bonds on fullerene. Fullerene modifications and derivatives of these modifications are seen in several studies. Accordingly, fullerene can be used to develop biosensors and sensors after being modified.

Apart from their use for modification material, another interesting feature of fullerene and fullerene-like materials is their photocatalytic advantage. C60 shows a semiconductor diode–like behavior and shows photoactivity when illuminated at a value close to 1.4 eV. This photocatalytic feature shows that it can be used as a photocatalyst in optical sensors and biosensors.

3.3 Synthesis Methods of C_{60} Fullerene

Several methods based on the top-down approach have been employed to synthesize fullerenes, such as electric arc heating of graphite, resistive arc heating of graphite, laser vaporization, and laser irradiation of polycyclic hydrocarbons (PAHs). Among these, laser vaporization was the first method through which fullerenes were synthesized in a very small amount. For large quantities, however, water laser along with arc heating of graphite are applied [5].

It was initially shown that the production of fullerene is achievable by means of an irradiating laser beam on a graphite rod placed in a helium atmosphere. However, the overall yield rate of fullerene was insufficient for its potential applications in various industrial fields. Therefore, different production methods have been developed for the sufficient production of fullerene. The second proposed method is based on laser ablation of graphite in a helium atmosphere. In the laser ablation method, materials are removed from a solid surface by irradiating it with a laser beam. During the laser irradiation of graphite, materials are evaporated and their vapors are converted to plasma. Upon cooling the gas, the vaporized atom tends to combine and form fullerene. The arc discharge process is an alternative method where the vaporization of the input carbon source is achieved by the electric arc formed between two electrodes. They can also be produced by the non-equilibrium plasma method, where a non-equilibrium gas phase in the glow discharge is induced by the non-equilibrium plasma, and fullerene is generated without the need for high temperatures.

3.3.1 Huffman–Krätschmer Method

Three main methodologies for the production of fullerenes have been utilized: evaporation of carbon, incomplete combustion of benzene in oxygen, and microwave method. The first bulky production of fullerene, in 1990, was based upon evaporation and recondensation of graphite; its schematic is shown in Figure 3.4a. Since a requisite for fullerene formation is carbon atoms in gaseous phase, in this process, pure graphite was used as a source of carbon atoms. By heating graphite in helium atmosphere with 100–200 torr pressure, a light and condensate soot was produced which contained fullerene. In order to extract fullerene, the soot was dispersed in benzene in a Soxhlet extractor, and the benzenic solution of fullerene was percolated from the Soxhlet cartridge in the flask and so separated by the other components. An alternative method for fullerene extraction included heating the soot in an inert gas or under vacuum, followed by sublimation and formation of fullerene.

In order to vaporize graphite or other sources of carbon like coal, techniques such as arc evaporation, pyrolysis, and radio frequency plasma and laser ablation could be exploited. Although these methods provide a higher quantity of fullerene, the arc process results to be the best-established technique for production of carbon soot, and it is more efficient and appropriate for commercial use. Regardless of the method used to produce carbon soot, fullerene must be purified, most of the time by extraction with organic solvents, and because of the limited solubility of fullerene in these solvents, large volumes of solvents are needed to produce an acceptable yield of fullerene.

3.3.2 Combustion Method

Another technology for producing fullerenes is based upon incomplete combustion of hydrocarbons in sooting flames. Significant yields of fullerenes have been extracted from laminar sooting flame of premixed mixture of benzene and oxygen at low pressure. The schematic of the premixed chamber is shown in Figure 3.4b. In this method, flame conditions like pressure, C/O ratio, residence time, and gas velocity in the combustion of benzene influence fullerene amount and composition. Among them, pressure is an influential factor, and the formation of fullerene could be done at low pressure, like the astrophysical atmosphere at temperatures lower than 1,700 K. Furthermore, combustions methods, including laser pyrolysis of vapor hydrocarbons and laser irradiation of polycyclic aromatic hydrocarbons (PAHs), have been used to produce fullerene.

3.3.3 Microwave Method

In addition to the well-known methods mentioned earlier, there are technologies exploiting microwave in order to synthesize fullerene.

Another use of microwave for the production of fullerene has been investigated recently to transform graphite powder to fullerenes. The microwave method possesses advantages over

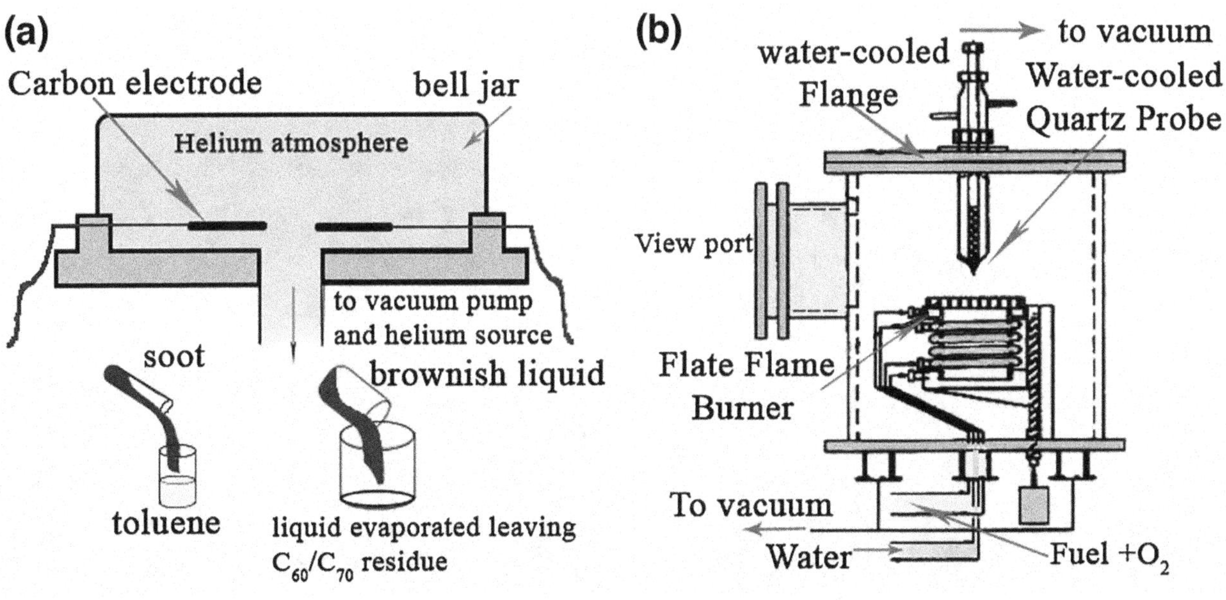

FIGURE 3.4 Schematic of fullerene synthesis methods: (a) Huffman–Krätschmer method based on evaporation of graphite and (b) premixed chamber in combustion method.

conventional heating methods, providing a homogenous heating of the precursors. It was found that time and temperature did not affect the production of fullerene, while the amount of graphite powder and microwave intensity led to a higher yield of synthesized fullerene.

3.4 Functionalization of Fullerene

Early studies on the C_{60} molecular structure showed that this carbon allotrope could undergo electron-deficient polyolefin reactions. The [6, 6] bonds have greater double bond character and are shorter than the bonds and, thus, used to functionalize C_{60} by nucleophilic, radical additions, as well as cycloadditions. Many reactions have been developed for the functionalization of C_{60}, which consists of cyclopropanation (the Bingel reaction), [4 + 2] cycloaddition (the Diels–Alder reaction), and [3 + 2] cycloaddition (the Patro reaction), [2 + 2] cycloaddition. The Bingel reaction has been frequently used to prepare C_{60} derivatives in which a halo ester or ketone is first deprotonated by a base and subsequently added to one of the double bonds in C_{60}, resulting in an anionic intermediate that reacts further into a cyclopropanated C_{60} derivative. In addition, cyclopropanation reactions have shown to be an efficient method for the preparation of fullerene derivatives with wide application in material science and in biological applications (Scheme 3.1a). Additionally, the double bonds that exist in C_{60} can react with different dienes with the Diels–Alder reaction (Scheme 3.1b). The main drawback of the Diels–Alder reaction is the low thermal stability of formed product. In another reaction (the Prato reaction), an azomethine ylide, generated in situ by the decarboxylation of iminium salts derived from the condensation of α-amino acids with aldehydes or ketones, reacts with fullerene to produce [3 + 2] cycloadduct (Scheme 3.1c). A wide variety of functionalization of fullerene molecule is possible by means of the Patro reaction. In another way, the addition of benzyne to C_{60} leads to the formation of [2 + 2] cycloadducts (cycloaddition) (Scheme 3.1d). However, among the available methods for functionalization of fullerene, cycloaddition reactions have emerged as very useful for functionalization of one or several of the fullerene double bonds.

The presence of double bonds is the most effective feature exploited to functionalize fullerene. In fact, they can be involved in addition reactions; therefore, the outer sphere of the carbon cage can be modified, and derivatives containing various functional groups can be synthesized. Also, pristine fullerene contains no hydrogen atom and cannot involve substitution reactions; however, fullerenes are oxidizing agent and, in particular, when exposed to UV-visible irradiation, can produce active oxygen forms.

Two approaches have been used to modify fullerenes: (1) use of solubilizing agent to partially mask fullerene surface, and (2) chemical modification of fullerene via covalent functionalization. The first can take advantage of linking polymer chains to fullerene, entrapping this molecule in cyclodextrins or calixarenes, incorporating into artificial lipid membranes, and inducing co-solvation with polyvinylpyrrolidone in organic solvents. Numerous functionalization routes have been used to enhance fullerene hydrophilicity and also extend its biological and pharmaceutical applications. The alteration of carbon atoms' hybridization from sp^2 to sp^3 is the driving force for the addition to fullerene. Various free radical reactions, cyclopropanation, or cycloaddition reactions, such as [1 + 2], [2 + 2], [3 + 2], and [4 + 2] reactions, can covalently conjugate various molecules to C_{60}. Due to the electron-deficient nature, fullerene behaves as 2p electron-deficient dienophiles and 1,3-dipolarophiles, which experience a variety of cycloaddition, reactions such as [1 + 2], [4 + 2] (Diels–Alder reactions), [3 + 2], and [2 + 2]. A large number of fullerene derivatives have been prepared using different types of cycloaddition reactions.

The latter approach, that is, chemical modification, is an advanced and effective method which results in a variety of fullerene derivatives with attached amine ($-NH_2$), hydroxyl

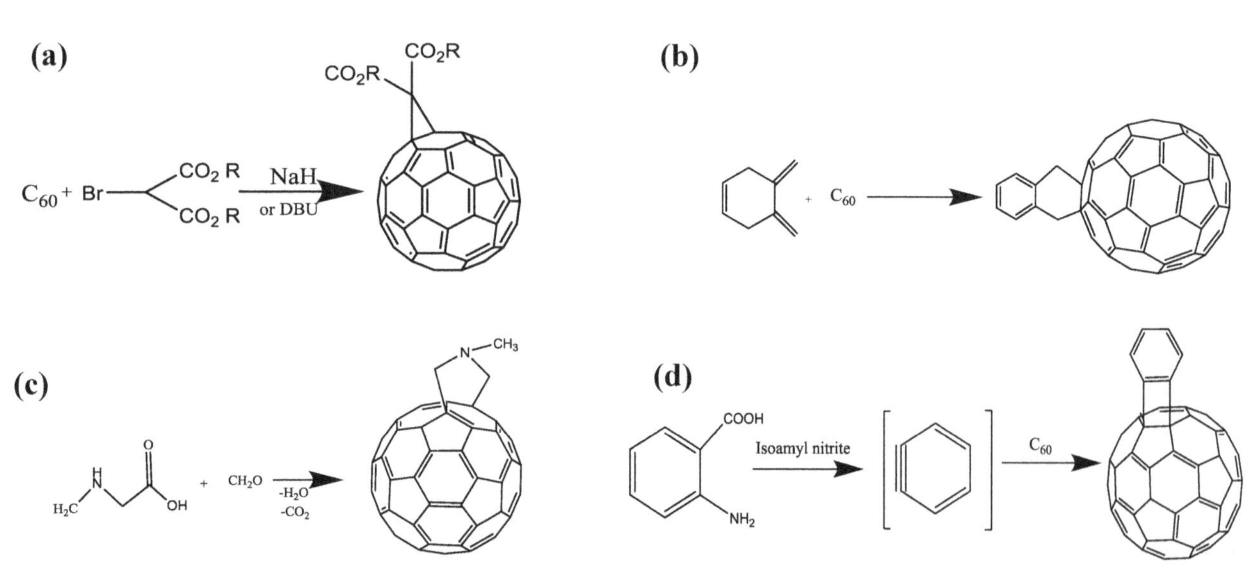

SCHEME 3.1 (a) The Bingel reaction; (b) the Diels–Alder reaction; (c) the Prato reaction; and (d) the cycloaddition reaction.

(–OH), and/or carboxyl (–COOH) groups and examples of some of the so-obtained derivatives. In addition, carboxyfullerenes have been exploited in the treatment of neurodegeneration caused by amyotrophic lateral sclerosis (ALS).

3.4.1 Synthesis of Endohedral Fullerenes

The fullerene hollow cage allows to use this carbon nanostructure as a container for various atoms, ions, and molecules, and the term "endohedral" is used to indicate such fullerene species. Endohedral metallofullerene is a captivating class of fullerenes which modifies the electric and magnetic properties of fullerene cage and extends the applications of this carbon allotrope in different fields, especially in the realm of biomedicine.

Until now, various methods have been developed for the production of endohedral fullerenes in macroscopic scale, similar to the fullerene preparation strategies, with the creation of carbon-rich plasma in the atmosphere containing inert gas like He or Ar. These techniques include vaporization of graphite with arc discharge, laser ablation, radio frequency furnace and resistive heating, implantation of the atoms through the carbon cages' walls via ion bombardment, high-pressure treatment, and the last technique, chemical routes by opening orifices in the fullerenes. Among these methods, arc discharge is the most favorable for the production of endohedral fullerene.

Initially, endohedral metallofullerenes (EMFs) were produced by laser ablation. In this process, a composite disk containing graphite and metal oxide is located in a furnace at 1,200°C. By irradiation of 532 nm laser onto the composite, EMFs and empty fullerenes are generated and flow through the tube with inert gas, and then they deposit on the tube wall. Nonetheless, this method is expensive, and the production rate is really low, so the large-scale production of EMFs with this method is limited. Contrary to laser ablation technique, the contact arc developed by Krätschmer and Huffman could be applied for mass production of EMFs. A schematic image of its process is shown in Figure 3.5.

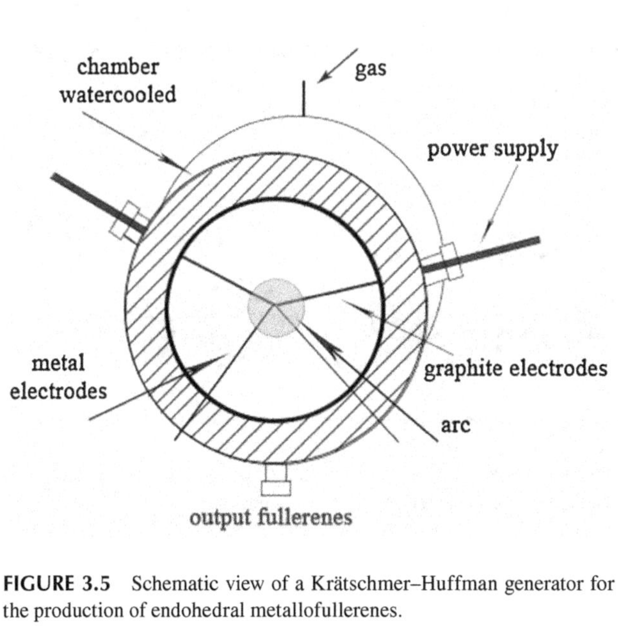

FIGURE 3.5 Schematic view of a Krätschmer–Huffman generator for the production of endohedral metallofullerenes.

In here, metal/graphite composite rods are used as anode and are exposed to a temperature above 1,600°C in order to form metal carbides in the composite rod for the efficient production of EMFs. Then, composite rods are arced in direct current in the range of 300–500 A and under flowing He as a cooling gas. In the further step, the produced soot can be collected. This method is proficient and cost-effective for the production of EMFs. There are two main obstacles in the extensive research regarding the structural properties of EMFs. First, the difficulties in the separation of EMFs culminated in the low availability of pure and symmetric single crystal of endohedral metallofullerenes. Second, because of the intrinsic features of EMFs, their investigation with standard tools is faced with numerous limitations. In addition to low amount of single crystals of endohedral metallofullerenes, X-ray diffraction investigations of single crystals impede the rotational disorder of the single crystal of fullerene molecule.

3.4.2 Fullerene-Based Nanomaterials

Self-assembly is a technique which has been used for synthesizing functional molecules with a variety of nanostructures. Nano-sized fullerene crystals have intermediate size, between molecules and bulk materials. Various methods exploited this characteristic in order to prepare 1D or 2D fullerene-based nanostructure.

Self-assembled fullerene nanostructures with disparate shapes could be synthesized by vapor-driven crystallization, liquid–liquid interfacial precipitation (LLIP), drop drying process, and template-assisted dip drying. Fullerene fine fibers, which contain single-crystal C_{60}, present diameters ranging from 100 nm to a few microns, and their lengths are hundreds of microns. They are called C_{60} nanowhiskers and represent a 1D fullerene nanostructure (Figure 3.6a). Fullerene nanowhiskers are crystalline thin fibers and can contain pristine C_{60}, and/or endohedral and/or functionalized fullerenes. The nanowhiskers could be synthesized by the liquid–liquid interfacial precipitation (LLIP) method, which is the most convenient procedure for the preparation of fullerene nanowhiskers, and it was developed. In this method, a solvent, in which fullerene presents low solubility, such as ethanol, isopropyl alcohol (IPA), and isobutyl alcohol, is mixed with a solvent able to properly dissolve C_{60}, such as toluene, *m*-xylene, benzene, and CCl_4. The liquid–liquid interface between these two types of solvents is the nucleation site for fullerene crystals. The increase in fullerene solubility in one of the solvents will enhance the liquid–liquid interfacial pressure, which is required for polymerization of fullerene molecules. Fullerene nanowhiskers with lengths in hundreds of microns and diameter in several nanometers possess a high aspect ratio and also a Young's modulus higher than those of pristine C_{60}. The schematic model of a body-centered tetragonal crystal fullerene nanowhiskers and its growth direction are shown in Figure 3.6b.

In order to improve the characteristics of fullerene nanowhiskers and prepare FW/PAni hybrid material, a polyaniline emeraldine base dissolved in N-methyl-2-pyrrolidone (PAni/NMP) was added to fullerene nanowhiskers by direct-mixing technique. Despite fullerene nanowhiskers, this hybrid

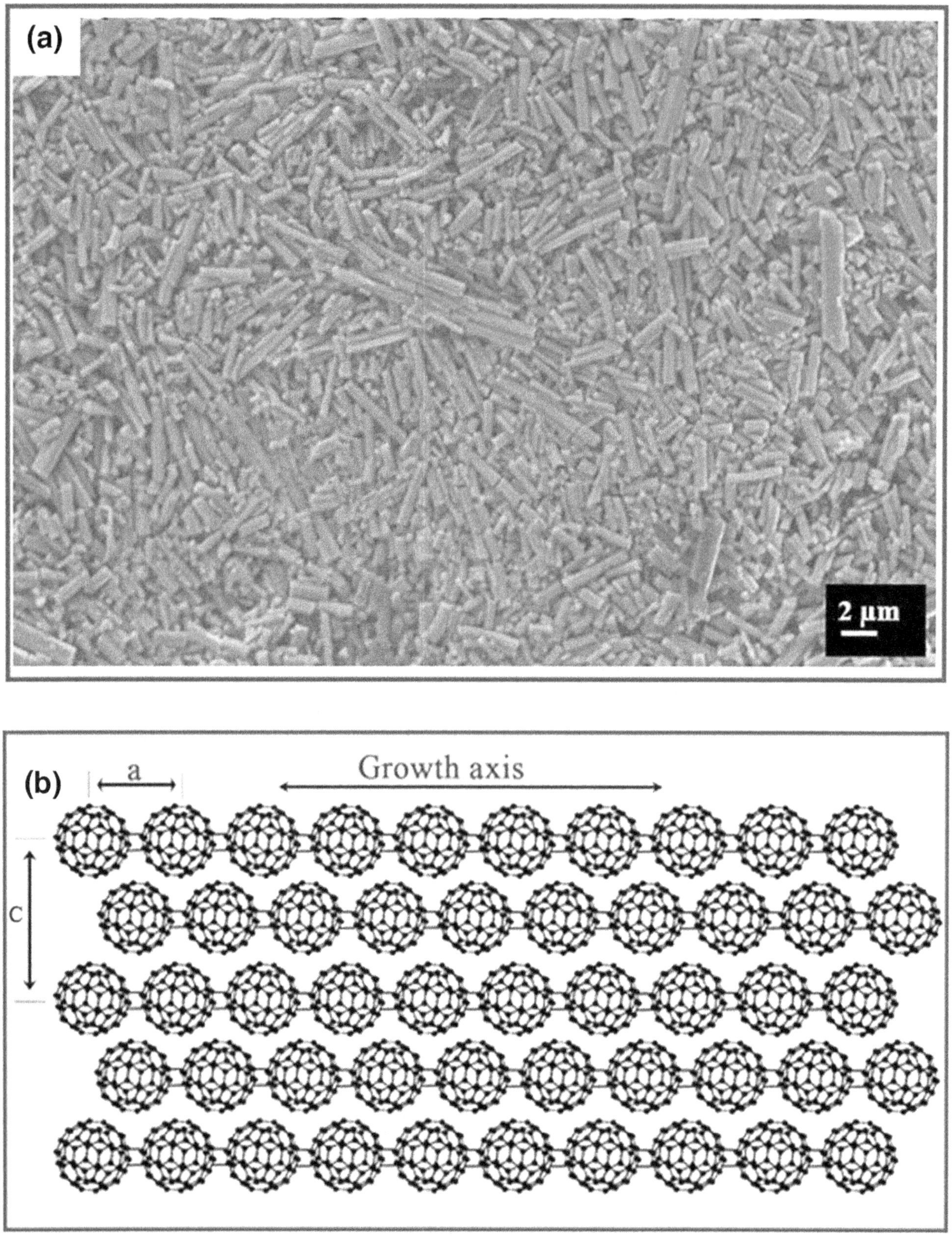

FIGURE 3.6 (a) SEM image of fullerene nanowhiskers showing the morphology of the nanowhiskers. (b) Model of one-dimensional fullerene nanowhiskers with body-centered tetragonal crystal structure, where *a* and *c* are lattice constants relative to the growth axis.

material has a tubular structure with a pleated surface morphology and, consequently, has a higher aspect ratio. The possible mechanism for the formation of this tubular structure is charge-transfer (CT) complex between the electron-rich polyaniline to the electron-deficient fullerene nanowhiskers. In another study, C_{60} nanowhiskers have been prepared by the LLIP method, and vortex flow–induced alignment method has been used for the alignment of C_{60} nanowhiskers. In this method, the mechanical stirring of the medium induces a vortex flow which aligns fullerene nanowhiskers. The aligned C_{60} NWs on a glass substrate were used as a scaffold for the culture of human osteoblast MG63 cells. The results of the study demonstrated that cell growth orientation was compatible with axis of C_{60} NWs, and these nanowhiskers were a significant substrate for adherence and growth of MG63 cells.

In addition to fullerene nanowhiskers, recently, fullerene cylindrical nanotubes with improved semiconducting and electronic properties were synthesized via LLIP method. In this procedure, *m*-xylene and TBA (tetrabutyl alcohol) were used as a saturating solvent and precipitation agent, respectively. In 2007, a flexible, porous, and transparent fullerene hexagonal thin crystalline nanosheet via LLIP method, using alcohol and CCl_4, has been synthesized. In this technique, the number of carbon atoms and the polarity of alcohols influence the particle size of the supramolecular structure, and high-polarity alcohols culminate in the formation of uniform hexagonal nanosheets. However, despite these indications, it is really hard to obtain a nanostructure with certain morphology in the self-assembly of fullerene because of the presence of many influential factors.

A hybrid hexagonal nanosheet containing C_{60} and ferrocene has been prepared via LLIP method. Recently, pressure-induced transformation of ferrocene-doped C_{60} nanosheets was investigated by in situ Raman spectroscopy in order to examine their controlled polymerization and form new planar polymers. By increasing pressure, orientation and polymerization of C_{60} layers happened. The presence of light irradiation in this polymerization process makes it a more controlled process and increases the formation of new layers.

The synthesis of an assemble fullerene nanocrystal at the liquid–liquid interface of C_{60} solution in butylbenzene and IPA. Low solubility of C_{60} in IPA and slow diffusion of IPA to fullerene promote the nucleation of small fullerene clusters and the further growth of crystals in hexagonal bipyramid and flower-like shape at liquid–liquid interface. Later, the same group investigated the effect of natural non-ionic surfactants diglycerol monomyristate ($C_{14}G_{12}$) and diglycerol monolaurate ($C_{12}G_2$) on the crystallization of C_{60} and the morphology of fullerene crystals. Based on their report, the applied surfactants caused a morphological transition in fullerene crystals from a 1D faceted rod to a unique zero-dimensional nanostructure called "konpeito-like" fullerene crystals, while in the absence of surfactants, the ultimate morphology was the one-dimensional nanorod with hexagonal close-pack structure.

One of the most recent fullerene crystal morphologies is fullerene flower, which has been prepared via solution-phase crystallization of fullerene molecules. The presence of mesitylene as a good solvent, ethanol as a poor solvent, and C_{60} and C_{70} molecules as the solute, and the difference between C_{60} and C_{70} solubility as the main factor for the occurrence of a two-step crystallization, resulted in a unique nucleation process and formation of flower-shaped crystals. By controlling the crystallization procedure and changing effective factors, different fullerene flowers can be obtained.

Another group of fullerene nanomaterials are polymer/fullerene nanocomposites, which can present novel physicochemical properties. Numerous polymers, such as polystyrene (PS) and polyethylene glycol, have been used as matrices for these nanocomposites. They integrated fullerene derivative 1,2-(1′,1′,2′,2′-tetracyanomethanoxymethanol) C_{60} (TCNEO-C_{60}) into polycarbonate (PC), the structure of which is shown in Figure 3.7a; moreover, they covalently linked N-methyl-pyrrolidone [60] fullerene to polycarbonate chain (MPYLDC60-PC, Figure 3.7b).

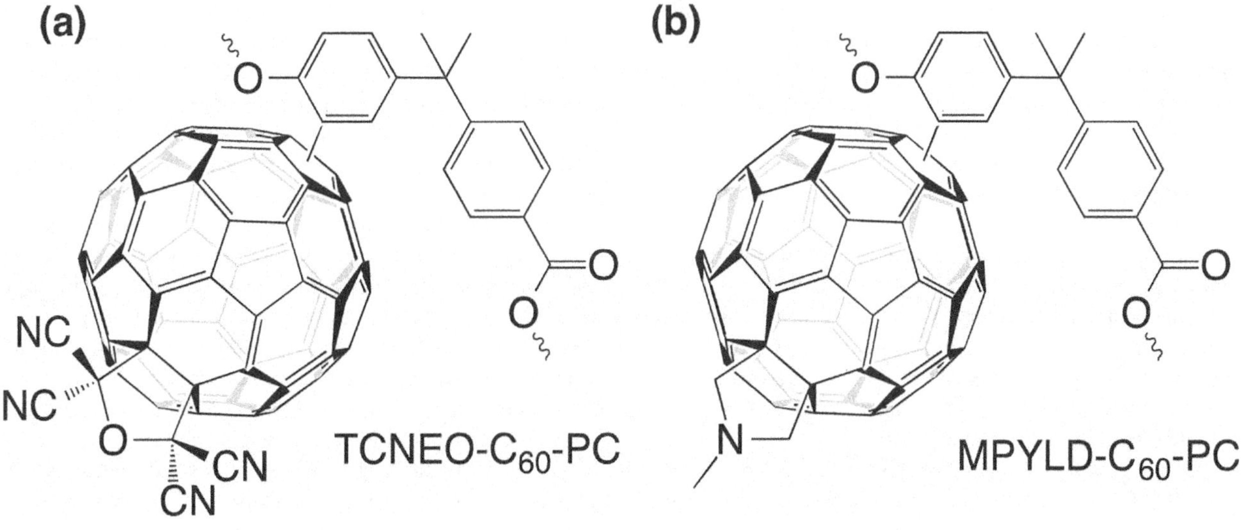

FIGURE 3.7 Polycarbonate containing fullerene derivatives.

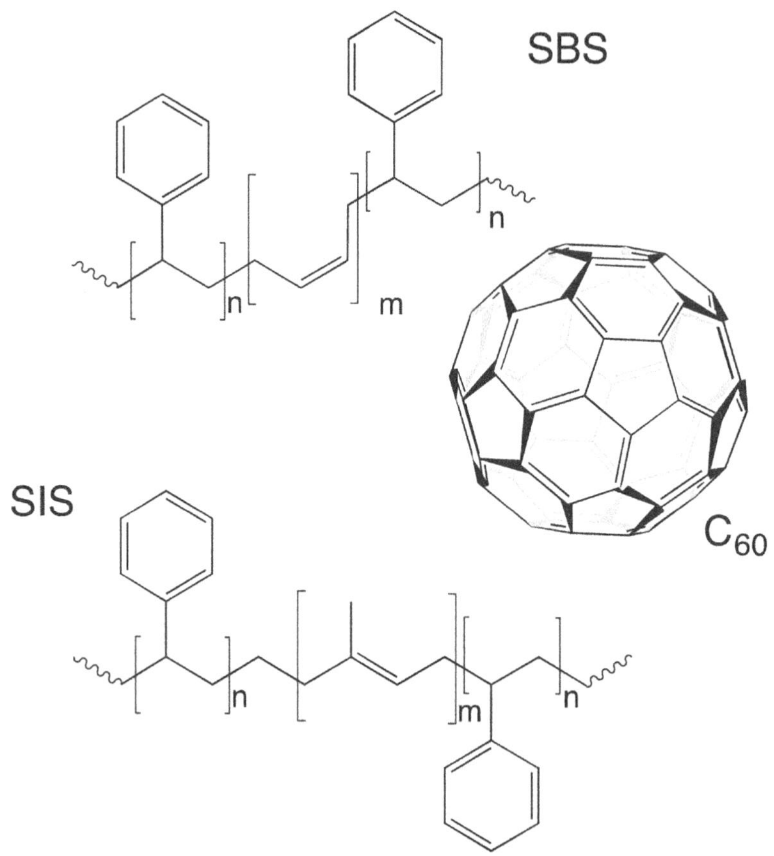

FIGURE 3.8 Chemical structure of SBS, fullerene, and SIS.

In 2007, a nanocomposite containing fullerene and polystyrene-polyisoprene-polystyrene (SIS) and polystyrene-polybutadiene-polystyrene (SBS) copolymers was synthesized (Figure 3.8), and their characteristics were investigated, finding that with the increase in fullerene content, the nano-tack adhesive forces decrease, and the bulk forces also showed results similar to those of nanoforces. Another nanocomposite containing fullerene was synthesized by Ag nanoparticles embedded in C_{60} matrix via thermal co-deposition, and the effect of temperature and nanoparticles percent in silver–fullerene nanocomposites was examined.

A polymer/fullerene nanostructure with a defined morphology and polymer fiber orientation via a novel technique based on no-covalent interactions between copolymer and fullerene derivative has been developed. Another group of fullerene nanocomposites are gel nanocomposites, in which fullerenes are embedded in the fibrillary gel networks. The incorporation of fullerene boosts the stability of the gels and their melting point. One example of these composites is fullerene-PEG gel, which has acceptable thermal stability and solubility in solvents like methanol, water, and THF.

Another group of polymer/fullerene nanostructure is polymer/fullerene core–shell composite nanofibers (NFs), which can be applied in solar cells and can enhance the performance of polymer-based solar cells. A novel composite containing conjugated polymer (poly[2-methoxy-5-(2-ethylhexyl-oxy)-p-phenylenevinylene], MEH-PPV) nanoparticles and fullerene phenyl-C_{61}-butyric acid methyl ester (PCBM) has been developed for applications in photodynamic therapy (PDT), in which MEH-PPV/PCBM nanoparticles generate ROS (reactive oxygen species) and exert toxicity toward cancerous cells. Conjugation of glycol chitosan (GC) grafted with 2,3 dimethylmaleic acid (DMA) and C_{60} (GC-g-DMA-g-C_{60}) is a self-assembled polysaccharide nanogel containing hydrophobic (C_{60}) and hydrophilic (GC and DMA) parts that can be used as a photosensitizer prodrug in PDT.

Fullerene hybrid macromolecular structures were synthesized by aggregation of C_{60} and terpolymer colloids in isopropyl alcohol and the mixture of isopropyl alcohol and water. The results demonstrated that fullerene macromolecular hybrid nanostructures in isopropyl alcohol were spherical structures with uneven surface, while in isopropyl alcohol–water mixture, clusters of crystalline nature of fullerene were observed. Recently, a group reported the preparation of a nanostructure containing fullerene C_{60} and carbon composite film via thermal sublimation in a vacuum of C_{60} powder, and then the films were deposited onto substrate materials.

The development of more fullerene-based nanostructures provides opportunities for enhancement of fullerene applications in various fields, like biomedical science, and can make fullerene a more biocompatible and applicable material.

3.4.3 Fullerene-Containing Polymers (Polyfullerenes)

Since immediately after fullerene discovery, fullerene-containing polymers emerged in the materials world, being able to associate extensive and favorable properties of polymers with the exceptional characteristics of fullerenes. Therefore, many efforts have been allocated to the synthesis of fullerene-containing polymers or polyfullerenes, and a large number of publications have reviewed those materials. Polyfullerenes can be classified into certain groups, including all-C_{60} polymers, cross-linked polymers, organometallic polymers, C_{60} dendrimers, end-capped polymers, star-shaped polymers, main chain polymers, side chain polymers, and supramolecular polymers. All-C_{60} polymers, also named "intrinsic polymers," can be synthesized via covalent linkage of fullerene units. Organometallic fullerenes can be considered as a kind of all-C_{60} polymers which contains a metal or element in their structures. The most favorable properties were attained via palladium copolymerization. Cross-linked polymers are a group of poly-fullerenes which can be synthesized by random reactions with assistance of C_{60}. Preparation of these cross-linked C_{60}-containing polymers can be performed by reaction of polymers with C_{60} randomly and in three dimensions. Another class of fullerene-containing polymers called fullerene dendrimers has regular branches and at least one fullerene molecule. Fullerene molecules can be located at the center, at the surface, or in the connection points of the dendrimer.

The end-capped polymers are considered a fascinating group of polyfullerenes which possess one or two fullerene molecules placed on the end of the polymer backbone and alter its properties. Fullerene units can be added after polymer synthesis, or otherwise, the growth of the polymer chain can start from the fullerene molecule itself. Star-shaped polymers containing a fullerene unit present from 2 to 12 long flexible chains with a topology similar to sea stars. These polyfullerenes can be prepared sing two approaches: (1) polymer chains can be linked to a fullerene unit, or (2) polymer chains can be grown from the surface of a fullerene unit.

Another class of C_{60}-containing polymers is the one in which fullerene units are placed in the backbone of a polymer and form a structure similar to a necklace. This polyfullerene can be synthesized by direct reaction of difunctionalized monomers and fullerene cage, and also by polycondensation between a fullerene bisadduct and difunctionalized monomers. The most studied group of C_{60}-containing polymers is side chain polymers. These polymers can be prepared in two ways, by direct reaction of fullerene units with preformed polymers or by functionalization of fullerene in order to be able to copolymerize with other monomers.

According to the synthetic method, supramolecular fullerenes are divided into four types: (1) interaction between fullerene and functionalized polymers; (2) fullerene derivative self-assembly; (3) multifunctionalization of C_{60} and complementary polymeric backbones; and (4) supplementary interactions between pristine fullerene and ditopic concave guests.

3.5 Toxicity and Biocompatibility Evaluation of Fullerenes

Since pristine and derivatized C_{60} can access intracellular space and accumulate into cell membrane and cytoplasm, they might be a threat to cell functioning and integrity. Physiochemical properties, ROS-related behavior, and toxicity of fullerene can generate different results, depending on the techniques employed for the solubilization of pristine C_{60}, including mechanical processing, long-term stirring in water, and chemical modifications that can change the general properties of pristine fullerene.

3.5.1 In Vitro Toxicity of Pristine and Derivatized Fullerene

The toxic effects of a fullerene colloid prepared with tetrahydrofuran (THF/nC_{60}) on different mammalian cells have been proven in a number of studies, which demonstrated ROS production, mitochondrial depolarization, and lipid peroxidation, resulting to necrotic cell death. One investigation to determine how THF affects fullerene toxicity *in vitro* has been done in 2009. The authors found that, in mouse macrophage cell line, the supernatant of THF/nC_{60} induces toxicity; rather, fullerene aggregates because of the presence of THF by-products, including γ-butyrolactone and formic acid. In fact, these by-products cause intracellular Ca^{2+} release, Ca^{2+} increase in mitochondria, and their perturbation. Therefore, the toxicity of THF/nC_{60} seems to be related to the method used for fullerene preparation rather than to the intrinsic properties of pristine fullerene. Another study also showed that THF peroxide is the main factor in the oxidative reactivity of THF/nC_{60}, and also, this THF derivative plays a significant role in the antibacterial activity of THF/nC_{60} toward *Escherichia coli*. In further studies, it has been confirmed that neither fullerene nor THF is responsible for toxicity, and indeed, THF by-products, such as γ-butyrolactone and THF hydroperoxide, induced toxicity, so extra washing steps to remove these by-products led to the absence of toxicity of THF/nC_{60} in *D. magna* and A549 lung cells. It seems that the fullerene functionalization degree can affect its tendency to form aggregates, and monofunctionalized molecules have more tendency to be aggregated than polyfunctionalized fullerenes, which are more stable in solution. Commonly, there is a belief that derivatization of fullerene can induce considerable decrease in toxicity for functionalized fullerenes. Therefore, highly soluble fullerenes have less cytotoxic activity, since the increase in the number of functional groups covalently attached reduces the ROS-generating capacity in fullerenes. Polyhydroxylated fullerenes (named fullerols or fullerenols), when irradiated with UV and visible light, produce singlet oxygen; although fullerenols produce less ROS than polymer-coated fullerenes, they induce photo-oxidative stress in human cells. However, at sub-cytotoxic concentration, fullerenols are able to scavenge hydroxyl radicals. Similarly to fullerenols, carboxyfullerenes are antioxidative/cytoprotective agents that, under light irradiation, exhibit cytotoxicity.

As mentioned, the ability of fullerene to penetrate cell membranes extensively influences its toxicity: cationic fullerene derivatives that can easily enter cells are more toxic than neutral and anionic fullerene derivatives. Parental administration of fullerenes in diagnostic and therapeutic applications, pulmonary exposure, and inhalation of fullerene nanoparticles may lead to cardiovascular adverse effects; therefore, a number of studies have evaluated fullerene cardiovascular toxicity. While C_{60} preparations obtained by sonication elicited platelet aggregation in a lower extent than other carbon nanoparticles, not developing thrombosis, organic solvent–prepared C_{60} was found to adhere to platelets, which may result in thrombosis.

As previously mentioned, the water-stirred C_{60} and fullerenols were found to induce intracellular Ca^{2+} increase and cause arrest in G1 cell cycle phase in human umbilical endothelial cells, although in the case of water-stirred C_{60}, no cell death was observed, while fullerenols cause apoptotic cell death, which may encourage coronary artery diseases and atherosclerosis. In another study, it was shown that fullerenols caused an accumulation of polyubiquitinated proteins and autophagy, leading to a decrease in cell density. In contrast with other fullerene nanoparticles and derivatives, hexasulfobutyl-C_{60} is able to inhibit low-density lipoprotein (LDL) from oxidation, so it can be effective in atherosclerosis prevention.

In addition to cardiovascular toxicity, the blood compatibility of fullerene in vitro has been investigated in a number of studies. THF/C_{60} causes oxidative stress–mediated lysis of erythrocyte cells associated with shrinkage and loss of their normal shape, while no intentional photoirradiation was applied. When fullerenes enter the bloodstream, they will translocate to the liver; therefore, investigation on the toxic effects of fullerenes on the liver seems to be important. γ-Cyclodextrin/C_{60}, upon photosensitization, triggers singlet oxygen-dependent oxidative stress in rat liver microsome, inducing protein oxidation and lipid peroxidation. The results obtained using polyhydroxylated fullerenes were similar to γ-cyclodextrin/C_{60}.

Further studies showed toxic effects of $C_{60}(OH)_{24}$ under ambient light on rat hepatocytes, which induced lipid peroxidation and depletion of intracellular ATP, leading to cell death, while $C_{60}(OH)_{12}$ exhibited less toxic effects. These results demonstrated that the toxicity effects of fullerenols are dependent on the number of hydroxyl groups present on the fullerene carbon cage, and probably to their solubility too.

Another cell type which has been tested for THF/C_{60} toxicity are canine kidney cells, and also, mouse renal epithelial cells were used to determine some toxicity of sonicated C_{60}, which decreases the transepithelial electrical resistance, an indicator of epithelial barrier function. Polyhydroxylated fullerene caused cytoskeleton disruption, mitochondrial dysfunction, followed by ATP depletion. The applications of fullerenes as drug carriers in order to bypass blood ocular barriers nudge researchers toward assessment of ocular toxicity of fullerene and its derivatives. Upon UV irradiation, g-cyclodextrin/C_{60} induced oxygen-mediated protein peroxidation which led to apoptotic cell death, while in dark or ambient light, no toxic effect was observed. The more aggregated γ-cyclodextrin/C_{60}, the less singlet oxygen production; therefore, fully aggregated fullerene showed no toxicity effect on lens cells. In an investigation of fullerenol toxicity, it has been observed that lower fullerenol concentrations caused oxidative damage to human lens epithelial cells under UV and visible light irradiation, while higher concentrations showed toxicity even in the dark. Another study reported that the toxic effect of fullerenol on retinal pigment epithelial cells was similar to its toxicity to human lens epithelial cells, indicating that the use of fullerenols in ocular application, especially in the presence of sunlight, may result in lens and/or retinal damage.

Solvent exchange–prepared THF/C_{60} nanoparticles, and also polyvinyl pyrrolidone/C_{60} complexes, can be immediately internalized by human keratinocytes and then accumulated in cytoplasm near the nucleus. It has been shown that THF/C_{60} nanoparticles decreased the growth of human keratinocytes, and under the light, its effect increased somewhat. However, further studies reported the toxic effect of THF/C_{60} nanoparticles on human keratinocytes, and also human dermal fibroblasts.

The complexes of C_{60} with γ-cyclodextrin, sodium dodecyl sulfate, or polyvinyl pyrrolidone prepared by mechanochemical approach have no cytotoxicity *in vitro*. In addition, they can reduce ROS generation, melanin production in human keratinocytes, and melanocytes under UV irradiation; this characteristic makes them applicable in skin care products, though γ-cyclodextrin/C_{60} under UVA irradiation caused oxidative stress in keratinocytes. In contrast to reports related to cytotoxic evaluation of polyhydroxylated fullerene, it has been found that $C_{60}(OH)_{32}$, unlike $C_{60}(OH)_{24}$ and $C_{60}(OH)_{20}$, in the absence of light, killed human keratinocytes, while other studies showed that, in human keratinocytes, polyhydroxylated fullerenes blocked DNA damage and oxidative stress induced by UV irradiation, so the increase of hydroxyl groups elevated the cytoprotective activity.

The reported results demonstrated that both antioxidant activity and toxicity in the dark rise with the increase in functionalization groups attached to fullerene cage, even though, in general, the definitive effect probably depends on the concentration. Polymer-coated fullerenes, in the absence of overt light irradiation, exhibited no toxicity towards neuronal cell lines. Carboxylated fullerene and hydroxylated fullerene also showed no toxicity to neural cell lines; however, they decreased the viability of primary mouse neurons.

Recently, an investigation has been accomplished in order to study the cytotoxicity of two types of fullerene solutions on Chinese hamster V-79 cells. Two fullerene solutions, one prepared via solvent exchange method and the other prepared via N-methylpyrrolidone (NMP), in which cluster size is smaller, were prepared and tested, and in both cases, no toxicity was reported in *in vitro* tests, demonstrating that N-methylpyrrolidone can be exploited as a solvent in preparing aqueous fullerene solutions.

3.5.2 In Vivo Toxicity of Pristine Fullerene and Derivatized Fullerene

Since nanoparticles are able to enter systemic circulation and exhibit systemic and local toxicity, *in vivo* evaluation of their toxicity seems to be significant. Moreover, *in vivo* tests can demonstrate fullerene toxicity more accurately than *in vitro*, as this approach simulates the body environment in a more satisfactory way. The first *in vivo* study was accomplished in

1996 by injecting an aqueous suspension of micronized C_{60} to rodents. In these experiments, C_{60} was demonstrated to be not deadly and did not show acute or sub-acute toxicity to this animal species.

Fullerenes are able to localize in lipid-rich regions like cell membranes, based on *in vitro* experiments, and they are redox-active. Additionally, as fullerene can form colloidal aqueous solution, the oxidative damage caused by fullerene has been studied in aquatic species, such as bass. The results have shown that, despite change in protein oxidation in any tissue, changes were observed in lipid peroxidation, in gill and liver lipid peroxidation, with their decrease, while, in contrast, the brain showed a trend of increased lipid peroxidation. These differences might be attributed to superior antioxidant defenses of gill and liver with respect to brain tissues, or fullerenes might reach the brain before the dissociation of colloids. Although this selective localization of fullerenes in cell membrane is fascinating, a balance between advantageous therapeutic and potential toxic effects can be avoided by coating the fullerenes.

Further studies have been performed on the animal exposure to atmosphere containing fullerene in order to investigate the effects of fullerene existing in urban atmospheres.

According to these results, C_{60} nanoparticles induce only transient lung inflammation and no pathologic changes in lung and also other tissues.

In order to evaluate fullerenol as a photodynamic therapy agent, it has been injected to mouse, and similar to pristine C_{60}, it was rapidly cleared from circulation and accumulated in liver, lung, and spleen. Moreover, the results demonstrated that fullerenol uptake by tumor cells was higher than normal tissue, and so it can be used as a photosensitizer in photodynamic therapy of some types of tumors.

A fullerene ammonium salt is also rapidly cleared from circulation; however, its rate is lower than that of pristine C_{60}. Most of it accumulates in the liver, and the rest in the lung, muscle, and skin. Similarly to pristine C_{60}, it did not reach the brain.

In addition to systemic administration of fullerene, a number of studies investigated the oral administration of fullerene. From these studies, it emerged that the gastrointestinal adsorption of fullerene and its consequent toxicity is low; however, in a number of experiments, oxidative damage of DNA mediated by pristine C_{60} has been reported, and this deserves substantial consideration.

Also, dermal toxicity of fullerene deserves special attention due to the cosmetic application of fullerene relating to its antioxidant activity. The penetration of C_{60} on pig skin depends on fullerene vehicle.

3.6 Types of Fullerenes and Their Specific Uses (C_{60}, C_{70}, Fullerenols)

Fullerene has many areas for use:

1. **Pharmaceutical:** Diagnostic reagents, superdrugs, cosmetics, nuclear magnetic resonance (NMR) with the developer, DNA affinity
2. **Energy:** Solar battery, fuel cell, secondary battery
3. **Industry:** Wear-resistant material, flame-retardant materials, lubricants, polymer additives, high-performance membrane, catalyst, artificial diamond, hard alloy, electric viscous fluid, ink filters, high-performance coatings, fire-retardant coatings, manufacturing bioactive materials, memory materials, embedded molecular and other characteristics, composite materials, etc.
4. **Information industry:** Semiconductor record medium, magnetic materials, printing ink, toner, ink, paper for special purposes
5. **Electronic parts:** Superconducting semiconductor, diodes, transistors, inductor, optical materials, electronic camera, fluorescence display tube, nonlinear optical materials.

3.6.1 Fullerenes C_{60}

In 1985, Professors Kroto and Smalley conducted experiments on the conversion of gaseous carbon into particles (soot), a phenomenon that occurs in stars. During the experiment, they found new stable structures, of which the most abundant was a molecule, C_{60}, which constitutes a new form of carbon; together with it, C_{70} was obtained to a lesser extent.

In C_{60}, each carbon atom is attached to three other atoms using sp^2 orbitals with an electron in each orbital. The fourth valence electron of each carbon would be in an orbital *p* perpendicular to the spherical surface. In this way, the orbitals overlap, forming a continuum of orbitals with electrons *p* inside and outside the sphere in the same way as it takes place in benzene with the six *p* electrons that give it the aromatic character. This means that we can consider fullerenes as an aromatic and stable sphere.

The structure of the C_{60} is similar to that of a soccer ball. It is shaped like a truncated icosahedron with 60 vertices, in each of which is carbon. It has 32 faces, of which 12 are pentagons, and the remaining 20 are hexagons; in addition, each pentagon is surrounded by five hexagons so that two pentagons cannot be adjacent to each other, but the six links of each hexagon are alternately fused to three pentagons and three hexagons.

As for the chemical behavior of this type of compounds, even though they are not aromatic in the sense of benzene, they experience double bond addition reactions (they cannot undergo substitution reactions since they do not have hydrogens). It is also able to react with chlorine at higher temperatures (>300°C).

It is important to keep in mind that the C_{60} carbons are equivalent (as in benzene), but not the bonds. C60 has two types of links, links 6–6 shared by adjacent hexagons and links 5–6 shared by a pentagon and a hexagon. Links 6–6 are shorter (1.39 A) than links 5–6 (1.43 A) and are more similar to double bonds, whereby most of the additions are carried out on link 6–6.

3.6.2 Applications of Fullerenes C_{60}

The importance of the discovery of these types of molecules is that it opens a new field of possible applications in the elaboration of new types of polymers, superconductors, structures with metals or with other atoms trapped within these carbon clusters, as well as new catalysts, pharmaceutical products, and other possible industrial applications. In the midst of other exciting applications, the electronic battery must be emphasized. The basis of these batteries is lithium cathodes. C_{60} fullerenes may also be used as additives for synthetic diamonds' high-pressure methods. Fullerenes may also be used in pharmacy for the creation of new pharmaceuticals. In addition, fullerenes found use as additives in fire-retardant paint.

3.6.3 Fullerenes C_{70}

C_{70} fullerene is the last of the three allotropic forms of carbon, after diamond and graphite. The molecule of fullerene that consists of 70 atoms of carbon is known as C_{70} fullerene. The "C" in code number (C_{70}) associated with fullerene denotes the atom of carbon, and the number 70 denotes the number of atoms present in a single molecule. C_{70} fullerene has a closed, hollow fused-ring structure that looks like a cage. The overall structure of C_{70} fullerene resembles a rugby ball; that is why they are often and commonly called "buckyball." These "buckyballs" are interconnected with 12 pentagons and 25 hexagons, in which the atom of carbon is present at each hexa- and pentagon's vertices, with a bond at each edge. A single atom of carbon is attached to the other three adjacent carbon atoms, bonded with single *s* and two *p* orbitals (sp^2 hybridization), which makes them stronger than the original ones, making them capable of making even stronger bonds. These formed molecules can undergo a variety of chemical reactions by accepting or donating an electron/s instantly.

C_{70} fullerene is a granular powder physically, dark brown in color. When sublimed, it changes its appearance to needle-like structures up to 5 mm in length, deep blue-black in color, with outer diameter of approximately 1 nm. Due to very bad delocalization of the electrons, C_{70} fullerenes are not "superaromatic." This is also a reason that it acts as an alkene, deficient in electrons, and reacts with an electron-efficient molecule rapidly.

3.6.4 Applications of Fullerenes C_{70}

C_{70} fullerenes find their applications in many domains. They are usually utilized as organic photovoltaics (OPVs). C_{70} fullerenes are powerful antioxidants which react instantly and at a great rate with free radicals, which are mostly a reason for cell death or damage. They are also deployed as catalysts in various chemical reactions, in the purification of water, protection of biohazard materials, production of portable power, and the field of medicine and vehicles.

3.6.5 Fullerenol

The derivatives of fullerenes that are soluble in water are called fullerenol. These molecules have the ability to remove free radicals. Fullerenols are commonly called "radical sponges" due to their characteristics of removing free radicals. They have great antioxidant properties due to the delocalized double pi-bond in the cages of fullerenes. They are mostly synthesized by the addition of the hydroxyl groups to C_{60} fullerene. Fullerenols possess a hollow spherical shape, like fullerenes.

3.6.6 Applications of Fullerenols

Fullerenols find the widest application in the field of science and technology. The ability of fullerenols to be soluble in water extends its uses in medical applications. They can be transformed into triplet state with the help of ultraviolet or visible light. The transformed material is very reactive and can rapidly react with oxygen or other biomolecules and finds its applications and uses in photosensitization. They are excellent antioxidants as well. Their dual nature enables them to act as cytotoxic materials in the diagnosis of tumors cells and as an immunity agent in normal cells to protect them.

Due to their spherical structure, they can be used for carrying contrast agents, drugs, and radiopharmaceuticals. They are also used to reduce oxidative stress during the transplantation of small intestine in dogs. They are used to protect the human lungs against oxidative damage. For their excellent pro-medical features, they are used in chemotherapy, radiobiology, and the diagnosis of neurodegenerative diseases. Due to their application in chemotherapy, they are excellent agents in the diagnosis and treatment of cancer and cancerous cells and tumors.

In brain tissue, biological oxidation is the most common. Biological oxidation occurs due to free radical formation. Fullerenols, or "radical sponges" are well-known agents to remove free radicals. They are utilized in the biological oxidation of brain tissue to remove free radicals, hence protecting the brain tissues from oxidation.

As the days and years pass by, more and more applications and reports on the utilization of fullerenols in various fields are coming out. But despite all the proven applications and advantages of fullerenols, there is still very insufficient knowledge of their mechanism of action and any of their side effects.

3.6.7 Other Types of Fullerenes

C_{60}, C_{70}, and fullerenol are not the only possible forms of fullerenes. There are, in fact, many types of structures that can be constructed with hexagons and pentagons. The interesting thing is that each type of structure must always contain 12 pentagons, whatever the number of hexagons. Pentagons are necessary to have a closed structure. The number of vertices in any form of fullerene is necessarily even. The smallest fullerene is the C_{20}, which contains 20 pentagons and no hexagons. However, this type of structure has strong internal tensions because the shape of each carbon molecule is strongly non-planar. Other possible fullerenes are C_{28}, C_{32}, C_{44}, C_{50}, C_{58}, C_{70}, C_{76}, C_{84}, C_{240}, C_{540}, C_{960}, and many others, as shown in Figure 3.9. Of the forms of fullerenes, the most common are C_{60} and C_{70}; the others are very rare.

Ju et al. presented a relationship between the Fowler–Manolopoulos hexagon indices and a particular hexagon structure count to provide a graphical interpretation. The complete list of different pentagon and hexagon combinations up to three connected faces is shown in Scheme 3.2.

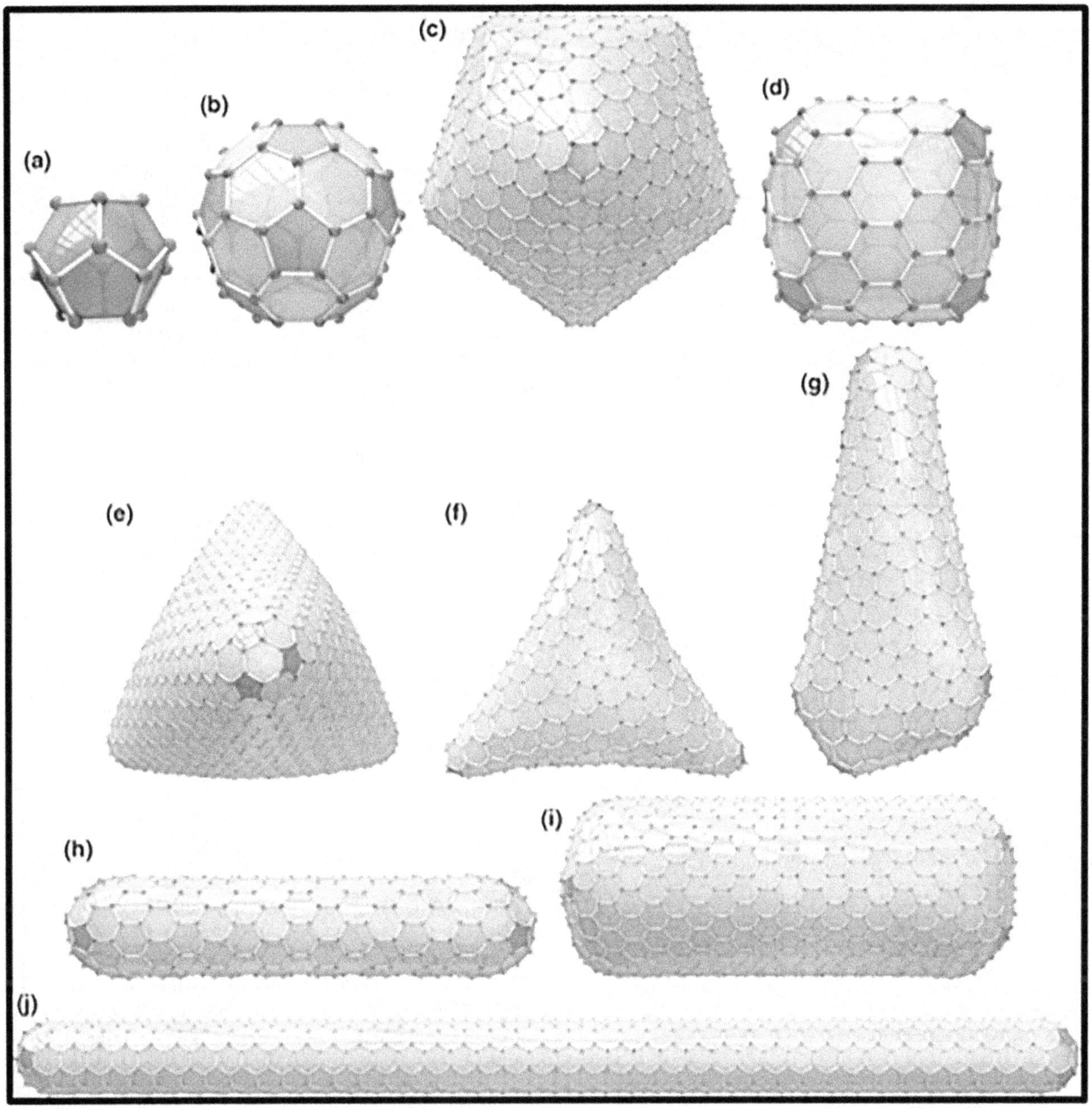

FIGURE 3.9 A selection of different 3D shapes for regular fullerenes (distributions of the pentagons DP are enclosed in parentheses). "Spherically" shaped (icosahedral), for example: (a) C20-Ih, (b) C60-Ih, and (c) C960-Ih (DP = 12 × 1); barrel shaped, for example: (d) C140-D3h (DP = 6 × 2); trigonal pyramidally shaped (tetrahedral structures), for example: (e) C1140-Td (DP = 4 × 3); (f) tetrahedrally shaped C440-D3 (DP = 3 × 4); (g) nano-cone or menhir C524-C1 (DP = 5 + 7 × 1); cylindrically shaped (nanotubes), for example: (h) C360-D5h, (i) C1152-D6d, (j) C840-D5d (DP = 2 × 6). The fullerenes shown in this figure and throughout the chapter have been generated automatically using the fullerene program.

Thus, fullerene is a carbon compound having a variety of types, of which the three important ones are C_{60}, C_{70}, and fullerenols. The fullerene carbon 60 consists of 60 carbon atoms which form a spherical surface of pentagons and hexagons. It looks like a football. These three forms of fullerenes have a wide range of applications, ranging from the medical sector to electronics. It was discovered by scientist Harold Kroto. He was awarded the Noble Prize for Chemistry for discovering this revolutionary material. Researchers are working on discovering more of their applications and aim to benefit from its unique characteristics in the future.

3.7 Uses of Fullerene

Fullerene has a variety of applications ranging from the medical sector to the electronic industry. It has excellent antioxidant and antibacterial properties, which encourage its use in

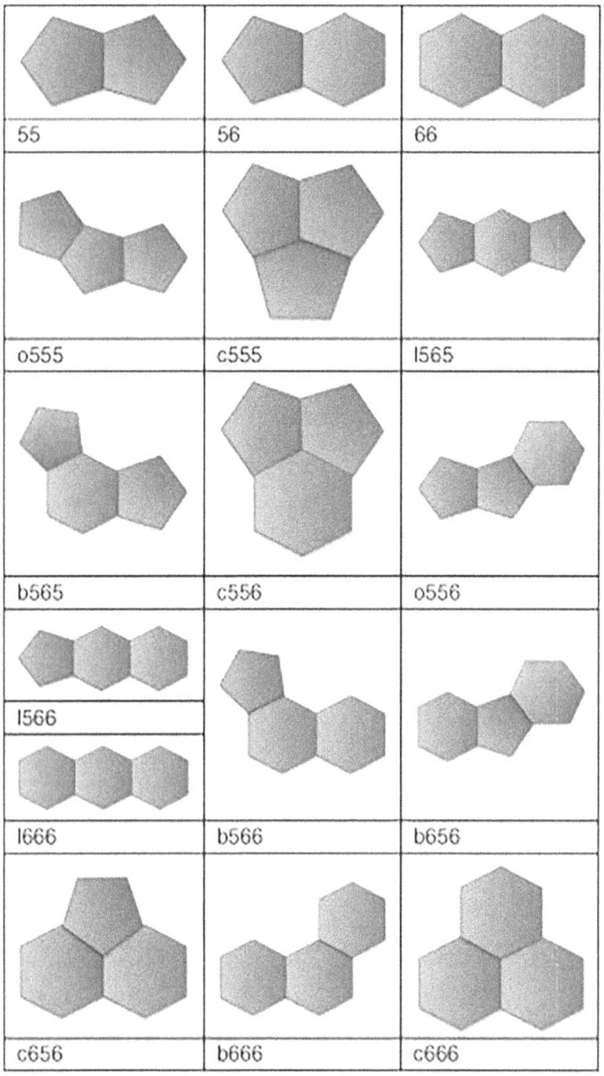

SCHEME 3.2 The 15 basic shapes for the two- and three-ring (face) adjacencies on the surface of a fullerene: denotes (a) linear, (b) bent, (o) open, and (c) closed ring patterns.

the medical sector. One of the important medical applications of fullerene is the controlled release of drugs. In the electronic industry, its applications can be found in solar cells, diodes, and semiconductors. Fullerene has great potential in the pharmaceutical sectors; its use in nanomedicine as well is of great importance. Fullerene may be used in pharmacy for the creation of new pharmaceuticals. The researchers are still busy in discovering more of its applications, and with the passage of time, the demand for various kind of fullerene will increase.

The applications of fullerenes range from molecular electronics, where they have interesting properties as rectifiers, to biomedicine, where, taking advantage of the fact that they are hollow, gadolinium atoms have been enclosed inside, which, thanks to their magnetic properties, increases the signal in resonance studies. Although these applications seem very promising, we have a molecular recycling problem. Nowadays, it is known how to enclose atoms within fullerenes and how to direct them towards a specific point of the organism, where they will perform their reparative work.

Fullerenes have been a focus of attention in the different fields of science since their discovery. Their properties and the physical characteristics that make them unique are the factors that make them unusual and appreciable materials. Fullerene has been used in the industry in different ways. For example, Bardahl used this material to include it in its oils, specifically in the manufacturing of the Technos C_{60} oil that provides a triple protection layer. It has various applications, such as surface coating, conductive devices, and the creation of molecular networks. In addition, within the field of medicine, a water-soluble fullerene showed activity against human immunodeficiency virus that causes AIDS; it can even be used as an antioxidant.

3.7.1 Fullerene as a Material for Semiconductor Technology

The molecular crystal of fullerene is a semiconductor with a bandgap of ~1.5 eV, and its characteristics are almost similar to those of other semiconductors. It has conventional applications in electronics, such as in diodes, transistors, photocells, etc.

3.7.2 Uses of Fullerenes in Solar Cells

Fullerenes, as spherical three-dimensional allotropes, are another class of the magic carbon derivatives with interesting properties and applications in nanoscience, medicine, and industry based on their remarkable electronic property. The world has now become a place where a lot of unexpected events take place day in and day out. As fullerenes show excellent antiviral behavior, their use can extensively be supported to fight viral attacks, which have been claiming millions of lives.

Due to its electronic characteristics, one of the most advanced applications is its use in solar cells. Since the 1990s, light-induced processes in supramolecular and multicomponent systems involving C_{60} molecules have been the subject of intensive research. Such interest is due to the property that fullerene has to accept electrons; in this way, if the C_{60} binds to a molecule that yields these electrons when it is exposed to light, we can manufacture devices that mimic the photosynthetic processes that occur in plants and thus obtain solar cells.

Using organic polymers composed of fullerenes, attempts are made to emulate the processes of photosynthesis of nature. There is a possibility that paints composed of fullerenes can be applied on any surface and become photovoltaic, generating electricity, but integrated into the environment. Instead of uncomfortable and aesthetic plates, electricity is generated by painting, for example, the exterior walls of buildings. It is also tried to draw electronic circuits with simple techniques similar to graphic printing, instead of the expensive and complex current systems.

3.7.3 Fullerenes in Electronic Battery

The electronic battery must be emphasized in the midst of other exciting applications which use fullerenes. The bases of these batteries are lithium cathodes. Fullerenes can also be used as additives for synthetic diamonds' high-pressure method. It increases the output by 30%.

3.7.4 Fullerenes for Photovoltaic Applications

Fullerenes' strong electron-accepting qualities with lower energy electron transmission process have made them potential and considerable components in artificial photosynthetic applications. They have found emerging attraction in electronics, photocatalysis, and photovoltaic devices since they interact well with electron donor groups, forming a donor–acceptor system to generate long-lived charge-separated electronic states. Some common organic donor groups linked to fullerenes cage are phthalocyanines, ruthenium complexes, metalloporphyrins, cyanines, boron-dipyrrins, and tetrathiafulvalenes. Also, polymer organic field-effect transistors as a class of polymer transistors that have shown to adopt improved performance.

3.7.5 Fullerenes in Fire-Retardant Paint

In addition, fullerenes found use as additives in fire-retardant paint. Due to the introduction of fullerenes, paint, under the influence of temperature, swells in case of fire; there is a fairly dense layer which builds up a couple of times while being heated to a critical temperature of the protected structures. Fullerenes and its different chemical derivatives are used in combination with semiconducting polymers for the production of solar units.

3.7.6 Incorporation of Fullerenes in Polymers

Due to the incorporation of fullerenes in the polymers, electroactive and optical-limiting properties would be achieved. This could mainly be applied in surface coating, conductive devices, and the creation of new molecular networks.

Once again, fullerenes' exceptional electronic behavior makes them qualified agents to be used in the polymer industry. Fullerene-based polymers are synthesized by angular attachment of fullerenes to a polystyrene through Friedel–Crafts reaction or indirect biding of fullerene C_{60} groups like Pt (aba)2, Pt (cad)2, and Pd2(aba)3 $CHCl_3$. The reaction with each one of these spacer agents displaces the ligands in order for them to be insoluble PtC60, which are originally reduction-oxidization active polymers based on fullerenes. Moreover, these polymers can also be produced through reducing fullerenes under cathodic conditions in an electrochemical method.

3.7.7 Growth Potential of Fullerenes

Harold Kroto, awarded the Nobel Prize in Chemistry in 1996 for the discovery of Mr. Fuller's balls, is still active and has surprised the entire scientific community with his latest publication in the journal *Nature Communications*. It describes the discovery that fullerenes are self-assembling through a closed network growth mechanism, that is, the trick of the formation of buckyballs was in their growth, by incorporating or absorbing carbon atoms and molecules. This discovery was not simple; it required a lot of ingenuity and a bit of luck, since the fullerene formation happened in an instant. They started with a few fullerene molecules mixed with carbon and helium and shot them with a very powerful laser, and instead of destroying the fullerenes, they were surprised to find that they had actually grown.

3.8 Fullerene in Biomedical Applications and Its Role in Drug Delivery

Fullerenes are hollow, inert, and indefinitely modifiable. They are not absorbed in water-soluble form when given orally, but they get quickly distributed to various tissues of the body when given through IV. They are excreted by the kidney without any change. Fullerenes are widely used for many biomedical applications, like in photodynamic therapy, gene and drug delivery, etc.

Comprehensive research on the biomedical applications of this molecule has been underway since its discovery. The greatest challenge that scientists faced in doing so was their insolubility in aqueous media and their tendency to form aggregates. This was overcome with the use of several techniques, such as encapsulation of fullerenes with hydrophilic molecules, suspending this molecule with other solvents, and conjugating it with other hydrophilic molecules.

A lot of biomedical applications have been suggested for fullerene mainly in biomedicine, including photosensitivity, antioxidation, antiviral activities, drug carrying, and tissue engineering and antioxidation. In a study, the gap in HIV-1 protease was tightly packed with C_{60} buckyball to form a protease–fullerene complex capable of eliminating and inactivating the activities of viruses. The C_{60} and fullerene family derivatives can bind to protease and trigger antiviral activity. In particular, fullerenes' amino acid complexes cause the inhibition of viral replication through fullerenes binding to divalent metal ions and subsequently penetrating bilayer lipids, changing the effect of membranes' enzymes. Fullerenes are hollow, inert, and indefinitely modifiable. They are not absorbed in water-soluble form when given orally, but they get quickly distributed to various tissues of the body when given through IV. They are excreted by the kidney without any change. Fullerenes are widely used for many biomedical applications, like in photodynamic therapy, gene and drug delivery, etc.

3.8.1 Fullerenes' Use in Nanomedicine

Another important field of use is nanomedicine. It is about enclosing beneficial molecules for the organism inside fullerene balls and directing them to bacteria or cancer cells. Upon reaching the destination, the spheres are dissolved, releasing all their content at the appropriate points, thus displaying all their effectiveness without being lost along the way.

3.8.2 Fullerenes against Viruses

In oxygen-rich environments, fullerenes can be excited from the ground state to rich a high energy level. Later, the fullerene energy can be transferred to oxygen to generate singlet oxygen.

This causes given viruses to lose the ability to infect and harm a tissue. The superoxide onions and singlet oxygen are incredibly reactive with DNA, which can, in turn, facilitates tumor cells killing and termination due to cytotoxicity properties. Fullerenes can attract electrons and free radicals since there is an abundance of carbon–carbon double bonds and LUMO orbitals, which make them very interactive to free radicals. Fullerenes can also engage in reactions with superoxide compounds in the case of an illness and recognize the free radicals within mitochondria to sustain their membrane integrity, with the subsequent cell protection from apoptosis and toxins [6].

3.8.3 Therapeutic Effect of Fullerenes in Nervous System

Fullerenes have therapeutic effects when the nervous system is vulnerable to damage by oxidizing agents and free radicals and has a limited capacity for regeneration. It has been found that fullerenes can protect neurons in the central nervous system [5].

3.8.4 Tumor Research and Antitumor Drugs

In cancer research, HeLa cells were used in recent experiments. This includes the production of new photosensitizers, which get absorbed by cancer cells and still trigger the death of the cell. To prevent damage to the cell, the body should not contain a new photosensitizer in it for long. When cancer cells absorb them, they get exposed to light radiation, creating reactive oxygen that damages the lipids, proteins, and DNA that make up the cancer cell. The cellular-level damage leads to the cancer cell going through apoptosis, which causes a reduction in tumor size. When the light radiation treatment ends, free radicals will be reabsorbed by the fullerenes to prevent tissue damage. The treatment may penetrate deeper into the body and be absorbed effectively by cancer cells in the near future.

Monoclonal antibody usually targets melanoma tumors. By combining a monoclonal antibody with multiple fullerenes, multiple drugs can be delivered to different tumors. Normally, multiple targeting agents are used in other methods to deliver individual drug-loaded nanoparticles to malignant cells, but the new way is better. It is proved that melanoma tumors get anticancer drugs delivered inside them through gp240, which is a tumor protein, and *ZME-018* binds itself to this protein, while the Rice group has been developing fullerenes as drug delivery agents.

3.8.5 Crossing the Blood–Brain Barrier

The blood–brain barrier is made of tight endothelial junctions that inhibit paracellular permeability, thus creating a big task to deliver drugs into the central nervous system. Fullerene and its water-soluble derivatives have a high potential to complete that task. In research, fullerene and hexamethonium complex systems were established, and it was compared with the delivery system of only hexamethonium. Forty times boosted potency was shown as a result of a complex delivery system of drugs. Also, neurodegeneration because of amyotrophic lateral sclerosis (ALS) can be treated by carboxyl-fullerenes. The brain's tight complex structure does not allow any chemical to pass through the barrier naturally, but delivery systems that are fullerene-based do not obey this and deliver the drug through their tight complex structures.

3.8.6 Fullerenes for Topical Drug Delivery and Controlled Release of Drugs

Fullerenes are used in cosmetic applications and transdermal delivery because of its antioxidant activity and its interactions with epidermal keratinocytes, which provides many spectacular abilities to them. Due to these properties, different forms are used often, like anti-inflammatory substances, moisturizers, cytoprotective and barrier-repair agents, UVB inhibitory agents, antimelanoma-genesis agents, and hair growth stimulators. In the drug delivery area, fullerene-based peptides showed satisfactory penetration, in comparison with mechanical flexion. Isopropyl myristate/Transcutol formulations with basic cosmetics without tough organic solvents proved to be good for cosmetics and biopharmaceutical applications. There are also a few publications on the use of fullerenes and noncovalently adsorbed drugs (fullerenes displaying stability at room temperature); that is why, when at optimum concentration, efficient and acceptable transdermal drug delivery is presented.

Due to selectivity, controlled release, and the decent biocompatibility of fullerenes, they are regarded as potential drug carriers for cells. If the right hydrophilic groups are attached to the fullerenes, they turn water-soluble and act exceptionally in gene and drug delivery. Studies have shown that DNA-functionalized fullerenes have remarkably been effective in lipid-based vectors.

Fullerene is an interesting element for the controlled release of drugs. Because they can be multifunctional, they can act as "absorbents" of drugs to form particles on a nanometric scale. An example of this is the derivative of the fullerene called methanofullerene, which, together with certain drugs that are used against cancer, has demonstrated an important activity in tissues and the slow and prolonged release of the drug.

Among the conventional methods for delivering drugs, oral and injection administration are the most used. In addition to these methods, there are some alternative approaches, including pulmonary, transdermal, transmucosal, ocular administration, and implantation. By using drug delivery systems, including nanoparticle carriers, the pharmacokinetics can be dramatically improved. Transferring bioactive elements like proteins, DNAs, and also various small molecules through the membrane into cells (cellular delivery) has drawn considerable attention due to its essential role in medicine and drug delivery, and the possibility to reach the cell nucleus is even more limited by various barriers and really challenging. Numerous nanoparticles can be used for targeted drug delivery and controlled release due to their biocompatibility and incredible characteristics, and fullerene exhibits a great potential in drug delivery systems.

Geometry, size, and surface of the fullerene cage seem to be appropriate for this application, considering its diameter in the range of 1 nm, approximately half of the average diameter of a DNA helix. Despite the hydrophobicity of fullerene cage, as already mentioned, it can be functionalized by hydrophilic moieties, achieving water solubility, and be used as drug carrier for bioactive molecules in the biological environment. The first attempt in this field has been accomplished by Nakamura et al., who synthesized two-handed tetraamino fullerenes which bound duplex DNA; therefore, these DNA–fullerene nanoparticles are capable of entering COS-1 cells. Foley et al. demonstrated that a fullerene derivative, $C_{61}(COOH)_2$, can cross the cell membrane and also localize into mitochondria; therefore, it can be used in organelle-targeted drug delivery. A fullerene derivative bearing two diamino side chains was used for gene delivery to mammalian cells, entering the cell by endocytosis. Rouse et al. proved that fullerene-based peptides are able to penetrate intact skin and, accordingly, can be applied in drug delivery; moreover, the authors also found that mechanical flexion can increase the penetration rate of the nanoparticles into the dermis.

The main positive point in fullerene-based drug delivery systems is their ability to carry multiple drug payloads like Taxol plus other chemotherapeutic drugs. This approach is really beneficial in cancer treatment, since cancer cells are easily drug-resistant, and effective treatment often needs the combination of more than one type of drug to overcome the resistance mechanism.

A drug delivery system containing fullerene and paclitaxel ranging in about 120–145 nm was proposed in order to perform aerosol liposome delivery of paclitaxel for lung cancer treatment. The half-life of paclitaxel in bovine serum was 80 min, and paclitaxel release took place by enzymatic hydrolysis.

Buckysomes, the spherical nanostructure made of amphiphilic fullerenes which present many hydrophobic regions, can embed hydrophobic molecules like paclitaxel, a very hydrophobic anticancer drug, inside its hydrophobic pockets. This spherical nanocarrier has been synthesized in aqueous environment and presents a diameter in order of 100–200 nm. Buckysomes were compared to Abraxane, which has also been used for delivering paclitaxel to suppress MCF-7 breast cancer cells. The results demonstrated that paclitaxel-embedded buckysomes can deliver higher amount of paclitaxel than Abraxane.

A new class of water-soluble fullerene-based transfecting agents has been synthesized using Hirsch–Bingel chemistry, and its ability in gene delivery has been evaluated: these derivatives can complex DNA, deliver it into cells, and evoke gene expression.

Doxorubicin, as mentioned previously, is a precious anticancer drug but induces acute and chronic side effects. In order to mitigate its side effects, one strategy is the use of drug delivery systems. Fullerenes, due to their antioxidant and radical scavenging activity, have the potential to be conjugated with DOX and to mitigate the DOX side effects triggered by ROS. The challenge in this approach is that DOX is water-soluble while fullerene is hydrophobic, so Sun et al. used ethylene glycol spacers for conjugating methano-C_{60} with DOX, improving the water solubility of the vector. In a similar attempt, fullerenols were conjugated to doxorubicin through a carbamate linker in order to promote an efficient delivery. This conjugation repressed the cancer cell proliferation *in vitro* by blocking G2-M cell cycle, causing apoptosis. In addition, the fullerenol–doxorubicin conjugate exhibited high antitumor activity *in vivo* in a murine tumor model, without causing systemic toxicity like free DOX.

An "on–off" drug delivery system for cancer treatment has been developed by the conjugation of DOX and fullerene (C_{60}) following attachment of the hydrophilic shell (distearoyl-sn-glycero-3-phosphoethanolamine-PEG-CNGRCK2HK3HK11, DSPE-PEG-NGR) to the outer surface of the conjugation. This drug delivery system has strong stability in physiological solutions even with pH around 5.5 in the "off" state; in contrast, in the "on" state, the generation of ROS by C_{60} results in the breaking of the ROS-sensitive linker, which enables the exploding release of DOX. In this innovative drug delivery system, the combination of photodynamic therapy and chemotherapy could be applied against tumor cells.

Furthermore, fullerenes were conjugated to other species, like nitroxide radicals, to preserve normal tissue and cells against chemotherapy; they can also be conjugated to metal complexes, such as cisplatin, which is widely used for cancer chemotherapy. Also, in this case, the anticancer activity against Lewis lung carcinoma cells of the conjugate was more efficient than the free drug.

In line with fullerene drug delivery applications, porphyrin adducts of cyclohexyl-fullerene were prepared for targeted delivery of Mg^{2+} to heart muscles, which resulted in 80% recovery of tissue hypoxia symptoms less than 24 hours after a single injection. Release of Mg^{2+} by nanoparticles stimulated ATP overproduction in oxygen-depleted cells. Since these smart nanoparticles release Mg^{2+} cations just in reaction to the metabolic acidic shift, the positive changes in heart cell energy metabolism can help the treatment and prevent local myocardial hypoxic disorders and protect heart muscles in different hypoxia-caused clinical situations.

Fullerenes have also been used in delivery of bioactive molecules like warfarin, a coumarin anticoagulant drug. Conjugation of warfarin to fullerene can alter its biological profile and prevent variation of its concentration in the blood. Erythropoietin (EPO), a hormone mainly produced by kidneys, can also be linked to fullerenes and carbon nanotubes. EPO usually is administered through intravenous injection, although its biological activity is reduced abruptly in this route. Nanoparticulate systems can be used for the effective administration of EPO: for example, EPO was absorbed on porous materials containing fullerene, and its bioavailability was intensely enhanced compared to conventional administration.

The highly water-soluble and non-cytotoxic fullerene derivative malonodiserinolamide C_{60} (C_{60}-Ser), was investigated as a delivery system. The internalization of PF-633 fluorophore conjugated with C_{60}-Ser (C_{60}-SerPF) within living cancer cells was observed. In addition, *in vivo* experiments in mouse bearing liver tumor demonstrated that C_{60}-SerPF permeated through the vasculature of the tumor and was detected in many tissues. In another study, PEI-derivatized C_{60} was prepared by cationic polymerization of aziridine on the surface of C_{60}-NH_2. Then, PEI-C_{60} was decorated with folic acid (FA) via amide linker, and docetaxel (DTX) was conjugated to C_{60}-PEI-FA, resulting in a complex drug delivery system able to cross cell membranes and to cause apoptosis in tumor cells, exhibiting higher antitumor efficacy than free DXT, without toxic effects on normal tissues. Recently, another fullerene-based drug delivery system has been prepared via grafting hyaluronic acid (HA) onto fullerene and combining this with transferrin (Tf), which has antitumor efficacy and also can be used in photodynamic therapy. Artesunate, an iron-dependent antimalarial drug, which is cytotoxic against tumor cells, was loaded into HA-C_{60}-Tf with a high loading efficiency. The *in vitro* and *in vivo* evaluation of this system demonstrated its high antitumor efficacy.

3.8.7 Nucleic Acid Delivery and DNA Photocleavage

C_{60} derivatives cytotoxicity was mediated by its DNA-cleaving capability. So other usages of fullerenes are related to its easy photoexcitation; that is why photodynamic compounds, which are fullerene-based, are being established for cancer treatment.

Targeted delivery to cells that has a deficiency in a nucleic acid is important. Mostly, viral delivery is used. In some research, due to their high efficacy, low cost, and non-immunological reactions, fullerenes, especially cationic ones, were used to transport small molecules. These complexes form micrometer particles by agglutinating in the bloodstream further with plasma proteins. The agglutinate rapidly clogs capillaries of lungs, releasing siRNA into cells of the lung to silence the targeted cancer gene expression, and after delivery of siRNA, it is rapidly cleared from the lung. It is proved that conjugated nucleic acids are used with fullerene-based delivery systems to increase the efficacy in a target-specific manner.

3.8.8 Cancer Treatment and Photodynamic Therapy

Cancer nanotechnology, using nanoscale materials or techniques to overcome the fatal hurdles in cancer treatment or detection, is a newly emerging area.

PDT is important in the treatment of diseases from a small infection to cancer. PDT's key limitation is that many photosensitizers have poor water solubility. Fullerenes have great advantages, some of them including their PDT potential—visible light's absorption combined with an efficient intersystem crossing to a long-lived triplet state which, on illumination, causes fullerenes to generate ROS and act as photosensitizers. In past years, many substances have been produced that are conjugated with fullerenes. The major problem was that the effects on cancer cells and on healthy cells were equal, but delivery systems based on fullerene increase the absorption in cancerous cells and decrease it in healthy cells, thus solving the problem.

Targeted delivery is required when it comes to cancer therapy; fullerenes offer that more efficiently. One other drawback in normal cancer therapy is that the use of multiple drugs is needed, but fullerene's remarkable structure gives it the capability to carry a payload of multiple drugs, which could solve many of chemotherapy's side effects. Doxorubicin side effects, like cardiomyopathy, make it an applicant for conjugation with fullerene, and then after conjugation, their outer surface attaches with the hydrophilic shell, developing a new strategy of "on–off" for delivering drug which causes the formation of novel, new drug delivery systems which are very stable in physiological solutions even in the "off" state, with pH 5.5; by contrast, ROS generation by fullerene leads to two types of treatment in the "on" state: first, oxygen species generation, which causes cell death (PDT), and, second, ROS-sensitive linkers getting broken, which enables doxorubicin's exploding release (chemotherapy).

As will be discussed in the next item, fullerenes have been known as radical scavenger and antioxidant agents, but paradoxically, they can also act as oxidants. In fact, they are able to promote the production of ROS within cells and consequently can stimulate the development of oxidative stress in some circumstances.

It was assumed that covalent bonds of fullerene react with ROS and form covalent bonds; however, this assumption made difficult to explain how fullerenes produce ROS during photodynamic therapy. Andrievsky et al. reported that hydrated fullerenes can inactivate ROS by the ordered "water coat" rather than covalently scavenging free radicals, considering that the ordered "water coat" can trap two hydroxyl radicals for enough time to react with each other and generate less-reactive hydrogen peroxide species.

One of the cancer treatment strategies using fullerenes is light-based therapies, such as photodynamic therapy and photothermal therapy (PTT). Photodynamic therapy is a noninvasive and nonsurgical treatment for some type of tumors and some non-malignant diseases. Photodynamic is a photochemical method that uses photosensitizing agents (photosensitizer [PS]) and light irradiation to produce reactive oxygen species in tumor tissue to induce damage and apoptosis. The schematic of this process is shown in Figure 3.10.

Fullerenes can be applied as possible PS for photodynamic therapy. Functionalization of the fullerene molecule can promote its capability to produce reactive species which can mediate PDT in medicinal applications. When C_{60} is irradiated with visible light, it can be excited from S_0 ground state to a short-lived state, S_1, excited state. S_1 quickly decays to lower-lying triplet state T_1, which has a long lifetime (50–100 μs; eq. (1)).

$$C_{60} + h\nu \rightarrow {}^1C_{60^*} \rightarrow {}^3C_{60^*} + {}^3O_2 \rightarrow C_{60} + {}^1O_{2^*} \quad (1)$$

In the presence of dissolved oxygen (${}^3O_2$), existing as a triplet in its ground state, fullerene T_1 is quenched to produce singlet oxygen (${}^1O_2$). So pristine and functionalized fullerenes are able to catalyze ROS production upon light irradiation. *In vitro* studies for the evaluation of fullerene in photodynamic therapeutic applications were implemented in the 1990s. Tokuyama et al. proved the phototoxic effect of fullerene functionalized with carboxylic acid on human cervical carcinoma cells. The toxicity and superoxide production ability of water-soluble polyethylene glycol fullerene derivative under visible light were demonstrated. The phototoxicity of pristine and functionalized fullerene has also been demonstrated in carcinoma cells by ROS generation: the phototoxicity of dendritic C_{60} monoadduct and TMA-C_{60} derivatives was investigated on Jurkat cells (T-lymphocytes) under UV irradiation, and the results

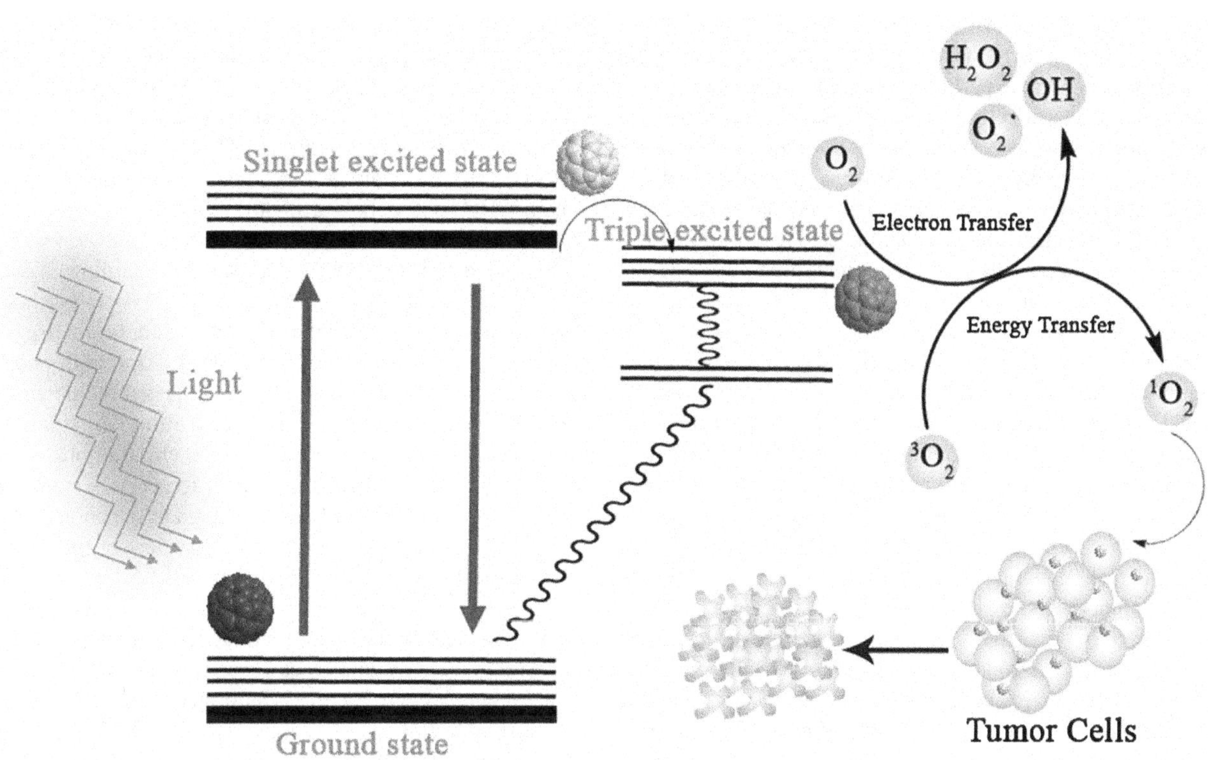

FIGURE 3.10 Schematic of photodynamic therapy with fullerene as photosensitizers.

showed that tris-malonic acid derivative is more phototoxic than dendritic one in killing Jurkat cells. The biodistribution and tumor uptake of $C_{60}(OH)_x$ has also been investigated in five kinds of mouse bearing tumors, demonstrating the utility of this derivative as a photosensitizer in photodynamic therapy of some tumors.

One of the most soluble fullerene copolymers, C_{60}-N vinylpyrrolidone, under visible light irradiation, demonstrated its potential as a photodynamic therapy agent. Mroz et al. studied the photodynamic activity of cationic and hydrophilic functionalized fullerene toward mouse cancer cell lines. They showed that the fulleropyrrolidinium salt could be used as an efficient photosensitizer for killing cancer cell by inducing apoptosis under illumination with the-already mentioned mechanism. The phototoxic activity of porphyrin-C_{60} dyad (p-C_{60}, its schematic shown in Figure 3.11) on Hep-2 human larynx-carcinoma cells was assessed. The dyad has the potential to form photoinduced charge-separated state and can act as a photodynamic agent for cell inactivation. The mechanism by which P-C_{60} induced apoptosis was caspase-3-dependent. Zhao et al. evaluated the phototoxicity of four different forms of fullerene prepared by solvent exchange and using dispersant agent: the results showed all four preparation have potential in photogeneration of singlet oxygen and superoxide. While in the dark no cytotoxicity was observed, the main photoinduced cytotoxic activity was due to singlet oxygen rather than superoxides. The photodynamic activity of fullerene toward HeLa cells has been investigated.

In vitro experiments to evaluate the photodynamic therapeutic applications of pullulan-fullerene derivative showed that it can prevent the growth of HepG2 hepatoma cells, while experiments via intravenous injection exhibited stronger antitumor activity in comparison with C_{60}-PEG conjugate or saline. Nobusawa et al. developed pH-sensitive

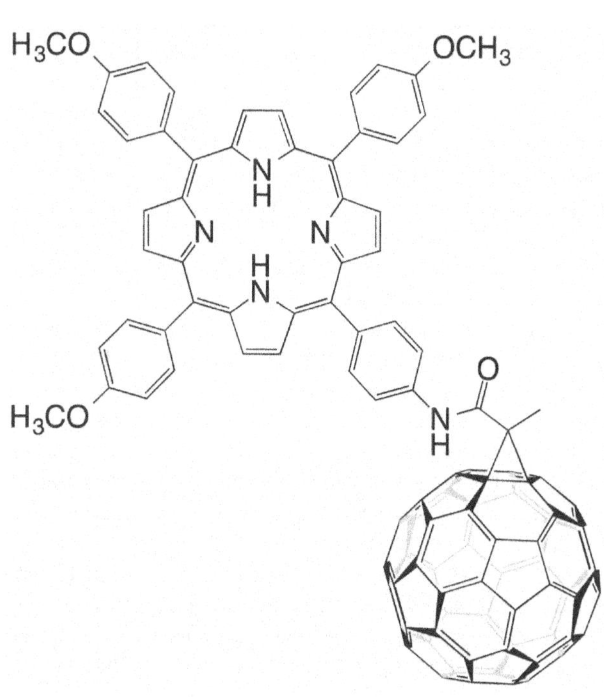

FIGURE 3.11 Molecular structure of PS porphyrin–C_{60} dyad.

6-amino-g-cyclodextrin (ACD) as carrier for C_{60} in order to release it for photodynamic activities on the acidic surface of cancer cells. In vitro experiments showed that ACD/C_{60} can be taken up into cancer cells. In the same year, a fullerene derivative has been synthesized using L-phenylalanine, L-arginine, and folic acid in order to alter fullerene's limited solubility, which leads to lower singlet production in photodynamic therapy. The results demonstrated that the uptake of this fullerene derivative in HeLa cells was higher than in normal cells, and the subsequent photoirradiation raises $^1O_2/O_2^{\bullet-}$generation and induces cell apoptosis.

A newer approach for cancer treatment implies the combination of C_{60} derivatives with other molecules. For instance, Shi et al. coupled iron oxide nanoparticles with C_{60} and functionalized it with PEG in order to improve its solubility. This nanocomposite can be used for photodynamic therapy and MRI, and also as a drug delivery system if in combination antitumor drug hematoporphyrin monomethyl ether (HMME). In this case, the photodynamic effect is higher than for free HMME. Also, a complex of C_{60} with γ-cyclodextrin polymer has been synthesized in order to improve phototoxicity of fullerene and make it more water-soluble, with higher efficacy in producing singlet oxygen and killing cancer cells under UV irradiation.

Later, a drug delivery system including C_{60}-PEI, a fullerene derivative loaded with doxorubicin (DOX, an anticancer drug), was developed to combine chemo- and photodynamic therapy for cancer treatment. The DOX release in this system is greatly dependent on pH values and in acidic condition (as in tumor cells). DOX was released with higher speed, with good inhibition of B16-F10 cell growth *in vitro*, and in *in vivo* experiment, good tumor suppression in murine melanoma cancer. Moreover, the side effects were lowered than in free DOX. The results gave credit to C_{60}-PEI-DOX to be used as a nanomedicine for cancer treatment. In other studies, a C_{60}-DOX combination was developed as an antitumor complex. At first, Prylutskyy et al. examined the structural and physiochemical properties of fullerene–DOX complex for tumor inhibition, and in a later study, they compared the antitumor activity of a fullerene–DOX combination with pristine fullerene and DOX themselves, used separately, in the treatment of Lewis lung carcinoma in male mice. Based on their results, the combination of fullerene and DOX was more efficient in inhibiting the tumor growth in *in vivo* models, and it could be used as an effective approach in antitumor therapy.

Additionally, a fullerene–DOX complex was investigated for its cytotoxic activity in tumor therapy, and the results revealed that the presence of fullerene improved the cytotoxic effect of DOX toward tumor cells by increasing hydrogen peroxide cellular production, although in *in vivo* model, the effect was more noticeable than that in *in vitro* experiments. These results are somewhat in contrast with a foregone study that has been carried out in 2005 which demonstrated that fullerenol has modulating effects on three antitumor drugs (DOX, cisplatin, and Taxol) when administered in combination. Further research and investigation on C_{60}–DOX complex have been developed, and recently, Prylutskyy et al. proved that C_{60}–DOX heterocomplexation is responsible for their synergy in physiological media. Recently, it has been proven that fullerene acts as an interceptor for DOX, and the hetero-complex of C_{60}–DOX performs as a nanocarrier for delivering doxorubicin to target cells. The attractive point is that the conclusion derived from these experiments can be generalized to other aromatic drugs, like actinomycin D, mitoxantrone, and topotecan.

The conjugation of Hoechst 33258–hyaluronate fullerene (Ho-HF) was examined to evaluate its antitumor activity against HCT-116 cells via photodynamic treatment *in vitro*, exploiting Ho–HF conjugation to improve the PDT efficacy of fullerene. Self-assembled microspheres containing fullerene-phenylalanine-polylactic acid (C_{60}-Phe-PLA) were synthesized in order to carry mitoxantrone (MTX), an antitumor drug. The combination of sustained release of MTX and high photodynamic activity of C_{60}-Phe-PLA demonstrated the potential of effective cancer treatment along with minimum side effects on normal tissues. In a recent study, a chitosan oligosaccharide was grafted on fullerene in order to generate endogenous ROS in mitochondria in human malignant melanoma (A375) cells, and results demonstrated that a low dose of fullerene can encourage the generation of endogenous ROS.

The influence of fullerene nanoparticles on the effectiveness of microwave heating for cancer treatment has been reported in this study; the combination of microwave heating and C_{60} was encapsulated in Pluronic F127-chitosan nanoparticles, a highly water-soluble fullerene derivative which can be taken up by the cells and improve the outcomes of microwave hyperthermia for killing cancerous cells. Various fullerene derivatives, separately or in conjugation with other materials, were utilized to assess their efficacy in the photodynamic treatment of cancers: the overall results showed that fullerenes are promising nanoparticles used in different cancer therapeutic approaches. Moreover, the combination with a number of antitumor drugs suggested that these constructs could be a promising approach in cancer therapy, even though further developments in this field require more advanced investigations.

3.8.9 Free Radical Scavenging and Antioxidant Activity

Fullerene compounds have a unique cage structure, combine in the core with numerous conjugated double bonds, interact with biomolecules, and have avid reactivity with free radicals. Fullerene derivatives' protective effect is explained in numerous systems, containing reduced injury on the ischemia-reperfusion intestine, protecting different types of cells from going through apoptosis, reducing the free radical level in organ perfusion, and neuroprotective effect. Derivatives of fullerene have shown good results in pre-toxicity studies. Also, both water- and lipid-soluble derivatives are possible, and this point has increased their importance as an antioxidant in health and personal care products, for example, in burn creams, nutritional supplements, and skin creams.

Fullerenes are highly reactive to free radicals through oxidizing them due to the double bonds and lowest unoccupied molecular orbital. This reactivity has once been challenged by adding some 34 methyl radicals onto a C_{60}, making it the world's most capable radical scavenger and oxidizing agent [5].

Fullerene C_{60} is a great antioxidant, and for us, it is the most important thing to highlight. Fullerene C_{60}, due to a large number of double bonds, behaves as a powerful antioxidant. But its ability to easily penetrate inside the cells, in its nucleus and its mitochondria, makes it a more effective existing intracellular free radical hunter. It is a great promise against neurodegenerative diseases, and at a scientific and medical level, it cannot go unnoticed.

Fullerene C_{60}, due to its small size, can easily cross the so-called blood–brain barrier. This wonderful property entails numerous medical applications, especially in the field of nanomedication, through the development of new active compounds that the brain can use. Fullerene C_{60} is discovered as a very effective and hopeful substance in the treatment of various neuronal problems.

Ongoing studies also show that it delays the symptoms of amyotrophic lateral sclerosis (ALS), and its antioxidant abilities reveal that it has neuroprotective effects against degenerative diseases of the Parkinson type and the like. In fact, fullerene C_{60} has the ability to remove superoxide and peroxide anion (H_2O_2) and effectively inhibit lipid peroxidation.

Fullerene can somehow be considered as an active element in the treatment of Alzheimer's disease, as researchers have shown that it fights the aggregation of beta-amyloid proteins and the degeneration of pyramidal neurons of the hippocampus. This could lead to the development of new medications for the brain, associating its antioxidant and antiplatelet properties.

Antioxidant activity and the body's balanced oxidation are to avoid diseases and toxicities that are caused by excess free radicals, for example, atherosclerosis and cancer. Fullerene cage has many double bonds inside, which makes them capable of reacting with free radicals, for example, hydrogen peroxide, hydroxyl radicals, and superoxide. Recently, C_{82} and C_{60}, two fullerenes, were used as an antioxidant when conjugated with three transition metals (gold, copper, and silver). Results showed that in the presence of metal, fullerene's antiradical capacity was boosted. Fullerenes antioxidant abilities are also applied in skin care products and cosmetics as an anti-aging agent. One of the major problems today is oxidative stress, which the fullerene-based systems are expected to balance. The fact that fullerenes can reduce apoptosis in cortical neurons and can also block receptors of glutamic acid has been reported. Trimesic acid (TMA) fullerenes and hexa(sulfobutyl) fullerenes also displayed their capability of trapping free radicals and efficiently help in the treatment of neurodegenerative diseases, such as Alzheimer's disease. Various studies revealed that fullerenols and malonic acid fullerenes, which are water-soluble derivatives, can react with superoxide free radicals and hydroxyl, lessening the degeneration of neurons related to ROS.

Free radicals are produced by normal cellular metabolism as well as abnormal reactions, encouraged by some disorders. They can trigger tissue abnormalities along with toxicities and disease processes, damaging biological molecules like proteins, lipids, and DNA. This leads to cell damage and, in some cases, to diseases, such as cancer and atherosclerosis.

One of the main characteristics of C_{60} is its exceptional free radical scavenging ability, which makes it favorable "free radical sponge" in order to protect biological systems against cell damage and tissue abnormalities. The presence of several double bonds in fullerene cage makes it able to react with free radicals.

Fullerenes, as the most efficient scavenger, can react with free radical species, like superoxide ($O_2^{\bullet-}$), hydroxyl radicals (OH), and hydrogen peroxide (H_2O_2), without being consumed; moreover, they can localize within the cells and inhibit free radical production. On the other hand, based upon reported studies, it can be hypothesized that radical scavenging capability of fullerenes may not be entirely attributed to the fullerene cage itself but can also be related to the functional groups attached to the carbon cage; therefore, free radical deactivating capacity of various fullerenes is different. Because of its insolubility in water, derivatized fullerenes are more favorable for radical scavenging; moreover, derivatized fullerene can interact with the cellular and subcellular environment more efficiently. Wang et al. evaluated the antioxidant activity of C_{60}, of three of its derivatives, and of vitamin E, determining the inhibition of lipid peroxidation. They reported that fullerene derivative can efficiently prevent peroxidation and membrane breakdown triggered by free radicals, and liposoluble fullerene derivative was more effective in inhibiting lipid peroxidation than vitamin E, which is a natural antioxidant. Their results also showed that both fullerene derivatives, liposoluble and water-soluble, can potentially be used as antioxidant derivatives. This property has been investigated also for other water-soluble fullerene derivatives, such as $C_{60}(OH)_n$, carboxyfullerenes, $C_{60}(ONO_2)_{7\pm2}$, and hexa(sulfobutyl) fullerenes, finding good radical scavenging abilities.

Derivatization of fullerenes with polar groups like polyhydroxylated fullerenes and tris(malonic)acid-C_{60} (TMA-C_{60}) makes them able to enter mitochondria, where free radicals are generated, and also, TMA-C_{60} showed strong neuroprotection in several cell culture models of neurological diseases like Parkinson's.

The assessment of radical scavenging properties of aqueous fullerene suspension has been studied by Gharbi et al., who demonstrated the prevention of free radical–related damage in the liver. The antioxidant properties of dendrofullerene and TMAC$_{60}$ derivatives have been investigated, together with amino acid derivatives of fullerene. For the latter case, fullerene-bearing seven β-alanine demonstrated antioxidant properties against hydrogen peroxide and prevented induced apoptotic cell death, since alanine-fullerene impeded ROS accumulation in extra- and intracellular environment. The α-alanine fullerene derivatives also showed efficient radical scavenging capability against superoxide and hydroxyl radicals. Also, another amino acidic fullerene derivative bearing five cysteines inhibits apoptosis induced by hydroxyl and superoxide free radicals.

Fulleropyrrolidines bearing one or two 3,5-di-tert-butyl-4-hydroxyphenyl units, reported by Enes et al. [7], have also confirmed the antioxidant properties. Lin et al. [8] have investigated the antioxidant activity of carboxyfullerene by *in vitro* study, and the iron-induced lipid peroxidation and autooxidation of brain homogenates were suppressed. Moreover, the *in vivo* studies showed that carboxyfullerene antioxidant activity preserves nigrostriatal dopaminergic system from iron-induced oxidative damage.

Another study investigated the antioxidant potential of carboxyfullerene for cells of immune system, with protection of inactive human peripheral blood mononuclear cells (PBMCs) from apoptosis induced by TNF-α plus cycloheximide or 2-deoxy-d-ribose(dRib) agents. In summary, along with other biological applications, fullerenes can be used as powerful antioxidants and are more active than currently used compounds, like vitamin E.

The radical scavenging kinetics of four fullerene polymeric systems, including C_{60}-PAA-C_{60}, PAAC_{60}, PDMA-C_{60}, and PEO-b-PAA-C_{60}, has been investigated. The radical scavenging process of these fullerene polymeric systems contained two-stage kinetic trends which relate to unimers and micelles existing in aqueous solution of fullerene polymeric system. Moreover, they reported that in free radical scavenging process, micelles and unimers react with radicals. Increasing the number of fullerenes in larger micellar cores results in faster reactions of radicals. In fact, they concluded that the nanostructure has an effect on the antioxidant activity of fullerene polymers.

3.8.10 Anti-HIV Activity of Fullerenes

Several reports are made on fullerene's ability to inhibit the activity of HIV-1 protease. Fullerene enters into the pocket and then, through van der Waals interactions, attaches to the active site, causing antiviral activity. Some fullerene derivatives inhibit the HIV-1 viruses that have resistance against multiple drugs. During treatment with these compounds, no toxicity occurred. That is why they should be the next generation treatment of HIV. Pyridine/pyridinium-type fullerene derivatives with no carboxylic acid inhibit HIV-1 reverse transcriptase in an environment that is cell-free. Results displayed fullerene cage's important role without any cytotoxicity sign.

Wudl et al. hypothesized that carbon 60 has almost the same radius as the cylinder, which explains the HIV protease active site; a chance exists for a strong hydrophobic interaction between the active site surfaces and C_{60} derivatives. HIV protease inhibition in C_{60} presence was explained through experimental observations and molecular modelling studies. Inactivation of virus assays proved fullerene derivatives' activity against HIV-2 and HIV-1.

HIV protease is the basic enzyme which assures virus survival and is specific for HIV proteins, so it is one of the main targets for antiviral treatment. The active site of HIV protease is a semi-opened hydrophobic ellipsoid with Asp-25 and Asp-125 standing out on the surface of the cavity and catalyzing the protease function on the scissile peptide bond of the substrate. The diameter of cavity is 10 Å, close to the diameter of C_{60} cage. The antiviral activity of fullerene derivatives is mainly related to its molecular structure. It has been reported that HIV protease can be inhibited by introducing a fullerene molecule into the catalytic cavity. Embedding C_{60} sphere in the center of the cavity allows van der Waals interactions. The evaluation of antiviral activity of amphiphilic fullerene bisadducts prepared by Prato and coworkers showed different inhibition of HIV-1. They also reported that this inhibitory activity in fullerene derivatives is strongly related to functionalization sites. Marchesan et al. synthesized bis-fulleropyrrolidium salts (Figure 3.12) in order to evaluate their inhibitory activity against HIV-1 and HIV-2, finding that the position of the side chains influences antiviral activity, and trans-fullerene

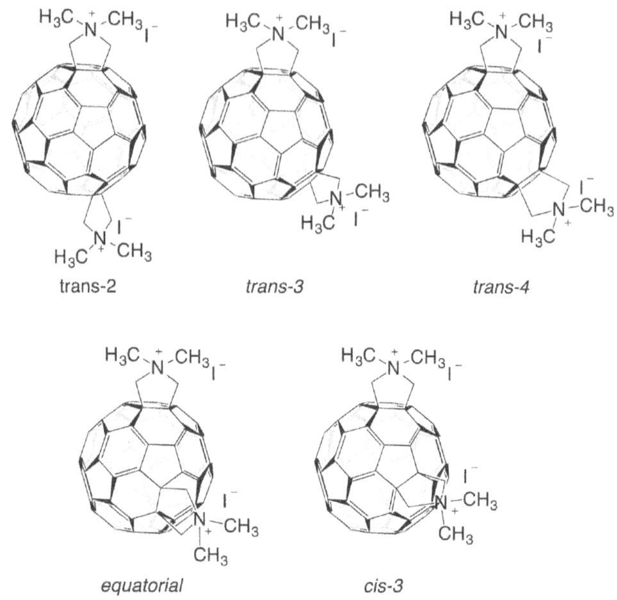

FIGURE 3.12 Structures of fulleropyrrolidinium salts [18] to evaluate their inhibitory activity against HIV.

bisadducts are more active than the *cis* one. Also, Kotelnikova et al. reported that amino acid derivatives of fullerene are able to inhibit HIV.

Amino acid fullerene derivatives (ADFs) carrying bivalent metal ions penetrate through the lipid bilayer of liposomes, insert to hydrophobic domains of proteins, and therefore change the function of membrane-bound enzymes. Cationic, anionic, and amino acid derivatives of fullerene have been tested for antiviral activity by Mashino et al., and their results demonstrated that amino acid derivatives are the most active derivatives. The authors also compared HIV inhibition activity of fullerene derivatives with nevirapine (a clinically used HIV inhibitor), and they found that the fullerene derivative is even more effective than nevirapine itself. The anti-HIV activity against both HIV-1 and HIV-2 of fullerene derivatives of multiple carboxylic acid moieties was also evaluated. They reported a fascinating approach using fullerene–sugar hybrid for photodegradation of HIV-1 protease. The role of the sugar was to promote the interactions between hybrid and HIV-1 protease via hydrogen bonding. The UV/vis irradiation of hybrid-HIV-1P complex led to viral degradation, which is attributed to the generation of ROS by fullerene. The enzymatic inhibition activity of TMA-C_{60} was also investigated and proved; however, this inhibition probably did not have any relation to ROS production.

In summary, fullerene derivatives can complex and inhibit HIV protease based upon their structure, being able to bind in the cavity regions of HIV protease and inhibit virus replication significantly [9], and also on their ROS generation activity.

3.8.11 Fullerenes' Antibacterial and Antiviral Action

One of the medical applications of fullerenes is the antibacterial and antiviral activity that these molecules possess. The first reports of the antibacterial activity of fullerene derivatives were reported in 1996. The main mechanism of action of fullerene when introduced into a bacterium is the rupture of the cell membrane of the bacterium, due to the large volume of the sphere, which seems to not adapt to a flat cell surface. In addition, since fullerenes have the particularity of reacting with oxygen, when they convert into hydrogen peroxide, they can inhibit the respiratory chain of the bacteria.

Amino fullerenes and fullerols, which are the hydrophilic derivatives of fullerenes, have been proven to exhibit antibacterial behavior with an application in water treatment. This property of fullerenes can come from their ability to create singlet oxygen and superoxide when interacting with organic solvents [5].

But without a doubt, one of the most important possible applications of fullerenes in the area of medicine is the report published in 1993 by a group of scientists from the University of California in Los Angeles, which was about the possible inhibition of human immunodeficiency virus (HIV) proteases by the interaction of fullerene with the enzyme's hydrophobic active site. Although many of the mechanisms of bacterial and viral inhibition are not fully understood, the use of fullerenes in medicine represents one of the most attractive, encouraging, and promising research fields of the moment.

Many functionalized fullerene derivatives demonstrated satisfactory effects of inhibition on bacteria. Carboxy-fullerene suppresses *S. pyogenes* growth, and its administration can prevent 1/4 of the mice from dying. In addition, more activity was exhibited against gram-positive bacteria, and none on gram-negative bacteria. Fullerenes can interact directly with biomolecules, for example, anticancer drugs or aromatic mutagens.

3.8.12 Fullerene Increases Life Expectancy in Rats

In science, there are many casual discoveries that seem impossible to believe. As long as there is no convincing explanation, we must be skeptical. A study published in the journal *Biomaterials* from Elsevier states that orally administering oil containing buckyballs (spherical C_{60} fullerenes) manages to double life expectancy in rats. Researchers at the University of Paris and their colleagues suggest that the reason is the effect of C_{60} as an antioxidant. Pharmacokinetic studies conducted over the past 25 years have shown that dissolved C_{60} is absorbed by the gastrointestinal tract and removed within a few hours, so its toxicity is very low. Therefore, its use had been proposed for the encapsulation of certain drugs (in biomedical applications, such as cancer therapies and neurodegenerative diseases). But from there, that the oral administration of C_{60} dissolved in olive oil (0.8 mg/mL) in repeated doses can double the life expectancy of the rats is an enormous step.

3.9 Other Biomedical Applications

3.9.1 Fullerene for Osteoporosis Treatment

Fullerene derivatives in bones, that is, polyfluoro-bi-phosphonated derivatives, are being considered as a bimodal drug for osteoporosis. Osteoporosis is a disease which makes bones brittle and prone to fracture even with mild stresses. This happens when the bone density decreases and the bone tissue has become weaker and causes fracture in the hip, spine, and wrist commonly. It is well-known that hydrophilic bisphosphonate groups have affinity toward the prominent bone mineral hydroxyapatite, which is applicable in osteoporosis and other bone-related diseases. Fullerene was coupled to bisphosphonate to prepare a tissue-vectored compound, namely, $C_{60}(OH)_{16}$AMBP. The *in vitro* experiments demonstrated that this compound possesses good affinity for hydroxyapatite and reduces its mineralization by 50% at 1 mM concentration. Also, $C_{60}(OH)_{30}$ reduces mineralization of hydroxyapatite (28% crystal growth rate) and exhibits affinity for hydroxyapatite. Some studies reported that the reactive oxygen species that contribute in osteoclast differentiation begins with RANK-RANKL signals. Therefore, controlling ROS can help in the treatment of osteoclast hyper-resorption on osteoarthritis. It has been proved that, in rat model, fullerene can reduce joint destruction and suppress bone resorption caused by osteoclasts. Fullerenols can also stimulate osteogenesis in bone marrow, via eliminating ROS in models which experience oxidative stress caused by dexamethasone [10].

3.9.2 Antimicrobial Activity of Fullerenes

Monomethoxy triethylene glycol (mTEG)–substituted fullerene-pyrrolidines show inhibition of *M. tuberculosis* and *Mycobacterium avium*. Carboxy-fullerenes inhibit *E. coli*–induced meningitis by lessening the damage which is caused by infiltrating neutrophils on the blood–brain barrier. Later, it was observed that carboxy-fullerenes could insert into gram-positive cocci's cell wall, disrupt its cell wall structure, and cause the death of the bacteria. The gram-negative organisms' cell wall has an outer membrane consisting of lipopolysaccharides, phospholipids, and lipoproteins. Fullerenes cannot assess it. This advises that carboxy fullerenes could be taken against gram-positive cocci as new antimicrobial agents.

In the 1990s, fullerenes have been evaluated for their antimicrobial activity, and promising results on the suppressive effects on bacteria, including *Bacillus subtilis*, *Candida albicans*, and *E. coli*, were obtained. The study on carboxy-fullerene revealed that it can be exploited as an antimicrobial agent to suppress group A streptococcus infection. The antimicrobial activity of carboxyfullerene was examined against *Streptococcus pyogenes* infection. *In vitro* experiments showed that this derivative can suppress the growth of *S. pyogenes*, and its administration to mice protects 33% of them from death. A fullerene peptide has been fabricated via solid-phase peptide synthesis from functionalized fullerene-containing free amino group and *N*-Fmoc-$_{L}$-glutamic acid a-tert-butyl ester (Figure 3.13), and its activity against bacteria *Staphylococcus aureus* and *E. coli* was tested.

Photodynamic inactivation is an emerging antimicrobial approach that fullerene derivatives, especially water-soluble cationic ones, can facilitate upon irradiation, and in this case, the compounds exhibit their activity both against gram-positive and gram-negative bacteria.

The results displayed that the smaller the fullerene aggregates, the higher the antibacterial activity; this phenomenon

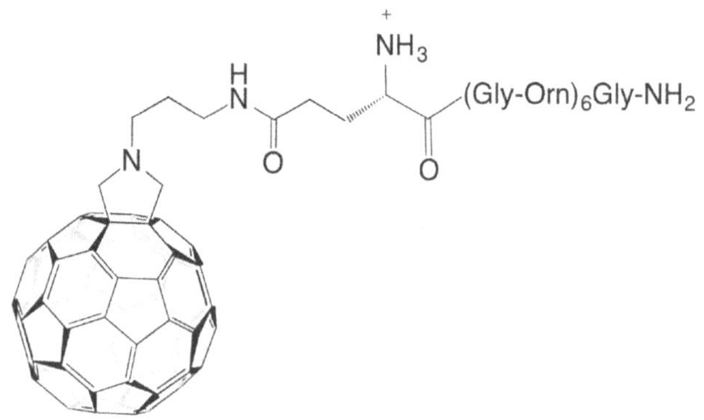

FIGURE 3.13 Schematic of functionalized fullerene–containing free amino group and N-Fmoc-L-glutamic acid a-tert-butyl ester.

could be related to the surface area that, in suspensions with smaller fullerene aggregates, is greater and provides higher antibacterial activity.

The genotoxicity of fullerene on bacteria has been investigated in two distinct studies. Therefore, these results are not conclusive, and DNA damage of fullerene was not caused by covalent DNA adducts formation; but there is an indirect mechanism which needs further investigations.

3.9.3 Fullerenes as Neuroprotective Agent for Cells

Hyperproduction of reactive oxygen and nitric oxide species, due to overexcitation of glutamic acid receptors, can cause cell death, resulting in chronic neurodegenerative diseases like Alzheimer's and Parkinson's. The neuroprotective activity of fullerene derivatives is similar to their radical scavenging activity. As mentioned earlier, fullerene and fullerenols have outstanding antioxidant activity. Their ability to reduce apoptosis in cortical neurons and also to block glutamic acid receptors has been reported. Also, the effectiveness of carboxyfullerenes in the treatment of amyotrophic lateral sclerosis (ALS) has been studied. Hexasulfobutyl fullerenes and TMA fullerenes also demonstrated their ability to trap free radicals and play an efficient role in neurodegenerative diseases treatment. Zha et al. investigated the correlation between fullerenes concentration and their activity. At low concentrations, fullerenols exhibit neuroprotective effect and increase hippocampal neuronal viability, while at high concentrations, opposite results were observed and hippocampal neuronal viability was reduced, with consequent apoptosis.

The experimental allergic encephalomyelitis (EAE) has been used as an animal model to investigate the effect of fullerenes in neuroprotection. It has been reported that a water-soluble fullerene derivative (ABS-75) bearing adamantyl units as NMDA receptor antagonist can block axonal damage and decrease progression in a chronic and progressive EAE model. The role of fullerene in suppressing EAE suggests that the compound can be used as a therapeutic strategy in controlling human multiple sclerosis [9]. Based upon various studies, water-soluble derivatives such as fullerenols and malonic acid fullerenes can react with hydroxyl and superoxide free radicals and reduce neuronal degeneration related to ROS.

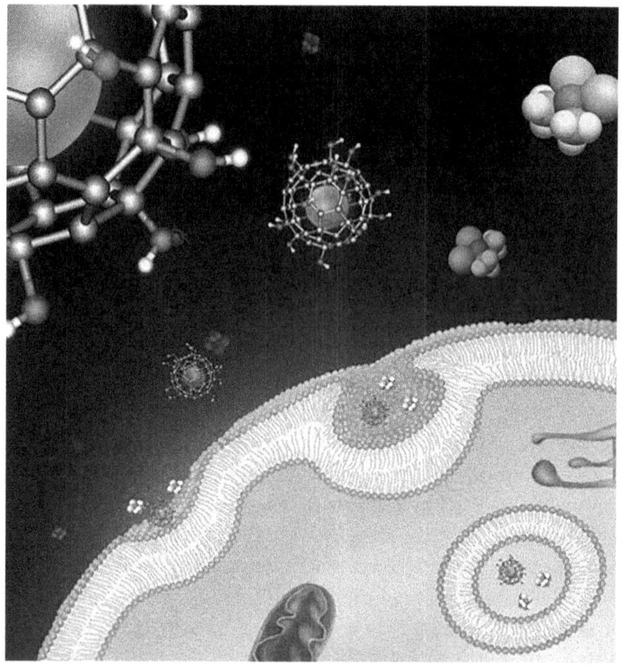

FIGURE 3.14 Nanoparticles activate endocytosis in the human chemotherapy-resistant cancer cells. Multihydroxylated metallofullerene nanoparticles are composed of an amphiphilic fullerene derivative that encapsulates gadolinium as a core. The metallofullerene nanoparticles may circumvent cancer cells' resistance to chemotherapeutical drugs by NP-enhanced endocytosis, thus increasing intracellular concentrations of the drugs.

Source: Photo from CAS Key Lab for Biomedical Effects of Nanomaterials and Nanosafety.

The application of C_{60} fullerene in biological, pharmacological, and medical areas has been very promising. For example, it has been observed that C_{60} fullerene is an effective free radical scavenger, so it can be used as a protective agent for cells or to reduce oxidative stress. In addition, when photo-irradiated, C_{60} fullerene can produce radicals, so it can also be used in photodynamic therapies (Figure 3.14). Nanoparticles activate endocytosis in the human chemotherapy-resistant cancer cells.

3.9.4 Fullerenes as MRI Contrast Agent for Diagnosis

Endohedral metallofullerenes have metal ion fixed inside the cage of fullerene. Water-solubilized forms are used as magnetic resonance imaging (MRI) and X-ray contrast agents and radiopharmaceuticals. One of these derivatives has been studied in detail as a radioactive tracer for diseased organ imaging and to kill the cancerous tumors. Inside the carbon shell, there is a stable, radioactive metal that is very resistant to the body's metabolism. Metallofullerenes are not toxic, and they allow imaging of the circulatory system by staying in the body for at least an hour.

Magnetic resonance imaging is a technique which uses gadolinium-based contrast agents. Fullerenes with their hallow cage can be used for encapsulating gadolinium in order to address challenges related to the use of Gd chelates for MRI, considering that after injection, C_{60} distributes in tissues and relocates in selected organs without detectable and acute toxicity. Endohedral fullerenes, which entrap metal atoms in the molecular cage without releasing them even in vivo, are good candidates as contrast agent both in magnetic resonance imaging and X-ray imaging.

The first approach in using fullerene endohedrals in MRI was reported. $Gd@C_{60}[C(COOH)_2]_{10}$ is water-soluble, and it has easy uptake in the reticuloendothelial system (RES). Later on, Toth et al. also investigated the MRI applicability of $Gd@C_{60}(OH)_x$. They showed that, being water-proton relaxivities dependent on temperature, magnetic fields, and also pH, these gadofullerenes possess the potential of pH-sensitive MRI contrast agent. Moreover, Liu et al. investigated the potential of Gd^{3+}-PEG-C_{60} in both photodynamic therapy and magnetic resonance imaging (MRI); the presence of Gd^{3+} converts PEG-C_{60} to a photosensitizer with dual application in diagnosis and treatment. Shu et al. synthesized gadofullerene MRI contrast agents, starting from higher fullerenes, as $Gd@C_{82}O_6(OH)_{16}(NHCH_2CH_2COOH)_8$, to evaluate its capability in magnetic resonance imaging, and also, in this case, it was demonstrated that they have promising characteristics in this field.

3.9.5 Fullerenes in Cosmetics

Personal care and skin care products are intricately intertwined with chemical industries. The emergence of nanotechnology in cosmetics was triggered about 40 years ago with the use of liposomes in moisturizing creams. Fullerenes, thanks to their antioxidant activity, are used in moisturizers. For the first time, Inui et al. investigated the clinical efficacy of fullerenes for treating acne. A fullerene-based gel was used in this study, decreasing the inflammatory lesions. Fullerene derivatives were reported to exhibit antioxidant activity, and also anti-melanogenesis, without any detectable cytotoxicity, and so they also have been used for anti-aging products. A water-soluble fullerene complex consisting of PVP and C_{60} has been proven for its cytoprotective activity against oxidative stress and its ultraviolet absorption proficiency. PVP/C_{60} is able to prevent the inhibitory effect of UVB on keratinocyte proliferation by its antioxidative effect, which suggests that PVP/C_{60} could be applied in cosmetic products due its free radical scavenging and as a barrier repair agent for promoting keratinocyte differentiation. Despite these commercials uses, fullerenes may cause undesirable side effects, since the application of fullerene in cosmetic products increases human exposure, and much more has to be investigated about this application.

An interesting role of fullerene nanomaterials which has been examined by the researchers is stimulation of hair growth. In this study, a fullerene derivative has been developed, and its role in the treatment of hair loss has been examined. The results of experiments exhibited that in fullerene-treated mice, hair growth and also the number of hair follicles have increased compared to mice receiving only vehicle. The production of reactive oxygen species as a possible underlying reason for aging and hair loss can describe the mechanism in which fullerene treats hair loss and increases the number of hair follicles; in fact, fullerene as a free radical scavenger is an attractive therapeutic option for the treatment of diseases involving reactive oxygen species. The various applications of fullerene derivatives in biomedicine are summarized in Table 3.1.

3.10 Applications of Fullerenes in Biosensors

A *biosensor* is an analytical device which can sense the presence and determine the amount of biomolecules, enzymes, microorganism, organelles, antibodies, and receptors by combining a biological sensing element or a recognition site with a transducer. The recognition site responds to the presence of the biomolecules, and the transducer converts this to signals which are measurable.

Fullerenes can be used as mediator between recognition site and biosensor electrode, amplifying the electron transfer rate created by biochemical reactions of analyte and biological component in recognition site. Considering that an efficient mediator should be hydrophilic and possess functional groups, which help it to conjugate the biomolecules in order to promote electron transfer at the reaction site, pristine fullerene does not seem to be the most advantageous mediator, being hydrophobic and insoluble in polar media. However, fullerene derivatives can be an effective material for use in biosensors. Intensive research accomplished on C_{60} derivatives demonstrated that functionalization imparts characteristics which improve the efficacy in biosensor applications. Among the other groups, carboxylic acid, amine, and hydroxyl groups are beneficial in allowing the interactions between fullerenes and biomolecules. C_{60}-containing supported bilayer lipid membranes (s-BLMs) as molecular device have been investigated. The results showed that C_{60} inserted in BLM is an efficient electron mediator which can be used in biosensors. Following this investigation, Szymańska et al. used this method in an electrochemical sensor for the detection of neutral odorant and demonstrated that functionalized fullerene facilitates charge transmission. Fullerenes have been also used in glucose biosensing and overcome some limitations which exist in glucose determination. The first attempt in this field was done in 2000, and various amounts of fullerene, from 0.6 to 1.7 μm, were immobilized to amperometric biosensor against glucose oxide enzyme. The results showed that, with the increase of the fullerene amount, sensitivity of biosensor also improved. Later, a fullerene-cryptand-22-coated sensor was applied for sensing gluconic acid, which is produced via glucose oxidation. The experiments demonstrated that this biosensor is selective to glucose, and no interferences caused by biological samples were observed. Furthermore, fullerene-cryptand-22 was used to coat piezoelectric quartz crystals along with immobilized C_{60}-urease membrane for sensing ammonium ions deriving from the catalytic hydrolysis of urea by urease. Similar to this study, C_{60}-coated piezoelectric quartz crystal sensor with immobilized C_{60}-lipase silicate plates was applied in order to detect the optical isomer of amino acid esters. The synthesized sensor was capable to distinguish between L- and D-amino acid esters.

Zhilei et al., with an inventive approach, developed a glucose biosensor exploiting fullerene along with ferrocene (Fc),

TABLE 3.1

Fullerene Derivatives and Their Various Applications in Biomedical Engineering

Fullerene Derivatives	Applications	Refs.
Fullerenol or fullerenol, $C_{60}(OH)_{12}$	Antioxidant and reducing apoptosis in cortical neurons cultures	[11]
Carboxyfullerene, $C_{63}((COOH)_2)_3$	Inhibiting neurodegeneration involved in ALS	[12]
$C_{60}(ONO_2)_{7\pm2}$	With antioxidant activity, can prevent oxidant-induced pulmonary diseases	[13]
Amino acid derivatives of fullerene	Antiviral activity	[14]
Hexa(sulfobutyl)fullerene, $[C_{60}(CH_2\text{-}CH_2\text{-}CH_2\text{-}CH_2SO_3Na)_6;(FC_4S)]$	Antiproliferative agent in arteriosclerosis and inhibition of plasma lipid peroxidation	[15]
Fullerenol	Non-invasive image-guided cancer therapy	[16]
Fullerenol	Tumor inhibitory activity	[17]
Bis-fulleropyrrolidines	Inhibitory activity against HIV	[18]
Fullerenol	Anti-metastatic activity, cancer treatment	[19]
$C_{60}(Nd)$ nanoparticles	Inducing autophagy in cancer cells and enhancing chemotherapeutic killing of cancer cells	[20]
$C_{60}[>M(C_3N_6+C_3)_2][>M(C_3N_6C_3)_2]\_(—I)10$	Antimicrobial photodynamic inactivation	[21]
Tris-Malonic acid fullerenes	Radical scavenging	[22]
Dendrofullerene	Antioxidant activity	[23]
C_{60}-PEI-FA	Drug delivery system	[24]
Fulleropyrrolidines bearing 3,5-di-tert-butyl-4-hydroxyphenyl	Antioxidant	[7]
Porphyrin-C_{60}	PDT cell inactivation	[25]
C_{60}-PEG-Gd	Antitumor activity	[26]
Pd@Cys-C_{60} nanoparticles	Glucose biosensor	[27]
Cucurbit[8]uril–fullerene	Photodynamic therapy	[28]
Gd@$C_{60}[C(COOH)_2]_{10}$	MRI contrasts agent	[29]
6-Amino-g-cyclodextrin (ACD)/C_{60}	Photodynamic therapy	[30]
Hexasulfobutyl fullerenes	Treatment of neurodegenerative diseases via radical scavenging	[31]
Fullerene-cryptand-22	Urea biosensor	[32]
Carboxyfullerene	Antimicrobial and antibacterial activity	[33]
$C_{60}(OH)_{16}$AMBP	Osteoporosis treatment	[34]
$C_{60}[C(COOH)_2]_2$/glucose oxidase (GOx)/TMB	Glucose colorimetric biosensor	[35]
Carboxyfullerene	Targeted drug delivery	[36]
Carboxyfullerene	Urea biosensor	[37]
Hoechst 33258–conjugated hyaluronated fullerene	Photodynamic tumor therapy	[38]
Fullerene-phenylalanine-poly lactic acid	Drug carrier—photodynamic therapy	[39]
Cystine C_{60} derivative	Inhibiting apoptosis	[40]
Amphiphilic fullerene bisadducts	Inhibiting HIV	[41]
DNA-fullerene nanoparticles	Carrying drug	[42]
Porphyrin adducts of cyclohexyl fullerene C_{60}	Targeted delivery of paramagnetic Mg 2+ isotope	[43]
Fullerenol	Stimulate osteogenesis in bone marrow	[10]
Fullerene containing free amino group and N-Fmoc-L-glutamic acid a-tert-butyl ester	Antibacterial activity	[44]
Malonodiserinolamide derivatized fullerene	Drug delivery system	[45]
Carboxyfullerene	Antioxidant activity	[8]

chitosan (CS), and ionic liquid (IL). The efficacy of this biosensor was evaluated by chronoamperometry, cyclic voltammetry, and impedance spectroscopy. The fast response of this biosensor and the minimum value of the Michaelis–Menten constant (k_m) among other glucose biosensors demonstrated the high sensitivity and great performance of this biosensor. In this, fullerene supports the oxidation of glucose molecules and stimulates the electrochemical reaction that results in the most applicable response in amperometric biosensors. In 2012, novel Pd@Cys-C_{60} nanoparticles were developed via in situ spontaneous reduction process, which was exploited for sensing glucose in glucose solution and human serum. The results showed that this biosensor has a linear range from 2.5 μM to 1 mM, and also, no interferences from other biomolecules were reported. A carboxyfullerene bisadduct, $C_{60}[C(COOH)_2]_2$, possesses peroxide-like catalytic activity and can catalyze the reaction of peroxidase substrate 3,3′,5,5′ tetramethylbenzidine (TMB) in the presence of H_2O_2. Therefore, $C_{60}[C(COOH)_2]_2$/glucose oxidase (GOx)/TMB system was designed to be a colorimetric sensor for glucose, which showed a detection range of 1.0–40 μM. In addition, this highly sensitive colorimetric biosensor can be exploited for quantitative measurement of glucose in human serum. In similar studies, functionalized fullerene was used as a mediator in glucose biosensors, exhibiting a convenient electron transfer between glucose oxide and glassy carbon. Also, Saeedfar et al. synthesized a urea biosensor using carboxyfullerene derivatives. This biosensor contained fullerene–urea bioconjugates on an acrylic-based hydrogen ion–sensitive membrane and demonstrated acceptable sensitiveness and response time.

In a recent study, a novel nanocomposite consisting of 3-aminocapto-1,2,4-triazole functionalized fullerene C_{60} coated by gold nanoparticles dispersed on a glassy nanostructured carbon electrode has been developed in order to investigate non-enzymatic sensing properties. This nanocomposite revealed excellent catalytic activity that is promising for application in glucose sensors with a really low detection limit. However, considering the attractive properties of fullerenes, extensive investigations are needed to better exploit fullerene derivatives in the fabrication of biosensors, which remains an important field of application.

3.11 Modification of Electrodes with Fullerenes

The idea of introducing C_{60} chemically modified electrodes (CME) was first reported by Compton and coworkers in 1992. They prepared C_{60}-based CMEs by immobilizing C_{60} films by drop coating onto surfaces of the electrodes, which were then coated with Nafion as protecting films. It was observed that the current signal improved compared to those using C_{60} dissolved in solution. Afterward, the electrochemical behavior of the C_{60}-CMEs, in non-aqueous and aqueous solutions, has been widely investigated, suggesting the possibility of their electroanalytical applications. Currently, fullerene-based CMEs are prepared in several different ways. The most common method is drop coating the electrode by using a fullerene solution of a volatile solvent. Electrochemical deposition is another technique of the fullerene film preparation. Moreover, fullerene-based CMEs can be prepared by electropolymerization, where the formed fullerene units are connected by polymer side chains or via epoxide formation. An alternative method for C_{60} films preparation is the self-assembled monolayer (SAM) film using either thiols or silane derivatives of C_{60} on the electrode surfaces.

In addition, fullerene C_{60} is widely used for the construction of electrochemical biosensors. Generally, electrochemical biosensors are analytical devices which consist of a bioreceptor, an electrochemical active interface, a transducer element which converts biological reaction to an electrical signal, and a signal processor. The principle of the electrochemical biosensors is based on the specific interaction between the analyte and biorecognition element, which is also associated with better correlation between the bioreceptor and the transducer surface. Utilization of different kinds of nanomaterials leads to important improvements in these aspects, and nanomaterials integrate widely in the construction of biosensors in order to improve the sensing performance of the biosensors. The ability of signal mediation, easy functionalization, and light-induced switching leads to the fact that fullerene is considered as a new and attractive element in the fabrication of biosensors.

Different biomolecules or organic ligands can be immobilized to the shell of fullerenes by adsorption or covalent attachment.

Carbon nanotubes (CNT) were also widely used to chemically functionalize electrodes due to their remarkable electrical, chemical, mechanical, and structural properties. It was shown that CNT which is chemically modified with different functionalized groups would make the electrodes more sensitive and selective in detection applications. Furthermore, CNTs have advantages over other carbon nanomaterials as they exhibit superior electrocatalytic properties.

3.11.1 Fullerene (C_{60})–DNA Hybrid

In general, combining two or more different materials via interaction forces leads to the appearance of novel hybrid materials with unique properties. Taking advantage of nanoscale properties of biomolecules holds great promise, since their characteristic is different from their bulk complements. Biomolecules hold great compatibility and suitability to form bionanohybrid structures, and significant efforts have been made to form nanobiohybrid systems for various applications. There are various approaches available to create hybrid materials consisting of biomacromolecules and nanomaterials. One approach is based on connecting the molecules through covalent bonding, and the other approach is adsorption (or wrapping) of a material onto the surface of other materials *via* supramolecular interactions, encapsulation, or groove of the other molecule.

Among the various biomolecules, DNA has attracted great attention due to its superior properties, such as structural regularity, biocompatibility, and unique double helix structure, which lead to a range of outstanding properties that are hard to find in other biomolecules. Furthermore, DNA is a potential material for combining with other chemicals, especially with nanomaterials, by different interactions. Taking into account the advantages of DNA and carbon nanomaterials, the combination of DNA and carbon nanomaterials offers unique advantages for different applications. Hence, the combination of DNA with new carbon allotropes is a skillful and challenging area that can lead to the development of novel nanobiomaterials with exceptional properties for a variety of potential applications, such as gas sensors and catalysts, as well as in electronic and optical devices, sensitive biosensors, and biochips.

3.11.1.1 Interaction of DNA with Fullerene

The interaction between DNA and other species plays an important role in life science since it is in direct contact with the transcription of DNA, mutation of genes, origins of diseases, and molecular recognition studies. Cassell et al. studied the interaction between DNA and fullerene. C_{60}-N,N-dimethylpyrrolidinium iodide is used as a complexing agent to form DNA/fullerene complexes through phosphate groups of the DNA backbone, which was imaged by TEM. It was shown that the complexation of free fullerene with DNA is sterically permitted, and surfactants can be used in order to prevent the DNA/fullerene hybrids from aggregation.

Later on, the interaction of DNA with fullerene C_{60} was studied in depth. The method used was based on the double-stranded DNA (dsDNA)–modified gold electrodes (dsDNA/Au) in combination with electrochemical method for investigation of the interactions between C_{60} derivatives and DNA. When fullerene is electrically neutral, the electrostatic interaction with the dsDNA vanishes, and the π–π interaction is present. In addition, it was shown that the binding and dissociation of $H_{10}C_{60}(NHCH_2CH_2OH)_{10}$ to the dsDNA are a reversible process.

So far, it is believed that the water-soluble C_{60} molecules only bind to the major grooves and free ends of the double-stranded DNA, but extensive simulations indicate that the association of hydrophobic C_{60} can also occur at the minor groove sites and no complexation occurs at the major grooves. It is stated that the free ends of the double-stranded DNA fragment are the hydrophobic regions which favor the diffusion of hydrophobic fullerenes toward their docking sites. Calculation of binding energy shows that the hybrid C_{60}-DNA complexes are energetically favorable compared to the unpaired molecules. The self-association of C_{60} molecules in the presence of DNA molecules reveals that self-association between C_{60} molecules occurs in the early stages of simulation. However, after 5 ns of simulation, one of the C_{60} molecules binds to one end of the DNA. Visual observation of the obtained results from simulation shows that the overall shape of the dsDNA molecule is not affected by the association of C_{60}. However, the association of C_{60} has more impact on the DNA structure when more hydrophobic contacting surfaces are exposed at the end of the double-stranded DNA. The binding between the C_{60} and the DNA molecules is attributed to the hydrophobic interaction between the C_{60} and the hydrophobic sites on the DNA. In another study, it is reported that the C_{60} molecule binds to the ssDNA molecule with a binding energy of about −1.6 eV, and the results are in close agreement with those given in many references. However, it is stated that the mobility of DNA and their interaction with water molecules, which often present in real physical systems, were not taken into these calculations.

3.11.1.2 Fullerene for DNA Biosensing

The preparation of DNA hybridization sensors involves the attachment of oligonucleotide probes on the surface of electrode, and the DNA immobilization step has been considered as a fundamental step in the fabrication of DNA biosensing. Various electrode materials, such as gold, carbon paste, glassy carbon, carbon fibers, and screen-printed electrodes, have been utilized to immobilize the DNA, despite carbon nanomaterials such as C_{60} being compounds that have attracted much interest as materials for DNA sensors and biosensors because of their unique properties. Shiraishi et al. demonstrated a new procedure of immobilizing DNA onto a fullerene-impregnated screen-printed electrode (FISPE) for detection of 16S rDNA, extracted from *Escherichia coli*. The integrated FISPE was the mixture of ink and fullerene solution which is modified with probe DNA in the next step. The efficiency of the developed method was tested by detecting 46S rDNA of *E. coli* by means of the modified electrode with perfectly matched probes. It is shown that the reduction peak of $Co(phen)_3^{3+}$ is enhanced only on the perfectly matched probes–modified electrode after hybridization. This fact was ascribed to the accumulation of indicator into the hybrid between perfectly matched probe and rDNA of target. In addition, it was observed that the electrochemical response of $Co(phen)_3^{3+}$ accumulated in the hybrid was better when using FISPE, which, based on the author's opinion, shows that the probe DNA was immobilized onto the PA-FISPE surface in a high concentration.

Other carbon nanomaterials were also used for the development of new (bio)sensing systems for application in the food industry, environmental monitoring, and clinic diagnostics. For example, recently, CNT-modified arrays have been used to detect DNA targets by combining the CNT nanoelectrode array with $Ru(bpy)_3^{2+}$-mediated guanine oxidation. In another study, a MWCNT-COOH-modified glassy carbon was used in combination with an amino-functionalized oligonucleotide probe and pulse-voltammetric transduction. Recently, an indicator-free AC impedance measurement of DNA hybridization based on DNA probe-doped polypyrrole film over an MWCNT layer was reported. A fivefold sensitivity enhancement was observed compared to analogous measurements without CNT. However, most of the examples suffer from the feasibility of scale-up conditions due to the low yield and expensive experimental procedures. Inhomogeneity in CNT samples due to the different production procedures limits their application.

3.11.1.3 Fullerene as an Immobilization Platform

Nano-sized materials can be used as potential building blocks to construct higher-ordered supramolecular architectures for designing highly sensitive biosensing platforms. The working electrode modified with partially reduced fullerene C_{60}–modified electrode had exceptional properties, such as high electroactive surface area, excellent electronic conductivity, and good biocompatibility. Zhang et al. have developed a technique to disperse fullerene C_{60} nanotubes (FNTs) homogenously into aqueous solution by forming a kind of complex with ssDNA. The FNT/DNA was modified onto the surface of the GCE by air-drying/adsorption, enabling the electrochemical analysis of the modified electrode with voltammetric technology. The electrochemical detection of dopamine (DA) in the presence of ascorbic acid was performed. The interaction of FNT with DNA was studied by UV-vis measurements. The observed redshift was attributed to the weak binding between the two, and it was shown that π–π stacking and hydrophobic interaction contribute to the formation of FNT/DNA hybrid. It is believed that the strong physisorption of DNA onto the FNTs via a wrapping mechanism prevents the FNT/DNA from precipitation upon adding water or organic solvent. Obtained SEM images of the surface FNT/DNA–modified electrode proved the formation of uniform films.

In another study, Gugoasa et al. investigated the influence of dsDNA which is physically immobilized on the multiwalled carbon nanotubes (MWCNT), synthetic monocrystalline diamond (DP), and fullerenes-C_{60} on the detection of three different neurotransmitters, namely, DA, epinephrine, and norepinephrine [46]. Optimized working condition for dsDNA biosensors was found to be a value of 4 for pH and the 0.1 mol/L KNO_3. It has been shown that the highest improvement of the signal for the DA was recorded when dsDNA was immobilized on DP. However, the larger working concentration and the lowest limit of detection were obtained when dsDNA was immobilized on MWCNT. In addition, immobilization of dsDNA on fullerene C_{60} decreases both the limit of detection and the limit of quantification. This occurrence is attributed to the fact that the immobilization matrix has a very important contribution to the biosensor performance. It was shown that not only the nature of the material but also the geometry of the substances at the molecular level has an effect on the behavior of the biosensors [46].

However, the obtained fullerene C_{60} by simply stirring or ultrasonication treatments was not suitable for biomedical applications because of their aggregation properties. To solve these limitations, the covalent binding of nano-C_{60} to amino acids, hydroxyl groups, carboxyl groups, etc., which can increase the nanoparticle's ability to interact with the biological environment, can be performed. On the other hand, synthesis of the functionalized C_{60} with non-covalent interaction based on supramolecular chemistry would preserve the original structure and electrochemical properties of C_{60}. Supramolecular chemistry is the chemistry of the intermolecular bond that aims to develop highly complex chemical system components in interacting with non-covalent intermolecular forces. A new supramolecular method is developed by Han et al. for the preparation of thiol and amino-functionalized C_{60} nanoparticles with better water solubility and larger active surface area. They used amino-functionalized 3,4,9,10-per ylenetetracarboxylic dianhydride (PTC-NH_2) as a π electron compound which can be bound to the surface of C_{60} via supramolecular interaction. Prussian blue-carried gold nanoparticles (Au@PBNPs) were interacted with $FC_{60}NPs$. In the next step, the detection aptamers for platelet-derived growth factor B-chain (PDGF-BB) as a model target were labeled by Au@PB/FC_{60} and coupled with alkaline phosphatase (AP) for electrochemical aptasensing (Scheme 3.3a). The combinations of fullerene C_{60} and AuNPs have been used for the immobilization of a large amount of captured aptamers on the surface of the electrode. The obtained SEM and TEM images showed that Au@PBNPs was adsorbed uniformly and tightly on the $FC_{60}NPs$. The performance of developed aptasensor was investigated by detecting PBGF-BB standard solutions (Table 3.2) [47].

Electrochemiluminescence (ECL) is a powerful analytical tool for the detection of clinical samples. A peroxydisulfate/oxygen ($S_2O_8^{2-}/O_2$) system is widely used for amplification of ECL signals, where the dissolved O_2 can serve as a co-reactant. The enzymatic reaction can catalyze in situ generation of the dissolved O_2 [50]. Zhuo et al. [50] developed a sandwich-type aptasensor based on mimicking bi-enzyme cascade catalysis to in situ generate the co-reactant of dissolved O_2 for signal amplification to detect thrombin (TB). Au nanoparticles (HAuNPs) were utilized as carriers to immobilize glucose oxidase nanoparticles (GOxNPs) and Pt nanoparticles (PtNPs). GOxNPs could catalyze glucose to generate H_2O_2, which could be further catalyzed by hemin/G-quadruplex and PtNPs, in order to in situ generate dissolved O_2 with high concentration. In this study, the detection aptamer of thrombin (TBA2) was immobilized on the PtNPs/GOxNPs/HAuNPs, and hemin was intercalated into the TBA2 to obtain the hemin/G-quadruplex/PtNPs/GOxNPs/HAuNPs nanocomplexes, utilized as signal tags (Scheme 3.3b). The surface of glassy carbon is modified with C_{60} and electrochemically deposited Au nanoparticles for further immobilization of thiol-terminated thrombin capture aptamer (TBA1). TBA1, TB, and TBA2 make a sandwich-type structure. The zero-dimensional nano-C_{60} was shown to enhance the immobilization of nanoparticles but also amplified the ECL signal, owing to its large specific surface area. The developed aptasensor is characterized by the ECL measurements. The bare GCE showed relatively low ECL intensity in the low-concentration level of dissolved O_2. The ECL intensity of the bare GCE was enhanced in the presence of dissolved O_2. The ECL intensity was increased when using nano-C_{60} coated onto the electrode, due to the enrichment effect of nano-C_{60}

TABLE 3.2

Comparison of Different Fullerene C_{60}–Modified Biosensors

Receptor	Analyte	Linear Range	Sensitivity	LOD	References
ssDNA	Dopamine	2–160 μM	—	0.6 μM	[48]
ssDNA	PDGF-BB	0.002–40 nM	—	0.6 pM	[49]
ssDNA	Thrombin	1 μM–10 nM	—	0.3 fM	[50]
ssDNA	16S rDNA	—	—	—	[51]
dsDNA	CD	0.1–25.0 nM	0.0235 μA·nM^{-1}	0.03 nM	[52]
dsDNA	Dopamine	10^{-5}–10^{-2} M	100 nA.nM^{-1}	1.2 μM	[46]
dsDNA	Epinephrine	10^{-6}–10^{-2} M	100 nA.nM^{-1}	0.1 μM	[46]
dsDNA	Norepinephrine	10^{-5}–10^{-2} M	0.1 nA.nM^{-1}	2.3 μM	[46]
Anti-IgG	IgG	—	1.25 × 102 Hz/(mg/mL)	—	[53]
Anti-Hb	Hb	—	1.5 × 104 Hz	<10–4 mg/mL	[53]
Anti–*E. coli*	*Escherichia coli* O157:H7	3.2 × 101 to 3.2 × 106 CFU/mL	—	15 CFU/mL	[54]
GOD-Chit	Glucose	0.05–1 mM	—	694 ± 8 μM	[55]
Cobalt(II) hexacyanoferrate-GOD	Glucose	0–8 mM	5.60 × 102 nA/mM	1.6 μm	[56]
Glucose oxidase	Glucose	—	5.9 × 102 Hz/Δlog M	3.9 × 10–5 M	[57]
Urease	Urea	1.2–0.042 mM	59.67 ± 0.91 mV/dcade	—	[58]
AuNPs-TVL	Laccase	0.03–0.30 M	—	0.006 mM	[59]

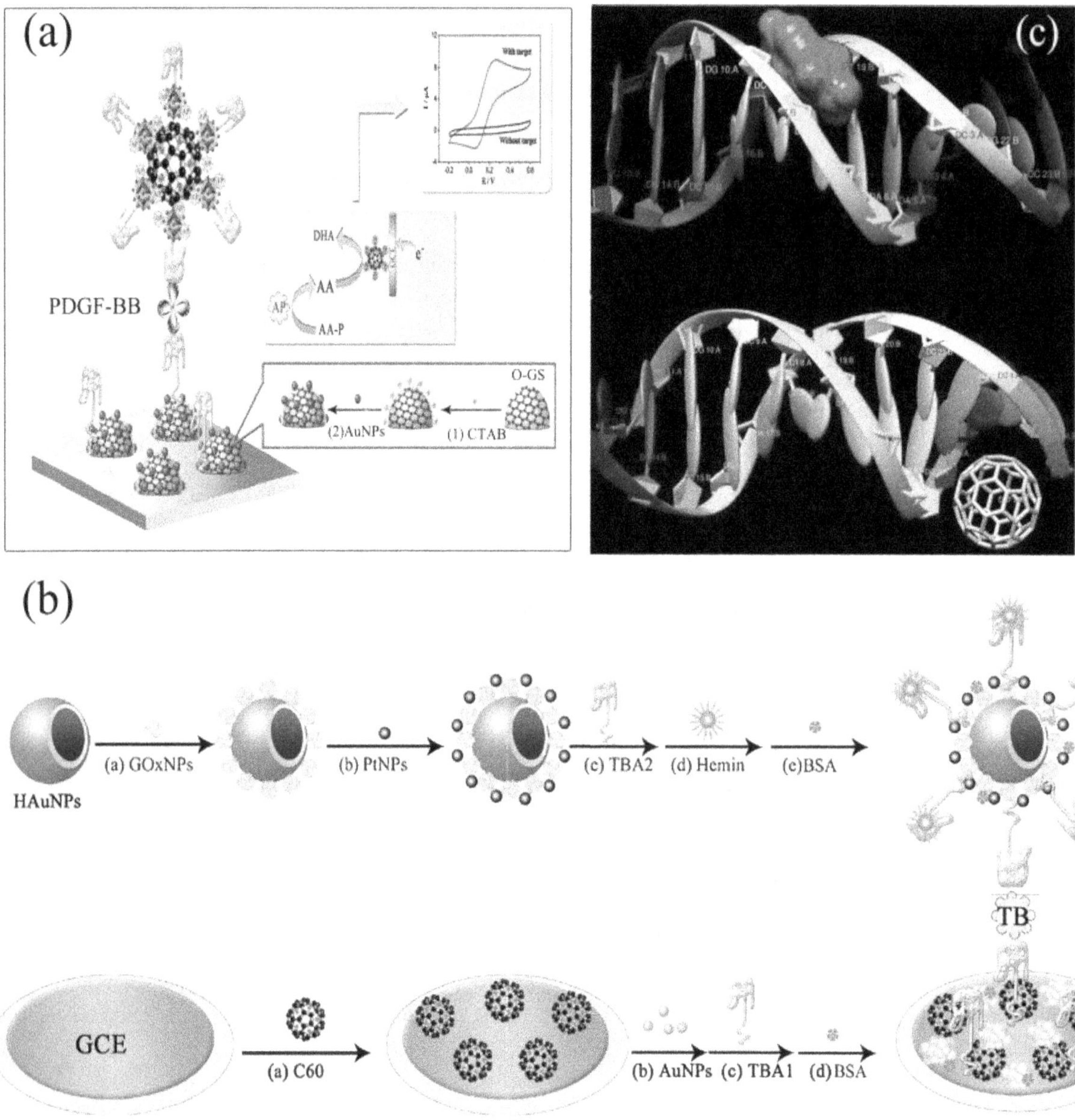

SCHEME 3.3 (a) Schematic illustration of the stepwise aptasensor fabrication process and the dual-signal amplification mechanism. (b) Schematic diagram of the fabrication and detection of the ECL aptasensor. (c) Results of molecular modeling related to (A) groove binding of small molecules to the minor groove of dsDNA and (B) groove binding of fullerene C_{60} to the major groove of dsDNA.

Source: (a) adapted from [49]; (b) adapted from [50]; (c) adapted from [52].

on peroxydisulfate luminescence. Electrodepositing AuNPs further enhanced the ECL intensity since it accelerates the electron transfer in ECL reaction. However, the ECL intensity decreased successively when TBA1 was immobilized onto the electrode. The ECL signal dropped again after the incubation of modified electrode with the target analyte of TB. The ECL aptasensor was also evaluated by CV in 0.1 M PBS. While the relatively low CV intensity was obtained at bare GCE, CV intensity was reduced when the electrode was coated with C_{60} due to its low electrical conductivity (Table 3.2).

In another report, Gholivand et al. studied the mechanism of the prevention of Parkinson's disease by means of carbidopa (CD) drug at a double-stranded DNA (dsDNA) and fullerene C_{60}–modified glassy carbon electrode (dsDNA/FLR/GCE) by cyclic voltammetry [72]. They have used multivariate analysis to distinguish the complex system. Firstly, the effect of pH on the electrochemical system has been studied, and a value of 4.0 for pH resulted in higher sensitivity of the system. It has been shown that the oxidation of CD was controlled by adsorption at the dsDNA/FLR/GCE. In addition, the CV recorded at different electrodes showed that the electrocatalytic behavior for oxidation of CD at FLR/GCE is improved noticeably in comparison with the bare GCE. When dsDNA was added to the CD solution, both oxidation and reduction peaks decreased markedly and shifted to less and more positive potentials, respectively, which indicates that CD interacts with dsDNA. They have used electronic UV-vis absorption spectroscopy to characterize the interaction between dsDNA and small molecules. In the obtained spectra, no redshift was observed, which represents that the binding mode is not the intercalative binding, and it could be groove binding [52]. By means of all these observations, it has been suggested that small molecules, such as CD, interact with the minor groove, while large molecules (fullerene C_{60}) tend to interact with the major groove binding site of DNA. This phenomenon was earlier reported and further proved by molecular modeling, which is performed in this study (Scheme 3.3c).

3.11.2 Fullerene (C_{60})-Antibody Hybrid

Conventional immunosensors suffer from drawbacks, such as intrinsic complexity and the requirement for signal amplification, large sample size, and high cost. By using nanoscale carbon materials, most of these limitations can be solved. Especially, fullerene C_{60} with conjugate π electrons can be considered as an electrophilic molecule, which can be attacked by electron-donating molecules, such as amines, antibodies, and enzymes.

A sensitive immobilized C_{60}-antibody-coated piezoelectric crystal sensor, based on C_{60}-anti-human IgG and C_{60}-anti-hemoglobin, was developed to detect IgG and hemoglobin in aqueous solutions (Scheme 3.4a) [53]. For this purpose, a fullerene C_{60}-coated piezoelectric quartz crystal has been used to investigate the interaction between C_{60} and the antibody, and the change in the resonant frequency of the crystal is recorded, which is directly related to the deposited mass. The frequency change responds sensitively to the adsorption of anti-IgG onto the C_{60}-coated crystals. The interaction between C_{60} and anti-IgG is found to be chemisorption with good reactivity. The effect of the C_{60} coating load on the frequency response of the C_{60}-coated PZ crystal for anti-IgG in water was investigated. The PZ quartz crystal with more C_{60} coating exhibited a larger frequency shift, but the frequency shift of the C_{60}-coated PZ sensor tends to level off with larger amounts of C_{60} coating, suggesting that C_{60} can only adsorb IgG on its surface to some extent. The obtained results revealed that the concentration of antibody, temperature, and pH have an impact on the response of the biosensor.

The immobilized C_{60}-anti-hemoglobin (C_{60}-Hb)–coated piezoelectric quartz crystal hemoglobin biosensor was also developed to detect hemoglobin in solutions. The partially irreversible response of the C_{60}-coated piezoelectric crystal for anti-hemoglobin was tested, suggesting the chemisorption and the good reactivity of anti-hemoglobin on C_{60}-coated crystal. The immobilized C60-Hb-coated piezoelectric crystal sensor exhibited linear response frequency to the concentration of hemoglobin, with sensitivity of about 1.56×10^4 Hz/(mg/mL) and detection limit of <10−4 mg/mL to hemoglobin in solutions (Table 3.2).

Recently, Li et al. reported the development of a sensitive and efficient electrochemical immunosensor for amperometric detection of *Escherichia coli* O157:H7 (*E. coli* O157:H7) [54]. The immunosensing platform was first composed of fullerene,

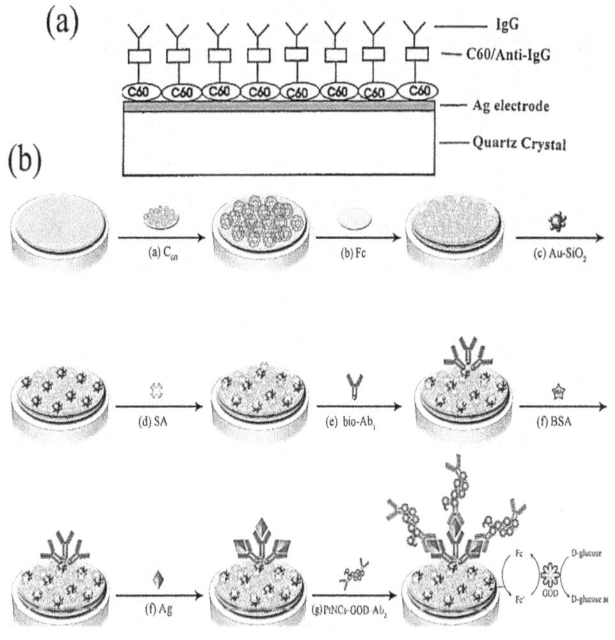

SCHEME 3.4 (a) Diagrams of the C_{60}-anti-human-IgG-coated quartz crystal electrode for IgG, and (b) the fabrication of the electrochemical immunosensor for *Escherichia coli* O157:H7.

Source: (a) Adapted from [53]; (b) adapted from [54].

ferrocene, and thiolated chitosan composite nanolayer (C_{60}/Fc/CHI–SH), and then Au nanoparticle–coated SiO_2 nanocomposites were assembled on the thiolated layer. Next, the large amount of avidin was coated on the Au-SiO_2 surface, which was used to immobilize biotinylated capture antibodies of *E. coli* O157:H7 (bio-Abl). For signal amplification, the glucose oxidase (GOD)–loaded Pt nanochains (PtNCs) were used as a tracing tag to label signal antibodies (Ab2) (Scheme 3.4b). It has been shown that Au-SiO_2-embedded C_{60}/Fc/CHI–SH provide a biocompatible platform for increasing the surface area to capture a large amount of SA/bio-Abl and Ab2 and GOD multifunctionalized PtNC nanocomposites as amplified signals.

3.11.3 Fullerene (C_{60})-Protein Hybrid

Direct electron transfer of biological redox proteins plays an important role in elucidating the intrinsic thermodynamic characteristics of biological systems and designing new kinds of biosensors or biomedical devices. Fullerenes (C_{60}) are ideal nanomaterial for absorbing energy, taking up electrons and releasing them to the transducer. They are small enough to locate at the closest distance to the active site of the catalytic enzyme, which makes the electron transfer easier. Moreover, they are not harmful to biological materials and proteins. The interaction between the enzyme and the nanomaterial surface could be a covalent or non-covalent bond. The improved stability, accessibility, and selectivity, as well as the reduced leaching, can be achieved through covalent bonding because the location of the biomolecule can be controlled. Moreover, several types of immobilization methods have been developed for biomolecules. These methods include entrapment, encapsulation, covalent binding, cross-linking, and adsorption.

3.11.3.1 Enzymes

Glucose oxidase. The determination of glucose is medically important for the diagnosis of diabetes, since the low absorption of glucose can lead to diabetes. In general, glucose is detected by an electrochemical method with an immobilized glucose oxidase (GOD) enzyme. Glucose oxidase (GOD) is a glycoprotein which catalyzes the electron transfer from glucose to oxygen with the by-product of gluconic acid and hydrogen peroxide [55,56]. The preparation of the immobilized GOD enzyme surface is a crucial step in the development of electrochemical glucose sensors. In most cases, GOD enzymes were immobilized by the entrapment of GOD in polymers or macromolecules, for example, polyvinyl alcohol, agar, collagen, cellulose triacetate, gelatin, and Nafion. On the other hand, the covalently coupled enzymes result in the formation of highly stable bonds between enzyme and matrix. Electron-releasing molecules such as amines can attack fullerene C_{60} with 60 π electrons. Therefore, the NH group–containing enzyme molecules is expected to bond chemically to the fullerene C_{60} molecule, resulting in the formation of stable, immobilized C_{60} enzymes [56].

Chuang et al. reported fullerene C_{60} glucose oxidase–immobilized enzyme platform to catalyze the oxidation of glucose and produce gluconic acid, which was detected by a C_{60}-coated PZ quartz crystal sensor for glucose [57]. Fullerene C_{60} was used as a coating material on the quartz crystal of a PZ crystal glucose sensor. The C_{60}-glucose oxidase platform was characterized by FT-IR spectroscopy with absorption peaks at 1,148 cm^{-1} and 1,600 cm^{-1} of glucose oxidase and 525–570 cm^{-1} for fullerene C_{60}. The activity of the synthetic C_{60}-glucose oxidase was investigated by means of the oxygen electrode detector and to catalyze the oxidation of glucose, which results in the consumption of oxygen. The effect of the amount of the immobilized glucose oxidase on the oxidation rate was investigated. It was shown that the consumption of oxygen is linearly proportional to the number of pieces of immobilized enzymes. The obtained results showed that only C_{60}-coated crystals with immobilized enzyme responded sensitively to glucose. The studies on the effect of the amount of C_{60} coating on the frequency response of the PZ glucose sensor with the immobilized enzyme C_{60} glucose oxidase show that the thicker C_{60} coating exhibits a better response, but with a larger amount of coating, it is leveled off. The pH and temperature effect on the activity of the immobilized enzyme C_{60}-glucose showed that an optimum pH of 7 and 30°C for temperature are suitable for the glucose oxidase activity (Table 3.2).

In another report, direct electrochemistry of glucose oxidase (GOD) was achieved with GOD-hydroxyl fullerenes (HFs)–modified glassy carbon electrode protected with a chitosan membrane [55]. The formed GOD-HFs nanoparticles in the chitosan membrane were characterized with TEM images, which showed the average size of 20 nm for GOD-HFs nanoparticles. It has been shown that while no redox peak was observed at bare GCE, Chit/GOD/GCE, and Chit/HFs/GCE, a pair of well-defined redox peaks was observed at the Chit/GOD-HFs/GCE. The CVs remained unchanged after successive potential cycle, showing that the formed Chit/GOD-HFs was stable on the GC electrode. In addition, the obtained Kappm value was lower than that of conventional values, which shows a strong interaction and higher affinity of glucose for the modified electrode.

Lin et al. developed a mixed-valence cluster of cobalt (II) hexacyanoferrate and fullerene C_{60}-enzyme-based electrochemical glucose sensor [56]. The C60-GOD was synthesized and applied with mixed-valence cobalt (II) hexacyanoferrate for analysis of glucose. Glucose in solution can be oxidized by C_{60}-GOD-modified glassy carbon electrode, which is followed by the oxidation of the reduced C60-GOD by oxygen in the solution and formation of H_2O_2. On the other hand, cobalt(II) hexacyanoferrate $(Co_3[Fe(CN)_6]_2)_{(Red)}$ can be oxidized by means of produced H_2O_2. At the end, the oxidized $Co_3[Fe(CN)_6]_2)_{(Ox)}$ was reduced with an applied electrode voltage at 0.0 mV (vs. Ag/AgCl), and the reduced current can be traced for the detection of glucose (Scheme 3.5a).

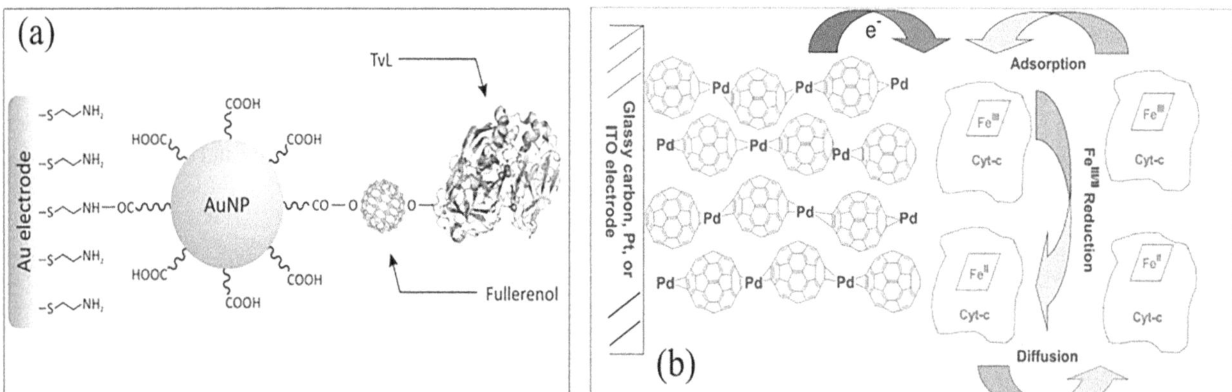

SCHEME 3.5 (a) Au-SAM/AuNPs-Linker/Fullerenols/TvL composite material assembly, and (b) proposed mechanism of cyt *c* immobilization and electrochemical reduction by C_{60}-Pd polymer film–modified electrode.

Source: Adapted from [59].

It has been shown that the electrodes with immobilized enzymes (C_{60}-GOD) show better responses than the electrode with free enzyme. In addition, it was demonstrated that the electrode with a thicker cobalt (II) hexacyanoferrate coating produces a larger current response for H_2O_2. However, the current response apparently tends to level off with larger amounts of cobalt (II) hexacyanoferrate coating. The C_{60}-GOD/cobalt(II) hexacyanoferrate-modified electrode in solutions at a higher stirring rate exhibited a larger current response to the same concentration of glucose. However, the current response apparently tends to level off at a higher stirring rate. Moreover, an optimum current response is obtained around pH = 6.2 and 30°C.

Urease. Urea is one of the by-products of protein metabolism. The precise detection of urea is crucial in various biomedical applications, glomerular filtration rate determination, and renal function tests. The enzyme urease could be employed for urea determination, whereby the urease catalyzes the hydrolysis of urea to form alkaline reaction products of NH_4^+ and CO_3^{2-}. The detection is based on pH changes resulting from the enzymatic reaction:

$$NH_2CONH_2 + H_2O \quad \underline{\text{Urease}} \quad NH_4^+ + CO_3^{2-} \tag{2}$$

Fullerenes have been used in the fabrication of certain biosensors with enzymes such as lipase and urease. Integrating fullerene molecule for the construction of biosensing devices may enhance the sensitivity of the analytical method when it is combined with urease because it provides high surface-area-to-volume ratio for urease immobilization.

A new way to construct a urea potentiometric biosensor has been developed by Saeedfar et al. [58]. The fullerene nanomaterial was functionalized with carboxyl groups by sonication, heat, and ultraviolet (UV) radiation. N,N′-dicyclohexylcarbodiimide (DCC) or N-(3-dimethylaminopropyl)-N′-ethylcarbodiimide hydrochloride (EDC) was utilized to immobilized urease enzyme onto carboxylic-modified fullerenes (C_{60}-COOH). It was observed that a lower sensitivity of the urea biosensor was obtained using water-insoluble DCC as a cross-linking agent instead of EDC. The immobilized urease catalyzed the hydrolysis of urea in the sample, which resulted in the production of OH^- ions. When the concentration of urea is low, the OH^- ion reacted with the buffer, and the concentration of the buffer became important. Therefore, buffer capacity could not maintain the pH, and the sensitivity increased. When the concentration of buffer is high, the sensitivity of the biosensor is decreased because the OH^- ion reacted with the buffer. The optimum pH range of the biosensor was obtained between pH 6.0 and 8.0. In another study, a fullerene C_{60}–coated piezoelectric quartz crystal urea sensor based on either solvated or immobilized urease was developed and applied to detect urea in aqueous solutions. However, the immobilized C_{60}-urease urea detection system shows lower sensitivity than that of the solvated urease detection (Table 3.2).

Laccase. The high stability and bioactivity of the bioelectrochemical interfaces play a crucial role in the performance of laccase-based biosensors. The immobilization of enzymes on solid supports is one of the effective approaches meeting the requirement for a highly sensitive and stable biosensor. There is extensive interest in the construction of laccase biosensors in combination with nanomaterials, due to their unique properties [56]. The fullerene C_{60} nanoparticles provide a suitable microenvironment for enzyme immobilization, maintaining their bioactivity, and accelerating the electron transfer between their redox-active center and transducer surfaces [59]. An electrochemical biosensing platform based on the coupling of two different nanostructured materials (gold nanoparticles and fullerenols) has been developed and characterized by Lanzellotto et al. [59]. The proposed methodology was based on a multilayer material consisting of AuNPs, fullerenols, and Trametes versicolor laccase (TvL) assembled layer by layer onto a gold electrode surface (Scheme 3.5b).

Linear dependence has been obtained between the voltammetry peak currents and the potential scan rate, which attributed to the immobilization of the redox protein. The calculated electron transfer rate constant (ks) values show a higher amount of immobilized TvL on nanostructures-modified electrodes compared to the gold electrode due to the increased roughness of the electrode surface. It was believed that the presence of nanostructured material increases protein loading due to high surface activity and provides an ideal microenvironment for proteins. Microscopic characterization of the electrode surface before and after modification with TvL has been performed by scanning tunneling microscopy. Before enzyme immobilization, several nanoparticles of 15 nm size are observed, and after modification with TvL, a huge increase of particles size is detected (35 nm). In addition, it was observed that Michaelis constant (KMapp) decreases after several introductions of AuNPs and fullerenol, showing an increase of enzymatic affinity for the substrate. It is ascribed to the fact that the fullerenes provide a suitable microenvironment for protein immobilization and induce protein molecule mobility in order to correctly orient its redox centers in order to achieve a proper electron transfer.

Single-walled carbon nanotubes (SWCN) and multi-walled carbon nanotubes (MWCN), with high surface area, high adsorption capacity, and rapid desorbability, are widely used for the construction of enzyme electrodes. One of the most recent examples is reported by Barberis et al., where simultaneous amperometric detection of ascorbic acid (AA) and antioxidant capacity has been performed based on fullerenes-C_{60}/C_{70} or nanotubes-modified graphite sensor-biosensor systems and ascorbate oxidase. It was found out that the combination of fullerene and ascorbate oxidase resulted in complete AA shielding and in the highest selecting capacity toward AA, while nanotubes only increased sensitivity without the ability to discriminate between different compounds. It has been hypothesized that fullerenes absorb more enzyme during dips so that they can oxidize more AA before it reaches the transducer surface.

3.11.3.2 Redox-Active Proteins

Two types of fullerene film–modified electrodes were utilized for immobilization of cyt *c*. One involves an electrochemically conditioned fullerene drop-coated film electrode, and the other an electropolymerized fullerene cross-linked with palladium acetate complex film electrode. The immobilization of cyt *c* on the fullerene film–modified electrode was examined by piezoelectric microgravimetry at a quartz crystal microbalance (QCM). It was shown that upon the addition of cyt *c*, the frequency decreased to reach plateaus. In addition, the blueshift and the broadness of the bands observed in UV-vis spectra were attributed to the cyt *c* molecules, which are tightly packed on the electrode surface. The proposed mechanism of the cyt *c* immobilization is illustrated in Scheme 3.4c. It is believed that site c is immobilized by one or more of the following ways: (1) electrostatically binding the electron-deficient C_{60} molecules with the cyt c molecules; (2) negative charge on the C_{60} film electrostatically binding with positively charged parts of cyt c protein; and (3) surface structure of C_{60} or C_{60}-palladium possibly affecting the immobilization of cyt *c*.

The CV behavior of cyt *c* immobilized on the C_{60} drop-coated film GCE and the C_{60}-Pd polymer film–modified electrode shows that upon the addition of cyt c to the solution, a cathodic peak appeared at Epc = −400 mV vs. Ag/AgCl. When the potential scan was reversed, an anodic peak at Epa = 50 mV vs. Ag/AgCl was also observed, indicating the reversible and slow electron transfer process. When the equilibrium occurs at C_{60}-Pd polymer film–modified GCE in the cyt *c* buffer solution, the CV peaks were still present, showing the stable immobilization of cyt *c* onto the C_{60}-Pd polymer film–modified electrode. In addition, the presence of partially reduced fullerene films stabilized the electrochemical reaction of cyt *c*. The response on the reduced and then oxidized films was also investigated. The oxidized film was still apparently coherent and did not show any signal of cyt *c*. A better response was observed if the films were porous and partially charged. Neutral fullerene films lack the charge, and fully reduced or oxidized films lack the porous character. If the fullerene film reduction was carried out in the presence of Na^+, it resulted in a completely inactive electrode, because it converts the films mainly to semiconducting Na_6C_{60}, which cannot participate in the reaction of cyt *c*. If the film reduction is carried out in the presence of K^+, the electrodes show short-lived transient responses again, as on bare electrodes or with neutral fullerene films.

3.12 Fullerene-Based Modified Sensors and Biosensors

Sensor and biosensor technology is an important starting line in the development of miniature analyzers. This technology is divided into two classes, depending on the interaction of the sensor and analyte molecule: if the analyte molecule is transformed on the sensor surface, it is called a catalytic-based sensor/biosensor, and if the analyte interacts with the surface, it is called an affinity-based sensor/biosensor. The measurement can be performed electrochemically, optically, and piezoelectrically. In electrochemical sensors, electrodes are used as transducers. Different types of electrodes can be used according to the modification and measurement principle. The electrodes can be gold, carbon, platinum, and their derivatives. It is desired to create a modification layer over the self-assembly monolayer; thiol-containing chemicals can be used for gold and gold derivative electrodes [60]. Carbon derivative electrodes can be used for polymer production and adsorption-type studies. Thus, measurement is carried out with electrodes modified with the immobilized recognition agent. If the recognition agent is a catalytic agent (enzyme or nanoparticle), the electroactive species are released as a result of the target molecule that is transformed by recognition receptor. The method of measurement may also vary depending on the type of these species. For example, an amperometric technique is used if an electroactive species is formed, or a potentiometric measurement method is used if an ion is formed. In addition, interaction-based measurement is desired without a reaction between the analyte molecule and the recognition receptor on the electrode surface (DNA, antibody, MIP, polymer, etc.), and impedimetric techniques can be used [60,61].

Optically designed sensor and biosensor systems use optic systems with optic sensitivity as transducers or surface plasmon resonance systems, which are a highly sensitive system that is used quite frequently today with laser canteen systems. The photons detected by the transducer with chemical reaction light-sensing capability that occurs in optic systems can be converted into meaningful signals. In cantilever systems, measurement is performed by creating differences in the angle of the reflected laser signal as a result of the analyte molecule, which is attached to the surface of the cantilever, whose laser signal is reflected under a lever, changing the oscillation of the lever. In surface plasmon resonance–type sensors, the laser signal reflected behind the gold bit surface changes with the binding of the target molecule to the dielectric constant of this gold surface. Here, too, the main purpose is the interaction between the analyte molecule and the recognizing receptor. If there is a catalytic effect, a photon-sensing transducer is used; if there is an affinity-based measurement, cantilever or SPR sensor systems are used.

Apart from these two techniques, piezoelectric systems, which are mass detection systems, can be designed as affinity-based instead of catalytic in biosensor and sensor systems. The method principle is that the analyte molecule interacts with piezoelectric crystals used as transducers, generating signals by changing the oscillation of the piezoelectric systems.

3.12.1 Fullerene-Based Modified Sensors

Sensor systems can use molecularly imprinted polymers, nanocomposites, and other polymeric or dendrimer materials as recognition agent, instead of a biomolecule from biological source, and measurement basis can be formed with it. In this section, examples of this type of sensor technologies are given with the use or modifications of fullerene nanoparticles.

Zhong and colleagues performed the fullerene nanoparticles for catalytic activities; fullerenes were covalently modified with cysteine, and then palladium nanoparticles were added to this spherical structure to create Pd@Cys-C_{60} structure to glucose detection without enzyme. Firstly, the fullerene covalently bonded with the alpha amino group of cysteine on the nucleophilic attack basis in the medium containing the nanoparticles NaOH and EtOH. Then, palladium cation was added, and Pd@Cys-C_{60} nanocomposite material was obtained. As is known, palladium is a highly effective catalytic material in nanoform. In this way, the researchers modified the glassy carbon electrode with this nanocomposite and developed a sensor system that can measure glucose between 2.5 µM and 1 mM, at the lowest detection limit of 1 µM. In selectivity studies, it gave 4.8% signal to substances such as fructose and ascorbic acid. As a result, sensitive and stable signals were obtained with fullerene, such as glucose sensors modified with previously made palladium nanoparticles.

Anusha et al. used fullerene nanomaterials with bimetallic nanoparticles to develop electrochemical sensors for vitamin D3 determination [62]. Copper and nickel metal nanoparticles were used in this study. Glassy carbon electrode was used as the working electrode, and this electrode was modified by dropping C_{60} in toluene. The C_{60} was further reduced in the KOH solution, and then the solutions containing CuNPs, NiNPs, and nanoparticles were deposited electrochemically on this electrode, through the respective electrodeposition steps. Modifying the electrode with these nanoparticles is due to their surface area–enhancing and catalytic effects. $VitD_3$ was measured by cyclic voltammetry by the electrochemical oxidation on NiNPs-CuNPs-C60-GCE. With the development of the method, 1.25–475 µM linearity and 0.0025 µM LOD values were achieved. As a result of the study, a more sensitive method than similar methods was developed [63].

Saha and Das have developed a moisture sensor with C_{60} nanoparticles immobilized on thick alumina layer [64]. In that study, they created nano-sized cavities on the sensor surface with the use of fullerene nanoparticles. With these gaps, they have improved the surface area and have developed a sensor that can detect even trace amounts of moisture not in literature by fullerene advantage. The sensor was briefly prepared by heating a ceramic layer at 900°C after being modified with fullerene, alumina, and polyvinyl alcohol, respectively. The sensor enables capacitive measurements to detect moisture at the ppm levels, in the range of 1–25 ppm. Supported with fullerene, it has the potential to be used successfully in the gas, oil, and food drying industries; due to the small pore size, a highly selective sensor has been developed for other volatile liquids.

Shetti and colleagues have developed a fullerene-modified GCE biosensor for electrochemical acyclovir (ACV) determination. GCE modification with fullerene was carried out according to the drying process on the previously mentioned GCE method. In that study, fullerene was dissolved in dichloromethane instead of toluene, dried by dropping on GCE, and reduced in KOH. Afterward, the electrode was immersed in ACV, and the accumulation of ACV on the electrode surface was carried out electrochemically. ACV measurement was carried out with DPV, and real sample experiments were carried out by adding ACV to the real samples as spike. With this sensor, ACV linear measurement was achieved between 90 nM and 6 µM and 1.48 nM lower limits. The sensor gave more sensitive results compared to other ACV measurement methods by modification with fullerene. Tartaric acid made the most interference on the sensor with 11.6%. In real sample experiments, a matrix effect of less than 3% is observed.

Ertuğrul Uygun and colleagues have developed an impedimetric sensor system modified with cortisol-imprinted polymers on fullerene for the determination of cortisol in saliva [65]. In this study, fullerene C_{60} was dispersed in dimethylformamide and dried on a carbon screen-printed electrode. COOH groups were then formed on fullerene by oxidation process in 2 M H_2SO_4. Afterward, acrylamide was polymerized with APS around cortisol via these COOH groups, and cortisol-imprinted polymers were synthesized on the electrode surface. After removing cortisol with acetic acid, the CE-C_{60}-polyAcry sensor is ready for the determination of cortisol. In that study, which was performed in real saliva samples and compared with tandem mass spectrometry, the cortisol measurement was performed between 0.5 and 64 nM, and the lowest detection limit of 0.14 nM was achieved. Modification of fullerene with carboxyl groups facilitated the synthesis of polymers and increased surface area. Sensor regression analysis compared to tandem mass spectrometry was found to be 0.9778.

Another sensor study developed the preparation of molecularly imprinted polymers by making them more advantageous with fullerene for the determination of ATP by Sharma and his colleagues. In this study, fullerene C_{60} nanomaterials were primarily modified with amide derivatives. After this modification, fullerene derivatives assembled around ATP by cross-linking them with Pd nanoparticles (Figure 3.15). The fullerene derivatives used herein are amide-, carboxyl-, and uracil-functionalized fullerene nanomaterials. This sensor is characterized by complex measuring systems. Concentration determination was carried out capacitively, and characterization of the polymer layer was performed piezoelectrically and voltammetrically. The ATP measurement was carried out piezoelectrically; 0.062 to 1.0 mM linear ATP was measured capacitively, and the lowest detection limit was 0.31 mM.

3.12.2 Fullerene-Based Modified Biosensors

Biosensor systems use biorecognition agents from biological origin as the recognizing agent. These systems can also be catalytic and affinity-based, just as mentioned before. Enzymes are used in catalytic biosensors. The important point here is, a catalytic biosensor system can measure the electroactive species or mediators released by enzymatic reaction. In affinity-based biosensors, the basis of the measurement is the measurement of the interaction between the biorecognition receptor and the target molecule. These interactions are DNA–DNA, DNA–protein, antigen–antibody, or protein–ligand. In this section, fullerene-modified biosensor systems are discussed.

Pan and Shih fullerenes have developed a piezoelectric-based immunosensor system with C_{60} nanomaterials. In this system, piezoelectric quartz crystals were modified by spin-coating the toluene solution containing polyvinyl chloride and fullerene onto these crystals. An adsorption-type modification was carried out by adding anti-immunoglobulin G on this modification. In this biosensor, IgG determination reached the determination range between 0.0001 and 0.01 mg/mL and the lowest detection limit below 0.0001 mg/mL and has shown a very high selectivity.

Suresh and colleagues have developed another C_{60}-modified immunosensor [66]. With this sensor, prostate-specific antigen was determined, and the lower measurement limit of 0.002 ng/mL was reached. The biosensor can detect PSA in a measure

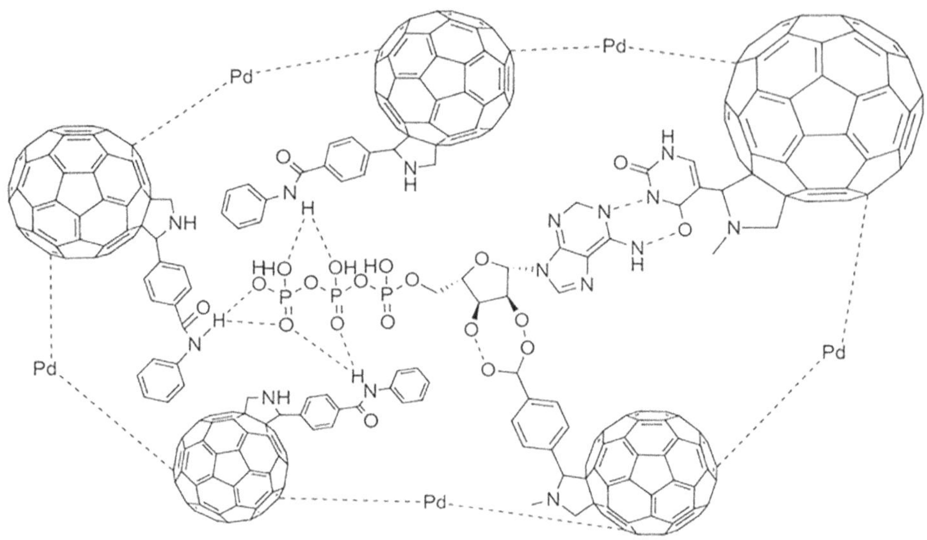

FIGURE 3.15 Amide-, carboxyl-, and uracil-modified fullerene polymers for ATP-imprinted sensor.

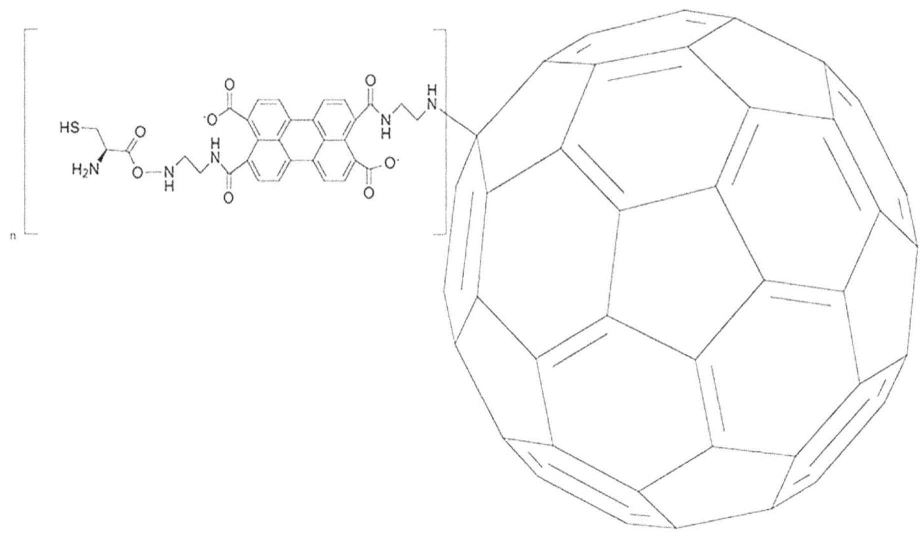

FIGURE 3.16 SH- and NH_2-modified PTC-NH_2-C_{60}.

ranging from 0.005 to 20 ng/mL. GCE was used as the working electrode in the study. The C_{60} was dissolved in toluene and dried on GCE. CuNPs were then deposited electrochemically on fullerene, which was electrochemically reduced in NaOH. Then, the electrode was immersed in hydroquinone (HQ) solution and electrochemically bound to the surface by the application of potential. After that, HQ-modified electrode was activated with EDC/NHS, and anti-PSA was covalently immobilized to this surface. PSA was determined by measuring the hydrogen peroxide reduction of HRP by forming layer by layer on electrode, by blocking the active ends exposed with BSA and the secondary antibody labeled with PSA and HRP, respectively. Electrochemical characterization was performed by CV and EIS. The measurement was carried out with the CV method by the principle of measuring the reduction of the HQ. The biosensor in the serum showed a more sensitive result than similar studies with its fullerene modification, showing a 2% matrix effect [67, 68].

Zhou et al. performed an ultra-trace amount of miRNA-141 measurement in another fullerene-modified biosensor study [69]. In this study, a new method has been developed that provides a double signal increase. G-quadruplex, which is complementary with miRNA-141, was combined to form the DNA–RNA hybrid. The DNA fragment was then cut with a duplex-specific nuclease, and miRNA-141 was released, triggering the next step and measuring. The reason of the system's ultra-sensitivity is that by C_{60}-modified gold electrodes modified with amino and thiol groups, fullerene dissolved in toluene, then passed to the water phase by removing toluene. PTC-NH_2 was obtained by adding anhydrous ethylenediamine to the solution containing 3,4,9,10-perylenetetracarboxylic dianhydride (PTCDA) (Figure 3.16). PTC-NH_2 was mixed with fullerene in the aqueous phase to form amid groups on the fullerene. Afterward, more active groups were formed by adding EDC/NHS on C_{60} by activated Cys. Gold electrode modification was carried out by forming the Au–SH bond of SH groups on the modified C_{60}. Electrochemical characterization of the biosensor was carried out by EIS and CV, and differential pulse voltammetry (DPV) was used as the method of analysis. The target miRNA-141 was determined with this biosensor to measure between 0.1 pM and 100 nM, and the lowest detection limit of 7.78 fM was achieved. As a result of increasing the surface area with fullerene on developed biosensor, the researchers have reached a very low detection limit.

Uygun et al. have developed an impedimetric Fetuin-A biosensor modified with Fullerene-PAMAM (G5) [60]. In this study, the gold electrode, as a working electrode, was first modified by forming self-assembly monolayer of 4-aminothiophenol (4-ATP). Then, activated by EDC/NHS, poly-hydroxylated fullerene was firstly dropped to this surface. Au-4ATP-C_{60}-OH was modified by PAMAM (G5) dropped to the surface, and anti-Fetuin-A antibodies were dropped to the surface, respectively (Figure 3.17). The biosensor compared to ELISA provided linear measurement between 5 and 400 ng/mL and the lowest 1.44 ng/mL measurement opportunity. The fullerene-PAMAM modification has shown that the biosensor is more advantageous than ELISA due to its 3 min determination and high surface area.

At present, we see a wide range of biosensors based on different physicochemical detectors used for recognition and classification, remote sensing of bacteria in the air, detection of pathogens, and other human and environmental healthcare applications. Since its discovery, biosensors have attracted a great deal of interest by researchers. However, in the development of biosensors, the discovery of the fullerene (C_{60}) has made a breakthrough. The reason for this is the nature of fullerene's unique properties. These features include wide light absorption in the UV-vis region, a combination of nucleophilic and electrophilic dual properties, structural angle tension, singlet oxygen production, the ability to be doped with multiple electrons and endohedral metal atoms, photothermal effect, long-life triple state, the ability to act as an electron acceptor. Due to these unique functions, fullerene has the advantage of offering high sensitivity to various biological and biomedical analysts, improved sensitivity, high selectivity, real-time responsiveness, and rapid signal transmission. Moreover, fullerenes that are not dangerous to biological systems and materials are sufficiently small so that they can detect close distance in the active areas of the biomolecules. They can also easily exchange electrons to species surrounding the biomolecules. Furthermore, they serve as an ideal substrate to receive and release electrons to a transducer. Consequently, it possesses a high potential for biosensor applications [70].

In the part of the identification of a biosensor, biological constituents such as antibodies, cells, microorganisms, organelles, enzymes, and tissues are utilized. Fullerenes are used as a mediator between the identification part and the electrode of a biosensor to increase the speed of electron transfer generated by reason of the biocatalytic or biochemical reaction of the analyte in contact with the biological element at the identification field (Figure 3.18).

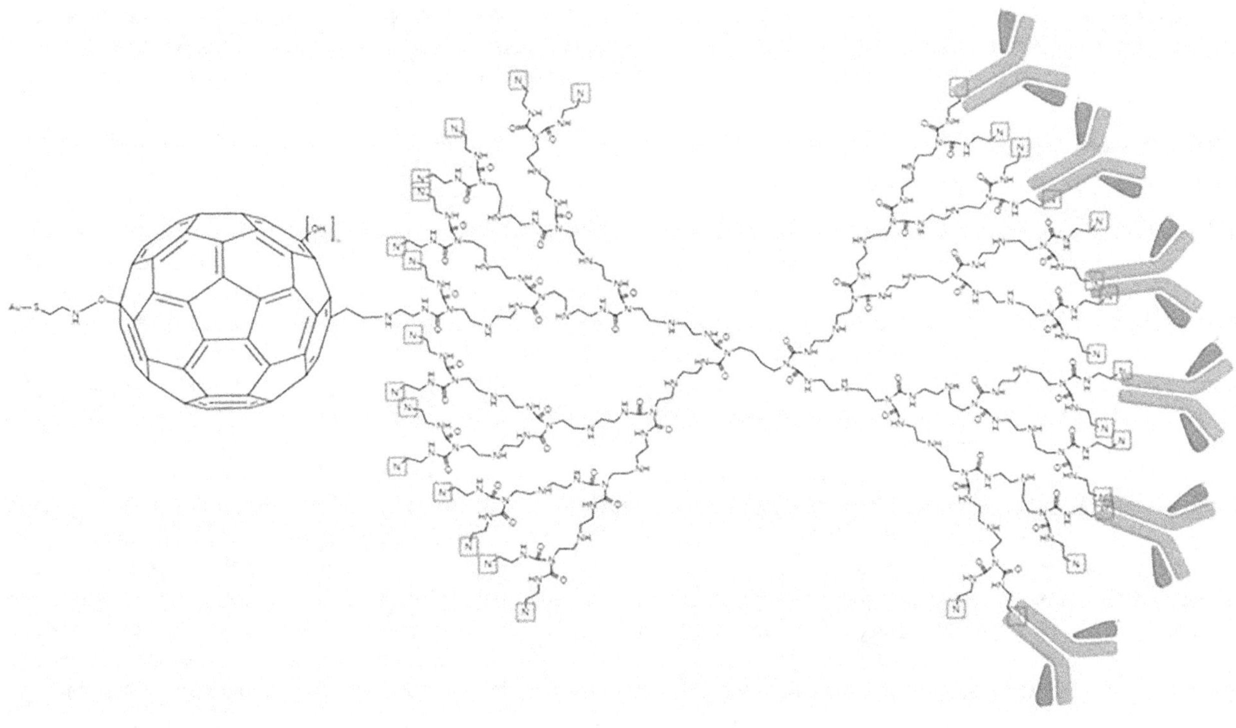

FIGURE 3.17 Modification layers of the fullerene-PAMAM-modified anti-Fetuin-A biosensor (red indicates nitrogen groups represent the active immobilization residue).

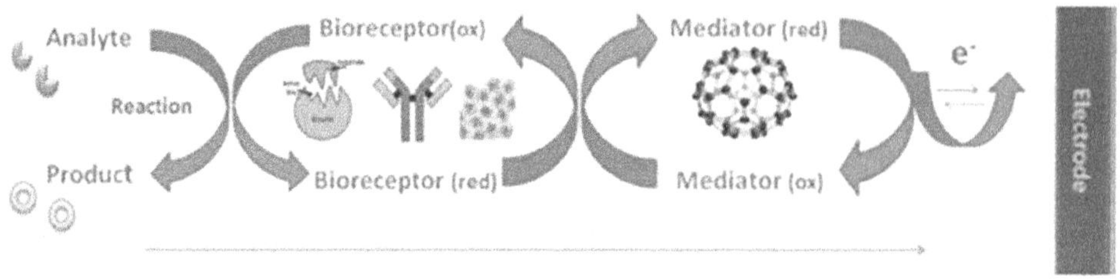

FIGURE 3.18 Biochemical signal to electric signal: role of fullerene.

TABLE 3.3

Comparison of the Fullerene-Modified Sensor and Biosensor Technology

Analytical Method	Modification	Analyte	Linear Detection Range	LOD	Reference
Chronoamperometry	Pd@Cys-C_{60}	Glucose	2.5 μM–1 mM	1 μM	[71]
Cyclic voltammetry	NiNPs-CuNPs-C_{60}	Vitamin D_3	1.25–475 μM	0.0024 μM	[62]
Capacitive	C_{60}.alumina	Moisture	1–25 ppm	1 ppm	[64]
Differential pulse voltammetry	ACV-C_{60}	Acyclovir	90 nM–6 μ M	1.48 nM	[72]
Electrochemical impedance spectroscopy	C_{60}-poly-acrylamide	Cortisol	0.5–64 nM	0.14 nM	[65]
Capacitive	Amide-C_{60}, carboxyl-C_{60}, uracil-C_{60}	ATP	0.062–1 mM	0.31 mM	[73]
Piezoelectric	Anti-IgG-PVA-C_{60}	IgG	0.0001–0.01 mg/mL	0.0001 mg/mL	[74]
Cyclic voltammetry	C_{60}-CuNPs-HQ-anti-PSA	PSA	0.005–20 ng/mL	0.002 ng/mL	[66]
Differential pulse voltammetry	C_{60}-PTC-Cys	miRNA-141	0.1 pM–100 nM	7.78 fM	[69]
Electrochemical impedance spectroscopy	4ATP- C_{60}-polyOH-PAMAM-anti-FetuinA	Fetuin A	5–400 ng/mL	1.44 ng/mL	[60]
Piezoelectric	C_{60}-GOx	Glucose	100 μM–10 mM	39 μM	[75]

Sensor and biosensor studies have shown that the use of fullerene has been an advantage in these systems. It is summarized in Table 3.3 with complete examples.

3.13 Fullerene-Based Polymers

Fullerenes and their derivatives have many remarkable chemical, electronic, and optical properties, but to date, few of these properties have been exploited in commercial products. One reason is that C_{60} and the other fullerenes do not easily lend themselves to processing. Pure fullerenes are insoluble in water, which is a problem when it comes to potential applications in medicine and other areas. Although water-soluble fullerenes can be produced by functionalization with groups such as –COOH and –OH, the dissolved fullerenes have a tendency to clump together rather than remain as separate molecules. Moreover, in order to solubilize fullerenes, it is often necessary to add more than one functional group. Not only can this change the chemical and physical properties of the carbon molecules, but the derivatives fullerenes also often contain a mixture of regioisomers, and these are difficult to separate. An alternative approach which avoids some of these problems is to incorporate fullerenes into polymers. In many cases, a single attachment between the fullerene and the polymer is sufficient to create solubility in water. As well as making fullerenes soluble, incorporating them into polymers generally enhances the processibility of these extraordinary molecules, thus facilitating their application in a wide variety of areas.

This section reviews the ways in which C_{60} and other fullerene molecules can be incorporated into polymeric structures. Firstly, polymers in which the fullerenes are incorporated into the structure by covalent or non-covalent bonding are discussed. These include "pearl necklace" structures, "charm bracelet" structures, organometallic polymers, cross-linked polymers, end-capped polymers, star-shaped polymers, and supramolecular polymers. Secondly, all-carbon polymers, which are produced by fusing fullerenes together, are covered. The synthesis and properties of each class of fullerene polymer are outlined, and the prospects for commercial applications considered.

The fullerene polymers described in this chapter can be divided into two broad classes. In the first class, covered in Sections 3.13.1–3.13.7, fullerenes are incorporated into the polymers by covalent or non-covalent bonding. In the second category, covered in Section 3.13.8, the fullerenes are fused together in all-carbon structures. Great ingenuity has been shown by synthetic chemists in finding ways to prepare the first class of polymeric structures, and many different varieties have been synthesized. The simplest to prepare, and the most widely studied, are charm bracelet, or side chain, polymers, where the fullerenes are attached to an existing polymer backbone. Among the potential applications of charm bracelet polymers has been in solar cells, where the use of a polymer enables the fullerene derivatives to be dispersed throughout the bulk, thus avoiding the issues with aggregation that can result when individual fullerene-based molecules are used. Pearl necklace or main chain polymers, in which the fullerenes are joined together by linking groups, have not been as extensively studied as charm bracelet polymers, as they are more difficult to synthesize. However, several pearl necklace polymers have been prepared, and like charm bracelet polymers, they have been considered as components of photovoltaic devices, as well as for other applications. The other members of the first type of fullerene polymers all have potentially useful applications. Thus, organometallic C_{60} polymers may be useful in catalysis and electrochemistry, while star-shaped polymers might be valuable as components of membranes for gas or water purification. Despite these many possible applications, however, it appears that there are no currently available commercial products which incorporate fullerene polymers. The reason may be the relatively high cost of these materials. The price of pure C_{60} is currently around USD 100 per gram, and the preparation of polymeric structures would add considerably to this cost. Until these prices can be reduced, the potential of fullerene polymers may continue to be unrealized.

Work began on the preparation of fullerene polymers shortly after the bulk synthesis of C_{60}. Since that time, the study of these polymers has grown into a significant sub-discipline of fullerene science [76]. Many different kinds of polymer have been synthesized, including the so-called "pearl necklace," or main chain, structures, in which the fullerene molecules are joined together with short bridging groups, as shown in Figure 3.19a, and the "charm bracelet," or side chain, polymers, where the fullerenes dangle from the backbone of existing polymers, as in Figure 3.19b. Other structures in which fullerenes are linked to existing polymers include random cross-linked and end-capped ones. Organometallic C_{60} polymers, which can be one-, two-, or three-dimensional, have been quite widely researched, while star-shaped polymers, in which a single fullerene molecule is joined to a number of polymer chains, have also been studied. Supramolecular polymers, where the fullerenes are incorporated into to the structure by weak intermolecular interactions rather than covalent bonds, have been prepared, and some have been shown to be soluble in water.

A quite separate class of fullerene polymers is produced by fusing fullerenes together to form all-carbon polymers. These structures can have interesting electrical properties, and they can display extreme hardness. The aim of the current section is to give a brief overview of the various forms of fullerene polymer, with references up to 2020 [77].

3.13.1 Pearl Necklace Polymers

An assembly consisting of two linked C_{60} molecules was synthesized. This could be considered the first step toward a pearl necklace polymer. The synthesis involved reacting C_{60} with the diazomethanes derived from m-phenylenebis (benzoyl) and p-phenylenebis (benzoyl). Early attempts to prepare extended pearl necklace polymers often resulted in intractable, insoluble mixtures. For example, in 2000, Geckeler et al. reported the synthesis of the first water-soluble C_{60} main chain polymer. Here, the linking groups were shielded inside cyclodextrin cavities with the fullerene, as shown in Figure 3.20. They showed that the fullerene retained its ability to cleave DNA nucleotides via a singlet oxygen transfer at the guanosine base sequence when attached to this polymer.

Main chain C_{60} polymers have also been considered as components of photovoltaic devices. The fullerene derivative most frequently employed in such devices is phenyl-C_{61}-butyric acid methyl ester (PCBM), but Hiorns and colleagues suggested that copolymers which incorporate fullerenes as alternating repeated moieties in a conjugated polymer structure might have advantages in this application [78]. The idea was that nanodomains of well-organized copolymers parallel to the electrodes

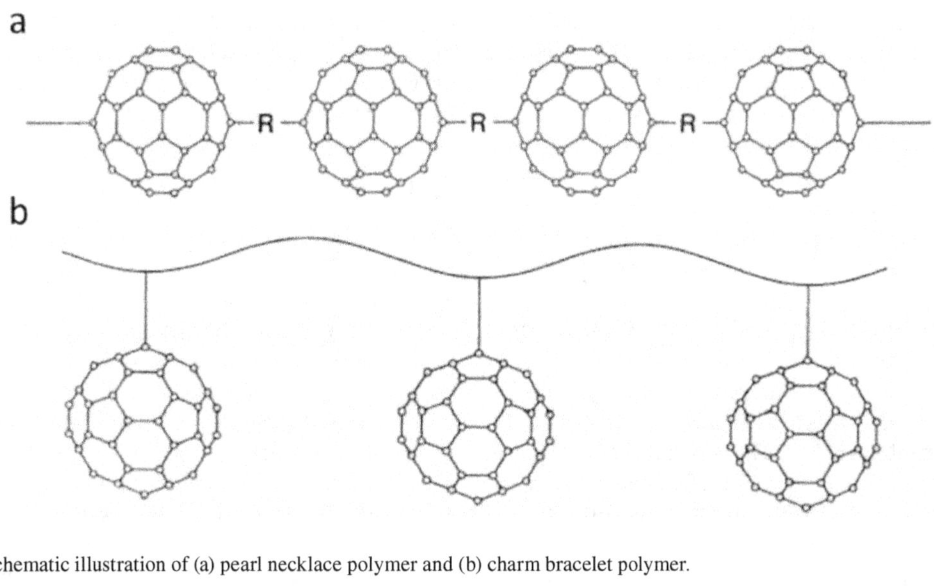

FIGURE 3.19 Schematic illustration of (a) pearl necklace polymer and (b) charm bracelet polymer.

Source: Adapted from Winkler and Balch (2006).

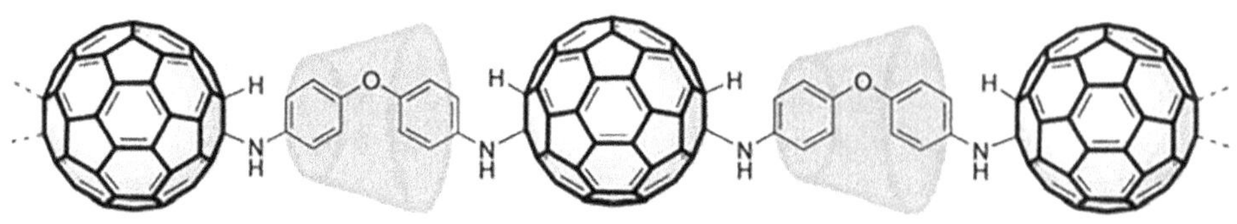

FIGURE 3.20 Water-soluble main chain fullerene polymer with supramolecular cyclodextrin shielding of linking groups.

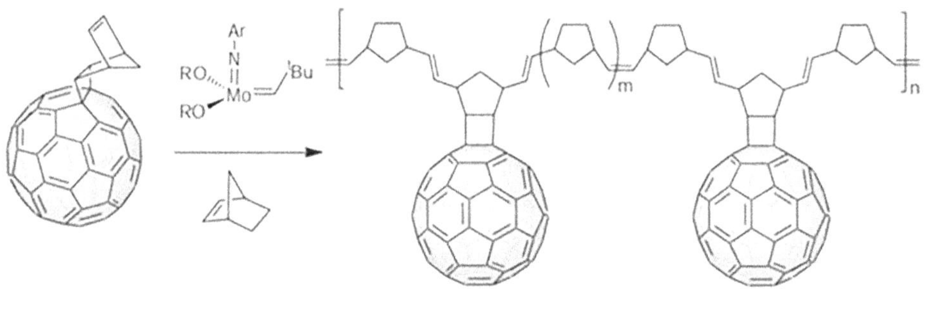

FIGURE 3.21 Polymerization of norbornene-modified C_{60} using ring-opening metathesis polymerization.

might enhance interface interactions and increase current flow. This group prepared bis-benzyl C_{60} polymers through atom transfer radical addition (ATRA) of 1,4-bis(bromomethyl)benzene intermediate to the fullerene. A solar cell containing such a polymer was shown to have an efficiency of 4.2%.

3.13.2 Charm Bracelet Polymers

Most of the common polymers have been functionalized with C_{60} in this way, including aminopolymers, polycarbonates, polysaccharides, polysiloxanes, and polyesters. A popular method for attaching C_{60} to polymers has involved cycloaddition to azido groups on the polymer chains. Hawker prepared polystyrene-C_{60} polymers using this method in 1994 and demonstrated that the copolymer retained both the electronic properties of the fullerene and the solubility and processability of the polystyrene. Other routes to charm bracelet C_{60} polymers include nucleophilic addition and ATRA.

As well as attaching fullerenes to pre-existing polymers, charm bracelet polymers have also been prepared by catalyzed polymerization of fullerene-bearing monomers. The involved polymerizing norbornene-modified C_{60}, in the presence of an excess of norbornene and a catalyst, using ring-opening metathesis copolymerization (ROMP), is shown in Figure 3.21. Other groups have subsequently used the technique.

A number of charm bracelet C_{60} polymers with water solubility have now been prepared. In 2006, Iwamoto and Yamakoshi synthesized a C_{60}-N-vinylpyrrolidone (NVP) copolymer using radical polymerization. This was found to have one of the highest water-solubilities (7.8 mM) of any fullerene derivative. In 2014, the same authors, with colleagues, prepared a soluble C_{60}-polyvinylpyrrolidone (PVP) copolymer and investigated its ability to generate photoinduced reactive oxygen species. A Russian group prepared fullerene-containing copolymers using radical polymerization in 2017. They suggested that the copolymers might find applications as photo- and electroactive materials.

It was noted earlier that main chain C_{60} polymers with potential use in solar cells have been prepared. Side chain polymers have also been prepared with this application in mind. Block co-polymers have often been favored, owing to their tendency to self-assemble into ordered structures. In 2005, Drees, Sariçiftçi, and colleagues described the synthesis of the fullerene derivative C_{61}-butyric acid glycidol ester (PCBG), which they then polymerized. Introducing this into the poly(3-hexylthiophene) (P3HT) active layer resulted in a network of fullerene molecules dispersed throughout the bulk, thus avoiding the issues with aggregation that can result when individual molecules of phenyl-C_{61}-butyric acid methyl ester (PCBM) are used in such cells. The device produced in this way had an energy conversion efficiency of 2%. Other groups have prepared side chain C_{60} polymers for photovoltaic devices. For example, polymerizable C_{70} derivatives have also been considered for this application [79].

3.13.3 Organometallic Polymers

Organometallic C_{60} polymers have attracted significant interest. The first example of such a polymer was a pearl necklace structure synthesized in 1992. By mixing C_{60} with $Pd_2(dba)_3$, where *dba* is dibenzylideneacetone, with 1:1 stoichiometry, these workers obtained a linear $C_{60}Pd$ polymer. They also showed that changing the Pd:C_{60} ratio or heating the one-dimensional polymer could produce three-dimensional polymers. Since this early work, many further polymers with fullerenes covalently bonded to palladium, platinum, and other transition metals have been synthesized. The polymers can be one-, two-, or three-dimensional. Figure 3.22 shows a linear organometallic polymer. A theoretical analysis of the interactions between Pd and fullerenes in polymers has been

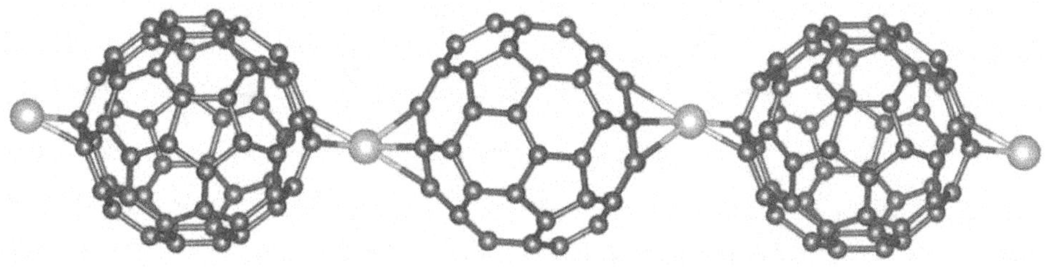

FIGURE 3.22 One-dimensional Ru–C_{60} polymer. Ru atoms are in gray.

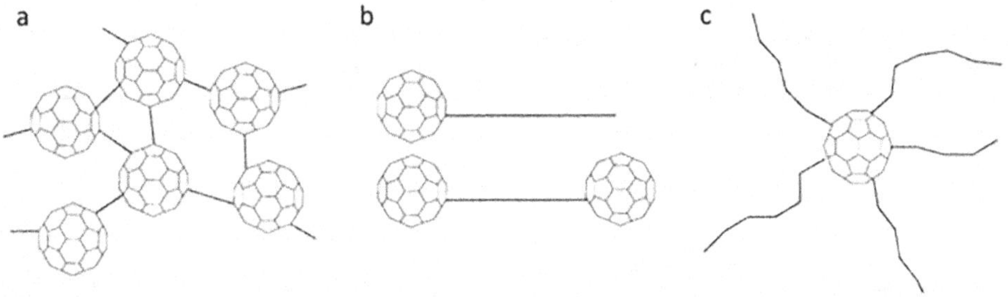

FIGURE 3.23 Schematic illustrations of (a) cross-linked C_{60} polymer, (b) end-capped polymers, and (c) star-shaped polymer.

given by Goclon and colleagues, who found that the most stable polymer structure is one in which the C_{60}s are bonded via the [6, 6] position of the fullerene molecules with Pd in a distorted tetrahedral coordination. Organometallic C_{60} polymers may have potential applications in catalysis [80], electrochemistry, and other areas.

3.13.4 Cross-Linked Polymers

Many of the early attempts to prepare extended pearl necklace and charm bracelet polymers resulted in intractable, cross-linked mixtures. However, a few groups have succeeded in introducing some control into the synthesis of cross-linked polymers in order to prepare potentially useful products. A schematic illustration of a cross-linked C_{60} polymer is shown in Figure 3.23a. In 2016, Sugawara et al. described the preparation of cross-linked polymer–fullerene networks by reacting a tetrazole-functionalized polymer with C_{60} under UV irradiation. They suggested that the networks may have applications in bulk heterojunction solar cells. Chen and colleagues synthesized a cross-linked composite by reacting C_{60} with an aromatic polyamide with pendent furan groups [81]. They demonstrated improved high-temperature shape memory behavior of the composite compared to the pure polymer. As a final example, Zhou et al. incorporated C_{60} into the conducting polymer poly(3,4-ethylenedioxythiophene) (PEDOT), with the aim of producing photo-responsive thermoelectric materials [82].

3.13.5 End-Capped Polymers

End-capped polymers are polymers with a fullerene bonded to one or both ends (see Figure 3.23b). An advantage here is that the exact number of fullerene molecules attached to the polymer is known: it is either one or two, as shown in Figure 3.23b, depending on the synthesis method.

In 2010, Karsten and coworkers prepared diketopyrrolopyrrole-based small-bandgap oligomers, capped at both ends with C_{60}. Upon photoexcitation of the oligomer, ultrafast energy transfer to the fullerene occurs, followed by an electron transfer reaction, suggesting that the assembly could be a useful component of photovoltaic devices. The polymer was added to the P3HT:PCBM active layer of a solar cell, resulting in enhanced performance and air stability of the cell. Hiorns and colleagues have also explored the application of end-capped fullerene polymers in solar cells. In 2017, Topham and colleagues described a method of linking chains of poly(3,4-dimethoxystyrene), generated by reversible-addition fragmentation chain transfer (RAFT) polymerization, to single C_{60} molecules. Their relatively simple approach should be applicable to the preparation of a wide range of different fullerene end-capped polymers.

3.13.6 Star-Shaped Polymers

The so-called star-shaped polymers usually consist of a single-molecule C_{60} joined to a number of polymer chains, as shown in Figure 3.23c. Another potential application for fullerene-containing star-shaped polymers might be as components of membranes for gas or water purification [83–85].

3.13.7 Supramolecular Polymers

In supramolecular polymers, the fullerenes are incorporated into the polymer by weak intermolecular interactions rather than covalent bonds. This has been used as a route to producing

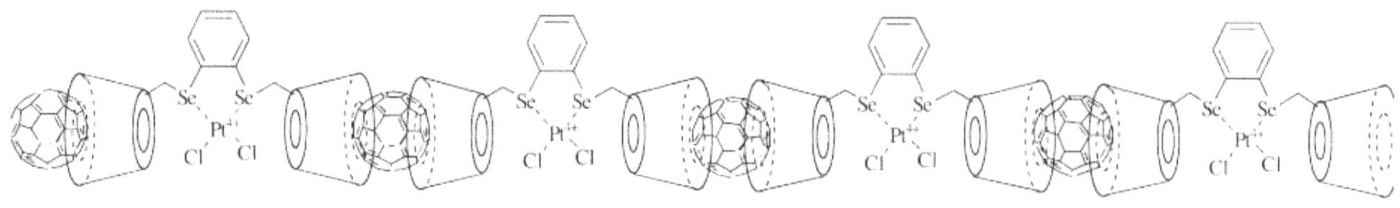

FIGURE 3.24 Supramolecular fullerene polymer mediated by metallobridged β-cyclodextrins.

Source: From Liu et al. (2004).

water-soluble fullerene materials. For example, in 2004, Liu and coworkers prepared the polymer shown in Figure 3.24, where C_{60}s are held within dimeric cyclodextrin units with coordinated metal centers. Assemblies of 60–80 units were prepared and imaged by scanning tunnelling spectroscopy and transmission electron microscopy. The polymer was water-soluble and displayed DNA-cleavage ability under light irradiation. As with the work by Geckeler et al. mentioned earlier, the DNA cleavage involves the generation of excited singlet molecular oxygen by the fullerene.

A high degree of polymerization has been reported, reaching molecular weights greater than 150 kDa in the solution, which was believed to be higher than any fullerene-based supramolecular polymer reported at that time. The authors suggest that these materials might find use in the construction of self-organized optoelectronic devices. Haino and colleagues have recently synthesized fullerene-terminated polymethyl methacrylates (PMMAs) and demonstrated that calix [76] arene hosts can bind to the fullerene moieties of the PMMAs, inducing interesting shape transformations in the polymers [86].

3.13.8 All-Carbon Polymers

As well as incorporating fullerenes into a polymer chain, or attaching them to a polymer via functional groups, it is also possible to prepare all-carbon fullerene polymers. It has been shown that irradiating fcc C_{60} films, in the absence of oxygen, with visible or ultraviolet light produced a phase transformation. Analysis of the new structure showed that the fullerene molecules within the film had been photopolymerized. Work published in the following year showed that polymerization could also be induced by the application of pressures above 1 GPa at moderate temperatures. A theoretical analysis of this process by a group from Grenoble suggested that it involves [2 + 2] cycloadditions between two 6–6 double bonds of neighboring C_{60}s to form cyclobutene rings connecting the fullerenes, to form a one-dimensional chain, as shown in Figure 3.25a. It is now established that a number of different polymeric phases, including two-dimensional and three-dimensional as well as one-dimensional phases, can be produced under different pressure and temperature conditions. Examples are shown in Figure 3.25. Davydov and colleagues have shown that there are two distinct one-dimensional phases, both orthorhombic: a phase formed at low pressure, which could be transformed to a new phase through the simultaneous action of pressure and X-rays. At higher temperatures and pressures, two-dimensional phases form. There are two different phases of these: tetragonal and rhombohedral.

The application of still higher pressures, above 8 GPa, can result in the formation of 3D polymers, and these have been very widely studied, both experimentally and theoretically. In many cases, the poor crystallinity of the 3D polymers means that X-ray crystal structures have not been obtained. One structure which has been established is shown in Figure 3.25d. This was prepared by a group led by Yamanaka in 2006 by applying a pressure of 15 GPa to 2D C_{60} polymer single crystals at 600°C. Single-crystal X-ray diffraction revealed that the 3D polymer crystallized in a body-centered orthorhombic structure, with the C_{60} monomer units substantially deformed to rectangular cuboidal shapes, each unit being bonded to eight cuboidal C_{60} neighbors via [3 + 3] cycloaddition. The structure contains both sp^3 and sp^2 carbon atoms. The polymer shown in Figure 3.25e is taken from work by Marques and colleagues [87]. This is an fcc polymeric C_{60} phase obtained at 9.5 GPa and 550°C. This phase was reported previously by Talyzin et al., but not structurally characterized. As a result, it is not possible to describe the polymer in terms of a defined crystallographic structure. Instead, they proposed a "frustrated" structure, where there is random bonding within the lattice while maintaining the cubic symmetry. Three-dimensional C_{60} polymers have been shown to have a range of interesting properties. In contrast with the nonconductive behavior of 2D polymers, 3D C_{60} polymers are electrically conductive, and they can possess extreme hardness. Research on C_{60} polymers and on the effect of high pressures on fullerenes has been reviewed [87, 88].

3.14 Conclusions and Future Prospective

Fullerenes have become important molecules in different health-related subjects during the last three decades. The biomedical applications presented in this manuscript represent potential uses of this class of carbon family, due to its extraordinary properties (see Table 3.1). As more applications of these nanomaterials become available, the demand for different forms of fullerenes will increase. For future works, functionalized fullerenes will considerably change the face of biological applications, and the credits go to the collaborative efforts of scientists who focus on both chemistry and medicine. These collaborative efforts are critical for introducing the most effective modifications on the carbon cage for successful diagnosis and therapeutic outcomes in different biomedical applications.

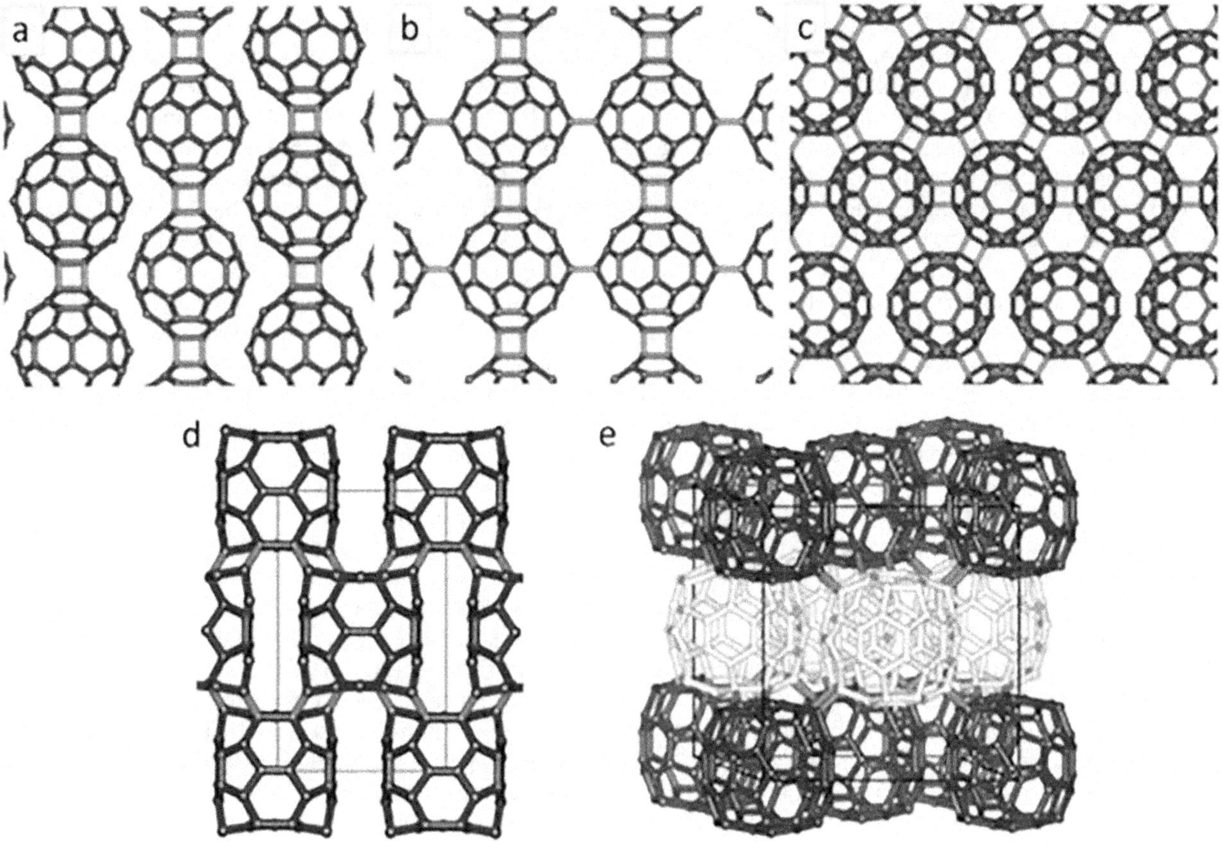

FIGURE 3.25 All-carbon polymerized C_{60} structures: (a) 1D, (b) 2D-tetragonal, (c) 2D-rhombohedral, (d) 3D cuboidal, (e) 3D AuCuI-type.

Source: Adapted from [87].

Here, we have provided an overview of the ever-expanding research on fullerenes in biomedical engineering applications ranging from drug delivery to non-invasive imaging in the human body. These studies are mostly limited to *in vitro* and *in vivo* researches and have not reached the final stages of clinical trials yet. It is expected that, with the rapid technological advancement in this field, this trend could change in the coming years so that the unique features of fullerenes could be exploited in clinical use. Although there are still major issues to overcome, the use of fullerenes for biomedical engineering will certainly have a bright future.

Nanomaterials are becoming more important and interesting day by day, and their usage areas are increasing. In this chapter, the sensor and biosensor systems modified with fullerene are explained; how fullerene is adapted to these systems and how it is modified are explained with examples as well. As a result, fullerene has successfully completed the task and contributed significantly to the development of these systems. The use of fullerene enabled the development of sensitive sensors by increasing the surface area. At the same time, its contribution to being an indestructible immobilization material and providing durability cannot be ignored.

Recently, nanostructured materials have been significantly used to create state-of-the-art electrochemical biosensors with enhanced performance. They provide analytical devices with the ability of miniaturization and reduced response time and cost-effectiveness for application in clinical diagnosis. Among different nanomaterials, carbon nanomaterials hold potential promise as a material for designing a new generation of biosensors due to their unique characteristics. Recently, fullerene C_{60} contributed greatly to the field of biosensing and bionanotechnology. The unique electrochemical and physicochemical properties, together with biocompatibility characteristics of fullerene, allow its wide use for designing the highly sensitive chemical/biosensors (www.webofknowledge.com).

Concerning all-carbon fullerene polymers, these are fascinating materials which continue to be the subject of intensive research. One-, two-, and three-dimensional structures have been synthesized, and many more potential all-carbon polymers are possible. The polymers which have been produced display a wide range of electronic and elastic properties, but as with the other forms of polymer discussed here, the high cost of fullerenes remains a serious problem when considering commercial applications.

Fullerene has the advantage of offering high sensitivity to various biological and biomedical analysts. Moreover, fullerenes that are not dangerous to biological systems and materials can also easily exchange electrons to species surrounding the biomolecules. Furthermore, they serve as an ideal substrate to receive and release electrons to a transducer. Consequently, it possesses a high potential for biosensor applications.

In this chapter, fullerene and many of its derivatives have been stated along with their uses in different pharmaceutical applications. Fullerenes have a specific structure, and it helps in the treatment of some diseases. What makes fullerene good for delivering the drug is the ability to cross the blood–brain barrier, carry the load of multiple drugs, deliver it to the targeted cells, and not dissolve before reaching the targeted cells. Fullerenes are used to deliver antitumor drugs, drugs for cancer therapy, and drugs that need to enter the brain. They can inhibit HIV-1 and also gram-positive bacteria. Fullerenes and their derivatives are widely used in the medical field.

In this chapter, we presented the most recent applications of fullerene C_{60}-based electrochemical biosensors, which employed various kinds of biomolecules. Especially, electrochemical biosensors based on the interaction between fullerene C_{60} and DNA has been reviewed in depth. It has been shown that fullerene C_{60} has been widely utilized for improving the sensitivity of electrochemical biosensors. Not only do they provide a suitable immobilization platform for DNA and antibodies, but they also have the ability to induce in redox-active proteins a proper orientation, which leads to better electron transfer properties. Therefore, fullerene C_{60} can be easily extended to immobilize and obtain direct electrochemistry of enzymes and proteins.

However, the range of applications is still limited, and further investigation is required. Easy functionalization and high surface area of fullerene can be utilized for designing more sensitive biosensing devices with high stability. The recent developments of electrochemical biosensors based on fullerene C_{60} may bring many researchers to use other analogues of fullerene C_{60} in the construction of electrochemical biosensors. Furthermore, multiple functionalizations of these kinds of nanomaterial may lead to the improved performance of biosensors. On the other hand, taking into account the biocompatibility of fullerene C_{60}, different kinds of biomolecules, such as microorganisms, organelle, and cells, can be easily integrated into biosensor fabrication. Moreover, fullerene-based biosensors could be integrated within bio-chips with onboard electronics. This will lead to fabricating devices which are small, low-cost, with simple operation procedure. Therefore, electrochemical biosensors based on fullerene C_{60}, with their cost-effectiveness and suitability for microfabrication, can be expected to become increasingly popular in the near future.

In conclusion, the interaction between the target molecule and the recognition receptor on sensor and biosensor systems can be measured with electrical, optic, and piezoelectric systems. The important point in these measurements is the characteristic of the modification layer on which the recognizing receptor is immobilized. As we mentioned earlier, the usage of nanomaterials in biosensor and sensor systems is to increase the surface area and electrical conductivity, to create a more stable layer for immobilization, and to use nanomaterials catalytically by generating electroactive signals from the electrical characteristics of nanomaterials. With the advantages of these materials, more sensitive and selective sensor and biosensor systems can be developed.

4

Computational Simulation Optimization and Pharmaceutical Role of CNTs-Based Development of New Target Drug Delivery Systems (DDSs) for Enhanced Efficacy in Anticancer Therapy

4.1 CNTs on Molecular Dynamics Simulation-Based Development of New Drug Delivery Systems

Carbon nanotubes (CNTs) are widely used in drug delivery systems (DDSs) due to their unique chemical and physical properties. Investigation of interactions between biomolecules and CNTs is an interesting and important subject in biological applications. The interactions in the CNT functionalized with polyethylene glycol (PEG) are more than the other investigated systems. Furthermore, it was found that the solubility of CNTs in aqueous solution is increased by functionalization. This is related to the intermolecular hydrogen bonds between functional groups and solvent molecules. The PEG group has the greatest effect on the solubility of the CNT in aqueous solution due to more polar interactions.

Cancer remains among the world's top devastating diseases, with millions of lives been affected each year. Conventional anticancer therapies are often far from ideal due to non-selective biodistribution. Therefore, carbon nanotube (CNT) has been developed as a drug carrier for targeting specific cancer cells. Computer modeling approaches have been applied to investigate the interactions of single-walled carbon nanotube (SWCNT) with three different anticancer drugs: doxorubicin (DOX), bendamustine (BEN), and carmustine (CAR).

Recently, physicochemical characteristics have been found from the ligands that can contribute to a higher affinity toward CNT, such as the presence of halogen substituents and the positively charged cation. On the other hand, the presence of anions groups, such as carboxylate, can decrease the interaction of the ligands and CNT. The binding free energy results indicate SWCNT (15,15) with a diameter of 20.3 Å as the most favorable for encapsulating drugs ranging from 12 to 39 heavy atoms. The basic knowledge obtained from this study [1] is expected to contribute to the molecular understanding of drug-loaded SWCNT for the development of a more efficient anticancer drug carrier. Figure 4.1 represents the molecular modeling and dynamics simulations of carbon nanotube as a drug carrier.

We conclude with some thoughts on the role that molecular dynamics simulation can grow to play in the development of new drug delivery systems (Figure 4.1) [1].

The exponential advance of the computational power available to us has led to related approaches attaining a prominent—one can argue, now dominant—position within pharmaceutical research. The majority of these toolkits, as we will elaborate later, are methodologies that fit experimental data to a mathematical model that provides a numerical answer, for example, a specific drug molecule structure or delivery system formulation. A subset of computational methodologies provides something further: mechanistic understanding; in place of just an answer, that is, an optimum value or set of values, *mechanistic understanding* means an elucidation of what is actually occurring in the system that produces the results: in simple terms, a model of the system, expressed as a cartoon in three dimensions, of what is happening. Such an output, often referred to as a simulation, has power far beyond that provided by a mere result of what is optimal for the specific application sought; it can lead to an informed design process that is more efficient, allows for broader intuitive leaps from its interpretation, and provides insight that transcends the specific application studied.

An extremely successful computational scheme for attaining mechanistic understanding is molecular dynamics simulation (MD), a methodology that models the system as a set of particles that interact through classical mechanics. An intuitive choice for these particles, particularly for those with a background in chemistry, is for them to represent atoms, with interactions between the atoms producing the intramolecular forces that govern the structure of molecules and the intermolecular forces that govern interactions between molecules. This is, however, not the only choice that can be made, as particles can be chosen to represent larger structures than single atoms; they can represent groups of atoms, whole molecules, or even groups of molecules. Such models can obtain insight into the system on a larger length and timescale than can be achieved through a model with atomistic resolution and are known as coarse-grained.

In this chapter, we will highlight the growing role that MD has played and will continue to play in drug delivery, what has been referred to as computational pharmaceutics by Ouyang and Smith, using computational methods to address issues related to drug delivery, including dissolution, solubility, protection from the body's defense mechanisms, controlled release, and targeted delivery. The development of advanced mechanisms for drug delivery based on nanoscale drug delivery vehicles, a field known as nanomedicine [2], is a particular area where MD methods have borne fruit. This review chapter has two target audiences: (1) pharmaceutical researchers intrigued by the rapid rise of computational methods applicable to their research, who are interested in learning what kind

DOI: 10.1201/9781032635989-4

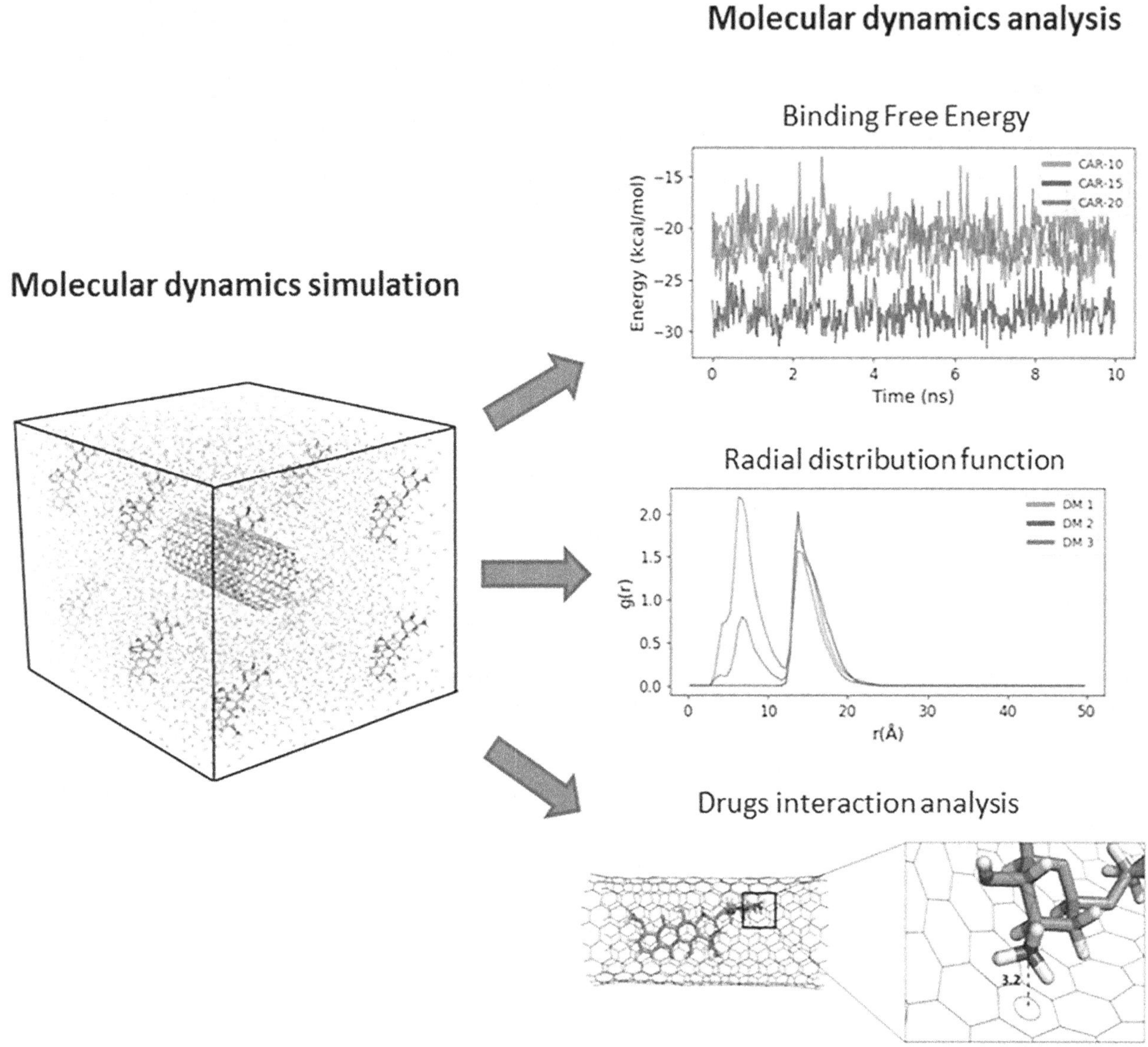

FIGURE 4.1 Molecular modeling and dynamics simulations of carbon nanotube as a drug carrier.

Source: [1].

of insight MD can provide, and (2) computational physicists and chemists with a background in MD methods, atomistic and coarse-grained, who, for reasons I most probably do not need to inform the reader of, realize that at this point in history pharmaceutical applications are an extremely desirable context for their research. Both of the target audiences will find certain elements of this chapter to be trivially basic and may even bristle at some oversimplifications; one should keep in mind the dual-audience-focused nature of this chapter. As the subject matter is extremely broad, with several areas covered by comprehensive reviews themselves, this publication can, to some extent, be seen as a meta-review, to be used as an initial jumping-off point leading to many further review papers, in addition to original work.

At its core, pharmaceutical science is roughly (1) the search for small molecules that, over the scale of the entire organism, do more good than harm under certain conditions (drug design) and (2) the development of the means by which these molecules can enter the body and reach their target tissue intact (drug delivery or pharmaceutics). Pharmaceutical science begins with Paracelsus, the man who is to pharmacy what Isaac Newton is to physics, and his maxim "the dose makes the poison"; substances exist that, at too high a dose, are a poison that will kill you but, when taken at a certain dose, can actually help you. The substance enters the body, dissolution occurs, and the drug molecules within the substance are freed and diffuse through the body; enough reaches, intact, the desired location in sufficient quantity to induce the desired effect. Any drug molecule will reach other parts of the body and have different effects which are undesirable: the toxicity, that is, side effects, of the drug. The conventional drug design paradigm is thus a balancing act between efficacy, toxicity, and solubility. A very efficacious drug can be found that either has intolerable toxicity or too poor solubility to be carried through the bloodstream, or due to the nature of the target tissue, insufficient quantities of the drug reach it to have the desired effect.

Initially, drugs were found through trial and error; however, the search space is gigantic: the number of different small organic molecules that are theoretically possible to synthesize is ~1,063 a number that dwarfs such quantities as Avogadro's number and the number of stars in the universe; drug design can be seen as searching this discrete "drug structure space." The latter half of the 20th century saw the onset of a systematic approach to searching this space based on the "lock and key" paradigm: drug molecules were designed to fit a certain active site on a certain protein to either inhibit or activate them. This was propelled by advances in three areas: (1) robotics, to enable massive simultaneous parallel screening experiments; (2) increasing numbers of high-resolution protein structures, determined first through X-ray crystallography but now increasingly through cryo-EM; and (3) the computational power and advanced algorithms to analyze the massive datasets produced. The computational component of this computational drug design can be divided into two methodologies: (1) ligand-based, where the target protein structure is not known, and (2) structure-based, where the binding free energy of potential drug molecules is calculated using the experimentally determined high-resolution protein structure, a calculation known as "ligand docking and scoring." Ligand-based methods use pattern recognition, now trendily referred to as "machine learning," algorithms where elements of the structural properties are mapped to either (1) high-throughput screening results for activity, that is, efficacy and other desirable properties, for example, solubility parameters (quantitative structure activity relationship/quantitative structure property relationship [QSAR/QSPR]) [3], or (2) elements of three-dimensional structure of the molecule (pharmacophore modeling).

Apart from the pharmacological research to determine appropriate target protein active sites, the aforementioned methodologies for drug discovery together are a fixed, simplified, purely empirical paradigm: fitting data without insight. As is the case with research carried out using a fixed paradigm, metaphorically speaking, continuing to turn the crank on the same machine, one reaches a point of diminishing returns; this is exactly what has occurred for the case of pharmaceutical research: as the resources spent globally on pharmaceutical research increase exponentially, the number of new drugs approved each year remains constant, a phenomenon referred to as "Eroom's law," the reverse of the famous Moore's law regarding the exponential increase in computational technology we have witnessed over the past half century: pharmaceutical research is slowing down exponentially; moving forward requires moving beyond this oversimplified model.

The situation for drug delivery, that is, pharmaceutics, is similar. When a given molecule is designed, using the preceding methodology, a set of rules of thumb is applied regarding its properties, known as "Lipinski's rule of 5." This determines whether the molecule is "drug-like," that is, a molecular structure likely to have a sufficiently optimal solubility profile, or not. Behavior of the drug in the body apart from its drug action, known as its absorption, distribution, metabolism, and excretion (ADME) properties, is a critical aspect that partially determines both efficacy and toxicity. This is modeled using numerical solutions to complex sets of coupled differential equations that represent the interactions of drugs and drug metabolites, as their distribution varies in time in the different tissues of the organism; this form of numerical computational modeling is known as pharmacokinetic/pharmacodynamics modeling [4]. While this form of modeling is not entirely empirical, as it is dependent on known metabolic relations, it still remains a method to calculate a quantitative result from experimentally measured parameters.

Given that the global pharmaceutical industry is estimated to have a turnover in excess of 1 trillion USD, there is obviously a substantial continuing effort to break out of the rut of diminishing returns it finds itself in. Regarding pharmaceutics, the last 30 years have seen the development of increasingly sophisticated mechanisms for enhancing the solubility profile, carrying/protecting drugs in the bloodstream and targeting them to the desired tissue: the aforementioned nanomedicine [2]. These involve either covalently bonding the drug to a molecule or packaging the drug into a nanoscale (diameter 100 nm or less) vehicle that performs this function. As this field has developed, these means have become increasingly complex and intricate, and as a result, this avenue has also become stuck: while increasingly complex devices make for engaging narratives, leading to well-cited publications, the greater the complexity, the more that can go wrong, resulting in a field of research that is far better at producing publications than real approved therapies. As Venditto and Szoka have put it, "so many papers and so few drugs!" The resulting system, coupled with the human physiological environment, is far too complex to be developed through the previously described limited, mostly empirical, paradigm.

It can be argued that what is missing is mechanistic understanding: insight into what is actually physically happening, that is, what the molecules are actually doing. The previously described computational methods do not provide this; what they provide is a numerical answer. Mechanistic understanding is obtained by a computational method that can, given knowledge of the structure of molecules, provide insight into how the molecules interact, that is, what structures they form and how they move with respect to each other with time: a three-dimensional movie of what is happening on the molecular length scale. A molecule, or system of molecules, is a set of nuclei and electrons interacting in a specific way. How this interaction affects the motion of the atoms, that is, the physics of the system, is quantum mechanics. Exact calculation is impossible; however, the discipline of theoretical quantum chemistry has developed many methods for approximating the behavior of molecules governed by quantum mechanics. While these calculations can be simplified through the use of semi-empirical methods, we are still left with a calculation that is too computationally intensive to simulate the length and timescales that are of interest to us. Making a set of approximations and accepting certain limitations of the variety of phenomena that can be observed, we arrive at the molecular mechanics paradigm: the molecule modeled as a set of particles with their interactions governed by classical mechanics.

The target-specific delivery of drugs or other molecular cargo by using carbon nanotubes (CNTs) has emerged as one of the most promising biomedical applications of nanotechnology. The ability of functionalized CNTs to become ingested into specifically targeted cells to release their contents in response has created a substantial impact for the treatment of patients suffering from various diseases. In particular, CNT-based targeted drug delivery has gained much attention for the improvement of cancer treatment to circumvent the unwanted side effects associated with nonspecific chemotherapy, which tends to kill normal healthy cells as well. Several research articles, reviews, and books have been published, highlighting the various insights based on experimental investigations on the biocompatibility, toxicity, functionalization, loading, unloading, and cellular uptake of CNTs. However, the remarkable physical, chemical, and mechanical properties of CNTs enable them to be useful for the applications of various drugs and proteins, as well as gene delivery.

One of the key advantages of CNT-based target-specific drug delivery is that a highly toxic drug can be used at a lower dosage, thus reducing side effects. Moreover, CNTs provide the perfect isolated environment for the drug while protecting it from degradation and reaction with healthy cells, as well as allowing the drug to circulate for a long period in the blood until it reaches and is delivered to the target site with minimal side effects. Thus, CNT-based drug delivery offers a promising alternative for the treatment of various diseases, such as infections, metabolic diseases, and autoimmune diseases, as well as for use in gene therapy. Recent advances in computer-aided drug design (CADD) strategies provide a great opportunity to efficiently build and simulate (in silico) the interactions of CNTs with drugs, as well as cell membranes, to gain insight into the various physicochemical requirements for engineering effective site-directed, CNT-based drug delivery.

Today, cancer is one of the key causes of mortality in modern societies. A variety of anticancer drugs has been employed in cancer treatment, but most of these drugs have systemic toxicity and low therapeutic effectiveness with acute side effects. PTX is a strong anticancer drug for the treatment of a wide range of cancers. However, the use of this drug is limited due to very low solubility in aqueous solutions and high severe side effects.

Today, many systems based on drug delivery have been developed to enhance bioavailability and reduce side effects of anticancer drugs. There are several types of nanoparticles, such as polymeric nanoparticles, CNTs, and nanocrystals, that can be used as DDSs for the PTX drug molecule. The encapsulation of PTX in these biodegradable and non-toxic nano-DDSs can enhance PTX solubility, improve PTX pharmacokinetic profiles *in vivo*, and decrease its side effects. Generally, one of the best carriers for drug delivery is CNTs, as they can bind to the drug molecules through covalent or non-covalent interactions. This type of DDS can improve the therapeutic performance of the drug molecules. Since pristine CNTs are chemically inert and do not dissolve in solvents, covalent or non-covalent functionalization is usually required to render them soluble, and also to attach other chemical moieties. These modifications can alter the CNT properties, such as the selectivity, biocompatibility, solubility, and decrease toxicity and retention in the tumor.

Lay et al. reported that modification of CNTs with PEG groups leads to improved cytotoxicity of PTX in cancer cells and enhances their solubility. They also found that modified CNTs can be used as DDSs to improve bioavailability and efficacy of insoluble drugs.

Arsawang et al. performed MD simulation to provide more insight into the structural properties of the encapsulation of gemcitabine in single-walled carbon nanotubes (SWNT). Their obtained results indicated that the drug molecule prefers to locate inside the SWNT, and the formation of π–π stacking interaction between the cytosine ring of drug and CNTs is the main interaction in the encapsulation of the drug. Li et al. reported MD simulation results for the vinblastine (VLB)–CNT interactions in different conditions. Free energy results reveal that the drug molecule can take three stable orientations on the CNT sidewall under the attachment of loading mode. Furthermore, they found that functionalization of the CNT with ester groups enhanced the biocompatibility of drug with biological systems and reduced the toxicity of the CNT.

Mousavi et al. performed steered molecular dynamics (SMD) to investigate the penetration mechanisms of carbon nanotube (CNTs)–encapsulated PTX, through the phospholipid bilayer membrane. They found that the CNT facilitates targeted delivery of the polar PTX molecule through the lipid bilayer since it has the ability to penetrate into the cell membrane. Their results show that the van der Waals and hydrogen bond (HB) interactions are the main interactions in the delivery of PTX molecules.

Despite the existence of numerous experimental studies on the CNTs (the pristine and modified CNTs) based on PTX delivery, there are few theoretical reports that investigate the interactions between this drug and CNT. Therefore, it is necessary to provide a thorough understanding of these systems and improve the performance of the DDSs. Such theoretical studies can provide fundamental knowledge for the design and optimization of CNT-based carriers for PTX delivery. The results of this work can give an insight into the effect of functional groups on CNT-based DDS, which could be helpful in future experimental studies by medical scientists.

4.1.1 The Molecular Mechanics Paradigm and Molecular Dynamics Simulation

The molecular mechanics paradigm is based on a combination of insight from the quantum mechanical interactions of atoms and empirical physical chemistry. The resulting model, illustrated in Figure 4.2, can be intuitively pictured as a set of sticky rubber balls (the short-range attractive van der Waals and repulsive Pauli exclusion forces modeled through what is known as the Lennard–Jones potential term) that are charged (electronegativity of atoms and H-bonding behavior modeled through partial charges) connected by springs (the bond forces) with hinges (angular interactions), axels (proper dihedral potentials), and other four-body interactions to produce the correct structure (improper dihedral potentials); the atoms and molecules follow Newton's equations of motions, knocking into each other and rattling about in response to these forces. The result is a three-dimensional movie of the system

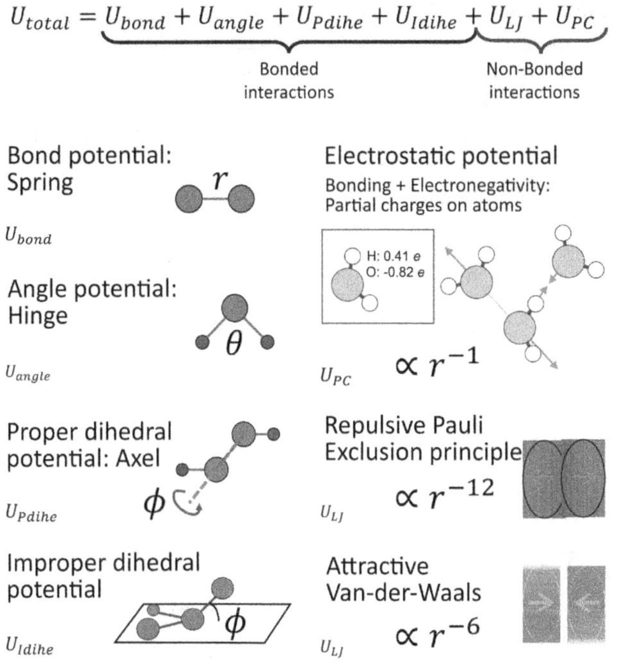

FIGURE 4.2 The set of interactions that are the molecular mechanics paradigm that defines the forces that drive the motion of atoms in a molecular dynamics simulation with all atom resolution. The bond, angle, and dihedral potentials are the intramolecular interactions that define molecule structure and the interactions between covalently bound atoms. Each atom has a partial charge that interacts with all other atoms through electrostatic forces to model electronegativity and H-bonding behavior; short-range attractive and repulsive forces due to the van der Waals and Pauli exclusion principle, respectively, are modeled through the Lennard–Jones interaction.

with atomistic resolution: molecular dynamics simulation. This has been referred to as a "computational microscope"; however, we feel this analogy is misleading, as this is not a visualization of a piece of a real system but rather the isolation and study of a specific aspect of the system that we have assembled the appropriate set of models of molecules to study. A discussion of the methods used to determine the parameters of this model can be found elsewhere.

Several competing potential sets exist, and for simulating any system with new molecules that have never been simulated before, often the case in pharmaceutical as opposed to biological research, since we deal with unique man-made molecules, quantum chemistry calculations must be performed; choosing and building potential sets for the model to obtain the correct result requires significant expertise. While molecular dynamics simulation with an all-atom model has seen significant success in the study of a wide range of biophysical systems, it is still limited to length scales of ~15 nm and timescales of ~1–2 µs: too small to obtain insight into several phenomena we wish to study. Here we return to the aforementioned coarse-grained models (Figure 4.3). While several phenomena cannot be observed, as they are dependent on specific interatomic interactions, for example, salt bridges and H-bonds, with good judgment, such models allow for the metaphorical camera to zoom out and study behavior on larger length and timescales, however with reduced resolution.

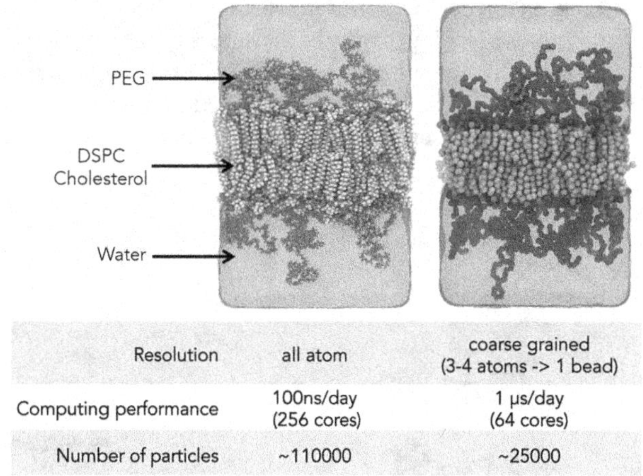

FIGURE 4.3 Illustration of coarse-graining: the same system, a PEGylated membrane, modeled with an all-atom and a MARTINI model is shown along with the decrease in the number of particles and acceleration in the simulation time.

While several schemes for the development of coarse-grained models have been proposed [5], the two that have been most frequently used are the MARTINI potential set, where the coarse-grained particles are groups of ~3 atoms with the potential sets developed based on the solubility parameters of these groups, and dissipative particle dynamics (DPD), where the degree of coarse-graining is greater still, where the particles are soft "momentum carriers" and temperature is controlled through a thermostat designed to conserve local momentum as the effects of hydrodynamics become important at this larger length and timescale. Another scheme is incorporating the effect of the solvent through adjustment to the interactions between particles in the molecules of interest, that is, simulating with adjusted potentials in a vacuum; this is known as the "implicit solvent" model. An ideal that is often sought and discussed is "multiscale simulation"—combining the insight from simulations carried out with different methodologies on different length and timescales. In 2013, the Nobel Prize in Chemistry was awarded to Arieh Warshel, Martin Karplus, and Michael Levitt for the "development of multiscale models for complex chemical systems" (The Nobel Prize in Chemistry 2013, 2013) [6]. From the literature search for this chapter, it can, however, be surmised that this ideal, for the most part, remains an ideal: for the recent original research found, in our literature search for this review, that applied MD simulation in the field of drug delivery, the number of publications that use more than one methodology remains a small minority. Several reviews cover the use of coarse-grained methods for the simulation of systems composed of lipids, polymers, and proteins [7].

Now that we have this three-dimensional movie of the system, known as a trajectory, beyond just visualization, there are several techniques to analyze this result and obtain useful insight into the system. Here we provide a few examples [8] of frequently calculated properties from the trajectory. Considering pharmaceutical applications of MD simulations, a description of a binding mode (hydrogen bonds, salt bridges, stacking interaction, and hydrophobic interactions) of a drug in the protein-binding cavity is the first key information to examine. Unlike binding modes obtained from experimental structural studies or docking predictions, MD simulations provide a dynamic description of the interaction between drug and protein (e.g., [9]); this allows additional insight regarding the importance of individual interactions. Moreover, simulations provide explicit information concerning water participation in the binding mode (e.g., [10]; Figure 4.4a), typically not resolved in structural studies and not considered in docking

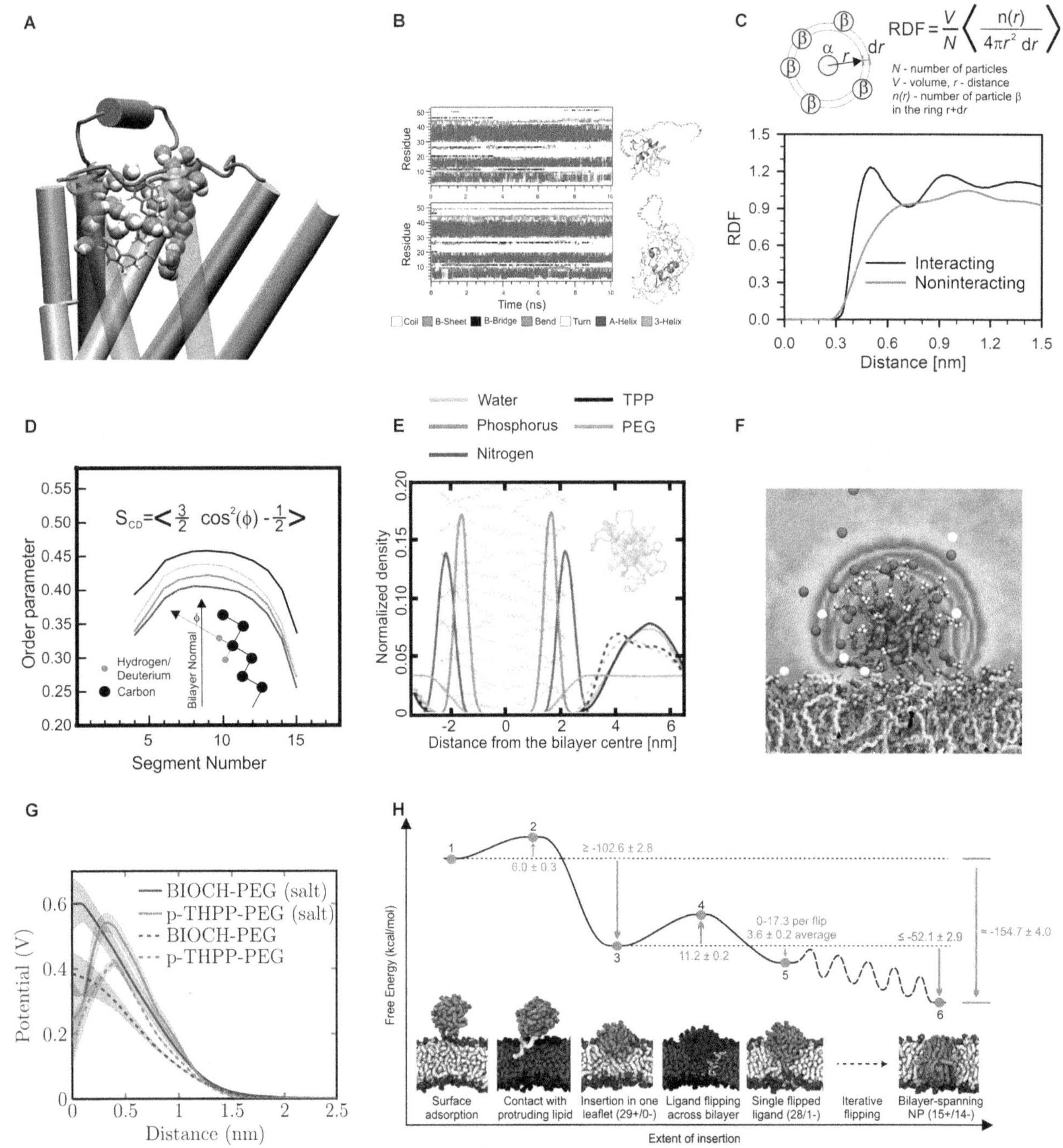

FIGURE 4.4 Results of MD simulations: (a) Snapshot showing involvement of water in binding mode of nebivolol to β2-adrenergic receptor. (b) Time evolution of secondary structure of PEGylated insulin molecules. (c) An example of radial distribution functions (RDF) for interacting particles (black line) and non-interacting particles. (d) Example of order parameter profile along the lipids acyl chain. (e) An example of density profile showing position of atoms of lipid headgroups (phosphorus and nitrogen) and PEGylated tetra-phenyl-porphyrin (PEG and porphyrin densities are shown separately), at the presence (dashed line) and absence (solid line) of salt in solution. (f) Distribution of counter ions around gold nanoparticle functionalized with hydrocarbons capped with amine group. (g) Electrostatic potential profile around PEGylated biochanin (BIOH) and tetra-phenyl-porphyrin (p-THPP) in the presence and absence of salt in solution. (h) Free energy landscape for the process of insertion of dendrimer into the lipid bilayer.

calculations. Analysis of intermolecular interactions is not limited to drug–protein interactions but can also be performed for any type of molecule/macromolecule studied, for example, drug–lipid interactions are frequently studied [11].

Additional observable properties used to evaluate intermolecular interactions are the radial distribution function (RDF) (Figure 4.4c) and the number of contacts. The RDF for the pairs of particles P1 and P2 gives us the normalized density of particle P2 at a given distance from particle P1. For the shortest distances, the RDF value is 0 due to steric repulsion and converges to a constant value in the limit of infinite distance; for homogenous systems, this value will always be 1. For an interacting pair of two particles, the RDF value initially rises with increasing distance to a maximum, followed by a subsequent minimum (Figure 4.4c). For example, for a pair of heavy atoms that form an H-bond, the maximum position is at ~0.25 nm, and the minimum at ~0.325 nm. The number of contacts is the number of pairs of heavy atoms of two molecules located at a distance shorter than the selected cutoff. The most frequent choice for a cutoff length is the position of maximum or minimum at the RDF for carbon atoms in the liquid hydrocarbons. Calculations of numbers of contact are useful to evaluate equilibration in the simulations where self-assembly is studied. When a stable number of contacts is reached, one can assume the end of the self-assembly process.

For interactions of larger molecules, MD simulations provide an area of contact (Acont). To obtain this, the solvent accessible surface area (SASA) for the considered molecule is first calculated separately (*Amol1* and *Amol2*), and next, the same calculations are performed for the dimer (*Adimer*); this results in an area of contact:

$$A_{cont} = \left(A_{mol/1} + Amol2\right) — A_{dimer}) / 2 \qquad (1)$$

Extensive MD simulations, either performed over a long time [12] or in as many multiple parallel simulations [13], are capable of elucidating the process of ligand entry into the binding pocket; however, the most frequent steered MD simulation methods or randomly accelerated MD (RAMD) simulations [14] are used to reveal the entry/exit patch as they are more computationally efficient. For the case of functionalized proteins, their stability can be evaluated via calculations of secondary protein structure (Figure 4.4b). Other standard measurable properties provided by MD simulations include root mean square deviation (RMSD) and root mean square fluctuations (RMSF). The RMSD describes the similarity between the structures at the given time with the initial structure; thus, a large increase of this parameter can indicate a lack of protein stability. In studies of the interaction of drugs and nanoparticles with lipid bilayers, one can obtain insight into the xenobiotic degree of membrane perturbation.

The most frequently used tools to study lipid bilayer properties are surface area per lipid molecule, bilayer thickness, and the order parameter. The most frequently calculated order parameters are the deuterium order parameter, SCD, and molecular order parameter S_{mol} (Figure 4.4d). The position in the membrane of any given xenobiotic molecule is quantitatively described by so-called density plots, which show the density of selected atoms, atom groups, or whole molecules, along the bilayer normal. As a reference point, selected atoms of lipid molecules can be used, for example, head groups, glycerol moiety, or the last carbon of the acyl tails (Figure 4.4e). The next parameter describing drug behavior in the lipid bilayer is the drug molecule orientation with respect to the bilayer normal. Location and orientation of the drug in the lipid bilayer can be important for the entry of the drug into a protein-binding cavity (e.g., [15]). Next, simulations describe the physicochemical properties of nanoparticles, including their size (quantitatively measured as the radius of gyration), nanoparticle hydration, interaction with ions (see Figure 4.4f), and electrostatic potential at the given distance from the nanoparticle center (Figure 4.4g). Finally, one should consider the statistical significance of results to avoid overinterpretation [16], carefully validate results against experimental data, and be critical, as simulations are prone to methodological artifacts.

Sometimes, the unbiased trajectory is not sufficient to obtain the insight we seek. The phenomenon we wish to study may occur in a region that is not sampled so frequently or we wish to calculate the free energy difference between two separate conformations of the system. For this, we need the ability to apply a bias to the simulation to push it artificially toward a certain region of conformation space that we wish to examine. From calculating the bias needed along a path between two conformations, one can obtain the free energy difference between them, an important measure of such quantities as the binding affinity of a drug for a specific active site of a protein. Two methods to calculate this free energy are umbrella sampling (Figure 4.4h), where the path taken is through conformation space and what is known as a potential of mean force (PMF) is calculated along this path and thermodynamic integration, an analogous calculation, but where the path is through parameter space. The free energy calculations are computationally demanding and sensitive to force field details. Also, one should consider possible artifacts due to a bias force, for example, deformation of the lipid bilayers was observed in a few studies during umbrella sampling calculation of the profile of PMF of the studied compound along the bilayer normal. *Metadynamics* [17] is an adaptive means to explore conformation space in an enhanced fashion by constantly biasing the system away from the regions of conformation space that has already been explored.

The remainder of this chapter will cover examples of how this tool, molecular dynamics simulation, has been, and can continue to be, used in the context of drug delivery research (pharmaceutics). We will discuss applications across the breadth of the field, including obtaining insight relevant to dissolution and solubility; however, the majority of the discussion will cover the recent explosion in publications that use molecular dynamics simulation to study the more advanced drug delivery mechanisms, collectively known as nanomedicine.

4.1.2 Mechanistic Insight into Drug Dissolution and Solubility from MD Simulation

The simplest application of MD simulation in drug delivery is gaining mechanistic insight into the universal processes of dissolution and solvation (Figure 4.5). Drugs often enter the body

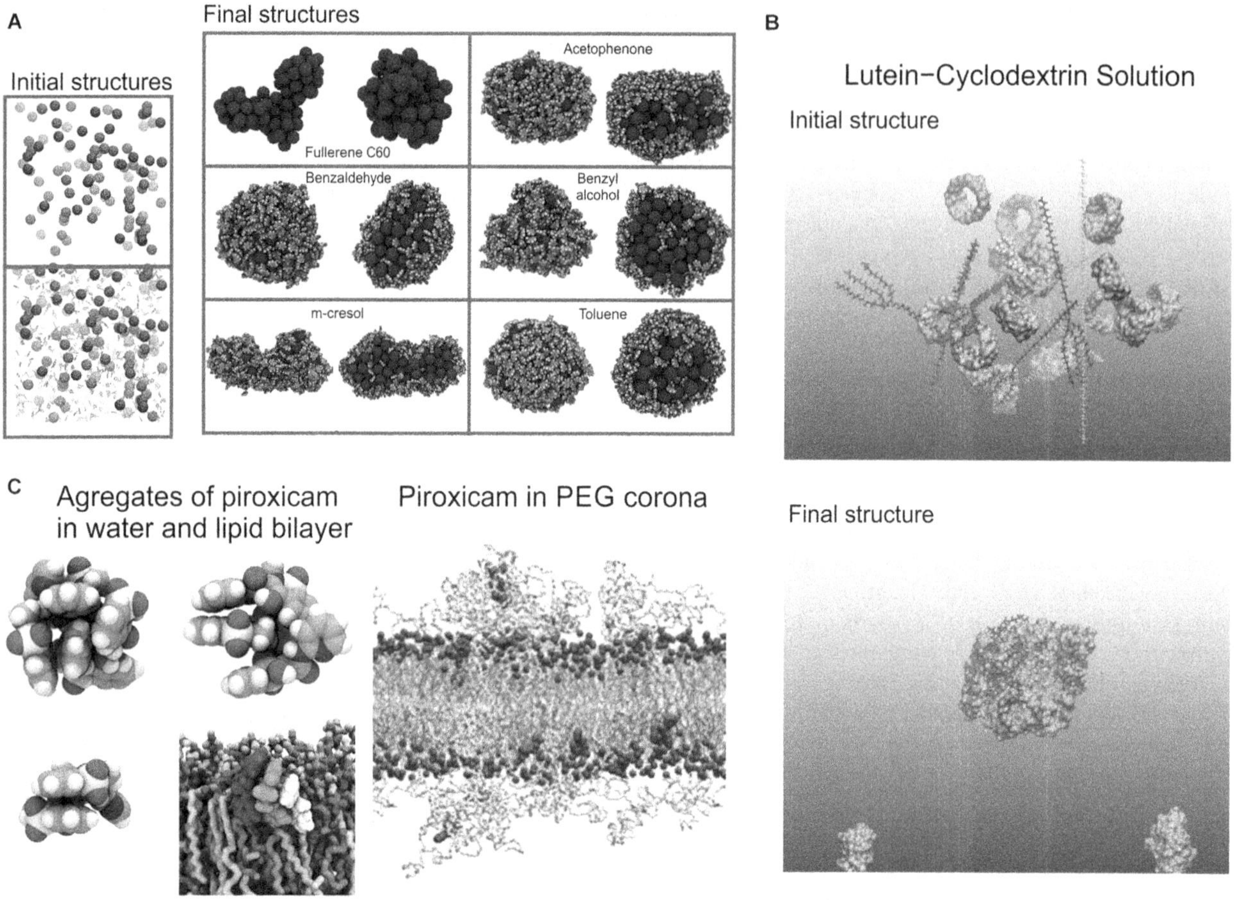

FIGURE 4.5 Dissolution and solubility. (a) Formation of clusters of fullerene with organic solvents. The final structure's clusters full view (left side) and its cross section (right side) are shown. Organic solvent covers fullerene from outside and is present in small quantities inside the cluster. (b) Formation of lutein and cyclodextrin complexes. (c) Aggregates of piroxicam formed in water and lipid bilayer, and piroxicam molecules dispersed in PEG corona of PEGylated lipid bilayer.

Source: (a) reproduced from Lehto, Karilainen, Roìg, Cramariuc, Vanhala, Tornaeus et al. (2014), Copyright: 2014; (b) reproduced from [29] Zhao et al. (2018), Copyright (2018) American Chemical Society; (c) reproduced from [12] Poojari et al. (2019).

in crystalline form, and dissolution of these crystals is the first steps. [18] have used MD simulation to study alteration to the crystal structure with varying levels of hydration. For systems with long-range order such as this, a more accurate and computationally intensive COMPASS force field is required, instead of the potential sets normally used for simulations of systems in the liquid state. The Ouyang group has studied the dissolution of drug molecules complexed with solid dispersions as a remedy for poor solubility using MD [19,20] in addition to machine learning techniques [21]. Coarse-grained simulations using the DPD protocol have been used by Otto et al. to study the release of the drug quercetin from poly(ethylene-glycol) (PEG) solid dispersions.

As stated earlier, simplified QSAR/QSPR [22] or related machine learning models [23] are generally used to correlate drug structure to solubility using pattern recognition to relate structure to experimental solubility data; MD simulation can, however, be used to obtain both a more accurate result and, additionally, provide mechanistic understanding. The partition coefficient between water and octanol can be calculated for the specific molecule through MD simulation using the aforementioned techniques for free energy calculation, either by (1) using umbrella sampling to physically pull the candidate drug molecule structure through the boundary between a water and an octanol phase and calculate the free energy change along this path, the aforementioned PMF (example of a PMF calculation shown in Figure 4.4H), or (2) performing thermodynamic integration between the drug solvated in water and the drug solvated in octanol. Such a calculation is not the mechanistic insight advertised in the introduction; here we are using MD simulation as a tool to obtain a numerical estimate of a quantitative result. It is possible, however, to examine the MD simulation output further to obtain mechanistic insight regarding the relation between the structure of the molecule and the solvent; for example, Zhang et al. have investigated the H-bond network of the drug ibuprofen in water and ethanol [24]. Erlebach et al. (2020) [25] have used a different technique, combining simulations with atomistic resolution with solubility calculations based on the Flory–Huggins theory. Other examples of MD used for solubility prediction also exist [26]. To aid in the delivery of drugs that are otherwise too lipophilic, they are administered not alone but in a formulation with other molecules, known as excipients. Optimizing this drug formulation can be performed through combining screening experiments with pattern recognition and optimization algorithms; however, here, too, MD simulation can play a powerful role in complementing other computational methods [27], for example, MD simulations of cyclodextrin–drug complexes [28,29]; cyclodextrin is a common agent for assisting the delivery of poorly soluble drugs. MD simulation has been used to study drug solubility in excipient formulations, and MD has been used to study polymeric excipients. MD has been used to study self-emulsifying drug delivery systems, and Hathout et al. have modeled drug loading in the gelatin matrix [30]. Several comprehensive review papers have been written on the synergistic use of MD with other computational techniques to determine the solubility and dissolution characteristics of drugs and drug formulations [31].

Describing the ease with which a drug travels through the body to reach its target through this one parameter, solubility, alone, is of course an extreme oversimplification: in addition to dissolving in the blood, drugs must traverse a variety of biological barriers; in particular, cell membranes and perfect solubility will not ensure this [32]. Building systems to deliver drugs through these barriers requires an extra level of complexity; we now cross from simple formulation with the goal to optimize solubility into nanomedicine: nanoscale vectors designed to transport the drug through the bloodstream while protecting it from the body's defense mechanisms and targeting the desired tissue.

4.1.3 Pharmaceutical Applications of Nanoparticle Design and Function in Drug Delivery Systems

Nanomedicine is officially defined as the pharmaceutical applications of nanotechnology. Since "nanotechnology" is a meaningless buzzword quickly fading from fashion [33], this is not a concise definition; in practical terms, this encompasses all drug delivery systems that involve packaging the drug in structures with diameters = 100 nm but larger than a single drug molecule: one or more drug molecules combined with one or more carrier molecules. For example, even merely grinding a crystal of the drug into pieces smaller than this size officially fits this definition, the result known as "nanocrystals," and recognized as the simplest form of nanomedicine. A very broad range of mechanisms has been developed that fits this definition, and the nomenclature is cluttered, that is, the language used to define different varieties, and how components are described, is inconsistent. We will now describe the nomenclature and definitions we intend to use, but be warned: when you read the cited publications, the nomenclature may not be consistent.

When the drug and carrier are combined, the result is referred to as a nanoparticle. Nanoparticles are formed in one of two ways: (1) directly functionalizing a molecule to the drug, that is, chemically bonding a molecule to the drug to alter its behavior in the bloodstream [34], or (2) combining one or more drug molecules with one or more carrier molecules that self-assemble to form the nanoparticle. I will refer to this as the functionalization and self-assembly routes of nanoparticle formation. The functionalization route to nanoparticle creation can also lead to the formation of a nanoparticle composed of more than one drug molecule, for example, functionalizing a hydrophobic drug with a polymer could result in the formation of micelles with the drugs at the core. In most cases, the direct functionalization is to a polymer, a long unstructured molecule, which, as a result, forms a protective sheath around the drug molecule in the bloodstream; however, functionalization to a smaller molecule is also possible, for example, folic acid [35, 36] or glycine [37]. A particularly ingenious idea is functionalization to amphiphilic "molecular umbrellas" that aid the transfection of hydrophilic drugs through the hydrophobic core of cell membranes. Drugs functionalized to polymers where the drug is activated by enzyme cleavage of the polymer are also referred to as "prodrugs" [38]. Functionalization to peptides or small proteins can result in very specific fine-tuning of the behavior of the drug as it interacts with its environment. Functionalization of lipids for a variety of applications is reviewed, and specifically for drug delivery. Regarding nanoparticles formed via the self-assembly route, a rigorous literature search leads to a subdivision of the majority according to topology and choice of carrier molecule into roughly the following nine categories: (1) solid inorganic, (2) micelles, (3) vesicles (Figure 4.6A), (4) lipoprotein-based structures (Figure 4.6C), (5) other lipid–polymer structures, (6) carbon architectures (Figure 4.6B), (7) dendrimers (Figure 4.6D), (8) protein/peptide, and (9) the aforementioned nanocrystals. The list of FDA-approved forms of nanomedicine has been compiled as of 2016.

Solid inorganic nanoparticles are rigid structures formed from inorganic substances. These include gold, silver [39], titanium dioxide [40], silica nanoparticles, and boron nitride oxide nanoflakes [41]. Gold and silver nanoparticles are solid structures that can be associated with drugs or can be functionalized themselves to perform a specific function: the nanoparticle itself is a drug. For the case of silica nanoparticles, they can be porous and contain drugs and can even have complex multi-compartment structure, carrying many different drug molecules [42–44], for example, for applications like theragnostics. In the same fashion as solid inorganic nanoparticles, carbon architectures are contiguous solid structures; however, due to its unique chemistry, composition from carbon allows for a wide variety of forms, including carbon dots, nanotubes, nanodiamonds, nanographene [36,45,46], and graphene oxide [41,47].

Nanoparticles have been developed to assist in drug delivery in a very broad range of pharmaceutical contexts, for example, treating atherosclerosis [48,49] and other neurodegenerative diseases, cardiovascular disease, diabetes, infections disease, protein drugs [50], and vaccine delivery—in fact, vaccine adjuvant development involves many of the same mechanisms as nanomedicine [51]. It can be argued that it is only for historical reasons that it is not referred to as nanomedicine. The main application of nanomedicine is, however, cancer therapy [52], particularly chemotherapy agent delivery, as this involves

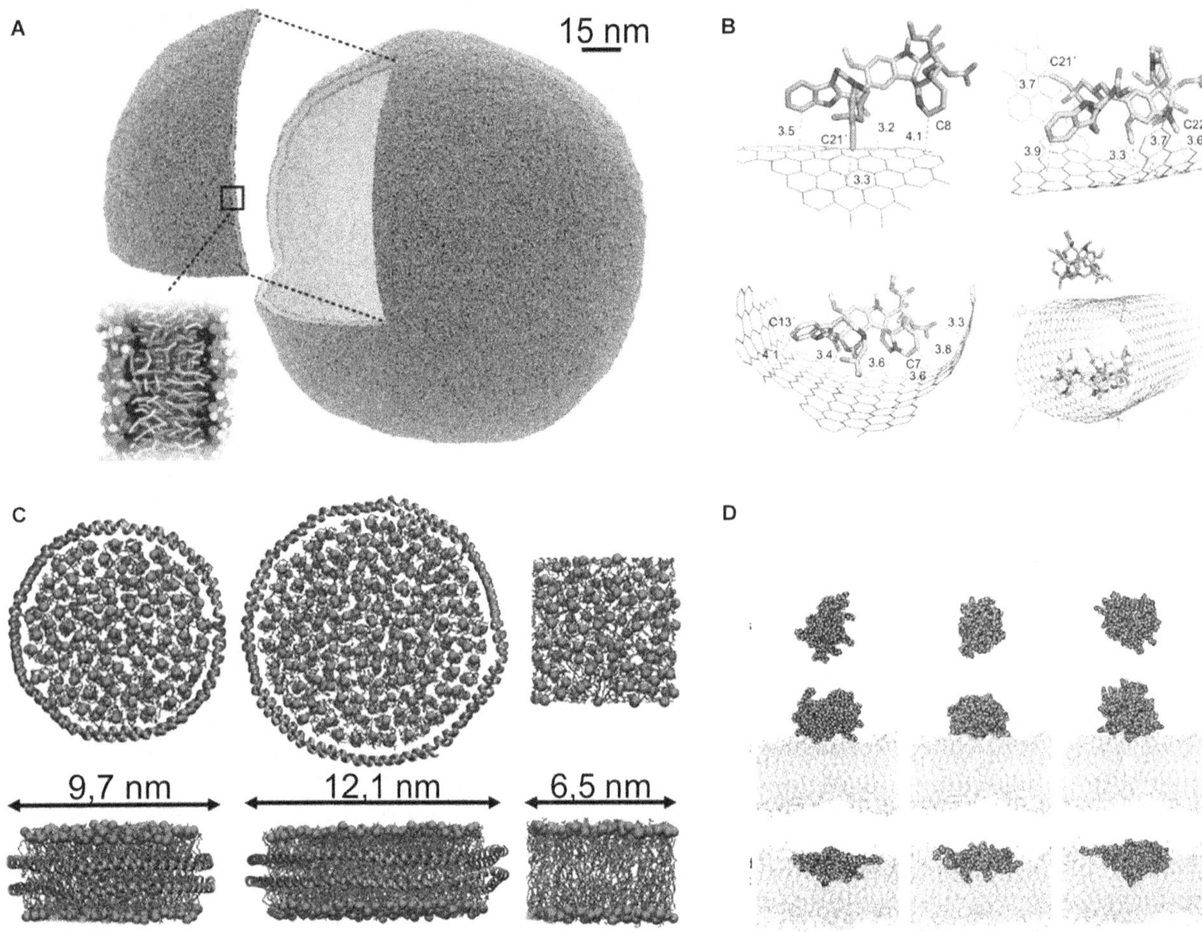

FIGURE 4.6 Nanoparticles: (A) Liposome simulated with dry MARTINI model. (B) Carbon nanotube used for delivery of vinblastine. (C) Nanodiscs formed of POPC and membrane scaffold protein MSP1D1 (left), MSP1E3D1 (middle), and lipid bilayer (right). Protein is shown as blue ribbon, phosphate groups of lipids shown as red sphere, and acyl tail as gray sticks. (D) PAMAM dendrimer in water phase (top), at the lipid bilayer in gel phase (middle), and at the lipid bilayer in fluid phase (down).

drugs with extremely high toxicity; targeted delivery, where the drug is kept from the rest of the body and the greatest possible fraction is delivered to the target tissue, in this case the tumor, is extremely desirable. The nanoparticle is designed to have features that protect the drug, in the context of nanomedicine commonly referred to as the "payload" of the nanoparticle. Targeting is achieved through either active or passive means. Active targeting [53] involves a specific ligand functionalized to the nanoparticle exterior that binds to receptors that are overexpressed in the outer cell membrane of cells of the target tissue, and passive targeting involves global properties of the nanoparticle that lead to a greater percentage becoming lodged in the target tissue in comparison to other tissues. An example of passive targeting is what is referred to as the enhanced permeability and retention (EPR) effect; liposomes can be designed to take advantage of the leaky vasculature of tumor tissue to become preferentially lodged there. PEGylation is a common means to achieve this. It must, however, be stated that whether or not the EPR effect is an effective passive targeting strategy in practical nanomedicine applications has recently been brought into question.

The nanoparticle thus carries and protects its drug payload through the bloodstream and preferentially delivers it to its target tissue. In the bloodstream, foreign particles in the size range of nanoparticles are removed (uptaken) by the mononuclear phagocyte system (MPS); this involves an extremely complex and specific cascade of proteins: complement activation. The efficiency with which a nanoparticle is removed through complement activation is determined by its surface properties. The nanoparticle can be designed to have a surface that inhibits uptake, thus prolonging circulation in the bloodstream and, as a result, the amount of the drug that reaches the target tissue per administered dose; such a nanoparticle surface is referred to as a "stealth sheath," and the aforementioned PEGylation is the gold standard to achieve this [54]. While PEGylation is an extremely successful strategy, it is not perfect, and the investigation of alternate polymers to PEG is an active field of research. Alternatives that have been proposed and studied include polyoxazolines [55], PASylation® [56], zwitterionic polymers, hydroxyethyl starch, and polypeptides [57].

PEGylation, or the creation of an alternate polymer stealth sheath, is achieved though functionalizing the polymer to a component of the nanoparticle. For the case of the functionalization route to nanoparticle creation, functionalization to the protective polymer itself can be the nanoparticle. It is also possible to functionalize the drug to a copolymer where one of the copolymer constituents is the hydrophilic stealth sheath and the other performs another function, for example, a hydrophobic polymer that encapsulates the drug. Examples of this include PEGylated boron nitride [58], folic acid [59], interferon [60], insulin, other PEGylated peptides (Figure 4.7F) and protein drugs ([60,61]; Figure 4.7B); the broader context of polymer-protein drug molecules is covered in several reviews [51]. As far back as 1977, long before "nano" was a word, functionalizing PEG to proteins was proposed to alter their immunological properties. For the

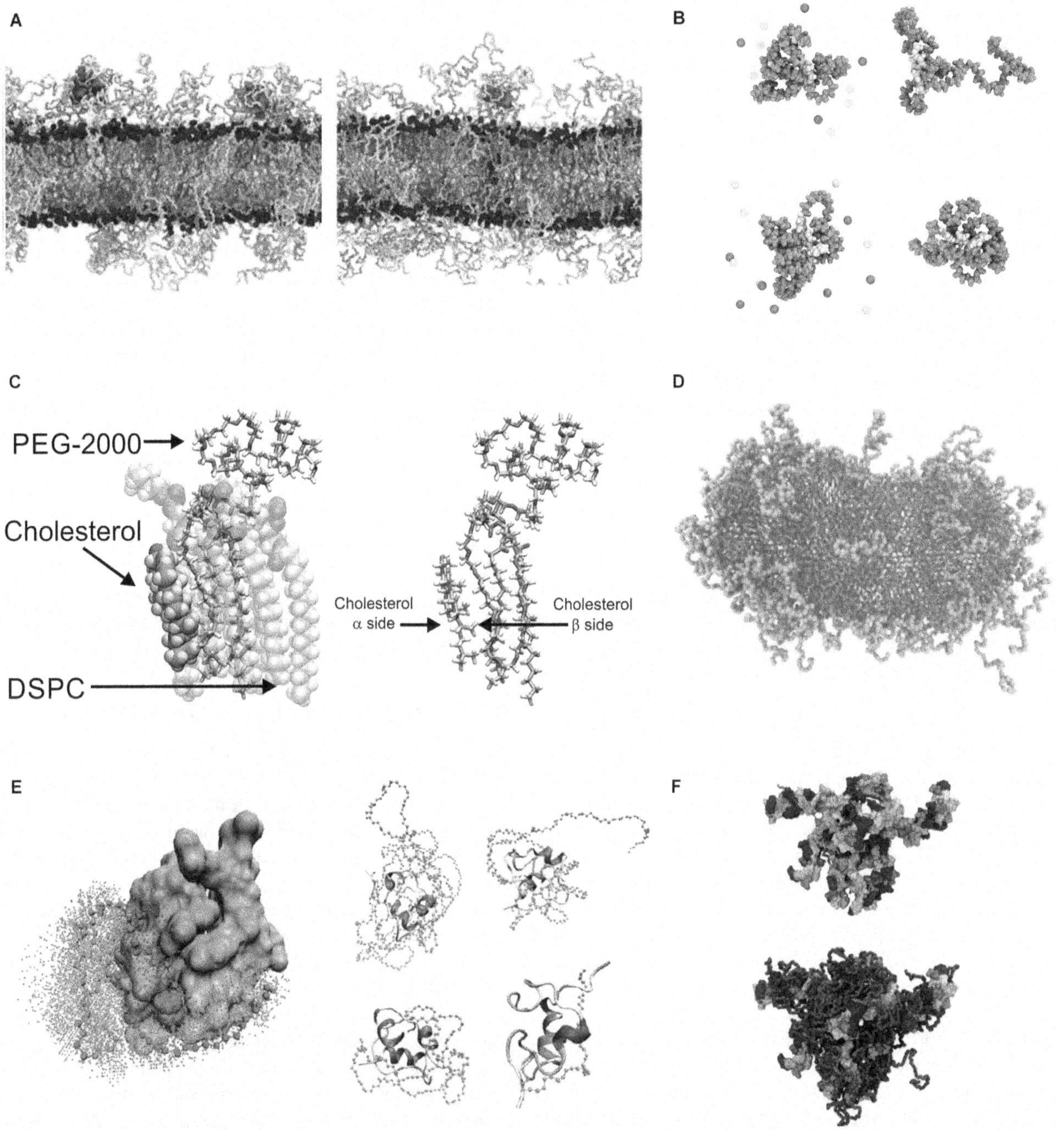

FIGURE 4.7 PEGylation: (a) snapshot showing PEGylated lipid bilayer; (b) PEGylated biochanin (upper) and tetra-phenyl-porphyrin (lower), with salt (left) and without salt (right); (c) snapshots showing DSPC, cholesterol, and DSPE-PEG molecules; (d) PEGylated bicelle containing 10.5 mol % DSPE-PEG, reproduced from Viitala et al. (2019); (e) PEGylated insulin: left panel shows position of PEG atoms during simulations, right panel shows snapshots of insulin PEGylated with PEG of various length.

Source: [65] copyright 2019.

self-assembly route to nanoparticle creation, the polymers are functionalized to constituent molecules of the nanoparticle. PEGylation has been proposed for virtually every one of the nanoparticle types described in the previous section. This includes PEGylated carbon nanotubes, gold nanoparticles [62], silver nanoparticle [63], silver–graphene nanoparticles, nano-graphene [64], lipid micelles ([65]; Figure 4.7D), nanodiscs, dendrimers, and a topic covered comprehensively in liposomes (Figures 4.7A,C).

Altogether, we see that the landscape of nanomedicine is extremely complex, both with a wide range of directions that nanoparticle design can take and the extremely complex environment of human physiology and the body's natural defenses. While *in vitro* experimental insight and clinical studies can make some progress, one quickly reaches a dead end in a sea of complexity without the rational design approach made possible by a mechanistic understanding. The next section shows how molecular dynamics simulations, alongside complementary experimental analysis techniques, to some extent, provide this.

4.1.4 Molecular Dynamics Simulation Applied to Nanomedicine

Now that we have outlined the different forms of nanomedicine and the issues encountered by nanoparticles in their context as drug delivery agents, we can proceed to showcase many examples where molecular dynamics simulation, using different degrees of coarse-graining, has provided mechanistic insight that complements the research program to develop new nanoparticle-based drug delivery mechanisms. The amount of work carried out in this area has exploded in the past decade, with molecular dynamics studies being applied to virtually every variety of nanoparticle discussed earlier in their context as drug delivery vehicles, including dendrimers, gel nanoparticles, polymeric micelles, other polymeric forms of nanoparticles, solid lipid nanoparticles, other micelles, nanocrystals, carbon dots, carbon nanotubes, nanographene, DNA nanotubes, nanodiamonds, peptide nanoparticles, gold nanoparticles, silver nanoparticles, silica nanoparticles, latex nanoparticle, and vesicles, of which the application of molecular modeling to liposome-based drug delivery systems is covered comprehensively in the previous review; there has, however, been a significant amount of work performed since its publication, and molecular modeling has now been applied to the study of other vesicle-based drug delivery systems, including niosomes, ufasomes, polymeric vesicles (polymersomes), and glyceryl monostearate vesicles. A list of publications that feature the use of molecular dynamics modeling to study each of these systems is found in [8]. One intriguing omission by the scientific community is lipoprotein-based nanoparticles, including nanodiscs. Nanodiscs have been studied in the context of their possible use as a drug delivery mechanism and have been studied, in a general context, using molecular dynamics simulation; however, molecular dynamics simulation has never been applied in the context of their possible use in drug delivery.

Regarding the functionalization route to nanoparticle development, there has also been a considerable amount of computational study carried out using molecular dynamics modeling. Protein structures can be downloaded, and their potentials have already been parameterized; attach a polymer to the protein, solvate in water, and you can study its behavior. Both PASylated and PEGylated human recombinant erythropoietin have been simulated; [66] used molecular dynamics simulation to study conjugation of PEG to a hydrophobic pocket of bovine serum albumin using a model with atomistic resolution and used a coarse-grained model to study site-specific PEGylation of the protein lysozyme. Atomistic MD has been used to study the effect of PEGylation on the stability and potency of interferon [60] and insulin and the steric shielding effect that results from the PEGylation of staphylokinase. A recent comprehensive overview of the application of molecular simulation to the study of protein–polymer conjugation has been written by Lin and Colina (2019) [67].

In terms of the delivery of specific drugs using nanomedicine, a very large number has been simulated and incorporated into a wide variety of nanoparticle types. These drugs include Alzheimer's medication, anti-worm drugs, antibiotics, anticancer drugs, including chemotherapy agents, antiviral agents, antifungal drugs, anti-inflammatory drugs, antimicrobial peptides, drug used for diabetes treatment, immunomodulators and immunosuppressants, local anesthetics, and others; a list is found, with citations, in [8]. Altogether, it becomes clear that there is simply too much work that has been carried out to concisely summarize in its entirety in this chapter. We will instead focus on a few key areas where MD modeling has provided important insight and discuss review papers that focus on certain aspects of the use of molecular dynamics in the context of nanomedicine and some key examples of original research that demonstrate the power of the technique. The discussion will include key examples where we show concrete insight gained by molecular dynamics simulation.

4.1.4.1 Drug Loading and Controlled Release

The ability of nanoparticles to hold drugs and release them with an external trigger has been studied for several nanoparticle forms by several groups. In most cases, the drugs being considered are hydrophobic and sit within a non-polar region. Nanoparticles that have been simulated carrying their drug payload include carbon nanotubes, nanographene, peptide carriers, PAMAM dendrimers, polymeric nanoparticles, polymeric micelles, hydrophobic drugs within the membrane of liposomes, other issues related to drug loading of liposomes, and polymersomes [8, 68]. Drug cargoes studied include cucurbitacin, carmustine, 5-flouracil, chalcone, picoplatin, porphyrins, ibuprofen, paclitaxel, and albendazole; however, the most popular drug for these model systems is doxorubicin [8]. In many cases, these nanoparticles are designed to release their drug payload in response to a pH change trigger [8]; MD simulation is able to model the effect of pH change. In an MD simulation, pH is modeled through the partial charges on the atoms, so the system can be equilibrated with the partial charges corresponding to neutral pH, and then the partial charges can be changed to model pH change, and the behavior of the system in response to this, that is, the drug release, can be modeled. One interesting aspect of the work carried out using MD simulation in this area is that the use of all three levels of coarse-graining is represented: atomistic MD, MARTINI model, and DPD [8]. Reading this literature with this in mind provides a very good case study of the strengths and weaknesses of each model and the aspects of the system each are most ideally suited to investigate.

Studies of itraconazole in a liposome, combining MD simulation with experiment, provide an example of where MD simulation was able to provide concrete insight not obtainable experimentally. Itraconazole is an antifungal drug characterized by low solubility, which limits its bioavailability. One possible solution to overcome low solubility is incorporating drugs into liposomes, which was achieved in a few independent studies. To optimize the liposome properties, cholesterol is frequently used as a molecule known to increase the stability of lipid bilayers. In fact, cholesterol is used in 9 out of 15 liposome-based formulations approved for clinical use. Thus, the incorporation of cholesterol into the liposome–itraconazole formulation was the next step. MD simulations showed that this is not the right choice, because cholesterol and itraconazole do not mix well and separate into small domains [69]. This observation was next validated in experimental studies, which showed decreased affinity of itraconazole toward liposomes containing cholesterol [69]. The observed behavior of the itraconazole may be explained by its structure: it is a long rigid molecule with a few weak polar groups distributed along the molecule backbone. Due to this structure, itraconazole molecules locate to the water membrane interface oriented parallel to the membrane surface and, in turn, orient other molecules in the same fashion [12]. On the other hand, cholesterol has strong preferences to adopt an orientation perpendicular to the membrane surface and affect the orientation of neighboring molecules; these opposite preferences lead to the observed demixing of drugs and cholesterol.

4.1.4.2 Nanoparticle Interaction with the Lipid Membrane

Once the nanoparticle has reached the cell, surviving the journey through the bloodstream with its payload still contained and intact, there is one final barrier that must be crossed for the drug delivery system to be efficacious: the cell membrane [32]. It is possible for nanoparticles, particularly if they are hydrophobic, to directly transfect, also referred to as translocation, through the cell membrane, and many nanoparticles enter the cell through this route. There is, however, an alternative: the nanoparticle can be designed to cross the membrane via receptor-mediated endocytosis. When a nanoparticle is taken up via endocytosis, it is possible to take advantage of pH-triggered release due to the lowered pH environment on the interior of the endosome. Valuable insights in both the contexts of direct membrane transfection and endocytosis have been obtained through MD simulation. As is the case with drug loading and release, MD simulation of nanoparticle–lipid membrane interactions has been carried out for different nanoparticle forms, including carbon dots, graphene, dendrimers, gold nanoparticles [8], and nanocrystals; examples can be found of all levels of model resolution being used, including atomistic MD, MARTINI model, DPD, and implicit solvent [8]. An overview of MD simulation of nanoparticle–lipid membrane interactions has been studied.

For nanoparticles that enter the cell through direct transfection, the issue is the direct physical reaction between the nanoparticle and the membrane; this phenomenon can be studied directly through an MD simulation of the nanoparticle interacting with the membrane [70,71]. When nanoparticles translocate through the membrane, the membrane structure can be disrupted and leakage and even pore formation can occur; this has been studied directly using MD [72]. The effect of size, shape [73], and surface properties of the nanoparticle on membrane transfection has also been studied, including effect of PEGylation [74], and other polymer coatings [75] as well as protein and, for the study of inhaled nanoparticles, pulmonary surfactant corona [74] and other issues related to translocation across the pulmonary surfactant monolayer [76]. Additionally, Gupta et al. used MD simulations to study transdermal delivery of interferon-alpha using gold nanoparticles [77].

Regarding receptor-mediated endocytosis, the interaction is more complex; while direct simulation of nanoparticle endocytosis has been performed and gained important insight, this only tells part of the story, as many aspects of the specific interaction between the ligand and the receptors are not elucidated by such a simulation. Nanoparticles can be designed to actively target specific cell types through functionalizing targeting ligands onto the nanoparticle surface. These targeting ligands bind to the specific receptors that induce endocytosis. There are two issues that govern the efficacy of this binding: (1) the distribution of the targeting ligands on the surface, that is, the pattern of where they are located, and (2) the orientation and, as a result of orientation, the extent of exposure at the nanoparticle surface, and thus availability to the target receptors. The effect of ligand distribution has been studied by Liu et al. (2016) through direct MD simulation of nanoparticle–membrane interactions, and ligand density has been studied through a different computational modeling technique: Monte Carlo simulation.

Thus, ref. [8] focuses on three areas: (1) behavior of the nanoparticle in the bloodstream and the protective polymer corona, (2) drug loading and release, and (3) nanoparticle interaction with lipid membranes and entry into the cell. We would like to alert the reader to the fact that there are other reviews of aspects of the use of computational modeling for nanoparticle design [78].

Regarding the orientation, and thus exposure, of the targeting ligand to the receptor that induces receptor-mediated endocytosis, one needs chemically accurate atomistic simulations of the nanoparticle surface to investigate the degree to which the targeting ligand is exposed and available to the receptor. We have performed such simulations for the case of liposome-based delivery systems, with targeting ligands, in several previous publications. Liposomes functionalized with stearylamine arginine ligands have also been studied. A comprehensive review of the theoretical and computational investigation of nanoparticle interactions with biomembranes has been written.

4.2 Structural Properties and Functionalization of CNTs

The unique electrical, chemical, and one-dimensional structural features of CNTs help them become the most significant leading molecular platform in a variety of applications, such as nanobiosensor devices, nanoelectronic applied catalysis, and energy storage devices. Moreover, the capability of CNTs in cell's piercing can confirm the capabilities of CNTs as nanocarriers for the delivery of drug molecules, proteins, and peptides.

Several features of carbon nanotubes, such as size, chirality, surface modification, van der Waals forces, and dosage, play an important role in defining their biocompatibility or cytotoxicity for application in biomedical systems. Beside these facts, it is shown that individualized CNTs which retain superior intrinsic properties, such as high specific surface areas, can be more applicable in nanobiomedicine fields, although pristine CNTs may have toxicity for use in biological systems. Therefore, surface modification is a useful tool for biomedicine studies. SWCNTs can be surface-functionalized and easily coupled with biomolecules through adsorption, chemical conjunction, or encapsulation.

The advantage of functionalized CNTs for biomedical systems is the ability to change their hydrophobicity characteristics in order to enhance their solubility in biocompatible aqueous media. It has been reported that after hydrophobic functional group attachment, f-CNT solubility is increased significantly and alters their cellular interaction pathways, resulting in a significant reduction of cytotoxic effects. As a result, bioactive molecules can be delivered into the cell nuclei or passed through the cell membrane by using functionalized SWCNTs. Several studies have approved the benefits of applying SWCNTs–drug delivery coupled systems, which result in enhanced efficiency in tumor targeting due to an improved permeability and retention effect of the carbon nanotube [79].

In addition, using CNTs as a drug delivery system to target cancerous tissues has confirmed that the side effects of chemical drug have decreased in several case studies. Functionalization of CNTs via covalent and non-covalent interactions (van der Waals and hydrogen bonds interactions) plays a critical role in the yield of systems containing drug delivery.

This chapter covers the physical and surface properties of CNT structure that affect interactions with drugs and biomolecules. Various mechanisms and the factors affecting internalization of CNTs within the cell membrane are also described. Among the various CADD strategies, molecular dynamics (MD) simulation is the most common approach to gain insight into the CNT interaction with biomolecules, including cell membranes. However, owing to the huge size of the CNT molecular system, several approaches that were developed to reduce the degrees of freedom and to simplify the intermolecular interactions are also emphasized here.

Carbon nanotubes are cylindrical wrapped graphene sheets of hexagonally arranged sp^2-hybridized carbon atoms. They exist as a single cylinder, known as single-walled carbon nanotubes (SWCNTs), and multi-cylinders with coinciding centers, known as multi-walled carbon nanotubes (MWCNTs). SWCNTs have diameter ranges of 0.4–3.0 nm and length of 20–1,000 nm, whereas MWCNTs have an average central cylindrical tube diameter of 1–3 nm and external cylindrical tube diameter of 2–100 nm, with length varying from one to several micrometers (Figure 4.8a). Based on the arrangement of the graphite layer, MWCNTs can be categorized into two types: "parchment-like" structures, consisting of a graphene sheet rolled up around itself, and "Russian doll" models, with multiple graphene sheets arranged within a concentric structure. Another important physical property of CNTs, in particular for SWCNTs, is chirality, which represents the axis around which the graphene plane is wrapped. The two main configurations of CNTs are zigzag and armchair, and several subconfigurations can be obtained by shifting the wrapping axis from the zigzag plane toward the armchair plane (Figure 4.8b).

Therefore, chirality can be simply represented as n and m indices. Knowing the indices for a CNT, it is possible to deduce other parameters, like diameter and chiral angle, as shown in eqs. (2) and (3). The influence of thickness, diameter, and chirality on the elastic properties of CNTs is properly explained by Tserpes and Papanikos.

$$d=\frac{\alpha}{\pi}\left(n^2+nm+m^2\right)^{\frac{1}{2}} \tag{2}$$

$$\theta=\tan^{-1}\left(\sqrt{3m}\,/\,(m+n)\right) \tag{3}$$

CNTs are mainly synthesized by following three standard techniques, namely, chemical vapor deposition (CVD), arc discharge, and laser ablation. The former method is conducted at comparatively low temperature (<800°C), whereas the latter two methods require high temperature (>1,700°C). Certain non-standard methods, such as pyrolysis and hydrothermal treatment, have also been used for the synthesis of CNTs.

The surface of CNTs in their original form (pristine CNTs) is a "bald" one. Pristine CNTs are highly hydrophobic and cannot be directly introduced to the human body because that could lead to various undesirable and severe toxicities, including cell-cycle arrest, apoptosis, and necrosis. Therefore, the functionalization of the CNT surface is of paramount importance before exposing them to the biological environment. Functionalization of CNTs helps increase the aqueous solubility, dispersion, and efficacy of insoluble drugs, as well as to improve the biocompatibility to reduce the nonspecific interaction with cell membranes and related toxicities. Functionalization is carried out by either covalent or non-covalent bonding of different functional groups on the surface or at the open ends of CNTs, depending upon specific application.

There are various chemical reactions involved in the covalent functionalization of CNTs, such as oxidation, hydrogenation, amidation, halogenation (F/Cl/Br), thiolation (SH), and addition of carbenes or nitrene. An example of covalent functionalization is the oxidation of the CNT surface to produce –COOH functional groups that can be used to link other molecules by amidation or esterification. Covalent functionalization results in altered hybridization from sp^2 to sp^3 on carbon atoms of CNTs, simultaneously blocking the p-electron transition, which is found to be favorable for pharmaceutical drug delivery because it causes slow release of therapeutic agents.

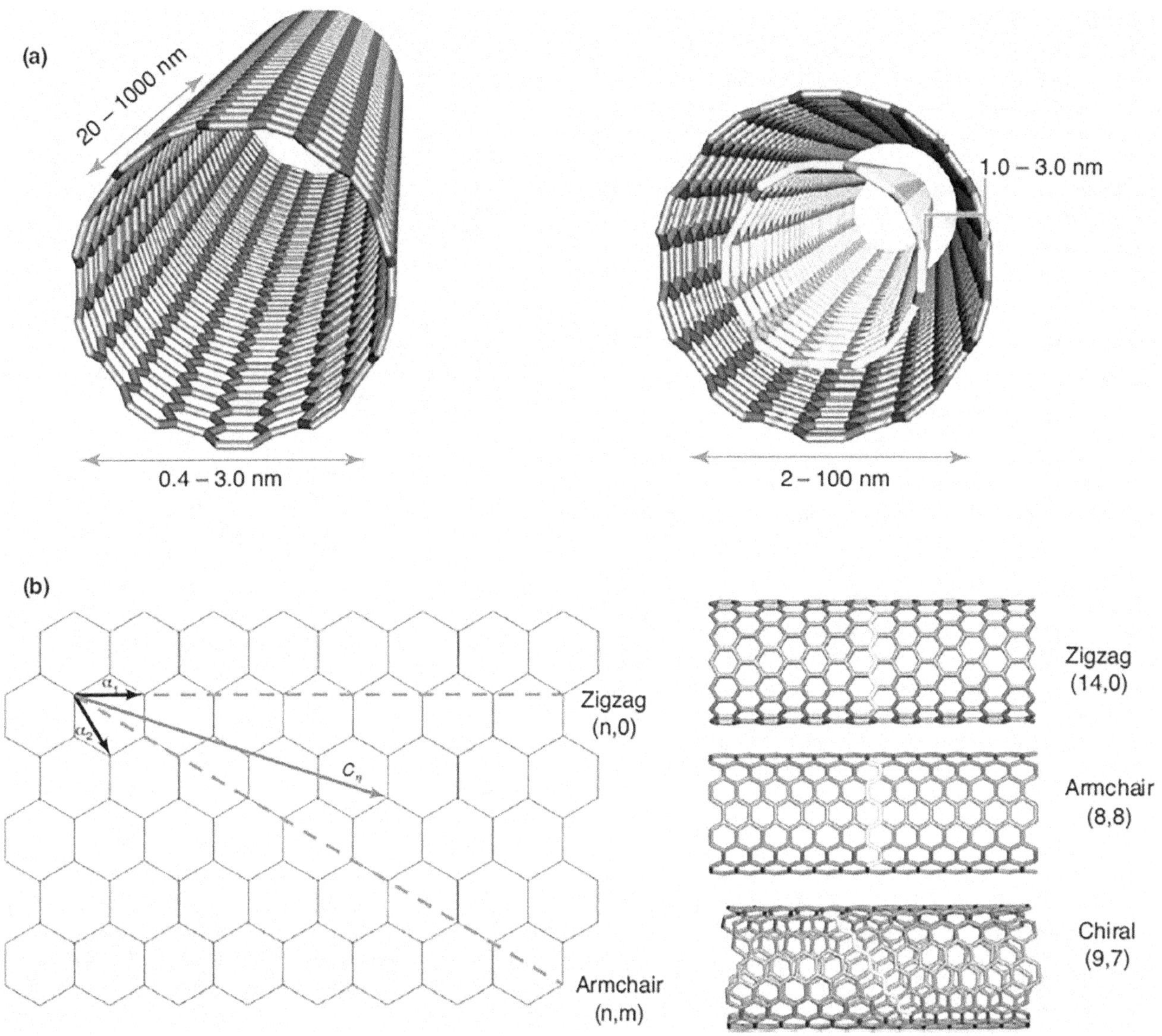

FIGURE 4.8 (a) The dimensions of a single-walled carbon nanotube (SWCNT) on the left and multi-walled carbon nanotube (MWCNT) on the right. (b) Schematic representation of graphene sheet showing zigzag and armchair configurations (represented as dashed lines). Any arbitrary configuration represented by C_h vector can be made by summation of integer multiplicand of a_1 and a_2a^2 vectors.

Hence, covalent functionalized CNTs are considered to be the most promising for diagnosis and pharmaceutical drug delivery. It is worth mentioning that the damage of the p-network is a big concern for fluorescence imaging applications because it shows a detrimental effect on fluorescence quantum efficiency.

Non-covalent functionalization of CNTs mainly includes supramolecular adhesion of polymers, biomolecules or amphiphilic surfactants on the CNT surface through van der Waals, pi–pi (π–π), or hydrophobic interactions. Non-covalent functionalization can also significantly enhance the solubility and dispersibility of CNTs, but in contrast to covalent functionalization, it has the limited capability of drug delivery owing to the presence of weak van der Waals forces. The functionalized CNTs have been efficiently used to deliver proteins, nucleic acids, and small drug molecules inside the cell-specific targets.

Recent advances in computer modeling approaches, in particular MD simulation [80], significantly help investigate the physicochemical properties required for functionalization and improving solubility, as well as gaining insight into the adsorption mechanisms of various drugs on pristine as well as functionalized CNTs. For example, Arsawang et al. investigated the structural properties required for encapsulation of anticancer drug gemcitabine in SWCNTs by employing MD simulation and found that the drug molecule preferred to reside inside the SWCNTs by forming π-stacking interactions between the CNTs and the cytosine ring of the drug. Similarly, Hashemzadeh and Raissi performed MD simulation to compare and gain insight into the adsorption mechanism of the anticancer drug paclitaxel (PTX) on pristine and three types of functionalized CNTs. Functionalization of CNTs was carried out by using polyethylene glycol (PEG), carboxylic (COOH), and amine (CH_2NH_2) groups. The results showed that PTX adsorbed on pristine CNTs by forming π–π interactions, whereas the maximum adsorption of PTX took place on the surface of PEG-CNTs by forming more polar interactions as compared with other functionalized CNTs. Moreover, the PEG-CNT system also showed the highest aqueous solubility by forming polar intermolecular H-bonds. There are many such examples of successful exploration of computer modeling of CNTs reported in the literature, indicating its potential for the design and optimization of various parameters required for the functionalization as well as improvement of pharmacokinetic properties to enhance biocompatibility while reducing the toxicity of CNTs.

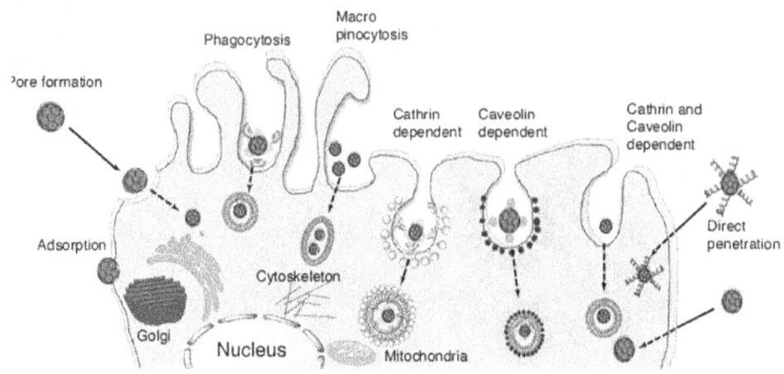

FIGURE 4.9 Schematic representation of the nanoparticle–biomembrane interaction mechanism. Four mechanisms, including adsorption onto the membrane surface, pore formation, direct penetration, and endocytosis, are involved in nanoparticle–biomembrane internalization.

4.3 Interactions of Carbon Nanotubes with the Cell Membrane

One of the major concerns in the development of nanoparticle (NP)–based drug delivery is to ensure their capability to interact and penetrate biological membranes successfully. To predict CNT-based drug delivery at the cellular level, the interaction between the cargo CNT and the cell membrane needs to be studied. Several mechanisms were proposed and experimentally approved for the cellular internalization of CNTs. It is important to note that some internalized CNTs can also lead to toxic effects on the cells, owing to their high reactivity as well as various other incompatible surface chemistries, as evident mainly from the cellular interaction of pristine CNTs. Therefore, the parameters governing the cellular internalization of CNTs should be accurately optimized during the design process to achieve efficient and selective drug delivery.

4.3.1 Mechanisms of Internalization of Carbon Nanotubes by the Cell Membrane

CNTs can be administered into the human body by various methods, such as oral, intravenous (IV), transdermal, subcutaneous, intraperitoneal injection, and inhalation routes. Cellular internalization of CNTs is related to several factors, such as surface characteristics, interactions with the medium, and biomolecules. The surface properties of importance include chemical composition, roughness, functionalization, shape, porosity, surface crystallinity, and heterogeneity, the angle of curvature, and hydrophobicity or hydrophilicity. Experimentally, it has been suggested that pristine CNTs can be internalized within cells either by endocytosis or spontaneous insertion and diffusion across the cell membrane. It is important to note that CNT internalization is not completely dependent on surface functionality. Several mechanisms of internalization of CNTs by cell membranes have been proposed (Figure 4.9).

4.3.1.1 Direct Penetration or Nanopenetration

This is an energy-independent passive process of CNT internalization either through membrane–transport protein channels or pores or directly through the cell membrane. Direct penetration offers the advantage of avoiding endosomal entrapment and the potential for lysosomal degradation. It has been postulated that energy-independent cellular internalization of CNTs is similar to passive diffusion of nano-needles and also similar to the process of polycationic cell-penetrating peptides (CPPs). In this regard, a study of passive penetration of fluorescein-isothiocyanate-linked CNTs and G-protein-coupled CNTs into keratinocytes and fibroblasts, respectively, suggests that functionalized CNTs resembling the morphology of CPPs and possessing overall charge might prefer to undergo penetration to the cellular membrane rather than endocytosis.

4.3.1.2 Endocytosis

Endocytosis is one of the most common methods for cellular internalization of functionalized CNTs by energy-dependent active transport in which the cytoplasmic membrane engulfs them by enclosing them in vesicles or vacuoles inside the cell. It is worth mentioning that this process of energy-dependent endocytosis might be hindered at low temperature, as well as in a low-ATP environment. Internalization of CNTs within the cell by the formation of endosomes can lead to lysosomal degradation of the CNT delivery system. Occasionally, the cargo CNT can escape from the endosomal trap by pore formation, proton sponge effect, or fusion in the endosomal membrane. The endocytosis process follows different mechanisms that often involve interaction with membrane receptors (Figure 4.10).

Clathrin-mediated endocytosis (<300 nm) is the most important route for internalization of NPs inside the cells (even exploited for uptake of pathogens like viruses and bacteria). In this method of internalization, transmembrane receptors undergo sorting upon binding to their extracellular ligand. The sorted receptors activate the formation of "coated pits" due to the assembly of several cytoplasmic proteins, leading to the formation of a clathrin cage (Figure 4.11). This energy-dependent clathrin-mediated endocytosis (CME) is also known as receptor-mediated endocytosis (RME). This process can facilitate the endocytosis of positively charged (e.g., plain gold) and negatively charged (e.g., PEG-coated gold) NPs.

Caveolae-mediated endocytosis (<80 nm) is used for cell signaling, vesicular transport, as well as virus entry. Caveolae are membrane invaginations 50–80 nm in size, containing the cholesterol-binding protein caveolin and sphingolipids. Caveolae-mediated endocytosis also plays an important part in

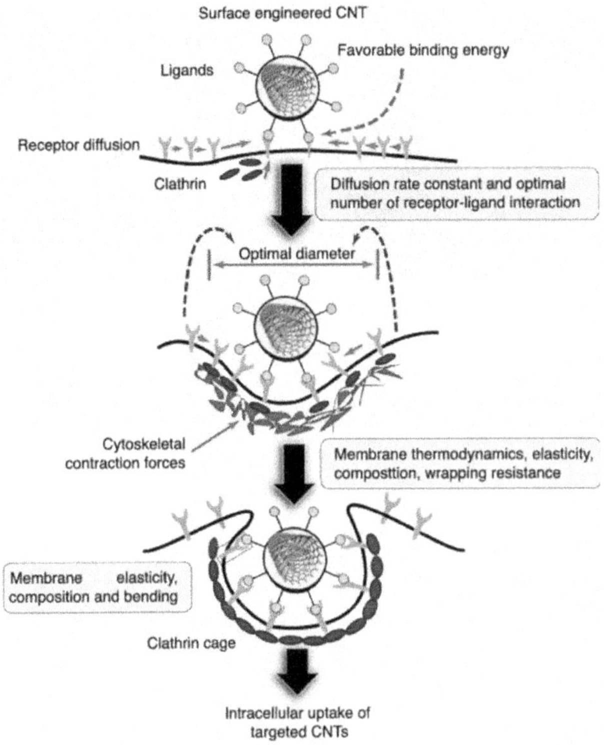

FIGURE 4.10 Scheme showing nanoparticle wrapping at the cellular surface membrane. The particle uptake starts with binding to the membrane through specific (ligand–receptor) or nonspecific (for example, hydrophobic, coulombic) interactions. The interactions should be strong enough (decrease free energy of the system) to overcome resistive forces (such as membrane bending). The blue beads represent clathrin, an example of an endocytic component that engages in the energy-dependent uptake of the particle through interaction between ligands (yellow dots) on the particle surface and membrane receptors (Y-shaped).

the cellular uptake of positively and negatively charged NPs, particularly in endothelial cells.

Macropinocytosis (>200 nm) is a process where cellular internalization takes place by the formation of waving sheet-like extensions of the plasma membrane due to actin-regulated movement. The mechanism most probably involves no interactions with transmembrane proteins. Macropinocytosis is found to play an important part in the cellular uptake of mainly positively charged NPs like plain gold NPs.

Phagocytosis (>750 nm) is a process of cellular internalization that is only performed by specialized cells like immune cells (monocytes, macrophages, and neutrophils) to engulf huge particles with diameter >750 nm, such as pathogens, dead cells, and cellular debris. It involves binding to specific membrane proteins. Here, the particle needs to be first coated by proteins (e.g., antibodies) to be recognized by membrane proteins.

4.3.2 Toxicities of Carbon Nanotubes

Pristine CNTs with highly hydrophobic surfaces tend to aggregate in cell culture medium, which results in binding to various biological species, including protein, via hydrophobic interactions, leading to cellular toxicity. Several mechanisms of CNT-induced cytotoxicity have been proposed, including penetration of cell membrane, oxidation of intracellular components, DNA damage, interruption of electron transfer, and formation of reactive oxygen species (ROS). CNTs can disrupt the cell membrane during penetration, leading to cytotoxic effects. Such disruption is related to the physicochemical properties that promote cell membrane penetration, such as CNT dimensions, surface properties (functionalization), and formation of corona with biomolecules. Several review articles have been published to highlight the various parameters responsible for CNT-induced toxicity. *In vitro* and *in vivo* experimental results of CNT toxicity studies reveal that various factors such as size, shape, composition, impurities, or residual metal (cobalt, nickel, molybdenum, etc.), as well as preparation methods, incorporate the toxicities in CNTs. Further, the methods of administration of CNTs (oral, inhalation, transdermal, subcutaneous, intraperitoneal, and IV injection) to the human body affect the toxicity elicitations of CNTs and must be considered judiciously. Some studies revealed that oral, dermal, and IV administration of CNTs might cause mild inflammation, whereas inhalation of CNTs can lead to severe inflammation. For example, depending upon the method of administration, the exposure of NPs (mainly pristine CNTs) to the respiratory system can lead to asthma, bronchitis, or lung cancer, whereas entry through the gastrointestinal tract (GIT) might result in Crohn's disease and colon cancer. Similarly, long exposure to the systemic circulation might cause blood clotting and various heart diseases.

4.3.2.1 Mechanism of Cytotoxicity by Carbon Nanotube Exposure

Cellular damage in response to various types of CNT exposure takes place by following any of the three types of cell death programs: apoptosis, autophagy, necrosis. It has been observed that CNT exposure to cells can result in lysosomal damage and consecutive release of digestive enzymes, leading to apoptotic and necrotic cell death. Several experiments also revealed that CNTs could decrease mitochondrial membrane potential (MMP), leading to the formation of ROS. High levels of ROS are an indication of oxidative stress, which can damage the cell by disrupting DNA, altering gene transcription, protein structure, and/or cell signaling. It was evident that the treatment of rat lung cells with varying concentrations of MWCNTs (0.5–10 mg/mL) resulted in apoptosis through mitochondrial damage. Although functionalization of CNTs reduces the toxicity, one of the studies showed that the COOH-linked SWCNTs induced autophagy in lung adenocarcinoma A549 cells.

4.3.2.2 Strategies to Circumvent Carbon Nanotube Toxicity

The functionalization of CNTs is one of the major approaches to improve aqueous solubility and biocompatibility while reducing the toxicity, as well as aggregation, in contrast to hydrophobic pristine CNTs. Although there are many ways to chemically functionalize CNTs, one of the most promising results was observed with PEG functionalization of CNTs,

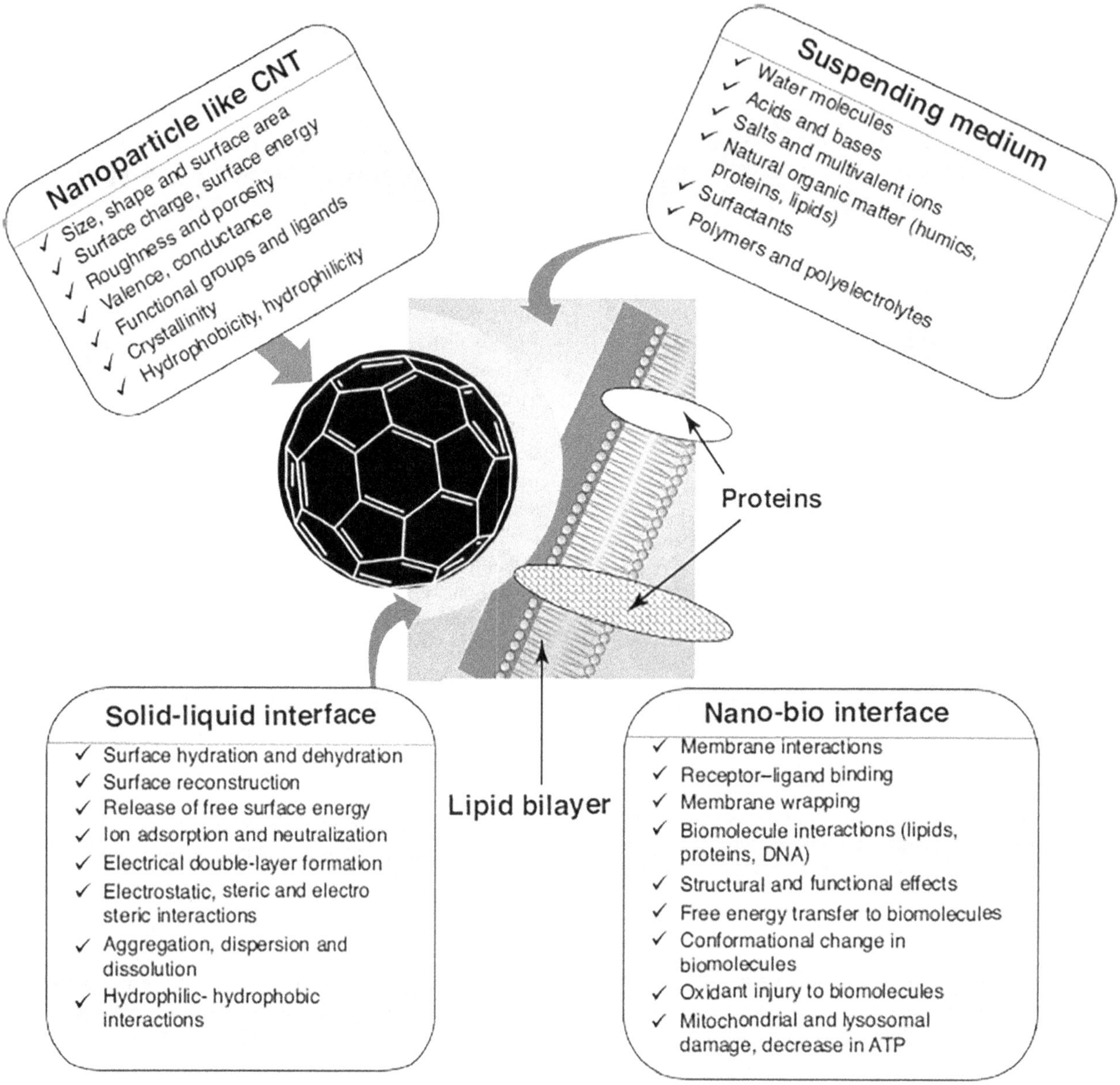

FIGURE 4.11 Representation of the interface between a nanoparticle and a lipid bilayer. The factors that affect the nanoparticle internalization belong to the nanoparticle surface, suspending medium, and dynamic interactions between the solid–liquid interface and the biomolecules and cellular compartments.

where PEG-CNTs were found to reduce the toxicity and reticuloendothelial system (RES) capture while improving the pharmacokinetic properties, including the prolongation of blood circulation half-life. A very low PEG-CNT-induced toxicity was found to be associated with very high doses of CNTs. Similarly, other studies demonstrated very low cell inflammation and mitochondrial destruction at very high doses of ammonium-functionalized CNT and tau-linked CNT, respectively, as compared with pristine CNTs.

It has been observed that residual impurities of metal catalysts (Co, Fe, Ni, and Mo) encapsulated in graphene layers following CNT synthesis can result in cell death through mitochondrial destruction and oxidative stress. In this regard, purification of CNTs by ultrasonication is another important approach that can significantly reduce cytotoxicity by promoting the release of metallic impurities into the solution.

4.3.3 Effects of Biophysical Parameters on Carbon Nanotube Interaction with the Cell Membranes

The cell membrane is mainly composed of lipids (saturated and unsaturated), cholesterol and embedded proteins. The interactions between cellular, environmental, and NP factors determine the CNT internalization within the cell (Figure 4.11). For example, the composition of the cell membrane can affect CNT penetration. The attachment of viral glycoproteins (e.g., hemagglutinin) with cell membrane receptors is important to initiate fusion. Such a technique can also be followed to design CNTs for intracellular delivery of drugs and genetic materials. The force required to rupture the cell membrane by CNTs is related to several factors of the membrane composition. For example, the presence of cholesterol (up to 30%) reduced the bending of the membrane, as a result of which the force required to puncture the membrane by CNTs is increased by 15 kcal/mol, and higher lipids were extracted during CNT penetration.

4.4 Molecular Dynamics Simulation of CNT-Cell Membrane Interactions

The interaction between CNTs and biomolecules can be studied experimentally. However, molecular simulation studies offer a detailed description of the process over time. MD simulation can be used to study various drug nanodelivery systems, such as those based on dendrimers, polymer micelles, liposomes, and CNTs. The computational study of a drug–CNT–cell membrane complex is essential for the rational design of CNT-based nanodelivery systems. There are trials to reproduce the experimental adsorption of aromatic compounds on pristine and functionalized CNTs using MD simulation. The MD simulations correlated with experimental results can explain the mechanism of drug delivery, rate of drug release, the observed aggregations of CNTs on cell membranes, and the selection of proper suspending medium for CNTs.

Therefore, computer-aided simulation studies can be used to find out the optimum parameters required for designing nanodelivery systems. In this regard, MD simulations provide valuable information about the thermodynamic convergence of the system over time using classical Newtonian mechanics. Classical mechanics can represent a CNT–membrane system as a set of charged atoms (balls) connected by flexible bonds (springs). However, several less-important representations for atoms, interactions, as well as bond flexibilities and vibrations can be omitted to simplify the calculations. Owing to the large molecular size of the CNT–cell membrane system and the need to run the simulation for a long time (up to milliseconds) to achieve convergence, several approaches have been introduced to reduce the computational costs with minimal effect on precision. Such approaches include the use of constraints and restraints.

For constraint, a fixed value is given for a known variable during simulation, such as for bond length and angle size, which can also extend to turn a whole flexible functional group or molecule into a rigid bead, or by setting a weak, long-distance interaction to zero. In restraint, an energy penalty or external force is applied to the system to perturb the conformational ensembles and direct the convergence toward a specific point. Specific sets of constraints and restraints are implemented in coarse-graining and steered MD, respectively. However, coarse-graining MDs obey a Newtonian or Hamiltonian equation of motions, whereas steered MDs do not. Therefore, the energy calculation is different in both the cases (discussed later).

4.4.1 Types of CNT-Membrane Models Used for Molecular Dynamics Simulation

Owing to the large sizes and complexity of the systems (CNT–membrane model), several techniques are used to tackle the problems of computational cost by using simplified MD. As discussed previously, the simplifications include the use of the simplified model (addition of constraints), which is mechanically governed by a simplified force field; however, such simplifications are consistent with the original model and force field. Whether atoms are treated individually (all-atomistic), as groups (coarse-grained), or both (hybrid systems), the force fields are available to carry the system toward convergence. Accordingly, CNT interactions with biomolecules can be studied by following various MD approaches, such as all-atomistic molecular dynamics (AAMD), coarse-grained molecular dynamics (CGMD), hybrid all-atomistic/coarse-grained molecular dynamics (AA/CGMD), and dissipative particle dynamics (DPD).

4.4.1.1 All-Atomistic Molecular Dynamics

In this system, all atoms are represented explicitly, including water molecules (if water is not represented implicitly). The interatomic interactions (whether bonded or nonbonded) can be represented by several force fields of different principles, such as *ab initio*, semi-empirical, and empirical force fields. The first two force fields are computationally expensive and help simulate bond breakage and formation during dynamics. However, the empirical force field is the most commonly used in MD simulation for biomolecular systems. The empirical force field equation includes terms for nonbonded interactions, such as van der Waals, H-bonds, and electrostatic, as well as terms for molecular mechanics, such as bond stretching, bending, angles, and dihedrals. More-complex force fields include additional terms accounting for atomic polarizability. Each term in an empirical force field is multiplied by a coefficient value that can be adjusted to reproduce the experimentally observed energy.

The AAMD simulations can be run with implicit or explicit water models. Most of the AAMD simulations with explicit water models use nonpolarizable and orientation-independent water models that have lower computational costs, such as TIP3P, SPC/E, and TIP4P, respectively. TIP4P is an improved water model; however, it shows anomalous movement inside the CNT which is not perceived with the TIP3P model. Also, water viscosity within CNTs seems to increase in direct relation to temperature and size of CNTs during MD simulation. These observations necessitate the precise choice of water model during CNT simulation. Although the implicit water model adds approximations on the calculations, the reduction in computational cost is not guaranteed.

Among the most commonly used empirical force fields are CHARMM, AMBER, united-atom GROMOS, and COMPASS. These force fields have been used to model the systems of molecular interactions between CNTs and proteins, nucleic acids, and drug molecules. Despite being computationally expensive, AAMD can also be used effectively for studying CNT interactions with the cell membrane.

4.4.1.2 Coarse-Grained Molecular Dynamics

CGMD methodology is used to simulate the mechanics of mesoscopic systems (<1 mm), depending on the statistical coarse-graining description. This technique depends on reducing the number of degrees of freedom as compared with the AA description, thus eliminating the fine interaction details. In this approach, the atoms are united together by merging nonpolar hydrogens bound to carbon, the addition of constraints to remove the highest frequency motion from the system, or simplifying a group of atoms into a single bead. Some types of coarse-grained models add restraint to preserve the conformation for a macromolecule (e.g., protein domain) during MD simulation.

The coarse-grained model for cell membrane phospholipids can include three types of particles: tail particle to represent four methylene groups [-$(CH_2)_4$-], water particle to represent four water molecules, and a head particle to represent the part of the head of the phospholipid, as shown in Figure 4.13 for the DPPC lipid. CGMD is usually used for large molecular systems where the interaction types are limited but repeated like the system of CNTs with cell membranes, polymers, solvent/detergent/lipids. Owing to the low computational cost of CGMD as compared with AAMD, the simulation period can be extended up to microseconds. Moreover, CGMD can also be used in simulating CNT interactions with proteins, carbohydrates, DNA, and other NPs. Several types of phospholipids with their atomistic and coarse-grained representations as well as chemical names are provided in Figure 4.12.

There are several types of force fields used in CGMD. The coarse-grained force field commonly used for CNT–membrane systems, such as the MARTINI force field, is a parameterized form of AA force field. This force field follows top-down approaches (i.e., a parameterizing classical AA force field) to reproduce some experimental observations using coarse-particle representation for the system. The MARTINI force field uses Lennard–Jones interactions, but with adjusted well depth (ε) to reproduce observed partition coefficients. The electrostatic interactions are also included in this force field as simple Coulombic potentials, whereas harmonic potentials define the length and angle for the bonded interactions. Although the MARTINI force field works well for several systems, it is not efficient in describing some interactions, such as water behavior at the water–solid interface, where abnormal

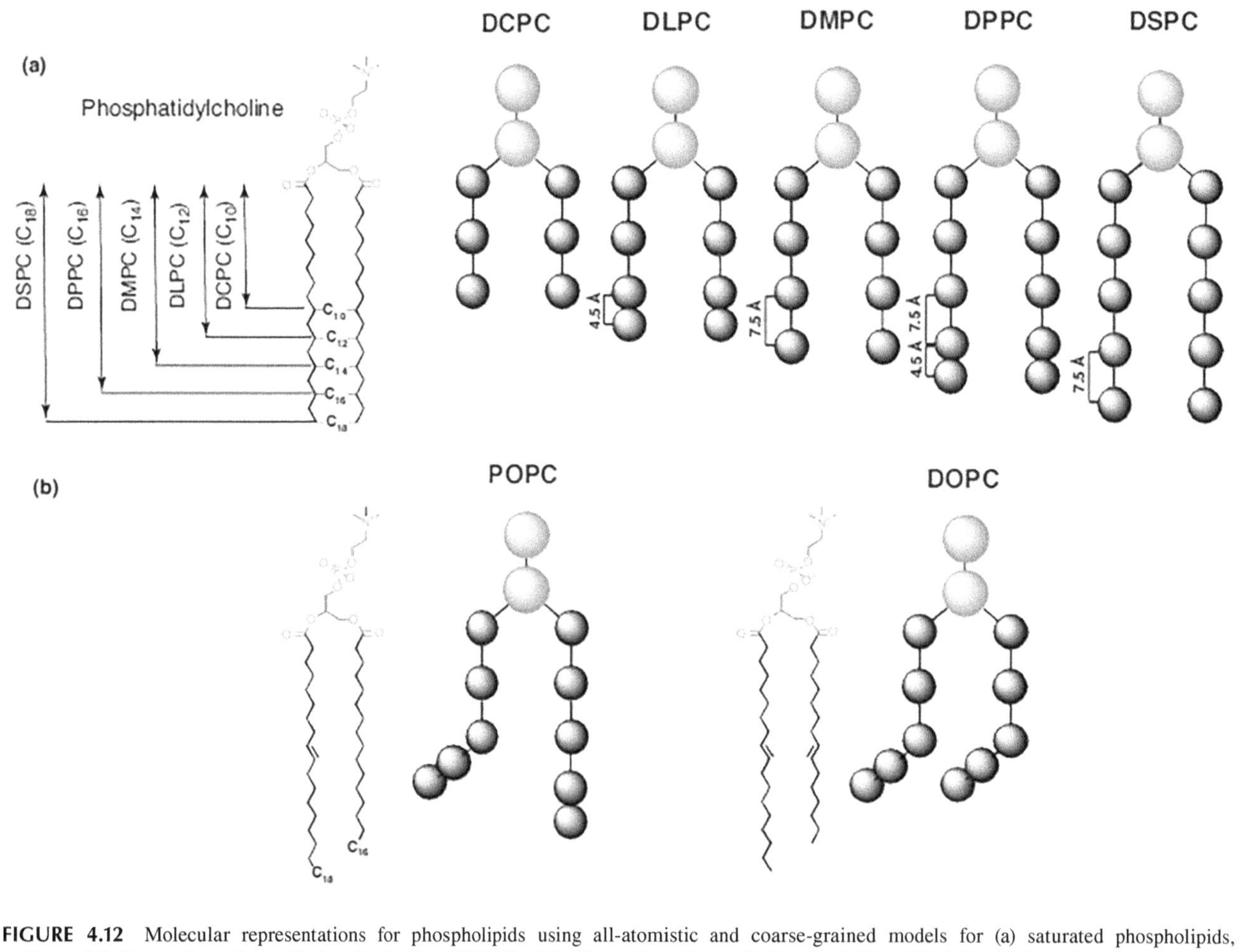

FIGURE 4.12 Molecular representations for phospholipids using all-atomistic and coarse-grained models for (a) saturated phospholipids, such as 1,2-dicaproyl-sn-glycero-3-phosphocholine (DCPC), 1,2-dilauroyl-sn-glycero-3-phosphocholine (DLPC), 1,2-dimyristoyl-sn-glycero-3-phosphocholine (DMPC), 1,2-dipalmitoyl-sn-glycero-3-phosphocholine (DPPC), and 1,2-distearoyl-sn-glycero-3-phosphocholine (DSPC), as well as (b) unsaturated phospholipids, such as 1-palmitoyl-2-oleoyl-sn-glycero-3-phosphocholine (POPC) and 1,2-dioleoyl-sn-glycero-3-phosphocholine (DOPC). Orange beads correspond to hydrophilic groups, and gray beads correspond to hydrophobic groups.

freezing can take place. However, this unwanted freezing can be minimized by using special large particles known as anti-freezing particles. Like AAMD, implicit water models are currently used with the coarse-grained force field, such as the new dry MARTINI force field, which was reported to produce significantly quicker calculations.

4.4.1.3 Hybrid All-Atomistic and Coarse-Grained Molecular Dynamics

In this methodology, some regions of the system are modeled as AA, and others as coarse-grained, like mixed quantum mechanics/molecular mechanics dynamic simulations. The AA/CG hybrid system requires the description of the interaction at the interface, such as those of electrostatic and van der Waals interactions. The force field required to represent the AA/CG hybrid system is derived from the force field representing the AA system (AA–AA), which is then mapped on to CG–CG interactions. At the interface, the AA molecules are mapped to coarse-grained particles, and the center of the mass is recalculated. Thus, a simple CG–CG interaction is being computed. The force generated from the interaction is then distributed on the atoms comprising the particle using mass-weighting. Such a technique is preferred in cases where full atomic details are required at the interaction site, such as for CNT–membrane or, more importantly, for protein–membrane systems. Some experiments use AA and coarse-grained models, but as a non-hybrid system, where the model is switched between AA and coarse-grained models during MD simulation. After convergence using CGMD, the AA details can be restored, and the simulation can be continued with AAMD. Various algorithms are available to map AA to coarse-graining, and vice versa.

4.4.1.4 Dissipative Particle Dynamics

This the simplest and computationally cheapest type of simulation, in which a single particle represents a group of molecules. It can be used for colloidal systems, where particles undergo Brownian motion within the solvent. The approach is similar to MD, where the forces acting on the particles are divided into conservative force (i.e., pair-wise potentials), dissipative force (i.e., due to friction), and random force. The frictional as well as random forces in Brownian dynamics do not conserve momentum. However, in DPD, the frictional and random forces obey action-equals reaction, as a result of which the model conserves momentum. The implicit solvent modeling in DPD was also reported to increase the speed of calculations. The DPD technique is more grained than the coarse-grained model and frequently used to simulate hydrodynamic behavior for CNTs with other materials, such polymer mixtures, surfactants, and water, as well as studying the macroscopic physical behavior of CNTs.

4.4.2 Free Energy Calculations from Molecular Dynamics Simulation Studies

MD simulation can be performed under constant pressure, temperature, and number of particles to achieve thermodynamic equilibrium. However, achieving equilibrium for large complex systems (such as CNTs and cell membrane) is computationally costly. Therefore, for extremely large systems, the simulation is usually accelerated toward convergence by applying an external force to cross the energy minima. However, this leads to non-equilibrium simulation, known as steered MD simulation.

The free energy for systems based on equilibrium or quasi-static simulation can be calculated using thermodynamic integration and umbrella sampling. Regarding non-equilibrium simulation, the affinity of ligand interaction to the receptor can be estimated from the energy essential to pull the ligand out of the receptor, which is an analog for atomic force microscopy. Thus, rather than binding free energy, the rupture force is measured as the maximum on the force-time/displacement profile and used as a scoring function, known as the potential of mean force (PMF). The PMF can be determined using Jarzynki's equation (eq. (4)) under constant temperature and pressure:

$$e^{-\beta\Delta G} = e^{-\beta W} \tag{4}$$

where $\beta = 1/k_\beta$ T, k_β is the Boltzmann constant, T is the temperature, G is Gibbs free energy, and W is the work done. The integration of force along the direction of steering gives the free energy.

For example, the PMF required for CNTs to penetrate the cell membrane is about tens of pN before the start of membrane curvature. Membrane curvature is a defect observed in the membrane due to the exposure of hydrophobic tails of lipids to water those results in the elevation of PMF to thousands of pN. However, PMF reduces when hydrophobic tails start wrapping around CNTs.

4.4.3 Molecular Dynamics Simulation Studies of Cell Membrane Internalization of CNTs

Many observations in physics, chemistry, biology, and other material sciences can be simulated using MD simulation. The accuracy of simulation results depends on the proper molecular representations of ligand, receptor, and medium, as well as a selection of valid force field and sufficient sampling. The cell membrane is composed of different lipid molecules, such as phospholipids, cholesterol, and glycolipids. However, only a single type of phospholipid is represented during MD simulation. The MD simulations usually follow the framework of the isobaric–isothermal ensemble (NPT), which is known as a favorable ensemble for membrane simulations. As the size of the system increases, a longer simulation time is required to achieve convergence (up to microseconds). Therefore, to extend the simulation time for the system, the number of atoms, degrees of freedom, and interactions of short range need to be reduced by grouping atoms into particles (coarse-grained) that interact with each other by a modified force field over long integration time steps (CGMD simulation). Such CGMD simulation can be used to simulate huge systems up to the size of fully enveloped influenza A virus in the microsecond timescale. The loss of accuracy owing to the coarseness can be reduced if atomistic detailing is applied at important interaction sites, as in AA/CGMD simulation.

Usually, the simulation of CNT–membrane interactions requires the use of CGMD. Using a single snapshot of an AA model, the coarse-grained model is generated, which usually involves 4:1 atom mapping of the carbon atoms in order to preserve the hexagonal symmetry of the CNT lattice. Recently, coarse-grained models compatible with the popular coarse-grained MARTINI force field can be automatically generated based on atomistic simulation trajectories, rather than fitting to a single snapshot, thus providing more accurate representation for the model. In their review article, Ingolfsson et al. discussed in detail the various developed coarse-grained force fields. The MARTINI coarse-grained force field was initially developed for lipids; however, the use of this force field was further extended and explored for proteins, carbohydrates, DNA, polymers, and other NPs. The experiments commonly conducted for CNT interactions with cell membranes are either thermodynamically equilibrated (i.e., penetration is driven by force field interactions only) or non-thermodynamically equilibrated (i.e., injection mainly driven by an external force).

4.4.3.1 Cell Membrane Penetration

In this method, the MD simulations are usually carried out by manually placing CNTs at a reasonable distance from the interacting molecules like membrane or protein, among others. For non-functionalized CNTs, van der Waals and hydrophobic interactions are the dominant interactions to be simulated, usually with explicit water representation.

The MD simulation can provide insight into the effect of length and chirality of CNTs on cell membrane penetration. If MD is allowed to run without constraints, the CNTs (~6 nm in length) can tilt during membrane embedding until the tube is completely buried within the hydrophobic part of the bilayer. Interestingly, the chirality of CNTs affects the rate of membrane penetration. For short CNTs (less than one membrane thickness), the rotation (tilt) during penetration is obvious, and the effect of chirality on penetration is minimal. However, if the length of CNTs equals twice the membrane thickness, the effect of chirality becomes pronounced, and the penetration of the membrane gets faster with lower chiral indices (higher aspect ratio), owing to lower adhesion to the membrane. Accordingly, the MD simulation can be used to adjust the physical properties for CNTs for customized drug delivery.

MD simulation can complement the transmission electron microscope to describe the mechanism of cell membrane internalization for amino-functionalized CNTs. The hydrophilic and positively charged functional groups of the surface guide the CNT orientation to be parallel concerning the membrane axis to maximize the interaction with the negatively charged membrane. Subsequently, the CNTs adopt a perpendicular orientation during internalization as mediated by CNT hydrophobicity. The degree of functionalization affects the penetration angle. The length of the CNTs is another important factor; CNTs <1 mm in length have a higher ability to penetrate the cell membrane than longer ones. Simulations and experiments showed incomplete uptake of long CNTs by lysosomes, which could eventually lead to activation of apoptotic signals and cell death. Moreover, different mechanisms of internalization are observed for capped and non-capped CNTs.

MD simulation can provide optimum conditions for drug loading into CNTs and unloading at the cell membrane. Larger-diameter CNTs are favored as drug carriers, and the π–π interaction is the main interaction between the CNT aromatic rings and lone pair electrons of the drug, such as those of oxygen atoms. MD can simulate the effect of other parameters on drug loading, such as temperature, solution composition, as well as the unloading parameters, like water effect and interaction with the cell membrane. For example, the loading of vinblastine on CNTs was favored with terminal esterification of CNTs with armchair chirality. For cisplatin, the insertion within CNTs and release at the cell membrane was dependent on water dynamics [74]. CNTs can also function as mediators for liposomal package fusion with the cell membrane by reducing the energy barrier. The effect of covalent and non-covalent functionalization of CNTs by PEG on cell membrane penetration and the aggregation of CNTs was studied using MD simulation. The results showed that covalent functionalization with PEG enhanced dispersion, but not membrane penetration, whereas the opposite was observed for non-covalent functionalization. The enhancement of membrane penetration by proper selection of type and density of non-covalent functionalization can also be simulated.

4.4.3.2 Cell Membrane Injection

This type of simulation study can help determine the structural properties in CNTs that are required for proper penetration with minimal damage to the cell membrane as well as for delivering the attached drug molecule at the site of penetration. The penetration of CNTs through the membrane can be enforced by using steered MD where external force and restrain are applied. For example, a spring connects CNTs to a dummy point moving with constant velocity across the membrane using a constant of 5–10 kJ mol^{-1} Å^{-2}, and the orientation of CNTs can be restrained with 10 kJ mol^{-1}Å^{-2} during the movement. The speed of the dummy atom can be 0.025–0.1 Å/ps, which gives a force of pulling CNTs through the lipid membrane ranging from 1,400 pN at the insertion or leaving stages to 400 pN when the tube is midway within the membrane. During the insertion, the hydrophobic CNT surface is resisted by the hydrophilic phase of the membrane; in addition, lipid molecules move upward to wrap the CNT surface exposed to the aqueous medium. During the leaving phase, the hydrophobic CNT surface is detached from the hydrophobic core of the membrane, and some lipid molecules are extracted from the membrane. Therefore, different forces are measured according to CNT displacement concerning the cell membrane.

The force acting on the dummy atom (PMF) can be calculated from the potential energy using eqs. (5) and (6):

$$F = -\nabla U \tag{5}$$

$$U = \frac{1}{2} K \left[vt - (r - r_0).n \right]^2 \tag{6}$$

Where ∇U is the potential energy gradient, k is the spring force constant, v is the velocity of pulling, t is the current time, r and r_0 are the instantaneous and initial positions, respectively, and n is the vector direction of the dummy atom.

TABLE 4.1
Molecular Dynamics Experiments for Carbon Nanotube–Membrane Interactions

MD Type	MD Software	MD Force Fields	MD Steering	Lipid	CNT Placement	Refs
AAMD	NAMD	CHARMM	Yes	POPC	Manual; 1 nm above membrane	[81]
AAMD	NAMD	CHARMM36	Yes, only CNT orientation is constrained	DOPC	Manual	[82]
AAMD	TINKER	CHARMM27 + MM3	No	DPPC	Manual above membrane by 2 Å	[83]
AAMD	GROMACS	GROMOS43A1	Yes	DPPC	Manual; 1 nm above membrane	[84]
AAMD	AMBER	AMBER	No	DOPC	Manual above membrane	[85]
CGMD	GROMACS	MARTINI	No	DPPC	Manual above membrane	[86]
CGMD	GROMACS	MARTINI	No	DOPC	Manual above membrane	[87]
CGMD	GROMACS	MARTIN-like	Yes, only CNT orientation is constrained	DPPC	Manual	[88]
CGMD	GROMACS	MARTINI	Yes	DPPC	Manual above membrane by ~30 Å	[89]
GCMD	GROMACS	MARTINI	Yes	DPPC, DHPC, b LPC	Manual; 3 nm above membrane	[90]
AA/CG MD	OCCAM	Specifica	No	DPPC	Manual above membrane	[91]
DPD	Unknown	Specifica	Yes	General	Manual; 1.6 nm above membrane	[92]

Although steered MD does not represent the real thermodynamic behavior of the system, it can be used to simulate the behavior of frequently employed nano-injectors. It has been observed that a higher speed of penetration (up to 50 Å/ns) can provide lower membrane perturbation in the direction antiparallel to the pulling force, as well as less CNT blockage during insertion into the lipid membrane, especially for small-diameter CNTs (<25 Å). The force required to inject CNTs (14–50 Å diameter, 50–100 Å in length) was computed to be almost 600 pN. The MD simulations can provide information about stress points on CNTs, optimum chirality (tilt angle), and the speed that promotes penetration, with minor destructive or deflective effects on the cell membrane and CNTs. Examples of recently conducted experiments for CNT–membrane interactions using different types of models, force fields, and lipids (with or without steering) are provided in Table 4.1. Although several commercial and noncommercial software packages are available to handle MD simulation for CNT systems, GROMACS is regarded as the most commonly used because it implements AA force fields (AMBER, CHARMM, GROMOS, and OPLS), as well as coarse-grained force fields (MARTINI).

A workflow for a CNT–membrane MD experiment is shown in Figure 4.13. The free energy, potential energy, or potential of mean force is determined.

4.4.4 Limitations of Carbon Nanotube–Membrane Molecular Dynamics Simulations

Limitations of the MD approach in general include lower precision in force fields to represent experimental observations, size limits for the system being simulated, and computational demands. CGMDs on their own, however, have limitations of being not transferable (i.e., not able to efficiently address atomistic model); the force fields are only parameterized for specific classes of molecules, and they are too coarse to capture certain behavior, such as H-bond directionality. Improvements in force fields and multiscale automatic transferability between AA and coarse-grained modeling are recommended to reduce the CGMD inaccuracy and to enable experimental data reproducibility. Improvements in algorithms and computational speed are required to achieve system convergence easily. With previous improvements, the MD simulation is expected to be a standard step in rational design of CNT-based nanodelivery systems.

4.5 Computational Aspects of Solvent and Co-Solvent Effects on the Interaction of Flutamide as Anticancer Drug Delivery System with CNT

Flutamide is used together with a luteinizing hormone–releasing hormone agonist, a type of hormonal injection such as leuprolide, goserelin, or triptorelin, to treat certain types of prostate cancer. Flutamide is in a class of medications called nonsteroidal antiandrogens. Ethyleneimine is used in polymerization products, as a monomer for polyethyleneimine, as a comonomer for polymers, and in paper and textile chemicals, adhesives, and binders. Ethyleneimine has been applied to modify the flutamide as anticancer drug. Therefore, investigation of the adsorption behavior and electronic properties of carbon nanotubes and nanocones against flutamide @ ethyleneimine was carried out by calculation of the density functional theory. The *N* atom of flutamide @ ethyleneimine helps its adsorption on the nanotubes and nanocones, showing adsorption energies of around –30.1 and –20.5 kcal/mol, correspondingly. Chemical activities of the nanocomplexes were specified through electronics parameters, such as electronegativity, electroaffinity, softness, and hardness. All calculated data obtained good behavior of flutamide @ ethyleneimine with nanotubes and nanocones adsorption as carrier.

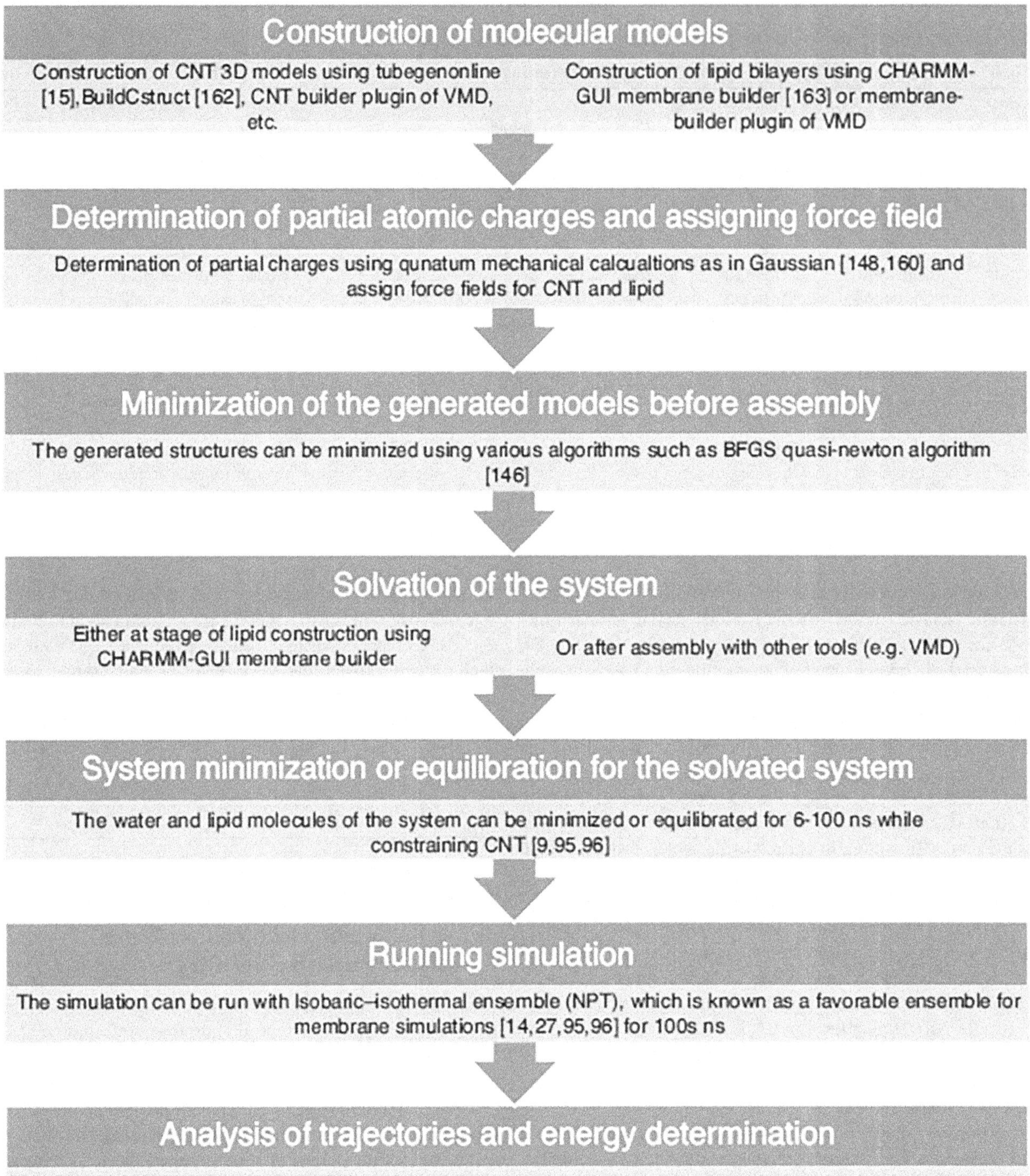

FIGURE 4.13 Workflow to set a CNT–membrane MD experiment.

4-nitro-3-trifluoromethyl-isobutilanilide, known as flutamide (FLU), is one of the most effective antiandrogenic agents which have antiandrogenic characteristics in genitalia organs. It is widely used in prostate cancer and mainly considered an antiandrogenic drug which lacks a steroidal structure. Recently, drug delivery has been considered a promising technique to directly send chemical drugs to target regions in order to minimize different aspects of drug toxicities.

Furthermore, nanoscience has revealed their unique and effective treatment behavior in medicine, specifically for the treatment of cancer, while applying the promising nanomaterials, such as carbon nanotubes (CNTs).

Carbon nanotubes draw the attraction of researchers in different areas due to their unique and extraordinary structure, electrical, and mechanical properties, which make them undoubtedly applicable for a wide range of applications, such as detection sensors, different types of transistors, thermal, and pressure sensors. In addition, the mentioned uncommon physicochemical properties of the nanotubes introduce them as very suitable and promising options for controlling biological delivery systems, like intracellular transport of nucleic acids, proteins, antibodies, and different chemical drug molecules. Moreover, single-walled carbon nanotubes (SWCNTs) have approved advantages, including their potential to carry a high cargo loading, their chemical and mechanical stability, and their structural flexibility, which could extend the circulation time. However, the stability of the SWCNT–other molecule complexes in biomedical media is a critical challenge that has developed their applications in drug delivery systems experimentally. Also, various techniques have been developed for CNT production, for instance, laser vaporization or chemical vapor deposition of hydrocarbons and thermal decomposition of C60 in the presence of transition metals.

To analyze the adsorption characteristics of the flutamide molecule onto the exterior surface of the single-walled carbon nanotube, density functional theory (DFT) has been applied in the gas phase and the water solution. Moreover, the effects of the drug adsorption on the structural and electrical properties of the pristine SWCNT are examined. Also, the effect of ethanol (ETOH) co-solvent on the interaction between the drug molecules and SWCNT is explained by molecular dynamics (MD) simulation.

4.5.1 Quantum Mechanics Calculations

The adsorption behavior of the FLU molecule on the surface of armchair (5,5) single-walled CNT has been investigated in the gas phase and water solution. It is known that the encapsulation in the nanotubes is influenced by drug diameter, according to Dalili Mansour's investigation [93]. Consequently, regarding the small size of the carbon nanotube diameter in comparison with FLU drug molecule, the selected (5,5) SWCNT is unfavorable for FLU drug encapsulation. All calculations on the pristine SWCNT and different configurations are performed using density functional theory at Becke, 3-parameter, Lee–Yang–Parr (B3LYP) functional, along with 6–31G(d,p) basis set as implemented in the Gaussian 03 program package. Furthermore, the effect of dispersion interactions on the adsorption properties of the studied configurations has been evaluated using the density functional theory in an extended framework with newly implemented Grimme corrections (DFT-D). For each system, the DFT-D total energy is equal to the sum of the corresponding conventional DFT energy and the correction value based on a damped atom-pairwise potential.

It is worth noting that the adsorption energy (E_{ads}) is considered a suitable and applicable tool to understand the interaction between different species in a selected complex. Furthermore, the adsorption energy is defined by the following expression:

$$E_{ads} = E_{CNT/FLU} - (E_{CNT} + E_{FLU}) + E_{bsse} \quad (7)$$

Where $E_{CNT/FLU}$ represents the energy of the nanotube with the adsorbed FLU molecule over its wall, E_{CNT} is the energy of the pristine nanotube, and E_{FLU} is the energy of a single FLU molecule, respectively. E_{bsse} is the basis set superposition error (bsse) correction included to eliminate the effect of basis set incompleteness, which is achieved by counterpoise correction method. According to this equation, the negative value of the E_{ads} reveals the exergonic characteristic of the adsorption process.

The effects of water solvation on the nature of interactions are included using self-consistent reaction field (SCRF) with Tomasi's polarized continuum (PCM) model. As water plays a major role in our body, it has been selected as a solvent in order to identify the interaction of FLU molecule with carbon nanotube while passing through human bodies.

Furthermore, in order to determine the stability of FLU/SWCNT complexes, solvation energy ($\Delta E_{solvation}$) has been calculated by applying the following equation:

$$\Delta E_{solvation} = E_{sol} - E_{gas} \quad (8)$$

Where $\Delta E_{solvation}$ refers to the solvation energy; E_{sol} and E_{gas} are also the total values of the energy in the selected systems in the solvent and gas phase, respectively.

The quantum molecular descriptors, like energy gap (E_g), the chemical potential (μ), and global hardness (η), are calculated according to the method proposed by Koopman [94] as follows:

$$Eg = E_{LUMO} - E_{HOMO} \quad (9)$$

$$\mu = E_{LUMO} + E_{HOMO} \quad (10)$$

$$\eta = E_{LUMO} - E_{HOMO} \quad (11)$$

Where E_{LUMO} is the lowest energy level of the unoccupied molecular orbital and E_{HOMO} is the highest energy level of the occupied molecular orbital, respectively.

The role of the chemical potential in chemistry has been analyzed by Parr and Pearson. They suggested that the chemical potential plays an important role in explaining chemical reactions through the charge transfer process.

In order to investigate the properties of the bond critical points (BCP), their electron densities (ρ) and their Laplacians (∇2ρ) atoms in molecule (AIM) calculations are carried out using the AIM2000 program. The natural bond orbital calculation (NBO) is carried out using the NBO 3.1 program. Additionally, to study the effects of the FLU attachment to the nanotube on its electronic properties, density of state (DOS) analysis is carried out. In order to explore the direction of the electron transfer between the FLU molecule and SWCNT in the adsorption process, the parameter ΔN, which determines the fractional number of electrons transferred from a system *A* (acceptor) to system *B* (donor), is defined as:

$$\Delta N = (\mu_B - \mu_A)/(\eta_A + \eta_B) \quad (12)$$

Where μ and η are the chemical potential and the chemical hardness of donor (*B*) and acceptor (*A*), respectively. The positive value of ΔN reveals that electron flows spontaneously from B to A, or otherwise, it is in the reverse direction.

Moreover, the reactivity descriptors, such as the overall stabilization energy ($\Delta E_{SE(AB)}$), the individual energy change of acceptor ($\Delta E_{A(B)}$), and the individual energy change of donor ($\Delta E_{B(A)}$), are applied to understand the stability of the resultant compounds, as follows [95]:

$$\Delta E_{A(B)} = \Delta N\left(-\mu_A + \frac{1}{2}(+\eta_B)\right) \tag{13}$$

$$\Delta E_{B(A)} = \Delta N\left(-\mu_B + \frac{1}{2}\eta_B \Delta N\right) \tag{14}$$

$$\Delta E_{B(A)} = \Delta N\left(-\mu_B + \frac{1}{2}\eta_B \Delta N\right) \tag{15}$$

4.5.1.1 Molecular Geometry and Adsorption Energies

In order to obtain the most stable model, different configurations have been investigated. In the considered configurations, the FLU molecule is approached to the exterior surface of SWCNT from the N-H, F, CH_3, and C = O terminals perpendicularly, and also in parallel mode to the z-axis of the nanotube. The graphical pictures of the optimized structures of the FLU drug and SWCNT, as well as initial and final forms of the FLU/SWCNT complexes, have been illustrated in Figures 4.14 and 4.18. After the optimization process, re-orientation of the drug molecule has been observed in the selected configurations; after all, stable configurations are obtained (see Figure 4.15). Table 4.2 illustrates the adsorption and solvation energies as well as the interatomic distance for the considered complexes in the gas phase and the water solution. The length and diameter of the optimized carbon nanotube are 11.68 Å and 7.47 Å, respectively.

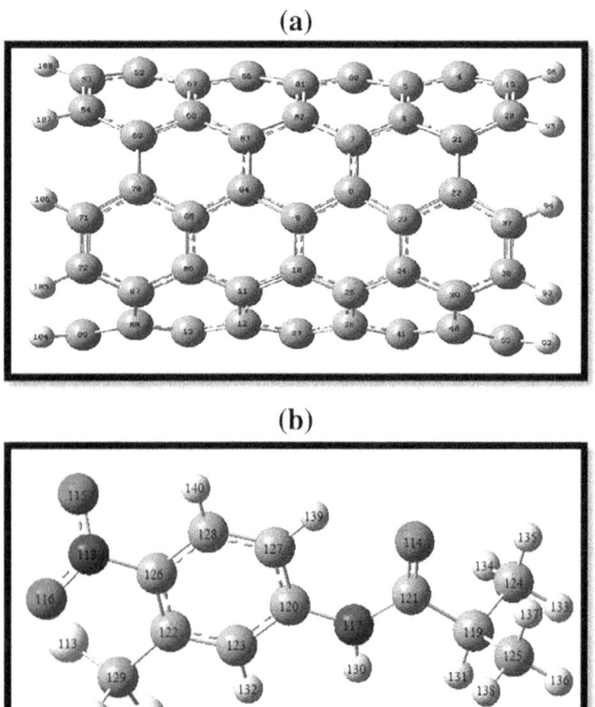

FIGURE 4.14 The optimized structures of (a) SWCNT and (b) free FLU drug.

The obtained values of the adsorption energies vary from −1.959 to −16.854 kJ/mol and from −1.551 to −5.991 kJ/mol in the gas phase and water solution, respectively (Table 4.2). These results [96] reveal that the FLU molecule can be adsorbed on the exterior surface of the SWCNT physically. Moreover, the negative Eads values verify that the drug adsorption process is exothermic. A close inspection of Table 4.2 shows that the sequence of the adsorption strength in the studied configurations without including the solvation effects decreases in the order 3 (−16.854) > 1 (−15.495) > 2 (−9.949) > 5 (−5.242) > 4 (−1.959). The inclusion of solvent effect changes the order of binding preference to be 3 (−5.991) > 1 (−5.002) > 4 (−3.778) > 5 (−2.541) > 2 (−1.551). As shown in Table 4.2, it is found that in going from the gas phase to the solvent phase, the adsorption energy values decrease. Close inspection of these results shows that the adsorption energy for configuration 2 changes so much between the water and vacuum system. In the optimized structure of the configuration 2 in the gas phase, the N = O terminal group of the adsorbed drug molecule is doubly hydrogen-bonded with the SWCNT edge, that is, $O_{115}\cdots H_{106}$ (2.773 Å) and $O_{115}\cdots H_{107}$ (2.786 Å), respectively. In this structure, the oxygen atom of the FLU drug as a Lewis base interacts with hydrogen atoms of the carbon nanotube as Lewis acids. On the other hand, there is no intermolecular hydrogen bond interaction in the optimized structure of configuration 2 in the water solution. It can be concluded that the highest adsorption energy of FLU molecule with SWCNT at configuration 2 in the gas phase is due to the presence of HB interactions. Therefore, a significant enhancement in the adsorption energy of the drug molecule and the carbon nanotube is observed in the gas phase for this configuration.

The obtained results reveal that the most stable configuration is configuration 3, with the most negative adsorption energy in both water solution and gaseous phase (Table 4.2). The large adsorption energy of this configuration is in accordance with the shortest intermolecular interaction distance between the nanotube and FLU molecule (Table 4.2). In most cases, stronger interactions well correlate with shorter bonds. In this configuration, the H130 atom of FLU molecule prefers to attach to C69 of the nanotube by the equilibrium distances of 3.00 Å and 2.90 Å in the water solution and gas phase, respectively. Analysis of the structural parameters indicates that the N117–H130 and C68–C69 bond lengths of the adsorbed molecule and the nanotube remain nearly constant at the most stable model (see Table 4.3). These results confirm that the interaction in this configuration is a type of weak interaction. Also, the obtained results reveal that the geometry of the drug adsorbed on the surface of the SWCNT in the studied configurations does not change appreciably when solvent effects are taken into account (see Table 4.3) [96].

From the adsorption energies presented in Table 4.2, it can be seen that the adsorption energies depend on the locations and orientations of the drug molecule. In other words, the calculated adsorption energy for those cases in which the FLU

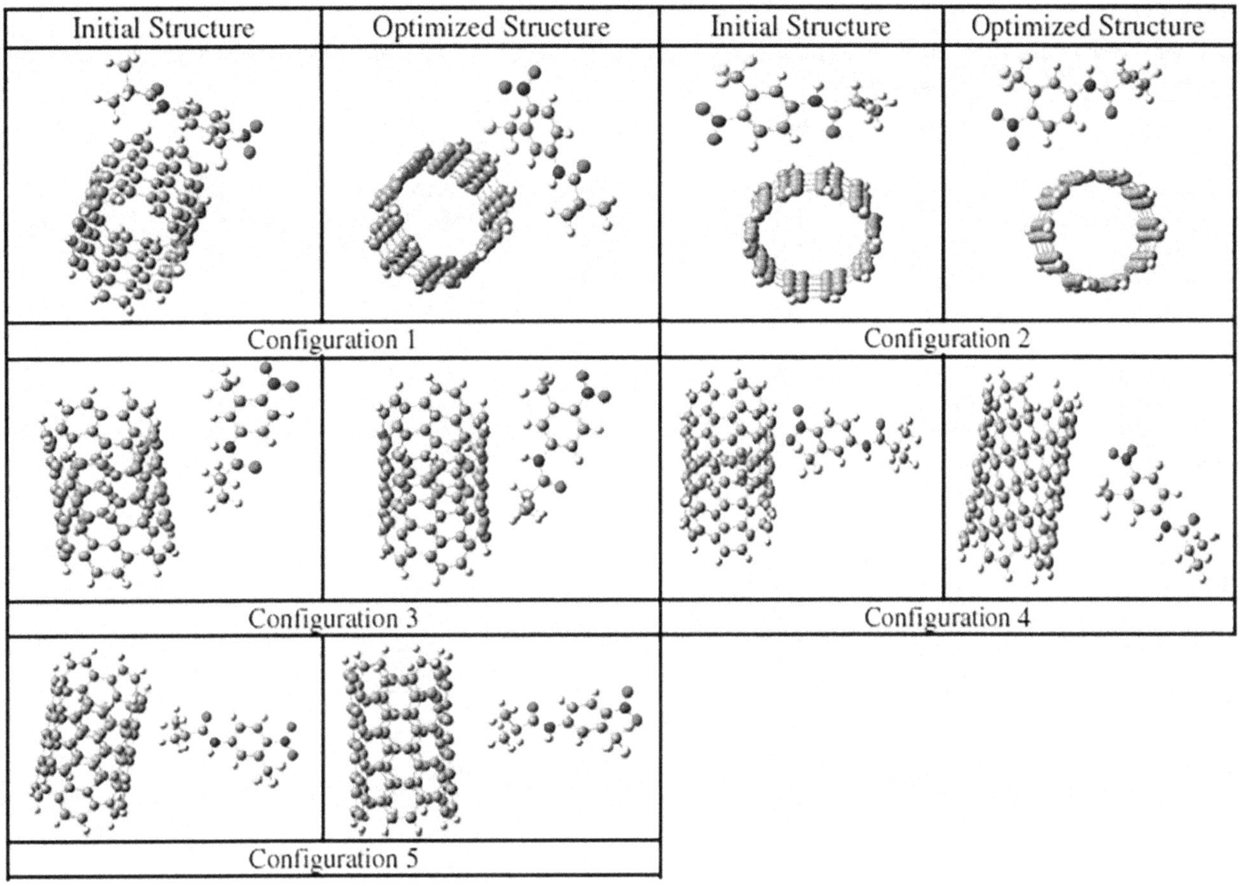

FIGURE 4.15 Initial and the optimized structures for different configurations.

TABLE 4.2

The Calculated Intermolecular Distances (Å) between the Adsorbed Drug and CNT, Dipole Moments (μ°) (Debye), the Adsorption (E_{ads}) and Solvation ($\Delta E_{solvation}$) Energies (kJ/mol) for the Considered Configurations Calculated at the B3LYP/6–31G** Level

	E_{ads}	Interatomic Contact	μ°	$\Delta E_{solvation}$
PCM				
Configuration 1	−5.002	C85–H134 = 3.095	9.224	−60.606
Configuration 2	−1.551	C68–H140 = 3.263	9.423	−62.701
Configuration 3	−5.991	C69–H130 = 3.000	10.417	−60.236
Configuration 4	−3.778	C84–F113 = 3.282	9.464	−72.917
Configuration 5	−2.541	C84–H136 = 3.255	9.740	−68.397
GAS				
Configuration 1	−15.495	C85–H134 = 3.375	8.803	—
Configuration 2	−9.949	H106–O115 = 2.773	6.481	—
		H107–O115 = 2.786		
Configuration 3	−16.854	C69–H130 = 2.900	9.705	—
Configuration 4	−1.959	C84–F113 = 3.302	7.485	—
Configuration 5	−5.242	C84–H136 = 3.261	8.593	—

drug is adsorbed on the SWCNT via its N–H terminal is more notable in comparison with other considered cases.

Furthermore, in order to investigate the effect of dispersion on the adsorption energy and geometry parameters, DFT-D calculations are performed for all investigated systems. It is found that the adsorption energy varies from −2.725 to −17.620 kJ/mol and from −1.924 to −6.238 kJ/mol in the gas and water phases, respectively (see Table 4.4).

These results [96] indicate that by including the dispersion correction, the adsorption energy value will increase for all configurations. Therefore, it can be stated that the dispersion energy acts as an important attractive interaction in the studied

TABLE 4.3

The Geometrical Parameters (Bond Lengths (R) Is in Å) for the Adsorbed Drug Molecule and CNT Before and After the Adsorption Process in the Gas Phase and Water Solution

	Bond	R_{inCNT}	$R_{incomplex}$	Bond	R_{inFLU}	$R_{incomplex}$
PCM						
Configuration 1	C85–C70	1.417	1.418	C124–H134	1.094	1.094
Configuration 2	C67–C68	1.435	1.435	C128–H140	1.082	1.082
Configuration 3	C68–C69	1.417	1.419	N117–H130	1.011	1.013
Configuration 4	C83–C84	1.424	1.423	F113–C129	1.347	1.347
Configuration 5	C84–C85	1.438	1.439	C125–H136	1.094	1.093
GAS						
Configuration 1	C85–C70	1.417	1.417	C124–H134	1.095	1.094
Configuration 2	C67–C68	1.434	1.434	C128–H140	1.083	1.082
Configuration 3	C68–C69	1.417	1.419	N117–H130	1.01	1.013
Configuration 4	C83–C84	1.424	1.423	F113–C129	1.341	1.343
Configuration 5	C84–C85	1.438	1.439	C125–H136	1.094	1.093

TABLE 4.4

Lenard Jones Parameters Applied for CNT and Functional Groups in This Study

	Atom	Sigma (A°)	Epsilon (kj/mol)	CNT
CNT	CA	0.35500	0.29288	
	HA	0.24200	0.12552	
PEG	CR	0.38754	0.23012	
	HC	0.23520	0.09205	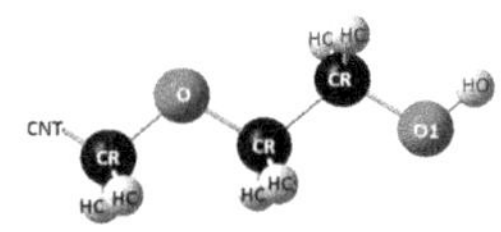
	O	0.31538	0.63639	
	O1	0.29578	0.66567	
	HO	0.04000	0.19246	
AMINE	C	0.35635	0.46024	
	H	0.23520	0.09205	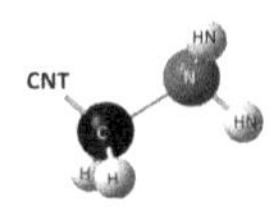
	N	0.32963	0.83680	
	HN	0.04000	0.19246	
COOH	C	0.35636	0.46024	
	O	0.30291	0.50208	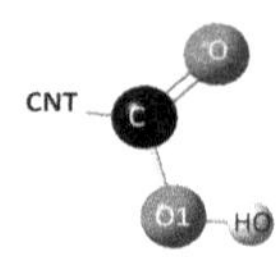
	O1	0.31538	0.63639	
	HO	0.04000	0.19246	

configuration. Also, the results indicate that the geometries calculated with the DFT-D method are the same as the ones obtained from conventional DFT.

Furthermore, dipole moments of the FLU drug molecule and the studied configurations are calculated by DFT method and provided in Table 4.2. The dipole moment is the first derivative of the energy with respect to an applied electric field as a measure of asymmetry in the molecular charge distribution. As can be seen from Table 4.2, the dipole moments of the selected configurations increase by changing the gas phase to the solution medium. Moreover, the enhancement polarity suggests the possible solubility of these complexes in the presence of the water solvent. Also, it is observed that greater dipole moment is associated with higher absolute values of the adsorption energy (see Table 4.2). Indeed, the high dipole moment illustrates the great reactivity and suggests the contribution from resonance.

In order to investigate the degree of solubility of the studied complexes in water media, the solvation energy parameter has been calculated, and the obtained results are tabulated in Table 4.2. Negative values of the solvation energy denote that the solvation is spontaneous, and it signifies the solubility of the considered systems in the aqueous environment.

The kinetic aspects of the interaction between the carbon nanotube and FLU drug molecule are investigated by using $\Delta E_{B(A)}$, whereas $\Delta E_{A(B)}$ and $\Delta E_{SE(AB)}$ are exploited to understand the thermodynamic stability of the studied complexes. By considering the calculated theoretical results, it can be concluded that the SWCNT is B (i.e., donor) and the FLU is A (i.e., acceptor). It is worth mentioning that the numerical value of ΔN easily defines the donor and the acceptor involved in the process of interaction. The values of ΔN and $\Delta E_{B(A)}$ are positive, which indicate that the electron flow is spontaneous from the SWCNT to FLU (see Table 4.5). The interaction is a "normal electron demand" (NED) reaction due to the direction of electron flow from the donor B to the acceptor A. Furthermore, the negative value of $\Delta E_{A(B)}$ confirms that the SWCNT–FLU complex is energetically stable. Also, the $\Delta E_{SE(AB)}$ value is negative

TABLE 4.5
The Values of the Overall Stabilization Energy ($\Delta E_{SE(AB)}$), the Individual Energy Change of Acceptor ($\Delta E_{A(B)}$), and the Individual Energy Change of Donor ($\Delta E_{B(A)}$) (All in eV) and Charge Transfer (ΔN) within the Reacting FLU Drug Molecule and SWCNT

	PCM	GAS
$\Delta E_{SE(AB)}$	−0.248	−0.291
$\Delta E_{A(B)}$	−1.868	−1.934
$\Delta E_{B(A)}$	1.619	1.643
ΔN	0.435	0.456

for the favorable intermolecular interaction between the drug molecule and the carbon nanotube (see Table 4.5).

4.5.1.2 HOMO and LUMO Analysis

In order to illustrate the ability to donate or obtain electron, the HOMO and LUMO profiles of the desired structures, that is, FLU molecule, pristine SWCNT, and the most stable configuration, are shown in Figure 4.16. As is illustrated in this figure, the HOMO and LUMO of the FLU molecule are not located on the CH_3 and CF_3 groups, but they cover the other parts of the drug molecule. This kind of profile implies that C = O and N–H terminals of the drug molecule are more reactive in comparison with CH_3 and CF_3 groups. Moreover, close inspection of Figure 4.16 shows that the frontier orbital plots of the pristine SWCNT are distributed in the uniform states. Furthermore, it is found that in the most stable configuration, the LUMO is localized on the FLU drug, while HOMO is placed at the surface of the nanotube. This suggests a charge transfer from the HOMO to the LUMO.

Moreover, different quantum chemical parameters for the FLU molecule, SWCNT, and the studied configurations have been analyzed and presented in Table 4.6. The direction of electron flow will be distinguished by electronegativity (χ) or electronic chemical potential. χ is the Mulliken electronegativity for atoms, which is called the absolute electronegativity ($\chi = -\mu$). When the FLU molecule and the nanotube are brought together, electrons will flow from that of lower χ (SWCNT) to that of higher χ (FLU) (see Table 4.6). Besides, considering the amount of chemical potential values of Table 4.6 confirms that electrons will flow from a particular occupied orbital in SWCNT into a definite empty orbital in FLU molecule. Indeed, the electron is transferred from higher chemical potential (SWCNT) to the lower electronic chemical potential (FLU), until the electronic chemical potentials become identical. Based on the Pearson's maximum hardness

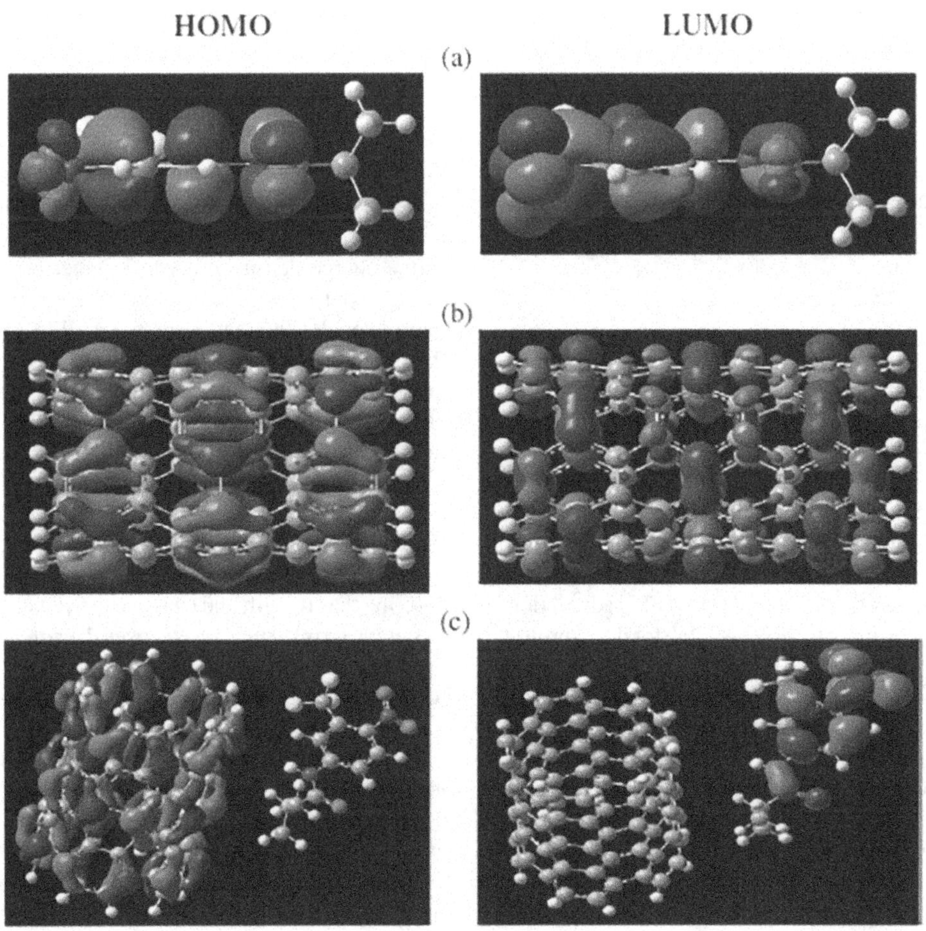

FIGURE 4.16 Orbital depiction of HOMO and LUMO in (a) FLU molecule, (b) SWCNT, and (c) the most stable configuration.

TABLE 4.6

The Values of the Highest Occupied Molecular Orbital Energies (EHOMO) and the Lowest Unoccupied Molecular Orbital Energies (E_{LUMO}), Energy Gap (E_g), Chemical Potential (μ), Global Hardness (η), and Electronegativity (χ) (All in eV) for FLU, the Pristine (5,5) Armchair SWCNT, and Different Models in the Gas Phase and Water Solution

	E_{HOMO}	E_{LUMO}	Eg	μ	η	χ
PCM						
Configuration 1	−4.162	−3.045	1.117	−3.604	0.558	3.604
Configuration 2	−4.158	−3.043	1.116	−3.600	0.558	3.600
Configuration 3	−4.187	−3.071	1.116	−3.629	0.558	3.629
Configuration 4	−4.151	−3.034	1.116	−3.593	0.558	3.593
Configuration 5	−4.165	−3.048	1.117	−3.606	0.558	3.606
FLU	−6.806	−2.677	4.129	−4.742	2.064	4.742
CNT	−4.159	−3.043	1.116	−3.601	0.558	3.601
GAS						
Configuration 1	−4.258	−3.146	1.111	−3.702	0.556	3.702
Configuration 2	−4.267	−3.158	1.109	−3.713	0.553	3.713
Configuration 3	−4.025	−2.919	1.106	−3.472	0.554	3.472
Configuration 4	−3.887	−2.778	1.109	−3.333	0.554	3.333
Configuration 5	−4.166	−3.055	1.111	−3.610	0.555	3.610
FLU	−6.990	−2.506	4.483	−4.748	2.242	4.748
CNT	−4.026	−2.916	1.110	−3.471	0.555	3.471

principle (MHP), it is found that the chemical hardness value of the SWCNT is smaller than that in the FLU molecule, indicating that this compound is softer than the FLU drug molecule, therefore the greatest polarizability there will be. As a result, FLU molecule has the capability to accept an electron from SWCNT, which is in agreement with the previous results.

As can be observed from Table 4.6, the largest reduction of E_g is predicted when the FLU molecule is adsorbed on the SWCNT at configuration ***3***, which would result in an electrical conductivity change of the nanotube according to the following equation:

$$\sigma \ \alpha \ \exp\left(\text{-}E_g = kT\right) \tag{16}$$

Where σ and k are the electrical conductivity and the Boltzmann's constant, respectively. This equation suggests that smaller E_g values result in the larger electric conductivities at a given temperature.

It is observed that when FLU drug is adsorbed on SWCNTs, the electronic chemical potential values of the most considered configurations are decreased, which indicates that the reactivity of these systems is increased (see Table 4.6).

In addition, in order to study the effect of FLU adsorption on the electronic properties of the SWCNT, the total and projected electronic density of states (DOS and PDOS) have been measured. The DOS plot of configuration ***3*** has no distinct changes compared to that of the pristine nanotube. Moreover, for the considered complex, the red curve (PDOS of SWCNT) is high and nearly approaches the black line (TDOS of the most stable model). Hence, it can be concluded that the nanotube has a significant contribution toward HOMO. Also, this figure demonstrates that no significant hybridization between FLU and SWCNT orbitals occurs during the adsorption process.

Moreover, it is found that the values of EHOMO, ELUMO, and HOMO–LUMO energy gap of the studied configurations in solvent phase have less deviation with respect to those corresponding values in the gas phase (see Table 4.6).

There is electron density overlap between SWCNT and FLU molecule for configuration ***3***, which represents the flow of the electronic charge between the drug molecule and nanotube.

4.5.1.3 AIM Analysis

Since the geometrical and electronic parameters may not be sufficient to have a comprehensive study of the analyzed the intermolecular interactions at the studied configurations, a study of the charge density properties is performed. Furthermore, in order to have a deeper knowledge about the nature of the intermolecular interaction between FLU drug molecule and the carbon nanotube, performing such calculations seems to be necessary. Therefore, AIM analysis is carried out on the basis of the distribution of electron densities in order to detect the bond critical points and to determine them according to the values of electron densities (ρ) and their Laplacian ($\nabla^2\rho$). The existence of BCP is the evidence for a transfer or partitioning of electron density between the atoms and consequently forming a chemical bond between them. The ρ and $\nabla^2\rho$ values describe the strength and characteristic of a bond, respectively. Different terms, such as *electron densities*, *Laplacians*, and other characteristics, such as the local kinetic electron density (G_C), the local potential electron energy density (V_C), and the total electron energy density (H_C), for all considered models are calculated and presented in [96]. Furthermore, the molecular graph and contour map of configuration **3** are illustrated, where the positions of all critical points are indicated, as well as the bond paths between attractors.

The character of the interaction could be classified as a function of H_C with Laplacian of electron density at BCP. This means that for strong interaction ($\nabla^2\rho < 0$ and $H_C < 0$), the covalent character is established; for medium strength ($\nabla^2\rho$

> 0 and $H_C < 0$), their partially covalent character is defined; and weak ones ($\nabla^2\rho > 0$ and $H_C > 0$) are mainly electrostatic.

Close inspection of the calculated electron density properties for the desired models shows that intermolecular contacts between the drug molecule and SWCNT have the small value of ρ, $\nabla^2\rho > 0$, and $H_C < 0$, which indicates that the nature of these interactions is partially covalent [96].

Analyzing the topological parameters for the most stable configuration reveals that because of the weak interaction between FLU molecule and the nanotube, the electron density at the BCP of N117–H130 and C68–C69 bonds of this complex did not undergo noticeable changes in comparison to the free drug molecule and the pristine nanotube [96]. These obtained results are in agreement with the obtained geometrical parameters for this complex.

4.5.1.4 Natural Bond Orbital Analyses

One of the important parameters that facilitate the adsorption of an adsorbate on an adsorbent is electron charge transfer. In this study, with a specific focus on the adsorption process, the charge transfer of the nanotube–drug molecule in the equilibrium FLU/SWCNT geometries is evaluated by the natural bond orbital calculations [95]. Also, quantitative assessments of the origin charge transfer between the individual orbitals at the studied configurations are executed by the NBO method, and the results of NBO analysis are tabulated in Table 4.7.

From Table 4.7, it is obvious that the values of the second-order perturbation energy ($E^{(2)}$) for the different configurations are in the range of 0.06–0.92 kcal/mol. It is worth noting that the greater amount of the $E^{(2)}$ is an indication of the strong interaction between FLU and the nanotube and more tendency of the nanotube to provide the electron to the FLU molecule during the adsorption process. Based on the obtained results from NBO analysis, the most important donor–acceptor interaction for configuration ***3*** in the gas phase is $\pi_{C68}–C_{69} \rightarrow \sigma *_{N117–H130}$ interaction. Thus, πC68–C69 acts as a donor, but σ * N117–H130 plays the role of an acceptor in the intermolecular charge transfer interactions by showing the stabilization energy value of 0.75 kcal/mol. Furthermore, the main reliable donor–acceptor interaction in configuration ***3*** in water solution is $\pi_{C53–C54} \rightarrow \sigma *_{C123–H132}$ interaction, with the intermolecular charge transfer value about 0.92 kcal/mol. As a result, the FLU molecule plays the role of an electron acceptor.

A close inspection of the NBO analysis reveals that the interaction between the FLU molecule and SWCNT in configuration ***3*** is stronger than the other complexes due to more total charge transfer energy. In addition, it is found that the greatest stabilization energy for configuration ***3*** is in accordance with the shortest intermolecular interaction (see Tables 4.2 and 4.7).

TABLE 4.7

The Second-Order Perturbation Energy ($E^{(2)}$, kcal/mol) Corresponds to Charge Transfer between SWCNT and FLU Molecule Computed at the B3LYP/6–31G** Level of Theory

	Donor → Acceptor	E(2)
PCM		
Configuration 1	π C70–C85 → σ * C124–H134	0.25
Configuration 2	π C68–C69 → σ * C127–H139	0.22
Configuration 3	π C53–C54 → σ * C123–H132	0.92
Configuration 4	—	—
Configuration 5	π C8–C9 → π * C124–H133	0.06
GAS		
Configuration 1	π C8–C9 → σ * N117–H130	0.57
Configuration 2	π C22–C23 → σ * C125–H137	0.11
Configuration 3	π C68–C69 → σ * N117–H130	0.75
Configuration 4	π C83–C84 → σ * F113–C129	0.06
Configuration 5	π C83–C84 → σ * C124–H133	0.11

4.5.2 Molecular Dynamics Simulation

In this section, the main purpose is obtaining physical insight into the effect of EtOH concentration levels as co-solvent on the interaction of FLU molecules with the SWCNT in aqueous media.

In the first step of analyzing a simulation, it is attempted to determine the equilibrium state of the studied systems by monitoring the quantities, such as the potential energy and root mean square deviation (RMSD) curves. It appears that the potential energies fluctuation curves have flat trajectories, indicating that all simulation systems have reached equilibrium. Moreover, the evolution of the root mean square deviation between FLU molecules and the SWCNT surfaces confirms that the equilibrium state is achieved after 1.5 ns of MD simulations.

In evaluating the structural features of the adsorption systems, the best concept of the adsorption process is obtained by the radial distribution function (RDF) for SWCNT-FLU interactions in the water and water/EtOH solution. The radial distribution function of the FLU drug molecules around nanotube surface vs. distance is studied.

It is found that the intense interaction between the adsorbed molecules and nanotube surface is at a distance of 0.5 nm. Close inspection [96] reveals that the strength of the g(r) profile between the SWCNT and FLU molecule in the presence of EtOH co-solvent at the concentration of 0.5 M is higher than the g(r) magnitude at the mentioned interaction in the other concentrations of EtOH co-solvent. This result approves that there is a strong interaction between SWCNT and FLU molecules in water/EtOH solution at the concentration of 0.5 M. Also, visual inspection of the RDF patterns of the studied systems reveals that the position of the highest peak is unchanged by varying the concentration of the co-solvent. The van der Waals energy calculation between FLU molecule and SWCNT in the water and water/EtOH solution has been investigated [96]. It is worthwhile to note that by the adsorption of FLU molecules on the SWCNT surface, the van der Waals interaction energy decreases; more especially, this decreasing trend becomes intense in the presence of 0.5 M EtOH co-solvent. This result is also an indication of the existence of the more tendency of the FLU molecule for the adsorption on the nanotube surface at the 0.5 M concentration of EtOH, which is in agreement with the RDF results.

The numbers of contacts of the drug molecules with the SWCNT wall within the pure water and mixture (water/

EtOH) solutions have been calculated [96]. It is found that the numbers of contacts for the simulation systems reach an approximately steady state at 14,000 ps. The close inspection of curves [96] shows that there is the maximum number of contacts between FLU molecules and SWCNT at the concentration of 0.5 M EtOH. Also, the study reveals that in all simulation systems, at first, there are a few interactions between SWCNT and FLU molecules; then, by approaching more drug molecule toward the nanotube surface, the van der Waals energy decreases.

The average number of hydrogen bonds per molecules for all systems has been studied. Close inspection of the curves figure shows an enhancement of the number of hydrogen bonds between water and drug molecules as a function of EtOH concentration. Since both drug molecule and SWCNT contain conjugated aromatic rings, therefore, the existence of partial π–π interactions between the drug molecule and the nanotube is expectable.

In general, the results indicate that the more interaction of the FLU drug molecule with the surface of the carbon nanotube at the concentration of 0.5 M EtOH could be attributed to the van der Waals energy, the partial π–π interaction, and the hydrogen bond formation between the studied fragments. Also, the performed simulation results show that drug binding inside the nanotube is impossible.

4.6 DFT Interaction of Flutamide Drug with COOH- and COCl-Functionalized CNTs

A study on the interaction between drugs and DNA represents a great interest in many aspects of today's biochemical research, not only in understanding the mechanism of action of the drug, but also for the design of new drugs. However, the mechanism of interactions between drug molecules and DNA is still relatively little-known. It is necessary to introduce more simple methods for investigating the mechanism of DNA–drug interaction. The understanding of the mechanism of interaction will promote designing of new DNA-targeted drugs.

In recent years, there has been a growing interest in the investigation of interaction between anticancer drugs and DNA-targeted molecules. This research is currently under intense investigation, owing to their therapeutic value as anticancer agents. Cancer, in which cells grow and divide abnormally, is one of the primary diseases with regards to how it responds to drug delivery.

Flutamide (4-nitro-3-trifluoromethylisobutylanilide), a synthetic antiandrogenic compound with therapeutic use in prostatic cancer, has been electrochemically studied to propose a new electroanalytical alternative for its quantitative determination in pharmaceutical forms. Flutamide is used as antineoplastic and antiandrogen drug. It is a powerful nonsteroidal androgen antagonist which is used to treat prostate cancer and is believed to block androgen receptor sites. Photochemistry and phototoxicity studies of flutamide, a phototoxic anticancer drug, have been investigated. The synthesis and biological activity of ferrocenyl derivatives of the non-steroidal antiandrogens flutamide and bicalutamide have been studied as well. Previously, the interaction of the flutamide (FLU) anticancer drug molecule with the four nucleobases, namely, cytosine (C), thymine (T), uracil (U), and guanine (G), has been investigated at different levels of density functional theory [97]. The molecular electrostatic potential (MEP), as a helpful criterion in research of molecular structure with its physiochemical property relationship, is evaluated based on the potentials created in the space around a molecule by its nuclei and electrons. The MEP surfaces of the single pyrimidine bases and drug molecule are shown in Figure 4.17. It is obvious that there is an extensive region of negative electrostatic potential around the oxygen atoms of the bases, whereas the regions around hydrogen atoms in the case of the considered bases have positive electrostatic potential (see Figure 4.17) [97].

On the other hand, as shown by the MEP plot in Figure 4.17, in FLU molecule, the oxygen atoms are negatively charged (red colors), while the hydrogen atoms are positively charged (blue colors). The negative regions of MEP, shown in red, correspond to electrophilic reactivity, and the positive regions, shown in blue, are responsible for nucleophilic reactivity. Therefore, hydrogen bonding in complexes formed between nucleobases and FLU drug is expectable. No significant changes occur in bases and FLU drug structures when we reoptimize them in the water phase.

The DFT results exhibit that interaction of the drug molecule and the nucleobases is favorable, and all the designed complexes are stable.

It is attempted to scrutinize the non-covalent interaction and two mechanisms of covalent between the flutamide anticancer drug (FLU) and functionalized carbon nanotubes (*f*-CNT) employing density functional theory (DFT) calculations regarding their geometries, binding energies, and topological features of the electron density in the water solution. For designed non-covalent interactions, binding energies, natural bond orbital (NBO), atom in molecule (AIM), and quantum molecular descriptor analyses were applied for further understanding of the adsorption process. The computed theoretical results [98] confirmed that binding of the flutamide molecule with functionalized CNT is thermodynamically suitable, and among two considered systems containing COOH-functionalized CNT (NTCOOH) and COCl-functionalized CNT (NTCOCl), NTCOOH revealed more binding energy value, which suggests it as a favorable system in drug delivery within biological and chemical systems (non-covalent). NTCOOH and NTCOCl can bond to the NH group of flutamide through OH (COOH mechanism) and Cl (COCl mechanism) groups, respectively. Finally, in order to obtain the values of activation energies, the activation enthalpies, and the activation of Gibbs free energies of two considered pathways, different calculations were performed, and the results have been compared with each other. Numerical studies for calculating activation parameters related to the COOH mechanism show higher values than those related to the COCl mechanism, and therefore, the COOH mechanism can be suitable for non-covalent functionalization. These results could be generalized to other similar drugs.

Among different types of cancers, one of the frequent cancers in men in most of the countries all over the world is prostate cancer. For curing this type of cancer, flutamide (FLU) is

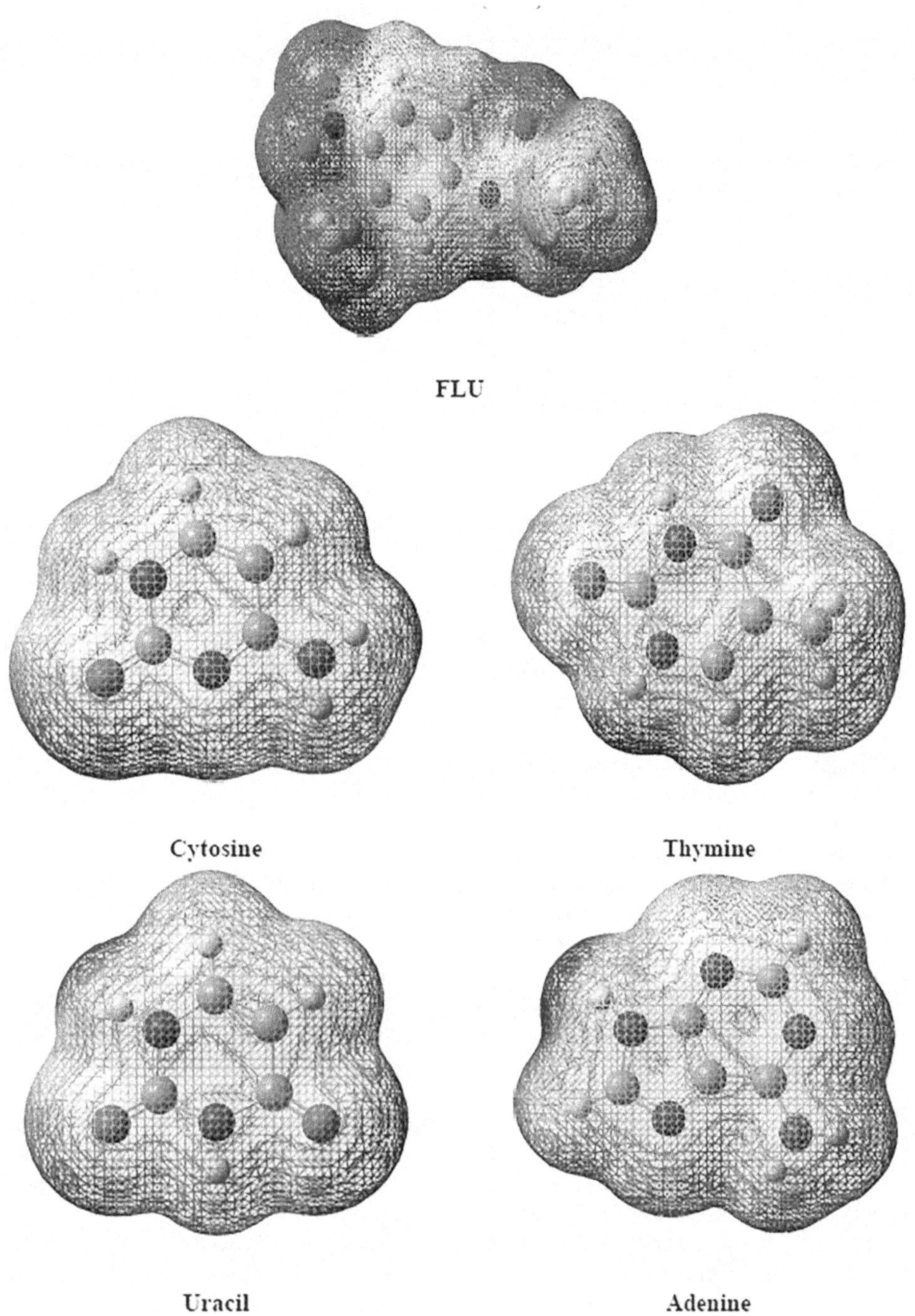

FIGURE 4.17 The molecular electrostatic potential surface of the FLU drug, cytosine, thymine, uracil, and adenine.

already one of the best-nominated antiandrogen drug which is widely applied.

In order to find out the adsorption behavior of the FLU molecule onto the exterior surface of the single-walled carbon nanotube and the mechanism of approaching functionalized flutamide drug to the surface of CNTs, density functional theory (DFT) in the water solution has been applied in this study. For better evaluation, quantum theory of atoms in molecules (QTAIM) and natural bond orbital (NBO) are used. To study the electronic properties, using Koopmans' theorem, quantum descriptors are also calculated. Notwithstanding several computational investigations on CNTs, there are few surveys focusing on the functionalization mechanism.

In this theoretical study [98], the characteristics of flutamide (FLU) molecule via the adsorption process onto the exterior surface of a functionalized armchair (5,5), single-walled carbon nanotubes have been deeply studied in solution phase.

To elucidate the importance of the functionalization of SWCNT on the strength of FLU adsorption, two functional groups of COOH and COCl are applied to modify the SWCNT surface. In order to simply note, the SWCNT with COOH group is shown as "NTCOOH," and the other with COCl group is denoted as "NTCOCl." The optimized molecular structures of FLU, NTCOOH, and NTCOCl in solution phase with their atom labeling have been investigated.

Furthermore, the *f*-CNT/FLU model in which FLU is adsorbed into the surface of the NTCOOH is called the "NTCOOH/FLUR" reactant (R); the other, in which FLU is adsorbed into the surface of the NTCOCl, is called the "NTCOCl/FLUR" reactant. The optimized structures of both *f*-CNT/FLU complexes are studied [98].

All DFT computations are performed using B3LYP functional at 6–31G(d,p) basis set as implemented in the Gaussian 03 program package. The solvent plays a crucial role in chemical systems explicitly or implicitly. Water solution was designed by using the SCRF keyword with Tomasi's polarized continuum (PCM) model.

In order to figure out the orbital interactions and charge delocalization during the course of the hydrogen bond (H-bond) formation between the drug molecule and the adsorbent surfaces [99], the natural bond orbital (NBO) method is done. The Bather quantum theories of atoms in molecules (QTAIM) methodology were carried out by the AIM 2000 program to analyze the electron densities of the considered systems. The molecular orbitals, along with the highest occupied molecular orbital (HOMO) and the lowest unoccupied molecular orbital (LUMO) energies, are examined in order to determine the quantum chemical parameters, such as energy gap (Eg), chemical hardness (η), electronic chemical potential (μ), and global electrophilicity index (ω), according to Koopmans' theorem. Moreover, GaussSum program has been used to obtain the density of states (DOS). The calculations were done on flutamide, COOH (in water), and COCl (in DMF) functionalized armchair (5,5) SWCNT comprising 114 atoms (10 Å) with the ends terminated by hydrogen atoms.

4.6.1 Non-Covalent Interaction

4.6.1.1 *Molecular Geometry and Adsorption Energy*

The obtained results in our last investigation by means of density functional theory calculations confirmed the acceptable drug delivery performance of the (5, 5) single-walled carbon nanotube with FLU molecule in both the gas phase and the water solution. However, screening of the geometries, adsorption energies, and topological features of the SWCNT as one of the potential carrier for flutamide anticancer drug led to this point that some modifications are needed to enhance the activation of the SWCNT surface for efficient adsorption of the FLU molecule. Therefore, this study has been performed to focus on the effect of functionalized carbon nanotube in the solution media.

It is worth noting that the obtained results in the previous study show that the most stable structure can be constructed when the drug molecule approaches the surface of SWCNT from the N–H terminal perpendicularly to the z-axis of the nanotube. Therefore, in the current work, the interaction between FLU molecule and functionalized CNTs through the NH group, which forms a hydrogen bond, has been selected to investigate further.

TABLE 4.8
The Adsorption Energy (ΔE, k/mol), the Stretching Frequencies (Δv, in cm^{-1}), and the Calculated Intermolecular Distances (Å) of the *f*-CNT . . . FLU Complexes in the Water Solution

Model	ΔE	$R_{CNT...FLU}$	Δv
NTCOOH/FLUR	−23.96	O112. . . H134-N121 = 1.99	vN–H: 3621.32 → 3513.24
NTCOCl/FLUR	−7.73	C111-O112. . . H134 = 2.44 N119-H132. . . Cl143 = 2.87	vN–H: 3621.63 → 3595.08

As is obvious, several key parameters of the investigation, such as the binding energy (ΔE), the stretching frequencies (Δv), intermolecular equilibrium distances, and the structural properties consisting of the bond lengths, are represented in Table 4.8.

Also, it is suitable to note that the binding energy discussion is normally an appropriate and useful means to better understand the interaction between different species in considered structures. Furthermore, the binding energies of FLU with NTCOOH (in water) and NTCOCl (in DMF) are defined by the following expression:

$$\Delta E = E_{NTCOOH(NTCOCl)/FLUR} - \left(E_{NTCOOH(NTCOCl)} + E_{FLU}\right) \quad (17)$$

It can be easily figured out that the contribution of the binding energy for the selected systems demonstrates the physical and energetic intrinsic of FLU adsorption on the functionalized nanotubes (NTCOOH and NTCOCl) in water and DMF solvent (see Table 4.8). By comparison of the values of the obtained binding energy for two configurations, it can be concluded that the configuration related to NTCOOH is more stable than that of the NTCOCl configuration.

As can be found out from [98], the drug molecule has the capability of performing an interaction in a vast range of intermolecular conventional (N–H . . . O and NH . . . Cl) and nonconventional (C–H . . . O) hydrogen bonds with the functionalized CNTs.

Considering NTCOOH/FLUR stable configuration, the interaction of H_{134} atom of the FLU drug with the O_{112} atom of the COOH group of the CNT results in the formation of hydrogen bond at the situation of perpendicular FLU molecule existence to the surface of the nanotube, which shows the value of intermolecular O . . . H distance being equal to 1.99 Å in the aqueous media. Furthermore, it can be claimed that in the N–H···O hydrogen bond in this system, FLU drug acts as a proton donor, and the oxygen atom of the carboxylic group of the NTCOOH behaves as a proton acceptor.

Based on our theoretical calculations, the weakest interaction between FLU molecule and the functionalized CNT has appeared in NTCOCl/FLUR reactant, with the O_{112} . . . H_{134} distance being equal to 2.44 Å in the DMF solvent. In this reactant, the hydrogen atom of the drug molecule as Lewis acids interact with oxygen atom of the functionalized group of the nanotube as a Lewis base and lead to C–H···O containing HB complexes.

Moreover, the interaction of the H atom of the adsorbed FLU as proton-accepting center with the Cl atom of the -COCl group of CNT as proton-donating molecule resulted in the N–H···Cl interaction with a distance of 2.87 Å obtained in the NTCOCl/FLUR reactant.

Several studies have been confirmed that the HB distance can play a critical role in the determination of the hydrogen bond strength. A close inspection of Table 4.8 reveals that less intermolecular hydrogen bond length in NTCOOH/FLUR reactant results in a stronger interaction within the NTCOCl/FLUR reactant. Moreover, the conventional hydrogen bond in NTCOOH/FLUR reactant is shorter than the nonconventional HB in NTCOCl/FLUR reactant. Consequently, it can be confirmed that this kind of intermolecular hydrogen bond has more strength than the other HB which exists in the NTCOCl/FLUR structure.

Based on the obtained results, no notable changes on the structural parameters of the adsorbed drug have been detected in the intermolecular interaction between FLU molecule and functionalized nanotubes (see Table 4.4). For instance, within the NTCOOH/FLUR stable structure, the N–H bond length of FLU drug has been changed from 1.01 to 1.02 Å; thus, it can be revealed that f-CNT can act as a structurally stable drug carrier.

In addition, in order to better clarify the hydrogen bond strength, for both reactants depicted in Table 4.8, vibrational frequencies are calculated. It is understood that mainly based on the formation of intermolecular HB between f-CNT and FLU molecule, the N–H stretching mode shifts from 3,621.32 (3,621.63 cm^{-1}) in the FLU drug to the low bands of 3,513.24 (3,595.08 cm^{-1}) in the NTCOOH/FLUR (NTCOCl/FLUR) reactant. Especially, it can be mentioned that the largest shift value of N–H vibrational frequency in NTCOOH/FLUR reactant indicates high interaction ability between FLU molecule and the exterior surface of functionalized nanotube.

4.6.1.2 Electronic Properties

Several definitions can be presented for better expressing the performance of a suitable drug delivery system, but the verified expression is the ability of delivering the drugs into the cells without any significant change in its intrinsic properties during the delivery process. Subsequently, theoretical analysis has been performed in this study to obtain the influence of the FLU molecule adsorption on the behavior of nanotubes.

Thus, first, the frontier orbitals of CNTs and the FLU molecule are calculated to predict the effects of FLU molecule and nanotubes analyzed. The isosurfaces of the frontier orbitals of the FLU molecule, *f*-CNT, and the nanotubes have been investigated, which are interacted with the FLU molecule. It can be elicited that the HOMO and LUMO of the isolated FLU are both distributed mainly over the whole molecule. Considering the NTCOOH/FLUR model, which contains the FLU-attached functionalized CNT, the HOMO are mainly located on the NTCOOH, while the LUMO are mainly distributed on the FLU molecule, indicating *f* CNT is an electron donor species and the FLU molecule is an electron-accepting one in this reactant. This proposes a charge transfer from the HOMO to the LUMO. Furthermore, it is interesting to see that both frontier orbitals are distributed over the surface of the nanotube at the NTCOCl/FLUR reactant of the pristine functionalized nanotubes. The DOS of a system demonstrates the number of states per interval of energy at each level of energy available to be occupied by electrons.

According to reference [98], and comparing the E_g (difference between LUMO and HOMO) values, it can be found that after the adsorption of FLU molecule on NTCOOH and NTCOCl, the HOMO–LUMO energy gap of nanotube has not been changed moderately. Considering the analysis of the DOS plots, it can be revealed that both their valence and conduction levels are altered very slightly by about 0.01 eV, which is negligible, and thus, the DOS plots of FLU-adsorbed functionalized nanotubes are close to that of the pristine nanotubes. As well, it can be suggested that *f*-CNT can carry FLU drug. Furthermore, the density of state (DOS) is plotted for two studied complexes and compared with that of the high interaction ability between FLU molecule and the exterior surface of functionalized nanotube.

In order to have a better understanding of the intrinsic interaction between FLU and *f*-CNT, the chemical reactivity and stability of the considered complexes have been investigated. Three DFT-based chemical descriptors, namely, μ, η, and ω, for FLU (H_2O and DMF), NTCOOH, NTCOCl, NTCOOH/FLUR, and NTCOCl/FLUR are tabulated in Table 4.9.

In these quantities, μ is analyzed as the average of HOMO and LUMO energies. η shows the resistance of one molecule against the change in its electronic structure, and it is calculated as half of the differences between the HOMO and LUMO energies. A decrease in η causes a depletion in the reactivity and an enhancement in stability. The electrophilicity index,

TABLE 4.9

The Values of the Highest Occupied Molecular Orbital Energies (E_{HOMO}), the Lowest Unoccupied Molecular Orbital Energies (E_{LUMO}), Energy Gap (Eg), the Chemical Potential (μ), Chemical Hardness (η), and Electrophilicity Index (ω) (All in eV) for FLU, the Pristine NTCOOH, NTCOCl, and the Studied Complexes in the Water Solution

Model	E_{HOMO}	E_{LUMO}	Eg	μ	η	ω
FLU (H_2O)	−6.81	−2.68	4.13	−4.74	2.06	5.45
FLU (DMF)	−6.81	−2.67	4.14	−4.74	2.07	5.43
NTCOOH	−4.04	−2.74	1.30	−3.39	0.65	8.86
NTCOCl	−4.07	−2.82	1.26	−3.45	0.63	9.45
NTCOOH/FLUR	−4.05	−2.76	1.29	−3.40	0.65	8.96
NTCOCl/FLUR	−4.08	−2.83	1.25	−3.46	0.63	9.55

which is mentioned earlier, can be calculated according to the equation:

$$\omega = \mu^2 / 2\eta \tag{18}$$

The ω is a useful tool in predicting the reactivity of the molecule. It has been found that there is a correlation between the electrophilic index of various chemical compounds and the rate of reaction in the biochemical system. Analyzing the obtained results, η and *Eg* related to the FLU drug are higher than those of NTCOOH/FLUR and NTCOCl/FLUR, an indication of the FLU stability reduction in the presence of COOH (COCl)–functionalized SWCNT and an enhancement in its reactivity. The electronic chemical potential displays the direction of electron flow. As can be seen in Table 10.9, the functionalized SWCNT has the higher chemical potential (μ) compared to FLU, hence the transfer of electrons from the nanotube to drug because electron flows from high chemical potential to low chemical potential. Also, the value of ω for FLU has been increased in the presence of COOH (COCl)–functionalized SWCNT, showing that FLU acts as an electron acceptor. Consequently, for non-covalent interactions, a deep look into COOH– and COCl-functionalized CNTs suggests that applying the COOH-containing complex can be more acceptable based on a stronger interaction between FLU and CNTCOOH.

4.6.1.3 AIM Analysis

In order to have further understanding of the intrinsic intermolecular hydrogen bonds in the considered complexes, the topological characteristics of electron charge density are analyzed by the theory of AIM [100,101]. The molecular graphs are represented, in which the positions of all bond critical points (BCPs) between the drug and the functionalized nanotubes are indicated. The formation of a chemical bond between the pairs of interacting atoms can be interpreted by the existence of BCPs. Moreover, it can be seen that there are CO···HC, CO···HN, and CCl···HN intermolecular interaction in the selected complexes. In both reactants, hydrogen bonds can be detected between the two interacting atoms.

The values of electron density (ρ), Laplacian ($\nabla^2\rho$), kinetic energy density (G), potential energy density (V), and total energy density (H) are given in Table 4.10. The QTAIM theory, and with respect to these parameters, provides information about the bonds at bond critical points. The electronic energy density (H) is the sum of G and V parameters and helps in more accurate descriptions of the nature of the bonds. Positive $\nabla^2\rho$ and H values denote weak interactions (electrostatic), negative $\nabla^2\rho$ and H values refer to strong interaction (covalent bond), and medium-strength ($\nabla^2\rho > 0$ and $H < 0$) is defined as partially covalent. Moreover, the intermolecular interactions have lower ρ and positive $\nabla^2_{\rho BCP}$ (see Table 4.10) with respect to the calculated electron density and Laplacian properties in the considered complexes. These properties are typical for the closed-shell interactions. On the other hand, negative value of ΔEA(B) specifies that the *f*-SWCNT/FLU complex is more stable than the *f*-SWCNT and free drug molecule.

The electron densities at BCP of X···H contact are well correlated with the hydrogen bond energies strength (E_{HB}), which are calculated by the Espinosa method. This method reveals the relationship between HB energy (E_{HB}) and the potential energy density at the bond critical point (V_{BCP}) as $E_{HB} = 1/2\ V_{BCP}$. All E_{HB} energies which are calculated from the potential energy densities of the intermolecular HB contacts are also included in Table 4.10. The strong hydrogen bond is found to be related with maximum electron density at bond critical point and higher stability, which is observed for the conventional $O_{112}\cdots H_{134}–N_{121}$ at the NTCOOH/FLUR reactant.

The reduced density gradient (RDG) analysis can determine more details about the nature of intermolecular interaction between the drug and the carrier molecules. The RDG plot allows us to identify the interacting regions as well as assess the type of interaction. From the color-filled RDG isosurface, different interactions can be identified based on their color. In this plot, the blue region implies strong attractive interactions, such as HB interaction, the green region relates to weaker attractive interaction, and the strong steric effects are represented in red. The RDG plot for complex NTCOOH/FLUR was calculated by Multiwfn program. The intermolecular HB between the drug and the carrier is clearly identified. Moreover, the interaction in the blue region is related to interactive interaction, approving hydrogen bond between H atoms with oxygen atom of the COOH group of nanotube. Another distinctive feature of the RDG plot is a wide red region in positive values of sign (λ2)ρ, which can be related to intramolecular steric effects in NTCOOH.

TABLE 4.10

The Density of the Total Energy of Electrons (H) and Its Two Components, the Kinetic (G) and Potential (V) Electron Energy, the Topological Parameters of Intermolecular Interactions Densities (All in a.u.) between FLU Drug and f-CNT for the Studied Complexes in the Water Solution

Model	f-CNT . . . FLU	ρ	$\nabla^2\rho$	G	V	H	E_{HB}
NTCOOH/FLUR	$O_{112}–H_{134}$	0.02103	0.06804	0.00176	−0.00778	−0.00602	−10.22
	$O_{112}–H_{136}$	0.00730	0.02584	−0.00029	−0.00104	−0.00133	−1.36
NTCOCl/FLUR	$O_{112}–H_{134}$	0.00952	0.02996	−0.00002	−0.00183	−0.00185	−2.40
	$Cl_{143}–H_{132}$	0.00588	0.02067	−0.00031	−0.00067	−0.00098	−0.88
	$Cl_{143}–H_{133}$	0.00463	0.01474	−0.00024	−0.00043	−0.00068	−0.56

4.6.1.4 NBO Analysis

The NBO analysis is a useful tool for applying a better understanding of intra- and intermolecular interactions in addition to preparing a good foundation for finding out the charge transfer (CT) in molecular systems [102,103]. The NBO second-order perturbation stabilization energy ($E^{(2)}$) for all investigated complexes is provided from NBO calculations and included in Table 4.11.

Including data from the NBO, it can be easily found that the oxygen lone pair (LP) of the NTCOOH overlaps with the LP* hydrogen atom of the NH terminal of the FLU drug molecule at the NTCOOH/FLUR reactant. This overlap results in a transfer of electronic charge from the LP O112 to LP* H134 with the second-order perturbation energy ($E^{(2)}$) value of 4.58 kcal/mol. As interparticular viewpoint of interaction, the oxygen atom of the –COOH functional group of the nanotube acts as a proton donor, and the NH terminal of the drug molecule acts as a proton acceptor in the NTCOOH/FLUR reactant.

It is obvious from the obtained data in Table 4.11 that electron is transferred from the NTCOCl to FLU, in which electrons are provided by the interaction of the LP (1) Cl_{143} of the NTCOCl with the LP*(1) H_{132} of the FLU molecule with $E^{(2)}$ energy value of 1.06 kcal/mol. Furthermore, the maximum $E^{(2)}$ value can make the NTCOOH/FLUR reactant more stable than the NTCOCl/FLUR reactant. The NBO analysis data approve that the intermolecular interaction of this reactant is stronger than that of the other reactant, mainly due to more total charge transfer energy. Also, it is found that the greatest stabilization energy for the NTCOOH/FLUR reactant is in accordance with the shortest interaction distance (see Tables 4.8 and 4.11). Results indicate that in both reactants, the charge transfer occurred from nanotube to drug. In order to confirm this result, the fractional number of electron transferred between the FLU molecule and *f*-CNT is evaluated. The FLU molecule acts as an electron acceptor/donor when ΔN has positive/negative value. The positive value of ΔN confirms that the charge is transferred from f-CNT to the FLU drug.

Parameters such as positive energy component ($\Delta E_{B(A)}$), negative energy component ($\Delta E_{A(B)}$), and the stabilization energy ($\Delta E_{SE(AB)}$) are computed to compare the interaction between drug and *f*-SWCNT and ordered. Analyzing the data from the listed parameters in the tables shows that the positive value of $\Delta E_{B(A)}$ means that the process is favorable from the energetic viewpoint, while a negative value of $\Delta E_{A(B)}$ specifies that the *f*-SWCNT/FLU complex is more stable than the *f*-SWCNT and free drug molecule. Moreover, $\Delta E_{SE(AB)}$ is negative, meaning, that the studied complexes are stable.

TABLE 4.11

The Electron Donors, Electron Acceptors, and the Corresponding Second-Order Perturbation Energy ($E^{(2)}$, kcal/mol) in the Water Solution

Model	Donor	Acceptor	E (2)
NTCOOH/FLUR	LP (1) O_{112}	LP* (1) H_{134}	4.58
NTCOCl/FLUR	LP (1) Cl_{143}	LP* (1) H_{132}	1.06

4.6.2 The Covalent Functionalization Mechanisms

For the covalent functionalization, NH group attacks the carbon atom of COOH or COCl to transfer its protons to the OH (Cl) group. We studied these two possible mechanisms for NTCOOH(Cl)/FLUR. The mechanism for the formation of covalent bond between FLU and NTCOOH (COOH mechanism), where k1 is rate-constant and K_1 and $^{K}{}_1$' are equilibrium constants, has been studied. In this mechanism, NTCOOH/FLUR is converted into the product NTCON by losing H_2O.

According to the study, in COOH mechanism, OH from NTCOOH is substituted by N from FLU to give product NTCON. The optimized structure of the product NTCON/H_2OP has been investigated.

Using reactant NTCOOH/FLUR and product NTCON/H_2OP, the transition state of k1 step was optimized, which we call TSk1. The optimized structures of TS_{k1}, TS_{k2}, and the N–H and C–O bond lengths increase (decrease) from 1.01 Å and 1.33 Å (3.61 Å and 3.05 Å) for NTCOOH/FLUR (NTCON/H_2OP) to 1.62 Å and 1.84Å for TS_{k1}, respectively, which have been investigated.

The relative energies for optimized structures in all pathways have been calculated in Table 4.12 by considering the electronic plus zero point energy (E), enthalpy (H), and Gibbs free energy (G) of reactants (NTCOOH + FLU) equal to zero.

The activation energy (Ea), activation enthalpy (ΔH‡), and activation Gibbs free energy (ΔG‡) for k1 step are 206.62 k mol^{-1}, 204.24 k mol^{-1}, and 217.47 k mol^{-1}, respectively. The total rate constant for overall reaction (COOH pathway) is equal to k1 × K1, so the total activation energy, the total activation enthalpy, and the total activation Gibbs free energy can be calculated by the following equations:

$$\left(\text{Ea} = \text{Ea}(\text{k1 step}) + \Delta\text{E}(\text{K1 step})\right) \quad (19)$$

$$\left(\Delta\text{H}\ddagger = \Delta\text{H}\ddagger(\text{k1 step}) + \Delta\text{H}(\text{K1 step})\right) \quad (20)$$

$$\left(\Delta\text{G}\ddagger = \text{"}\,\text{G}\ddagger(\text{k1 step}) + \Delta\text{G}(\text{K1 step})\right) \quad (21)$$

The mentioned parameters for COOH mechanism are 184.31 k mol^{-1}, 187.93k mol^{-1}, and 236.58 k mol^{-1}, respectively (Table 4.12). The other reaction for the covalent functionalization of FLU onto COCl-functionalized carbon nanotube has been studied (COCl mechanism).

In this reactions, NTCOOH was firstly converted into alkyl chloride using $SOCl_2$ (NTCOCl) in DMF. FLU then reacts with NTCOCl to form a covalent bond. COCl mechanism begins with the attack of NH of FLU to Cl in the NTCOCl to form products NTCON/HClP.

Using NTCOCl/FLUR and NTCON/HClP, a transition state is optimized, which we call TS_{k2}.

The C–Cl and N–H bond lengths increase (decrease) from 1.84 Å and 1.01 Å (3.99 Å and 3.26 Å) for NTCOCl/FLUR (NTCON/HClP) to 3.77 Å and 2.90 Å for TS_{k2}, respectively. Ea, ΔH‡, and ΔG‡ for k_2 step are 62.32 k mol^{-1}, 59.20 k mol^{-1}, and 80.17 k mol^{-1}, respectively. The total activation energy, the

TABLE 4.12

Relative Energies (k/mol) for Different Species in COOH and COCl Mechanisms

Species	E	H	G
In water		COOH mechanism	
NTCOOH + FLU	0	0	0
NTCOOH/FLUR	−23.96	−16.31	19.13
TS_{k1}	184.31	187.93	236.58
NTCON/H_2OP	106.06	113.67	157.03
In DMF		COCl mechanism	
NTCOCl + FLU	0	0	0
NTCOCl/FLUR	−6.1	0.33	28.59
TS_{k2}	56.22	59.53	108.74
NTCON/HClP	23.14	28.4	71.24

Note: *E*, *H*, and *G* are electronic plus zero-point energy, enthalpy, and Gibbs free energy, respectively.

total activation enthalpy, and the total activation Gibbs free energy for COCl mechanism are 56.22 k mol^{-1}, 59.53 k mol^{-1}, and 108.74 k mol^{-1}, respectively (Table 4.12).

The total activation energy, the total activation enthalpy, and the total activation Gibbs free energy for COCl mechanism are lower than those of COOH mechanism by 128.09 k mol^{-1}, 128.38 k mol^{-1}, and 127.84 k mol^{-1}, respectively.

Both mechanisms (COOH and COCl) are nucleophilic substitution reactions. Generally, these reactions proceed through a tetrahedral intermediate. A tetrahedral intermediate has been designed as input, and ultimately, a structure was optimized which is similar to the reactant NTCOCl/FLUR. This means that tetrahedral intermediate could not exist, probably due to the electronic and steric effects of carbon nanotubes.

4.7 Molecular Dynamics Simulation Study of the Functionalized CNTs to Enhance the Efficacy of the Anticancer Drug Paclitaxel

In the present section, the adsorption mechanism of the PTX anticancer drug on pristine and functionalized CNTs has been investigated and compared. Functionalization of the CNT was done using carboxylic (-COOH), CH_2NH_2 (-AMINE), and -PEG groups. PEG is a biocompatible polymer which can be conjugated with CNTs and has attractive advantages, such as extension blood circulation time of CNTs, by reducing the amount of their uptake by the reticuloendothelial system (RES); it also enhances the dispersion and biocompatibility of CNTs. Furthermore, the adsorbed orientation of the PTX molecule on the sidewalls of CNT has been examined. Finally, comprehensive investigations have been done on the role of functional groups on the solubility of CNTs in aqueous solutions. The evaluation of the effect of several functional groups on the DDS performance and the PTX solubility distinguishes our study from other investigations.

4.7.1 Structures

An armchair (12, 12) SWNT with a diameter of 1.61 nm and a length of 4 nm was selected as the model carrier. CNT was first generated from the Nanotube Modeler package and then functionalized with -COOH, -PEG (contains 12 monomer), and -AMINE groups in four sites at two entrances of CNT (Figure 4.18 shows the structure of pristine CNT and *f*-CNTs from the front and side view).

The geometry of the PTX molecule has been optimized at the B3LYP/6–31G* level of theory, as implemented in GAMESS package, and partial charges on each atom have been obtained from these DFT calculations. The chemical structure of the PTX molecule is shown in Figure 4.19.

In all investigated systems (pristine CNT and *f*-CNTs), the PTX molecules were located around the outer surface of the CNT and separated sufficiently far away (>3 nm) to eliminate the effect of starting orientations.

4.7.2 Simulation

Molecular dynamics simulation was performed using the GROMACS 4.5.5 MD simulation package. Body temperature is 310 K, and for this reason, MD simulation was performed at this temperature. Temperature was maintained by applying the V-rescale thermostat, and pressure was kept constant at 1 bar using the Berendsen algorithm. The equations of motion were solved using the leapfrog algorithm under periodic boundary conditions, and the simulation was carried out for the total time of 150 ns.

For all systems, the dimensions of the simulation box were set as 7 nm × 7 nm × 13 nm. LINCS algorithm was used to constrain all bonds in all the systems. The particle-mesh Ewald (PME) method was used to treat long-range electrostatic interactions, while electrostatic interactions between charged groups Lenard–Jones (L-J) interactions were calculated with a 1.4 nm range cutoff. Grid algorithm was used to search neighbors. The visual molecular dynamics (VMD) program has been used for molecular visualization. The initial and final structures of investigated systems with 5 PTX molecules have been studied from top and side view.

4.7.3 Mechanism of Adsorption

The equilibrium state and the stability of the structure during MD simulations can be evaluated by several quantities, such as the potential and total energy, root mean square deviation (RMSD), the pressure of the systems, etc. RMSD for pristine CNT and f-CNTs and total energy curves, respectively, have been studied for all the investigated systems. The results indicate that all the systems reached equilibrium state after 1 *ns*.

4.7.4 Radial Distribution Function (RDF)

For all systems, the first 10 ns of simulations were calculated to analyze the characteristics of interactions. The RDF represents the probability of finding atom *i* at a spherical shell of

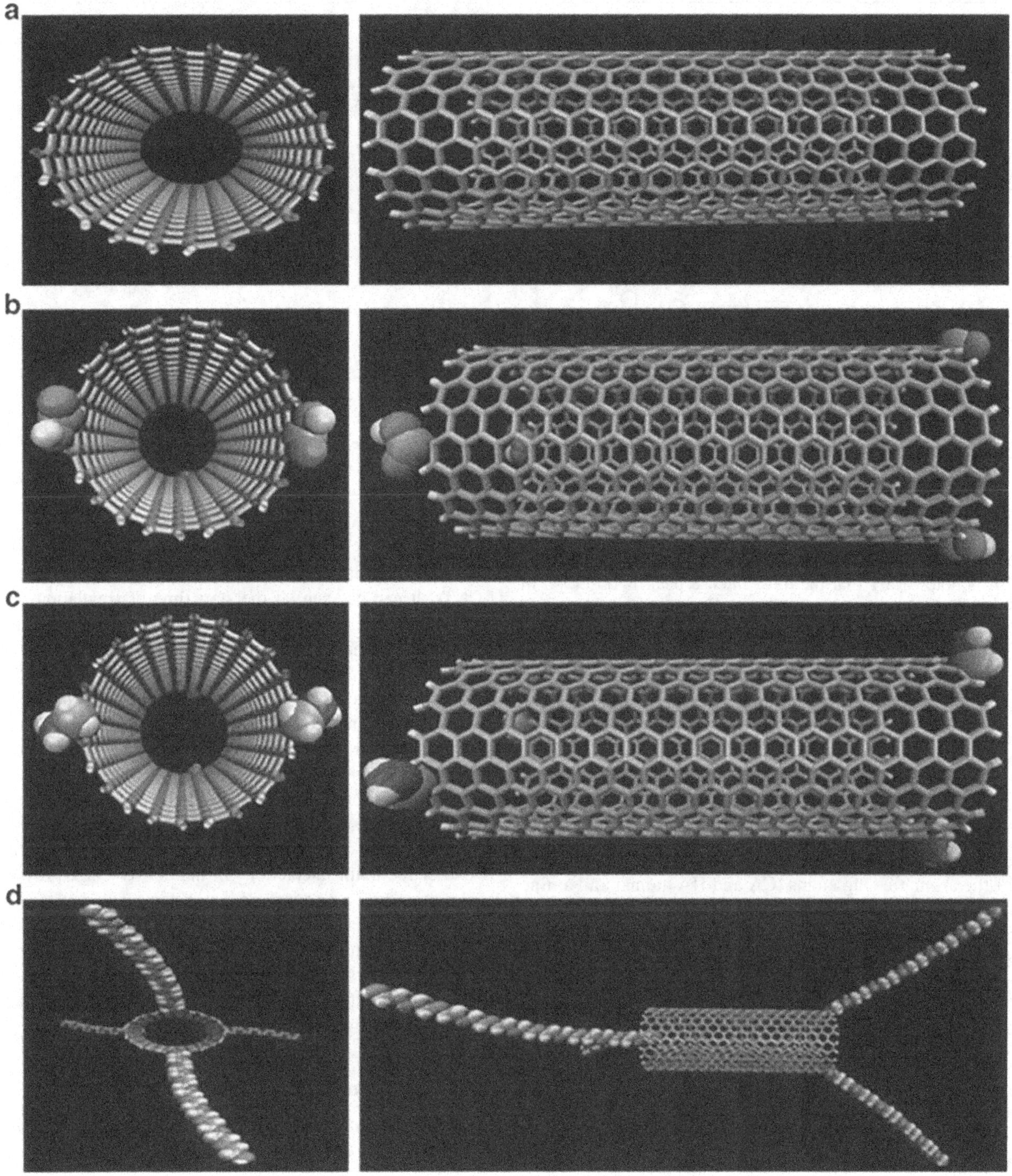

FIGURE 4.18 Schematic structure of the pristine CNT and *f*-CNTs from the front and side view: (a) pristine CNT, (b) COOH-CNT, (c) AMINE-CNT, (d) PEGCNT.

a certain distance (r) from atom j. A sharp peak in the RDF plots is attributed to the interaction between two groups. The RDF for PTX molecules around the surface of CNTs was calculated. According to the obtained results, the main amounts of interactions between PTX molecules and CNTs exist at a distance of approximately 0.5–2.2 nm, and the maximum interactions occur at 0.92 and 2.08 nm. Based on previous works, these peaks can be related to the formation of the π–π stacking interactions between aromatic rings of PTX molecules and sidewalls of CNTs. Also, the polar interactions, such as partial π–π interactions and hydrogen bonds (HBs), which can be formed between the functional groups of CNTs

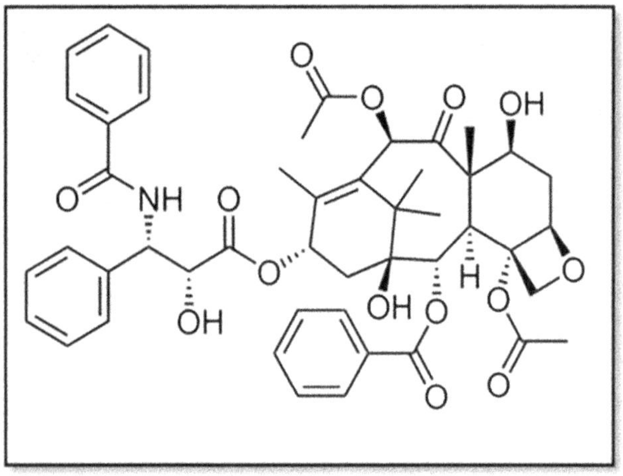

FIGURE 4.19 Paclitaxel (PTX) structure.

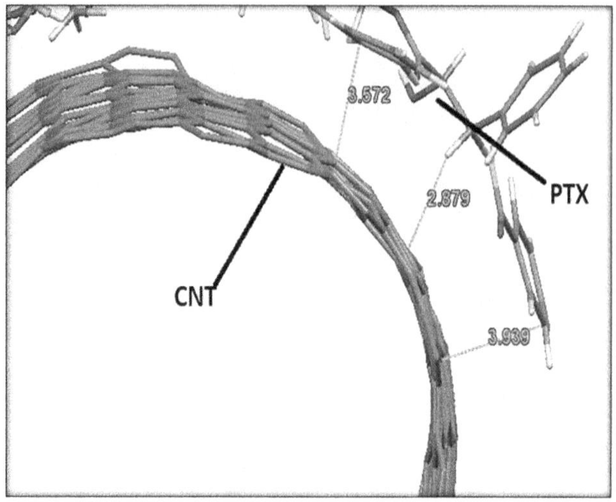

FIGURE 4.20 The π–π stacking interactions between PEG-CNT and PTX.

and the heteroatoms of PTX, are the other reasons for this observation.

It is noteworthy that the most intense peak is observed in the PEG-CNT system, which shows that this system has more interaction with PTX than the other systems. The RDF of water molecules around the surface of CNTs has been calculated. It is obvious that the lowest intensity peak is related to the PEG-CNT system. The result confirms that increasing the interaction of CNT and drug leads to the repulsion of water molecules from the CNT.

To understand the molecular orientation of PTX adsorbed on CNTs, we calculated the atomic RDF of drug molecules. The calculated atomic RDF for the drug molecules are given in Figure 4.26a. It is observed that the sharp peaks for the aromatic ring atoms (CA and HA atoms) and amine groups (N and HN atoms) are located at 0.50 and 0.70 nm, while the wide peaks for other atoms (CR, CO, OC, HO, and HC) are located between 0.80 and 1.10 nm. These results show that the PTX molecules with their aromatic rings are adsorbed on sidewalls of CNT, which emphasizes that the π–π stacking between the PTX and the CNT surface plays a major role in drug adsorption. Furthermore, it is interesting to note that the oxygen atoms of the drugs are oriented away from the CNTs and toward the aqueous phase to enhance the solubility of DDS in water solution. According to these results, the suggested schematic model for the orientation of adsorption of PTX molecule on PEG-CNT is shown in Figure 4.20.

To study the geometry of π–π stacking interactions, the distance between the CNT surface and the aromatic rings of PTX has been calculated. The schematic view of the distance between CNT and PTX is provided in Figure 4.20.

There are two types of π stacking interactions between aryl groups of PTX and CNT surface, T-shaped and parallel π–π stacking interactions with 2.87 Å and 3.57–3.93 Å from the CNT sidewall, respectively. In parallel orientation, the aromatic rings of PTX have an almost coplanar structure (torsional angle 6°).

4.7.5 The van der Waals Energy

It has been calculated between the PTX and pristine CNT and *f*-CNTs. It can be seen, at the start time of simulation, that there is little van der Waals attraction between PTX molecules and CNTs, but the van der Waals energy decreased when the PTX molecules approached the CNT surface. This finding confirms that the drug molecules can be adsorbed spontaneously on the surface of CNT in aqueous solutions. It also shows some representative conformations in the first 15 ns simulation of trajectories. These conformations clearly indicate that the absorption of the drug leads to a decrease in van der Waals energy.

Mousavi et al. mentioned that the van der Waals interaction is one of the main interactions in the delivery of PTX molecules. As a result, we conclude that systems with the lower LJ value have higher efficiency in drug delivery cellular uptake. It has been illustrated that the van der Waals interactions in the PEG-CNT system are stronger than in the other systems. It indicates that in this system, the PTX molecules interact more favorably with stronger affinity.

4.7.6 The Number of Atomic Contacts

The number of atomic contacts between the PTX molecules and the pristine CNT and f-CNTs was calculated by using:

$$N_c(t)=\sum_{i=1}^{N_{CNT}}\sum_{j=1}^{N_{PTX}}\int_{r_1}^{r_1+0.6nm}\delta\big(r(t)-r_j(t)\big)dr \qquad (22)$$

Here, N_{CNT} and N_{PTX} are the total number of CNT and PTX atoms, respectively, and r_j is the distance of jth atom of PTX from the ith atom of the CNT. The δ function ensures counting of all drug atoms within 0.6 nm from CNT atoms. The number of atomic contacts between the PTX molecules and the pristine CNT and *f*-CNTs has been studied. This study shows that by adsorption of drug, the number of contacts in all systems significantly increased, and at the end of the simulation, the number of these contacts for PEG-CNT, AMINE-CNT,

COOH-CNT, and pristine CNT are 7,900, 5,000, 4,900, and 4,300, respectively. These values show that the numbers of contacts with drug molecules in *f*-CNT systems are more than in pristine CNT, which suggest that the functional groups play an important role in drug adsorption.

There is a significant correlation between the number of contact values and other obtained results that have a good agreement with the results previously and vividly show that the PEG group can greatly enhance the efficiency of CNT in PTX delivery.

Furthermore, it should be mentioned that some adsorbed drug molecules can be desorbed from the CNT surface and then re-adsorbed to CNT later to take proper orientation. For this reason, the number of contact curves fluctuates in the first 5 ns of simulation and then stabilizes.

To further clarify the effect of functional groups on drug adsorption, we calculate the RDF and the number of HBs between functional groups and PTX. The RDF of PTX around the functional groups shows that the intensity of the interactions between this group and the drug molecules is markedly raised for the PEG group.

The numbers of HBs between PTX molecules and functional groups have been investigated. As expected, the HBs between the PEG group and PTX molecules are more than in COOH and AMINE groups. According to the theoretical and experimental evidence, these HBs can enhance the capacity of adsorbance and increase the stability of the drug.

4.7.7 Solubility

The main purpose of functionalization of CNTs is to improve the dispersion of CNTs in aqueous solutions. In the present work, CNT was functionalized by using three functional groups in four centers in the same sites at the end of the CNT (all *f*-CNT shown in Figure 4.18). These groups were selected because they represent a high water solubility and good biocompatibility. Different parameters, including the number of HBs between *f*-CNT and water molecules, solvation free energy, solvent-accessible surface area (SASA), and number of water molecules within 3.5 Å regions from the surface of CNT, have been calculated in order to evaluate the effect of functional groups on the solubility of CNTs.

HB undoubtedly is one of the most vital and interesting interactions that frequently occur in nature which can affect many biochemical processes. Hydrogen bonding leads to considerable change in the properties of liquids, solids, or large clusters. Since HB is a very important phenomenon in nature, there are many studies for understanding the nature of HBs. The solubility of organic structures can usually be controlled by forming intermolecular hydrogen bonds between water molecules and their functional groups. In our investigated systems, intermolecular HBs can be formed between heteroatoms of f-CNTs and water molecules, an overview of the intermolecular hydrogen bonding that occurs between PEG functional groups and solvent molecules. As can be seen, the PEG group in HB can act as both an acceptor and a donor so that its oxygen atoms act as acceptor and the terminal hydroxyl groups act as donor.

The number of HBs between the water molecules and the f-CNT was calculated. Comparison with fCNTs indicates that the number of HBs in the PEG-CNT system is greater than in COOH-CNT and AMINE-CNT. These results show that the PEG groups not only increase the adsorption capacity but also enhance drug solubility in the aqueous solution.

One of the most important developments in computational chemistry is solvation free energy calculations of molecules accurately using thermodynamic perturbation. Solvation free energy, ΔG_{sol}, for CNT and *f*-CNT was calculated and is represented in Table 4.13. Among the four systems, the highest solvation free energy was found in the PEG-CNT system due to greater HB formation between PEG and water molecules.

The SASA is the surface area of compounds, which is accessible to contact with solvent molecules. According to the first algorithm proposed by Lee and Richards, SASA of an atom is the area on the surface of a sphere of radius *R*, on each point of which the center of a solvent molecule can be placed in contact with this atom without penetrating any other atom of the molecule. The radius *R* is given by the sum of the van der Waals radius of the atom and the chosen radius of the solvent molecule. An approximation of this area is computed by this program using the formula:

$$SASA = \sum \left[\frac{R}{\sqrt{R^2 - Z_i^2}} \right] L_i \cdot D \tag{23}$$

$$D = \Delta Z / 2 + \Delta' Z \tag{24}$$

where L_i is the length of the arc drawn on a given section i, Z_i is the perpendicular distance from the center of the sphere to the section i, ΔZ is the spacing between the sections, and $\Delta' Z$ is $\Delta Z/2$ or $R - Z_i$, whichever is smaller. Summation is over all the arcs drawn for the given atom.

The hydrophobic SASA for all the investigated systems. Average values of the hydrophobic SASA for CNT, COOH-CNT, AMINE-CNT, and PEG-CNT are 59.45, 53.32, 51.99, and 62.92 nm^2, respectively. The higher values for the PEG-CNT, in comparison to the other CNTs, confirm that the PEG-CNT system has more surface area, which is available to interact with water molecules.

Furthermore, the study of hydrophobic SASA for pristine CNT and f-CNTs. The hydrophobic SASA for all systems is decreased by increasing the time. The reason for this decline can be related to the formation of π–π interactions between

TABLE 4.13

Computed Solvation Free Energies

Name	Free Energy (kJ mol−1)
CNT	−1,829.63
PEG-CNT	−2,159.35
COOH-CNT	−1,907.84
AMINE-CNT	−1,911.06

the hydrophobic surface of CNT and the aromatic rings of the drug molecules.

Finally, the number of water molecules within the CNTs for pristine CNT and f-CNTs as a function of time of simulation of water molecules within 3.5 Å of CNTs for all systems as a function of time is investigated. Water molecules form a hydration shell around CNT surfaces, which can be affected by the adsorption of drug on the sidewalls of CNTs. This means that the drug drives away the water molecules from the CNT surface, leading to the formation of strong π–π interactions. For this reason, the number of water molecules was decreased in all the investigated systems. Also, this figure shows that the number of water molecules in the PEG–CNT system is almost more than in the other systems. This result indicates that this system was more soluble in water solution.

The obtained results from the number of HBs, free energy, SASA, and water molecules are in agreement and show that functionalization of CNT increases its solubility. Also, these parameters confirm that the PEG–CNT system has the highest solubility.

4.8 Computational Simulation Study of CNT as a Carrier in Drug Delivery System for Carnosine Dipeptide

CNTs in the role of drug deliverer can be utilized to inactivate the drug until attaining the target. They must be able to transport drugs while remaining soluble in a biological system.

The biological application of carbon nanotube in drug delivery is our main concern in this section. For this purpose, the interaction of carnosine and carbon nanotube has been investigated in both gas phase and separately in aqueous media. Three possible interactions of carnosine dipeptide with (5,5) carbon nanotube in physiological media were considered. At first step, each species was modeled using quantum mechanical calculations; in the next step, their properties in aqueous solution were studied by applying Monte Carlo simulations. The results of density functional calculations in gas phase showed that interaction of zwitterion of carnosine with carbon nanotube via NH_3^+ had relatively higher interaction energy than the other complexes. Computation of solvation-free energies in water showed that functionalization with carnosine enhanced the solubility of carbon nanotube significantly, which improved the medicinal applications of these materials. The calculation of complexation-free energies indicated that zwitterion of carnosine with carbon nanotube via NH_3^+ produced the most stable complex in aqueous solution. This tendency could be observed in gas and liquid phases similarly.

Carnosine (β-alanine-L-histidine), known as an enigmatic dipeptide, is an effective anti-ageing compound. The formation of carbonyl groups in proteins due to oxidation and reduction induces cellular ageing. Protein carbonyl groups result from oxidation, glycation, and reaction with malondialdehyde, methylglyoxal, and finally, glycolytic intermediates.

During glycation (which happens simultaneously with ageing), some molecules attach to proteins. These unusual proteins might build up, forming agents that could react with free radicals to degenerate diseases associated with ageing. It has been found that carnosine possesses considerable antiglycating properties, and also a strong antioxidant property. Carnosine characters cause it to encompass several clinical applications. To mention some: antitumor actions and delayed ability to obtain ATP of cancer cells. Carnosine has been utilized by several kids with "attention deficit hyperactivity disorder" (ADHD), education problems, and autism. Another application of carnosine is in age-related skin creams. Creams including it have been used as a cosmetic to avoid or treat wrinkle-forming mechanism. The other properties of carnosine are membrane receptor alleviation and anti-apoptotic actions. Therefore, it has significant neuroprotective actions. Carnosine protects the action of neurons during stroke models.

Carnosine displays neuron protection, especially in Alzheimer's dementia. It protects against neuronal cell loss via a weakening of the oxidation process.

The existence of an enzyme with the ability to hydrolyze the peptide bond in carnosine has been demonstrated. They named the enzyme carnosinase (or β-Ala-His dipeptidase) and classified it as metalloproteases. Two isoforms of carnosinase have been characterized, a cytosolic form (named tissue carnosinase and strongly inhibited by Bestatin) and serum carnosinase (characterized by its distribution in the plasma and brain). Usually, carnosinase acts rapidly, with the serum levels of carnosine dwindling, thus reducing its clinical efficiency. Joining carnosine to a transporter can shield it against carnosinase degradation.

The development of new and efficient drug delivery systems has an impact on improving pharmacological science. One of those substances consists of a carbon nanotube (CNT), which has appeared as an efficient choice for carrying molecules. CNTs have recently become promising materials in various biological applications, such as drug delivery, tumor therapy, and biosensors. Two limitations of CNT usage in biological systems are their low solubility and toxicity. However, there are a number of conflicting reports about the toxicity of CNTs. Several groups of investigations have reported toxic effects, while others demonstrate very low or insignificant cellular responses. This contradiction is related to the usage of varying types of CNTs, different preparation and purification procedures, evaluation methods, and even different exposure conditions. Many factors, such as impurities and chemical and structural characteristics (surface modification, shape, length, agglomeration, or layer numbers), can affect CNT toxicity.

The surrounding environment is another important factor for evaluating CNT toxicity. As a consequence of low solubility, CNTs usually deposit on the cell surface without proper dispersion in the biological systems and generate some health concerns. Moreover, CNTs tend to aggregate due to their insolubility, and therefore, such toxicological responses are not surprising.

In fact, the solubility of CNTs in aqueous solutions is a precondition for biocompatibility, so CNT derivatives in therapeutic delivery should meet this basic prerequisite. Furthermore, CNT dispersions should be uniform and stable to attain accurate concentration information.

The hydrophobic character of CNTs, together with the strong interactions between the individual tubes causing

CNT assemblies, reduces their solubility. Solubility under physiological conditions is an important problem to work, in a compatible biological medium. Therefore, in the first step, applicability of CNTs as a drug delivery system is related to their solubility and wet ability in aqueous environments. Non-functionalized CNTs are poorly soluble in water.

Surface functionalization increases the solubility of nanotubes. A theoretical study of functionalization effects on the solubility of nanotubes has shown modifications in their properties due to the functionalization with some organic molecules. Among various species, functionalization of nanotubes with nucleic acids and proteins improves solubility in aqueous solution, hence alleviates the application of nanotubes in biotechnology and biomedicine. Theoretical studies on functionalized NTs with DNA bases indicate the augmentation of solubility of nanotubes in water.

CNT can be functionalized with peptides, proteins, drugs and exploited as a drug delivery system. Since functionalized CNTs display low toxicity and are not immunogenic, such systems have a great potential in the field of nanomedicine.

It was shown that CNTs can be used as templates to transport bioactive peptides to immune system. Functionalization of CNT with natural biomolecules has been made to improve nanotube solubility, and a significant reduction on toxicity and biocompatibility. Functionalization changes the CNT structure to attainable component of therapeutic agent appropriate for clinical use. Immunization studies using the CNT peptide in mice reveal that no antibodies are produced against functionalized CNT. This issue suggests that carbon nanotubes would not possess essential immunogenicity, and CNT peptide can be considered a biocompatible system.

The immunogenic structures of peptide–CNT are stable. Additional studies have shown that phenylalanine has an important role in the enhancement of the adsorption of the peptides on the CNTs. Peptide function has opened a new scope in the discussion of biological properties of CNTs. In fact, CNTs can be functionalized with peptides to transport them into different types of cells. Moreover, the interaction of peptide drugs with CNTs as a drug deliverer can enhance the solubility and biocompatibility of CNTs. In fact, functionalization of CNTs by these drugs can achieve both two aims. Therefore, an investigation of the interaction of carnosine dipeptide as a drug with CNT and the stability and solubility of the compounds were the aim of this study. Solvation free energies of complexes of CNT with carnosine dipeptide were studied in order to evaluate the effect of binding of dipeptide with CNT on solvation.

Solvation free energy is the free energy difference when a molecule is transferred from gas phase to solvent. The solvation energies of nanotubes are unattainable experimentally due to problems of low volatility. Therefore, the application of computational methods may be the best approach to achieve the solvation behavior of these nanomaterials. These methods have extensive applicability in studies of absolute solvation free energies and binding free energies. The importance of computational method is not only to reproduce experimental results but also to gain insight of probability of the interactions. Moreover, the important usage of theoretical methods is in cases where experiments cannot be performed.

Despite biological interest, there is not enough detailed theoretical study of interactions of CNTs with proteins and peptides.

In this section, the interaction of CNT and carnosine dipeptide in gas phase and aqueous solution has been investigated. Quantum mechanical calculations were used to estimate the interaction energies in gas phase, which is followed by Monte Carlo simulation of the structures in aqueous media in the following section. Biocompatibility of functionalized CNTs was then determined. The applicability of CNTs as drug delivery systems is related to their solubility and wet ability in aqueous environments. Therefore, it is vital to verify the solvation of CNT in physiological media after functionalization with carnosine. Perturbation methods were used to compute solvation free energies and evaluate the solubility of the complexes. To mention more, complexation free energies of carnosine–CNT complexes were computed to evaluate the stability of the structures.

The main purpose of this research section covered interactions of carnosine (drug) and CNT in aqueous media, followed by studies to monitor binding energies and solubility of related structures. The research included two divisions: (a) quantum mechanics (QM) and (b) Monte Carlo (MC) simulation. In the QM part, following optimization of isolated molecules, binding energies and stability of the structures were studied by quantum mechanical calculations. In the next step, MC simulation was applied for dilute solutions of nanotubes in water. Solvation free energies and complexation free energies of related structure were computed in this section.

4.8.1 Quantum Mechanics Part

All structural optimization were performed using GAMESS-US quantum chemistry package. For functionalized CNT, all the possible interactions of carnosine with CNT were considered. Carnosine dipeptide structure consists of β-alanine and L-histidine.

Among the possible isomers of the protonated and non-protonated forms of carnosine, zwitterion and its non-protonated form (containing NH_2 group instead of NH_3^+) were considered. Isoelectric pH of carnosine is 6.9, and the ideality of this compound as a buffer at physiological pH is underlined. It has the zwitterion form in isoelectric pH and, above this pH, has the non-protonated form. So we considered the interaction of these two structures with CNT. Three possible interactions with CNT have been studied: interactions via NH_3^+ and COO^- of zwitterion forms of carnosine and interaction via NH_2 group of non-protonated carnosine.

The optimized structures are proposed in Figure 4.21.

Natural bond orbital (NBO) theory was examined for optimized geometries in order to determine natural atomic charges. In the following calculations, quantum mechanical charges have been used.

The interaction of all possible sites of carnosine with (5, 5) armchair CNT has been studied. A carnosine dipeptide structure consists of β-alanine and L-histidine. It is known that the interactions of peptides and surfaces involve many types of covalent and non-covalent forces, including electrostatic,

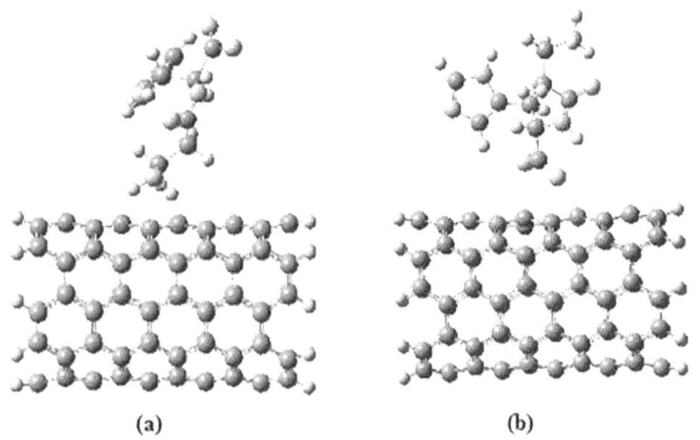

FIGURE 4.21 Interaction of carnosine with CNT: (a) via NH_3^+ of zwitterion, (b) via COO of zwitterion.

hydrogen bonding, hydrophobic, or entropic in nature. It has been shown that peptide binding to ester-functionalized SWNTs occurs via π–π interaction, and the ester group reacts with amine groups of peptides to form covalent amide linkages. However, certain proteins are found to bind to SWNTs even without sidewall functionalization, and their interactions were not similar. Interface of alanine and histidine (two amino acids that participate in carnosine dipeptide) with CNT was exercised, and the possible interactions were examined. The results indicated that π–π interaction via aromatic ring of histidine is impossible, and Alanine produces NH_3 interaction with CNT. It was found that the binding of β-alanine with CNT is stronger than histidine.

The carboxylate group of alanine and the amine group of histidine take part in the peptide bonding in carnosine dipeptide. Therefore, the amine group of alanine and the carboxylate group of histidine were free for the interactions with CNT. Orientations and positions were specifically chosen so that the amine group of alanine (Figure 4.21a) and the carboxylate group of histidine (Figure 4.21b) approach directly on top of CNT atoms.

The binding energies (E_b) were revealed as the energy variation of the energy summation of two individually optimized monomers and optimized complexes.

Their energetic properties (outcomes of two methods, B3LYP and wB97XD) were shown in Sepideh and Leila (2017). As mentioned before, zwitterion of carnosine with the NH_3^+ and COO^- groups and also that of non-protonated carnosine with NH_2 group were considered for the interaction with CNT. As illustrated, B3LYP binding energies of the interaction of NH_3^+ and COO^- groups with CNT were −1.6863 eV and −1.4208 eV, respectively. The same overall trend for wB97XD method has been observed. So the NH_3^+ group was preferred for interaction of zwitterion of carnosine with CNT. Interaction of non-protonated carnosine via NH_2 and CNT with binding energy of −0.0068 eV was very weak compared to NH_3^+ group of zwitterion. So it was predicted that the interaction of carnosine with CNT occurred via the NH_3^+ group of zwitterion rather than other possible sites and forms. The charged nature of amine and carboxylate groups promoted the adsorption of the peptide onto CNT. This result was previously attained about the adsorption of glycine amino acid onto CNT. Roman and his colleagues conclusively established that glycine zwitterions interact stronger onto the CNTs in comparison with their non-ionic species. They demonstrated that glycine bind CNT by its deprotonated carboxylate group. This configuration was a result of the interaction with both carboxylate oxygen atoms. The results presented that carnosine dipeptide adsorbs onto CNT with amine group rather than carboxylate with 0.2655 eV difference in B3LYP binding energy. The capability of functionalization depended on the reactivity of the functionalizing group, reactivity of the CNTs, steric factors, etc. The steric effect could affect the interaction of dipeptide with CNT. The steric hindrance of the imidazole ring of carnosine dipeptide on interaction of carboxylate group with CNT induced smaller binding energy than did the amine group.

Comparing the two DFT functional results, about 10% differences in binding energies were identified. It was apparently accepted that non-dispersive DFT functional tends to underestimate the interaction between sp^2-like materials. It should be emphasized that apart from the main interactions, there are other interactions existing in the system, such as the dispersion and CH–π interactions between aliphatic groups (CH_2 and CH_3) and CNT. However, these interactions were found to be much weaker than the main interactions. Hence, besides the differences of B3LYP and wB97XD energies, both methods pointed out that the interaction of CNT and carnosine via NH_3^+ group of zwitterion was energetically more favorable than other interactions. The QM structures were applied as the initial structures for MC calculations. In fact, our major concern was to evaluate the interaction of carnosine with CNT in aqueous solution by using MC simulation method. It was pointed out in computational details that to simulate interactions, a Lennard–Jones potential function was implemented (in addition to Coulomb potential). Therefore, the weak van der Waals interactions were also considered in the study to compute binding energies in aqueous media accurately.

Reaction-free energies of carnosine with CNT have been evaluated by means of thermodynamic cycle.

In this section (QM part), the possible interactions of carnosine and CNT as a drug delivery system were studied. The efficient drug delivery systems should transport and protect the pharmacological and therapeutic properties of a drug molecule. Therefore, besides the binding of carnosine to CNT as a drug transporter, protection of carnosine (toward hydrolysis) should also be discussed in this section. The wide range of protective properties, such as antioxidant agent, makes carnosine of great interest for scientific and commercial applications. Carnosine has been found as a bioactive peptide in several pathological conditions, but its rapid hydrolysis in blood limits its pharmacological application. In fact, carnosine efficiency as a drug is a dare due to the presence of carnosinase enzymes. Therefore, it would be a potential interest to inactivate carnosinase or design carnosine structures that are resistant to hydrolyzation by the carnosinase enzyme.

Inhibitors can inactivate carnosinase, and hence prevent hydrolysis of carnosine, followed by the interaction of carnosinase and carnosine. However, we used CNT as a drug delivery system that can interact with carnosine and prevent its hydrolysis simultaneously.

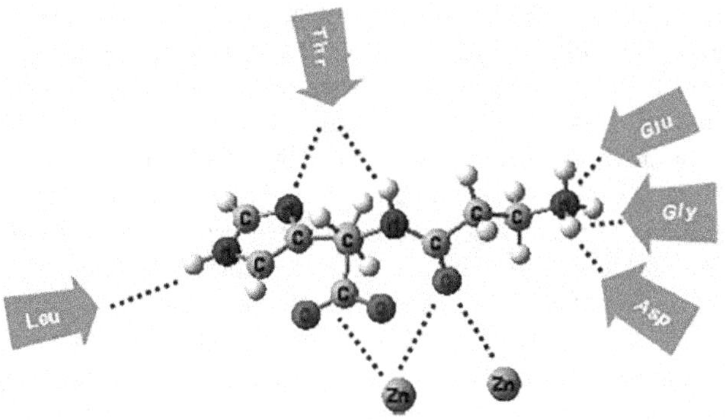

FIGURE 4.22 Interaction pattern between carnosinase and carnosine.

The molecular detection of carnosine by carnosinase performs better perception about the reason of conservation of the peptide bond after binding of carnosine to CNT. The structure of carnosinase consists of two separate domains: noncatalytic or lid domain and catalytic domain, with two Zn^{2+} ions at the active center. The catalytic domain contains a series of anti-parallel β-sheets surrounded by a crown of α-helices. A complex between carnosine and the catalytic site of human serum carnosinase has been suggested. Figure 4.22 depicts the interaction pattern between carnosinase and its substrate carnosine. It defines a recognition pharmacophore of serum carnosinase toward carnosine. As is seen, the enzyme binds the ammonium group, the carboxylate group, and the imidazole ring of carnosine. The ammonium group of carnosine interacts with carboxylates of aspartic acid (Asp) and glutamic acid (Glu) and with the backbone carbonyl of glycine (Gly) of carnosinase. Carbonyl and carboxylate groups of carnosine also interact with Zn^{2+} ions in the catalytic site of carnosinase. Polarization of the carbonyl group of carnosine is then increased and activates hydrolyses. Backbone carbonyl of leucine (Leu) forms a hydrogen bond with imidazole ring, and threonine (Thr) produces a set of interactions, a hydrogen bond with nitrogen, a second hydrogen bond with the amide group, and a hydrophobic interaction with the imidazole ring. Our computational results indicated that carnosine dipeptide interacts with CNT via NH_3^+ (more favorably than carboxylate). Therefore, at least one of the reactive groups of carnosine is covered by CNT and restrains its hydrolysis. As was mentioned before, the interaction of carnosinase with the NH_3^+ group of carnosine promoted the hydrolysis of the peptide bond. Vistoli et al. also explained the lower activity of serum carnosinase toward some carnosine analogue dipeptides. Carcinine lacks a carboxylate group, while N-acetylcarnosine does not have a charged ammonium, which prevents polarization and interaction of the carbonyl group with the zinc ions of carnosinase.

4.8.2 Monte Carlo Simulation

The objective of this part is to evaluate the possibility of CNT and carnosine interaction in aqueous solution. Solvation free energies and complexation free energies of carnosine–CNT structures have been calculated. Thermodynamic perturbation method was applied for all computations (for CNT, carnosine, and three complexes of carnosine–CNT in water). Appropriate steps were implemented to achieve the most accurate possible results with a molecular mechanical-based approach. In addition, the appropriate force field, the Monte Carlo simulation, including Metropolis sampling, and the NVT ensemble were utilized.

All simulations were carried out in a box with dimension 50 × 50 × 50 Å3 containing about 4,000 water molecules at the experimental density of water, 0.993 g/cm^3, at 37°C. In that study, a very low-concentration solution of each species was used, so one molecule of solute was merged in a cubic box of water, and by considering the size of the solute, some water molecules were put out from the box.

One molecule was selected and translated randomly on each move. An acceptance rate of 50% for new configurations was attained by using ranges of ±0.13 Å for the translations and ±15° for the rotation about a randomly chosen axis. Periodic boundary conditions were employed for the initial configuration, and each produced configuration energy computation, in translations and rotations. The system was thoroughly equilibrated using 10^7 configurations. The energy of a configuration was obtained from the pair-wise sum of interaction contributions of molecules. Every calculation was extended to include as many configurations as necessary to reduce the statistical error to a level at which calculated energy differences have quantitative significance.

The solvation of solute molecule in water could be presented as following:

$$\text{solute}\,(g) \rightarrow \text{solute}\,(aq)$$

A further discussion was the solvation of carnosine, CNT, and their complexes, in the presence of water. Monte Carlo simulations were used to calculate the average energies when one molecule of solute was merged in water. For instance, the snapshot of the simulation of carnosine–CNT complex in aqueous solution issued from MC simulation of carnosine–CNT complex in water is studied.

4.8.2.1 *Total Energies*

Total energies include three other parameters: number of solvent molecules (N_{H2O}) in the cubic box, STDEV (the standard deviation of the calculated average in the simulation of finite number of steps), and relative errors.

The results exhibited that CNT absolute total energies were less than carnosine–CNT complexes. Absolute energy of carnosine (NH_3^+)–CNT in water was larger than that of carnosine (COO−)–CNT. Moreover, absolute total energy of the carnosine (zwitterion)–CNT complex in water was larger than that of the carnosine (non-protonated)–CNT complex.

The electronic structure of the CNT is highly sensitive to its environment. Large changes in the properties of the CNT structure will occur in the presence of electrostatic charges and adsorption of various molecules on the surface. Intermolecular interactions (including electrostatic and van der Waals interactions) have an important role in E_{tot}, and atomic charges affect the electrostatic term of E_{tot} (eq. 25).

$$E^{AB} = \sum_{i}^{onA} \sum_{j}^{onB} 4\varepsilon ij \left[\left(\frac{\sigma_{ij}}{r_{ij}} \right)^{12} - \left(\frac{\sigma_{ij}}{r_{ij}} \right)^{6} + \frac{q_i q_j e^2}{r_{ij}} \right] \quad (25)$$

Quantum mechanics calculations showed that as a result of carnosine–CNT interaction, atoms in carnosine–CNT complexes carry partial charges. Therefore, interaction of the CNT complexes and water was larger than that of pure CNT. So CNT complexes had larger absolute total energy in water than pure CNT. The effect of van der Waals interactions in E_{tot} should also be considered. It should be noticed that in charged systems, van der Waals interactions' contribution in E_{tot} is not large. For better evaluation, electrostatic and van der Waals effect in potential energy was also computed, including electrostatic and van der Waals contributions in solute–solvent interaction energy.

Van der Waals contribution of CNT in intermolecular interaction with water was −0.302. As could be seen in carnosine–CNT complexes, electrostatic contribution of solute–water interaction energy was larger than van der Waals contribution due to partial atomic charges in complexes. Pure CNT had no atomic charges, and so electrostatic contribution in CNT–water interaction energy is negligible. Therefore, E_{soln} and E_{tot} of complexes must be larger than those of pure CNT. Between carnosine–CNT complexes, electrostatic contribution of solute–water interaction energy for carnosine (NH_3^+)-CNT (−203.263 kJ mol^{-1}) was greater than carnosine (COO−)–CNT (−119.432 kJ mol^{-1}). These results confirmed that absolute total energy of carnosine (NH_3^+)–CNT in water (208.522 kJ mol^{-1}) must be greater than carnosine (COO−)–CNT (123.842 kJ mol^{-1}). In fact, as an outcome of drug (carnosine) and CNT interaction, charge transfer between drug and CNT occurs, and so the electrostatic interaction of water and CNT is increased. To study drug effect in intermolecular interaction of CNT and solvent, drug contribution in solute–solvent interaction energy was also computed. As shown in Sepideh and Leila (2017), drug (carnosine) contributions on CNT–water interaction energy for solutes, carnosine (NH_3^+)-CNT, carnosine (COO−)-CNT, and carnosine (NH_2)-CNT were, respectively, −126.018, −41.547, and −5.736 kJ mol^{-1}. These results indicate that interaction with zwitterion of carnosine(a) via NH_3^+ was the most effective form for increasing the intermolecular interaction of CNT and water. So it was expected that from different candidates, carnosine (NH_3^+)-CNT must have the largest solubility in water. In order to confirm these consequences and to evaluate the solubility of the CNTs, we need to approximate solvation free energies of the structures. Therefore, solvation free energies of CNTs were calculated in the next step.

Simulation process creates enormous amount of data which need to be analyzed properly to extract appropriate properties and to check that calculation is performed appropriately. In order to consider the accuracy of Monte Carlo simulation, some important factors should be discussed, such as sample size effect and statistical fluctuations of calculated ensemble averages. The first factor was spotlighted because locating a limited number of molecules in a box, followed by subsequent implementing of periodic boundary conditions, brings in error into molecular correlations. For a given system, this effect diminishes with the sample size. In most cases which we were interested in, there is a lack of knowledge in choosing the size of the system in order to minimize the effect of periodic boundary conditions. A series of calculations in which the sample size is systematically increased until the calculated values remain stable has been carried out. The errors were reported in Sepideh and Leila (2017).

It could be observed that simulation error was under 1%.

4.8.2.2 Solvation Free Energies

For each of the solutes (that is, CNT, carnosine, and carnosine–CNT complexes), solvation free energy was calculated. To model solvation of CNT and its complexes, simulation was conducted on the system with the solute fully represented, and then its electrostatic and van der Waals parameters were decreased to zero.

Computed solvation free energies, ΔG sol, are shown in Table 4.14. It could be seen that CNT had the smaller solvation free energy than complexes. The results are compatible with the experimental studies. Synthesized amino acid–functionalized CNTs pointed out high solubility in aqueous solution. The CNTs carrying ammonium groups were very soluble in water and have potential application in the delivery of therapeutic molecules. Pantarotto et al. declared that biologically active peptides can also be easily linked through a stable covalent bond to CNTs, and then highly water-soluble CNTs can be obtained.

The computations of solvation free energies indicated that solvation of CNT in water would be increased with complex formation with carnosine. However, increase of solubility of CNT complex was not the result of carnosine solubility alone. As seen in Table 4.14, ΔG_{sol} of CNT–carnosine (all

TABLE 4.14

Solvation Free Energies (ΔG_{sol}) and Complexation Free Energies (ΔG_r) of Carnosine–CNT Complexes

Species	ΔG_{sol} (kJ mol−1)	ΔGr (kJ mol−1)
CNT	−12.426	–
Carnosine (a) (zwitterion)	−84.684	–
Carnosine (b) (non-protonated)	−52.794	–
Carnosine (a)–CNT (via NH3+)	−1,688.670	−1,591.560
Carnosine (a)–CNT (via COO−)	−914.769	−817.658
Carnosine (b)–CNT (via NH_2)	−554.828	−489.607

species) was >10 times of carnosine. In fact, the charge transfer between CNT and carnosine increases charge distribution on the surface of CNT and results in an increase of the electrostatic part of solvation free energy (as computed and shown in Table 4.14).

Although, sometimes, after the binding of ligand to nanotubes, the solubility decreased, it was found among DNA bases that only thymine and cytosine can increase the solvation free energy of SiCNT. Adenine and guanine decreased solubility due to a decrease of electrostatic interactions with water. Moreover, the effect of ligand on the solubility was different. Solvation free energy of CNT–carnosine was more than those of CNT–histidine or CNT–alanine.

Atomic charges in the solutes affect electrostatic terms of intermolecular energies directly. As mentioned previously, atoms in pure CNT had no atomic charge, and so solvation of pure CNT is lower than in carnosine–CNT complexes. It could be predicted that the drug has a large contribution in increasing the solvation of CNT. The solvation of CNT was increased significantly by the interaction with carnosine. In fact, due to the interaction of drug with CNT, solvation free energy increased from −12.426 up to −554.828, −914.769, and −1,688.670 kJ $mol^{-1}$for carnosine (NH_2)–CNT, carnosine (COO−)–CNT, and carnosine (NH_3^+)–CNT, respectively. This was related to the larger electrostatic contribution and also larger intermolecular interactions between solute–solvent molecules. Consequently, among the three possible carnosine structures, zwitterion (via NH_3^+) was the most effective form of carnosine for producing the best soluble drug–CNT species in aqueous solution. Therefore, it can be concluded that carnosine dipeptide increases the solubility of CNT, which leads to several applications of these materials in biotechnology.

Moreover, the calculation of solvation free energies was not only to study solubility but also to calculate complexation free energy and study the possibility of CNT–carnosine interaction in aqueous solution. The real goal was to study the possibility of carnosine carrier with CNT in aqueous media.

4.8.2.3 Complexation Free Energies

The complexation free energies (ΔG_r) in aqueous solutions have been computed using eq. 26:

$$\Delta G_{sol}(A)=G_{sol}(A)-\Delta G_{gas}(A)\rightarrow \qquad (26)$$

By using the FEP method, the solvation free energy of species A can be stated in terms of perturbations, where the species fade away in the gas phase ($\Delta G_{gas}(A\rightarrow 0)$) and in solution ($\Delta G_{sol}(A\rightarrow 0)$):

$$\Delta G_{sol}(A)=G_{sol}(A)-\Delta G_{gas}(A)\rightarrow \qquad (27)$$

The actual perturbations were divided into a sequence of steps that were attached to a linear parameter λ running from 0 to 1. Double-wide sampling was utilized, yielding a step size Δλ equivalent to 0.1.

Reaction free energies of carnosine with CNT have been evaluated by means of the thermodynamic cycle. By considering the thermodynamic cycle and eq. 28, the complexation free energy of carnosine (L) and CNT in solution is given by eq. 29:

$$\varepsilon ij = (\varepsilon i\ \varepsilon j)^{1/2} \qquad (28)$$

$$\Delta G_r=\Delta G_{sol}(L\rightarrow 0) + \Delta G_{sol}(CNT\rightarrow 0) - \Delta G_{sol}(\mathrm{LCNT}\rightarrow 0) \qquad (29)$$

For this purpose, three solvation free energies are needed: carnosine species, CNT, and carnosine–CNT complexes solvation free energies (Table 4.14). It could be seen that carnosine (zwitterion)–CNT complexation free energies were larger than in the carnosine (non-protonated)–CNT complex. So it was concluded that zwitterion of carnosine was the most appropriate form to interact with CNT in aqueous media. Complexation free energies of carnosine (COO−)–CNT and carnosine (NH_3^+)–CNT were −817.658 and −1,591.560 kJ mol^{-1}, respectively. The steric effect of an interacting group can affect the interaction of functionalization agent and CNT. So between the two sites of carnosine zwitterion, interaction through NH_3^+ makes the most stable complex in water. Furthermore, greater electrostatic interactions of water and carnosine (NH_3^+)–CNT enhance the stability of this complex in water when comparing with other complexes. This consequence seems to be compatible with the gas-phase result.

In addition, the reaction free energy of hydrolysis of carnosine-bound CNT to predict the possibility of the reaction toward the carnosinase enzyme has been computed, reactions for which $\Delta G_r > 0$ are not spontaneous. Regarding the hydrolysis process of carnosine by carnosinase, hydrolysis of CNT–carnosine can be considered as:

$$\mathrm{CNT-carnosine}\ \underline{\mathrm{carnosinase}}\ \mathrm{CNT\text{-}alanine + histidine}$$

Free energies of the hydrolysis of CNT–carnosine were calculated using the thermodynamic cycle and solvation free energies. Solvation free energies of CNT–carnosine (Table 4.14), CNT–alanine, and histidine were −1,688.670, −51.610, and −27.802 kJ mol^{-1}. Free energies of the hydrolysis of CNT–carnosine were then +1,609.258 kJ mol^{-1}. Therefore, hydrolysis of CNT–carnosine toward carnosinase is not spontaneous.

4.9 Computational Study of Leflunomide on SWCNT and SWBNNT

Leflunomide (HWA 486 or RS-34821, 5-methyl-N-(4trifluoromethylphenyl)-4-isoxazole carboxamide) is an immunosuppressive agent effective in the treatment of rheumatoid arthritis. Dihydroortate dehydrogenase (DHODH, EC 1.3.3.1) immobilization on the nanotubes was carried out, and biochemical characterization of free and immobilized enzyme was determined. The behavior of anticancer drug leflunomide adsorbed on the external surface of zigzag single-walled (6,0) carbon and boron nitride nanotubes (SWCNT and SWBNNT) was studied by means of DFT calculations at the B3LYP/6–31G* level of theory. The larger adsorption energies and charge transfer showed that the adsorption of leflunomide onto SWBNNT is more stable than the adsorption of leflunomide onto SWCNT. Frontier molecular orbitals (HOMO and LUMO) suggest that adsorption of leflunomide onto SWBNNT behaves as charge transfer compounds, with leflunomide as an electron donor and SWBNNT as an electron acceptor. Thus, nanotubes (NTs) have been proposed and actively explored as multipurpose innovative carriers for drug delivery and diagnostic application. The AIM theory has also been applied to analyze the properties of the bond critical points: their electron densities and their Laplacians. Also, the natural bond orbital (NBO) calculations were performed to derive natural atomic orbital occupancies and partial charges of the interacting atoms in the equilibrium tube–molecule distance.

In this research, the adsorption behavior of leflunomide on two representative models of the zigzag single-walled (6,0) carbon and boron nitride nanotubes with tube lengths of 9.27 and 9.34 Å, respectively, has been considered. The (6,0) carbon and BN nanotubes with 4.8 Å and 5.1 Å diameters are shown in Figure 4.23. The first model is the (6,0) SWCNT, consisting of 48 C atoms forming eight layer of atoms along the tube axis (Figure 4.23c). The second model is the (6,0) SWBNNT, consisting of 24 N and 24 B atoms, which could be divided into four layers of B and four layers of N atoms (see Figure 4.23b). In each of the models considered in this study, both portals were capped by 20 H atoms in order to avoid dangling bonds and to decrease calculation time. Firstly, the sites that a leflunomide molecule can adsorb into the nanotubes have been examined. Different adsorption sites on carbon and BN nanotubes, T1 (top of the carbon or boron atoms), T2 (top of the carbon or nitrogen atoms), and B (top of the axial C–C or B–N bonds), were considered for their interactions with leflunomide molecules (see Figure 4.23e and d). Fully optimized geometries and the properties of the electronic and structural properties of the (6,0) pristine and leflunomide adsorbed on pristine and vibrational frequency analysis were derived by means of density functional theory (DFT) method with the B3LYP functional (Becke's three-parameter hybrid exchange functions using the Lee–Yang–Parr gradient-corrected correlation). For all systems, a geometry optimization calculation was performed using 6–31G* basis set. Harmonic vibrational frequencies were estimated at the same level for checking the nature of optimized geometries for local minima and also to account for the zero point vibrational energy (ZPVE) correction. The calculations were carried out using G03 package.

The adsorption energy (Ed) of leflunomide molecule has been calculated by the following equation:

$$E_d = R_r\left(\frac{\text{leflunomide}}{\text{SWNTs}}\right) - E(\text{SWNTs}) - E(\text{leflunomide})$$

Where *E(leflunomide/SWNTs)* is the total energy of the adsorbed leflunomide molecule on the SWNTs surface, and *E(SWNTs)* and *E(leflunomide)* are the total energies of the pristine SWNTs and the leflunomide molecule, respectively. If the value of ΔE is negative, the complex is more stable relative to the precursors. The binding energies of the complexes were corrected separately for both zero-point energy (ZPE) and the basis set superposition error (BSSE) using the counterpoise correction scheme. The Bader quantum theory of atoms in molecules (QTAIM) was also included here. The analysis of the distribution of electron densities was performed to find the bond and ring critical points and to characterize them in terms of values of electron densities and their Laplacian.

The AIM calculations were carried out using the AIM2000 program. In addition, the natural bond orbitals (NBO) method

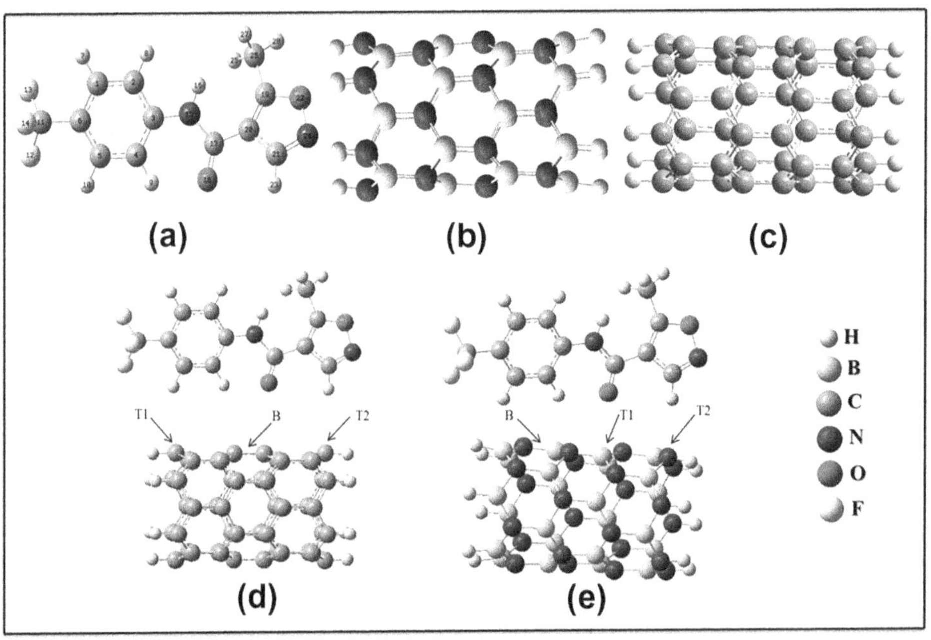

FIGURE 4.23 Optimized geometries for (a) leflunomide, (b) zigzag (6, 0) SWBNNT system, (c) zigzag (6, 0) SWCNT system, (e) leflunomide adsorbed on the SWBNNT, and (d) leflunomide adsorbed on the SWCNT.

was applied to calculate the second-order perturbation theory interaction energy. The contour plot for visualization of the NBO result is constructed by the NBOView (Version 1.1) software package using the standard keywords implemented therein. The molecular orbital (MO) calculations, such as HOMO–LUMO, are also performed on studied systems. Conceptual density functional theory provides insights into the popular qualitative chemical concepts, such as electronic chemical potential (μ), hardness (η), and electronegativity (χ). χ is defined as the negative of μ, as follows: $\chi = -\mu$. The chemical potential (μ) and global hardness (η) of the complexes using Koopmans' theorem have been calculated, as given:

$$\eta = \frac{E_{LUMO} - E_{HOMO}}{2}, \mu = \frac{E_{LUMO} - E_{HOMO}}{2}$$

Where E_{LUMO} is the energy of the lowest unoccupied molecular orbital and E_{HOMO} is the energy of the highest occupied molecular orbital. Hard molecules thus have a large HOMO–LUMO gap and soft molecules have a small one. The obtained values of χ and η are used to calculate the fraction of electron transferred, ΔN, transferred from a system A (leflunomide) to system B (SWNTs) and was calculated as follows:

$$\Delta N = \frac{X_A - X_B}{2(\eta_A - \eta_B)}$$

Where χ_A, χ_B and η_A, η_B are the electronegativity and chemical hardness of the systems A and B. A positive value of ΔN indicates that charge flows from B to A and A acts as an electron acceptor, whereas a negative value of ΔN indicates that charge flows from A to B and A acts as an electron donor.

4.9.1 Leflunomide Suppresses Cancer Cell Proliferation

DHODH is expressed in multiple myeloma cell lines, inhibits cell growth, and induces apoptosis in these cells. RPMI-8226 has therefore been incubated with clinically achievable concentrations of leflunomide or active metabolite for 48 and 96 h. MTT assays revealed that exposure to leflunomide concentrations >50 μM resulted in significant dose-dependent reduction in cell proliferation. MTT cell proliferation assay showed dose-dependent inhibition of RPMI-8226 cell growth in vitro. Cell line RPMI-8226 was incubated with 0, 10, 50, 100, and 150 μmol/L leflunomide for 6 days. The highest doses (150 μM) significantly suppress growth significantly by day 2. Dose- and time-dependent reduction in proliferation was observed. The experiments show that cell growth was totally abrogated upon incubation with 150 μmol L^{-1} leflunomide in the tested cell. Compared with control media and DMSO, 50 μM, 100 μM, and 150 μM drug treatments for 4 days reduced growth by 18%, 49%, 76%, and 82%, respectively.

It has been observed that for the leflunomide/SWBNNT system, the values of ρ(r) at B . . . O_{18}, N . . . H_9, and N . . . H_{23} BCP have been increased, whereas the values of ρ(r) at N . . . H_{10} BCP have been decreased in comparison with the corresponding values of the leflunomide/SWCNT system. For investigated systems, molecular graphs (including the critical points and bond paths, Figures 4.24 and 4.25) represent four critical points in . . . O_{18}, X . . . H_9, X . . . H_{10}, and X . . . H_{23} bonds (X = B, N, or C) in connection with the region of leflunomide to SWNTs. It is obvious that the leflunomide/SWBNNT system with the shorter N . . . H distance has greater ρ(r) at N . . . H BCP. The value of ρ(r) at N . . . H_{23} BCP in this complex is more than in others. As a result, the N . . . H_{23} bond in leflunomide/SWBNNT is stronger than in others. The values of ρ(r) at newly formed B . . . O_{18} and C . . . O_{18} contacts in leflunomide/SWBNNT and leflunomide/SWCNT are 0.0069 and 0.0044 au, respectively, which imply that the B . . . O_{18} bond in the former is stronger than in the C . . . O_{18} bond in the latter. This conclusion is in agreement with the greater binding energy obtained for the leflunomide/SWBNNT complex. From comparison of the values of ^{2}ρ(r) and H(r) at X . . . O_{18}, X . . . H_9, X . . . H_{10}, and X . . . H_{23} (X = B, N, or C) BCP, it can be concluded that the covalency nature of these bonds in the

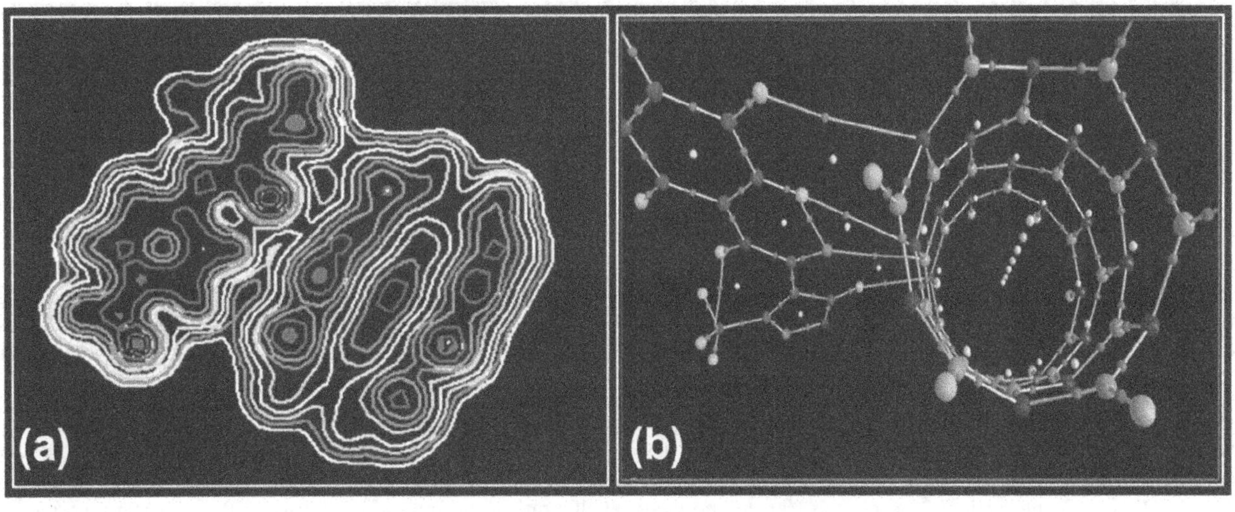

FIGURE 4.24 (a) The contour map of leflunomide/SWBNNT obtained from the DFT calculation. (b) The molecular graph of leflunomide/SWBNNT obtained from the DFT calculation.

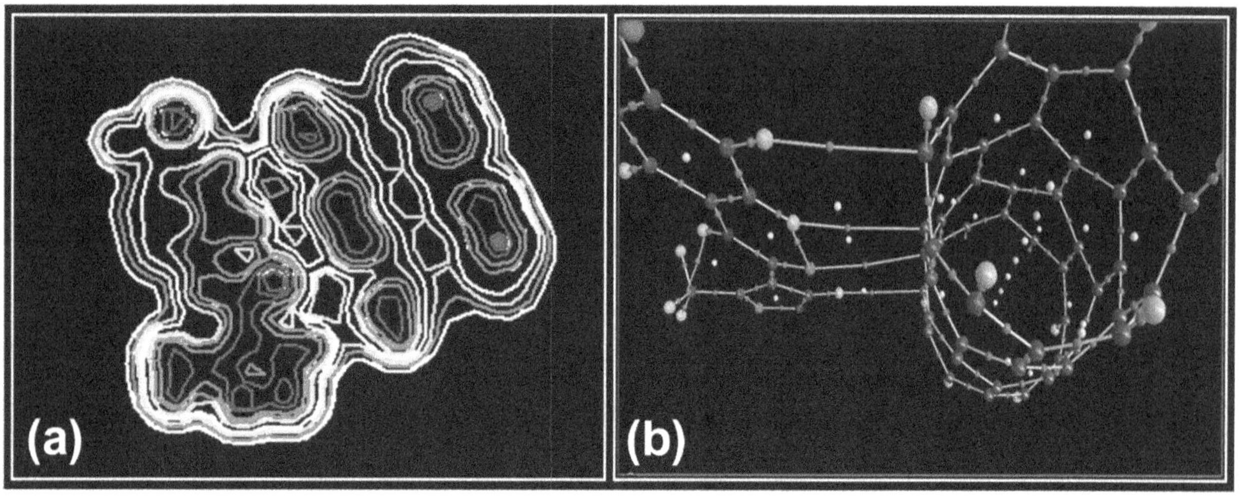

FIGURE 4.25 (a) The contour map of leflunomide/SWCNT obtained from the DFT calculation. (b) The molecular graph of leflunomide/SWCNT obtained from the DFT calculation.

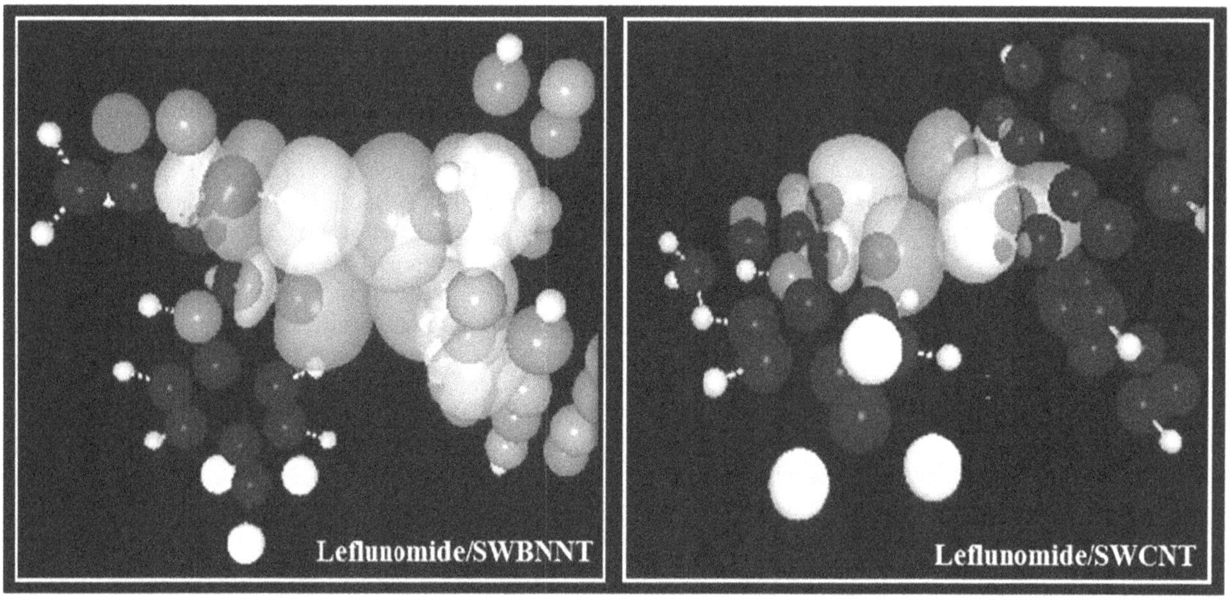

FIGURE 4.26 3D NBO contour plot illustrating the interaction between the electron lone pair of oxygen (O_{18}) and X (X = C or N) with an antibonding X–Y orbital (X–Y = B–N or C–C) in leflunomide/SWCNT and leflunomide/SWBNNT systems.

leflunomide/SWBNNT system is weaker than in leflunomide/SWCNT ones.

The NBO analysis reveals interesting details on the electron density transfer in donor acceptor interactions. The results of NBO analyses[42] were applied to evaluate X . . . O_{18}, X . . . H_9, X . . . H_{10}, and X . . . H_{23} (X = B, N, or C) interactions in the leflunomide/SWCNT and leflunomide/SWBNNT systems. Charge transfer from the B to N atom in pristine SWBNNT occurs. So the isolated BNNT could be considered as a unique tube that consists of the ionic B^+–N– bond. In the NBO analysis of X . . . H_9, X . . . H_{10}, and X . . . H_{23} (X = B, N, or C) interactions, the charge transfer between the lone pairs of N or C as proton acceptor and anti-bonds of the proton donor is most important. Our theoretical results illustrate that in the investigated systems, lone pairs of O_{18} participate as a donor and the π^* B_{30}–N_{31} and π * C_{30}–C_{31} interaction as an acceptor in intermolecular charge transfer interactions with the energy values of 3.41 and 0.06 kcal/mol, respectively. There is stronger intermolecular interaction in leflunomide/SWBNNT in comparison with leflunomide/SWCNT because of more total charge transfer energy associated with the intermolecular interaction. This implies that the properties of the charge transfer between the lone pairs of proton acceptor and anti-bonds of proton donor (ECT) could be very useful to estimate the strength of the intermolecular interaction. Figure 4.26 displays the 3D NBO contour plot illustrating the interaction between the electron lone pair of oxygen (O_{18}) and X (X = C or N) with an antibonding X–Y orbital (X–Y = B–N or C–C) in leflunomide/SWCNT and leflunomide/SWBNNT systems.

4.9.2 Electronic Properties

The final study in this section is to evaluate the reactivity of (6,0) SWNTs as drug delivery systems through analyzing the electronic structures for the most energetical configuration. The plots of the highest occupied molecular orbital (HOMO) and the lowest unoccupied molecular orbital (LUMO) for the leflunomide molecule, the SWBNNT and SWCNT models, and leflunomide/SWCNT and leflunomide/SWBNNT complexes are shown in Figures 4.27 and 4.28. It is obvious that, for the case of pristine SWBNNT, the HOMO is localized at the tube end, with most contributions at N atoms that are terminated by H atoms. The high coefficient of wave function for the nitrogen atoms in the HOMO indicates the large probability that the

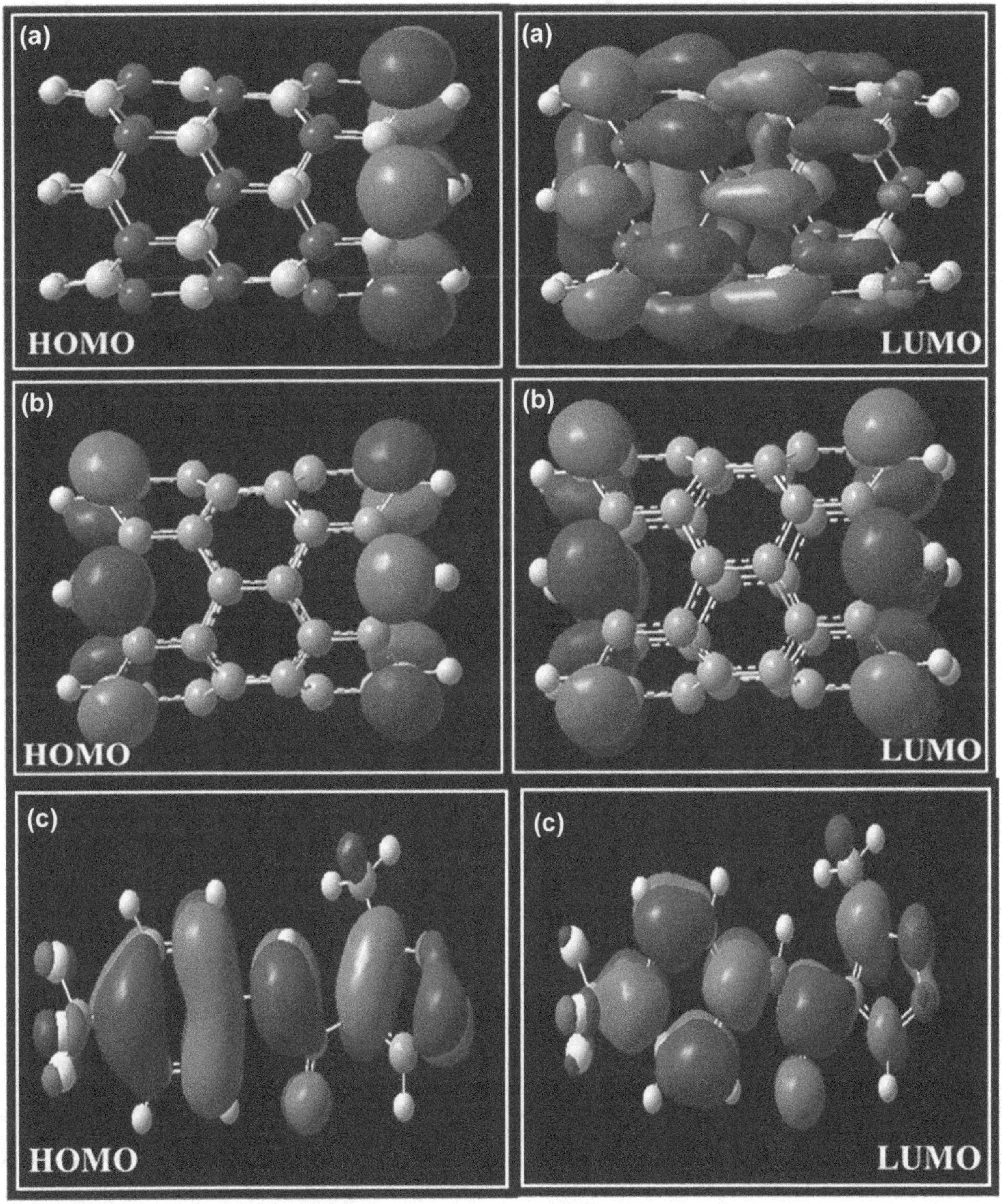

FIGURE 4.27 The calculated orbitals localized at (a) the topmost valence band (HOMO) and the lowest conduction band (LUMO) of isolated SWBNNT; (b) HOMO and LUMO of isolated SWCNT; and (c) HOMO and LUMO of isolated leflunomide molecule.

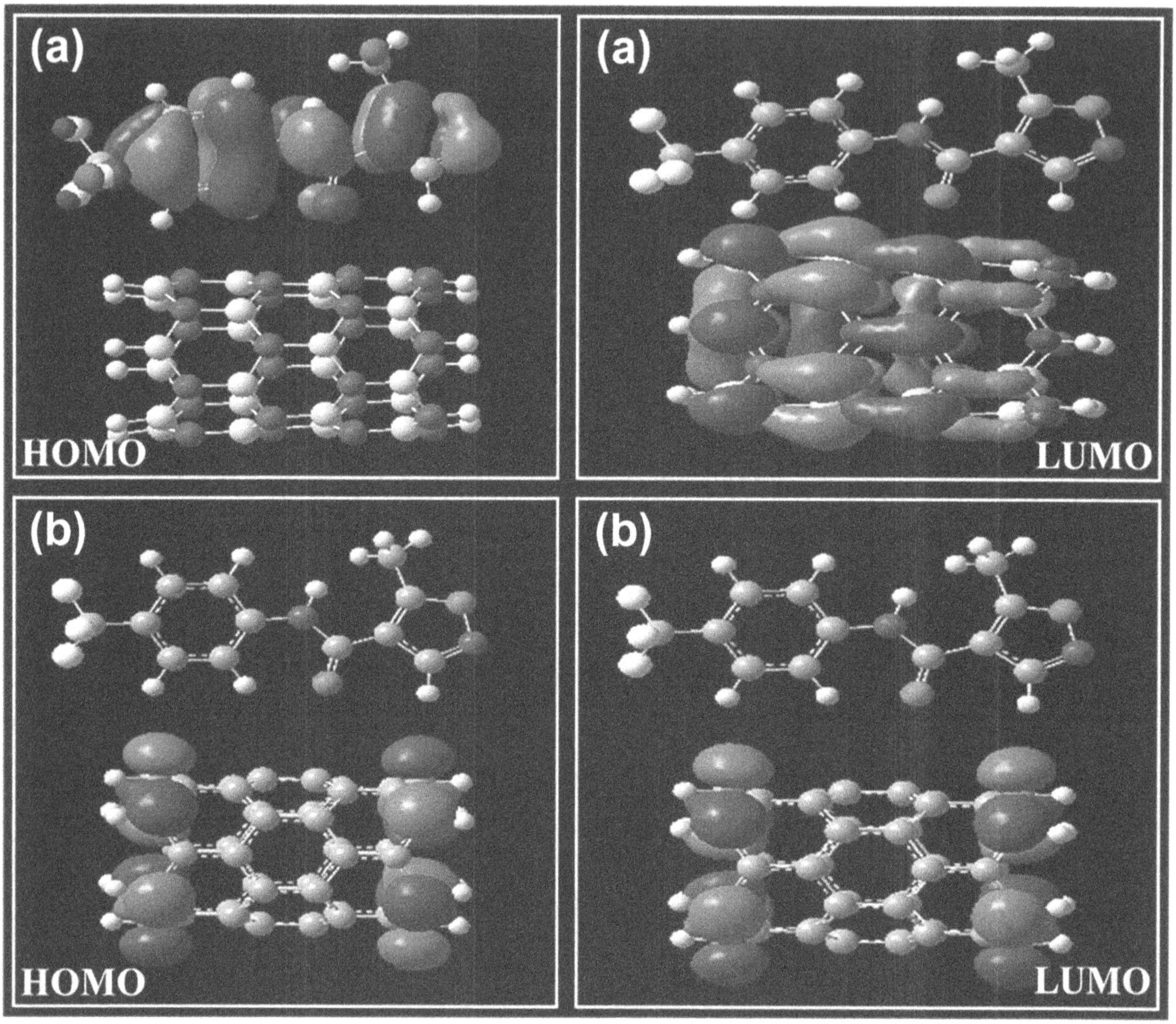

FIGURE 4.28 The calculated orbitals localized at (a) HOMO and LUMO of leflunomide/SWBNNT complex and (b) HOMO and LUMO of leflunomide/SWCNT complex.

molecule can undergo an electrophilic attack. In contrast, the LUMO is present as π states localized at the N–B pair along the tube axis (Figure 4.27a). In this model, the distribution of LUMO orbital seems more regular. It is also evident that for pristine SWCNT studied, the HOMO and LUMO are localized at the tube end, with most contributions at C atoms that are terminated by H atoms (see Figure 4.27b).

The leflunomide/SWCNT model shows similar HOMO and LUMO, which are mainly localized at the tube end, with most contributions at C atoms that are terminated by H atoms (see Figure 4.28b). No meaningful changes are seen between both molecular orbitals for leflunomide/SWCNT system. Figure 4.28b shows that the adsorption of leflunomide molecule onto the SWCNT has no significant effect on the HOMO and LUMO isosurfaces compared to those of pristine SWCNT system, informing the improbability of modification of the electronic properties of considered SWCNT by the leflunomide adsorption process. In leflunomide/SWBNNT system, the HOMO is localized on the leflunomide molecule and the LUMO on the SWBNNT, suggesting that, in these complexes, leflunomide molecule is an electron donor species and SWBNNT is an electron-withdrawing one. This suggests a charge transfer from the HOMO to the LUMO. Also, the energy gaps (ΔE_{H-L}) between HOMO and LUMO have been calculated. The calculated energy gaps (ΔE_{H-L}) of the perfect (6,0) zigzag SWCNT and SWBNNT are 0.4417 and 4.8843 eV, respectively, whereas these values decrease to 0.4401 and 4.8019, respectively, in the complexes. These results show that leflunomide adsorption on the pristine (6,0) zigzag SWCNT has more influence on the energy gap of the nanotube than the pristine (6,0) zigzag SWBNNT. The DEH–L characterizes molecular chemical stability, and it is a critical parameter in determining molecular electrical transport properties because it is a measure of electron conductivity. It is well-known that molecules with high LUMO–HOMO energy gap are kinetically stable. Closer inspection of the theoretical results denotes that the leflunomide/SWBNNT complex has higher ΔE_{H-L} value, which reveals greater stability of this complex.

The global indices of reactivity in the context of DFT χ is the Mulliken electronegativity for atoms, which is called the absolute electronegativity ($\chi = -\mu$); for an equilibrium system, it must be constant everywhere. The hardness need not be constant and can have local values, but η is the average or global value. When the leflunomide molecule and carbon nanotube are brought together, electrons will flow from that of lower χ to that of higher χ. On the other hand, electron is transferred to the lower electronic chemical potential until the electronic chemical potentials become equal. The difference in electronegativity drives the electron transfer, and the sum of the hardness parameters acts as a resistance. The electronic chemical potential and the hardness are molecular and not orbital properties. The amount of charge transfer between the leflunomide and the SWNTs is calculated using the ΔN method. A positive value of ΔN indicates that the leflunomide acts as an electron acceptor, while a negative value of ΔN indicates that the leflunomide acts as an electron donor. In the leflunomide/SWCNT system, the ΔN value is positive, indicating that leflunomide acts as an electron acceptor, whereas in the leflunomide/SWBNNT system, the DN value is negative, indicating that the situation is vice versa. Thus, electrons will flow from a definite occupied orbital in SWCNT and will go into a definite empty orbital in a leflunomide molecule. Moreover, due to Pearson's maximum hardness principle (MHP), which points out that the minimum energy structure has maximum chemical hardness, therefore, leflunomide/SWBNNT complexes are capable to create greater chemical hardness and chemical potential values with respect to leflunomide/SWBNNT complex.

For leflunomide/SWCNT complex, chemical hardness and chemical potential are less than in the leflunomide/SWBNNT complex, indicating that the former complex is softer than the latter. The electronic structures of leflunomide molecule adsorbed on the surface of considered SWNTs have been performed to discover the binding nature in these systems. Therefore, the calculations of density of state (DOS) for the combined system of leflunomide/SWNTs compared with the corresponding DOS for the individual parts (leflunomide and SWNTs separated) were carried out. The calculated density of states (DOS) for an isolated leflunomide, an isolated SWCNT, and SWBNNT, and the combination of the two at equilibrium geometry, has been investigated. It is obvious that the DOS of the combined system is almost the superposition of the DOS of the individual parts, and the DOS near the Fermi level is not affected by the adsorption of the leflunomide molecule on the surface of SWNTs; the entrance of the weak interaction was obtained quantitatively in terms of binding energies. Furthermore, the small difference in the Fermi level of the SWCNT and SWBNNT (E_F = 4.1652 and 3.7392 eV, respectively) and leflunomide/SWCNT and leflunomide/SWBNNT (E_F = 7.3717 and 7.5224 eV, respectively) clearly reveals a weak charge transfer between the considered species in the adsorption process. The peak position of the leflunomide/SWNTs is in accordance with those of pure SWNTs, but it seems that they are combined with the downshifted peaks of the leflunomide from their original positions. Similarly, the strong peaks of the leflunomide/SWNTs combine the peaks of the SWNTs, with those of the leflunomide downshifted. Again, based on analyzing the band structure and the DOS in which the characteristics of each component is still observed independently except for the shift of some energy levels, it is inferred that the interaction between SWNTs and leflunomide would be weak. The MEP is a useful property to study the reactivity that an approaching electrophile will be attracted to negative regions (where the electron distribution effect is dominant). In majority of the MEPs, while the maximum negative region, which is the preferred site for electrophilic attack, is indicated as red color, the maximum positive region, which is the preferred site for nucleophilic attack, is denoted as blue color.

The importance of MEP lies in the fact that it simultaneously displays molecular size, shape, as well as positive, negative, and neutral electrostatic potential regions in terms of color grading (Figure 4.29) and is very useful in the research of molecular structure with its physiochemical property relationship. The different values of the electrostatic potential at the surface are represented by different colors; red represents regions of most negative electrostatic potential, blue represents regions of most positive electrostatic potential, and green represents regions of zero potential. Potential increases in the order red < orange < yellow < green < blue. In MEP map of leflunomide, the surfaces over the O, N, and F atoms, representing maximum negative electrostatic potential, and the surfaces over the C and H with maximum positive electrostatic potential may be

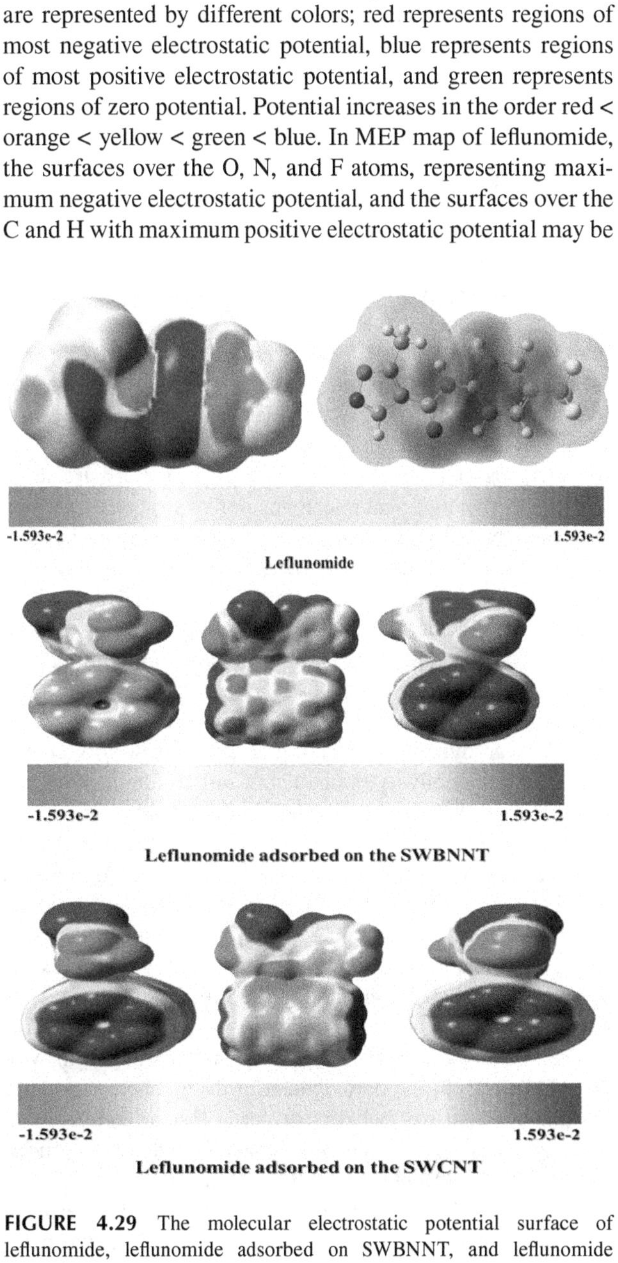

FIGURE 4.29 The molecular electrostatic potential surface of leflunomide, leflunomide adsorbed on SWBNNT, and leflunomide adsorbed on SWCNT.

sites of electrophilic and nucleophilic reactions, respectively (see Figure 4.29). For leflunomide adsorption on SWBNNT, the MEP plot shows a strong positive electrostatic potential (electron-poor, blue color) and weak negative electrostatic potential (electron-rich, red color) occurring at the end and opposite end regions of nanotubes, respectively, where the hydrogens are located. Moreover, the results of MEP show that the regions of negative electrostatic potential (denoted by red) are usually applied to identify hydrogen bond–acceptor sites, while for describing the hydrogen bond–donating sites, the regions of positive electrostatic potential (denoted by blue) are significant.

4.10 Concluding Remarks

In this chapter, we have attempted to summarize the role that molecular dynamics modeling can play as a tool in drug delivery research in a fashion that is hopefully comprehensible to both those with an expertise in molecular modeling who wish to pursue pharmaceutical applications of their research and pharmaceutical researchers interested in what insight this new tool can provide. All aspects of the journey that the drug molecule takes, from dissolution to solvation or transit through the bloodstream inside a nanoparticle to finally crossing the plasma membrane of the target cell, is a story of molecular interactions. The interactions involved, however, are not all interactions. Any chemist reading this review will have noticed an omission: chemical reactions; these play a very small role in the story, one dominated by intermolecular interactions. For this reason, MD simulation is the perfect tool to obtain molecular-level insight, as precisely the varieties of interaction it is best able to study are those which play the dominant role: formation of structure based on lipophilicity and H-bonding. Whether it is the hydration that occurs during dissolution, interaction between drug molecule and excipients, behavior of molecules at the surface of the nanoparticle in the bloodstream, or the interaction between the nanoparticle and the plasma membrane of the target cell, these are the interactions that determine the most important aspects of behavior.

Molecular dynamics modeling is still a new tool in the design of drug delivery mechanisms; only in the past decade have we seen the explosion in the number of publications that make use of this tool. Widespread adoption is hindered by the fact that, unlike computational drug design tools like ligand docking and QSAR/QSPR, the calculations involved are, as of yet, for the most part, too expensive to be carried out anywhere other than national-level supercomputing resources. As the widely available computational power continues to grow exponentially, this barrier may dissipate. Looking toward the future and the role that molecular dynamics modeling will be able to play in the development of drug delivery systems, the analogy that we feel is most apt is that of computationally assisted design (CAD), in mechanical and civil engineering. Before the advent of computational technology, engineers were forced to build scale models of systems and experiment with them, testing every aspect with real experimental models, and sometimes varying parameters empirically. Now, with widespread computational resources available to all engineers, CAD allows every aspect of a new machine, or structure, to be examined and tested in silico with all aspects of mechanical stress, heat dissipation, etc. of the system visible, and the change resulting from any design alteration straightforward to analyze entirely virtually. While we clearly do not mean to imply that human physiology is no more complex than designing a car or a bridge, we foresee that, in the future, drug delivery devices will be designed in an analogous fashion, with molecular dynamics modeling playing the role in pharmaceutics that CAD plays in mechanical and civil engineering. The studies of the AETP targeting moiety and itraconazole in liposome-based delivery systems show clear examples of how the design approach can be applied, using in silico modeling to test aspects of the delivery system design in an analogous approach to CAD. Alongside cutting-edge experimental techniques that complement it, molecular dynamics simulation has the potential to lead the way to a new era of rational design in the development of drug delivery systems. Finally, other complementary reviews that cover similar material can also be found [104–106].

The CNT-based target-specific delivery of drugs, or other molecular cargo, has emerged as one of the most potential biomedical applications of nanotechnology. To achieve efficient CNT-based nanodrug delivery, the interactions between the drug, CNT, and biomolecular target need to be properly optimized. Further, inappropriate physicochemical properties of CNTs can disrupt the nuclear or cellular membrane during penetration, leading to various cytotoxic effects. The CNT–bimolecular interactions can be optimized by adjusting the various physicochemical properties of drugs and fine-tuning several parameters of CNTs to achieve effective drug delivery while avoiding toxicities. Recent advances in computer-aided molecular design tools, in particular MD simulation studies, offer an appropriate low-cost approach for such optimization. This chapter highlights the various potential MD simulation approaches along with their strengths and weaknesses in current use for the simulation of CNT interactions with the cell membrane. An attempt has also been made to emphasize the various methods of internalization and toxicities of CNTs. The detailed analysis of several MD approaches discussed in this review will be useful to build new strategies to develop the necessary computational setup for designing rational CNT-based targeted drug delivery to circumvent the limitations associated with the clinically available various nonspecific therapeutic agents.

Due to the potential applications of CNTs in drug delivery and medical science, a study of the interaction of carnosine dipeptide with CNT in gas-phase and aqueous solution was the goal of this chapter. CNTs are poorly soluble in water, and this has initially limited their use as a delivery agent for medicinal purposes. Therefore, the solubility of carnosine–CNT complexes was also inquired. Two sections of this research chapter were dedicated to QM and MC computation. In the QM part, binding energies of carnosine and CNT were calculated in the gas phase. Three possible interactions with CNT were considered: carnosine zwitterion via NH_3^+, carnosine zwitterion via COO–, and non-protonated carnosine via NH_2. The calculations showed that carnosine zwitterion via NH_3^+–CNT had the highest interaction energy. Second division, which was MC constituted of estimation complexes solvation free energies by free energy perturbation method. Computations showed that solvation of carnosine (NH_3^+)–CNT complex in water was larger than in other complexes. In addition, solvation free energy computation results indicated that functionalization with carnosine increases solubility of CNT considerably. Therefore, these functionalized CNTs displayed low toxicity, and such systems held great potential in the field of nanomedicine. Computed complexation free energies of these complexes in physiological media pointed out that the carnosine (NH_3^+)–CNT complex had the larger complexation free energy. Therefore, it was the most stable compound in water. Our interim result can be summarized as: functionalization with carnosine dipeptide significantly improved solubility of CNT in biological fluids and so improve their biocompatibility. CNT can be considered as a promising drug delivery system for carnosine to transport it to target cells.

MD simulations were performed to investigate the adsorption mechanism of the PTX drug on a pristine CNT and *f*-CNTs in aqueous solution. In this chapter, CNT has been functionalized with COOH, PEG (with 12 monomers), and CH_2NH_2 in four centers in the same sites at the edges of the CNT. Radial distribution functions, van der Waals energy, the number of contacts, and the number of hydrogen bonds are analyzed to understand the nature of the main interactions between PTX molecules and CNTs. The obtained results show that the PTX drug can be adsorbed on CNTs by π–π stacking, which was formed between the PTX and surfaces of CNTs, and also by formation of polar interactions between drug and functional groups of *f*-CNTs. Results of van der Waals energy and the number of contacts indicate that the PEG-CNT system has the best performance in drug adsorption.

The number of hydrogen bonds, solvent accessible surface area, and water molecules around the CNT show that functionalization strongly increases the solubility of CNT. This fact can be attributed to the formation of hydrogen bonds between functional groups of CNTs and water molecules. Furthermore, the PEG-CNT system has the highest solubility in water solution.

In this chapter, quantum chemical calculations and molecular dynamics simulation provide an understanding into the nature of the interaction of anticancer flutamide drug molecule and the single-walled carbon nanotube surface. DFT calculations confirmed the energetic stability of the optimized geometries and showed that the interaction of the drug molecule with the outside of the nanotube is a spontaneous process. Moreover, the enhancement polarity of the considered configurations, which is a desired property for drug delivery systems in the human body, is observed by going from the gas phase to the water phase. The AIM theory has been used to analyze the properties of the bond critical points: their electron densities and Laplacians. Moreover, NBO analysis suggests that the nanotube plays the role of an electron donor and the FLU molecule acts as an electron acceptor for the FLU/SWCNT complex. Moreover, the interaction is explained on the basis of four reactivity descriptors (i.e., ΔN, $\Delta E_{B(A)}$, $\Delta E_{A(B)}$, and ΔE_{SE}). Moreover, the MD simulation is performed to study the dynamic adsorption process of the FLU molecule on the nanotube at the different concentrations of ethanol. Based on the RDFs and the van der Waals energy results, it can be concluded that the addition of EtOH molecule with the concentration of 0.5 M can increase the stability of the simulation system.

In summary, the non-covalent interaction of FLU drug molecule on functionalized nanotube surface with COOH and COCl functional groups is investigated using density functional theory. Several useful and applicable computational tools, such as the geometrical and electronic properties, NBO and AIM, were applied to study the details of the interaction. With respect to the calculations, the negative binding energy values illustrate and confirm the favorable interaction between FLU drug and f-CNT at the considered complexes. Also, the amount of the binding energy related to NTCOOCl is lower than that related to NTCOOH, indicating that NTCOOH/FLUR reactant is stabilized. The obtained information from AIM calculations confirmed the presence of the partial covalence interaction between FLU drug and *f*-CNT. In addition, it can be approved that the functionalized nanotube has the role of an electron donor and the FLU acts as an electron acceptor at the investigated complexes by the NBO analysis. The global hardness and HOMO–LUMO energy gap of NTCOOH/FLUR reactant are higher than those of NTCOCl/FLUR reactant, indicating that the reactivity of the FLU increases in the presence of NTCOCl and its stability decreases. In addition, covalent functionalization of the drug flutamide onto NTCOOH (COOH mechanism) and NTCOCl (COCl mechanism) has been investigated in detail. The obtained information shows that the activation parameters related to COOH mechanism are higher than those related to the next mechanism. Consequently, for covalent functionalization, a comparison between COOH- and COCl-functionalized CNT shows that using the second one is more suitable due to lower activation energy.

Dihydroortate dehydrogenase immobilization on the nanotubes was carried out, and biochemical characterization of free and immobilized enzyme was determined. In comparison with free enzyme, the immobilized DHODH showed improved stability and reusability for investigation of inhibition pattern of drugs such as leflunomide. The experimental data showed that DHODH was inhibited by the active metabolite of leflunomide, with a K_i and K_I of 0.82 and 0.06 mM, respectively. Also, adsorption of leflunomide on SWCNT and SWBNNT has been explored through a density functional theory–based method. The geometrical and electronic structures, density of state, and frontier molecular orbital were analyzed to predict the adsorption properties and mechanism of these complexes. For the leflunomide/SWBNNT system, our theoretical results showed that the N nuclei were relaxed outward and the B nuclei were relaxed inward of the nanotube after geometry optimization. Also, the tube diameters at the N- and B-ends were not equal in the zigzag model, where that of the N-end was longer than that of the B-end. The computations show that the adsorption of leflunomide on zigzag (6,0) SWBNNT is more stable than in leflunomide on zigzag (6,0) SWCNT. The current results clearly indicate that the adsorption processes for leflunomide molecule and SWNTs are physical in nature.

The calculated adsorption energies for leflunomide/SWCNT and leflunomide/SWBNNT complexes are about 0.0123 and 0.0126 eV, respectively. From the comparison of the values of adsorption energies, it can be concluded that the leflunomide adsorption capability of SWBNNT is higher than that of SWCNT. In the leflunomide/SWCNT system, DN value is positive, indicating that the leflunomide acts as an electron acceptor, whereas in the leflunomide/SWCNT system, DN value is negative, indicating that the leflunomide acts as an electron donor. Interestingly, NBO and AIM analysis revealed that the interaction of nanotubes with leflunomide is more electrostatic (ionic) in nature.

5

Cutting-Edge Nanobiotechnology in Advanced Drug Delivery Nanosystems for CNTs, Fullerenes, NDs, and Graphene-Based Materials

5.1 Introduction

Carbon is one of the most abundant elements on Earth. In nature, it occurs mainly as part of a huge amount of organic matter and, in the form of carbon dioxide, can be found in the atmosphere. Pure carbon occurs in nature in several crystallographic modifications, such as graphite, diamond, lonsdaleite, and chaoite. For example, fullerene C60, or the noncrystalline mineraloid shungite, can also be found in nature. Other allotropic modifications of carbon include graphene (and its various oxidized or reduced forms, including graphene QDs), graphyne, graphdiyne, and carbon nanotubes.

Since ancient times, carbon-based materials such as graphite, charcoal, and carbon black have been utilized for writing and drawing materials. As these materials possess excellent chemical, mechanical, electrical, and thermal features, they have been readily engineered into carbon-based nanomaterials (CNMs), such as carbon nanotubes, graphene oxide, graphene quantum dots, nanodiamonds, fullerenes, carbon nano-onions, and so forth. These materials are now widely explored in biomedical applications.

After carbon nanotubes (CNTs) were discovered [1, 2], their utilization is found to be in diverse range of applications, such as nanomechanical resonators and nanobiological sensors. The unique great physical properties of the carbon nanotube lead to various usage in different fields, such as nanoelectromechanical systems and actuators. The use of CNT in medical fields is enormous. The applications of CNT in electrochemical sensing [3], nanoactuators, and nanosensors are demonstrated in Scheme 5.1.

Nanomechanical resonators have been demonstrated in weigh cell, biomolecules, and gas molecules. There is an increasing attention of CNTs in biological applications. Difficulties of experimental and advantages of the theoretical modeling of nanoscale devices and CNTs are explained.

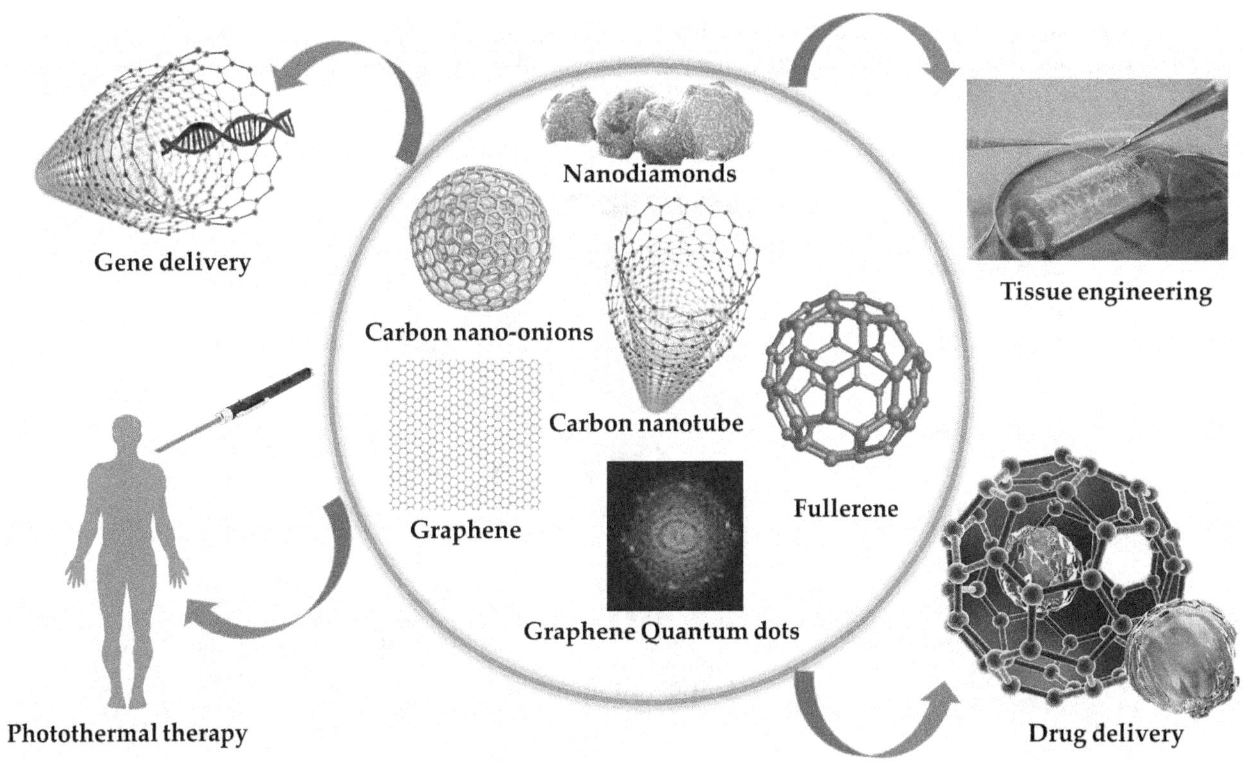

SCHEME 5.1 Applications of different carbon nanomaterials allotropes.

DOI: 10.1201/9781032635989-5

By using CNT-based sensors, the sensing of volatile organic compounds related to human diseases is demonstrated [4], glucose oxidase (GOD) sensing using CNT is performed [5], and the extraordinary low detection limit of CNT working electrodes is shown. Producing biosensors using CNT is an emerging trend. Many articles show the modeling techniques of elastic continuum mechanics concepts for analyzing the vibration of carbon nanotubes. The theory of the mechanical behaviors of materials dealing with continuous mass is called continuum mechanics. There are two significances for the continuum modeling approach. It needs less work of the computational process than the molecular dynamics modeling, and nanostructures behavior analysis is much cheaper through the continuum model. Continuum beam and shell models have been elaborately studied. The beam theory concepts implemented using the single-walled carbon nanotube are explored. The elastic material properties and continuum models of carbon nanotubes have been studied.

The theory of mass recognition using CNT resonators is on the basis of the proven fact that the resonant frequency is sensitive to CNT resonator mass, which includes self-mass of the CNT resonator and attached mass. The change of attached mass on the CNT resonator triggers a change to the resonant frequency. The sensitivity, defined as the ratio of frequency shift to unit mass loaded, is a linear function with the square of the mode number. Advantages of distributed mass load spanning the entire sensor surface in biological and chemical applications were discussed.

Innovations in microfabrication and nanofabrication technologies permit attaining significantly smaller mechanical transducers with micro-sized and nano-sized moving elements whose deformation and vibration are sensitively altered upon molecular adsorption. This type of mechanical biosensors is known as nanomechanical biosensors. The utilization of well-established semiconductor engineering allows the batch production of arrays of numerous nanomechanical systems. In general, all the nanomechanical biosensors are cantilever-shaped. So developing the cantilever or bridge-type mechanical nanobiosensor is getting an important role in emerging medical industry.

Nanotechnology has offered mankind various nano-enabled products or nanosystems, currently also serving various biomedical applications. These nano-constructs and assemblages with drugs, proteins, DNA/RNA, viruses, cellular lipid bilayers, cellular receptor sites, and antibodies (pivotal for immunology) are intricate in the arena of nanostructural scope. Carbon-based nanomaterials (CNMs) could be considered as such a class of nanosystems which have been explored for the delivery of therapeutics, biosensing, and bioimaging. Of late, they have been pragmatic in applications such as regenerative medicine, cancer therapy, and theranostics [6] (Figure 5.1).

Carbon is one of the most interesting elements that possess extreme qualities of forming a wide range of structures with different properties. Carbon is conventionally available in allotropes [7] as "hard" diamond and "soft" graphite, where atoms are pure sp^2 or sp^3 hybrids organized in a hexagonal or cubic lattice; owing to the valance of carbon atoms, other allotropes, such as zero-dimensional fullerenes and carbon quantum dots, one-dimensional carbon nanotubes [1], and two-dimensional graphene sheets (Figure 5.2 and Figure 5.3), have been discovered. Carbon nano-onions (CNOs) are another type of CNMs that are gaining considerable academic and industrial interest for their pertinence in various biomedical extents.

Graphene (GR, Figure 5.3a) [8] is formed by six-membered cycles arranged in planar carbon layers (sp^2 hybridization). In 2010, the Nobel Prize in Physics was awarded for the discovery of a two-dimensional GR material. The surface of graphene is hydrophobic. Graphene nanosheets are composed of more than ten graphene sheets below 100 nm in thickness. GR has very remarkable properties, which makes GR

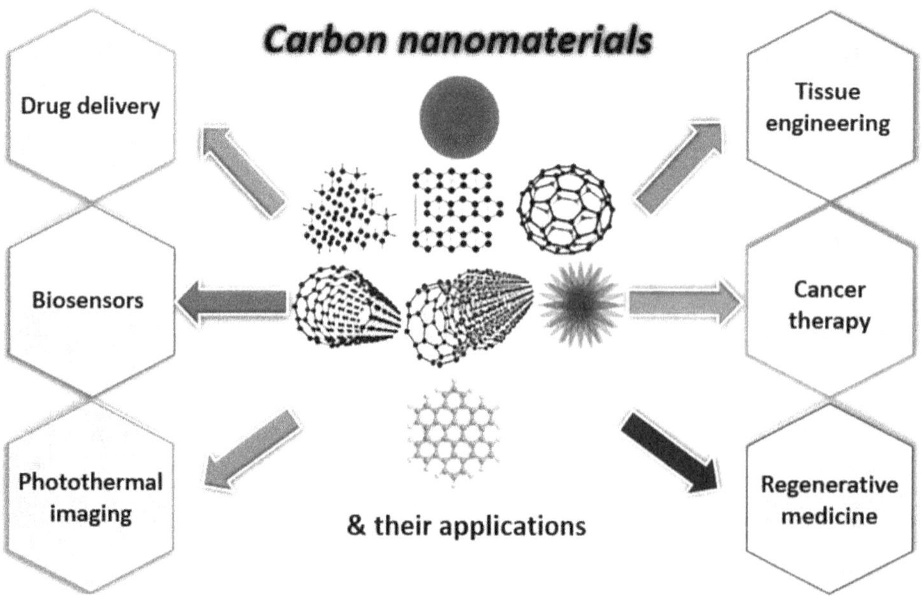

FIGURE 5.1 Carbon nanomaterials and their applications in the vast biomedical arena.

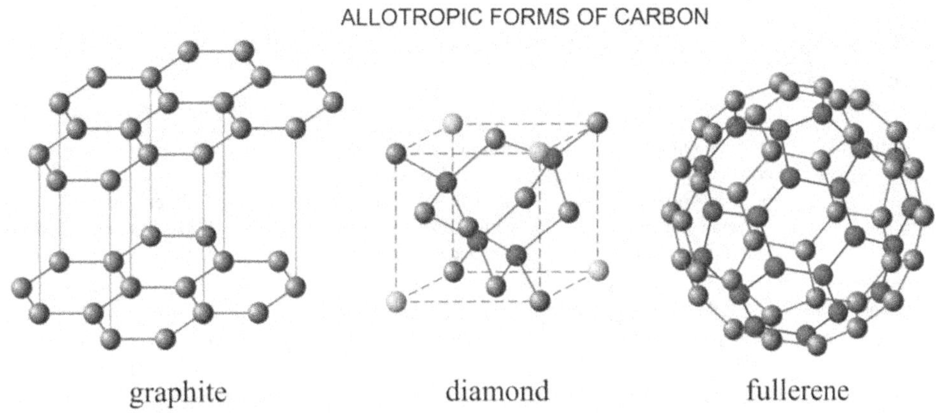

FIGURE 5.2 Various allotropes of carbon.

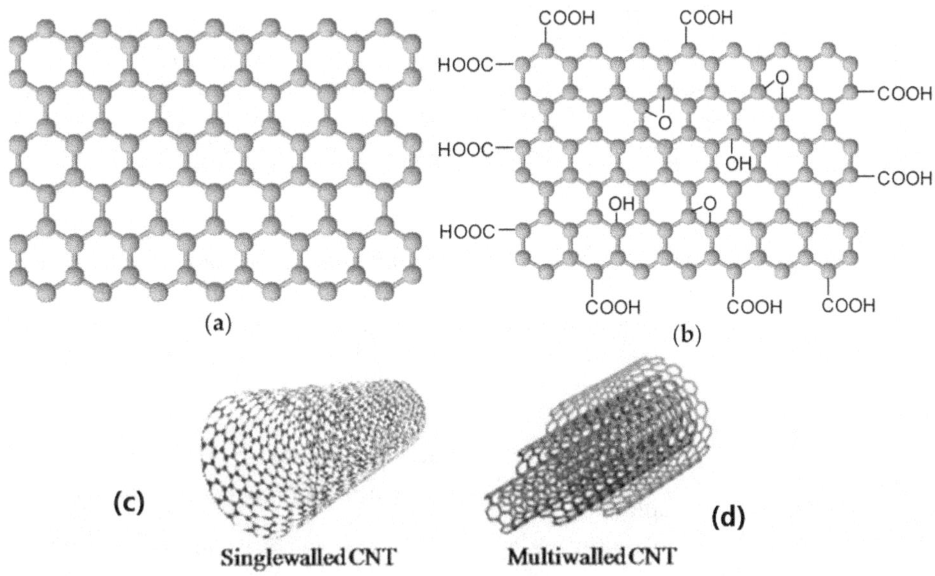

FIGURE 5.3 Structures of (a) graphene and (b) graphene oxide, (c) single-walled carbon nanotubes, and (d) multi-walled carbon nanotubes [8,9].

a very promising material for a variety of bioapplications [9]. Graphene oxide (GO, Figure 5.3b) [8] is prepared by oxidation of GR, that is, by introducing carbonyl, hydroxyl, and epoxide groups on planar surfaces and edges of GR carbon plates. These are carbon structures in the hybridization of sp^1 and sp^2. Graphyne forms monoatomic layers. Graphdiyne has a similar structure to graphyne, which is supplemented by diacetylene bridges [9]. Carbon nanotubes (CNTs) are carbon allotropes with a cylindrical structure with open or closed ends. They can be classified based on the number of concentric layers of rolled graphene sheets: single-walled CNTs (SWCNTs, Figure 5.3c) [9] generally showing an outer diameter of 0.8–2 nm, and multi-walled CNTs (MWCNTs, Figure 5.3d) [9] with outer diameters of 5–20 nm. Their lengths can range from 100 nm to several centimeters [8]. Other characteristics of GR, GO, rGO, and CNTs can be found, for example, in [8].

Carbon nanomaterials possess specific properties, such as high surface area and excellent mechanical and electrical properties, that promote their application also in the therapeutic and diagnostic fields. A few of the advantages of carbon nanomaterials are summarized as follows, and Table 5.1 gives a brief overview of different CNMs discussed in this chapter, with their benefits and limitations:

1. Their supramolecular π–π stacking attribute allows them to adsorb a high amount of drug.
2. As a result of their unique optical characteristics and facile amalgamation with luminous substances, CNMs can be utilized as theranostics materials.
3. CNMs possess excellent heat conversion capacity in the near-infrared region that could be well utilized for photothermal therapy.
4. Tunable surface chemistry can be used for the controlled release of therapeutics.

Colloidal stability in the aqueous suspension of CNMs is a major concern for their utilization in biomedical sectors;

TABLE 5.1

A brief Overview of Carbon Nano-Onions (CNMs), with Their Advantages and Limitations

S. No.	Carbon-Based Nanomaterials	Advantages	Limitations in Biomedical Applications
1.	Carbon nanotubes	Have good mechanical strength, aspect ratio, conductivity, and chemical stability. Offers tunable physical properties (e.g., diameter, length, single-walled vs. multi-walled, surface functionalization, and chirality), biocompatibility, and high surface area.	Lack of solubility in aqueous media, non-homogenous in size (diameter and length), and possibilities of metallic impurities. Pristine CNTs being a lightweight powder may enter into the respiratory tract.
2.	Graphene/graphene oxide/graphene quantum dots	Offers excellent electrical, optical, and thermal properties. The two-dimensional atomic sheet structure of graphene enables more diverse electronic characteristics than CNTs.	Colloidal instability, lack of reproducibility, limited synthetic control, poor chemical stability in the biological environment, susceptibility to the oxidative environment.
3.	Fullerenes	Peculiar photoelectrochemical properties, the possibility of surface modification, and superconductivity.	Low aqueous solubility, accumulation in cell membranes, susceptible to degradation in the presence of light and oxygen, susceptible to deactivation process, such as quenching.
4.	Nanodiamonds	Fluorescence and photoluminescence, biocompatible, smaller size compared to other CNMs, hard, corrosion-resistant, chemical inertness, high electrical resistance, and optical transparency.	Difficult to manufacture via covalent manner, tedious to remove toxic organic solvents while fabrication, abrupt drug release, and tendency to aggregate.
5.	Carbon nano-onions	Unique electronic and structural properties, including the ability to accept electrons reversibly, a high surface-area-to-volume ratio, and broad absorption bands.	Hydrophobic, low biocompatibility, aggregation, prone to oxidation, low surface chemical reactivity.

Source: [13–17].

however, this can be tackled by activating the CNM surface by covalent and non-covalent functionalization techniques. The functionalization of CNMs is one such unavoidable step that involves modification of the surface by introducing specific functional groups. Covalent functionalization approaches include oxidation, ozonolysis, plasma treatments, dehydrogenation, etc.

CNMs have been exploited extensively in the delivery of therapeutics owing largely to the functionalization of their surface, rendering them capable of, for example, crossing biological membranes. Functionalization with appropriate targeting ligand aids in the reduction of cytotoxicity of loaded drugs toward healthy cells and augments therapeutic efficiency. The addition of small targeting molecules—for example, folic acid [10] targeted against folate receptors expressed on the surface of a broad spectrum of solid tumor cells, ligands having affinity against a given receptor overexpressed on a specific tumor type, antibodies that identify tumor-associated antigens, and magnetic nanoparticles—can be associated with the drug-loaded CNMs. Via these methods, active targeting by receptor-mediated endocytosis or drug accumulation at the target site via an external magnetic field can be attained. Thus, functionalized CNMs have found applicability in the delivery of small molecules, peptides, proteins, and nucleic acids. For instance, CNMs have been utilized in the delivery of anticancer agents, fluorescent markers for tumor detection [11], cancer phototherapy [12], theranostics, and so forth.

In this chapter, we have compiled the recent developments attained in the field of CNMs for the delivery of biological and therapeutics, with an emphasis on carbon nanotubes, graphene oxides, graphene quantum dots, fullerenes, nanodiamonds, and carbon nano-onions as carrier materials. We have examined various CNMs employed for the treatment of different dreadful ailments and discussed the toxicity concerns along with their possible remedial approaches. Their fate for clinical use in the upcoming future has also been a focus. We expect that this chapter will assist researchers to focus on the possible designing of CNMs for future biomedical implementations.

5.2 Carbon Nanotubes-Based Drug Delivery

Carbon nanotubes are cylindrical large molecules that are composed of a hexagonal arrangement of sp^2-hybridized carbon atoms (C–C distance of approximately 1.4 Å). The wall of CNTs comprises single or multiple layers of graphene sheets. The single rolled sheets of graphene are termed single-walled carbon nanotubes (SWCNTs), while multi-walled carbon nanotubes (MWCNTs) are formed by the rolling of more than one graphene sheet. Both SWCNTs and MWCNTs are capped at both ends of the tubes in a hemispherical arrangement of carbon networks, known as the fullerenes, wrapped up by the graphene sheet (Figure 5.4). The graphene layers of MWCNTs are separated internally by 0.34 nm on average, which constructs an individual tube of a larger outer diameter of 2.5 to 100 nm, while SWCNTs have diameter in the range of 0.6 to 2.4 nm only. Single-walled CNTs own a well-defined wall structure in comparison to multi-walled CNTs, which have slight structural defects displaying somewhat-unstable nanostructure. CNTs, with their small size, high surface-area-to-volume ratio, and ability to contain biomolecules, are an ideal candidate for the delivery of various substances.

Carbon nanotubes have found enormous potential due to their size (1–100 nm), which can be considered 1,000 times thinner than human hair; still, they are 50 times sturdier than steel. Carbon nanotubes possess exclusive spectroscopic

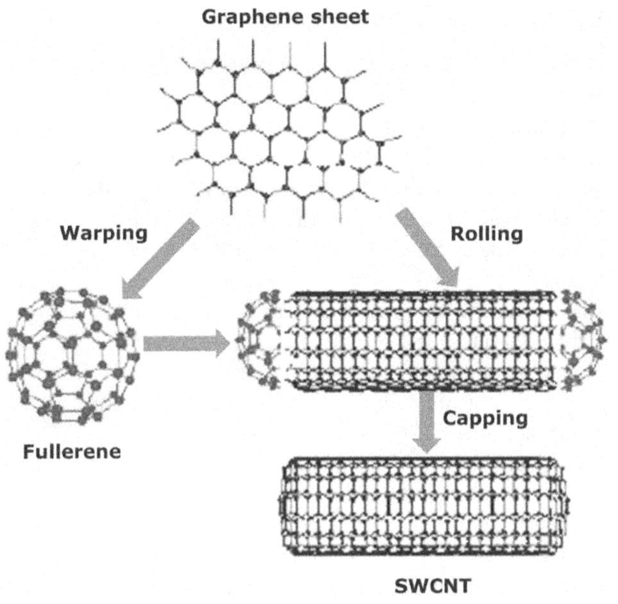

FIGURE 5.4 Preparation method of end-capped single-walled carbon nanotubes (SWCNTs).

properties; their end and sidewalls can be easily functionalized either covalently or non-covalently, and they can be fabricated with bioactive peptides, small-molecule drugs, proteins, or nucleic acids. Such agents can be easily conjugated to the nanotube through a cleavable bond. CNTs possess the potential for penetrating the cells, which enhances the cellular uptake of therapeutic agents and protects them during transportation and cellular permeation. The recent advancements made in the carbon nanotube–based delivery of various therapeutic agents are summarized in Table 5.2.

Drug loading to the end-capped CNTs can be attained during the synthesis or post-synthesis of the CNTs. Drug loading largely depends upon the melting point, reactiveness, surface tension, and sensitivity of the molecules to be inserted and the diameter of the CNTs. After synthesis, drug loading can be achieved by opening up the ends of the CNTs by passing electric currents through them, or by attacking the CNT with acid that corrodes the angled end parts of the tube, or by oxidization using carbon dioxide. The most appropriate method of drug loading is the attachment of a functional group to the CNTs. The functional groups can either be bonded inside or outside of the walls. Gao et al. reported that hydrophobic and van der Waals forces also play an important part in aqueous solutions during drug loading. After loading, CNTs are washed using a solution that dissolves the deposits left on the outer surface.

TABLE 5.2

Recent Advancement in Carbon Nanotube–Based Delivery

S. No.	Indication	Drug/Vaccines/ Genes	CNT Functionalization	Results	Refs.
1.	Cell proliferation	Tissue engineering	Hydrogels of PEG-CNTs	Pristine CNTs and PEG–CNT hydrogels enhanced the cytocompatibility, viability, and proliferation of L29 fibroblasts.	[18]
2.	Cancer	Gemcitabine–Lentinan	MWCNTs/Gemcitabine (Ge)/ Lentinan-Le	MWCNTs-Ge-Le showed augmented chemo and near IR-photothermal synergistic antitumor activity.	[19]
3.	Ischemic brain tissue	Dexamethasone	PEGylated vertically aligned MWCNTs	Low cytotoxicity was observed on the PC-12 cell line by the MWCNTs.	[20]
4.	Bladder cancer	Epirubicin (Epi)	Magnetic MWCNTs–Epi	Externally magnetic-guided MWCNTs showed enhanced sustained release, prolonged retention behavior, and better antitumor activity than the free epirubicin both *in vitro* and *in vivo*.	[21]
5.	Antileishmanial	Cisplatin (Ci)	Ci-SWCNTs, Ci-MWCNTs	Ci-MWCNTs showed potent *in vitro* antileishmanial activity at low concentrations on *Leishmania major*.	[22]
6.	Antibacterial activity	Curcumin	Glucose-modified calcium alginate single-walled carbon nanotubes (CA/ SWCNT-Gl)	CA/SWCNT-Gl nanocomposite showed better antibacterial activity against *Bacillus cereus* and *Escherichia coli*.	[23]
7.	Cancer therapy	Doxorubicin (DOX)	N-isopropyl acrylamide carbon nanotubes loaded with DOX	Smaller polymer chain length resulted in more hydrogen bonding with the drug, five mer N-isopropyl acrylamide–augmented DOX loading.	[24]
8.	Cancer therapy	Doxorubicin	A pH-sensitive conjugate of DOX-loaded SWCNTs and MWCNTs	Bonds between DOX and MWCNTs were stronger, which resulted in controlled drug release in cancer tissues in comparison to SWCNTs.	[25]
9.	Genetic engineering	Plastid genome	Chitosan-complexed SWCNTs utilizing the lipid exchange envelope penetration mechanism	Chitosan–SWCNTs selectively delivered plasmid DNA to the chloroplast in *Eruca sativa*, *Nasturtum officinale*, *Nicotiana tabacum*, and *Soiacia oleracea*, and isolated *Arabidopsos thaliana* mesophyll protoplasts.	[26]
10.	Peptide delivery	G_S-protein	The casing of SWNTs with polycationic and amphiphilic peptides [H-(-Lys-Trp-Lys-Gly-)7-OH]	Seven times more uptake in comparison with the SWCNT–peptide composite without PEGylation.	[27]

Post–drug loading, the caps are closed by passing a current that fuses the ends. Drug loading during synthesis yields low loading efficiency of around 10%, whereas, after synthesis, the drug loading percentage can reach up to 50–100%.

5.2.1 Techniques for the Fabrication of Carbon Nanotubes

Carbon nanotubes can be produced by various innovative methods, such as arc discharge, laser ablation (excluding carbon black), and chemical vapor deposition methods (Figure 5.5). The detailed fabrication methods of CNTs have already been extensively reviewed [28]. Also, the types and properties of these nanomaterials can be manipulated by altering fabrication conditions, such as reaction temperature, input gas concentration, or pressure.

5.2.2 Functionalization of Carbon Nanotubes

As a result of their innate hydrophobic nature, carbon nanomaterials are very difficult to disperse in the aqueous phase. Therefore, to augment their solubility and amalgamation with the biological environment, their surfaces are usually functionalized non-covalently with amphiphilic macromolecules, such as lipids, polymers, and surfactants, or covalently with hydrophilic functional groups.

5.2.2.1 Covalent Functionalization

Covalent modifications can be achieved by the direct sidewall functionalization or by defect group functionalization, which involves converting or rehybridization of sp^2 carbon into sp^3 configurations and, finally, forming covalency with attacking species. This is either accomplished by using halogenation, the cycloaddition of azomethine ylides, and the addition of radicals. The defect group surface modifications are finished by engendering defects by oxidation to yield carboxylic acid functionalities, which render them the functionality to attach various targeting groups, such as peptides, proteins, or antibodies, by employing amidation or esterification. Double and triple covalent functionalization is used for the fabrication of multifunctional CNTs that can be utilized for drug delivery. The double covalent functionalization can be achieved either by 1,3-dipolar cycloaddition and esterification/amidation and cyclopropanation, double arylation, arylation and amidation, amidation and cyclopropanation, double 1,3-dipolar cycloaddition, 1,3-dipolar cycloaddition and arylation, etc. The triple functionalization can be accomplished by simultaneous functionalization with different aryl diazonium salts [29].

5.2.2.2 Non-Covalent Functionalization

The covalent functionalization achieved by the aforesaid modifications may lead to the loss of electrical and optical

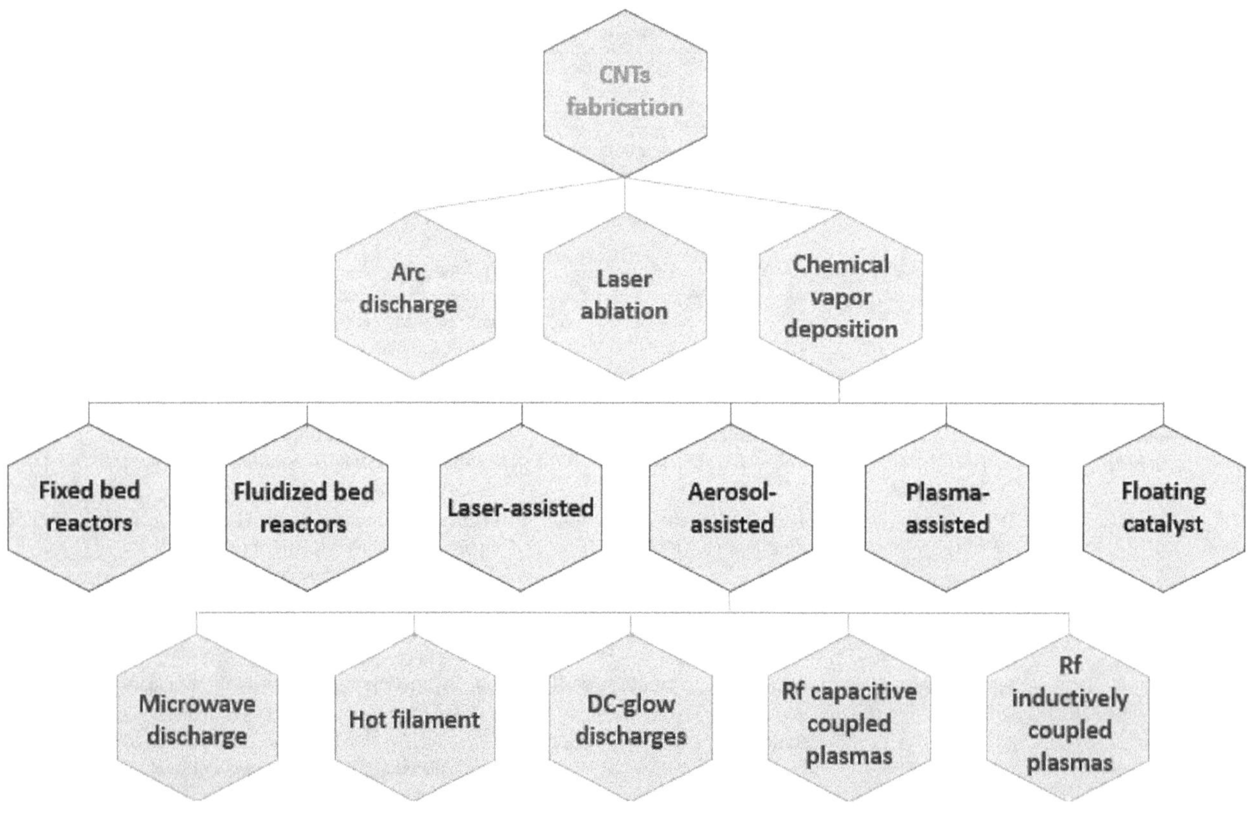

FIGURE 5.5 Fabrication methods of carbon nanotubes.

Source: Adapted from [29].

characteristics of carbon nanomaterials. Therefore, non-covalent functionalization methods were used that can avert the negative effects of the covalent modifications of CNTs. Non-covalent functionalization can be done by adsorption/wrapping biopolymers, surfactants, and polymers on the tubular surface via π–π stacking and van der Waals interactions. Polymers—for example, polyethylene glycol (PEG), poly(vinylpyrrolidone), tetraalkylammonium, poly (meta phenylene vinylene), etc.—are utilized to form a case around the single-walled carbon nanotubes when suspended in a solution of the polymer. Surfactants such as sodium dodecyl sulfate, sodium dodecylbenzene sulfonate (SDBS), Triton X-100, etc. aid in the improvement of dispersibility, solubility, and permeability through the gastrointestinal tract (GIT) by adsorbing on the surface of CNTs via π interactions.

5.2.3 CNTs for Drug Delivery

In the early 1990s, Ijima [30] developed a new allotrope of carbon using the carbon arc discharge method and named it the "multi-walled carbon nanotubes," which was needle-like and made up of several graphene sheets. A few years later, Prof. Ijima and Bethune established single-walled carbon nanotubes. Both single- and multi-walled carbon nanotubes hold exclusive mechanical, electrical, and structural properties which lend them higher forte, litheness, and electrical conductivity toward various biological entities that can be utilized for sensing, diagnosis, and drug delivery.

CNTs have unique electronic properties that are regulated by the quantum confinement of electrons, which propagates the electrons along the tube axis in the forward and backward direction, thus conserving energy and momentum. In addition, CNTs have a smooth density of states (DoS) and are characterized by several van Hove singularities. This DoS relies on the diameter and chirality of the nanotube. The conducting asset of CNT is an inverse function of its diameter, that is, the bandgap between the valence and conduction bands decreases with an increase in diameter. At a definite point, both the bands overlap to give rise to metallic nanotubes.

Pristine CNTs are generally hydrophobic, having poor aqueous and organic solubility, and this hydrophobicity can be attributed to the size, structure, and bundling effect that restricts the uptake and assimilation in the biological environment. Functionalization reduces this bundling effect that occurs due to the van der Waals forces between the adjacent nanotube surfaces, which aids in enhancing the biocompatibility and thus helps in cellular internalization and movement. Few studies reported that the functionalized nanotubes displayed improved biocompatibility with diminished *in vivo* and *in vitro* toxicity. The extent of functionalization relies on the behavioral characteristics and reactivity of sidewall (curvature), the number of functional groups that can be attached to the sidewall, and the steric hindrance between the functional groups and nanotube sidewall [31]. Drug entities can be attached to the functionalized CNTs' sidewalls through covalent or non-covalent bonding.

Saikia N. and Deka RC, in their studies, developed armchair (n, m) and zigzag (n, 0) SWCNTs loaded with 2-methyl heptyl isonicotinate and pyrazinamide, which were functionalized with PEG, and they investigated the structure, electronic properties, and reactivity of a series of 1,3-dipolar cycloaddition (DC) using first-principles density functional theory (DFT) calculations. The researchers reported that with an increase in sidewall functionalization, hardness, and the highest occupied molecular orbital–lowest occupied molecular orbital HOMO–LUMO energy gap decreases, which indicates a decline in the stability of the complex and localized deformation in the nanotube at the site of covalent attachment. They further reported that the solubility of pure isoniazid and pyrazinamide increased in the presence of SWCNTs. The researchers finally concluded that the optimum length and chirality of the CNTs are essential to comprehend the electronic characteristics of functionalized CNTs to understand the mechanism of the delivery of drugs [31].

Kang et al. tested the effect of temperature on the bovine serum albumin (BSA) release from chitosan-functionalized CNT with a thermosensitive polymer, poly-N-isopropyl acrylamide (NIPAAm), and 1-butyl-3-vinyl imidazolium (NIPAAm-co-BVIm). They reported that the release of BSA occurred just above the lower critical solution temperature of polyVBIm (38–40°C. Functionalized CNTs lead to PEGylation, which improves constancy in the body fluids. Both hydrophilic and hydrophobic drug materials can be conjugated with the PEGylated CNTs either on the terminal functional groups of CNTs or to the PEG chains. Prakash Chandra et al. fabricated thermally stable, highly electrically conducting polyaniline MWCNT (PANI/MWCNT) nanocomposites doped in two different protonic acids (i.e., hydrochloric acid and sulfuric acid) by surfactant-assisted in situ oxidative polymerization of aniline in the incidence of potassium persulfate as oxidant. The micellar structure of the surfactant abetted the dispersion of MWCNTs along with the development of PANI/MWCNT tubular structures and provided exceptional electrical and dielectric assets for microelectronic bids [32]. Shi et al. demonstrated ibuprofen release from a hybrid hydrogel composed of sodium alginate, bacterial cellulose, and MWCNTs using an electric field.

A dual-responsive drug delivery system was fabricated by Seyfoori et al. for the precise delivery of doxorubicin using MWCNTs functionalized with $MeFe_2O_4$ magnetic nanoparticles, which were coated with chitosan nanogel. The pH-responsive accelerated drug release was tested on U-87 glioblastoma cells, and the result suggested higher cell mortality in a time-dependent manner [33]. Meherjuoi et al. designed silver (Ag) nanowires as a stimulator for the release of cisplatin from the interior of the various types of CNTs. They compared CNTs, silicon carbide nanotubes, and boron nitride nanotubes and reported that drug release was fast and not dependent on the structural composition of nanotubes.

Gutiérrez-Hernández et al. fabricated functionalized MWCNTs in combination with bacterial cellulose as a three-dimensional (3D) scaffold for osteoblastic cell culture. They mixed the MWCNTs with innate bacterial cellulose (secreted by *Glucanocetobacter xylinus*) to strengthen the mechanical properties of the bacterial cellulose. The BC–MWCNTs scaffold reinforced osteoblast viability, adhesion, and propagation at higher levels in comparison to traditional culture substrates were reported. Finally, they concluded that the BC-MWCNTs scaffold holds the potential for bone regeneration.

Chemotherapeutic agents usually induce systemic toxicity and drug resistance and experience low cellular infiltration. Chemotherapy leads to the death of cancer cells along with normal cells instigating serious side effects. Considering these hindrances, CNTs can protect the chemotherapeutics and, in turn, lower their toxicity toward normal tissues by localizing the drug at the target site [34,35]. Their interaction with lipid membranes and intracellular transport mechanism is inadequately understood, but few studies have suggested that CNTs enter cells via various endocytic processes. During tumor progression, increased tumor vascular permeability and insufficient lymphatic drainage lead to enhanced permeability and retention (EPR effect), which allows these nanoparticles to deliver the anticancer drugs to tumor sites rather than exposing healthy cells to these, thereby reducing toxicity.

Many anticancer drugs have been successfully conjugated with CNTs, such as doxorubicin, flutamide, cisplatin, methotrexate, paclitaxel, etc. Chu et al. prepared integrin-binding arginine-glycine-aspartic acid (iRGD)–conjugated polyethyleneimine (PEI)–functionalized MWCNT conjugated with candesartan (CD). They assembled the formulation with plasmid AT (2) (pAT(2)). They targeted avb3-integrin and AT1R of tumor endothelium and lung cancer cells with iRGD-MWCNT-CD. The anticancer drug molecule displayed synergistic downregulation of vascular endothelial growth factor VEGF upon uniting with pAT (2) and inhabited angiogenesis effectually. Karimi and others fabricated multi-walled CNTs conjugated with folic acid through ethylenediamine coupling. They reported that high cancer cell death was achieved via thermal ablation induced by the CNTs. You and coworkers demonstrated the effective anticancer agent delivery to brain glioma as evident by in vitro and in vivo studies. *In vitro* studies were performed on rat glioma cells (C6) and human glioma cells (U87 and U251), whereas *in vivo* studies were conducted on mice with induced orthopedic brain glioma. From the cytotoxicity studies, they reported that the prepared complex is more cytotoxic than free oxaliplatin and suggested that functionalized MWCNTs can be a good carrier for orthotopic brain tumors [34].

Various herbal anticancer compounds, such as curcumin [36], paclitaxel [37], docetaxel, vinca alkaloids, camptothecin, quercetin, oridonin, etc., have been effectively combined with CNTs for their delivery to cancer cells. Zhao et al. also developed a multi-stimuli-responsive drug delivery system for combinational chemotherapy and photothermal therapy. They fabricated mesoporous carbon nanoparticles (MCN) that displayed high loading efficiency of DOX and used them as near-infrared-responsive drug carriers. Human serum albumin (HSA) was attached to the pore openings of MCN via disulfide bonds and was used as a concierge, owing to its biocompatibility and apposite molecular size. The dispersity and biocompatibility of the developed system were enhanced by PEG functionalization. The drug release was pH-responsive, and *in vitro* studies showed laser power and concentration-dependent photothermal conversion capacity. Biodistribution studies exhibited prolonged retardation of DOX at tumor sites. *In vivo* antitumor studies revealed that MCN/DOX with NIR irradiation displayed the highest tumor inhibition rate against 4T1 tumors in mice. They concluded that the fabricated MCN/DOX system could be discovered as a multi-responsive drug release platform for combinable photothermochemotherapy [38]. Mehra and Jain prepared DOX-loaded folic acid and estrone-anchored PEG-functionalized MWCNTs for the targeted release of drug. They reported the expanded survival period of the experimental model in comparison to the animals treated with free drugs.

5.2.4 CNTs for Vaccine Delivery

A vaccine must instigate a potent immune response at the cellular or humoral level. At the cellular level, it excites cytotoxic T cells, which mark and abolish infected cells, whereas at the humoral level, vaccines rouse the making of counteracting antibodies, which helps opsonization and the following pathogen removal. For diseases such as HIV or malaria, vaccines need both cellular and humoral responses for the deterrence of infection and the abolition of circulating pathogens. The immune system (innate and adaptive) comprises a collection of cells that circulate within the body as well as reside at the site of entry points, such as skin, respiratory, gastrointestinal, and genital tracts, waiting to counter invading pathogens. The innate immune cells, such as macrophages and neutrophils, identify pathogens instantly and abolish them through the activation of different antibacterial effector functions. T and B cells are crucial for the instigation of the cell-mediated and humoral immune system. T cells with CD4+ helper T cells stash various cytokines to control the functions of B cells, whereas CD8+ T cells identify and terminate virus-infected cells.

Vaccine delivery faces many issues, such as inappropriate absorption, the probability of antigen-caused hypersensitivity, anaphylactic responses, and adjuvant vaccine aversion. A lot of new tactics have been tested to boost vaccine delivery, and owing to the adjuvant action, CNTs have also been implied for vaccine delivery to improve the action of the vaccine. The structure of SWCNTs is 100% surface atoms, and thus, they allow the conjugation of various antigens onto their surface. The delivery of vaccines/antigens can be promoted by the engulfment of the system by phagocytic cells, inducing an immune response.

Various types of immune cells, such as macrophages, monocytes, natural killer cells (NK), dendritic cells, and T and B cells, are known to uptake CNTs. At the same time, CNTs did not hamper the health of these cells, due to their non-toxic nature. It is imperative to modify the surface of the single or multi-walled CNTs for the induction of diverse reactive moieties which later can be utilized for the addition of antigenic peptides and proteins as well as vaccines. Chemical modification of the CNTs renders a high dispersion of vaccines, thereby enhancing the performance of the antigen in terms of their pharmacokinetic and pharmacodynamic behavior [39]. Yang and coworkers demonstrated that MWCNTs and tumor lysate protein (tumor cell vaccine) conjugate specifically enhanced the efficacy of antitumor immunotherapy in a mouse model bearing the H22 liver tumor.

The characteristic feature of CNTs to link various antigens or immune stimulants enables them to be attached to bacterial, viral, and protozoal antigens. Pescatori et al. demonstrated a microarray profiling of THP-1 (a monocytic cell line) with both functionalized and non-functionalized CNTs, which activated several genes involved in monocyte response to infection or vaccination, such as nuclear factor kappa-light-chain-enhancer of activated B cells (NF-κB), interleukin-1β (IL-1β), IL-6, and tumor necrosis factor-α (TNF-α), along with others.

5.2.5 CNTs for Gene Delivery

The introduction of nucleic acids has created great curiosity in disease treatment to regulate, repair, restore, add, and/or seize a specific genetic site essential for disease indication. Gene therapy may well be utilized for the delivery of nucleic acids either through viral or non-viral vectors. Viral vectors have shown raised efficacies in transfection, but their clinical application is stalled by the glitches of immunogenicity and oncogenicity, lack of cell targeting potential, and low genetic payload. Non-viral vectors possess an upper hand over viral vectors as they are safe, can deliver genes, and are reasonably inexpensive. Several non-viral vectors (gene carriers), including nanoparticles, peptides, dendrimers, liposomes, carbon nanotubes, etc., have been investigated for gene delivery [40]. CNTs have been widely utilized for the delivery of nucleic acids. The chemical modification of pristine CNTs (single- or multi-walled CNTs), for example, aminated or carboxylated or strengthened CNTs using the proton-rich polymer polyethyleneimine (PEI), offers them litheness for gene therapy. SWNTs or MWNTs offer benefits of effectual surface modification for the designing of nanovectors for effective gene therapy. Varkouhi and his group investigated two cationically functionalized (CNT-PEI and CNT-pyridinium) CNTs for siRNA delivery. They reported that both functionalized CNT-complexed siRNAs showed 10–30% silencing activity and reduced cytotoxicity against H1299 cells. They stated that the type of functionalization of CNTs resulted in a non-cytotoxic CNT-based delivery system. Tan et al. non-covalently functionalized SWCNTs with PL-PEG-NH or PL-PEG-maleimide. They further conjugated the functionalized SWCNTs with a 5′-thiolated siRNA against GFP (siGFP) and RFP (siRFP). They evaluated the silencing of GFP and RFP expression by SWCNT–siRNA via fluorescence spectroscopy and reported a 50–80% GFP expression knockdown in H1299, HeLa, MCF-7, and 293T cells by SWCNT-siGFP. They also observed gene silencing despite incubation with inhibitors on different cellular internalization pathways. SWCNT–siRNA showed successful knockdown of GFP expression in different cell lines, indicating the release of siRNA into the cytoplasm, which silenced the gene expression.

Table 5.3 provides a list of various carbon nanovectors explored in the treatment of cancer.

5.3 Graphene/Graphene Oxide/ Reduced Graphene Oxide

Graphene and its derivatives are the material of thoughtful consideration because of their inimitable inherent assets, such as highly interesting photoluminescence properties, as well as easy surface functionalization, which leads to its applicability in various biological settings. The large surface area, chemical purity, and free π-electrons make graphene a suitable candidate for the delivery of therapeutics, whereby conjugation strategies can enhance the biocompatibility and residence time *in vivo*. These materials have been explored for the delivery of chemotherapeutic agents [54], genes [55], peptides [56], and tissue engineering [57]. The accurate chemical structure of GO has

TABLE 5.3
Various Carbon Nanovectors Used in the Treatment of Tumors

S. No.	Carbon-Based Nanovectors	In Vitro	Indication	Reference
1.	Hyaluronic acid–modified carbon dots	4T1 cells	In vivo antitumor activity	[42]
2.	Poly(ethylene glycol)-block-poly(β-benzyl-L-aspartate) (PEG-b-PBLA) polymers, octadecyl amine-p(Asp-API)10 (OAPI) polymers, and legumain-cleavable linker containing doxorubicin (DOX)–carbon quantum dots conjugations (CDs-C9-AANL-DOX)	Tumor cells	In vivo antitumor activity	[43]
3.	Tegafur-loaded graphene oxide nanosheet	Molecular dynamics simulation survey for drug release across the cell membrane	Antitumor activity	[44]
4.	Epirubicin-loaded multi-walled CNTs	T24 and 5637 cells	Bladder cancer	[21]
5.	Single-walled CNTs	4T1 cells	Chemophotothermal therapy	[45]
6.	Single-walled CNTs	Human breast cancer cell (MCF-7)	—	[46]
7.	Single-walled CNTs	A549 and NIH 3T3 cells	—	[47]
8.	Multi-walled CNTs	HeLa cells	Photothermal therapy	[48]
9.	Double network structured GO	HCT116 cells	Chemophotothermal	[49]
10.	Graphene QDs	BT-474, MCF-7 cells	—	[50]
11.	Graphene QDs	PANC-1, A-549, HepG2	—	[51]
12.	PEG-functionalized multi-walled CNTs	U87, U373MG, NHA	Brain tumor therapy	[52]
13.	Multi-walled CNTs	MCF-7 and MDA-MB-231 human breast cancer cells/rats	—	[53]

Source: [41].

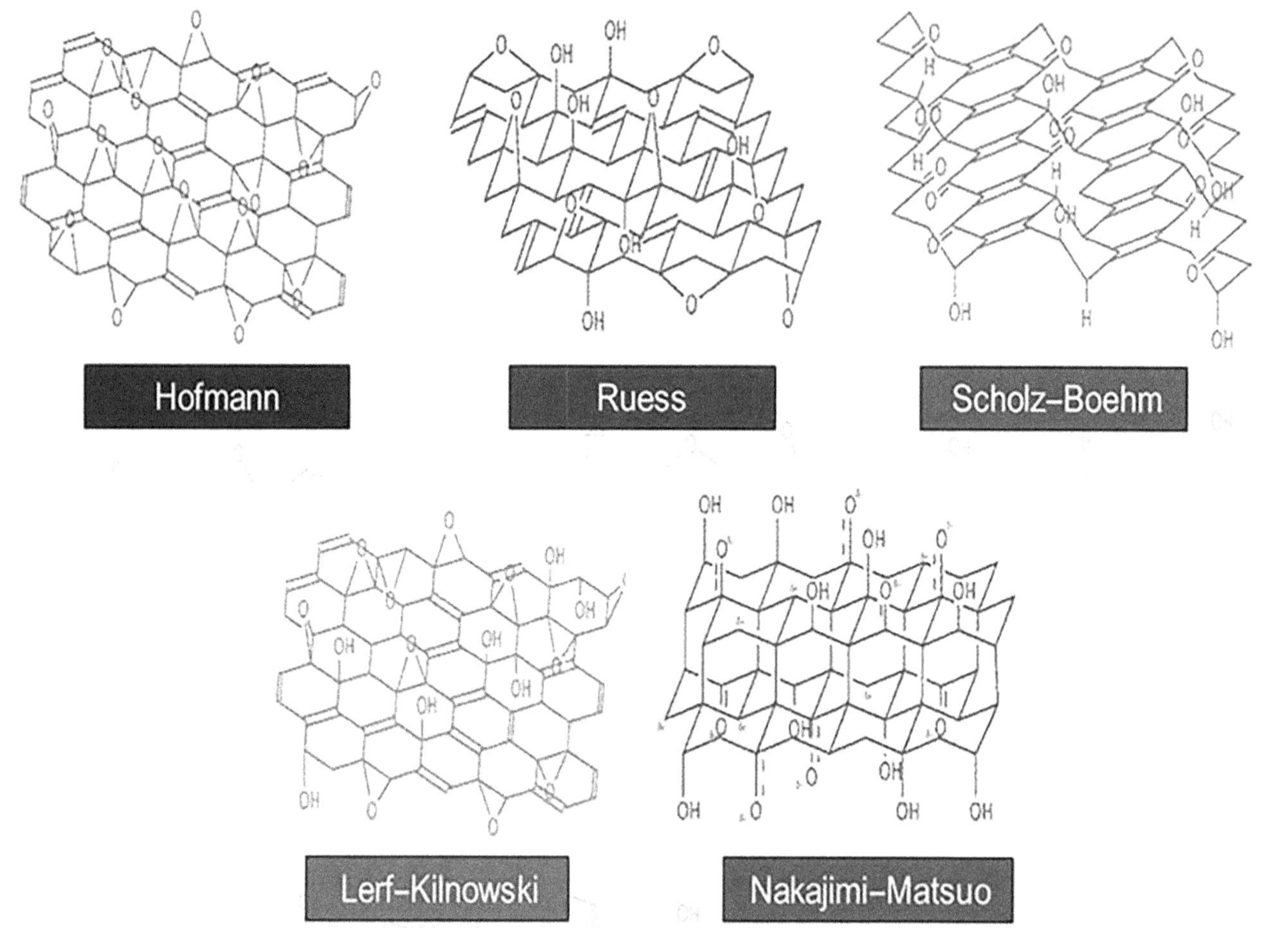

SCHEME 5.2 Different models of GO.

been considered uncertain over the years. The uncertainty is due to several reasons, such as complex amorphous structure of GO, nonstoichiometric composition of atoms, and nonavailability of precise characterization techniques for such materials. However, several old structural models (Scheme 5.2) have suggested a regular framework of GO consisting of distinct repeat units.

The GO structure is composed of epoxy groups (–O–) located diagonally on the basal planes of graphene oxide. The other chemical groups were not present in this model, so this model was not sufficiently informative. The earlier four models were characterized by reactivity, X-ray diffraction, and elemental analysis, whereas the Lerf–Klinowski structure was characterized by solid-state nuclear magnetic resonance spectroscopy. Based on material's reactivity, Lerf also prepared a number of GO derivatives.

Hummers (1958) developed graphene oxide by the vigorous oxidation of graphite. A schematic illustration of their use is given in Figure 5.6. Graphene oxide possesses unique structural features, such as large and planar sp^2 hybridization of carbon, high surface area, and augmented oxygen-containing groups. Oxygen groups offer biocompatibility, physiological solubility, and stability to GO, and a high payload of drugs/genes via chemical conjugation or physisorption tactics can be achieved. Graphene oxide used for drug delivery is generally one to three layers thick, with a size ranging from a few nanometers to several hundred nanometers [58].

5.3.1 Techniques for the Fabrication of Graphene

Graphene can be synthesized using two methods, namely, bottom-up and top-down synthesis methods. The synthesis methods lend excellent properties to these materials. The interaction between therapeutics and graphene-based materials depends on their properties, such as layer number, lateral dimension, chemical residual, surface charge, and surface functional groups.

Bottom-Up Synthesis: This method includes three procedures: (1) epitaxial growth on silicon carbide, (2) the chemical vapor deposition method (CVD), and (3) the plasma-enhanced chemical vapor deposition (PECVD) method. The first method uses the thermal decomposition of silicon carbide at

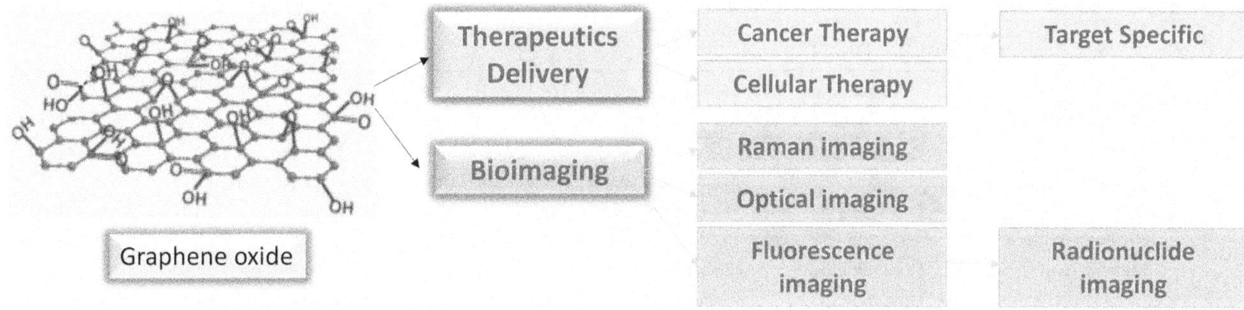

FIGURE 5.6 Various applications of graphene oxide in the biomedical arena.

Source: Adapted from Rowley-Neale et al. (2018).

high temperatures under vacuum or in inert gas. As carbon has negligible vapor pressure in comparison to silicon, graphene layers are formed on the silicon carbide surface after silicon sublimation. Large-surface-area graphene can be produced by the CVD method. In this method, a precursor gas (e.g., methane, acetylene, ethylene, propene) containing hydrocarbon molecules is charged into the reactor, in which the hydrocarbon molecules are catalytically decomposed into carbon radicals and arranged into graphene structures on the catalytic layer of the substrate (Ni, Cu, Rh, Co, or alloys). The properties of the fabricated graphene, such as layer number and crystal size, are largely affected by several factors, such as precursors, assistant gases, catalyst layer, and temperature. PECVD shows an advantage over CVD in the synthesis of graphene at a relatively low temperature with reduced deposition time. It also resolves the evaporation problem of a catalyst layer at high temperatures.

Top-Down Synthesis: This method helps in the segregation of graphene sheets from high-quality graphite, which contains stacked multi-layer graphene, using a mechanical or chemical method. It involves mechanical and chemical exfoliation methods and the GO reduction method. The mechanical exfoliation method is used to separate graphene from graphite using a scotch adhesive tape to break the van der Waals force between the layers of graphite by a repeated sticking-and-lifting process, producing high-quality graphene, but it lacks large-scale production ability. On a large scale, graphene can be fabricated using the reduction of graphene (rGO) method. This method involves GO production and GO reduction to rGO by the method described by Hummers. The oxidation process involves the reaction of graphite with sodium nitrate, concentrated sulfuric acid, and potassium permanganate, which introduces oxygen-containing functional groups onto graphite sheets. The graphene oxide layer can be separated by ultrasonication in a polar solvent, for example, water, because of the introduction of an enlarged layer space due to the insertion of functional groups.

5.3.2 Functionalization of Graphene

For their biomedical use, graphene-based materials should be functionalized for the same reasons mentioned earlier for CNTs. This can be achieved, for instance, via PEGylation or coating with dextran, both of which decrease their toxicity and augment their biocompatibility. Surface functionalization can be achieved by non-covalent and covalent binding.

Non-Covalent Functionalization: This method involves forces such as hydrophobic interactions, π–π stacking, or electrostatic binding between the graphene-based materials and the active molecules. The hydrophobic interactions are utilized to absorb the aliphatic parts of surfactants onto the graphene by the interaction of polar parts of surfactants, thus enhancing the stability of surfactant-functionalized graphene or rGO in polar solvents. Electrostatic interactions can also be used for the functionalization of these materials, since GO sheets are negatively charged, and consequently, a positively charged biomolecule can be electrostatically adsorbed to the surface of the GO surface. The same strategy can also be used to flexibly modify the GO surface with polymers and targeting ligands.

Covalent Functionalization: The functional groups, such as the carboxyl, epoxy, and hydroxyl groups, on the GO can be used for covalent functionalization. Similarly, the carboxylic acid group of GO can be utilized for the amidation reaction with the amine group in polymers. PEI functionalization was achieved on poly(acrylic acid)–modified GO upon the reaction of ethyl(dimethylaminopropyl) carbodiimide/N-hydroxy succinimide EDC/NHS with the carboxylic acid group. This covalent functionalization augmented the in vitro proliferation and focal adhesions in hMSCs of the GO–PEI nanocomposites [59]. Due to its highly cationic charge density, PEI can also be electrostatically adsorbed to the GO surface (as outlined earlier) and thus serve as a versatile platform for further functionalization based on amine chemistry.

5.3.3 Graphene Oxide for Drug Delivery

Several hydrophobic drugs, for example, doxorubicin and docetaxel, can be adsorbed onto graphene using simple physisorption via π–π stacking, along with antibodies for the selective targeting to cancer cells. π–π stacking and electrostatic or hydrophobic interactions of graphene provide a high carrying capacity of poorly soluble drugs deprived of conceding drug strength. Table 5.4 summarizes the application of GO-based drug delivery.

Boran et al. conjugated graphene oxide with zoledronic acid (ZOL-GO) and evaluated these *in vitro* on cells. They explored

TABLE 5.4
Application of Graphene Derivatives for Drug Delivery

S. No.	Graphene Derivative	Therapeutic Agents	Application and Outcomes	References
1.	GO	Zoledronic acid	Bone marrow–derived mesenchymal stem cells (BM-MSC), and Michigan Cancer Foundation-7 (MCF-7) breast cancer cells.	[60]
2.	Pristine graphene and graphene oxide	Doxorubicin	In vitro: pH simulation.	[61]
3.	Graphene oxide	Doxorubicin	In vitro: drug release.	[62]
4.	GO-FA-AuNPs	Doxorubicin	Significant in vivo tumor reversion in solid tumor model in Balb/c mice.	[63]
5.	GO nanosheets doped into ZnO NPs	Doxorubicin	GO-doped ZnO NPs displayed higher drug loading efficiency of 89% in comparison to 82% of ZnO. The developed system enhanced the dissolution of the drug.	[64]
6.	PEG-functionalized GO	Cephalexin	In vitro, CEF release exhibited burst release, followed by sustained release over the 96 h period, with a cumulative release of 80%. MIC values stated dose- and time-dependent antibacterial activity for GO-PEG-CEF against both gram-positive and gram-negative bacteria.	[65]
7.	GO-PVP	Quercetin and gefitinib	Dual drug-loaded GO-PVP nano-vehicles showed higher drug loading, and cancer cell cytotoxicity was more in contrast to an individual GO-PVP system in PA-1 ovarian cancer cells and compared to their effects on IOSE-364 ovarian epithelial cells.	[66]
8.	GO	Ampicillin, chloramphenicol, and tetracycline	GO potential as an antibacterial along with antibiotic drugs displayed synergistic effects against *S. aureus*, *E. coli*, *E. faecalis*, and *P. aeruginosa* and the toxicological effects of GO toward human epidermal keratinocytes (HaCaT).	[67]
9.	PEGylated GO	Doxorubicin	PEGylation of the GO efficiently augmented the average water density around the nanocarrier, which acts as a barricade, leading to the DOX migration to the solvated PEG-free part of the GO surface. The computational results exhibited the fact that increasing the PEG chain length aids DOX loading on the nanocarrier.	[68]

Source: [41].

the allied morphological changes of bone marrow–derived mesenchymal stem cells (BM-MSC) and MCF-7 breast cancer cells along with the effect of the drug on the mineralization of BM-MSCs. They reported that the nanostructured ZOL-GO facilitated the mineralization of BM-MSC cells, which was demonstrated by the formation of clusters around the cells. The Boran group concluded that the ZOL-GO nanostructures can be a promising drug complex for the treatment of osteoporosis and metastasis [60].

Islami et al. constructed efficient quercetin-loaded single-layer graphene oxide (GO) sheets grafted with hyperbranched polyglycerol (HPG) on the surface of GO through the ring-opening hyperbranched polymerization of glycidol. The fabrication was carried out using both a modified and improved Hummers method. HPG improved the stability of GO sheets in biological fluids with augmented drug-loading capacity and high encapsulation efficiency. HPG-GO displayed the controlled and sustained release of quercetin and suggested that an acidic pH could aid in the drug release. Moreover, the HPG-GO did not exhibit cytotoxicity on the MCF-7 cell line in diverse concentrations during 72 h incubation [69].

Yang et al. developed a magnetic and bio dual-targeting GO–Fe nanoparticle hybrid. From the in vitro experiments, they demonstrated that the drug delivery cargo not only enhanced the anticancer outcome but can also provide site-specific targeting of the SK3 human breast cancer cells by the magnetic field–guided GO–Fe nanoparticles. Yu et al. designed an α, β6-targeting peptide (HK-peptide)–functionalized and photosensitizer (HPPH)–coated graphene oxide (GO (HPPH)-PEG-HK), which triggered the dendritic cells and expressively barred tumor growth and lung metastasis by increasing the intrusion of cytotoxic $CD8^+$ T lymphocytes in the interiors of the tumors, as evinced by *in vivo* optical and single-photon emission computed tomography.

The Cheon group fabricated a doxorubicin-loaded BSA-functionalized graphene sheet for combinational chemo- and photothermal therapy in brain tumors. Fong et al. developed hyaluronic acid-chitosan-g-poly (N-isopropyl acrylamide) grafted DOX-folic acid-GO thermosensitive hydrogel for breast cancer therapy. Shao et al. fabricated a mesoporous silica nanoparticles coated with polydopamine functionalized with rGO, followed by modification with hyaluronic acid and loaded with DOX. The developed system was pH-dependent, which triggered the release of the chemotherapeutic agent and proved to be an effective carrier for cancer therapy.

5.3.4 Graphene Oxide for Gene Delivery

Graphene-mediated gene delivery has emerged as a novel technique where graphene derivatives have shown tremendous potential for gene transfection. However, it is essential to modify graphene derivatives with polymers to render them with cationic surface properties, which facilitate electrostatic interactions with anionic oligonucleotides. To date, PEI and poly(sodium 4-styrenesulfonates) have been well thought out for gene delivery via graphene derivatives [70].

Zhang et al. observed the use of PEI-conjugated GO to deliver DOX and siRNA. They demonstrated that the conjugate not only enhanced the therapeutic efficiency but also led to an increment in safety. Similarly, Feng et al. explored the effects of PEI (1.2 kDa and 10 kDa) on the cytotoxicity of PEI-GO. Cao and the group reported the role of lactosylated chitosan oligosaccharide LCO–functionalized GO in the removal of toxicity and the enhancement of loading efficiency of fluorescein amidites (FAM)-DNA to human hepatic carcinoma cells (QGY-7703). Liu and his group fabricated a graphene-based gene vector by employing graphene-oleate-polyamidoamine (PAMAM) dendrimer hybrids, owing to the high dispersion and stability of graphene in water solutions. The hybrid was developed by using oleic acid and covalent binding of PAMAM dendrimers. The group investigated the plasmid DNA transfection capacity and its cytotoxicity toward HeLa and MG-63 cells. They reported that the developed hybrid was biocompatible to HeLa cells, and cell viability retains about 80%, although the hybrid was cytotoxic to MG-63 cells at concentrations above 20 mg/mL.

5.4 Graphene Quantum Dots (GQDs)

Graphene quantum dots (GQDs) have found their place recently as the newest member of the carbon nanomaterial family. GQDs comprise a few layers of graphene, and its functional group has a lattice distance of about 0.24 nm with sp^2 hybridization, which is somewhat similar to a small flake of graphene. They can be differentiated from carbon quantum dots (CQDs), which possess a lattice distance of about 0.34 nm, and further, CQDs are amorphous with sp^3 hybridization. GQDs possess characteristic photoluminescence owing to quantum confinement. Also, GQDs hold the same features as graphenes, such as large surface area and free π-electrons availability, which makes them suitable for imaging, sensing, cancer therapy, etc.

5.4.1 GQDs for Drug Delivery

The oxygen-rich surface of the GQDs is the key feature that makes them suitable for drug adsorption and enhancing colloidal stability *in vivo*, along with the features of a single atomic layer and small size. The fluorescent characteristics of graphene quantum dots render them traceable when targeted to, for example, cancer cells. Tian et al. developed a framework of zeolite imidazolate (ZIF-8)–embedded DOX-loaded GQDs, which showed an acidic pH-responsive drug release behavior. Zheng et al. demonstrated intracellular drug delivery and real-time drug release from DOX-loaded aptamer/GQD-capped fluorescent mesoporous silica nanoparticles. Under extracellular conditions, the fluorescence of the fluorescent mesoporous silica nanoparticles (MSNs) remains off at a low ATP level. When the nanocarrier is recognized and internalized into the target tumor cells by an AS1411 aptamer, in the ATP-rich cytoplasm, the ATP aptamer causes the shedding of the GQDs from the nanocarriers, thus resulting in drug release, and at the same time, the fluorescence of MSNs provides real-time imaging possibility.

The Wei group developed DOX-loaded GQDs and conjugated them with Cy5.5 dye via a cathepsin D-responsive (P) peptide, which augmented tissue penetration and cellular uptake of the drug. The cell uptake in 4T1 cells and the drug release were monitored by confocal laser scanning microscopy. The GQD-treated cells displayed blue fluorescence, exhibiting the internalization of the developed formulation. They reported superior therapeutic performance both *in vitro* and *in vivo* due to the enhanced tissue penetration and cellular uptake. The developed system served as probes for programmed tracking of the drug delivery and release process, as well as drug-induced cancer cell apoptosis via the GQDs, doxorubicin, and Cys fluorescence. The Nigam group fabricated a GQD-conjugated gemcitabine-loaded HAS nanoformulation for the targeted delivery of the drug to the tumor cells with the help of albumin via the gp60 pathway.

5.5 Fullerenes Composition

Buckyball clusters, or buckyballs, also known as endohedral fullerenes, include fullerenes, buckminsterfullerene, and C60, which are composed of fewer than 300 carbon atoms. Fullerenes possess numerous functional points that permit the attachment of chemical groups of targeting ligands in three-dimensional orientations, which could facilitate cellular targeting. It is also possible to modify their allotropes to optimize pharmacokinetic characteristics, therapeutic effects, and other attributes, such as size, hydrophilicity, and colloidal stability in a biological environment.

5.5.1 Techniques for the Fabrication of Fullerenes

Fullerenes can be synthesized via the pyrolysis of polycyclic aromatic hydrocarbon as naphthalene, corannulene, or higher polycyclic compounds. These compounds are decomposed at high temperatures (around 1,000°C) with the cleavage of hydrogen bonds and production of mainly C60 and C70, in the presence of an inert gas (argon). Fullerenes can also be fabricated by an arc discharge method between two graphite electrodes by applying high voltage. The discharge induces vaporization of the graphite with the formation of plasma. Fullerenes are synthesized by condensation of the graphite plasma in particles that get deposited onto the reactor walls [71].

5.5.2 Functionalization of Fullerenes

Fullerenes are functionalized to overcome the problems of poor water solubility and low solubility in several organic solvents. Their surface can be functionalized by the use of a solubilizing agent complexation to partially mask the surface of the fullerenes and by covalent functionalization. The presence of double bonds in the fullerene structure lends them to be modified greatly by functional groups of choice. Fullerenes are comprised of carbon of erratic size and molecules that look like a hollow sphere or tube. They are composed exclusively of carbon in varying sizes resembling a hollow sphere, ellipsoid, or tube with a strong apolar character that enables them to develop into lipid-like systems that can easily cross biological membranes.

5.5.3 Fullerenes for Drug Delivery

Zhao's group prepared a fullerene-based (C82) DOX-loaded cyclic RGD (DOX-C82-cRGD) complex for lung cancer treatment that possessed probable clinical effectiveness. Hazrati and coworkers constructed a C30B15N15 heterofullerene carrier system by employing the density functional theory for the delivery of isoniazid. They reported that the interaction of the -NH_2 group of isoniazid with the boron atom of the fullerene engendered a high amount of energy, which altered the fluorescence emanation of the $C_{30}B_{15}N_{15}$ that caused the parting of isoniazid from the surface of the carrier by proton attack at a low pH of cancerous tissues.

Tan and coworkers fabricated a biocompatible and water-soluble fluorescent fullerene (C60-TEG-COOH)–coated mesoporous silica nanoparticle, which delivered the DOX in a pH-responsive manner, and the cellular uptake of nanoparticles was detected via the green fluorescent property of the C_{60}. Fullerenes have also found their application in the delivery of anti-inflammatory agents. Recently, C60 fullerenes have been recognized to persuade the suppression of Ag-driven type-I hypersensitivity through the prominent prevention of an IgE-dependent mediator. Hence, they can manage mixt mast-cell-dependent allergic inflammations, asthma, inflammatory arthritis, heart diseases, and multiple sclerosis. Also, fullerenes exhibit anti-inflammatory properties by stabilizing mast cells and peripheral blood basophils and inhibiting the release of proinflammatory mediators.

5.5.4 Fullerenes for Antibody/Antiviral Delivery

Fullerenes, due to their excellent surface structural properties, have also been utilized in the delivery of antibodies. Ashcroft and coworkers successfully conjugated antibodies to fullerenes by using a novel water-soluble C60 derivative as the fullerene scaffold. The scaffold was modified through the Bingel–Hirshc reaction, and an antibody, ZME-018, was covalently attached through the disulfide bridge exchange. ZME-018 explicitly targets the gp240 antigen present in over 80% of the human melanoma cells. Fullerenes were also functionalized to produce a photoactive stage for the distant deactivation of viruses and bacteria. Kim and his group fabricated a substratum of hot-pressed silica particles placed on a metallic substrate functionalized with 3-aminopropyltrietoxysilane and amine groups to covalently couple the fullerenes. The research group studied the inactivation of the MS2 bacteriophage at predefined distances from the irradiated surface and reported disinfection of the bacteria and virus by the immobilized C60 in the gas phase via photosensitization, contrary to singlet oxygen ($^1O_2$), which was effective up to around 10–15 cm from the surface [72].

5.6 Nanodiamonds (NDs)-Based Drug Delivery

Nanodiamonds (NDs) are the newest exposed allotropes of carbon with a large surface area and a single crystal size of 2–8 nm. NDs are mostly created by the detonation process and chemical vapor deposition methods. They are nanocrystals with tetrahedral carbon atoms in a 3D cubic trellis owning a diamond-shaped structure with electrical properties of diamond, coated with an onion-like graphite shell. Their surface comprises functional groups formed on the ND surface after purification stemming from the residual (non-diamond) carbon as a result of the detonation process, usually containing oxygen, such as hydroxyl, carboxylic acid, ketone, lactone, and ether. NDs with nitrogen vacancies in their center, thus exhibiting photoluminescence characteristics, are termed fluorescent NDs (FNDs) and have found highly interesting applications in bioimaging [73–75].

ND physicochemical properties, such as size and surface chemistry, are highly decisive for their fluorescence properties [76]. NDs are very seldom present as single crystals in solution, the aggregates of which determine their size during application. Nevertheless, these aggregates are often hydrophilic due to the functional groups and can thus still form a stable aqueous colloidal suspension [77], which is imperative for their biomedical applicability. Due to this property, NDs have also been proposed as drug carriers, whereby the large surface area is exploited for adsorbing or linking numerous drug moieties on the surface of the NDs by covalent and non-covalent functionalization methods. However, given the diversity of the ND surface, owing to the production method, the precise surface chemistry of ND is challenging to control and define. Another widely employed strategy to make use of the intrinsic photoluminescent properties of ND while increasing their drug-carrying capacity is by coating the ND with shells of other materials that can harbor drug molecules in much higher amounts than what can be adsorbed onto the native ND surface or otherwise improve their biomedical applicability. The drug adsorption onto native nanodiamonds depends on parameters such as maximal monolayer capacity, binding strength, and the degree of drug removal from the solution. The various applications and advantages of NDs are illustrated in Figure 5.7.

5.6.1 Nanodiamonds for the Delivery of Therapeutics

The Li group successfully treated the immunosuppression associated with glioblastoma with DOX-polyglycerol-ND composites. They developed cellular and animal GBM models by THP-1-derived dendritic cell and female athymic Balb/c nude mice correspondingly. The group reported that the nanocomposite could rouse the immunogenicity of glioblastoma cells both *in vivo* and *in vitro* by persuading autophagy and emanating antigens from the glioblastoma cells [10]. Roy et al. formulated -COOH-functionalized and -NH_2-functionalized NDs loaded via monolayer surface adsorption with efavirenz. They revealed that the bioavailability of the efavirenz was augmented, and non-functionalized NDs possessed higher

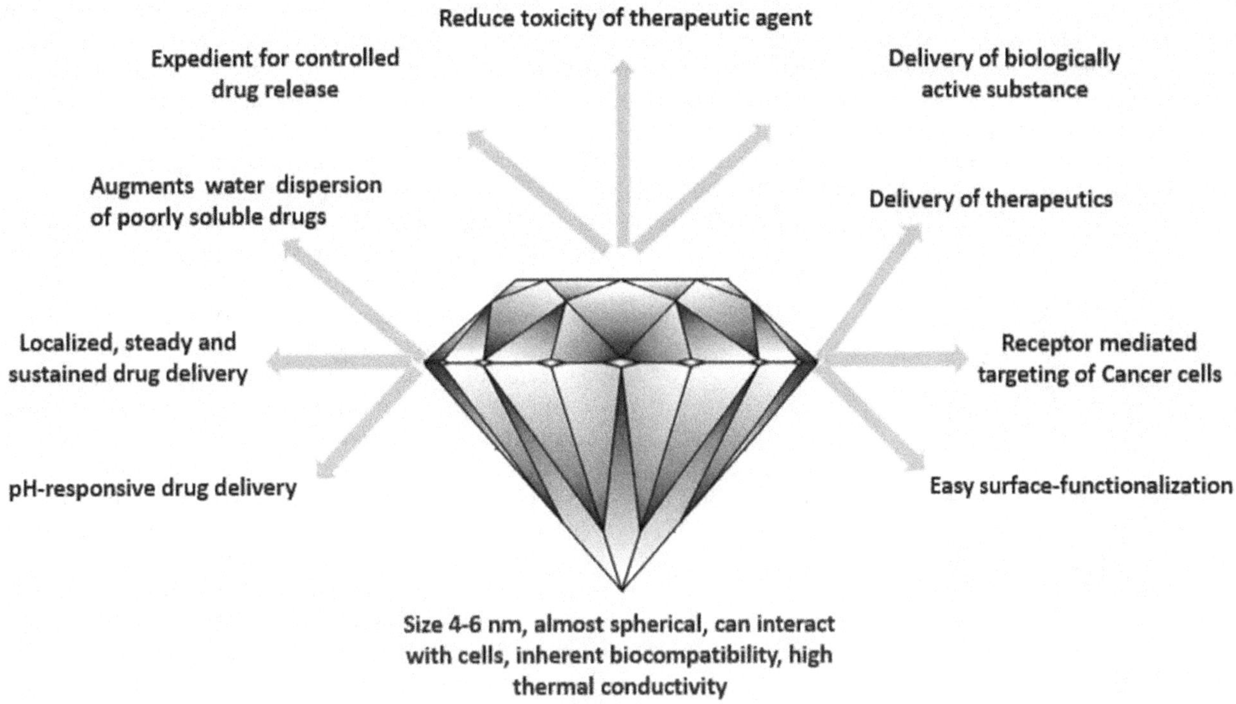

FIGURE 5.7 Applications and advantages of nanodiamonds.

Source: **Adapted from [16].**

drug-loading capacity than the functionalized NDs. They demonstrated that the functionalized NDs can infiltrate the blood–brain barrier and release the drug in the central nervous system using an *in vitro* BBB model of primary human brain microvascular endothelial cells and astrocytes. Neural stem cells can multiply and segregate into astrocytes, neurons, and oligodendrocytes. This differentiation of neural cells can be helpful in the treatment of neurodegenerative diseases, such as Alzheimer's and Parkinson's [78].

Nanodiamonds can boost neural stem cell adhesion and differentiation. In a trial, Taylor et al. demonstrated that the NDs support rodent neuronal outgrowth. They inspected the interaction of human neural stem cells with the NDs. Edgington and Jackman nurtured human neural stem cells with oxygen- and hydrogen-functionalized monolayers of NDs and evaluated neural stem cell adhesion and proliferation for seven days and stated that the adhesion and proliferation were higher with oxygen-functionalized NDs than in the hydrogen-functionalized NDs. It was reported that the ND monolayers can provide comparable physicochemical characteristics of extracellular matrix protein. Their report suggested that the NDs can be a substratum for neuronal growth and be a possible applicant in neurodegenerative brain disorders.

5.7 Carbon Nano-Onions (CNOs)-Based Drug Delivery

Carbon nano-onions (CNOs) are zero-dimensional carbon nanoparticles that are categorized by their multi-layered closed shells all encompassing one another, similar to that of an onion. These CNOs possess a diameter in the range of 1.4 to 50 nm, with an interlayer distance of approximately 3.4 Å, with a C60 or C80 fullerene at their core (Figure 5.8) [79]. Structural and dimensional variations are bound and vast, depending on the method of preparation. CNOs can be fabricated through various techniques, which results in the production of CNOs of various shapes and sizes. DC arc discharge [80], electron beam irradiation, underwater arc discharge, thermal annealing under high vacuum, thermal annealing under helium environment, catalyst-free synthesis through thermolysis under Ar or air environment, and thermal reduction are the methods that can be used for the production of CNOs with tunable sizes and shapes.

Pristine carbon nano-onions (p-CNOs) developed through the aforementioned methods are hydrophobic, which leads to their aggregation in aqueous and organic solvents, even after sonication. Their solubility and dispersibility can be amended via covalent and non-covalent surface modification. The covalent functionalization of CNOs, particularly by oxidation, renders them with augmented water dispersibility, extending the possibility of amidation and esterification reactions of the carbon nano-onions. CNOs can be functionalized by non-covalent interactions via electrostatic interactions, van der Waal forces, and π interactions.

5.7.1 Carbon Nano-Onions for Therapeutics Delivery

Utilizing the functionalization of the CNOs, their application in various biomedical sections, such as drug delivery, tissue engineering, bioimaging, sensing, CNOs as a drug for cancer, and CNS-related disorders have been vastly explored (Figure 5.9, Table 5.5) [41]. The supramolecular functionalization of CNOs via stimuli-responsive biocompatible polymers enables them to be an effective targeted drug delivery system. Narsimha and coworkers engineered 4-hydroxyphenyl methacrylate-carbon nano-onions (PHPMA-CNOs = f-CNOs) embedded bovine serum albumin (BSA) nanocomposite fibers

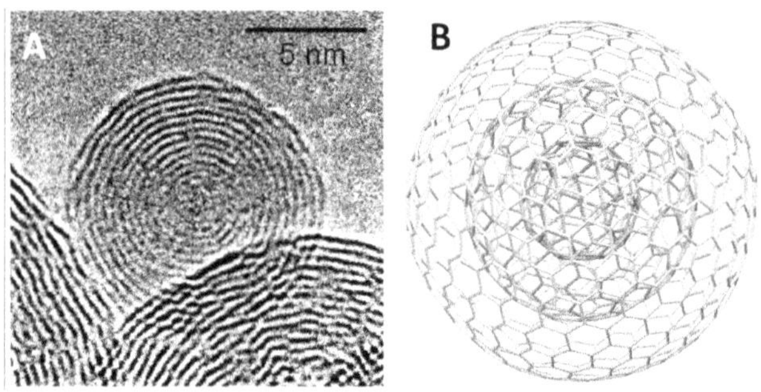

FIGURE 5.8 High-resolution TEM image of (a) carbon onion and (b) structure of carbon onion.

Source: Reproduced with permission from Camisasca and Giordani (2017).

by Forcespinning® (FS) technology for stimuli-responsive delivery of DOX. The group reported a slow and prolonged DOX release over a 15-day study along with augmented thermal properties and *in vitro* degradation. They tested the cytotoxicity of hydrogels with osteoblast cells that displayed good cell viability and cell growth. The developed system exhibited a pH-responsive sustained drug release over 15 days, which suggested that zein/f-CNOs hydrogel could be a potential drug delivery system for the colon [81].

D'Amora et al. functionalized CNOs non-covalently with hyaluronic acid–phospholipid (HA-DMPE) and successfully targeted CD44 overexpressed cancer cells. Functionalization augmented the solubility of the nanoconstruct, enhanced the *in vitro* cell toxicity in human breast carcinoma cells overexpressing CD44, and increased the uptake in comparison to human ovarian carcinoma cells with an imperceptible amount of CD44. They reported that the CNOs composite possessed high *in vivo* biocompatibility in zebrafish (*Danio rerio*) during the different stages of development and established CNO localization in the digestive tract of the zebrafish larvae [87].

Carbon nano-onion/surfactant (CNO/surfactant) composites facilitate the manufacturing of soluble nanostructures by utilizing the hydrophilic attribute of surfactants and robustness of carbon structures in the fabrication of CNO/surfactant composites, with enhanced solubility and other physicochemical

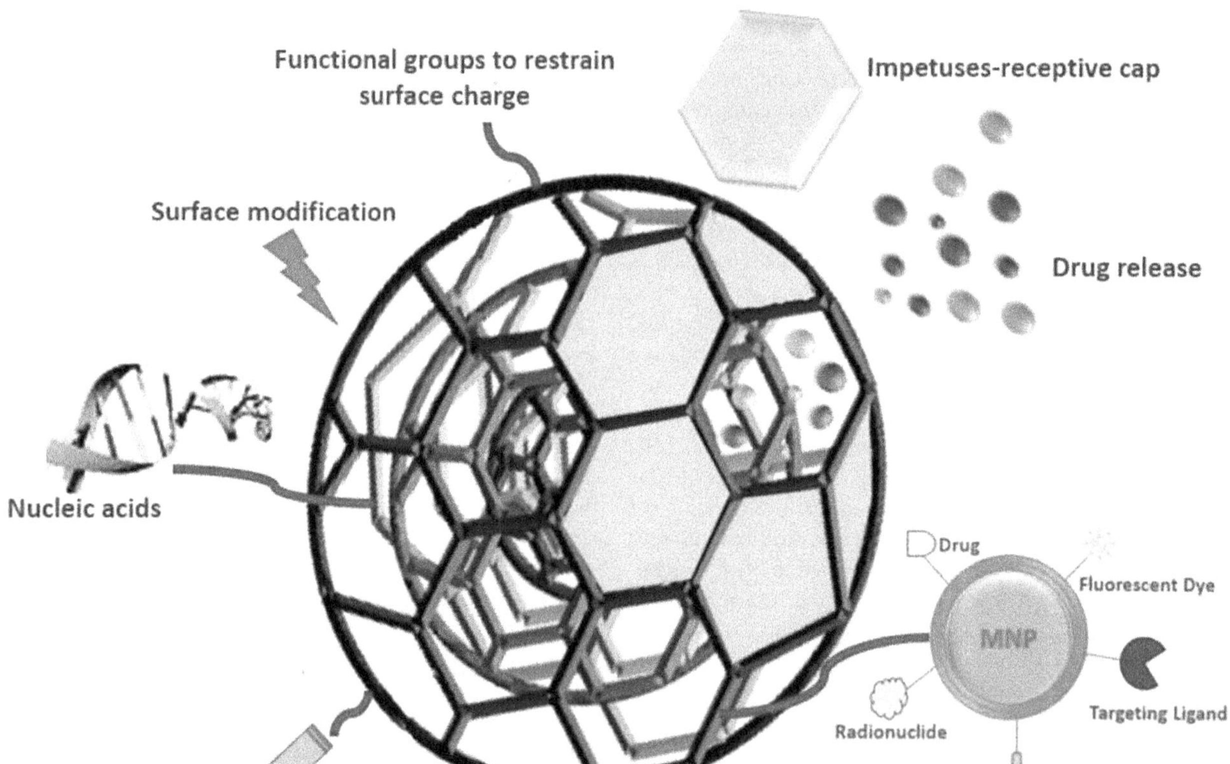

FIGURE 5.9 Graphic illustration of carbon nano-onion (CNO) functionalization and applications.

Source: Adapted from [17].

TABLE 5.5
Recent Progress of CNOs in Biomedical Applications

S. No.	Delivery System	Application	Results	Reference
1.	Polycaprolactone/f-CNO nanocomposite fiber	Anticancer drug delivery	DOX release from PCL/f-CNO nanocomposite fiber was pH-dependent. F-CNOs augmented the mechanical strength, hydrophobicity, and biocompatibility of the PCL nanofibers.	[82]
2.	f-CNO-reinforced zein hydrogels	Anticancer drug delivery	CNOs improved the mechanical strength of zein hydrogels. The delivery system exhibited good cytocompatibility against the osteoblast cell line. A pH-responsive sustained drug release over 15 days was observed.	[81]
3.	f-CNO/gelatin composite hydrogels	Anticancer drug delivery	5-FU/f-CNO/gelatin hydrogels exhibited augmented tensile strength in comparison to pristine gelatin hydrogels. A sustained release of 5-FU for over 15 days was observed, which indicated possible prospects in cartilage tissue engineering and drug delivery.	[83]
4.	Ox-CNO-loaded chitosan polyvinyl alcohol (CS/PVA/oc-CNO) nanocomposite film	Tissue engineering application	Ox-CNO enhanced the stability of the CS/PVA/ox-CNO scaffold. The nanocomposite film displayed no allergic response or pus formation in Wistar rats after subdermal implantation of the scaffold. The CS/PVA/oc-CNO scaffold exhibited tissue regeneration capability.	[84]
5.	Pristine CNOs (p-CNOs), ox-CNOs, far-red fluorescent-CNOs	Cellular imaging application	Ox-CNOS and Fluo-CNOs exhibited excellent cytocompatibility against MCF-7 and HeLa cells. Far-red fluorescent images indicated the internalization of fluo-CNOs by the MCF-7 cells, conforming that fluo-CNOs can be utilized as a high-resolution cellular imaging agent as an alternative for organic dyes.	[85]
6.	DNA sensor composed of glassy carbon electrode (GCE)/pristine-CNO	Sensing biomolecular interaction	The GCE/CNO nanocomposite DNA sensor sensed the human papillomavirus oncogene DNA sequence via amperometric detection. Modification via electrochemical grafting of the GCE/CNO surface with two different diazonium salts (4-aminophenylacetic acid) PAA and (4-aminophenylmaleimide) PM yielded GCE/CNO/PAA and GCE/CNO/PM nanocomposite. Both surfaces supported the attachment of thiolated or biotinylated short recognition DNA sequences (DNA probes). The large surface area and the enhanced electron transfer properties of this analytical sensor helped in the sensing of biomolecular interactions.	[78]
7.	CNO-based catalytic biosensor	Nanobiocatalyst for biosensing application	CNO-based catalytic biosensor (CNO/enzyme) conjugate retained optimum pH and temperature, displayed stability over a longer duration at 37°C. The CNO catalytic biosensor efficiently detected the immobilization of various enzymes, such as alkaline phosphatase, horseradish peroxidase (HRP), and glucose oxidase (≈0.5 mg of enzyme per mg of CNOs).	[86]

properties. Bobrowska et al. employed hexadecyltrimethylammonium bromide (CTAB), sodium dodecyl sulfate (SDS), sodium dodecylbenzene sulfonate (SDBS), Triton X-100, and Tween 20 to functionalize the CNOs by the non-covalent technique. This method produced a stable, well-dispersed CNO/surfactant nanocomposite structure that was evaluated for its *in vitro* biological activity against *E. coli*. Their study revealed that only the CNO/CTAB composite decreased the cell viability *in vitro*. They further reported that this activity could be allocated to the simple composite dissociation in water solutions, although antimicrobial assets of the composites are better to some extent in comparison to pure CTAB, indicating a synergistic effect of the CNO/surfactant nanocomposite when compared to pure surfactant.

Babar and coworkers reported an interaction between calf-thymus (CT) double-stranded DNA (dsDNA) and water-soluble carbon nano-onion (wsCNO) in water that followed denaturation of dsDNA (double-stranded DNA) to ssDNA (single-stranded DNA). The ssDNA concomitantly wrapped with the spiked surface of wsCNO and created a triangular aggregate confirmed by SEM images, which further aggregated to form a six-petal flowery arrangement hexagonally and reached a dead-end network, as evident by SEM and optical fluorescence microscopy. This dead-end network aggregate lacked the intrinsic optical property of DNA and displayed a loss of its activity (Figure 5.10) [41]. The researchers finally concluded that the wsCNO being non-toxic can be explored to control the unwanted proliferation of rouged DNA by interacting with wsCNO, which can be utilized for the prevention of such viral DNA replication in recognized diseases.

5.8 Carbon Nanotubes (CNTs)-Based Advanced Dermal Therapeutics

The search for effective and non-invasive delivery modules to transport therapeutic molecules across skin has led to the discovery of a number of nanocarriers (viz., liposomes, ethosomes, dendrimers, etc.) in the last few decades. However, available literature suggests that these delivery modules face several issues, including poor stability, low encapsulation efficiency, and scale-up hurdles. Recently, carbon nanotubes (CNTs) emerged as a versatile tool to deliver therapeutics across skin. This section expounds the state-of-art synthesis methodologies, skin penetration mechanism, drug liberation profile, loading potential, characterization techniques, and transdermal applications,

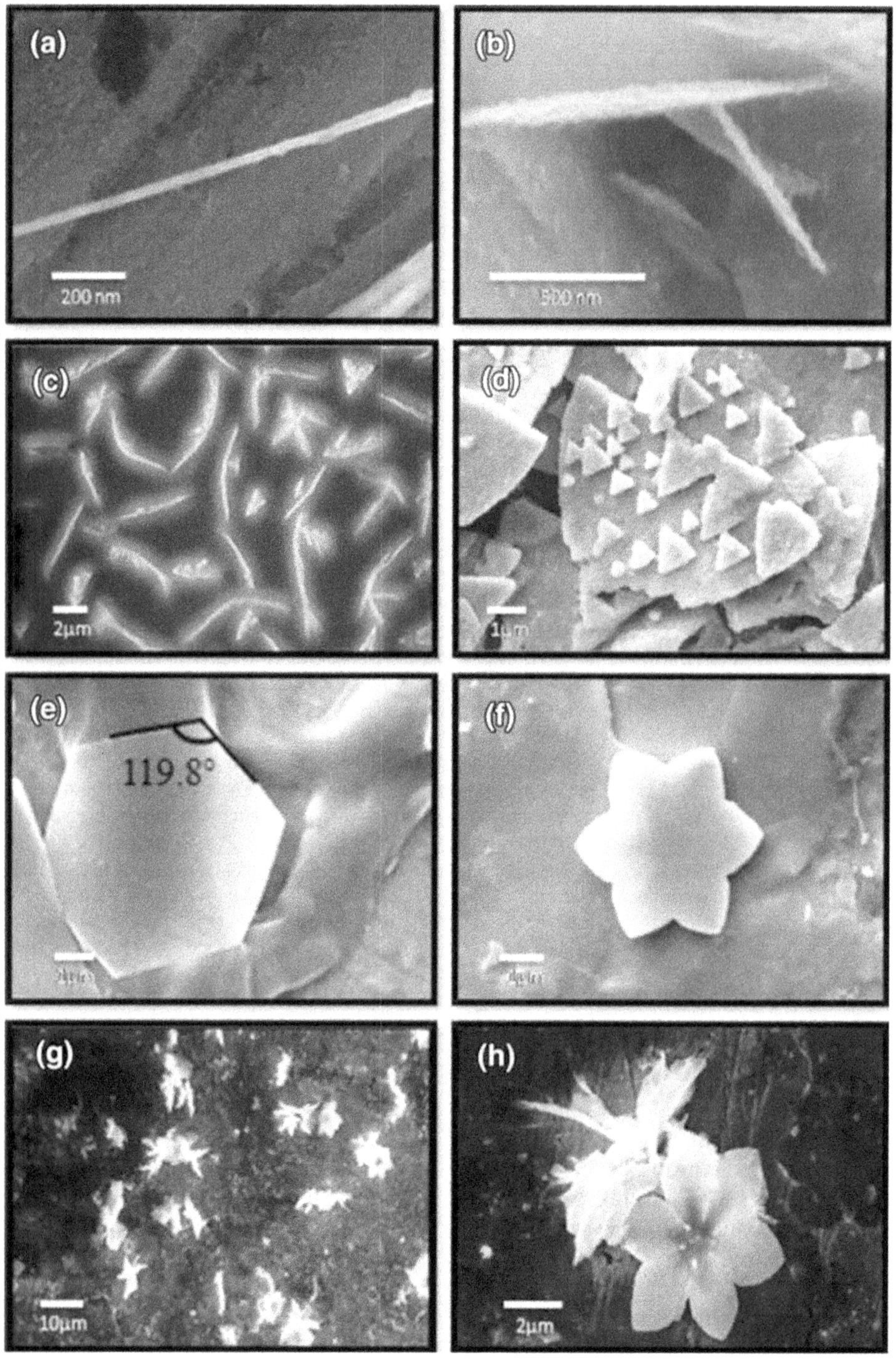

FIGURE 5.10 SEM photomicrographs of DNA composites: (a) DNA-water-soluble carbon nano-onion (wsCNO) at 1 h; (b) growth at 4 h; (c) aggregation at 4 h; (d) triangle formation at 16 h; (e) hexagon formation; (f) flower formation; (g) assorted flower formation; (h) selected six-petal flower.

along with a summary on patent/regulatory status and future scope of CNT-based skin therapeutics.

5.8.1 Dermal Disorders and Available Therapeutic Interventions

During the last decades, noteworthy changes have been observed in the treatment and management of dermal disorders as a result of better understanding of the molecular and cellular basis of many skin conditions and diseases. However, as per a recent report of the global burden of disease study, dermal disorders are found to be the fourth leading cause of nonfatal disease burdens. Monitoring the prevalence of skin disease/conditions is vital in the context of global dermatological health perspectives. Dermal disorders, including psoriasis, mycosis, acne, blister, bacterial infection, fungal infection, skin ulcer, rash, erythema, scabies, contact dermatitis, hives, allergy, and skin cancer, are posing significant challenges to the scientific community as they vary widely in symptoms and severity. A major obstacle in the treatment of dermal disorders is the barrier function of stratum corneum.

Among the possible treatment approaches like creams, gels, lotions, solutions, etc., transdermal patches have gained important attraction due to their effective clinical output and better patient compliance (as dose dumping is not a problem with patches). Some investigators concluded that patches are more advantageous over an oral delivery route due to their longer clinical effects and lesser adverse effects; for example, estradiol patches, which are known to be utilized by millions of patients yearly worldwide, and in contrast to oral dosage form, don't lead to liver damage.

In addition, patches formulated using clonidine, nitroglycerine, and fentanyl are reported to show minimal side effects compared to traditional oral formulations. In context, the emergence of nicotine-loaded transdermal patches (1991–1992) evoked people to quit smoking and thereby enhanced their quality of life. Investigations demonstrated four times better results in helping patients quit smoking by daily applications of patches continuously for two years in contrast to patients on placebo.

Also, novel transdermal approaches (i.e., photodynamic therapy and radiotherapy) are used to treat skin cancers. Collectively, all these approaches have hit the dermal market very significantly in the last few decades. Therefore, the next subsection sums up progression made in the dermal market over time.

5.8.2 A Quick Look at the Dermal Market

Nowadays, tremendous advancements in nanotechnology-based delivery systems have enabled an improvement in the performance as well as efficacy of skin delivery systems. The global nanotechnology-based product market is a fast-growing market valued at \$22.9 billion in 2013 and increased to about \$26 billion in 2014. This market is expected to reach about \$64.2 billion by 2019, a compound annual growth rate (CAGR) of 19.8% from 2014 to 2019. Nanostructured lipid carriers (NLC)– and solid lipid nanoparticles (SLN)–loaded dermal formulations are excellent examples of nanotechnology-based approaches to enhance skin delivery.

Lipopearls are one such dermal delivery system made up of pearlescent beads containing emollient oils and vitamins. Furthermore, skin delivery can also be enhanced with external triggers by iontophoresis, sonophoresis, and solid or hollow microneedles.

5.8.3 Drawbacks of Conventional Transdermal Therapeutics: A Call for Improvement

Effective transdermal delivery of therapeutics primarily depends on physicochemical properties of the therapeutic which is to be delivered, but they have some restricting values, that is, low atomic weights (~500), greater lipophilic values (high oil solubility), and low therapeutic dose (up to 10 mg/24 h). Currently, the lowest-molecular-weight patch available commercially is nicotine (0.162 kDa), and the highest-molecular-weight patch is oxybutynin (0.359 kDa).

Drugs with prominent hydrophilic characteristics are still one of the biggest challenges in their successful transformation into effective dermal products. Apart from properties related to a therapeutic to be delivered, a vehicle used must show optimum solubility for the therapeutic so that movement of the therapeutic entity from vehicle to the stratum corneum is possible at a desirable rate. This rate can be determined by calculating partition coefficients. Another important factor is the concentration of the drug, which, upon increasing, will give increased bioavailability, and the excess of the non-dissolved drug will maintain the equilibrium. Once the dissolved drug has diffused into the skin membrane, only then will the excess dissolve, thereby giving a sustained release. But higher drug concentration may also increase the size of the delivery system, which sometimes may be unsuitable.

Usually, delivery accomplished using traditional dosage forms like creams, ointments, and lotions share four constraining properties: bigger particle size (more than 1,000 nm), low permeation rate, high dose requirements, and multiple applications in a day. However, many investigators have adopted various approaches (e.g., iontophoresis and ultrasound) to overcome these problems and efficiently transfer the dermal formulation at the desired site (local/systemic).

Overall, constraints related to drug properties and delivery modules call for better understanding and improvement to effectively target skin diseases. The next section deals with skin-associated limitations and eventual progress of different generations of transdermal therapeutics to have a clear understanding of further developments and improvements of dermal therapeutics.

5.8.4 Transdermal Therapeutics and Skin Barriers: Leads from Existing Reports

Drug/therapeutic absorption through skin layers is a fundamental point to be considered for two reasons: first, the absorption of a drug into the skin is via passive diffusion, through a concentration gradient, and second, the vehicle used in a formulation can have wide effects because it determines rates and amounts of drug absorption.

A major prerequisite for efficient transdermal delivery is the potency of the drug that is required in low dose. Also, the surface of the transdermal delivery device is considered to be a vital aspect in controlling the rate at which the drug is delivered (area must not exceed 50 ms^2). The entry of the foreign particles into the body via skin is restricted due to the formidable barrier nature of skin. Thus, a dose of not more than 50 mg is allowed to effectively permeate through the skin in a day. Apart from its barrier function, skin also resists diffusion through its layers; thus, the therapeutic agent selected must be effective when delivered as a loaded cargo slowly over an extended period of time. Even if the delivery rate is enhanced by the addition of certain permeation enhancers, it does not show a pulsatile type of delivery, as in the case of an injection or pulmonary inhalation. Figure 5.11 illustrates various obstacles related to skin, drug properties, and delivery systems in relation to dermal deliveries of therapeutics.

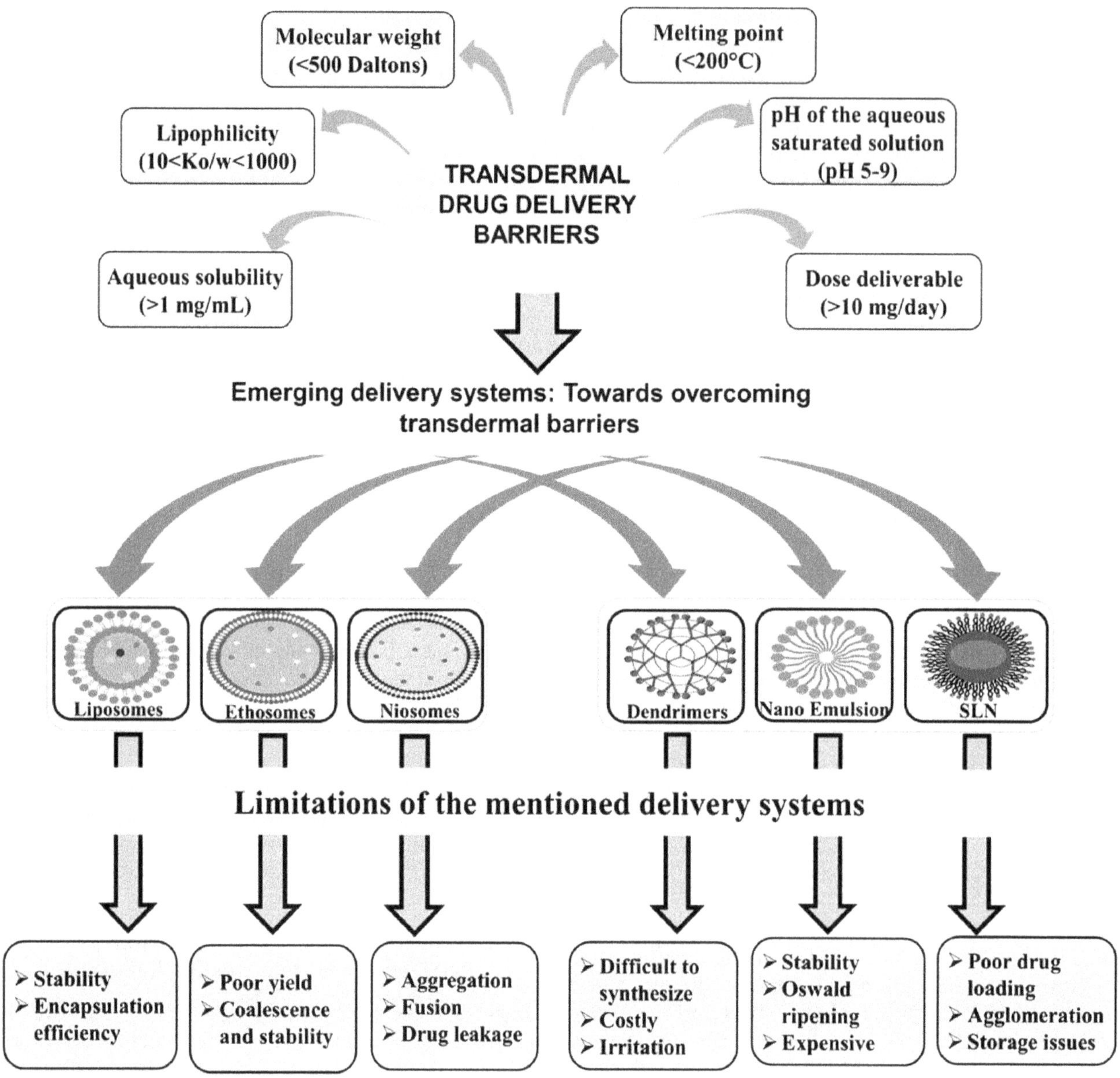

FIGURE 5.11 A diagrammatic representation of barriers to skin delivery of therapeutics presents a brief understanding of the parameters which behave as barriers for transdermal delivery, along with available systems of nanoformulations employed for transdermal deliverance, and also mentioning their limitations. Note: *SLN* = solid lipid nanoparticles.

From a global perspective, investigators categorized transdermal devices in three generations. The first generation involves systems that are nothing but the simple patches with a sensible choice of drugs which can cross the skin at therapeutic rates with little or no improvement. The major restriction for first generation, other than epidermis (avascular and 50 to 100 μm thick), is the stratum corneum, which has brick-and-mortar-like structures, indicative of a mixture of lipids which are systematized in bilayers. The hurdles posed by stratum corneum for delivery across skin shift the paradigm to develop second-generation therapeutics. The second generation of transdermal devices employed certain chemical permeation enhancers (surfactants, terpenes, laurocapram, fatty acid/alcohol, alcohols and glycols, pyrrolidones, sulphoxides, etc.) for enhanced delivery via stratum corneum. The methods of iontophoresis and non-cavitational ultrasound devices are also considered among the second-generation devices. However, the second generation created a less clinically meaningful effect on the delivery of macromolecules and therefore called for further improvement, that is, third-generation transdermal delivery devices. The third-generation delivery devices primarily involve microneedles, thermal ablation, and microdermabrasion to deliver macromolecules, which include therapeutic proteins and vaccines, across the skin, but they are still under clinical trials. These third-generation devices are actively involved in making use of nanotechnology. Programmable implants, nanomembranes, and hydrogels are a few examples of dermal deliverables of this generation based on nanotechnology. "Diclac lipogel" is an example of a diclofenac-loaded nanogel formulation commercially available (Sandoz, a private limited company in India), showing the potential of nanotechnology-based approaches. Another example is the liposomal formulation ("Daylong Actinica"), encapsulated with ultraviolet A– and ultraviolet B–absorbing agents, approved by the European Union as a medical device for the management of actinic keratosis in high-risk organ transplant recipients on a long-term basis. Considering the significant involvement of nanotechnology-based products, the next section is presented with the aim of exploring possible opportunities and thrust in developing nano-based transdermal medications.

5.8.5 Evolution of Nanotechnology in Transdermal Therapeutics: A Turnaround

In the current scenario, nanosystems are those which are rapidly establishing themselves in the field of nanomedicines due to their unique size-dependent properties along with optical and magnetic benefits. Figure 5.12 depicts several phases of a transdermal delivery system starting with the conventional formulations which lacked specificity and low skin penetration; these demand nanoformulations which have enhanced permeation and help transmit the drug to its site of action. These avenues of nanoparticles have now protracted toward early diagnosis and effective treatment of various dermal diseases by showing accurate targeting toward affected regions and also can bypass the tight epithelial junctions of skin.

A recent report published in *Nature Scientific Reports* indicates the successful development of a pregabalin-loaded niosomal-based topical hydrogel (hydroxypropyl methyl cellulose and Carbopol 934–based) formulation. The formulation was designed via quality-by-design (Qbd) approach to eliminate undesired factors and achieve effective therapeutic concentration across skin for the treatment of fibromyalgia syndrome (continuous and persistent pain lasting for months). The investigators concluded that the only formulations finally delivered via hydrogels were found to accumulate in deeper skin regions with controlled release profiles. This work created a paradigm for future investigations to benefit nanotechnology-based transdermal medications.

The increasing importance of molecular dynamics in context to skin permeation of nanotechnology-based approaches forms the root of the progress of advanced transdermal delivery devices. Considering this, investigators from India studied the effect of size and surface electric charge on gold nanoparticles with human skin permeation and published the data in *Nature Scientific Reports*. In this investigation, researchers performed coarse-grained molecular dynamic simulations to unveil the skin penetration ability of dodecanethiol-capped water-insoluble gold nanoparticles of different sizes (1–5 nm) and surface charges (positive and negative) via a human skin model. The findings suggest that maximum permeability was observed with 2 nm gold nanoparticles and minimum of 3 nm positively charged gold nanoparticles. This investigation provides an idea about engineering and developing gold nanocarriers for delivering targeted drug/proteins.

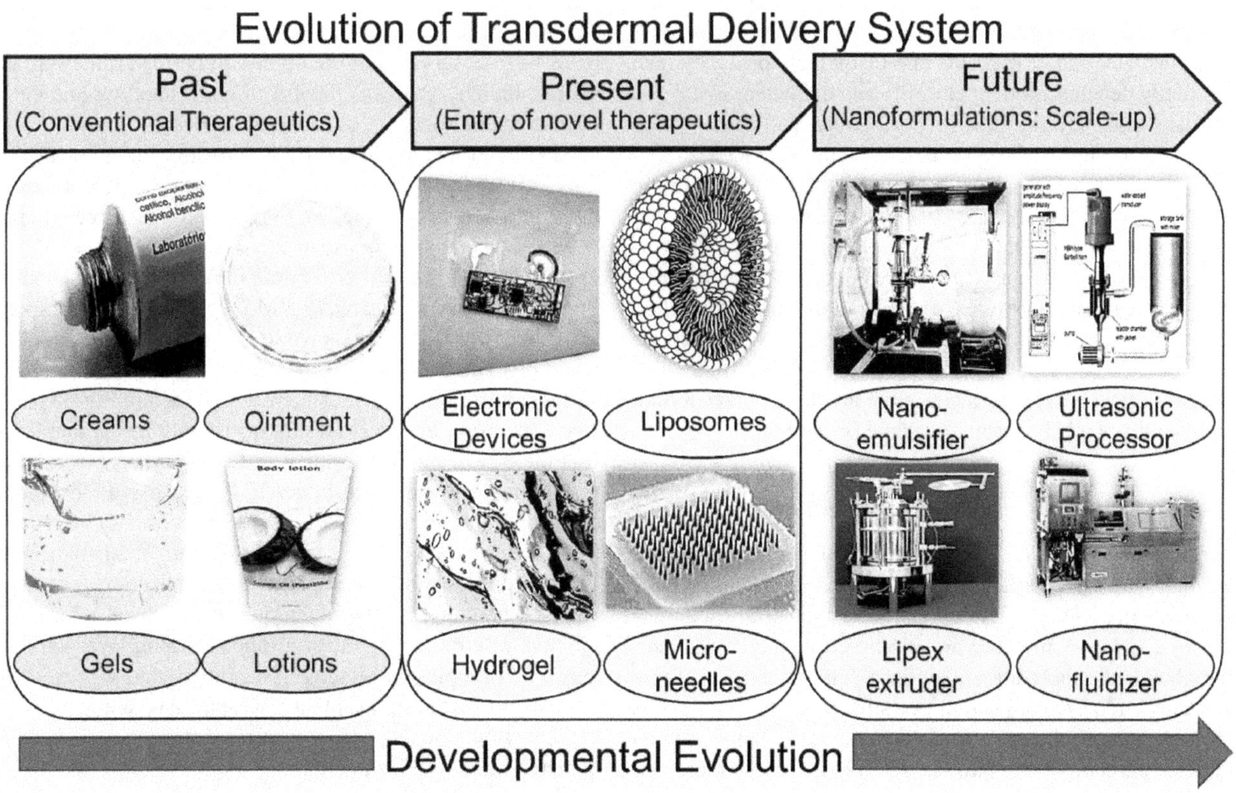

FIGURE 5.12 Schematic presentation of the evolution of dermal therapeutics. Past: Indicating the most widely used traditional marketed formulations. Present: Indicating the novel formulations for drug delivery. Future: Indicating the methods for scale-up of the nanoformulations.

However, the problem with most of these systems is with their scale-up; therefore, there is a need for advanced machinery which could solve this problem. Reports are also available on transdermal nanosystems primarily involving nanosuspension, nanoemulsion, liposomes, niosomes, ethosomes, hydrogels, microneedles, nanoparticles, and carbon nanotubes (CNTs). This section thus encompasses the criticality and the importance that CNTs have in transdermal applications.

5.8.6 CNTs-Based Things to Know about This Emerging Transdermal Nanocarrier

5.8.6.1 Historical Perspective

CNTs were first discovered by Iijima, and these belong to the family of fullerenes, in which carbon atoms are bound in the form of a hexagonal mesh [1]. One such carbon layer, called graphene, is wound in the shape of a cylinder to form CNTs. The CNTs that Iijima observed were so-called multi-walled CNTs (MWNTs); they named them "Russian dolls" as they "nested" like them, which had at least two graphitic layers having an inner diameter of around 4 nm.

Leading from this report, Iijima and Ichihashi and colleagues of the IBM Almaden Research Centre in California synthesized single-walled CNTs (SWCNTs) [2]. These SWCNTs were synthesized by the same route by which Iijima et al. used to fabricate MWCNTs, but with a slight modification. They added some metal particles to the carbon electrodes, and the appearance of these CNTs was quite different than that of the MWCNTs. Individual tubes possessed a very small diameter of ~1 nm, and each was curled and looped rather than being straight. The investigation concluded that SWCNTs can either be semiconducting or metallic, and that which form they take eventually depends on their chirality and diameter.

Meanwhile, several other reports were published which explained the innovative synthetic designs, characterization, prospective applications, and basic mechanical and electronic properties of CNTs. Because CNTs possess several interesting properties like strength, flexibility, carbons with sp^2 hybridization, and ability to arrange themselves in rope-like structures, they have grown to be one of the most intensively studied nanostructure materials. With the passage of time, several milestones were achieved, and notably, from the year 2010 onward, a significant increment in the number of transdermal applications of CNTs began to emerge (Figure 5.13).

5.8.6.2 Innovative Synthesis Techniques

During the past decade, major advancements have reported various synthesis methods of CNTs, and the major methods generally used to develop CNTs in industrial quantities are laser ablation method, arc discharge method, and thermal chemical vaporization technique. The majority of these techniques requires a vacuum pot still; however, continuous research and development for new catalysts is being carried out for continuous growth to make CNTs more commercially beneficial. For better understanding, we have summarized a few major techniques with characteristic remarks used for the synthesis of CNTs of either type (Table 5.6).

There are many other reported techniques that are generally used for the synthesis of CNTs, which include sonochemical/hydrothermal (fabrication of nanowires, nano-ions, nanobelts, and nanorod MWNTs), electrolysis (this proceeds in the condensed phase and employs graphite as the feedstock at relatively low temperatures), and solar energy (used mainly for fullerene and is based on solar light applications). Among them, a solar method proposes to use solar light to induce vaporization of the target and claims the possibility to regulate each synthesis parameter independently. Following the discussion on synthesis methods, one can select a method for manufacturing according to the need and application of CNTs required.

5.8.6.3 An Outlook of Characterization Approaches

CNTs, in any of their forms (i.e., SWCNT or MWCNT), need to be characterized and checked for the presence of impurities. The techniques most frequently used for this purpose include Raman spectroscopy (to confirm any possible interaction of other material with CNT and to confirm the functionalization and modification made to a CNT) and scanning electron microscopy (to understand the surface morphology).

The utility of SEM for characterizing CNTs and determining optimum concentrations can be properly understood by understanding a study conducted by Jandial et al., wherein by analyzing SEM images they observed aggregates which were self-organized in bundles when they used 20% concentration of SWCNTs. Also, a large amount of amorphous carbon and graphitic particles was observed. Further, when the concentration was reduced to 7.5%, large numbers of bundles in aggregates were observed, but the other carbon materials were not visible; thereby, this was helpful in understanding and determining the morphology of nanocomposites.

Another study conducted by Safarova et al. characterized SWCNTs using multiple techniques, such as SEM, transmission electron microscopy (TEM), atomic force microscopy (AFM), and energy-dispersive X-ray (EDX). TEM was used to gather internal structural information, as shown in Figure 5.14a and b, whereas AFM helped in the morphological analysis of CNTs, as shown in Figure 5.14c and d. Also, a result of EDX was used for the detection of metal impurities and the presence of other elements, as shown in Figure 5.14e. The conclusion drawn from this investigation was that TEM was the best technique to analyze CNTs because of its high resolution, whereas SEM and AFM were useful for understanding morphological results. It was observed by using SEM that there was a thin layer (0.1–0.5 μm) of an amorphous carbon film that further impeded the application aspects of CNTs. Therefore, a new technique was devised which was efficient in eliminating the amorphous carbon layer with the help of H_2O–plasma etching. The investigators proved via microscopic examinations that H_2O–plasma etching does not cause any major changes in the original structure of CNTs, as depicted in Figure 5.14f and g.

The study also revealed that over a prolonged etching time of the aligned CNTs, their tips were more reactive than the sidewalls; thus, after removing the graphite layer from the

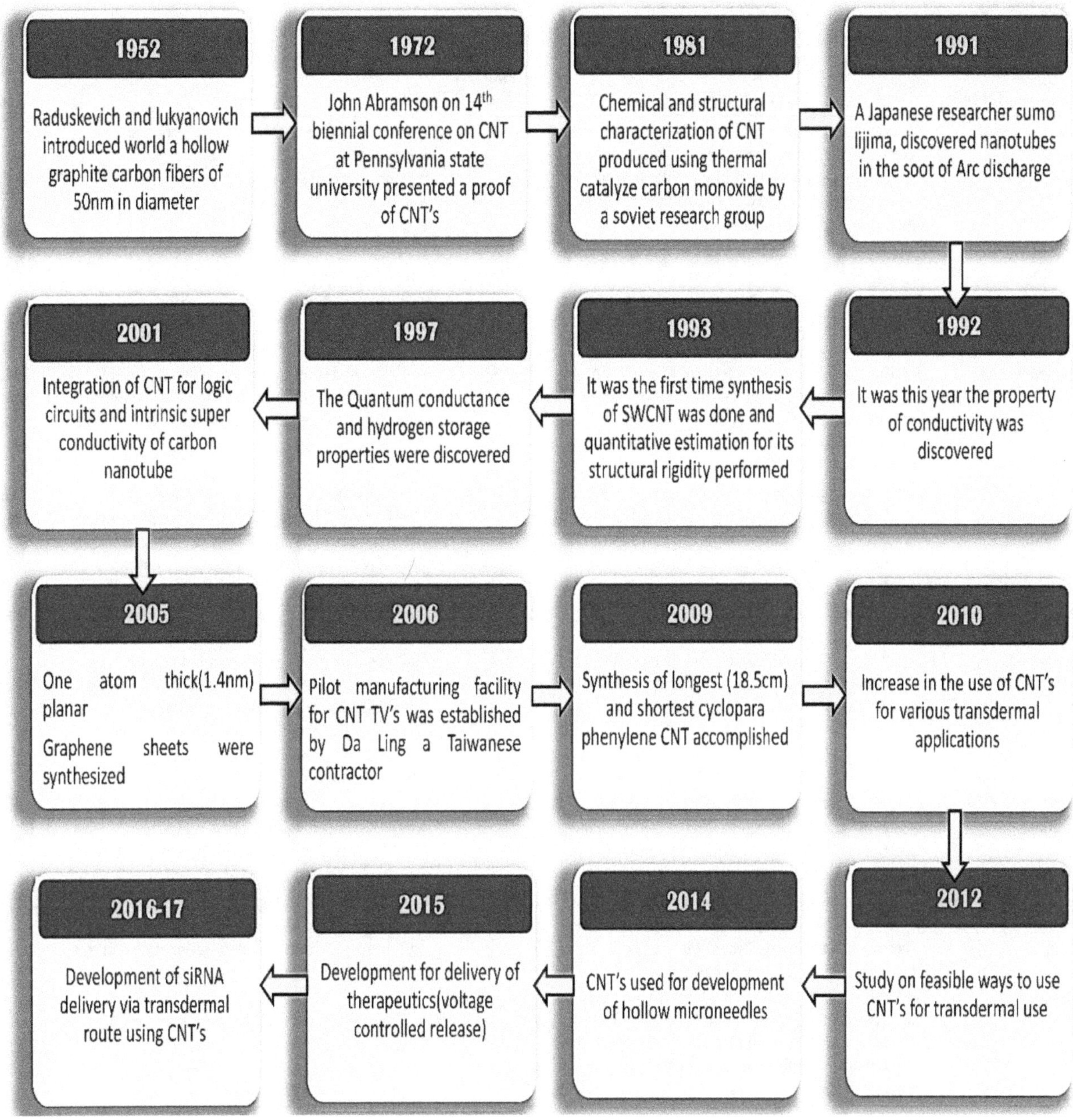

FIGURE 5.13 CNTs historical timeline. A brief depiction of the historical timeline mentioning the major developmental aspects that guided the applications of CNTs.

aligned CNTs, they opened after an etching time of 80 min due to over-reactivity of their tips. Therefore, it established that H_2O–plasma etching could be used for producing one-side-closed and one-side-packed nanotubes, thereby enabling the creation of miniaturized test tubes for experimenting with various physicochemical processes at the nanometer scale.

Another key technique used for characterization is EDX spectroscopy, which is used to estimate metal impurities in CNTs that tend to show up during a synthesis process. Collective compilation of such research papers related to the utility of this technique was well presented by Sunny et al. They used EDX to confirm the presence or complete absence of other contaminants in CNTs.

Another technique utilized for the characterization of CNTs and like composites, and to determine several elements and nanocompounds present in SWCNT and MWCNT, is X-ray photon spectroscopy (XPS). Also, it is employed to evaluate the compositional and structural properties of CNTs doped with N_2.

Next to characterization, loading of the therapeutic molecules in CNTs is of prime importance and is discussed in the following section.

TABLE 5.6
An Updated Summary of Synthetic Schemes for the Synthesis of CNTs

Name of Method	Process Applied	Reported Yield	Remarks	Ref.
Laser ablation method	Blast graphite with intense laser pulses rather than electricity to generate carbon gas, from which the nanotubes are formed, continue with various conditions until a process with required amount of SWCNTs is obtained.	Up to 70%	Good diameter control, fewer defects, the reaction product is pure, but is a costly technique, expensive power requirement.	[88] and [89]
Arc discharge method	Connect two graphite rods to a power supply and space them a few millimeters apart. And then complete the circuit, at 100 amps; carbon vaporizes and forms a hot plasma.	30–90%	An easy method to synthesize SWCNTs and MWCNTs; few structural defects, less expensive, open-air synthesis possible. Tubes tend to be short and of random sizes and shape and need a lot of purification.	[90]and [91]
Plasma torch	A gaseous combination of ferrocene, ethylene, and argon is passed through a plasma torch and atomized at atmospheric pressure to form a flame. The fumes that are formed because of flame contain the SWCNTs.	30–90%	The process is continuous and cost-effective; also proven to be ten times less in consuming energy when compared to graphite vaporization.	[92] and [93]
Thermal chemical vaporization technique	Substrate is placed in oven at a temp of 600°C, and then carbon-bearing gas (e.g., methane) is added slowly. As this gas decomposes, it forms carbon atoms which reassemble in the form of nanotubes.	20–100%	Easiest method to scale up; also, long-length CNTs can be synthesized. It is a simple process wherein diameter can also be controlled. Mostly are MWCNTs and often riddled with defects.	[94]and [95]
Plasma enhanced chemical vapor deposition (PECVD)	As compared to normal CVD, plasma processing is used, which results in dissociation to form high-energy electrons, and thereby, the substrate temperature can be reduced drastically as compared with normal CVD processing.	95–100%	Latest and upcoming technique for synthesis of CNTs. Very useful in the field of emitters and flat panel displays. It is a method employed to get controlled vertically aligned CNTs. CNTs can also be synthesized using different methods, like inductively coupled PECVD, microwave PECVD, hot filament PECVD, and glow discharge PECVD.	[96–98]
Condensed phase synthesis	Electric current is passed through an electrode made of graphite dipped in LiCl at 600°C in an inert atmosphere, which then forms a mixture of carbonaceous materials.	20–30%	Particles encapsulated by CNTs could be possible. Various salts, like KCl, NaCl, and LiBr, also have been utilized safely as electrolytes for the synthesis of CNTs.	[99]and [100]
Catalytic pyrolysis of hydro-carbon	Catalyst nanoparticles in colloidal suspension, or as an organometallic precursor along with carbon feedstock, are directly brought into a CVD chamber, where the organometallics undergo sublimation and thereby form catalyst nanoparticles which are then decayed by heat. Usually, a double-stage furnace is employed for organometallic sublimation and growth of the nanotubes	~95%	Commonly used for large-scale synthesis of CNTs. Also, the aligned CNT bundles can be synthesized within one step, and that also at low cost and without any pre-perpetrations.	[101]and [102]

5.8.7 Mechanistic Outlook on Loading of Therapeutics in CNTs

Both SWCNTs and MWCNTs are rolled graphene sheets which are capped with a hemispherical network of carbon termed as fullerenes [72]. Therefore, drug loading into CNTs can be done either during their synthesis or post-synthesis. However, loading of drugs during synthesis may result in decreased (~10%) loading, whereas loading after synthesis is better organized and yields of 50–100% are attainable. Also, due to the capping property, loading into CNTs provides the best solution for drugs which are easily decomposed or sensitive to the environment.

Post-synthesis loading includes two methods to entrap drug/therapeutics in CNTs: one is functionalization, and the other is capillarity. Functionalization is difficult because carbon is rather inert, so oxidization is used to produce a more reactive attachment surface. A functional group is either bonded to the inside or outside of the walls. The second method, which is the most widely used for entrapping in CNTs, is capillarity. The constraining factor in a capillarity method is the acquired diameter of the synthesized CNTs and surface tension of the material (the threshold material surface tension is approximately 200 mN m^{-1}). Certain forces, for example, hydrophobic and van der Waals forces of interaction, come into play when an aqueous solvent is used. In cases of chemicals with greater surface tension, a strategic synthesis of a suitable composite, which could be reduced back to its original substance after loading of CNT is completed, can be employed.

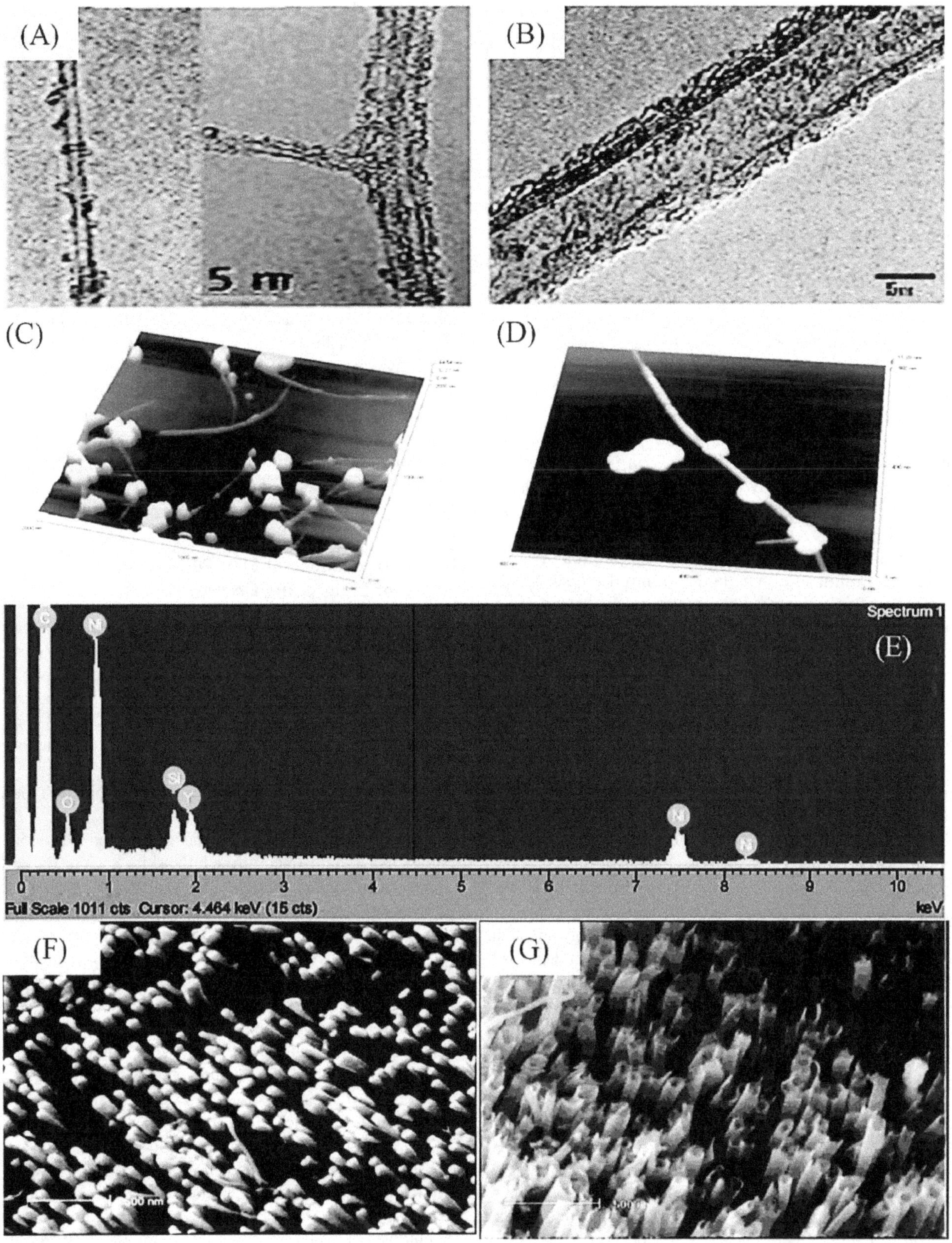

FIGURE 5.14 Pictorial and morphological images of CNTs: (a, b) TEM images of SWNCT and MWCNTs; (c, d) AFM images of SWCNTs; (e) EDX spectrum of SWCNTs, where Y and Ni are considered as a metal catalyst. (F) SEM image of aligned CNTs; (G) SEM image after H_2O–plasma etching with one end opened.

Source: (e) Adapted with permission, copyright 2007 Formatex. (g) Adapted with permission, copyright 2002 American Chemical Society.

Again, CNTs washed with such a solvent, which shows restricted solubility for the impregnating fluid, would result in only the deposits which are left outside being dissolved and washed off. Once the loading is completed, a predetermined current is passed, thus closing the ends of the tube via fusion. This process might sound systematically simple but is still considered tedious to perform; hence, loading of CNTs is still an area requiring further research.

5.8.8 Understanding Release Mechanism for Liberation of Drugs from CNTs

There are reports showing successful transportation and release of drugs, proteins, and additional pharmaceutically important molecules into cells for a variety of disease interventions.

One of the theories behind the release of drug molecules from CNTs is a pH-dependent stacking interaction. Liu et al. demonstrated an in vitro release of doxorubicin (DOX, an anticancer drug molecule) applying this approach. Structurally, doxorubicin is aromatic and therefore can interact with sp^2-hybridized sidewalls of SWCNTs, and then, upon pH change and pH-dependent stacking interaction, DOX would disengage to yield free molecules in an acidic medium.

An understanding of the release mechanism from a carrier system is of immense importance to unveil the subcellular mechanisms of this carbon-based nanocarrier to design and fabricate innovative delivery systems and modified-release approaches. For example, in the study carried out by Liu et al. using doxorubicin-capped SWCNTs, doxorubicin was expected to get released inside the lysosomes after undergoing endocytosis within the cells because of the acidic microenvironment generated due to proton pumps present on lysosomes. However, until now, the direct surveillance of this drug-release process within living cells has not been seen, and for tracking such a process in living cells, it is mandatory to identify location and movement of the CNTs and the subsequent drug loading or release, which is quite challenging to achieve and thus requires being explored on a molecular dynamic level.

Based on available reports and our survey of each available source, we revealed that many factors, including molecular structure of a drug, surface functionality, method of drug loading, proteins presents in the human body fluid, adsorption time at the time of synthesis of CNTs, attachment of targeting moiety on the surface of CNTs, and nature of bonding with drug (covalent or non-covalent), affect the release of biomolecules from CNTs.

5.8.9 Rationale and Designing of CNTs in Dermal Therapeutics

CNTs exhibit great surface areas, high drug loading, and high aspect ratios, enabling them to be suitable candidates for drug delivery. Owing to their excellent physicochemical properties and nano-size (~10–20 nm), CNTs can be utilized to facilitate transdermal delivery with external support, for example, by using electrical bias. Their nano-needle shapes enhance drug adsorption and thereby increase loading capacity. Thus, along with high loading efficiency, they also tend to offer increased transdermal permeation of a drug upon application of electrical bias, that is, electrically tunable systems, as widely reported in literature. Collectively, these factors provide a strong rationale for employing CNTs in delivering therapeutics across the skin, which allows users to control deliverance rate, through its application via the skin.

In the current scenario, transdermal delivery systems are gaining more attention and are an attractive route for the administration of bioactives, especially while treating patients for drug addiction, such as nicotine patches for limiting the habit of smoking and withdrawal symptoms upon opium cessation.

CNTs not only have a huge potential for utility in novel applications related to nanomedicines as a supportive and biocompatible substrate but could also be aids for creating a multifaceted drug delivery system.

We have summarized the various beneficial properties along with synthetic and transdermal applications in Figure 5.15. Collectively, CNTs present a good delivery option for a variety of drugs due to their immense properties. There are bountiful applications reported for transdermal delivery of therapeutics using CNTs, and that is an important part of our discussion in the following sections.

5.8.10 Mechanism of Skin Permeation of Drug Using CNT

The basic mechanism of delivering a drug from CNT-based formulations is either via an application of electric current through an applied potential across the transdermal application or by degradation of polymers used along with CNTs, or when a CNT itself transmits the payload across the skin. When administered via an intravenous route, functionalized CNTs show non-receptor-mediated endocytosis and receptor-mediated endocytosis, depending upon the type of functionalization.

Several reports are available on penetration behavior of CNTs when administered through the skin. Such a study was carried out by Rouse et al., wherein the investigators employed fullerene and conjugated it with peptides along with fluorescent markers in order to track its penetration. The findings revealed that the formulated complex did not show any penetration through the skin when no mechanical stress was applied, but significant penetration was observed when mechanical stress (like running, stretching, etc.) was applied. This investigation indicated that CNT itself does not likely stand a chance to show penetration unless physiology of the skin is modified.

Therefore, the application of an externally applied current is a promising approach to facilitate the delivery of drugs via CNTs across the skin. The rationale behind this approach is that CNTs are good conductors of current; thus, when a certain voltage or current is applied through the transdermal system, it leads to flow of electrons in a particular direction, which then causes the repulsion of an anionic drug from the CNTs–drug system and eventually forces the drug molecules into the skin, thus penetrating the stratum corneum. The general mechanism of skin penetration is briefly described for several CNT formulations in Figure 5.16a, wherein an electric current of almost 1.1 V was applied so as to force the drug molecules across the skin.

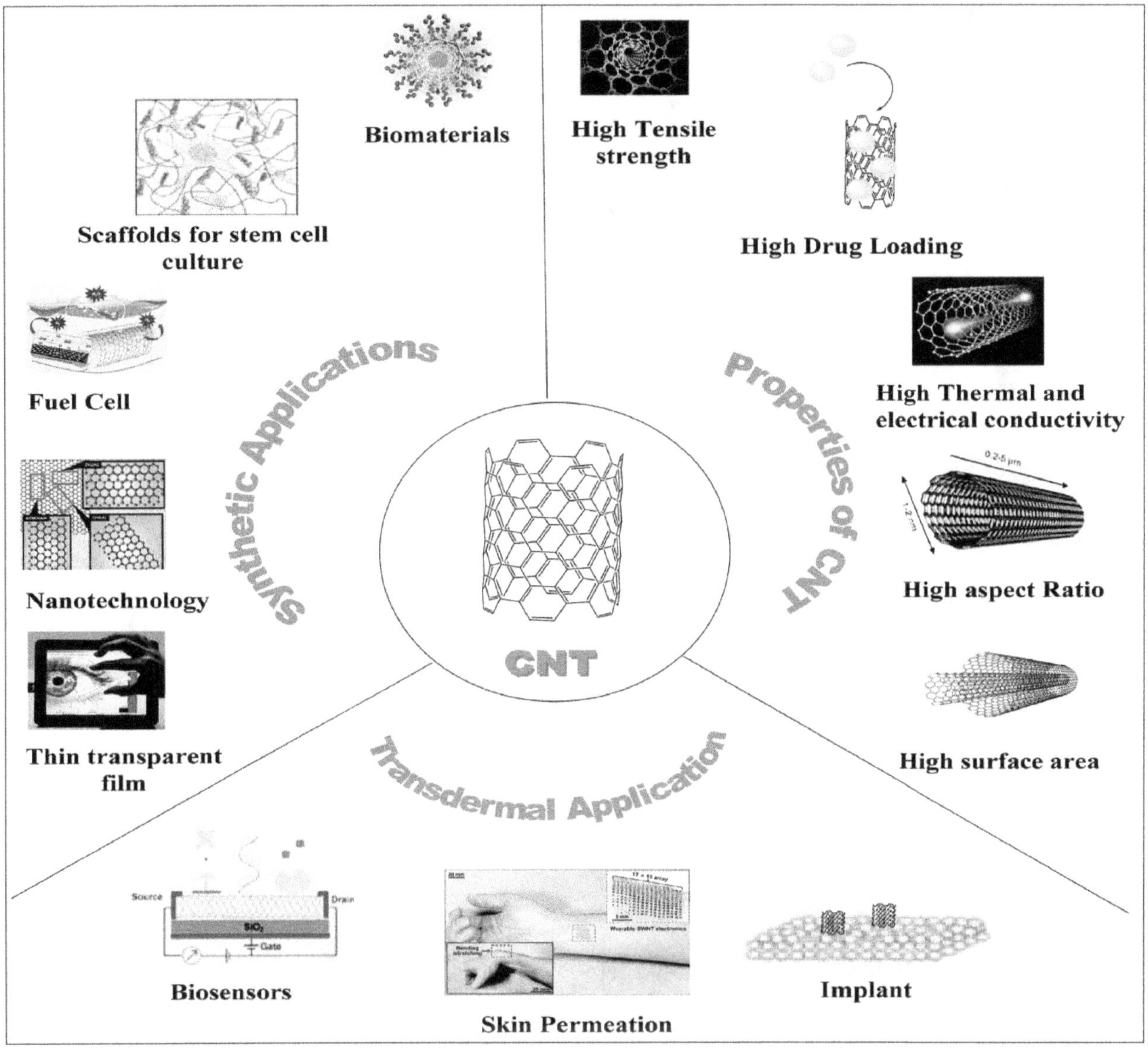

FIGURE 5.15 An overview of properties of CNTs and with synthetic and transdermal applications. Various properties of CNTs enabling them to be used in transdermal applications are depicted. Additionally, synthetic applications of CNTs are also depicted.

Similarly is the case with hydrogels, as hydrogels themselves do not possess an electrical conducting property, but upon loading with CNT fibers, conductance increases, thereby creating an electrical stimuli–based delivery system, as shown in Figure 5.16b. Recently, CNT has also been employed in the synthesis of microneedles with more mechanical strength, which makes them able to penetrate the skin with ease and without any breakage. In such cases, the microneedles can push the drug across the skin via the mechanism shown in Figure 5.16c.

In the case of CNT-polymer-drug-loaded microneedles, skin penetration of a drug can be achieved by the degradation property of a polymer over time (degradation rate) and also by the diffusion rate of the drug. The ratio of polymer and drug used with respect to CNTs will control the release of a drug via the skin. Figure 5.16 explains the basic mechanism of drug penetration and the usually applied method for delivering the payload across the skin. The hypothesis of drug permeation via CNTs across the skin is supported by many studies. Investigators mainly used some novel systems, such as tunable or hybrid hydrogel systems, programmable nanoporous membranes, electroactivated and electroresponsive devices, microneedles, and buckypapers, which we have covered in the later part of this section.

5.8.11 CNTs-Based Devices: Delivering and Monitoring Therapeutics across the Skin

5.8.11.1 Tunable and Hybrid CNT Hydrogels for High Transdermal Permeation

Hydrogels consist of hydrophilic polymeric materials and also bear the competency to hold a hefty amount of water into their 3D plexus. This makes them able to act as a good vehicle

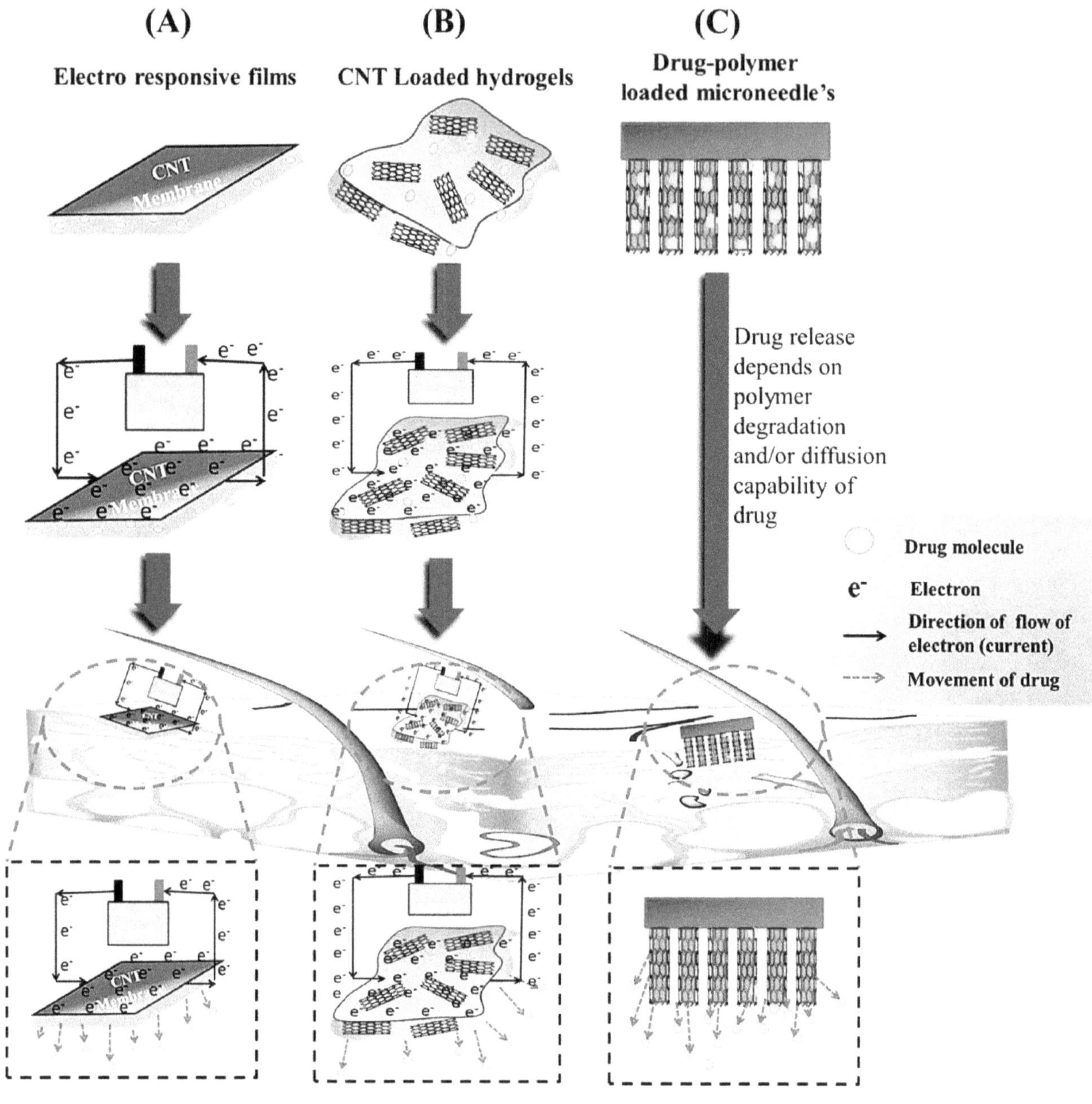

FIGURE 5.16 Schematic representation of delivery mechanisms associated with electrically tunable CNT films, hydrogels, and CNT polymer composite microneedles. (a) CNT membrane would be either covered or loaded with pure drug alone; upon application of voltage, it forces the drug to permeate through the tough stratum corneum. (b) In CNT hydrogels, the conductance capacity, which has been enhanced due to the incorporation of CNT, compels the drug to permeate through the skin, thereby reaching the desired site of action and showing its therapeutic effect. (c) CNT microneedles; the polymer–drug complex, which gets wicked within CNT needles, provides an excess mechanical strength to penetrate the skin, and it also governs the drug release profile, which is completely dependent on the degradation mechanism and kinetics of the polymer.

for delivery of drugs via a transdermal route. Their water-holding sufficiency depends on the availability of hydrophilic functional groups (amino, amido, hydroxyl, carboxyl groups, etc.) present inherently within polymer chains, and the aqueous content could vary from 10% to a few thousands folds the weight of dry polymer network.

Mostly, all the polymeric gels used for covered applications are either composed of synthetic polymers, such as (polyethylene glycol)(PEG), poly(vinyl alcohol) (PVA), polyacrylamide (PAM), poly(acrylic acid) (PAA), and poly(methyl methacrylate) (PMA), or natural polymers, like pectin, alginic acid, dextran and agarose, chitosan, and chitin. Some of these polymeric networks are dexterous and showcase phase transition and changes in their counterpoise state in response to external piquing (stimuli) and are hence also termed "stimuli-responsive" or "smart" hydrogels.

The role of a hydrogel in delivering drugs from CNTs can be understood by understanding the study done by Yun et al., who synthesized an electroresponsive delivery system via PVA/poly(acrylic acid)/MWCNTs, wherein hydrophobic MWCNTs were functionalized using oxyfluorination, which helped in the uniform dispersion of them in hydrogel matrices, and also were involved in affecting drug release and swelling characteristics. Changing the voltage applied resulted in altering the level of ionization of functional groups in the polymer matrices, thereby governing the release profile. Moreover, a uniform distribution of oxyfluorinated MWNT in the nanofibers was found to be crucial to their electroresponsive swelling and drug releasing behaviors. The amount of released drug increased by increasing the content of MWCNT, by using an oxyfluorination with higher oxygen content, and by applying the highest electrical voltage. The nanocomposite showed more than 80% cell viability, enough to be used as a non-toxic and biocompatible material.

In context, Servant et al. carried out a fascinating approach which involved free radical polymerization to create an electrosensitive hydrogel drug delivery system (radiolabeled sucrose was used as a model drug), which was able to obtain a pulsatile release showing peaks and valleys upon applying subsequent on/off applications of external voltage. However, almost 70% release was attained after the application of short electrical stimulation. The effect of pMWNTs and cross-linker concentration on the electrical and mechanical properties of these hydrogel hybrids was also investigated. It was observed that upon altering the concentration of pMWNTs, mechanical properties, like pore size and degree of swelling of hydrogel, were also altered. As a concluding remark, improved hydrogel efficiency can be achieved with enhanced conductance, along with (more than 70%) in 80 min. The pulsatile fashion achieved, as by on/off exposure to the electric field, was significantly better than the basic hydrogel system.

Later, the same group of researchers came up with slight modifications and radio-labeled [^{14}C]-sucrose with a similar formulation (hybrid gels; 0.2 mg mL^{-1} of pMWNT) for pulsatile drug release by an in situ radical polymerization method, wherein they studied *in vivo* levels of [^{14}C]-sucrose after subcutaneously implanting it in the dorsal region of CD^{-1} mice. The device showed a pulsatile release, and this versatility of electrically tuned hydrogels makes these materials very appealing for possible applications in transdermal systems, although no studies showing actual skin delivery was found; this creates a new avenue to be studied.

In recent literature, there are many reports for delivery of cationic and anionic drugs, but not non-ionic drugs for CNT-based hydrogels. Considering this, Cirillo et al. explored the performance of CNT-doped acrylate hydrogels (indicated for use in wound healing treatment) to match the hurdles of controlling the non-ionic drug curcumin (CUR) release by considering variables like the CNTs amount and strength of the applied external voltage. Varying amounts of CNTs in the prepolymerization feed were used in a range from 0.5 to 2.0% by weight to optimize their electric behavior and observe drug-to-carrier interactions.

Effects at different voltages from 12 to 48 V on release profiles were also studied. Outcomes clearly marked influence of the CNT's amount on material performance, and it also showed a strong relationship between drug partition and the polarization features of composite networks. CNT's amounts in the polymerization feed (1.25% by weight) allowed achieving the desired release rates, which matched well with various therapeutic needs. Versatility included low and prolonged dosages at 0 V, fast release at 12 and 48 V, and intermediate behavior at 24 and 36 V. Such degrees of versatility make CNTs an ideal material for utilization in the topical treatment of skin injuries using several active compounds which are from natural resources and are non-ionic in nature in personalized therapies.

5.8.12 CNTs-Based RNAi Therapeutics: Next-Generation Transdermal Therapeutics

RNAi produces a natural/biological mechanism that interferes with RNA which, upon delivery into a targeted cell, interferes with expression of certain proteins responsible for causing symptoms or a diseased condition. This therapy is considered to create new avenues in the field of nano-based medicines. Although applications of this technology in clinical trials have proven to be limited, the major problem for this is the delivery route or delivery system. Application of several therapeutics, which are intended toward treating certain cutaneous pathological conditions, topical delivery, may be the best choice for effective treatment therapy. Topical delivery allows self-administration, non-invasiveness, and selective targeting of products toward the pathological location; many reports are available justifying this statement.

Previously, it was established that CNTs could be used for the delivery of nucleic acids, including siRNA, which acts as a "nanoneedle" so as to internalize delivery into the cell. Although no proper reports explaining the diffusion of CNT–nucleic acid complex through the skin was found, a study done by Siu et al. showed topical application of functionalized CNT–siRNA complex for treating skin cancer. Investigators in this experiment demonstrated functionalized SWCNTs-based delivery of Braf siRNA based on non-covalent interaction for the treatment of cutaneous melanoma. For non-covalent conjugation of siRNA to the CNTs, the PEI was initially succinylated to form PEI-SA and to create a positive charge on the surface which forms the basis for electrostatic interaction. Following that, the PEI-SA conjugation of CNTs for functionalization was accomplished (cationization) and confirmed using zeta potential, SEM, and TEM imaging. Then, the formed conjugate of CNTs with PEI-SA was named IS/C and added in different molar ratios (1: 1, 1: 2, 1: 3, 1: 4, and 1: 5) to couple with siRNA. Among them, 1: 2 was found to be appropriate to condense all siRNA with CNTs, as 1: 2 did not show any unbound siRNA when evaluated with gel electrophoresis.

Transdermal delivery of siRNA-loaded IS/C was showcased by witnessing the fluorescence of Cy-3-labeled siRNA, which, due to the size of CNTs, effectively delivered siRNA across the skin. There was an intriguing observation noted, in which IS/C incubated with siRNA showed less penetration as compared to IS/C siRNA without incubation, although no rationale for such observation was drawn. There are other topical approaches for delivery of siRNA already made, but the method used was sonoporation. Authors generated a murine melanoma model by inoculating B16-F10 cells into C57BL/6 mice to study the delivery of IS/C-loaded siRNA into melanoma cells. As shown in Figure 5.17a, significant siRNA penetration was noted in tumors.

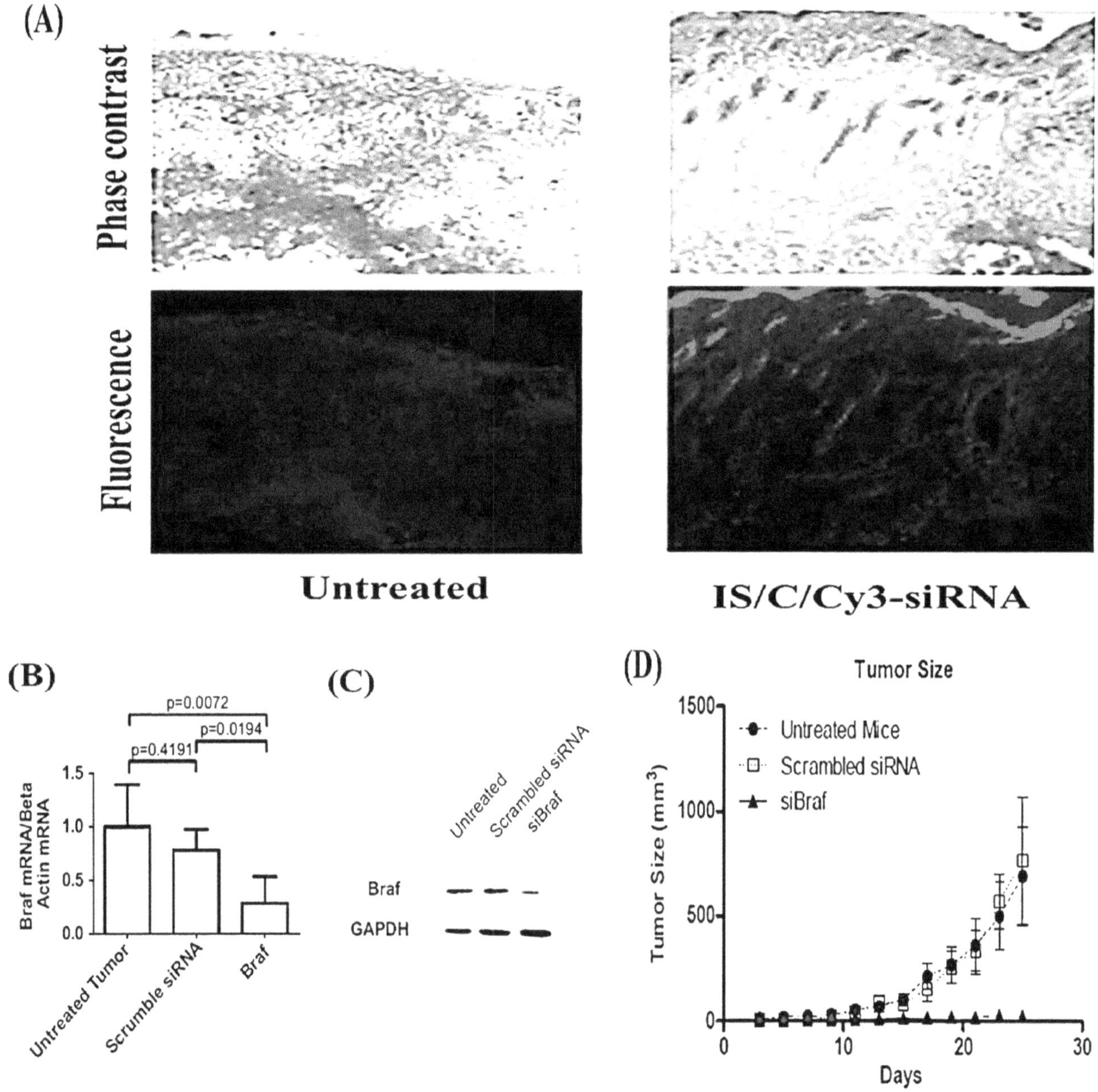

FIGURE 5.17 Topical administration of siRNA and genetic knockdown of the tumor: (a) Fluorescence microphotograph of ISC/Cy3–labeled siRNA complexes. Left-side images represent untreated tumor sample, while right-side images represent topically treated tumor. (b, c) Tumor-bearing mice were treated with IS/C/siRNA; two days later, the mice were sacrificed, and the tumor samples removed. The tumor samples were homogenized, and RNA was isolated by the Trizol method for qRT-PCR. The protein was isolated with RIPA buffer for Western blot. (d) Estimation of tumor size was done using Vernier caliper, using π ($l \times W^2$)/6 formulas, where l is length and W is width.

Source: Adapted with permission, copyright 2016 Springer Science and Business Media New York.

The investigation using qRT-PCR demonstrated gene silencing (over 72%) of Braf using siBraf, in comparison to the siScramble and untreated tumors (Figure 5.17b). Moreover, results of Western blotting exhibited similar findings (Figure 5.17c). Tumor growth was also found reduced with siBraf, as shown in Figure 5.17d. Therefore, the CNTs–Braf siRNA approach via dermal route demonstrated *in vivo* clearly revealed the reduction in tumor growth within 25 days. As a conclusive remark, authors stated that the use of CNTs for dermal delivery of siRNA is a potential field for treating diverse skin conditions/abnormalities, including skin cancer.

5.8.13 Programmable Nanoporous Membranes for "On Time" Delivery of Therapeutic Molecules

A nanoporous membrane can be characterized as one with pores which lie in the range of nanometers or even in sub-nanometers.

They are capable of distinguishing and separating liquids and gaseous mixtures and find their applications in separation of different size composites, which is considered as "mole sieving" and used for determination of adsorption selectivity and understanding wetting or steric hindrance. The selective materials for synthesis of such nanoporous membranes are amorphous metal oxides, carbon, and zeolites. Among them, carbon in the form of CNTs has shown a good potential as a material for nonporous membrane synthesis, owing to its electrical conductance, which allows control over flux through this nanoarchitect, and recently, it was reportedly used for the deliverance of several therapeutics through a transdermal route.

Production of CNTs-based nanoporous membranes utilized the slots which are present between the CNT's structure and are ingrained with a polymer substrate and a quartz backing engraved by employing hydrofluoric acid. Water plasma is latterly employed to eliminate additional polymer from the superficial surface of the film. This whole procedure yields a sturdy membrane with open-ended carboxylic acid (at tips)–functionalized CNTs.

Therefore, by applying a very minute electrical bias (approximately 50 mV) to the membrane, negatively charged end groups are either attracted toward the nanotubes, blocking the pore and permitting no entry through it, or are repelled from one surrounding nanotube, thus causing the functional group to remain elevated (away from a pore) and thereby permitting fluid passage and drug deliverance. Hence, incorporating such a CNTs-based controlling membrane in a transdermal system gives a programmable control of overdosing by a physician or by the patient himself or herself (patient-friendly approach).

Already-available systems (inhalants, chewing gums, tablets, patches, etc.) are deficient in controlling the release rate because they utilize the flux values of the drug for managing nicotine addiction and opioid withdrawal symptoms (nicotine for smoking cessation, clonidine for opioid withdrawal), which results in variable flux. This problem of variable flux can be resolved using functionalized CNT membranes, and the deliverance rate of a drug to the skin can be manipulated by the applying potential so as to develop a "programmable drug delivery system." Currently, available CNTs-based nanoporous membranes find their application in the treatment of nicotine addiction and opioid withdrawal symptoms.

Paudel et al. fabricated a portable transdermal nicotine patch device (Figure 5.18a) for showing *in vivo* effectiveness in a bald guinea pig (Figure 5.18b). The compact CNTs membrane–based device, equipped with 1.5 V batteries, is sufficient to power efficient pumping of nicotine at levels which are 6–8 times more than what is achievable in passive diffusion. The investigation revealed that the cotinine blood plasma concentrations in the model were enhanced from 5 to 11 ng mL^{-1}, and the release of therapeutics from a patch was altered from passive diffusion–based to an active pumping state–based system (Figure 5.18c).

Similarly, Gulati et al. quantified the variable fluxes of nicotine through a programmable device consisting of a CNTs membrane and validated its performance using an *in vitro* microdialysis method. The CNTs membrane in this device act as a rate-limiting membrane placed over the porcine skin, which contained a microdialysis probe underneath it and allowing quantification of nicotine flux across the skin membrane. In this investigation, authors created a programmable type of device wherein a desired level of nicotine can be achieved. It was demonstrated that if the device is set as "ON" state from "OFF" state through the application of bias fluxes, eventually, three times the nicotine level can be achieved as compared to that of commercial nicotine patches (21 mg/24 h, 14 mg/24 h, and 7 mg/24 h), suggesting an enhanced therapeutic efficiency of this programmable device. Another feature of it was its Bluetooth connectivity, which means that it could be programmable by a smartphone and could also be attached with a distant counseling application for an enhanced smoking cessation treatment.

In this programmable CNTs membrane–based transdermal nicotine device, the advantage of using CNTs is creating energy-effective pumping via a one-atom-thick graphitic core, allowing for high ON/OFF ratios using devices which are equipped with batteries. These batteries can last up to ten days continuously and eventually control the rate of pumping potent therapeutics, as in the case of nicotine.

In another investigation, wherein functionalization with an anionic dye at CNTs pore entrances was used, almost a fourfold greater rectification factor (magnitude of change in current in electrode upon a change in its applied amplitude of the voltage across the same electrode) for ionic current was witnessed in dye-functionalized DWCNTs membranes in contrast to the other membranes. It also validated that the flux through CNT cores is more suitable for utilizing them in switching devices. The collective nicotine release via a DWCNTs membrane employed in a flow cell and microdialysis membrane probe (the assay used by the authors for validation) was measured, and the results obtained showed differences in the magnitude of two cumulative curves obtained. The reason for this observation was a relatively small diffusion area (0.08 cm^2) of the microdialysis membrane as compared to the receptor compartment of the flow cell (0.3 cm^2). An interesting finding was that the shape of the two curves overlaid; this specified that the release of nicotine in the microdialysis membrane probe was comparative to the nicotine release profile in the flow cell. Apart from the benefits of delivering drugs through a transdermal route, several other advantages are also associated with these programmable devices, such as control through the smartphone-based application and counseling application, which further adds to its therapeutic success and prevents the reoccurrence of undesired events.

Another application of CNT membranes is mimicking, as Ilbasmis-Tamer et al. demonstrated with artificial skin, where they developed an artificial CNT-based membrane as an alternative to predict skin permeation. In that study, simultaneous diffusion studies were conducted with variable membrane compositions, including CNTs containing diclofenac, salicylic acid, and dexketoprofen, and compared with commercially available synthetic membranes.

Good correlations can be drawn between permeability values of compounds for human skin and the skin models (e.g., CNTs membrane, isopropyl myristate–treated CNTs membrane [IM-CNTs membrane], bovine serum albumin-cholesterol, and dipalmitoyl phosphatidyl choline-treated membrane [BSA-cholesterol-DPPC-IM-CNTs membrane]). Correlation revealed that in dexketoprofen-loaded CNTs,

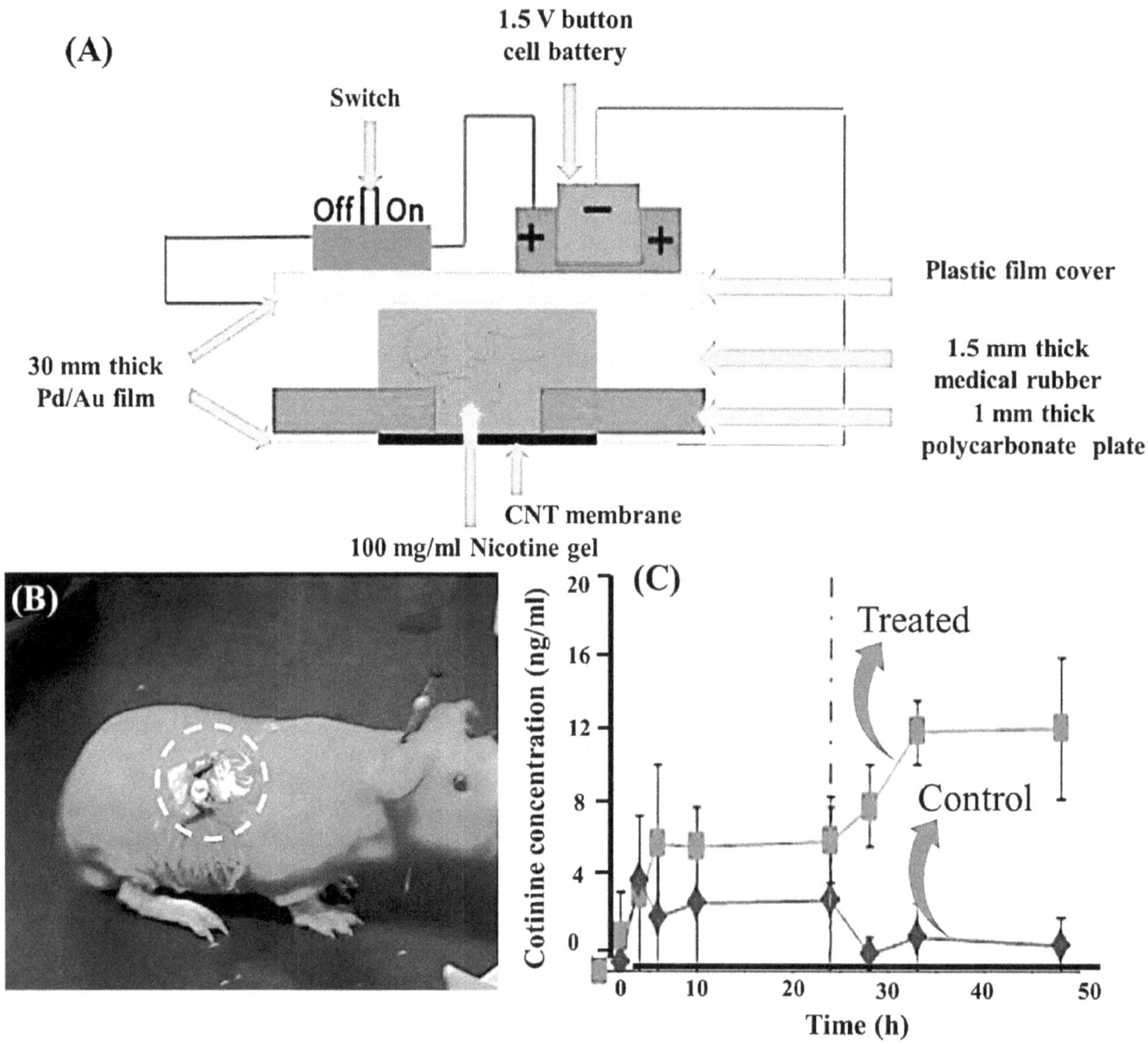

FIGURE 5.18 Programmable transdermal device for controlled release of nicotine from a delivery vehicle: (a) Representation of CNTs membrane transdermal patch construct employed for the *in vivo* programmable delivery of nicotine in bald/naked guinea pigs. (b) Optical picture of a guinea pig with the applied device (encircled as yellow) that is covered with bio-occlusive tape. (c) Release profile of cotinine in an animal model for the OFF/ON study. The patch was off for the first day and then was kept on for two days. As a control, the patch was kept off for those two days.

Source: Adapted with permission, copyright 2012 Wiley Periodicals.

membrane flux values of BSA-cholesterol-DPPC-IM-CNTs (371 ± 328 μg cm^{-2} h^{-1}), CNTs (148 ± 79.7 μg cm^{-2} h^{-1}), and cholesterol-IM-CNTs membrane (139 ± 69.4 μg cm^{-2} h^{-1}) were found to be close to human skin values (267 ± 216 μg cm^{-2} h^{-1}). This demonstrated that a CNT itself could be used as an alternative to predict permeability across skin, adding valuable information to transdermal delivery–based approaches.

Collectively, these findings suggest that CNT-based nanoporous membranes create a very flexible and reasonable solution to drawbacks in smoking cessations and opioid withdrawal symptoms. Also, the problem of therapeutic efflux was also being solved; just by applying electrical flux (or potential), one can adjust the flux of a patch. This technique not only improves patient compliances because of a transdermal route but also proves to be a superior therapy and has helped advance the quality of life of masses of addicted individuals. Finally, these nicotine patch devices possess great potential to be effectively used in clinical settings, with a programmable delivery function on a remote counseling, to empower smoking cessation treatments.

5.8.14 CNTs for Designing Electroactivated and Electroresponsive Transdermal Drug Delivery

The importance of dermal delivery routes increases manifolds when it comes to treatment and management of chronic pain, particularly with limitations of needle phobias and allied discomforts associated with conventional injections, and the present obstacles related with oral dosage forms. However, the development of patch-like devices employed with a mechanism like microelectronic processing, wherein the pharmaceutically active substance is placed in a compact switchable device, is much anticipated by pharma majors.

Primarily, such patch-like delivery devices can successfully deliver larger-molecular-weight molecules, which usually requires higher permeabilization and subsequent enlargement of the stratum corneum, which is possible through electrostimulation.

In support of the previous statement, Guillet et al. recently developed a device which works through "electropermeabilization" (enhancement of skin permeability for permeation of even larger molecules via modifying stratum corneum permeability through electrostimulation). Investigators designed a needleless device composed of DWCNTs-containing nanocomposite material. The fabricated device contains agarose hydrogel and DWCNTs to enhance its electromechanical characteristics. The authors evaluated the fabricated device for structural organization, storage capacity, electrical conductivity (Figure 5.19a and b), and release investigation (Figure 5.19c and d). They observed that DWCNTs were capable of storing agarose gel for a longer time. Also, agarose gel made using water as the only solvent was found to be very effective in dispersing DWCNTs. *Ex vivo* fluorescence investigation using mouse skin showed better accumulation of fluorescein isothiocyanate (FITC) dye in the presence of electric output (1 Hz–1 MHz, with an applied AC voltage of 100 mV at room temperature), in contrast to non-electric output (Figure 5.19e–j). These encouraging results provide good evidence that the use of DWCNTs improves transdermal delivery potentialities of the biocompatible polymer matrix.

Giri et al., in their studies, witnessed an enhanced drug release upon increased applied potentials, and the reason for this observation was the high electrical conductivity of CNTs. Investigators devised composites, including MWCNTs, with carboxymethyl guar gum, which showed ability to be a probable device which could be employed for obtaining a sustained release of NSAIDS via a transdermal route. The authors revealed that MWCNTs homogenously dispersed in carboxymethyl guar gum and marginally reinforced it at 0.5 and 1.0 wt% concentrations; however, the interaction level fell, especially at high temperature, when 1.0 wt% concentration was exceeded. The presence of MWCNTs increases diclofenac sodium retention efficiency inside a hydrogel; maxima have been shown at a 1 wt% level. Hybrid nanocomposites, excluding neat carboxymethyl guar gum and carboxymethyl guar gum 30/3.0, showed a steady and sustained transdermal drug release profile following a non-Fickian-type mechanism. A bursting effect with a high release rate was observed in CMG and, to some extent, in CMG30/3.0, which was due to low matrix viscosity. Finally, authors concluded that CMG30/1.0 gives the slowest release of diclofenac sodium because of its high viscous resistance, and has shown great promise toward future applications.

In a different study by Spizzirri et al., a composite electroconductive hydrogel (ECH) comprised of a natural protein along with MWCNTs was developed. The composite was prepared with an intention of controlling the electroresponsive discharge of diclofenac sodium salt from a hydrogel hybrid prepared from gelatine as a gel-forming agent and CNTs as electrical conducting material, and was synthesized by a simple synthetic approach based on a modified grafting approach.

Collectively, these newer technologies of electroresponsive switchable devices consisting of CNTs are very promising for applications in the arena of transdermal drug delivery. To take the ongoing research in this particular segment, some research groups try hard to optimize the electrostimulation conditions, as the idea of the inclusion of CNTs is also to be able to perform the delivery under much milder conditions, more compatible with a realistic clinical use.

5.8.15 CNTs Membranes as Protein Channel Mimetic Platforms

Biological protein canals are extraordinary systems that can judiciously propel essential chemicals and signals through cell walls at a multiple-fold faster rate than simple diffusion. Impersonating the mentioned function, in the case of drug delivery, by altering chemical conditions or by outside signaling, can expose pores to show a controlled dosing for the desired drug. Thus, complex dosing regimens, generally prescribed in case of addiction treatments, can be empowered by employing such technology.

A common problem of low flux rates has been experienced by all the nanometer-scale pores for selective chemical transport. Slow flux rates are observed as a consequence of Fickian diffusion and sluggish fluid movement in nanometer-scale pores in the case of Newtonian fluids. In this context, liquid movement through the cores of CNTs is expected to demonstrate improved conveyance of hydrocarbon gases and water; similarly, one revolutionary molecular dynamics study anticipated that aqueous movement through electron-rich "hydrophobic" SWCNTs would be possible and, in fact, would be intensely improved.

Transport of drug molecules via skin can be tempered by "gatekeeper" chemistry at the aperture entry by employing the concept of electrostatic attraction/repulsion, by steric hindrance, or by manipulating the biochemical state. Moreover, the exclusive shape construct of CNTs permits chemicals to be positioned exactly at aperture entries, permitting gatekeeper activity. The term "gatekeeper" is analogically utilized as a chemical layer at an aperture entry that precisely permits elements to pass through them, which is analogous to naturally available protein channels. Electro-osmotic movement is considered to be exceedingly effectual and could propel through regions of chemical selectivity. Thus, the essential necessities of imitating protein channels are inherited with CNT membrane.

The notion of an efficient "gatekeeper" which can propel out of or be taken in from an aperture entry could lead to creating the origin of considering it as a "pump" or the lively component of a transdermal drug delivery system. Getting an efficient "gatekeeper" activity employs small voltages, which can be applied using small watch batteries, to open and close membrane apertures so as to control drug release from the reserve. This will enable having programmed and desired medication

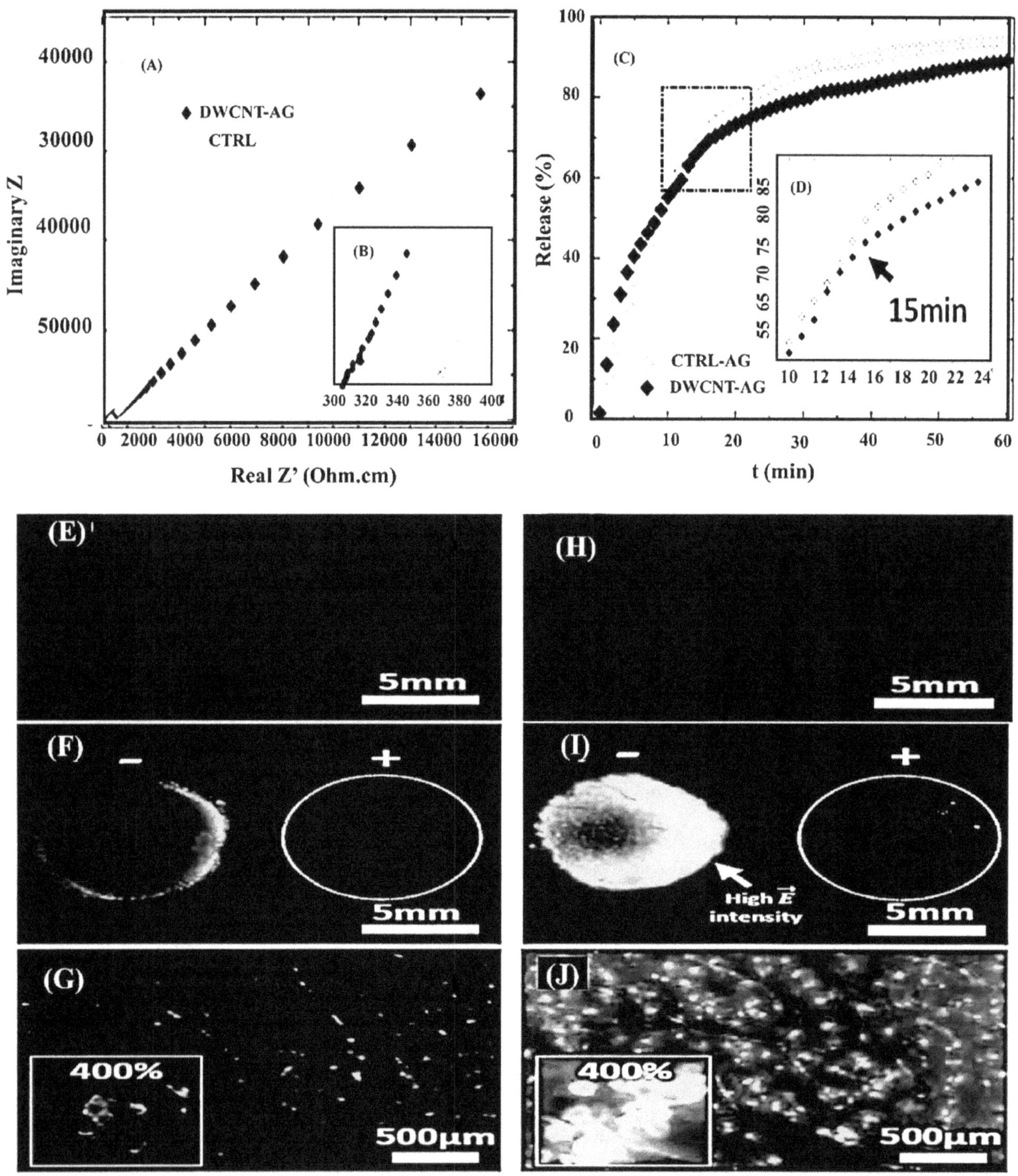

FIGURE 5.19 EIS characterization, release study, and skin visualization (mouse skin) of the CTRL-AG and DWCNTs-AG hydrogel (1 wt% DWCNTs) in the swollen state: (a) Investigation of ionic resistivity. (b) Zoom in the low Z' range. (c) FITC-D release due to release % *vs.* time from CTRL-AG hydrogel and DWCNTs-AG hydrogel nanocomposite (1 wt% DWCNTs). (d) Zoom on the transitory area. (e–h) CTRLAG and DWCNTs-AG without electrical stimulation in identical conditions at the same intensity level (X0, 57). (f, i) Images with electrical stimulation wherein the anode and cathode are positioned on the left- and right-hand side, respectively. (g, j) Images at resolution (×4) of the anode area of (f, h), respectively. The frame on the left side of (g, j) images represents a numerical magnification ×400.

Source: Adapted with permission, copyright 2017 Wiley-VCH Verlag GmbH and Co. KGaA.

regimes which could be easily altered, depending upon a prescribed procedure, so as to avoid any kind of dependency, especially in cases when narcotics are involved.

5.8.16 CNTs in Transdermal Reverse Iontophoresis for Advanced Monitoring

Transdermal reverse iontophoresis is one of the recent methods for therapeutic drug monitoring and is a non-invasive method that can detect drugs and biomolecules. Thus, due its non-invasive nature, it has great perspective in the field of analytical and diagnostic branches of medical science, although the concept of iontophoresis is not new and has been observed since the early nineties. Remarkably, in 2001, the GlucoWatch® G2 Biographer was launched, and it was the first-of-its-kind non-invasive device which could determine plasma sugar level accurately. The major concern for the letdown of the GlucoWatch® G2 Biographer was its incapability to produce suitable electrical signals (lack of sensitivity leading to misleading reports) in the case of hyper- and hypoglycemia; thus, as it could not stand up to the desired expectancy, it was terminated from markets in 2007.

In context, Sun et al. had attempted to resolve this issue by employing CNTs. They established a glucose biosensor which involved an epoxy composite of MWCNTs on a planner carbon electrode. This biosensor enjoys higher sensitivity (low detection potential) that also, within 25 s, shows a brilliant linear response for a series of glucose detections.

Limited reviews are available on the application of CNTs in painless or needle-free optical sensing of biomolecules. An excellent review on the uses of CNTs as an optical painless glucose-sensing tool that was published has been found. The review encompasses many milestone studies in the field, such as functional design of the device, fluorophore properties, advantages, and disadvantages of *in vivo* fluorescence detection of glucose using an SWCNTs-incorporated device, near-infrared optical sensors based on single-walled CNTs (a report published in *Nature Materials*), and the logical strategy of nitric oxide peculiarity toward SWCNTs in near-infrared fluorescence devices for biological molecules recognition (a report published in *Nature Chemistry*).

The preceding reports collectively concluded that the major obstacle in designing CNT-based biomolecule-sensing tools is recognizing and fabricating molecular receptors specific for glucose that will bind effectively in a CNT-detecting system. Another obstacle is to know the mechanism of transferring the glucose-binding proceedings into the modulation of CNT-based fluorescence to attain accuracy with *in vivo* determinations. CNT-based NIR optical sensing opens new paths to reply to significant biological queries concerning painless and needle-free transdermal monitoring of biomolecules. This technology also has potential to be extended to numerous *in vivo* detection systems.

5.8.17 CNTs in Designing Microneedle-Based Composites for Non-Invasive Skin Delivery

In the case of CNT-based microneedles, various researchers approached synthesizing functionalized CNTs using repeated etching and micromachines. However, these approaches increase the complexity of fabrication and therefore limit scale-up and industrial applications. The latest approach to using CNTs for transdermal applications is synthesizing hollow microneedles by employing vertically aligned CNTs (VA-CNTs) to obtain a quick transdermal delivery.

Therefore, the formation of microneedles with a novel approach using VA-CNTs seems to be a good option. These VA-CNTs introduce a whole new perspective on the fabrication of hollow microneedles. First, the VA-CNTs were utilized as a scaffold to guide the figure of the microneedle and then, later on, were used as fiber integral constituents in polymer composites in order to develop good strength which is quite proficient in piercing skin. To grow VA-CNTs, established methods were used, which involved (1) catalyst pattering and (2) thermal chemical vapor deposition (CVD), thereby forming the hollow microneedles.

When designing CNTs–polymer composites for microneedles, the final product must possess four mechanical properties: (1) sufficient mechanical strength when pressure is applied to attain skin penetration, (2) proportionate covering of VA-CNTs with a certain polymer base for easy relocation from growing substrate to drug delivery platforms, (3) attaching microneedles to a mutual polymer base for an uninterrupted relocation from the growth substrate to drug delivery platforms, and (4) reserving an unhindered hollow void for drug delivery. These objectives rely on each other. Hence, careful selection and application of a polymer must be done to fabricate functional microneedles.

Figure 5.20 demonstrates the method and steps for fabrication, beginning with CVD synthesis of patterned VA-CNTs and SU8–2025 (MicroChem, Newton, MA), a negative photoresist, as a polymer candidate. Investigators selected SU8–2025 due to its ability to form thick films through spin coating and the ability of high UV absorbance, which aids to selectively cure the microneedle device.

In the first step of a CNT–polymer composite, SU8–2025 is incorporated to create the microneedle composite. SU8–2025 was drop-cast on the VA-CNTs sample, and then it was inertly wicked into interspacing of the VA-CNTs. In the second step, the sample was spin-coated at 3,000 rpm for 1 min to get rid of additional material and, subsequently, to establish a base which is sufficiently bulky and dense, so as to allow the microneedles to become easily detached from the silicon substrate with minimum impairment to needles and polymer base.

However, SU8–2025 has a high viscosity that disables it from pooling in the internal voids of the microneedle. Then, curing is done wherein oblique UV/visible light was exposed, which selectively cured only the sample. The sample is selectively entrenched within the interspaces between VA-CNTs, but the SU8 which is in the inner cavity remains un-cured due to oblique incidence of UV that avoids direct exposure to internal voids. Consequently, the quantity of light reaching the internal void is further reduced by VA-CNTs in the CNTs-SU8 composite. In the fourth step, the sample was passed through a post-exposure baking of 3 min at 197.6°F, and then the microneedles were plunged in SU8 developer to remove the uncured photoresist from the internal void. The

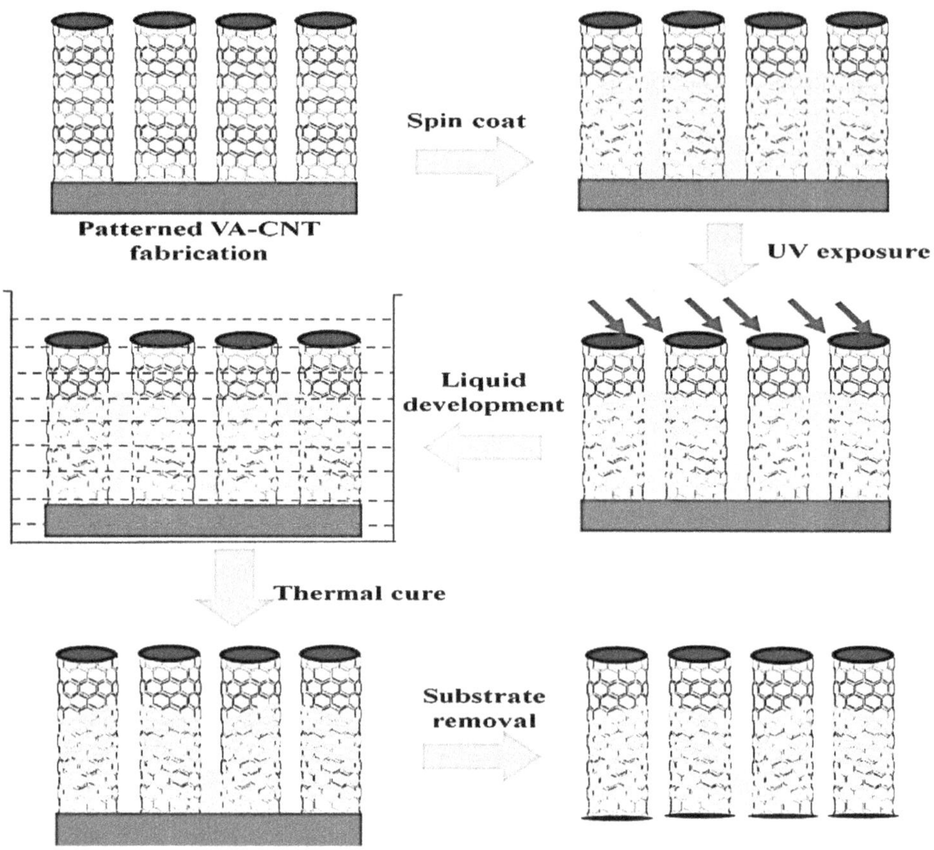

FIGURE 5.20 Schematic representation of the microneedle fabrication process. Microneedle synthesis process preliminary begins with CVD synthesis of patterned VA-CNTs.

plunged system was then placed on a shaker table. Following this, in step 5, the sample was washed with isopropanol and cured under vacuum in an oven at 302°F for 20 min. At this stage, the microneedles were completely formed, with an almost-clear internal void and with SU8 as a base. Thus, utilizing this advantage in step 6, microneedles were removed using a razor blade or tweezers. Next, the delivery stage that attaches the inner voids of microneedles to the liquid reservoir, allowing the drug flow, was connected and then could be used for delivery.

Thus, a new method of fabricating microneedles using VA-CNTs and SU8–2025, wherein there was a synthesis of a strong composite (due to SU8–2025) with VA-CNTs, created an ancillary base for the microneedle array. The early experiments also showed penetration of CNTs-SU8 needles through the skin in in vitro analysis and proved to be able to withstand greater flow rates of up to 600 μL min^{-1} per needle. The authors found that CNTs-SU8 fabrication of microneedles was much easier than silicon microneedles. Thus, further studies are yet to be buttoned up for scalability aspects of CNTs–polymer microneedles to properly recognize future applications and markets for this technology. Thus, such advancements have led to various research avenues which could be explored in context with CNT applications in several fields, especially in transdermal delivery.

5.8.18 Buckypapers: Thinnest Solution for Delivering Drugs

Buckypapers are thin microscopic sheets of randomly entangled CNTs, which are highly porous networks. They are composed of several aggregates of CNTs or carbon nanogrid paper or "buckytubes." In contrast to steel, buckypapers have one-tenth the weight of steel yet are almost 500 times stronger than steel when stacked to form composites. Owing to high surface area and drug loading capacity, buckypapers eventually found applications in transdermal drug delivery.

One such study which employed buckypapers for transdermal application conducted by Schwengber et al. included synthesis of buckypapers using diverse types of CNTs, followed by characterization and estimating their potential as a novel transdermal delivery system. In this study, the authors employed clonidine hydrochloride as their model drug. Then, they employed several variations in composition, along with functionalization of drug-loaded buckypapers; finally, its effect in *in vitro* release was studied. Thus, it was observed that the higher the degree of functionalization with hydroxyl or carboxyl groups, the slower the release of parameters that were found to influence the release rates, that is, drug mass ratio, the framework like the layers of CNTs, that is, monolayer or bilayer, and the chemical buildup of the drug that can affect the release profile. This shows a colossal future for CNT applications in drug delivery, as release profiles can be altered just by altering such parameters.

Now, to understand whether the nature of a drug affects the release profile, Schwengber et al. used two model drugs in which clonidine hydrochloride (CHC) and acidic drug flurbiprofen (FB) were loaded in electromodulated CNT-derived buckypapers. Figure 5.21a and b show the SEM images of ethanol-crystallized CHC and FB. Also, Figure 5.21c, when compared with Figure 5.21d and e, show how well CHC and FB dispersed within the interstices of the nanotubes.

The laboratory-synthesized MWCNTs were found to be thicker and straighter than commercially available MWCNTs, as can be observed from Figure 5.21F. Further, the authors observed a passive release profile which is dependent on the non-covalent interaction between the drug and the CNTs. Thus, the modulation of a drug release profile could be possible by applying electrical biases of proper polarity. Thus, in the future, such devices could be employed for controlling the release profile of several drugs which could be easily modified depending upon what the desired rates are.

5.8.19 Limitations of CNTs as a Transdermal Carrier

5.8.19.1 Dermal Absorption of CNTs: A Limiting Factor

Though investigations from several laboratories have generated extensive data related to the toxic nature of CNTs, there is very little literature available on how CNTs cross the skin and its permeation mechanism. The main hurdle for a CNT for its topical delivery is the stratum corneum, because it is hydrophobic in nature. But as CNT possesses a high aspect ratio and hydrophobicity, that increases the chance for a macromolecule to penetrate. Even though permeation of CNTs is

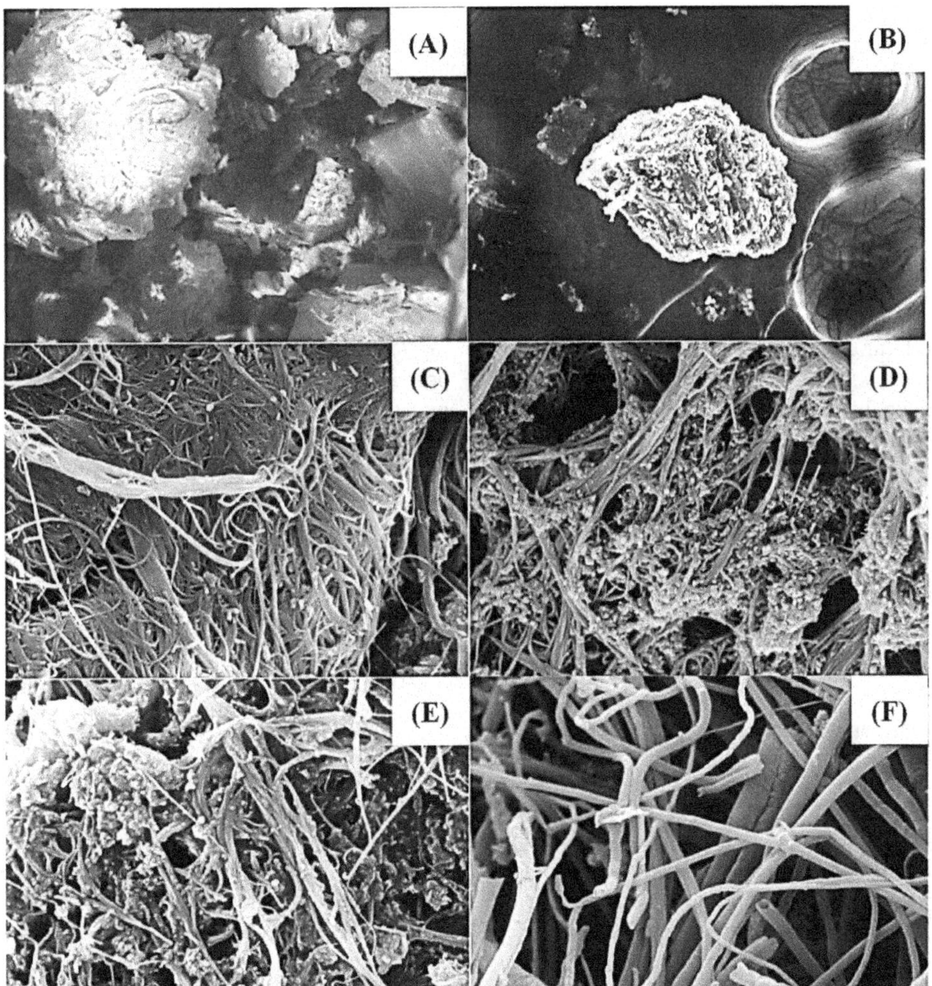

FIGURE 5.21 Scanning electron microscopic images of recrystallized drug and loaded and synthesized MWCNTs: (a) SEM image of recrystallized CHC using ethanol antisolvent. (b) Recrystallized FB using ethanol antisolvent. (c) Empty or unloaded buckypapers based on commercial MWCNTs. (d, e) Buckypapers loaded with CHC and FB, respectively. (f) Lab synthesized MWCNTs.

Source: **Adapted with permission, copyright 2015 Elsevier B.V.**

not yet properly understood, several studies have been conducted to look for the kinds of interactions shown by CNTs with keratinocytes.

Such findings revealed that MWCNTs which are neither derivatized nor optimized tend to exhibit localization within the epithelial cells and initiate irritation (IL-8 release) in the same, which constitutes a transdermal route; however, the study was carried out *in vitro* that lacked the mimicking of stratum corneum, and thus, the mechanism for penetration still remains to be elucidated.

Extending the observed findings, a similar group of investigators undertook another study aiming to discover a surfactant that precludes the development of bulky conglomerates formed of MWCNTs without producing toxicity to the HEKs. For this purpose, HEKs were prepared in serial dilutions (10% to 0.1% v/v) of L61, L92, and F127 Pluronic and 20 or 60 Tween for one day. Upon evaluation of viability, the viability of HEK was found to be proportional to surfactant concentration, which was set within a range from 26.9% to 97.9% with Pluronic F127; viability along with additional surfactants was lower than 11%. The decrease in the aggregation of MWCNTs in the medium was observed with all the tested surfactants. MWCNTs at 500 μg mL^{-1} in 6% or 2% Pluronic F127 were incubated with HEKs and then analyzed for the presence of interleukin 8.

There have been other findings which also revealed dermal irritation in humans when exposed to carbonaceous materials, as in the development of dermatitis or hyperkeratosis. Similarly, Shvedova et al. suggested that nanoparticles such as CNTs and the like may produce toxicity due to immortalized HaCaT human keratinocyte cultures. The obtained data pointed out that nanotubes which are not optimized for cellular delivery are liable to transform keratinocyte functions.

Moreover, various factors also have a significant impact on how the pattern and degree of absorption of CNTs through the skin surface will be. These generally include size, structural morphology, surface functionalization, and composition. Therefore, a prediction of dermal absorption of CNTs still requires many experimental data to prove using different size, shape, type, and functionalization methods, and so there are still thrust areas in the field of drug delivery.

5.8.20 Potential Risks with CNTs: Reports on Transdermal Toxicity

In explaining toxicity, the resemblance of CNTs with asbestos has provoked investigations to study their effects on the respiratory system, as there is a probability that CNTs can be delivered into the body through several routes which could be toxic in other unknown ways [103]. Moreover, in vivo toxicity studies of CNTs can play a significant role in risk assessment. These methods can be used to measure acute toxicity, chronic toxicity, developmental toxicity, genotoxicity, and reproductive toxicity. However, the mechanism of toxicity remains the same irrespective of the administration of CNTs into a body and is largely manifested as oxidative stress, inflammatory responses, malignant transformation, DNA damage and mutation, formation of granuloma, and interstitial fibrosis.

There are several *in vitro* assessments related to CNT toxicity, one of which was done by Witzmann et al., which concluded that MWCNTs, when exposed to human epidermal keratinocytes (HEKs) for 24 h, lead to dysregulation of 36 proteins (with $P < 0.01$). This was confirmed through 2D gel electrophoresis and mass spectroscopy, and almost 106 proteins were dysregulated when exposed for 48 h. Thus, this dysregulation of proteins could have direct effects on cell metabolism, cell signaling, cytoskeletal elements, and vesicular trafficking components.

Another study was done by Sato et al. wherein the role of the length of CNTs exposed to skin was deduced. *In vitro* studies done on human acute monocytic leukemia cell line THP-1 CNTs of 220 nm (220-CNTs) and CNTs of 825 nm (825-CNTs) in length showed no significant response in eluting distinctive inflammatory response, although *in vivo* 825-CNTs showed an inflammatory response in subcutaneous tissue more than 220-CNTs. This was because the macrophages could easily uptake 220 nm CNTs, but not the 825 nm CNT.

Although there are numerous factors which affect CNT's toxicity, such as intrinsic physiochemical properties of CNTs, there are also many external factors, like cell types, experimental conditions, and assays. Numerous in vivo experiments are being carried out to examine the consequences of dermal exposure to CNTs.

One such study claims that, when non-purified CNTs are placed on mice skin, it leads to oxidative stress and also causes depletion of glutathione and enhanced dermal thickness due to amplified dermal cell numbers. The metal (particularly iron) content of SWCNT has been demonstrated via the metal's ability to interact with the skin, initiate oxidative stress, and induce redox-sensitive transcription factors, leading to inflammation. The effects of SWCNT were assessed both *in vitro* and *in vivo* using EpiDerm FT engineered skin, murine epidermal cells (JB6 P+), and immune-competent hairless SKH-1 mice. Topical exposure of SKH-1 mice (five days, with daily doses of 40 g per mouse, 80 g per mouse, or 160 g per mouse) to unpurified SWCNT caused oxidative stress, depletion of glutathione, oxidation of protein thiols and carbonyls, elevated myeloperoxidase activity, an increase of dermal cell numbers, and skin thickening resulting from the accumulation of polymorphonuclear, leukocytes (PMNs), and mast cells. Topical exposure of un-purified SWCNT, that is, 60 μg per mice, revealed accumulation of polymorphonuclear leukocytes (PMNs) within the epidermis and dermis as compared to control-exposed skin (Figure 5.22A). The inflammation, that is, recruitment of PMNs, was localized around or within the hair follicles. Increased inflammation was observed in adipose tissue as well as in a few sebaceous glands of SWCNT-exposed mice. Also, the skin of mice exposed to unpurified SWCNT showed increased mast cell activity and degranulation that was not observed in the skin of control mice (Figure 5.22B).

The outcomes of this investigation signified that the purity of the CNTs is a critical factor in imparting toxicity when administered topically. Several metals, predominantly iron, are considered to be a type of impurity in CNTs, and the main reason to find such materials in CNTs as impurities is their employment during the synthesis process.

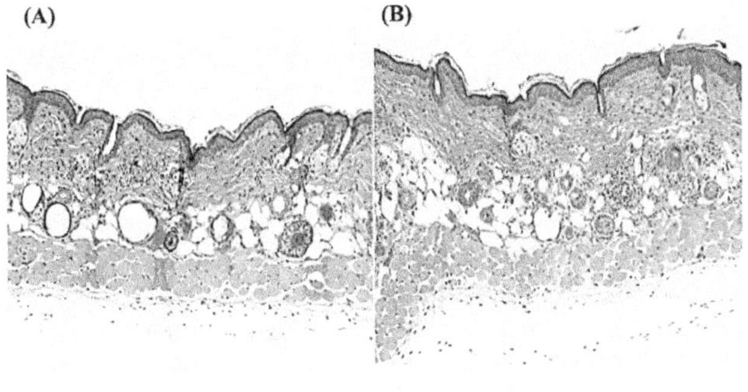

FIGURE 5.22 Photomicrographs of skins of SKH-1 mice upon treatment with (a) un-purified SWCNT (30% weight iron contamination; 160 g per mouse) and (b) control (PBS) daily for five days.

Source: Adapted with permission. Copyright 2009 Elsevier.

In a very recent report, Ema et al. compiled the outcomes of their investigations on sensitization of skin along with eye and dermal irritation upon exposure with CNTs. It is well-known that dermal and ophthalmic sites have the maximum risk of adverse biological reaction with CNTs. To understand the toxic effects, different CNT-based products from various manufacturers (Nikkiso-SWCNTs, Nikkiso-MWCNTs, Super-growth SWCNTs, and Mitsui-MWCNTs) were evaluated for skin and eye irritation employing rabbits, and skin sensitization employing guinea pigs. Upon skin/eye irritation tests, Nikkiso-SWCNTs, super-growth-SWCNTs, and Nikkiso-MWCNTs were not found as irritants to the skin/eyes. The Mitsui-MWCNTs was found to produce minor erythemas after one day of exposure, but nothing was observed on the third day after exposure; once the patch for dermal irritation was removed, conjunctival redness and blood vessel hyperemia were observed at 1 h, but nothing was observed after one day, in the eye irritation experiments. These results concluded that SWCNTs-based products, and one of the MWCNTs-based product, were safe, and only one of the MWCNTs products showed a little skin-sensitization effects.

Interestingly, in a recent investigation, Kishore et al. assessed the dermal and ocular *in vitro* and *in vivo* toxicity data on rabbits using two different sizes of commercially available MWCNTs (average diameter 135 nm and 12.5 nm). Results of acute eye irritation toxicity studies with two different sizes of MWCNT in rabbits demonstrated reversible conjunctival redness and discharge and exhibited minimal concern, while acute dermal irritation studies indicated that both the sizes of MWCNTs were non-irritating to the skins of rabbits. *In vitro* skin (EPISKIN) irritation studies revealed that two sizes of MWCNT were non-irritating to the skin. *In vivo* skin irritation studies revealed no dermal reactions like erythema and edema in rabbits when both sizes of MWCNTs were applied. The results [104] revealed cytotoxicity for HEK cells when exposed to MWCNTs, and this result was independent of the level of surfactant exposed. MWCNTs-induced IL-8 release declined when 2% or 6% Pluronic F127 was exposed. However, it was worth noting that MWCNTs and the surfactant, either alone or in combination, could enhance the IL-8 release, unlike that seen in control exposures at 12 and 24 h. The final outcome showed that there were several complex interactions observed between surfactant and MWCNTs, rather than just a simple dispersion alone, and hence, there is a call for further investigation to determine the mode of interaction. In conclusion, this work [104] purports that the future of alternative research lies in the validation of methodology for nanomaterials.

A study done by Koyama et al., wherein levels of $CD4^+$ and $CD8^+$ T cells were measured upon exposure of four different types of CNTs with varying length, diameter, surface area, iron content, and post-treatment after synthesis (SWNTs, MWNTs-I, MWNTs-II, and Cup-stacked CNT), described inflammation caused from CNT exposure. It was observed that all mice survived up to three months upon subcutaneous implantation of CNTs only. SWNCT showed higher $CD4^+/CD8^+$ values after one week via a major histocompatibility complex (MHC) class I pathway of antigen–antibody response system. Thus, after two weeks, significantly higher values in $CD4^+$ and $CD4^+/CD8^+$ without change in $CD8^+$ signified an activated MHC class II for all samples. The toxicological response was much lower in comparison to asbestos; hence, the authors concluded that such relatively lower toxicity observed for CNTs could lead to assert for its widespread application.

Still, a proper and in-depth understanding of the toxicological profile concerning CNTs is unclear; thus, more quantitative and robust data relating to dermal toxicity upon exposure of CNTs is required so that a path to successful application in skin therapeutics can be built.

5.8.21 Patents on the Use of CNTs in Transdermal Delivery

CNTs possess high charge density, small pore dimensions, and fast flow through CNT cores. Thereby, we can control the rate of drug release. Also, in the previous sections, they have been efficiently proven to deliver drugs transdermally with minimal skin irritation. Most of the patents in this arena are related to impregnation of CNTs with microneedles.

Gharib et al. received a patent for developing a transdermal patch comprising a substrate with an array of CNTs having two ends. One end of the CNT was attached to the substrate, and the other end protruded out through the substrate, facilitating the transfer of a substance from the substrate to tissues. Additionally, CNTs were grouped into bunches such that each bunch could efficaciously function as a needle. A drug can coat on the surface of CNTs. Such a nanotechnology-based patch can be employed to deliver through skin or to the superficial surface of an angioplasty balloon.

Similarly, Bosnyak et al. received a patent for developing open-ended CNTs dispersed in a polymer forming film as a transdermal drug delivery system. Investigators described the specification as CNTs having a length smaller than about 4 μm, preferably smaller than 2 μm, and an aspect ratio of about 10 to about 500 (preferably about 50 to 120).

Lyon et al. formulated a polymer CNT hollow microneedle array for transdermal application. Methods described by the investigator involved providing a plurality of CNT bundles in an array. Upon further substrate coating, the substrate bundles were impregnated with a liquid polymer (poly(3,3″,4,4″-benzophenone tetracarboxylic dianhydride-co-4,4″-oxydianiline/1,3-phenylenediamine)polyimide), which is

TABLE 5.7
Representative Various Patents for Transdermal Application Using CNTs

Patent No.	Patent Title	Patent Filing Date	Patent Publication Date	Ref.
US9050444B2	Drug delivery and substance transfer facilitated by nano-enhanced device having aligned CNTs protruding from device surface	Feb. 7, 2013	Jun. 9, 2015	[105]
WO2015103214A1	Transdermal patches with discrete CNTs	Dec. 30, 2014	Jul. 9, 2015	[106]
US20140296780A1	Polymer composite CNTs microneedle devices and their fabrication	Mar. 31, 2014	Oct. 2, 2014	[107]
CN105520905A	Preparation method and application of podophyllotoxin transdermal drug delivery preparation	Nov. 17, 2015	Apr. 27, 2016	[108]

Source: [104].

a thermosetting polymer resin. Curing the polymer produced polymer composite CNTs pillars embedded in a polymer base; the last step involved removing the base from the substrate.

One investigator prepared podophyllotoxin-loaded CNTs for transdermal application wherein each 100 g by mass consisted of 0.1–10 g of carboxylic CNT–loaded podophyllotoxin, 1–5 g of carbomer, 5–15 g of glycerol, 3–6 g of the zone, 0.1–0.5 g of triethanolamine, and 80–85 g of pure water. This podophyllotoxin CNT transdermal preparation can be formulated into a gel, which showed better stability compared to the podophyllotoxin gel. Additionally, skin penetration rate was found to be relatively low, and the amount retained in the skin was increased, so that the curative effect on condyloma acuminate was enhanced. Side effects and skin sensitivity were also reduced. Thus, CNTs have demonstrated the potential to be fabricated into transdermal drug delivery systems.

Thus, recent patents records reveal CNTs as emerging nanocarriers for transdermal delivery. Also, surface modification of CNTs is an additional attribute which enhances skin permeability. The diversity of CNTs may lead to many more patents in the arena of transdermal delivery. Table 5.7 [104] lists various patents on CNTs as vector for transdermal delivery.

5.9 Toxicity Concerns for Carbon-Based Nanomaterials

There have been a lot of concerns on the safety issues of the biomedical applications of CNMs. Many of the toxicity and long-term effect concerns are related to the persistence of CNMs in biological systems. A series of information on the pharmacokinetics, metabolism, long duration of CNMs *in vivo*, and toxicity is required. Several studies have been conducted reflecting the conflicting outcomes over the toxicity of CNMs, concerning their successful biomedical application [109]. It has been demonstrated that concentration, lateral dimension, surface properties, types, and presence of functional groups markedly affect their toxicity in the biological environment (Figure 5.23).

Tripathi et al. developed graphitic photoluminescent water-soluble carbon nano-onions (wsCNO) from the traditional pyrolysis of vegetable ghee without employing any metal catalyst through a simple oxidative treatment using nitric acid. The fabricated wsCNO possessed tunable photoluminescence behavior from the visible-to-near-infrared region. They further segregated small-sized wsCNO from the bulk via gel filtration, acquiring a highly fluorescent colored fraction, which they used for cell imaging of *E. coli* and *Pseudomonas putida* and the selective, immediate detection of glucose molecules based upon a simple fluorescence "turn-off"/"turn-on" technique. Pakhira and co-researchers demonstrated the successful crossing of small-sized wsCNO through the blood–brain barrier in the murine model of cerebral autosomal-dominant arteriopathy with subcortical infarcts and leukoencephalopathy (CADASIL), as well as in glioblastoma multiforme (GBM)–induced mice. They reported that the drug was readily eliminated from the animal model after a few days, signifying the probable use of water-soluble carbon nano-onions as a drug carrier.

The physical characteristics of CNTs, such as fiber shape, length, and accumulation, could affect the immunological responses and their accretion in tissues. Shorter CNTs were reported to be less toxic than longer CNTs when injected subcutaneously. Shorter CNTs were found in the cytosol of the macrophage after four weeks, but longer CNTs were found to be free-floating and caused inflammation. This study confirmed that the toxicity of MWCNTs was length-dependent and was comparable with that of asbestos toxicity.

Wang et al. exhibited a cell mapping curve for various cells under similar conditions and stated that GQDs having a size below 10 nm possess high cell viability. There are reports that the solubilizing agents also impacted the toxicity of CNTs. Jos et al. reported that COOH-functionalized SWCNTs induced greater toxicity in the human umbilical vein endothelial cell (HUVEC) lines in comparison to the non-functionalized SWCNTs. Metallic impurities such as metal ions incorporated during fabrication contribute a lot to the toxicity of CNTs. Graphene also has toxicity concerns that restrict its use in the biomedical field, and to lower it, coating with blood protein has been demonstrated by the Chong group. GQDs with smaller size seem to be less toxic than GO or CNT. Tian and the group reported that hydroxylated GQDs showed substantial toxicity on A549 and H1299 cells. Simultaneously, a study conducted by Nurunnabi et al. stated that carboxylated GQDs showed no acute toxicity on KB, MDA-MB231, A549, and normal cells, such as MDCK. They further reported in their in vivo studies that the GQDs did not affect the organs notably in long-term studies.

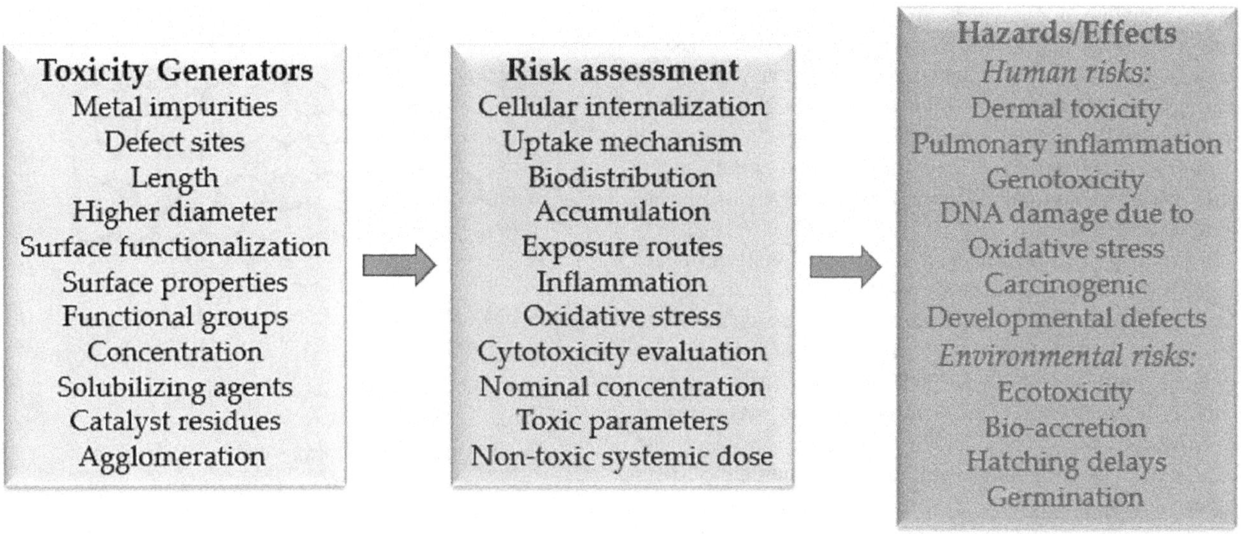

FIGURE 5.23 An insight on the factors causing toxicity, their risk assessment and deleterious effects on humans as well as the environment by carbon-based nanomaterials (CNMs).

Garriga et al. reported the cytotoxicity of the various carbon nanomaterials in their study. They developed multiple CNMs, such as carbon nanohorns (CNH), carbon nanotubes (CNT), carbon nanoplatelets (CNP), graphene oxide (GO), reduced graphene oxide (rGO), and nanodiamonds (ND). They tested the *in vitro* cytotoxicity of the aforementioned CNMs by the MTT assay in human epithelial colorectal adenocarcinoma (Caco-2) cells and human breast adenocarcinoma (MCF-7) cells. The cell viability was found to be in the following order: CNP < CNH < RGO < CNT < GO < ND for both Caco-2 and MCF-7 cell lines. They reported that ND and GO showed low toxicity, owing to the presence of oxygenated functional groups on their surface, which guards their hydrophobic domains. On the other hand, carbon nanohorns and carbon nanoplatelets induced Caco-2 and MCF-7 apoptosis/necrosis and increased ROS levels, which could be associated with the lowering of cell viability in comparison to carbon nanotubes and reduced graphene oxide [110]. Graphene has been evaluated for its toxicity in animals and cells [111]. A range of animal models has also been utilized in the investigation of, for example, ND biocompatibility and fate *in vivo* [112]. Various *in vitro* and *in vivo* studies have been reported to assess the cell viability, gene activity, and physiological behavior of the CNMs. In a study on mice, nanodiamonds, when administered within the trachea, exhibited low pulmonary toxicity. The amount of nanodiamonds decreased with time in the alveolar region, and the macrophages laden with nanodiamonds stayed in the bronchia for 28 days after exposure.

Toxicity issues of CNMs on humans are still not assessed. Few studies have indicated that pristine CNTs, similarly to asbestos, could be the possible source of lung disease in industrial workers.

Ali-Boucetta et al., in their studies, reported that the asbestos-like reactivity and pathogenicity reported for long pristine nanotubes can be reduced completely by surface modification and curtailing their length upon reacting with chemicals such as tri(ethylene glycol) (TEG).

By the functionalization of CNMs, toxicity can be lowered for their biomedical applications. Rungrotmongkol et al., in their studies, indicated that non-covalently functionalized chitosan-coated CNTs accumulated in the reticuloendothelial system (RES) and were slowly excreted through the bile without causing side effects to the mice. The so-fabricated CNTs displayed improved dispersion and biocompatibility. Similarly, Kam and the group non-covalently functionalized SWCNTs with amphiphilic phospholipid–polyethylene glycol (PLPEG). The developed system exhibited augmented solubility, biocompatibility, and stability in the aqueous phase, as the hydrophobic lipid chains of PLPEG were strongly adsorbed onto the CNTs surface, while the hydrophilic PEG chain enhanced the solubility and biocompatibility of the entire functionalized SWCNTs.

Russier et al., in their recent study on myelomonocytic leukemia, reported that few-layers graphenes (FLG) dispersions can attack monocytes, being non-toxic to the immune cells. They demonstrated that graphene holds targeting ability and boosted the necrosis of monocytic cancer cells. They further compared the FLG and etoposide chemotherapeutic potential, where FLG showed substantial anticancer activity.

5.10 Computational Investigations of Fixed-Free and Fixed-Fixed Types of SWCNT Mass Sensing Biosensor

Using carbon nanotubes for sensing mass in a biosensor has recently been proven as an emerging technology in the healthcare industry. This study investigates relative frequency shifts and sensitivity studies of various biological objects, such as insulin hormone, immunoglobulin G (IgG), the most abundant type of antibody, and low-density lipoproteins (LDL) masses, using single-walled carbon nanotubes as a biomass sensor via continuum mechanics. Uniform distributed mass is applied to the single-walled carbon nanotube mass sensor. In this study, fixed–free and fixed–fixed type single-walled carbon nanotubes with various lengths of relative frequency shifts are studied.

In this section, we developed a computationally efficient single-walled carbon nanotube as a biological mass sensor with the continuum mechanics method using the finite element method. Using biological objects such as insulin hormone, immunoglobulin G (IgG), and low-density lipoproteins (LDL) masses as a distributed load, the mass sensing investigations are carried out. In this study, fixed–free and fixed–fixed types of single-walled carbon nanotubes with various lengths of relative frequency shifts and sensitivity analysis are examined. Additionally, sensitivity analysis of fixed–free and fixed–fixed type CNT biological mass sensors is carried out.

5.10.1 Vibration Analysis of the CNT Model with Distributed Mass

The Euler–Bernoulli theory is used to model SWCNT as resonators via continuum mechanics. The motion of free vibration equation can be expressed as:

$$EI\frac{\partial^4 u(x,t)}{\partial x^4} + \rho A\frac{\partial^4 u(x,t)}{\partial x^4} = 0, \tag{1}$$

Where $u(x, t)$, E, I, and ρ are considered as the transverse deflection, Young's modulus, second moment of the cross-sectional area A, and the density of SWCNT, respectively. The fundamental frequency can be expressed as:

$$fn = \frac{1}{2\pi}\sqrt{\frac{k_{eq}}{m_{eq}}}, \tag{2}$$

Where keq is the equivalent stiffness, and meq is the first-mode vibration of attached mass with SWCNT mass. In this study, two different boundary constraints, named fixed–free and fixed–fixed type, are considered for the mass sensing analysis of the biosensor.

5.10.1.1 Analysis of SWCNT with Fixed–Free Boundary Condition

Figure 5.24 shows SWCNT with fixed–free boundary condition. By taking into account the length L of SWCNT is perturbed with the uniform mass M, that is, at $x=L$. The resonance frequencies of fixed–free SWCNT can be attained from:

$$fn = \frac{\lambda_j^2}{2\pi}\sqrt{\frac{EI}{\rho AL}}, \tag{3}$$

Where λ_j values are acquired and expressed the subsequent transcendental equation:

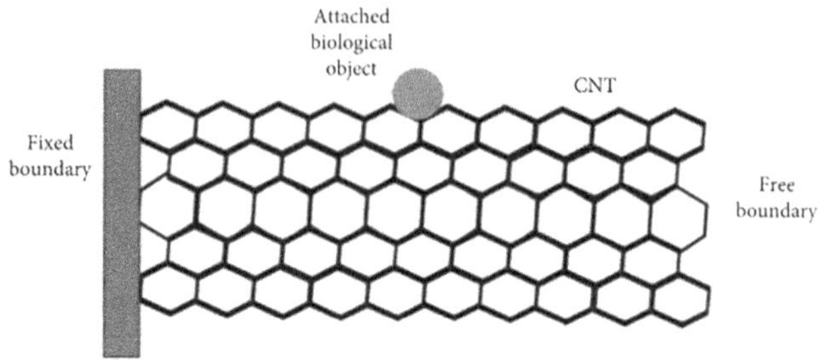

FIGURE 5.24 SWCNT with fixed–free boundary condition.

$$\cos\lambda \cos\lambda + 1 = 0 \tag{4}$$

The mode shapes of vibrations can be attained as:

$$Yj(\xi) = (\cosh\lambda_i\xi - \cos\lambda_j\xi) - \left(\frac{\sin\lambda_j - \sin\lambda_j}{\cosh\lambda_j - \cosh\lambda_j}\right) .(\sinh\lambda_i\xi - \sin\lambda_j\xi) \tag{5}$$

Where $\xi = x/L$ is the length of CNTs along normalized coordinate. The first mode of vibration is significant for the sensing applications, and the value is $\lambda_1 = 1.8751$. The value is attained by executing the transcendental (4).

$$k_{eq} = 12.36\frac{EI}{L^3}; \qquad m_{eq} = \rho AL + 4M. \tag{6}$$

Since we have applied distributed load, where:

$$M = m \times \gamma L, \tag{7}$$

$$f_n = \frac{1}{2\pi}\sqrt{\frac{k_{eq}}{m_{eq}}} = \frac{1}{2\pi}\frac{\alpha_k\beta}{\sqrt{1+a_m\Delta M}}, \tag{8}$$

Where $\alpha_k = 3.5$, $\alpha_m = 4$.

$$\Delta M = \frac{M}{\rho AL} \tag{9}$$

$$\beta = \sqrt{\frac{EI}{\rho AL^4}}.$$

5.10.1.2 Analysis of SWCNT with Fixed-Fixed Boundary Condition

For the fixed–fixed boundary condition shown in Figure 5.25, the motion and the natural frequency equations are followed by (1) and (2), respectively.

Moreover, the λj values are attained by executing

$$\cos\lambda \cosh\lambda + 1 = 0 \tag{10}$$

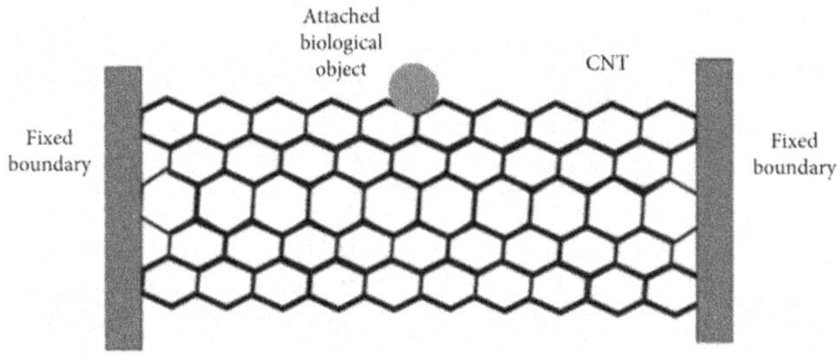

FIGURE 5.25 SWCNT with fixed–fixed boundary condition.

The mode shape of vibration is stated as:

$$Y_j(\xi) = (\cosh\lambda_i\xi - \cos\,\lambda_j\xi) - \left(\frac{\cosh\lambda_j - \cos\lambda_j}{\sinh\lambda_j - \sin\lambda_j}\right)(\sinh\lambda_i\xi - \sin\,\lambda_j\xi) \tag{11}$$

Where $\xi = x/L$, and the value of first-mode vibration is $\lambda 1 = 4.7300$. Using equation (6), the mode shape normalizing is carried out.

$$k_{eq} = 500.56\frac{EI}{L^3};$$
$$m_{eq} = \rho AL + 2.52M. \tag{12}$$

Since we have applied distributed load and $M = m \times \gamma L$,

$$f_n = \frac{1}{2\pi}\sqrt{\frac{k_{eq}}{m_{eq}}} = \frac{1}{2\pi}\frac{\alpha_k\beta}{\sqrt{1+a_m\Delta M}}, \tag{13}$$

Where $\alpha_k = 22.37$, $\alpha_m = 2.52$:

$$\Delta M = \frac{M}{\rho AL},$$
$$\beta = \sqrt{\frac{EI}{\rho AL^4}}. \tag{14}$$

5.10.1.3 Analysis of Mass Detection

For the free vibrations of CNT, substituting $\Delta M = 0$ in (8), the resonant frequency is attained as:

$$f_{0n} = \frac{1}{2\pi}\alpha_k\beta. \tag{15}$$

From (13) and (15), the resonant frequency shift attained due to the distributed attached mass can be expressed as:

$$\Delta f = f_{0n} - f_n = f_{0n} - \frac{f_{0n}}{\sqrt{1+\alpha_m\Delta M}}, \tag{16}$$

And the added mass actual value can be attained as:

$$M = \frac{\rho AL}{\alpha_m}\frac{\left(\alpha_k^2\beta^2\right)}{\left(\alpha_k\beta - 2\pi\Delta f\right)^2} - \frac{\rho AL}{\alpha_m} \tag{17}$$

Eq. (17) relates the added mass with the shift of frequency.

5.10.2 Model Validation

The fixed–free and fixed–fixed based CNT models' mode shapes for six fundamental frequency levels for the length-to-diameter ratio of 7.27 for getting the precision of the model have been studied. To find the accuracy of the present CNT model, initially, our finite-element CNT model is verified with previous molecular dynamics and commercially available finite element model for the same material properties and the dimensions.

The fundamental frequency comparison for the present FEM work with the existing work has been investigated. The results [113] are compared with those of the previous study and will be agreed with that study. The values of the existing work and present work are given in Table 5.8. From the table, it has been clearly demonstrated that our model CNT provides minimum discrepancy compared to the previous length-to-diameter ratio studies, and it provides the assurance to take on further studies as a biological mass sensor. The value of E and ρ is taken as 1: 0 TPa and 2: 24 g/cc, respectively.

The present work provided better error results than previous works.

5.10.3 Resonance Frequency Analysis for Fixed-Free Boundary

The continuum mechanics single-walled CNT is modelled as a fixed–free beam, where one end is to be fixed and the other end is to be free. Figure 5.26 shows the fixed–free type of CNT. Distributed load is uniformly applied on CNT. The fixed–free CNT is initially assumed straight and no extensile and loaded the distributed forces uniformly. From this technique, the mechanical behavior of the nanoresonator biosensor solutions provided is accurate and reliable. Using this system, the mode shapes analysis and frequency shift studies of the nanobiosensor are performed. SWCNT from fundamental frequency to six changes of frequencies without attaching any mass on CNT has been studied. In the fixed–free mode, the length of the carbon nanotube is changed from 2 nm to 20 nm to obtain the various results and mode shapes analysis up to six levels. The diameter of the carbon nanotube is 1.1 nm for all the studies in this work. The change of frequencies is in GHz. To understand SWCNT as a nanobiomass sensor, in this study, three biological objects—insulin hormone; immunoglobulin G (IgG), the most abundant type of antibody; and low-density lipoprotein (LDL) masses—are considered. The mass values of insulin hormone 9.644 zg, immunoglobulin G 249.081 zg, and low-density lipoproteins 4981.620 zg are taken into account for the analysis. Compared to different distributed uniform masses attached with fixed–free SWCNT, the frequency changes occurred reasonably. The mode shape and

TABLE 5.8
Fundamental Frequency Comparisons for the Present FE Work with Existing MD Work

L/D	Fundamental Frequencies	MD [114]	FE [115]	% Error	Present	% Error
3.727	F1	10.315	10.769	–4.40	**9.409**	**–8.78**
	F2	10.315	10.769	–4.40	**9.411**	**–8.75**
	F3	10.478	16.859	–60.90	**9.945**	**–5.08**
	F4	10.478	22.224	–112.10	**9.946**	**–5.07**
	F5	15.796	22.224	–40.69	**14.589**	**–7.63**
5.090	F1	6.616	6.683	–4.04	**6.561**	**–0.82**
	F2	6.616	6.884	–4.05	**6.561**	**–0.82**
	F3	9.143	12.237	–33.84	**8.329**	**–8.89**
	F4	9.143	14.922	–63.21	**8.333**	**–8.85**
	F5	11.763	14.924	–26.87	**10.986**	**–6.60**
7.272	F1	3.800	3.900	–2.63	**3.845**	**1.19**
	F2	3.800	3.900	–2.63	**3.845**	**1.20**
	F3	8.679	8.659	–0.23	**7.840**	**–9.65**
	F4	8.679	9.034	–4.09	**7.844**	**–9.61**
	F5	8.801	9.034	–2.65	**8.189**	**–6.94**

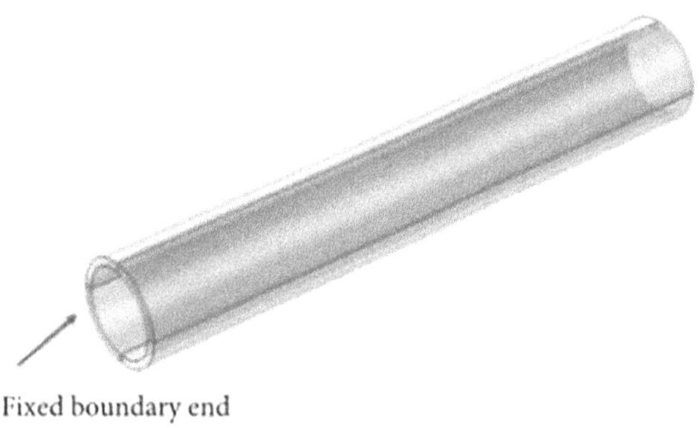

FIGURE 5.26 Fixed–free boundary fundamental frequency analysis (one end is fixed and the other end is free).

frequency shift changes have been investigated. From the results, it can be understood that the lower-dimensions CNT highly varied rather than the higher-dimensions CNT.

5.10.4 Resonance Frequency Analysis for Fixed–Fixed Boundary

Both the boundary ends of SWCNT are fixed and are investigated with the no mass and with the added mass of insulin hormone, immunoglobulin G, and low-density lipoproteins independently for the various lengths of CNT. While adding mass on the bridge-type SWCNT, mode shapes variations are very high. Figure 5.27 shows the fixed–fixed type of CNT. SWCNT shows resonant frequency with no mass and the insulin hormone, immunoglobulin G, (IgG), and low-density lipoproteins (LDL) masses [113].

From the results [113], compared to no mass CNT resonant frequency and the insulin hormone, IgG, and LDL masses, it can be understood that when the mass of objects increases, the resonant frequency of CNT reduces. The higher mass of the low-density lipoproteins (LDL) resonant frequency is lower than others.

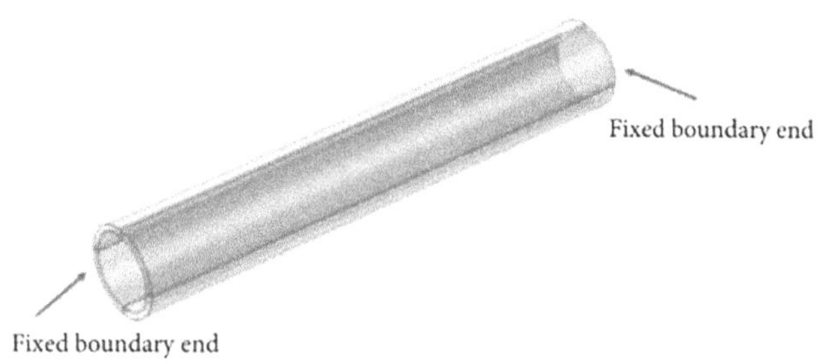

FIGURE 5.27 Fixed–fixed boundary fundamental frequency analysis (both ends are fixed).

5.10.5 Comparisons of Relative Frequency Shift Analysis for Fixed–Free and Fixed–Fixed Type of CNT

To identify various biomasses sensing for different biological objects, the frequency shift studies are carried out for fixed–free and fixed–fixed SWCNT. Figure 5.28 shows the frequency shift results of the insulin, IgG, and LDL biological sensing output on fixed–free SWCNT. Figure 5.28 [113] shows that when the length of the CNT is reduced, the frequency shift is increased. But the length of CNT at 6–12 nm provides better variation frequency shift for biosensing.

Figure 5.29 shows the results of the fixed–fixed type of SWCNT frequency shift for various biological objects. Since both the ends are fixed, the relative frequency shift results show the clear difference between all the lengths of CNTs and insulin, IgG, and LDL mass sensing. Reducing the length of the CNT provides higher shifts rather than higher-length CNTs.

5.10.6 Sensitivity Analysis for Fixed–Free and Fixed–Fixed Type of CNT

To investigate the accuracy of biomass sensing for different biological objects, sensitivity studies are important. Insulin,

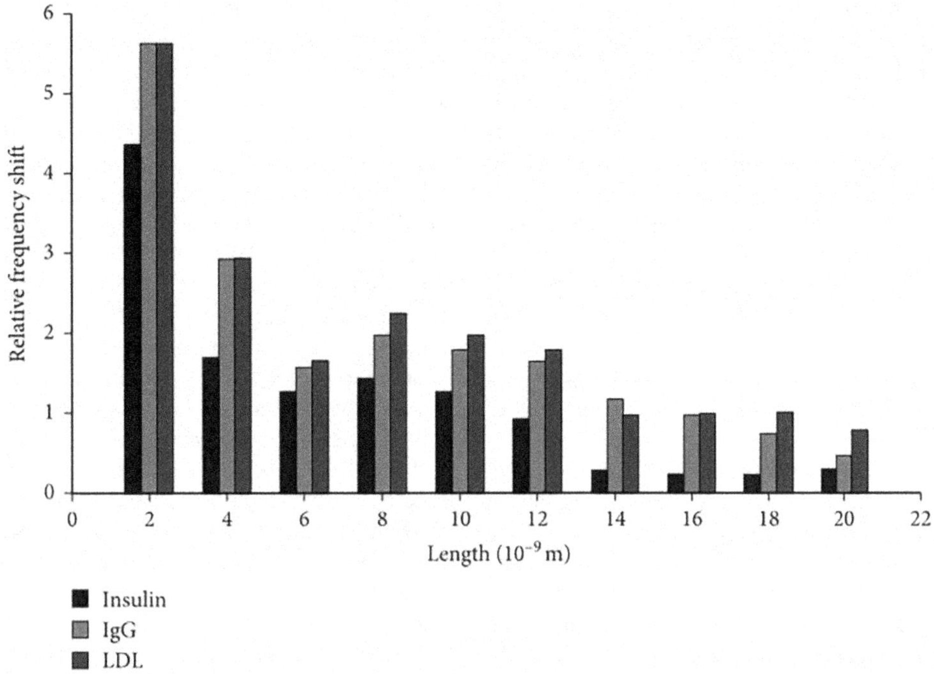

FIGURE 5.28 Comparisons of fixed–free boundary relative frequency shift analysis for CNT.

Source: [113].

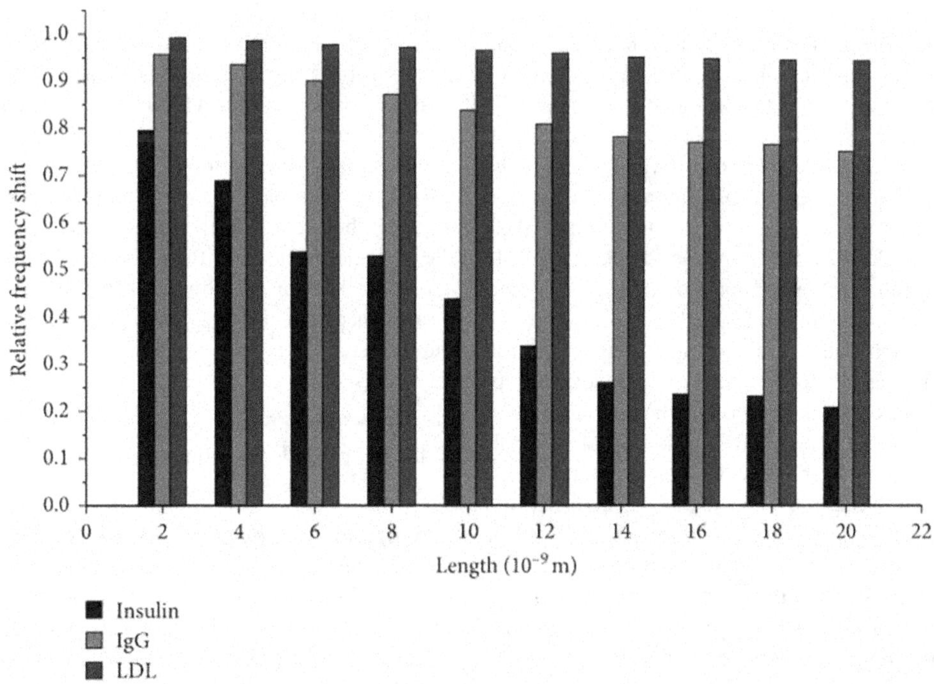

FIGURE 5.29 Comparisons of fixed–fixed boundary relative frequency shift analysis for CNT.

Source: **[113].**

IgG, and LDL sensing for the fixed–free CNT has been investigated [113]. Based on the mass of the insulin, IgG, and LDL, the sensitivity level has been varied, and it can be clearly identified. The sensitivity level gets high when the length of CNT is reduced. When adding the low mass of insulin, the zeptogram-level sensitivity is achieved, and when the mass increased for IgG and LDL, attogram sensitivity is attained.

Also, insulin, IgG, and LDL sensing for the fixed–fixed CNT have been investigated. Insulin sensitivity is lower than IgG and LDL. Compared to the fixed–free type, the sensitivity is reduced in the fixed–fixed type CNT.

5.11 Conclusions

The current market showcases more than 50 nanomedicine-based drug products that are positively affecting the health of humans, and there are hundreds of clinical trials that are ongoing for the treatment of ailments, such as cancer, rheumatoid arthritis, inflammatory bowel diseases, and diabetes [116]. Therefore, nanomedicine could be the frontier that could systematically curtail all the toxicity issues to utilize CNM's potential in biomedical applications.

Carbon-based nanomaterials have established themselves as promising materials within nanomedicine, having found applicability in the potential treatment of many ailments, such as cancer, genetic disorders, and the allowed inventive delivery of bioactive. CNTs (single- and multi-walled) have displayed excellent carrier properties for the effective delivery of chemotherapeutics, antibiotics, proteins, DNA, RNA, vaccines, genes, etc. Graphene derivatives such as functionalized nano-GO have been effective in delivering anticancer agents without affecting healthy cells. The combining factor for the success of CNMs finding their applicability in drug delivery is due to the excellent opportunity of surface functionalization. For instance, the first *in vivo* transfection example by using a poly-functionalized fullerene derivative has been recently reported, thus exhibiting their capability in the delivery of nucleic acids. However, toxicity-related issues are to be addressed before and after the CNMs have delivered their payload to finalize their biological fate in the delivery of therapeutics. Although CNMs have immense potential in their application, they have still to find their practical applicability in biomedicine.

Skin has been established as a challenging barrier for the deliverance of therapeutics into circulation, and several factors, for example, circulation of blood to the applied region, thickness of skin on the applied region, density of hair follicles, etc., must be considered before designing a transdermal delivery device. Exploring the history, there is a rise in the number of fields and applications where the involvement of CNTs has shown a great potential, and the fundamental reasons are the properties of CNTs which abet for such utility, that is, high encapsulation efficiency, stability, electrical conductance, mechanical strength, and flexibility.

A CNT-based hydrogel was utilized to control the release of a drug, and the polymer–CNT composites are being extensively investigated along with its application in creating an electrically tunable CNT hydrogel for the delivery of cationic, anionic, and non-ionic drugs. The fundamental use of CNTs in such devices is to regulate the release of loaded therapeutics by altering the voltage applied to the system. Another application of using CNTs is as a nanoporous membrane to control flux across the membrane and thereby control the drug delivery rate, and its application to develop a device for transdermal delivery of nicotine for cessation of the smoking habit.

As CNTs have inner diameters in the nanometer range and lengths in meters, they can be aggregated to form a thin film called buckypapers, which also has a wide range of applications through several fields, including the application of it for the delivery of small molecules. Transdermal applications are amongst the most flourishing field for various therapies for smoking cessation, opioid withdrawal symptoms, and other therapies, which include drugs with a low therapeutic index. A preliminary requirement of a potent drug is to show a controlled release to be safe and therapeutically beneficial. This issue of a controlled release is well resolved by the application of programmable transdermal devices which program the delivery rate depending on time but not the concentration.

Biological sensing with the one-dimensional nanostructure is one of the vital roles in clinical and healthcare industries. In this chapter, we have modeled computationally efficient single-walled carbon nanotube as a biological mass sensor with the continuum mechanics technique using a finite-element numerical package. The investigations are carried out using the resonance frequency analysis method. To prove the accuracy of the model, the SWCNT model is tested with the previous study [115]. Insulin hormone, immunoglobulin G (IgG), and low-density lipoproteins (LDL) masses are considered for analyzing as a biological mass sensor. In this study, fixed–free and fixed–fixed type of single-walled carbon nanotubes with various lengths of relative frequency shifts are studied for insulin, IgG, and LDL. Additionally, the sensitivity analysis of fixed–free and fixed–fixed type of CNT biological mass sensor is carried out. This chapter clearly shows that the change of biological object masses will change the frequency shift and the sensitivity of the SWCNT sensor. From the outcomes, it can be understood that SWCNT can be employed as a high-accuracy biological mass sensor for various biological objects when reducing the length of CNTs. While attaching the biological objects in the CNT nanobiosensor, the complications in measuring a high number of vibration modes and loss of mechanical energy in liquids have to be explored in the future.

5.12 Future Perspectives

Since the advent of CNMs about 30 years ago, they have established themselves as promising carrier materials in various biomedical sectors, such as biosensing, bioimaging, delivery of therapeutics, etc. Despite several advantages, their toxicity concern toward human cells has rung alarm bells for the researchers to seriously monitor this issue. Along with this, their fabrication takes a long time and is expensive, posing a challenge for large-scale production. Therefore, there is a strict need to find solutions to overcome the challenges of producing non-toxic carbon nanomaterials at a relatively fast pace on a large scale with low production costs.

Covalent and non-covalent functionalization has paved a way for CNMs to expand their applicability into the biomedical arena, but more has to be done to improve their biocompatibility, that is, interaction with biological surroundings (cells, or tissues, or organs) and biodegradability or elimination from the body. They are extensively used in aeronautics, space, automobile, textile, sports goods, and so on, yet their applicability on human beings for diagnostics and therapeutic use has not translated from the research laboratory to clinical trials. Their therapeutic use in humans is still waiting to surpass the regulatory hurdle of proving their compatibility, safety, and efficacy. There is a need to develop a systematic nanotechnology-based approach to build an environment for their use *in vivo* in serious and still largely untreatable ailments, such as brain tumors, cerebral stroke, or neurological disorders such as Alzheimer's or Parkinson's.

Future fabrications of CNMs should be amalgamated with some novel intuitive guiding moieties so that they could directly approach the target cells, or the researchers could devise such carbon nanomaterials that could be driven from the outside directly to the affected tissue/organ, thus circumventing the side effects of the CNMs on the neighboring healthy tissues. Functionalization techniques (covalent and non-covalent), modifying the shape and size, use of solubilizing agents, removal of metallic impurities, administration route, coating with polymers, and/or blood proteins, etc., could be the possible answer to improve the raw hydrophobic CNM's solubility and biocompatibility. Their cellular uptake (*in vitro*) and blood circulation and biodistribution (in vivo) largely rely on surface chemistry. Functionalized carbon nanomaterials with improved solubility, targetability, and biocompatibility could successfully find their way to the clinics for the improved delivery of biomolecules (such as RNA, DNA), small drug molecules, proteins, and peptides. As with any nanomaterials intended for drug delivery, a proper risk assessment evaluation of the toxicity concern of CNM-based delivery of therapeutics is required that should ultimately be extended to clinical trials. An array of safety assessments and *in vitro*/*in vivo* cytotoxicity evaluations is the need of the hour to test the effectiveness of CNMs. Hurdles such as the long-term fate of CNMs should be assessed carefully, and the published data from past studies should be thoroughly screened to bring CNMs further toward clinical translation, to be able to make proper use of the promising applications presented in this chapter.

The use of CNTs in hydrogels, nanoporous membranes, buckypaper, programmable transdermal devices, and microneedles has opened a new area of drug delivery and monitoring and is concluded to be applicable in numerous ways to overthrow many drug- and skin-related barriers. The market sector of CNTs is expected to grow more in the future as observed from 2010 to 2017 and discussed here. There has been a sudden tilt toward transdermal applications, thereby pointing out a vibrant future for transdermal applications. CNT membranes have proven to accelerate the flow of ions through them as compared to conventional membrane permeation due to the complete absence of friction at the carbon nanotube wall; thus, in the future, it could be used for several transdermal applications, including opioid withdrawal and smoking cessation therapy, which are current issues. However, reports on toxicity of CNTs are still insufficient, and additional exploration to completely answer the toxicological profile of this versatile nanocarrier is still awaited to designate them as generally regarded as safe (GRAS) nanosystems for transdermal use.

6

Bright Future of Carbon Nanomaterials for Cancer Nanomedicine-Based Enzyme Immobilization Conjugates

6.1 Introduction

Carbon nanomaterials (i.e., fullerenes, carbon nanotubes, and carbon dots) have attracted significant attention of researchers in various scientific fields, including biomedicine. Nanomedicine, as a new branch of science, is of interest for many investigators due to the important advances for cancer treatment. Early diagnosis and effective cancer therapies are required to treat cancer, with approximately 18.1 million new cases and 9.6 million deaths yearly worldwide [1]. *Nanomedicine* has been defined by the European Science Foundation (ESF) as follows: "Nanomedicine uses nano-sized tools for the diagnosis, prevention and treatment of disease and to gain increased understanding of the complex underlying pathophysiology of disease. The ultimate goal is improved quality of life." It involves diagnosis, imaging, and drug delivery with nanoparticles in the 1–1,000 nm range. Nanotechnology could overcome many limitations of conventional approaches by reducing side effects, increasing tumor accumulation, and improving the efficacy of drugs. Early pioneers in the modern era of nanomedicine can be traced back to Ilya Metchnikov and Paul Ehrlich, who jointly received the Nobel Prize for Medicine in 1908 for their work on phagocytosis and cell-specific diagnostics and cell-targeted therapies. They coined the phrase "magic bullet" and gave us immunotherapeutics and the first synthetic low-molecular-weight chemical entities. In the last 30 years, research on nanoparticles for nanomedicine has been increasing and includes studies with polymer–drug conjugates, polymer–protein conjugates, polymer nanocapsules, liposomes, [2] block-copolymer micelles, [3] antibody–drug conjugates, DNA–drug complexes, and albumin–drug conjugates. Nanotechnology has developed rapidly, allowing the incorporation of multiple therapeutics, and sensing and targeting agents, into nanoparticles, providing new devices with the ability to detect, prevent, and treat complex diseases, such as cancer [3, 4]. Nanotechnology represents a complementary strategy to be integrated with the information derived from the genetic and epigenetic characteristics of tumors. It is well-known that chemotherapeutic agents present severe side effects, including bone marrow suppression, cardiac and kidney toxicity, hair loss, and mucositis. In addition, these drugs are poorly soluble in biological fluids and quickly cleared from the body. The important properties for a drug delivery system with nanoparticles are biocompatibility and biodegradability, prevention of degradation and clearance of the drug by minimizing protein binding and escaping the immune system, and increasing tumor accumulation by passive or active targeting.

With the advancements in nanotechnology, the size, structure, composition, and surface properties of nanoparticles can be controlled during synthesis. In fact, these properties play important roles in the design of nanoparticle-based drug carriers with a high level of efficacy. The potential for surface functionalization to prevent agglomeration is considered as one of the most important factors of nanoparticle synthesis. For example, inorganic nanoparticles, such as gold or silver nanoparticles, can easily aggregate together in water due to their hydrophobic properties. Furthermore, when they are injected into the blood flow, the surfaces of inorganic nanoparticles generally bind with serum proteins through electrostatic interactions. Therefore, these particles can be recognized by the immune cells and eventually scavenged by phagocytosis. To overcome these problems, hydrophilic and biocompatible polyethylene glycol (PEG) polymers have been widely used to decorate the surface of inorganic nanoparticles. With a high grafting density, tethered PEG polymers form a brush on the surface of these nanoparticles, and thus, they can be well-dispersed in water, reduce the absorption of serum proteins, and increase the circulation time and the accumulation in tumor sites *in vivo* due to the enhanced permeability and retention (EPR) effect.

Nanomaterials could overcome many limitations of conventional approaches by reducing side effects, increasing tumor accumulation, and improving the efficacy of drugs due to their unique physical/chemical properties and biological compatibility and are among the most promising materials that have already changed and will keep changing human life. Among numerous types of nanomaterials developed in the past years, carbon nanomaterials have attracted particular interest in a large variety of fields, including biomedicine [5], owing to their distinctive physical and chemical properties. Based on the covalent bonds linking their carbon atoms, carbon nanomaterials may be classified into sp^2- and sp^3-carbon nanomaterials (Figure 6.1). Typical sp^2-carbon nanomaterials include zero-dimensional (0D) fullerenes, one-dimensional (1D) carbon nanotubes (CNTs), and two-dimensional (2D) graphene, all with well-defined structures. Carbon nanoparticles (CNPs) or carbon dots (CDs) are nanoclusters of amorphous carbon (or composed of small crystalline structures) with sizes smaller than 10 nm and can also be considered as a type of 0D sp^2-carbon nanomaterial.

Many carbon nanomaterials, including CNTs, graphene derivatives, and CDs, show interesting inherent optical properties, such as fluorescence, making them useful as contrast agents in optical imaging and sensing. The excellent electrical properties of CNTs and graphene allow them to be extensively

DOI: 10.1201/9781032635989-6

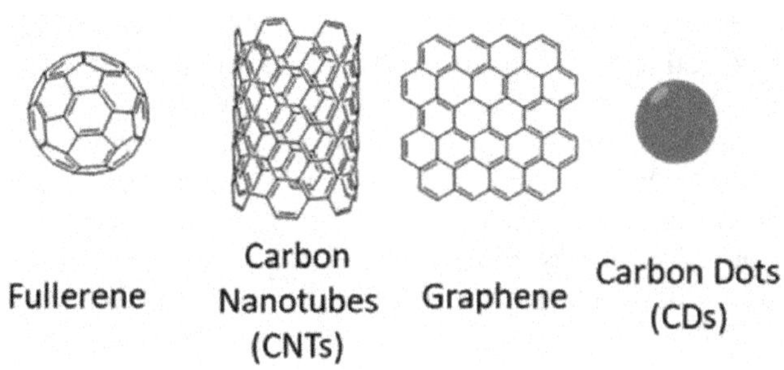

FIGURE 6.1 Different types of carbon nanomaterials explored for biomedical applications.

used in a wide range of biosensing platforms. Sp^2-carbon nanomaterials, especially single-walled carbon nanotubes (SWCNTs) and graphene with all-carbon atoms exposed on their surfaces, exhibit ultrahigh surface areas available for efficient drug loading and bioconjugation [6]. For fullerenes and CNTs with hollow structures, the inside space may be utilized to load other functional species for theragnostic purposes. CNTs and graphene derivatives with strong optical absorbance in the near-infrared (NIR) region are also useful for photothermal ablation of cancer [6]. Moreover, compared with many other inorganic nanomaterials, such as quantum dots (QDs), which usually contain heavy metals, carbon nanomaterials simply composed of carbon are relatively safe, at least in terms of elementary composition.

6.2 Nanozymes to CNM-Enzyme Conjugates

Carbon nanomaterials (CNMs) and enzymes belong to two scientific fields that have been traditionally widely separated, and research at their interface bears a number of challenges to overcome, both experimentally and culturally. Nevertheless, in recent years, a number of studies have allowed great progress in this research area, pushing the limits of what was considered possible and demonstrating great innovation potential for a wide number of applications. Enzymes can be covalently conjugated onto nanocarbons, adsorbed on their surface, or even encapsulated in those with a hollow structure, as reviewed elsewhere [7]. The interactions between proteins and nanocarbons can play an important role in determining their fate *in vivo*, including their biodegradation [8], formation of a biocorona [9], and consequent modulation of the immune response.

Besides the exciting area of biointegration of nanocarbons, for instance, for the regeneration of conductive tissues [10], and (flexible) bioelectronics' development [11], the fields of sensing and diagnostics [12] certainly benefit from the inclusion of both nanocarbons and enzymes. Finally, considering the current emergency we are facing in terms of environmental impact of human activities and climate change that requires urgent action, the use of enzymes is very attractive for the production, modification, and degradation of nanocarbons to render the relevant processes more sustainable.

To provide a general overview of the diverse members of each family, this chapter will briefly introduce the classification of enzymes and nanocarbons, followed by an overview of the literature describing their combination. We will then discuss the recent progress in a variety of applications, directing the reader to reviews of each topic, where older research can be found. Finally, we will conclude with a perspective toward the future of this exciting research area.

6.2.1 Enzyme Classification

Enzymes have attracted scientists' attention for a long time. It is imperative to adopt an unambiguous nomenclature and classification for this enormous and diverse group of biological catalysts to permit their rigorous study and accelerate scientific progress in this area. The International Union of Biochemistry and Molecular Biology (IUBMB) has introduced the IUBMB ExplorEnz website [13], where it is possible to navigate the Enzyme Commission (EC) system, which uses four-component numbers to identify each enzyme (i.e., EC X.X.X.X):

1. The first component refers to the general type of reaction being catalyzed. For instance, EC 1 indicates oxidoreductases that catalyze redox reactions, and EC 3 identifies hydrolases that catalyze hydrolytic reactions (Figure 6.2).
2. The second number indicates the subclass based on the type of compound or functional group involved in the reaction. For example, EC 1.13 refers to oxygenases that insert oxygen on the substrate, and EC 2.3 indicates acyl-transferases that transfer acyl groups, etc.
3. The third component denotes the sub-subclass, by further specifying the reaction being catalyzed, for instance, in terms of acceptors, or specific groups being transferred. As an example, EC 2.1.1 indicates methyl transferases.
4. The fourth component is simply a serial number that refers to the specific enzyme.

However, the system presents room for improvement, because it is not always unambiguous. In fact, new classes are constantly being added to the EC system, and it should also be noted that non-physiologically occurring enzymes are not included [14]. For these reasons, many other databases

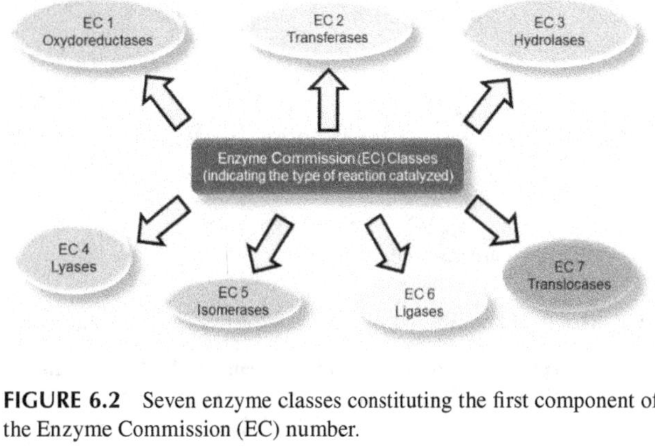

FIGURE 6.2 Seven enzyme classes constituting the first component of the Enzyme Commission (EC) number.

can be useful to complement the ExplorEnz information. For instance, helpful information can be found in the relevant metabolic pathways described on KEGG [15], kinetic data on BRENDA [16], thermodynamic data on NIST [17], and human gene names curated by HUGO [18] and NCBI [19]. New databases are continuously being created, including some that use different classification criteria, such as MEROPS for peptidases, and others that more generally collect various types of data pertaining to proteins, such as Expasy [20].

6.2.2 Carbon Nanomaterials (CNMs)

The family of CNMs is very diverse, with new members continuously being discovered. In this minireview, we will examine the most popular types of CNMs (Figure 6.3), as well as their general properties. Those features are briefly discussed in the following subsections, where readers are referred to reviews that describe in more depth the various CNM types that are mainly composed of carbon atoms, and their general properties. We will briefly mention their main features in the following subsections, where readers are referred to recent reviews that describe more in-depth the various CNM types.

Generally, sp^2-hybridized carbon allotropes share common features, such as high mechanical strength and electronic conductivity, together with low density, and a high surface area; these can be functionalized to tailor their properties ad hoc for the intended application, as reviewed elsewhere [12]. In particular, the various modes of interaction and conjugation with proteins are a widely covered topic in the literature, and thus, it will not be discussed here. CNMs composed mainly of sp^3-hybridized carbon atoms exist also, such as nanodiamonds (NDs); they find scope especially in sensing and catalysis [21], although they have not attracted scientists' attention to a great extent, likely due to their more limited accessibility relative to other CNMs.

Each carbon nanostructure has a specific size, morphology, curvature, and reactivity. However, despite the many research efforts on their modification for tailored applications, it is not always straightforward to predict a priori which one will give the best performance, with great variation across allotropes [22]. Nevertheless, their conductivity is particularly promising to enhance (bio)materials' properties [23] for the regeneration

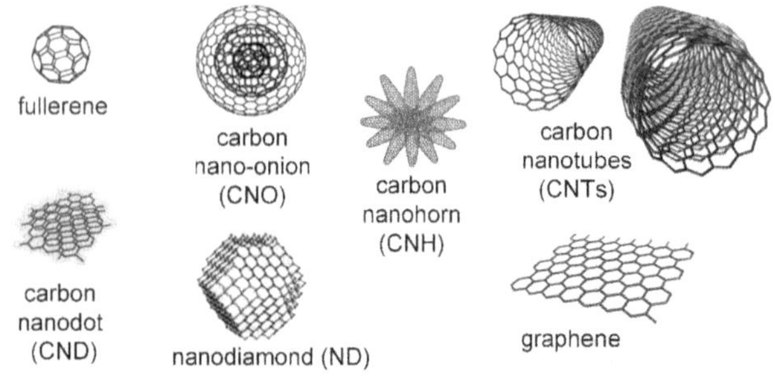

FIGURE 6.3 Main types of carbon nanostructures (not to scale).

Source: Reproduced from Adorinni, S.; Cringoli, M. C.; Perathoner, S.; Fornasiero, P.; Marchesan, S. "Green approaches to carbon nanostructure-based biomaterials." *Appl. Sci.* 2021, 11, 2490.

of conductive tissues, such as the challenging nerve [24] and cardiac tissues [25], in sensing [26] and various types of catalyses [27], and in the field of energy sustainable production, conversion [28], and storage [29]. Furthermore, the performance in the latter fields can be enhanced by the generation of highly porous materials. Indeed, carbon foams [30] and porous carbon [31] are highly advantageous since they can be produced at low cost and from a variety of precursors [32], such as polymers [33] and biomass [34], bearing high potential, especially in gas [35] and energy storage [36], and in catalysis. However, in this chapter we will focus on the traditional CNM types, as described in the following subsections.

6.2.2.1 Fullerenes

Buckminsterfullerene, a discrete molecule composed of 60 carbon atoms (C_{60}), was the first nano-allotrope to be discovered, in 1985. Fullerenes can also be composed of more carbon atoms, such as C_{76}, C_{84}, and C_{90}. After C_{60}, the rugby ball–shaped C_{70} is the second most known, and it is easier to isolate in sufficient amounts for research than higher fullerenes. The advent of 100 mg scale preparation of C_{60} opened the way to decades of research that have provided several routes for its chemical functionalization, as recently reviewed. Further tailoring of C_{60} properties can be attained through doping with heteroatoms. Molecular confinement also offers the possibility to encase other elements in their interior to provide endohedral fullerenes with interesting properties [37].

Fullerenes are fascinating molecules that have attracted researchers' interest as they can be formed in space [38]. On Earth, they have been proposed for various applications, including the targeted delivery of therapeutics [39] and innovative antiviral therapies [40]. Despite the many potential uses in medicine [41], especially in photodynamic cancer therapy thanks to their ability to generate and modulate reactive oxygen species (ROS) levels [42], their electronic properties thus far found translation mainly in the field of photovoltaics, thanks to their electron-acceptor nature [43] and electron-transport ability [44].

6.2.2.2 Carbon Nano-Onions (CNOs)

Multiple fullerenes can be organized one inside another in carbon nano-onions (CNOs). These concentric, multilayered fullerenes can have a size ranging from 2 to 100 nm, depending on the method of synthesis [45]. Generally, multi-fullerenes display a decreasing reactivity with increasing size, corresponding to decreasing curvature, and therefore, the associated strain on the CNO surface. Consequently, small CNOs present good reactivity, although it should be noted that also other factors, such as the production method and the consequent amount of defect sites, affect their reactivity.

In the last decade, their biological and electrochemical [46] applications have significantly expanded due to the favorable properties of the nanomaterial, including their small size, large accessible surface area, and high biocompatibility [47], especially once they are rendered soluble through covalent and non-covalent functionalization [48]. It is worth noting that recent findings described white-light luminescence arising when CNOs were produced through pyrolysis and underwent oxidative treatments [49].

6.2.2.3 Carbon Nanohorns (CNHs)

Carbon nanocones can form clusters termed *carbon nanohorns* (CNHs). Like many other CNMs, pristine nanocones unfortunately tend to aggregate in many solvents, and they do so in various morphologies, termed *dahlia-*, *bud-*, or *seed-like* CNHs. Despite this limitation, they can find promising applications in biosensing [50], medicine [51], and electrocatalysis [52], sometimes even outperforming other CNMs [53], and with relevance to clean energy and carbon dioxide fixation [54]. There are not many studies on CNHs relative to the other CNMs, possibly also due to a more limited number of commercial sources. As a result, this type of nanomaterial remains an underexplored opportunity for innovation in numerous fields.

6.2.2.4 Carbon Nanodots (CNDs)

In the last few years, luminescent carbon dots (CNDs) have emerged for their innovation potential, especially in sensing and biomedicine [55], thanks to their low toxicity, chemical inertness, ease of preparation, environmental friendliness, and interesting physicochemical properties [56]. Another key advantage relative to many other CNMs is the excellent solubility of CNDs in a large variety of solvents, both organic and aqueous, depending on their chemical nature [57].

These nanomaterials have attracted great attention for their cost-efficient and sustainable production, using, for instance, natural products [58] or biomass waste as carbon source [59]. However, the fine tailoring of their desired optical properties has been challenging. Indeed, the exact chemical structure of CNDs still poses many unanswered questions [60], and the thorough use of spectroscopic methods is key to providing an accurate characterization of the emissive species [61]. As we advance our understanding of CND's nature, further prospects open up [62], expanding their applications to organocatalysis [63], sensitizers for photocatalysis and pollutant degradation [64], and energy conversion and storage [65], as capacitor electrodes, for instance [66].

6.2.2.5 Nanodiamonds (NDs)

NDs are characterized by sp3-hybridization of their carbon core. NDs come in different sizes, morphologies, and surface types, depending on the method used for their preparation and functionalization [67]. They display attractive physicochemical properties, such as hardness, biocompatibility, and chemical inertness, leading to research on a variety of potential biological uses, especially delivery of therapeutics and imaging [68], but also sensing, tissue regeneration, skin products' formulations, and in polished or active coatings with antimicrobial, antifriction, and mechanical reinforcing properties [69].

Recently, NDs have been considered also for their use in theranostics as applied to neurodegenerative diseases, thanks to their additional benefit of crossing the blood–brain barrier [70]. Other emerging areas of application include primarily biological use in cells and *in vivo*, but also catalysis [71].

6.2.2.6 Carbon Nanotubes (CNTs)

Carbon nanotubes can be composed of one graphitic layer rolled up in single-walled CNTs (SWCNTs) or multiple coaxial graphitic nanotubes, called multi-walled CNTs (MWCNTs), which can be grown with branches also [72]. CNTs can have very different properties; for instance, they can be semiconducting or metallic, depending on their type and chirality [73]. Over the years, several functionalization strategies have been developed; oxidation is by far the most popular way to increase their polarity and dispersibility in various solvents, including water [74]. Therefore, fine control over their synthesis, purity, and thus, homogeneity is critical to enable their translation into large-scale use [75] and to fill the gap between their properties as individual CNTs and those of their bundled aggregates—often a practical limitation for industrial use [76].

CNTs have attracted great interest, although there are still challenges to overcome to enable a wider commercial use of their unique properties. Key areas of application include various types of high-performing composite materials, where demands of conductivity, robustness, flexibility, and mechanical resistance are high [77]. These include artificial neuromuscular prostheses [78] and, more generally, nanobioelectronics [79] and wearable electronics, but also sensing and imaging, orthopedic devices [80], tissue regeneration and biomedical use [81], electroactive materials for environmental and energy technology [82], electronics and computing [83], and various forms of catalysis [84].

6.2.2.7 Graphene (G) and Graphene-Based Materials

In the last decade, the most popular carbon allotrope has been graphene (G), which can be considered as a 2D layer of sp^2-hybridized carbon atoms arranged in a honeycomb lattice. It is worth noting that G can come in many forms, in terms of size, layers, level of oxidation, etc., which will all affect its physicochemical properties. In particular, graphene oxide (GO) [85], or its reduced form (rGO) [86], is often used for its improved dispersibility relative to pristine G. G properties have also been tailored through topology [87], such as twists and nanoribbons [88]. Given the large heterogeneity in size, number of layers, and defects of G flakes, the general term of graphene-based materials is preferred over just G, to refer to this subclass of CNMs.

Applications are similar to CNTs, and they include composite reinforcement [89], wearable [90] and flexible electronics [91], including memory devices [92], and even stretchable batteries [93], energy storage [94] and conversion [95], environmental remediation [96], varying types of catalysis [97], and innovative uses in the healthcare sector [98], such as regenerative medicine [99] and sensing [100]. In this case, large-scale, cost-effective production of high-quality G [101] and standardization are key for the translation of G properties into commodity products at a global level [102].

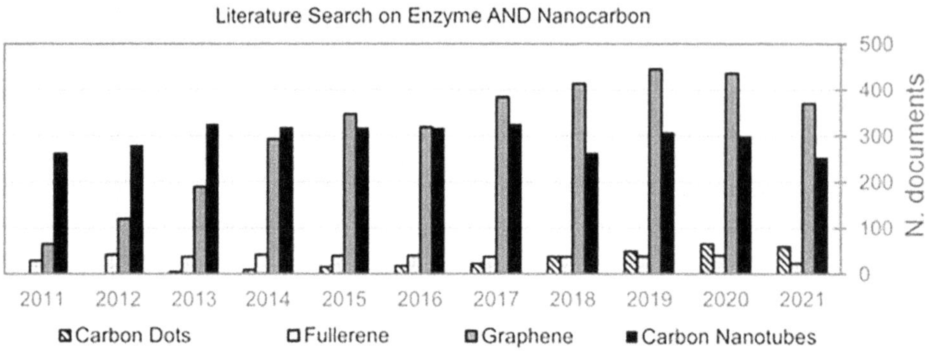

FIGURE 6.4 A literature search on carbon nanomaterials and enzymes focused on the last decade.

Source: Scopus, November 14, 2021.

6.2.3 Bibliometric Analysis of CNMs and Enzymes

A literature search for the term "enzyme" in conjunction with each one of the most popular CNMs shown in Figure 6.3, in the title, abstract, or keywords, has revealed that the vast majority of scientific articles pertain to CNTs (4.3×10^3 documents), followed by G (3.4×10^3 documents). However, in the last decade (Figure 6.4), scientific works on either one averaged about 300 per year, with a slight decrease for CNTs after 2017, as opposed to a continuous increase for G up to 2019, surpassing CNTs in 2015. This trend could be related to concerns over CNTs' toxicity, as suggested by the fact that scientific documents on this topic peaked at nearly 300 in 2015 and, since then, held steady. However, given their high innovation potential in medicine [103] and the high number of variables that affect their biocompatibility [104], alarming generalizations to ban their use are best avoided [105].

In comparison to CNTs and G, all the other CNMs lagged behind, each one reaching far less than 100 in total—with two exceptions—and representing today a missed opportunity for research. The first exception was fullerenes, possibly since they were the first to be discovered and thus have had more years of related research, reaching just over 600 records. The second exception was CNDs, which are among the most recent CNMs to be discovered. Scientific papers on CNDs have been increasing steadily year after year since the first ones appeared in 2004. Therefore, it is foreseeable that CNDs will keep rising in popularity in the immediate future, although there is still a long way ahead to approach the numbers seen for CNTs and G.

In terms of applications, most studies pertain to biosensing and biofuel cells [106], although biocatalysis and biomedical applications other than sensing have been pursued with these systems. Interestingly, CNMs have also been envisaged as enzyme mimics, inhibitors, or detectors. We will concisely cover the progress made over the last five years on all these topics in the following sections.

6.3 CNMs for Enzyme Mimicry, Inhibition, or Monitoring

6.3.1 CNMs for Enzyme Mimicry

A plethora of works describes the use of CNMs as nanozymes, meaning, nanostructures that mimic enzymes, as they display catalytic activity [107]. Research in this area is intended to overcome some of the common limitations of enzymes, particularly the limited physicochemical resistance against solvents and changes in temperature, pH, or other experimental conditions [108]. Potential applications range from various biomedical applications [109], including innovative therapy [110], biosensing [111], and disinfection, to environmental monitoring and remediation [112]. In particular, peroxidase mimicry by CNMs has been widely studied [113], especially for the development of glucose biosensors [114], although hydrolase mimicry is also attracting increasing interest (Figure 6.5) [115].

In particular, CNDs have been functionalized with Fe(III) to mimic peroxidases and exert antimicrobial activity through the generation of hydroxyl radicals [116]. In contrast, no hydroxyl radicals were generated when they were derivatized with glucose or cyclodextrin to mimic peroxidases, indicating a different mechanism [117]. The peroxidase mimicry activity can be correlated to the phosphorescence quantum yield and can inhibit bacterial growth under light irradiation, an activity that was envisaged for photodynamic antimicrobial chemotherapy applications [118]. Alternatively, the use of light

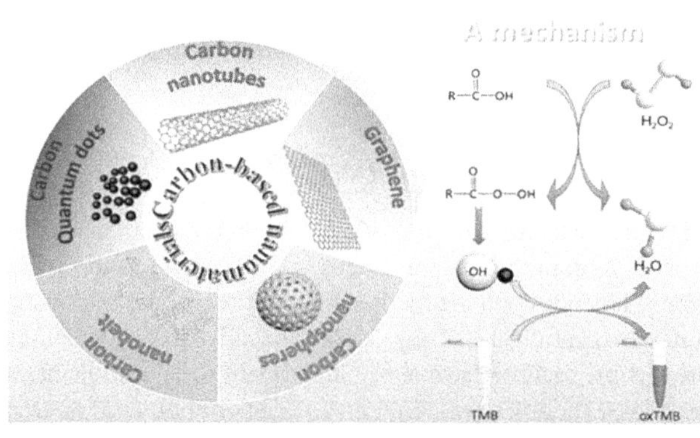

FIGURE 6.5 CNMs typically used for peroxidase mimicry (left) and a possible reaction mechanism that ultimately generates hydroxyl radicals for the oxidation of colorless 3,3′,5,5′-tetramethylbenzidine (TMB) to a colored product (oxTMB).

Source: **Reprinted with permission from [115]. Copyright © 2022, American Chemical Society.**

could trigger radical oxygen species generation by the CND nanozymes, in an effort to mimic nuclease activity and cleave DNA [119].

Chemical functionalization has been successfully employed to attain CNDs with switchable fluorescence too. In this case, the fluorescence of amino-derivatized CNDs can be quenched by chelation with Fe(II) ions as nanozymes and restored upon treatment with hydrogen peroxidase with a concomitant shift from yellow to green [120]. Furthermore, addition of other divalent metal cations can lead to additional advantages. For instance, Mn(II) extends the peroxidase mimicry by CNDs to neutral pH values, which is otherwise rather uncommon [121]. Despite the fact that mimicking enzymes' enantioselectivity is a grand challenge, recent reports are demonstrating it is possible, in topoisomerase mimicry, for example [122]. Heteroatom-doped CNDs have been developed for theranostics as well, thanks to nanozyme activity [123]. Many other examples of nanozymes based on CNDs have been reported, through addition of other components, such as hemin [124], metal nanoparticles (NPs) [125], co-doping with various elements [126], MOFs [127], carbon nitride [128], and metal oxides [127].

Both graphene oxide (GO) and its reduced derivative (rGO) have also demonstrated peroxidase-mimicking ability, which has been ascribed to the presence of carbonyl groups on the surface of the nanomaterial that get activated by hydrogen peroxide as a key step in the catalytic cycle [320]. Interestingly, rGO co-doping with N and B allowed the development of nanozymes for the selective mimicry of peroxidases (but not oxidases) with enhanced catalytic performance for the development of biosensors [129].

Analogously, oxidized CNTs demonstrated peroxidase-like activity, which was envisaged for the treatment of bacterial infections [130]. Different oxygen-bearing functional groups exert competing interactions with hydrogen peroxide (Figure 6.6), and thus, control over oxidation is important [130]. Combination of CNTs with other chemical components is a popular strategy to tailor nanozyme activity to the intended application. In a recent example, SWCNTs have been functionalized with a nickel complex for the biomimicry of oxidase for H_2 oxidation and subsequent integration in fuel cells. Alternatively, MWCNTs were coated with polypyrrole to introduce N-based ligands for Fe to be used in single-atom catalysis as peroxidase mimics [131]. CNTs were combined with hemin for peroxidase mimicry also [132]. They have been derivatized with polyoxometallate-based metal-organic frameworks (MOFs) for the selective sensing of cysteine [133], or with copper complexes [134], MOFs [135], and NPs [136] to develop nanozymes. For this type of application, many types of metal NPs have been used [137], as well as polymers to mimic phosphodiesterases [138].

CNTs can be further assembled into macroscopic materials, such as carbon nanofibers (CNFs), which find many uses, especially in high-performance composites and energy devices [139]. In this case, they have been decorated with Fe(III) complexes to mimic oxidases [140], peroxidases, and catalases for sensing and environmental technology [141]. Analogously to CNTs, CNFs can be oxidized, although gas-phase methods are preferable to the liquid-phase methods typically used for CNTs, to preserve the CNF macroscopic morphology, with the additional advantage of being virtually waste-free [142].

Peroxidase mimicry can be exerted by other CNMs as well, and for various uses. CNHs have been used as peroxidase mimics for the detection of drug traces as environmental pollutants [143]. They have been combined with nano-sized ceria to detect hydrogen peroxide in commodity products, such as washing liquids and milk. In the case of CNOs, nitrogen doping has been successfully applied to improve their catalytic performance in the electrochemical generation of molecular oxygen from hydrogen peroxide. Boron and nitrogen co-doped CNOs showed great performance as electrocatalysts for the oxygen reduction reaction [46]. Interestingly, in the case of NDs, they were envisaged for redox-enzyme mimicry, with an activity that could be selectively tailored depending on the pH.

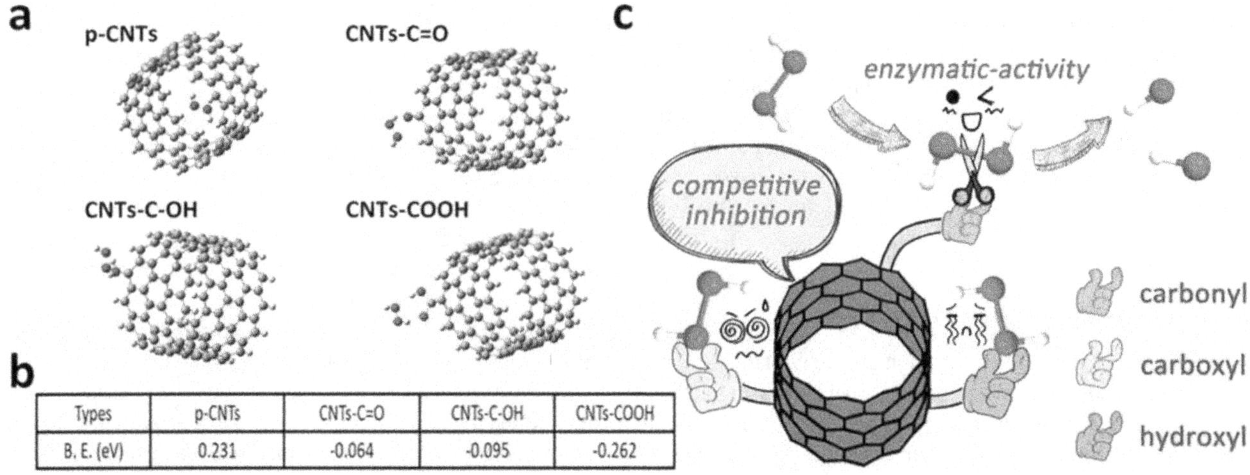

Types	p-CNTs	CNTs-C=O	CNTs-C-OH	CNTs-COOH
B. E. (eV)	0.231	-0.064	-0.095	-0.262

FIGURE 6.6 (a) Optimized binding modes between hydrogen peroxide and CNTs either in their pristine form (p-CNTs) or with different oxygen-bearing functional groups. (b) Binding energies between hydrogen peroxide and the various CNT types shown in (a). (c) Schematic illustration of peroxidase mimicry by oxidized CNTs.

At acidic pH, NDs catalyzed the reduction of molecular oxygen and hydrogen peroxide. At alkaline pH, they catalyzed the dismutation decomposition of hydrogen peroxide to produce molecular oxygen. It was proposed that the molecular mechanism of their peroxidase-like activity is electron-transfer acceleration, the source of which is likely derived from oxygen-containing functional groups on their surface.

Finally, besides peroxidases and, generally, redox-active enzymes, which represent the vast majority of nanozyme mimicry studies on CNMs, hydrolases have started to attract scientists' attention. In a recent report, fullerene derivatives were applied to this end through the presentation of multiple functional groups inspired from the natural enzymes' catalytic sites [144]. Analogously to the other CNMs, fullerenes could also act as peroxidase mimics at acidic pH and were thus envisaged for the eradication of *Helicobacter pylori* in vivo [145].

6.3.2 CNMs as Enzyme Inhibitors

Fullerene derivatives have been envisaged for the inhibition of a variety of enzymes, including recent examples of HIV-1 protease, ribonuclease A, glycosidases, ubiquitin-activating enzyme 1, and acetylcholinesterase. Their size, hydrophobic nature, and spherical morphology appear very suitable for hydrophobic interactions with lipophilic sites on the target enzymes, whilst C_{60} functionalization can add hydrophilic appendages for more specific interactions.

CNDs have been used to inhibit tyrosinase for cosmetic and food applications, thanks to hydrophobic interactions between the CNDs and the enzymatic surface, as well as chelation by the CND COOH groups of the enzyme copper ions. Tyrosinase is involved in the browning process of fruits and vegetables, and its overexpression has been linked to skin pigmentation disorders and tumorigenesis. Therefore, its inhibition could find several useful applications [146]. Furthermore, CNDs were found to tune glucose oxidase activity, depending on their functionalization type [147], and inhibit maltase, an effect that was envisaged as an innovative means to control physiological glucose levels.

Enzyme inhibition has been studied for CNTs also. SWCNTs demonstrated the ability to act as competitive inhibitors for proteases, such as chymotrypsin, thanks to the hydrophobic interactions between the curved CNT surface and a morphologically complementary crevice on the enzyme surface, without alteration of the enzyme secondary structure or active site [148].

6.3.3 CNMs for Enzyme Monitoring

CNMs can be engineered to monitor enzymatic activity. Several examples have been reported especially using CNDs, whose fluorescence is initially quenched through interaction with a second component, and then restored upon a chemical transformation triggered by the activity of the target enzyme [149]. To this end, graphene CNDs have been functionalized with a cobalt derivative to allow for redox-dependent fluorescence that can be used to detect alkaline phosphatase activity, in serum, through the dephosphorylation of a substrate on the CNDs that releases ascorbic acid, which restores fluorescence. Through a similar principle, silver NPs have been applied to quench the fluorescence of CNDs so that, in the presence of enzymatic activity that generates hydrogen peroxide as a by-product (e.g., through an oxidase), the silver NP structure decomposes and fluorescence is restored. Applications in the health sector were envisaged, in particular, for the monitoring of relevant biomolecules, such as glucose or cholesterol, that could act as substrates for the corresponding oxidase [149]. Alternatively, glycosidases could be monitored through a similar principle, by functionalizing the CNDs to favor interaction with p-nitrophenol, which is generated through enzymatic activity on a glycosylated derivative. Another target enzyme was thioredoxin reductase, overexpressed in many cancer cells.

SWCNTs have been applied to enzyme biosensing. Recently, SWCNTs were coated with a peptide to develop a biosensor for trypsin detection in urine samples, exploiting variations in CNT near-infrared photoluminescence upon enzymatic degradation of the peptide coating [150]. In another example, CNTs were envisaged for applications in cancer diagnostics, through the detection of matrix metalloproteinase-7, which is overexpressed in cancer cells [151]. Finally, CNT fibers have been used to develop highly sensitive (54 $\mu A \cdot cm^{-2} \cdot mM^{-1}$) photoelectrodes for the detection of NADH, which is a key cofactor in many biocatalytic processes; its quantification correlates to specific enzyme activity [152].

6.4 Applications of CNM-Enzyme Conjugates

6.4.1 Biosensing

Biosensors typically comprise three elements, which are (1) an element for biological recognition, such as an enzyme; (2) a transducer, to convert energy from the biorecognition event into another form (electrical, thermal, optical, etc.); and (3) a signal processing system for the response readout and/or recording [153]. Biosensors often rely on enzyme inhibition, thus being ideal to monitor inhibitors that are relevant to human health, such as drugs or pollutants. Enzymes are ideal components for biosensing, thanks to high sensitivity, specificity, low cost, and accessibility [153]. Coupling a semiconductor to enzymes can be exploited in photobiocatalysis, which is inspired by natural photosynthesis but does not necessarily involve light for activation. In general, inclusion of nanomaterials allows for better performance in a variety of analytical parameters, such as sensitivity, detection limit, stability, and response rate [154].

In particular, CNMs are ideal supports especially for biosensors that require multiple layers of enzymes, but also for providing a good electronic contact through the layers and with the electrodes. CNMs can be good active supports for oxidoreductases as they may facilitate electron transfer to enhance catalysis, whilst offering a high surface area for high-level loading of enzymes [155]. However, the occurrence of direct electron transfer (DET) is a matter of ongoing debate, depending on the type of enzymes under consideration, the accessibility of their redox-active site to the CNMs, and the type of direct or indirect contact between CNMs and enzymes [155]. The electronic properties of CNMs render them attractive building blocks for electrochemical biosensors, besides the more traditional optical alternatives [156].

Graphene is one of the most studied CNMs for a variety of biosensing devices (Figure 6.7) [157], thanks to its exceptional electronic and mechanical properties, as recently reviewed in detail elsewhere [157]. Other, less-studied CNMs, such as CNOs, can also make attractive electrode components for the development of low-cost, simple-to-use, and highly sensitive sensors [158]. CNOs (mean size of 30 nm) were employed as electrochemical sensors by covalently immobilizing the glucose oxidase enzyme (GOx) on their surface via carbodiimide chemistry. GOx selectively catalyzed the oxidation of glucose, giving a sensor with high sensitivity and selectivity. However, the catalytic activity of GOx on the sensor electrode was highly sensitive to environmental conditions, such as temperature, pH, and humidity. Furthermore, the performance of the sensor was limited by enzymatic stability. Thus, an enzyme-free glucose sensor was designed, using Pt-decorated CNOs (Pt@CNOs) that outperformed many other CNMs previously studied for the same application.

In 2020, Cumba et al. [158] described the preparation of the first ink that was based on CNOs to produce cheap and disposable electrodes, yielding sensors with elevated performance (Figure 6.8) [158]. Careful selection and optimization of all the components was a key step to attain a suitable formulation for the ink to be screen-printed. They included the conducting nanocarbons (i.e., graphite (GRT) and CNOs), the polymer binder, the plasticizer, and the organic solvent. The electrodes were screen-printed, and they consisted of a conducting network of interconnected CNMs with a uniform distribution. The system displayed a heterogeneous electron transfer rate constant corresponding to $1.3 \pm 0.7 \times 10^{-3}$ cm·s^{-1}, and also a current density that was higher than the ferrocene/ferrocenium coupled to a GRT screen-printed electrode that was commercially available. Furthermore, the CNO/GRT electrode allowed for the detection of dopamine in micromolar concentration (i.e., 10.0–99.9 μM), and with a 0.92 μM detection limit. The analytical sensitivity thus revealed a notable fourfold increase relative to the commercial reference electrode based on GRT. Overall, this study opened the way to the use of CNO-based electrodes for high-performance sensing, electrocatalysis, and battery research [158].

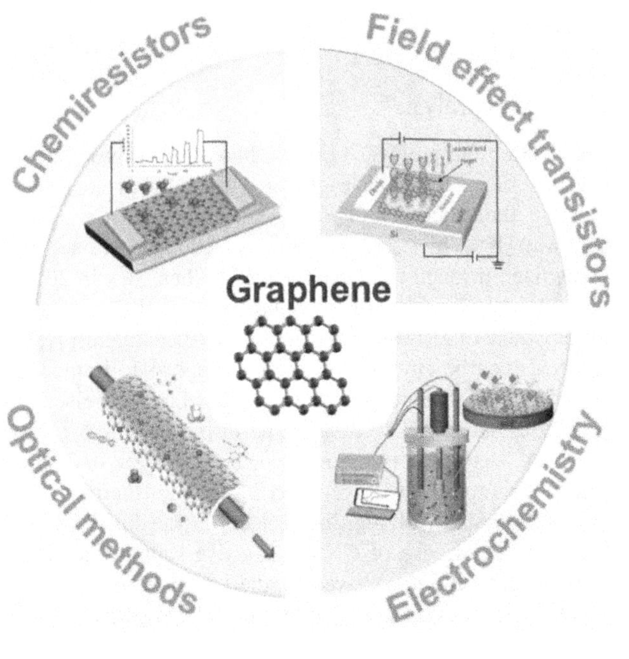

FIGURE 6.7 Graphene is one of the most popular CNMs, employed in a variety of biosensing devices thanks to its exceptional electronic and mechanical properties.

Source: Reproduced with permission from [157]. Copyright © 2022, American Chemical Society.

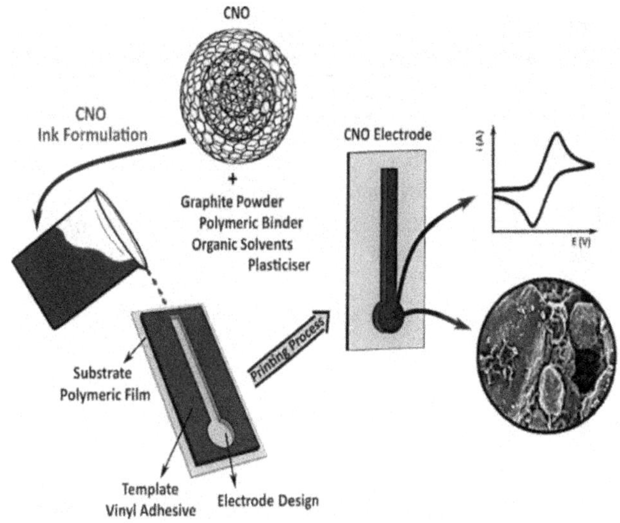

FIGURE 6.8 Screen-printed electrode preparation using a conductive ink based on graphite and CNOs.

Source: Reproduced from [158] under a Creative Commons license.

As can be seen from [106], the vast majority of CNM–enzyme conjugates have been studied for biosensing applications. The most popular target molecule is glucose for biometric health monitoring (Table 6.1) [147]. However, biosensors have been developed to detect many other bioactive compounds too, such as cholesterol [159] and triglycerides, lactose and lactate, neurotransmitters and hormones, various disease biomarkers [160], microRNAs drugs [161], pathogens and toxins, xanthine and caffeic acid [162], p-coumaric acid [163], ferulic acid [164], trace metals [165], and oxygen.

6.4.2 Biofuel Cells

Biofuel cells are electrochemical devices that typically use redox enzymes as sustainable catalysts for the conversion of chemical energy into electrical energy (Figure 6.9) [174]; they consist of two-electrode cells that are separated by a proton-conducting medium. At the bioanode, fuels are oxidized, freeing electrons that flow to the biocathode through the external electrical circuit. At the biocathode, oxidants such as oxygen or peroxide are reduced to water [174]. Redox-active enzymes have attracted great interest for their use in the electrochemical

TABLE 6.1
Comparison of Recent Reports (Since 2017) That Described CNMs-Based Sensors for Glucose Detection

CNM Type	Conjugation	Linear Range	Detection Limit	Sensitivity	Ref.
CNDs	Non-covalent	250–3,000 μM	n.a.	n.a.	[147]
		0.1–500 μM	65 μM	21.6 μA·mM–1·cm–2	[166]
	Covalent	0.1–500 μM	0.04 μM	n.a.	[167]
CNOs	Covalent	1,000–10,000 μM	210 μM	26.5 μA·mM–1·cm–2	[168]
CNTs	Covalent	100–6,000 μM	9.01 μM	n.a.	[169]
		n.a.	n.a.	0.27–3.7 μA·mM–1·cm–2	[170]
	Non-covalent	1,000–20,000 μM	n.a.	0.198 μA·mM–1·cm–2	[171]
		1–5,000 μM	0.36 μM	n.a.	[172]
		0–5,000 μM	50 μM	289 μA·mM–1·cm–2	[173]

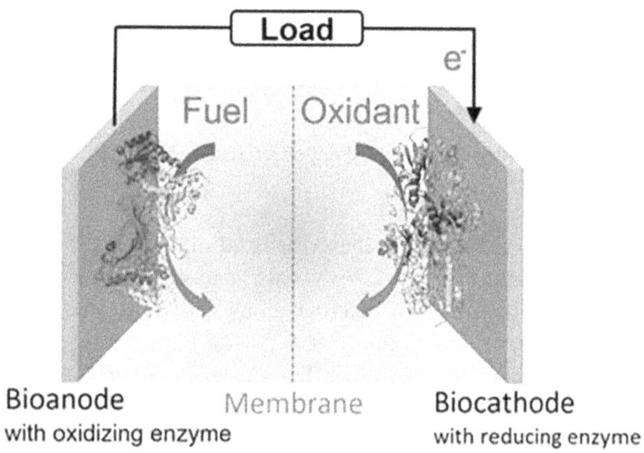

FIGURE 6.9 Schematic representation of biofuel cells with enzymes at the bioanode, where the fuel is oxidized, and the biocathode, where oxidants are reduced.

Source: Reproduced with permission from [174]. Copyright © 2022, American Chemical Society.

production of fuels as sustainable alternatives in the field of clean energy, such as water splitting reactions [175].

Conjugation with CNMs allows for high-performance devices. They have been coupled to enzymes to serve as anodes [176], cathodes [177], or both [178].

An electrochemical reaction of particular interest is the molecular oxygen reduction (ORR) at the cathode. In this case, use of CNT–laccase as biocathode allowed reaching current densities >1.8 mA·cm^{-2}, a direct electron transfer efficiency as high as 70–100%, and a turnover frequency of 5.0·103 s^{-1} [179]. When bilirubin oxidase was used, coupled to CNTs at the cathode, a maximum current density of 5.5 mA·cm^{-2} was found, and a power density of 1.85 mW·cm^{-2} at 0.6 V was attained, relative to 2.46 mW·cm^{-2} at 0.32 V with Pt/C as counter-electrode. The addition of catalase to a glucose oxidase (GOx)–CNT conjugate was thought to be another convenient strategy for ORR. In this case, GOx catalyzes the oxidation of glucose to gluconolactone, with the concomitant consumption of molecular oxygen to produce hydrogen peroxide, which is then converted by the catalase into water and molecular oxygen that feeds back into the GOx reaction. As a result, this type of catalyst reached a maximum power density of 0.18 mW·cm^{-2} and a current density of 59 μA·cm^{-2}. Another additive that can assist with catalytic performance in ORR is 2,2′-azino-di-(3-ethylbenzthiazoline sulfonic acid) or ABTS, which is a common substrate for hydrogen peroxidase and acts as an efficient electron transfer mediator between the enzyme and the electrode surface. With ABTS, a maximum power density of 1.12 mW·cm^{-2} at 0.45 V was obtained, which, after two weeks, had decreased just to 0.928 mW·cm^{-2}, indicating good stability over time.

Wearable CNT-based biofuel cells were developed on a cotton textile that allowed illumination of a LED on the cloth. Amongst the CNMs that have been used with enzymes in biofuel cells, as summarized in [106], CNTs are certainly the mostly studied [171]. Recently, scientists have recognized innovation opportunities also in other types of CNMs, such as CNDs, GO, or rGO, although reports in this direction are still very limited.

6.4.3 Biocatalysis

Thanks to great progress on biotechnology and protein engineering, biocatalysts have emerged as a green solution to increase the efficiency of industrial processes in a sustainable way [180]. Its importance and societal impact have been recognized through the Nobel Prize in Chemistry in 2018 to Arnold, who pioneered the directed evolution that enabled the development of resistant enzymes of industrial interest [181].

CNMs can be envisaged as active supports to immobilize enzymes and facilitate their recycling. Besides, their electronic properties may favor the catalytic performance of redox-active enzymes. To this end, enzymes have been coupled to CNTs to enable asymmetric hydrogenation in flow. Furthermore, bioelectrocatalysis involving direct electron transfer (DET) can benefit from the use of CNMs as active supports for redox enzymes, and the role played by their surface functionalization in the process has recently been reviewed [182].

6.4.4 Water Remediation and Environmental Monitoring

Enzymes supported on nanomaterials can be very convenient to detect pollutants for environmental monitoring through the development of sensitive sensors, but also for their removal from polluted waters. For example, CNMs coupled to enzymes can be applied for the electrochemical monitoring of chromium [183]. CNDs' fluorescence has also been envisaged for the optical detection of organic pesticides through coupling with an enzymatic reaction. In addition, rGO has been envisaged for the detection of pesticides through the immobilization of an esterase on a biocomposite containing fibrin and thrombin, which was assembled taking inspiration form the blood coagulation process. Finally, CNOs were coupled to a peroxidase in a cyclodextrin polymer matrix for the detection of herbicides, as tested in soil and river water samples [184].

6.4.5 Innovative Therapy and Theranostics

The rise of smart materials that can respond and adapt to stimuli and changes in the local microenvironment has opened new avenues that are enabling great progress, especially in the biomedical field [185]. Enzymes can be used as convenient stimuli for the design of responsive materials [186], with great potential in the development of combined therapy and diagnosis, for instance, through activation on a target pathological site characterized by the selective overexpression of certain enzymes. The coupling of enzyme-responsive materials with nanostructures can be convenient to develop photodynamic therapies for cancer treatment [187].

Alternatively, enzymes can be supported onto CNMs for combined chemodynamic therapy (CDT). For example, MWCNTs were functionalized with Fe_3O_4 and glucose oxidase so that the enzyme could convert glucose into gluconate and hydrogen peroxide. Conversion of the latter through the iron oxide–mediated Fenton reaction into hydroxyl radicals induces tumor cell death, and the reaction is favored by the lowered pH of the local microenvironment due to gluconate production. Finally, near-infrared (NIR) light irradiation can further boost the overall process at the target pathological site through generation of hyperthermia.

With the rise of biologics, enzymes have found applications also as therapeutic agents. As an example, laronidase can be used as replacement therapy for a type of mucopolysaccharidosis that is associated with deficiency of the natural enzyme, which hydrolyses glycosaminoglycans, causing their pathological accumulation in lysosomes. MWCNTs were thus envisaged as vectors for laronidase, which was covalently conjugated onto the CNMs. There are clearly many unexplored opportunities in this research area that are worth future investigation.

6.5 Enzymatic Biodegradation of CNMs

The possibility of biodegrading CNMs through enzymatic activity is very appealing for various reasons, including lowering their persistence in the environment after use, but also avoiding or reducing their bioaccumulation in living organisms. Furthermore, the breaking down of larger CNMs, such as GO, into smaller components can be envisaged as a green production method of graphene quantum dots (Figure 6.10) [188].

In general, the aromatic nature of CNTs renders them persistent in the environment, with little or no degradation by microorganisms, yet their oxidized forms appear to be biodegradable by microorganisms, whose enzymes are likely to use hydroxyl groups on the CNT surface as attackable sites that can be processed through enzymatic activity. Various peroxidases have been found to be able to biodegrade CNTs and G derivatives, as recently reviewed. They are mainly horseradish peroxidase (HRP), myeloperoxidase (MPO), manganese peroxidase (MnP), and lignin peroxidase (LiP). These four enzymes require hydrogen peroxide to participate in the degradation of CNMs. In the enzymatic degradation process of CNMs, molecular docking technology is used to predict possible binding sites, which helps to understand the degradation mechanism. Recently, oxidases were reported to biodegrade MWCNTs, CNDs [8], and fullerenes [189]. It is not surprising to see that nanozymes are being developed for the same purpose, for instance, as applied to the degradation of GO.

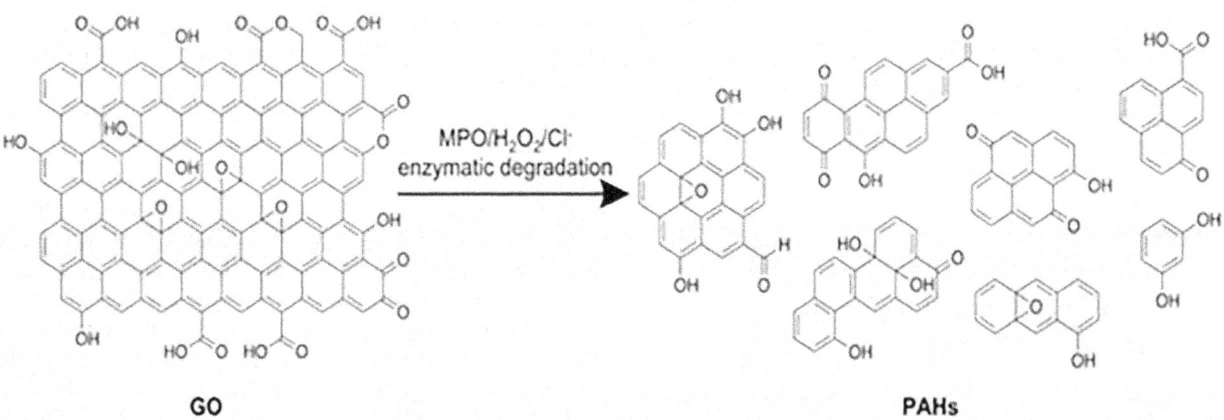

FIGURE 6.10 Enzymatic biodegradation of GO as a green production method of graphene quantum dots.

Source: Reproduced with permission from [188]. Copyright © 2022, American Chemical Society.

It is worth noting that besides the type of CNM, the level and type of functionalization is one of the factors playing a key role in determining CNM biodegradation. Whilst it is accepted that oxidation generally favors biodegradation [74], other types of functionalization can have the opposite effect. In particular, chemical reduction of GO and/or coating with bovine serum albumin or polyethylene glycol rendered the CNM resistant to peroxidase-mediated biodegradation.

CNM biodegradation mediated by bacteria typically involves electron-transfer processes, which lead to the breaking of C–C covalent bonds. As a result, numerous pores arise on the surface of CNMs, which lose structural integrity. Electrons can flow in either direction at the CNM–bacteria interface. In particular, cationic and anionic CNMs act as electron acceptors and donors, respectively. Furthermore, oxygen interference can occur at the point of electron transfer between bacteria and CNMs. In general, the functionalization of CNMs with anionic species on the surface of CNMs favors the electrostatic interaction with enzymes, which often display cationic amino acids on their surface, but also, the catalytically active heme group in redox-active enzymes plays a role in the interaction with CNMs. Clearly, pristine CNMs may be more challenging to degrade, and defect sites offer typical locations for the beginning of their structural deterioration.

Currently, fullerene biodegradation is still a largely unexplored research topic. It is known that this nanocarbon is challenging to degrade when exposed to soil bacteria. However, the situation is notably improved in the case of organics-rich clay, such that more than half of the fullerene present can be mineralized just over two months, and even more so in the case of functionalized fullerol. Its structural deterioration can be notably accelerated through the combination of biodegradation with photochemistry, which likely mediates the destruction of the stable aromatic core. Likewise, C60 photodegradation using UV light was facilitated by hydroxylation. In another study, fullerene aggregates decreased in volume upon exposure to bacteria, with occurrence of hydroxylation, although the structural deterioration of the nanocarbon was slow, and no significant production of carbon dioxide from C_{60} was noted, using isotope labelling. In general, the efficiency of photodegradation can be relatively high, but it should be noted that only UV light can degrade CNMs. In natural environments, CNMs will react with other substances too, and their degradation by UV light will be affected by all these factors. There is still a knowledge gap in the detailed understanding of biodegradation of several CNMs, especially in realistic experimental conditions pertaining to those found in the environment, including soil and water.

6.6 CNT-Based High-κ Dielectric Ion-Sensitive Field-Effect Transistor–Based Cholesterol Biosensor

Carbon nanotube (CNT)–based high-κ dielectric ion-sensitive field-effect transistor (ISFET)–based cholesterol biosensor has been realized using polyethylenimine (PEI)–doped CNT channel and nanocomposite of potassium-doped CNT with polypyrrole as sensing membrane. Device has been fabricated using solution method, and electrical characterization of the device has been carried out after immobilization of enzyme cholesterol oxidase (ChO_x) in the presence of PBS solution. Device has shown a wide dynamic range (0.5 to 25mM), a good sensitivity of 60 mV/decade, low response time (~1 s), low detection limit (0.23 mM), good stability (7 months), and high selectivity (interference ~1.8%) [190].

Biosensors based on the ion-sensitive field-effect transistors, so-called biologically modified field-effect transistors (BioFETs), have been intensively investigated because of their potential advantages, such as fast response, low weight, device miniaturization, better fabrication scopes and packaging, high selectivity and sensitivity, high reliability, low cost, on-chip integration.

Enzyme-modified field-effect transistor (ENFET) is a class of BioFET which is constructed by immobilizing an enzyme on the top of the gate insulator of ISFET. The simplest physics theory behind the working of this device is the exploitation of field-effect concept introduced by an electrolyte gate electrode, which is capacitively coupled through a thin dielectric layer. The enzyme reacts with the analyte of interest and generates or consumes protons which change charge at the gate surface in accordance with site binding theory. This change in charge at the gate surface modulates the channel conductance, and hence the channel current between the source and the drain of the ISFET. This output current can be related with the concentration of analyte under examination.

Referring to immobilization of enzyme on the top of the insulating surface of ISFET, various advanced materials, such as CNT, gold nanoparticles, and porous materials, have been used for firmed immobilization of the enzyme. In general, these materials cannot support enzyme directly, and hence, selection of an enzyme-loaded matrix compatible to both the insulating layer and the enzyme has importance in ENFET construction. In the present context, a nanocomposite of N-type carbon nanotube (prepared by doping potassium) with polypyrrole has been used as the enzyme-loaded matrix. In general, the compatibility of CNT with enzyme is very high, and when it is doped with potassium, it increases free high-mobility carriers. Due to this, electron transfer rate increases between the enzymatic reaction site and the oxide layer. Polypyrrole not only provides the support for the enzyme immobilization but also helps in better dispersion of CNT. These properties of the nanocomposite can therefore be used to improve the device performance as far as selectivity, response time, stability, and dynamic range are concerned.

In recent years, CNT-based ENFETS (CNTENFETs) have attracted great attention because they have been found as an ideal biosensor with high selectivity, real-time response, and the capability of label-free detection. In CNT-ENFETs, the silicon substrate of conventional BioFETs is replaced by semiconducting CNT channel. Polyethylenimine (PEI)–doped carbon nanotubes exhibit excellent n-type FET characteristics and have advantage over other types of n-doping techniques because it has the highest density of electron-rich amine amongst all the polymers. High-density electrons of n-type CNT result in better transconductance and, hence, improve the sensitivity of the device. The various intrinsic properties of CNT which are successfully utilized in biosensor development can be obtained elsewhere. One of the important properties of CNT that can be exploited to fabricate advanced miniature field-effect devices is its compatibility with high-κ dielectric materials. Such high-κ dielectric ENFETs have importance in "point-of-care" diagnosis systems and nanobiosensing areas.

Referring to cholesterol biomolecule, it is an essential steroid metabolite found in most of the human cells and is carried through blood by lipoproteins. Its importance in the design of structure of cell walls, synthesizing bile acids in intestine, production of vitamin D, and contribution in making steroid hormones are well-known. However, an elevated level of cholesterol is a biomarker for myocardial infarction, type 2 diabetes, thrombosis, high blood pressure, and cardiovascular diseases. Therefore, the development of a low-cost, integrated, disposable, and reliable technique for its detection is significant and essential in medical and clinical applications. In this communication, therefore, we have reported the fabrication and characterization of high-κ dielectric CNT-based ENFET for detection of cholesterol (CNT-Ch-ENFET) [190].

6.6.1 Device Fabrication and Characterization

Fabrication has been started with cutting of ITO-coated glass substrate (purchased from Sigma-Aldrich) using a conventional glass cutter tool (dimension ~5 mm × 2 mm). For removal of impurities, ITO-coated glass substrate has been washed using a solution of deionized water, ammonium hydroxide, and hydrogen peroxide in the ratio 2:1:1. Since ITO surface is a conducting surface, therefore, to block the conduction from CNT channel to ITO, a layer of ZnO (κ ~1.5) has been deposited on the top of the ITO substrate using the solution method, commonly known as electrochemical deposition (ECD) technique. This has been done by using a three-electrode electrochemical cell purchased from METROHM (http://www.metrohm.com/AUTOLAB PGSTAT128N). The details of preparation of the solution and its deposition methodology can be obtained in the earlier publication.

On the top of the ZnO dielectric layer, a thin film of PEI-doped carbon nanotube has been deposited by spin-coating technique. Doping of carbon nanotube with 30% polyethylenimine has been done in the presence of EDC-NHS cross-linker. The polymer-doped carbon nanotubes have been washed with deionized water and filtered using Teflon filter paper to remove unbounded particles. The doped CNTs have then been heated at 150°C for 1 h to remove moisture content. Solution has been prepared by adding 10 mg of PEI-doped CNTs in 20 mL of analytical-grade acetone. The solution has then been sonicated for 30 min using a probe sonicator (the amplitude of the sonicator has been set to 60% with a duty cycle of 50%). For better dispersion, the sonicated solution has been centrifuged using high-speed micro-centrifuge REMI RM 03 at 12,000 rpm for 20 min. CNT layer has then been deposited using the ECD technique. The sample has been heated at 150°C, and the process has been repeated until desired thickness of ~10 nm has been obtained. On the top of the channel region, a thin layer of zirconia has been deposited for serving as the top gate insulator. The cathodic deposition of zirconia layer has been carried out using the same workstation as used for bottom dielectric deposition. To deposit this ZrO_2 layer over channel region, a non-aqueous solution has first been prepared by dissolving zirconium tetrachloride in absolute ethanol in the ratio 1:5. The solution has then been sonicated at 20 KHz for 15 min. The deposition process has been carried out by applying constant working electrode potential −1.0 V for about 15–20 min. The deposited sample has then been dried using vacuum oven (LABFREEZ) at 250°C for 2 h. The thickness of this layer is ~10 nm. The source and drain region has been covered with Teflon tape to avoid deposition. Source (S) and drain (D) contacts have been fabricated by physical vapor deposition using metal aluminum. Aluminum (Al) metal has been deposited due to its suitable properties, such as low melting point, good adhesion with dielectrics, and low resistivity. Then, top sensing K/PPy/CNT layer has been deposited on the top of insulating ZrO_2 layer by spin-coating technique. The nanocomposite has been prepared by adding 10 mL of 1.0 M KOH to 5 mg of f-CNT. Then, 5 mL of pyrrole solution made in formic acid has then been added to the K/CNT. The solution has been sonicated for 20 min. using a probe sonicator and kept idle for 12 h. After the fabrication of the device, 10 μL of ChO_x has been immobilized on the sensing layer by physical adsorption technique (13). Passivation of the device has been done by coating a layer of polydimethylsiloxane (PDMS). The device has then been dried and kept in refrigeration until used. The schematic of CNT-based cholesterol ENFET (biosensor) is shown in Figure 6.11 [190].

Morphology of all the deposited layers has been investigated using SEM, FESM, and TEM results. The layers have been found to be uniform, and good adhesion was observed between the layers. The bonding structures of the CNT layer and K/PPy/CNT nanocomposite have been studied using Fourier transform infrared spectroscopy (FTIR) analysis, and the presence of carboxylic acid groups has been found.

6.6.2 Electrical Characterization

The measurement setup for experimentation is shown in Figure 6.12. Dual tracking power supply has been used for

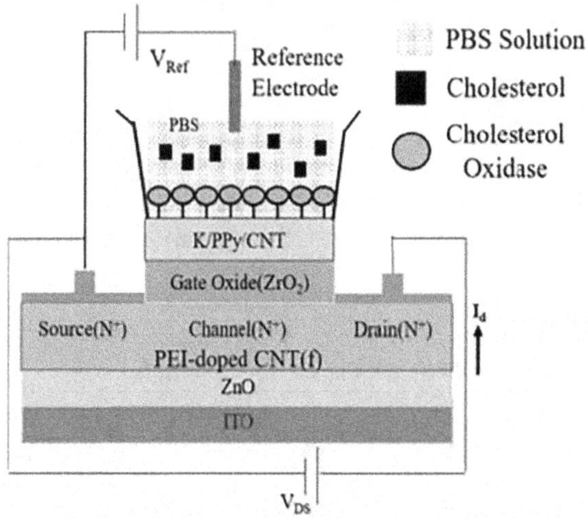

FIGURE 6.11 Schematic diagram of cholesterol ENFET.

Source: [190].

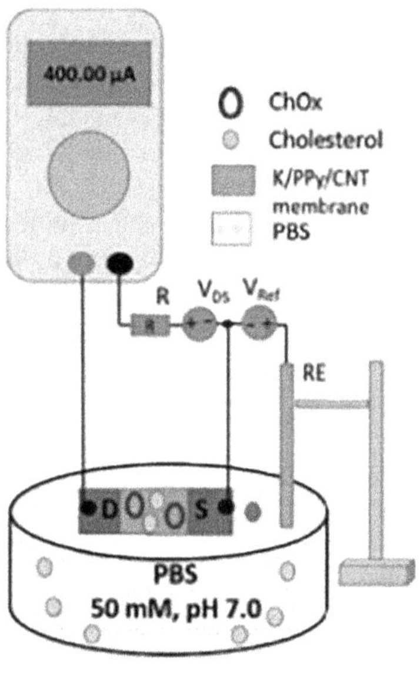

FIGURE 6.12 Cholesterol measurement setup.

providing desired voltages at drain and gate. The fabricated device is immersed in a PBS solution of 50 mM concentration and 7.0 pH. Ag/AgCl reference electrode is used for gate biasing.

Prior to being used as ENFET, the device has been biased for electrical characterization. It has been done at pH 7, and changing drain voltage in steps of 0.1 V, the biasing points have been fixed at $V_{GS} = 0.6$ V and $V_{DS} = 0.3$ V.

Threshold voltage of ENFET can be determined using extrapolation in linear region (ELR) technique. Using this technique, the ENFET threshold voltages have been calculated at different cholesterol concentrations from transfer characteristics curve.

As far as sensitivity of ENFET device is concerned, it is given by eq. (1). This equation implies that the sensitivity is given by the slope of the V_{TH} vs. concentration curve.

$$S = \frac{V_{TH}(ENFET)}{\Delta G} \quad (1)$$

Drain characteristics of the cholesterol ENFET have been determined using cholesterol stock solutions of different concentrations. The output characteristics at different concentrations and linearity curve of the device have been studied, respectively [190]. It is observed that the dynamic range of the device is 0.5–25 mM, and it is observed also that the device is linear from 1.8 mM to 19 mM, with regression coefficient of 0.9943. The current sensitivity has been found to be ~75.17 µA/mM.

Limit of detection is an important parameter in biosensor application. LoD is the least quantity of the analyte which can be detected by the biosensor. It is calculated using eq. (2) [191] and found out to be 0.23 mM.

$$LOD = \frac{3X\sigma}{S} \quad (2)$$

Where S is the slope between cholesterol concentration and response in terms of interfacial potential and σ is the standard deviation of the response.

Linweaver Burk plot has been used to find the Michaelis–Menten constant (K_m). The value of K_m is found to be 3.4 mM and 2.1 Mm for ohmic and saturation region of device output characteristics, respectively. The value of K_m shows that the device has high affinity toward the analyte.

The reproducibility test has been performed by characterizing five similar fabricated devices, and repeatability test has been performed by characterizing the same device for 5 times (once a week).

The fabricated device has been compared with other cholesterol biosensors and shown in Table 6.2 [190]. The measurements have been performed under similar conditions.

Temperature dependence of the device has been investigated. In the temperature range of 20–40°C, max response is obtained at 30°C. Degradation of enzyme activity is responsible for lowering of drain current at higher temperatures. The study shows that the interference of CNT-based cholesterol ENFET is negligible with other biomolecules, such as glucose, uric acid, urea, etc.

6.7 Bright Future of Carbon Dots for Cancer Nanomedicine

Carbon dots are a new class of carbon nanomaterials which have been acknowledged as quasi-spherical particles with sizes below 10 nm. The accidental discovery of these nanoparticles during the separation and purification of SWCNTs by Xu et al. in 2004 triggered subsequent studies to exploit their fluorescence properties to create a new class of viable fluorescent nanomaterials. Fluorescent CNPs were named carbon quantum dots (CQDs), or carbon dots (CDs), or carbon nanodots

TABLE 6.2

Comparison of Different Cholesterol Biosensors

Sensor Type	Sensing Material	Linearity (mM)	Km (mM)	Sensitivity	Ref.
Solution-gated FET	ZnO	1×10^{-3}–45 and 10 µA/mM/cm^2	—	—	[192]
Extended-gate FET	Ferrocenyl/alkanethiol	1.8–12.9	—	43.13 mV/decade	[193]
Potentiometric	ZnO/Ag	1×10^{-3}–10	—	35.2 mV/decade	[194]
Potentiometric	Co_3O_4	1×10^{-4}–1	0.039	94.031 mV/decade	[195]
CNT-ENFET	K/PPy/CNT	1.8–19	2.1	60 mV/decade	[190]

(CNDs), in 2006 by Sun et al., who proposed a synthetic route to produce CDs with enhanced fluorescence emissions via surface passivation. Over the past decade, a variety of additional terms have emerged in the literature describing different structures of the nanoparticles, such as graphene quantum dots (GQDs) or carbon nanoclusters. For more discussion about this topic, we recommend to the readers the recent contribution of Valcàrcel and coworkers. In this chapter, the term *carbon dots* (CDs) will be generically used to describe such nanoparticles without consideration of their actual morphologies.

Resulting from their tunable structure and diverse composition, CDs can have advantageous characteristics, such as excellent chemical stability, ease of modification, high water solubility, and tunable fluorescence with high quantum yield, good biocompatibility, and low toxicity. Particularly, CDs have wide application, including bioimaging, drug delivery, photodynamic therapy, sensors, optoelectronics, and photocatalysis. Furthermore, it has recently been found that CDs exhibit strong luminescence upon two-photon excitation in the NIR region, further expanding their applications in bioimaging. In fact, the colorful photoluminescence, high photostability, and low toxicity of CDs enable them to be strong competitors and potential alternatives to heavy metal–based semiconductor quantum dots (QDs) currently in use.

The following sections review the progress in the research and development of carbon dots (CDs) in nanomedicine. Compared to other reviews on this topic, the following sections focus their attention on synthetic strategies that could be employed for fabricating CDs and endowing them with particular characteristics that are essential for the design of efficient biological applications. The optical properties of these materials will be discussed, as well as their biological applications, with particular attention towards nanomedicine applications, such as bioimaging, drug carriers, gene therapy, thermal treatments, cancer diagnosis, and receptor-mediated therapy.

6.7.1 Synthetic Methods of Carbon Dots

In recent years, much progress has been made in terms of the synthesis, properties, and applications of CDs. Many methods have been proposed to prepare CDs, which can be roughly classified into "top-down" and "bottom-up" approaches. Top-down methods consist of arc discharge, laser ablation, and electrochemical oxidations, where the CDs are formed or "broken off" from a larger carbon structure. Bottom-up approaches consist of, for example, combustion/thermal/hydrothermal, microwave, or ultrasonication methods, during which the CDs are formed from smaller molecular precursors. Typically, their surfaces are oxidized by nitric acid (HNO_3) and further purified by centrifugation, dialysis, electrophoresis, or other separation techniques. Three potential issues related to the fabrication of the CDs should be taken into account: (1) Aggregation in larger clusters can occur, preventing the formation of the nanomaterials. This can be avoided by using electrochemical synthesis, confined pyrolysis, or solution chemistry. (2) Excessive heterogeneity of their dimensions should be avoided since the size strongly influences the luminescence and chemical properties. This can be performed by post-treatments, such as gel electrophoresis, centrifugation, and dialysis. (3) Control of the surface composition and derivatization leads to materials with different properties, such as solubility, photoluminescence, and QY. This can be tuned by varying the synthetic conditions and the post-treatment protocols.

6.7.1.1 Top-Down Approaches

6.7.1.1.1 Arc Discharge Methods

In 2004, Xu et al. isolated a fluorescent carbon nanomaterial while purifying SWCNTs derived from arc discharge soot. To improve the hydrophilicity of the material, the authors oxidized the arc soot with 3.3 M HNO_3 to introduce carboxyl functional groups, and then extracted the sediment with an NaOH solution (pH 8.4) to produce a stable black suspension. The suspension was separated by gel electrophoresis into SWCNTs, short tubular carbons, and a fast-moving band of highly fluorescent material which was composed of CDs.

6.7.1.1.2 Laser Ablation Methods

Sun et al. produced CDs via laser ablation of a carbon target in the presence of water vapor with argon as a carrier gas at 900°C and 75 kPa. Upon post–surface passivation with PEG_{1500N}, the final CDs emitted strong and tunable photoluminescence in both solution and solid states, depending on the excitation wavelength progressively changing from 400 nm to 600 nm. The synthesis and the passivation of fluorescent CDs by laser irradiation of a suspension of carbon materials in organic solvent have been reported. By selecting organic solvents, the surface states of CDs could be modified to achieve tunable light emission. Based on control experiments, the origin of the luminescence was attributed to the surface states related to the ligands on the surface of CDs. In this approach, a pulsed Nd–YAG laser was used to irradiate graphite or carbon black dispersed in diamine hydrate, diethanolamine, or PEG200N for 2 h while under ultrasonication to aid in particle dispersion.

After laser irradiation, centrifugation was used to precipitate residual carbon powder fragments while CDs remained suspended in the supernatant. These CDs averaged 3 nm in size, with lattice spacings varying from 0.20 to 0.23 nm, similar to that of diamond. Kim et al. reported the synthesis of nitrogen-doped CDs, starting from graphite flakes and employing EDTA as a doping agent. Laser ablation of ethanol solution of graphite and EDTA produced CDs with a relatively good QY (4.2–9.1%) and presented an N/C ratio of 7–15%, depending on the sonication power and a dimension around 2 nm [196].

6.7.1.1.3 Electrochemical Synthesis

Electrochemical synthesis of CDs was first demonstrated by Zhou et al. when they grew MWCNTs from scrolled graphene layers on carbon paper by chemical vapor deposition (CVD). These nanotubes were designed to serve as the working electrode in an electrochemical cell consisting of a platinum (Pt) wire counter-electrode and an $Ag/AgClO_4$ reference electrode with degassed acetonitrile solution containing 0.1 M tetrabutylammonium perchlorate ($TBA^+ClO_4^-$) as the electrolyte. This solution changed from colorless to yellow to dark brown, which indicated the formation of CDs with good solubility in various solvents.

Li et al. reported an alkali-assisted electrochemical method to prepare 1–4 nm CDs with controlled sizes. They were able to cut a graphite honeycomb layer into ultra-small particles, obtaining CDs with a narrow size range and thereby offering a straightforward and facile strategy to prepare high-quality CDs. Using graphite rods as both the anode and cathode and NaOH/EtOH as the electrolyte, they synthesized CDs with a current intensity of 10–200 mA cm^{-2}. The alkaline medium is the key factor, and OH− groups are essential for the formation of CDs by this electrochemical oxidation process since the same procedure performed in an acidic environment did not yield any CDs. Another facile electrochemical approach was reported by Ming et al. for the large-scale synthesis of high-quality CDs using only pure water as an electrolyte. The obtained CDs featured a highly crystalline nature, excellent water solubility, and remarkable down- and up-converted photoluminescence (PL) properties without extra purification. Moreover, they demonstrated that CDs possessed high photocatalytic activity under visible irradiation. The use of a microbial fuel cell (MFC) to produce CDs was exploited by Liu et al., who used a graphite rod as the cathode and carbon source. Such CDs contained a high amount of oxygen on the surface, improving their PL properties, and were exploited to prepare a photocatalytic ink to target pollutant degradation and for H_2 generation. The CDs adhered to normal paper and efficiently degraded Rhodamine B under visible light. When the CDs were instead employed in an MFC for hydrogen production, they showed good performance under visible light irradiation.

6.7.1.2 Bottom-Up Approaches

6.7.1.2.1 Combustion/Acidic Oxidation Methods

Liu et al. first reported that fluorescent CDs can be obtained from the combustion soot of candles after refluxing with oxidative acid. A glass plate placed over a burning candle was used to collect the hydrophobic soot, which could be turned hydrophilic by means of HNO_3 treatment. The suspension was purified by electrophoresis, revealing the presence of three bands, the first one consisting of nine fast-moving fluorescent smaller bands with different emission spectra. This study indicated that the fluorescence emission of CDs is size-dependent and/or charge-dependent.

This candle-burning approach was also followed by Ray et al. The candle soot was similarly collected and refluxed with 5 M HNO_3 for 12 h. The particle suspension was then precipitated by adding acetone and centrifuging at 14,000 rpm for 10 min. Size separation was achieved by fast centrifugation; the particles were centrifuged at different speeds, and the solids were collected every time. At 8,000 rpm, precipitate was no longer observed, and the supernatant contained CDs with particle sizes in the 2–6 nm range. Precipitates at lower centrifugation speeds contained large carbon nanoparticles of 201–350 nm in size. The 2–6 nm CDs were found to be graphitic, according to the lattice spacing in HRTEM images, and exhibited high PL quantum yields in comparison with the larger particles.

In a further study, Tian et al. purified CDs from the combustion soot of natural gas. By inverting a glass beaker above the flame of a natural gas burner, they were able to collect around 100 mg of soot, which was then refluxed in 5 M HNO_3 for 12 h, followed by centrifugation and dialysis to afford purified CDs. The purified CDs exhibited PL with a λ_{ex} maximum of 310 nm and an emission wavelength (λ_{em}) maximum of 420 nm. High-resolution transmission electron microscopy (HRTEM) showed CDs with an average diameter of 4.8 ± 0.6 nm and with crystalline lattices consistent with graphitic carbon.[13] C NMR and FT-IR measurements also revealed the presence of sp^2 carbon and carboxylic/carbonyl moieties, thus leading the authors to conclude that the CDs consist of a nanocrystalline core featuring graphitic sp^2 carbon atoms and a surface functionalized with carboxylic/carbonyl moieties.

Acidic oxidation is another popular method to prepare CDs. Typically, in this process, strong acid treatment of carbon precursors is conducted at high temperature. Leblanc's group reported an acidic oxidation route for converting carbon powder into CDs, in which a mixture of sulfuric acid, nitric acid, and carbon powder was refluxed at 110°C for 15 h. After cooling, CDs were successfully obtained as a black powder. Qian et al. reported a mild and facile synthesis of CDs from the mixed acid treatment of activated carbon. In their synthesis, a reaction temperature of 80°C was used, and the purified product could be obtained by dialysis.

More recently, our group synthesized CDs from black tea using acidic oxidation. This synthesis is simple and economical because of the selection of an inexpensive carbon source. CDs are synthesized with a narrow size distribution, tunable optical properties covering visible to deep-red absorption, non-toxicity, and easy synthesis for large-scale production. These CDs are utilized to label subcellular structures such as exosomes. More importantly, these new CDs can escape lysosomal sequestration and rapidly distribute in the cytoplasm to release doxorubicin (DOX) with better efficacy than the free drug at low pH, similar to the tumor microenvironment.

Park et al. employed a different acidic treatment for tuning the PL of the CDs employing tomatoes as the precursor. The biomass was first lyophilized and then treated with H_2SO_4 or H_3PO_4 at room temperature or at 80°. The syntheses yielded CDs with a blue, green, and yellow emission and a high biocompatibility toward HeLa cells. Furthermore, all the samples were employed as sensors for Fe^{3+}, with the blue CDs demonstrating the best performances, with a detection limit of 0.016 μM.

6.7.1.2.2 Thermal/Hydrothermal/Solvothermal Methods

For the synthesis of CDs, thermal/hydrothermal or solvothermal treatments are the most employed bottom-up procedures due to their low cost, easy feasibility, environmental friendliness, and applicability with various renewables carbon sources.

In general, with the thermal method, organic precursors are first pyrolyzed at high temperature (i.e., 200–400°C) without solvent for hours or days under air or inert gas, yielding a carbonized solid. Next, the CDs are recovered using water or other suitable solvents and purified by filtration or dialysis. However, this thermal method can only be applied for organic precursors having a melting point lower than the working temperature. Compared with this pyrolytic decomposition method, both the hydrothermal or solvothermal procedures are typically carried out in the presence of water or organic solvent in a pressure reactor at lower temperatures (i.e. 50–300°C) and shorter reaction times (minutes or hours). In the solvothermal carbonization, the CDs are recovered by extraction with an organic solvent, followed by a concentration/evaporation step. By using the solvothermal method, Bhunia et al. synthesized two kinds of CDs, hydrophobic and hydrophilic, with diameters <10 nm, from the carbonization of carbohydrates. The hydrophobic ones were produced by mixing the carbohydrate with octadecylamine and octadecene before heating to 70–300°C for 10–30 min. The hydrophilic ones instead were produced in water in a wide range of pH after heating at 80°C for 1 h, with the final materials presenting interesting yellow and red emissions. Generally, hydrothermal or solvothermal methods are simple, and the obtained CD suspension can be used without further purification.

Despite the difficulties to accurately rationalize the morphology and the photoluminescence properties of the CDs made by thermal or solvothermal methods, generally, large carbogenic structures with low luminescence are obtained by pyrolysis, while nanoscopic particles with strong photoluminescence are obtained with the hydrothermal or solvothermal methods. These differences can be ascribed mainly to the degree of carbonization reached during the synthesis and, therefore, to their different molecular-, amorphous-, or graphitic-like nature.

One of the first examples of the thermal synthesis of CDs was reported by Giannelis's group in 2008. The authors demonstrated the applicability of the pyrolytic procedure by heating different ammonium citrate salts or 4-aminoantipyrine at 300°C for 2 h in air, leading to the formation of both hydrophilic and lipophilic surface-functionalized carbogenic nanoparticles. These nanoparticles possessed an average size of <10 nm, were highly dispersible in organic or aqueous solvents (depending on their surface functionalization), and emitted light in the visible spectrum when excited at different wavelengths. By extending the procedure to neat citric acid, a completely insoluble carbogenic solid was obtained. Recently, Guo et al. developed a simple and low-cost approach to synthesize highly fluorescent CDs, by a one-step hydrothermal treatment of sodium citrate and ammonium bicarbonate in water. Experimental investigation confirmed that NH_4HCO_3 decomposed to CO_2 and NH_3, which conferred high pressure into the reaction medium and thus facilitated the decomposition of sodium citrate into small nanoparticles that produced the CDs. These CDs had an average size of 1.59 nm and exhibited a high PL quantum yield (68%) as well as good photostability. XPS confirmed the presence of carboxyl and hydroxyl groups on the surface of the CDs, and they were found to be very stable at a high concentration of ionic solution and could be used to detect mercury ions in aqueous solution with good selectivity and sensitivity. Generally, in all the preceding cases, the synthesis involves the carbonization of the reagents (via dehydrogenation, decarboxylation, and further polymerization reactions), leading to a complex carbonaceous material formed by amorphous aggregates and carbogenic structures having sp^2/sp^3 carbon domains decorated with -OH, -COOH, -COOR, and amino-derived functional groups [104]. Nowadays, citric acid is effectively considered the most common starting material for the thermal or hydrothermal synthesis of highly luminescent CDs, especially in combination with other heteroatom-doping reagents, such as nitrogen- or sulfur-containing compounds.

In 2014, Guo's group demonstrated the possibility of producing water-soluble CDs using only citric acid (treatment at 180°C for 2.5 h) as an organic precursor by suspending the resulting insoluble carbogenic solid in water, adjusting the pH to 7.0 using NaOH and thus forming Na^+-functionalized CDs.

Following these preliminary investigations, further improvements of this methodology have been carried out in Reisner's group by increasing the heating time up to 40 h at 180°C, thus avoiding the purification step to remove the residual citric acid. These amorphous CDs (a-CDs) had an average diameter of 6.8 ± 2.3 nm and low crystallinity, consisting predominantly of an amorphous carbon core with regions of graphitic carbon and carboxylate functionalities on the surface. Graphitic CDs (g-CDs) with an average size of 3.6 ± 1.0 nm were also prepared via a higher-temperature pyrolysis of citric acid. In brief, the precursor was heated in air at 180°C for 40 h, and then at 320°C for 100 h, during which full graphitization occurs. Furthermore, they extended this thermal procedure to produce graphitic nitrogen-doped CDs (g-N-CDs) with a narrow size distribution and a small average diameter of 3.1 ± 1.1 nm, by using aspartic acid in air at 320°C (required for the decomposition of the reagent) for 100 h. The resulting "nitrogen-doped" carbon dots are quasi-spherical, with a nanocrystalline graphitic N-doped core, with carboxylates as the primary surface functionality (Figure 6.13).

Very recently, Perosa's group synthesized amorphous and graphitic non-doped or N-doped CDs by two different preparation methods—hydrothermal and pyrolytic—and from two sets of reagents—neat citric acid and citric acid doped with diethylenetriamine (Figure 6.14) [197].

They demonstrated that the hydrothermal syntheses yielded amorphous CDs, either non-doped (a-CDs) or nitrogen-doped (a-N-CDs), while the pyrolytic treatment afforded graphitic CDs, either non-doped (g-CDs) or nitrogen-doped (g-N-CDs). The morphology, structure, and optical properties of the four different types of CDs were also determined, revealing significant differences, depending on the synthetic pathway. The CDs were then employed as photosensitizers in an organic

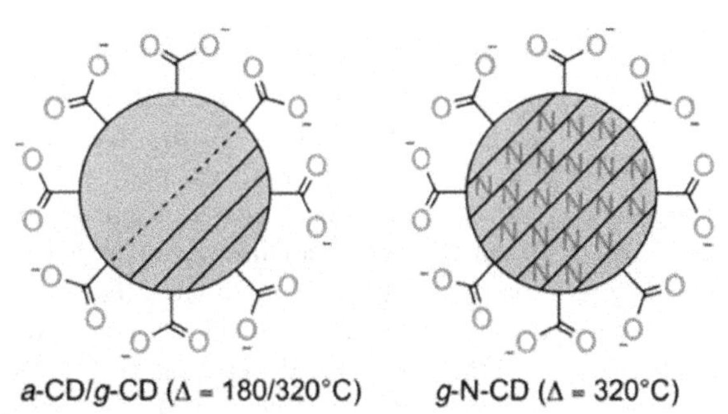

FIGURE 6.13 Schematic representation of amorphous or graphitic CD structures obtained by the thermal decomposition of citric (a-CDs and g-CDs) or aspartic (g-N-CDs) acids. Picture of different fractions of fluorescent carbon under 365 nm UV irradiation and TEM images of short tubule carbon and purified SWNTs.

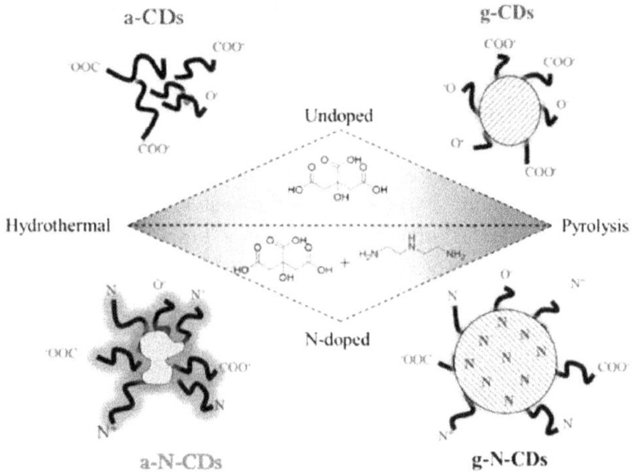

FIGURE 6.14 Schematic representations of the four CDs studied in this work: purely carbogenic (a-CDs, g-CDs) or N-doped (a-N-CDs, g-N-CDs) obtained by a hydrothermal method (180°C, hours, water) or thermolysis (220°C, days, neat) of citric acid with or without diethylenetriamine as a doping agent.

Source: **Figure reproduced from ref. [197] with permission from the American Chemical Society. Copyright 2018.**

reaction, demonstrating excellent performance, depending on their structure and synthetic pathway [198].

Zhu et al. fabricated nitrogen-doped citric acid–derived CDs by a hydrothermal method. Citric acid and ethylene diamine were dissolved in deionized water and heated at 200°C for 5 h in a Teflon-lined autoclave. The reaction occurred by first condensing citric acid and ethylene diamine, whereupon they formed polymer-like aggregates, which were then carbonized to form the CDs. The quantum yield of these N-doped CDs reached 80.6% at an excitation wavelength of 360 nm, nearly equal to that of most semiconductor QDs and fluorescent dyes.

More recently, Lu et al. synthesized N-CDs with an average size of 2.6 nm using a one-pot hydrothermal treatment with citric acid as the carbon source in the presence of polyethylenimine (PEI) as a simultaneous nitrogen dopant and surface passivation agent. N-CDs synthesized emitted a strong blue luminescence with a QY of 51%. The N-CDs exhibited excellent photostability and low cytotoxicity, making the N-CDs promising optical nanoprobes for real-time live-cell imaging. Moreover, their small size and the surface positive charge rendered by the polyethylenimine (PEI) endow them with the ability to cross the blood–brain barrier (BBB), making them potentially useful in traceable drug delivery in brain disorders.

The second prominent heteroatom which is included into the structure of CDs is sulfur. Aside from limited examples, where only sulfur was reported to be doped into CDs, most studies focus on their co-doping with nitrogen, in order to improve the optical properties of the CDs, in particular their PL QY. Dong et al. synthesized nitrogen–sulfur co-doped CDs via a one-pot hydrothermal treatment of citric acid and L-cysteine at 200°C (PL QY of 73%).

Aside from citric acid, another approach toward the synthesis of N-doped CDs was recently reported by Jiang et al., who synthesized color-tunable CDs by heating phenyl-diamines in ethanol at 180°C for 12 h. The difference in functional group configuration from ortho, to meta and para, changed the emission color of the resulting CDs from green to blue to red.

In recent years, more work has been carried out to find other bio-based precursors (glucose, sucrose, fructose, ascorbic acid, polyols, polymers, amino acids, proteins, natural products, and some wastes) to synthesize CDs. In this context, Zhang et al. reported a high-yield synthesis of hydrophilic CDs by controlled carbonization of sucrose. Green luminescent CDs and non-luminous CDs were effectively separated by dialysis. After surface functionalization with PEG_{2000N}, the non-luminous CDs emitted blue fluorescence. Another one-step synthetic route, in which the CDs were synthesized from the hydrothermal oxidation of carbohydrates (glucose/sucrose/starch) with acid/alkali additives, was reported. Addition of HCl enhanced emission of the CDs at longer wavelengths, while NaOH enhanced the emission of CDs at shorter wavelengths. The authors proposed that these additives induce different defects on the surface of the CDs, which act as surface energy traps that result into the different PL behaviors. These CDs exhibited NIR emission excited by NIR excitation, as well as up-conversion PL properties. The elemental analysis showed that they contained predominantly elemental carbon and oxygen. It was also revealed that the functional carboxyl and hydroxyl groups on the surface of these CDs made them dispersible in water.

Fluorescent CDs with a diameter of about 2.0 nm were prepared directly via a simple hydrothermal method by using L-ascorbic acid as a carbon source. The solvent used in the dissolution of the acid was investigated and proved to have a strong link with the CD PL. Ethanol proved to be the best as it provided a reaction medium for the uniform growth of the nanoparticles due to its ability to cap and inhibit the aggregation of the nanoparticles. In contrast to the previous methods, no strong acid or further surface modification was needed for the preparation. The CDs had uniform shapes and sizes in the range 2.0–2.5 nm and were water-soluble and exhibited λ_{ex}-dependent emission. Experiments revealed that the emission of these CDs exhibited good stability in reaction media of high ionic concentrations that could be tuned by adjusting the pH. Water-soluble and well-crystallized CDs with a lateral size of about 3.0 nm were also fabricated by a hydrothermal cutting method. The atomic force microscopy (AFM) observation of the CDs deposited on a mica substrate shows a narrow height distribution from 1.5 to 1.9 nm, suggesting that the CDs typically consist of 2–3 graphene layers.

In order to favor the formation of biocompatible nanostructures suitable for medical applications and to avoid the formation of harmful chemical compounds, Cailotto et al. hydrothermally synthesized monosaccharide-derived CDs starting from fructose, glucose, and ascorbic acid, without any passivating or doping additives. These CDs were characterized from a morphological, chemical, and toxicological point of view, and their potential application as drug nanocarriers was tested using doxorubicin as a model drug. Interestingly, the cytotoxicity of the CDs was affected by the choice of the starting materials; CDs synthesized from fructose were found to be toxic, while high biocompatibility was observed starting from glucose or ascorbic acid. Their drug loading capabilities were evaluated, indicating the crucial role of the CD morphologies, rather than the surface functional groups, in controlling the doxorubicin uptake. With the more suitable glucose-derived CDs, the authors found up to 28%w/w of drug loading.

Zhou et al. reported large-scale CD preparation starting from watermelon peel. The fresh peel was carbonized at 220°C for 2 h under an air atmosphere, filtered, centrifuged, and dialyzed, yielding highly luminescent CDs with a blue fluorescence, good water solubility, small particle size, and good stability in a wide range of pH values and at a high salt concentration. Passivation enabled their use in biological applications, such as *in vivo* bioimaging and as bioprobes, as it introduced specific function on the surface of the nanomaterial.

Sahu et al. prepared highly photoluminescent CDs with a quantum yield (QY) of 26% in a one-step hydrothermal treatment of orange juice, followed by centrifugation. These CDs with sizes of 1.5–4.5 nm were applied in bioimaging due to their high photostability and low toxicity. Yang et al. reported a one-step synthesis of amino-functionalized fluorescent CDs by hydrothermal carbonization of chitosan at 180°C for 12 h. These CDs are demonstrated as excellent probes as bioimaging agents.

6.7.1.2.3 Microwave Methods

Microwave heating has become important in synthetic chemistry. Compared with other methods, it is more convenient and rapid to heat the carbon precursors, and it simplifies the synthesis, yielding CDs readily within a few minutes and with higher yield. Multicolor luminescence has been achieved by microwave synthesis of CDs using dextrin as a starting material in the presence of sulfuric acid. This solution was microwave-heated for 2.5 min at 800 W, and a light-brown supernatant was obtained along with a black precipitate. The solution containing the CDs was centrifuged to obtain a clear solution. The obtained CDs were characterized using different techniques, and the luminescence spectra showed that the particles attained multicolor luminescence without any requirement for surface-passivating agents. The quantum yield was between 5 and 9%. This multicolor luminescence might be very helpful in the field of bioimaging. Wang et al. presented a facile one-step microwave-assisted approach to prepare water-soluble phosphorus-containing CDs with strong green fluorescence. In this synthesis, 2 mL of 70% phytic acid and 1 mL ethylene diamine were mixed in 25 mL ultrapure water and then heated for about 8 min in a domestic 700 W microwave oven. Notably, these CDs present two-peak emissions when excited at low wavelengths; however, at high-excitation wavelengths (360–460 nm), only one emission peak at 525 nm was observed. The highest quantum yield of the resulting phosphorus-containing CDs was about 21.65%.

Qu and coworkers reported a one-step microwave heat treatment of carbohydrates to synthesize multicolored photoluminescence CDs without any surface passivation reagents. Glycerol was mixed with phosphate solution and subjected to microwave heating for 14 min to generate the CDs. The PL showed that the emission spectra were broad and ranged from blue to yellow, depending on the excitation wavelength. The CDs possessed carboxyl and hydroxyl moieties that enhanced their hydrophilicity and stability in aqueous systems, shown by their ability to maintain PL intensity even with increased ionic strength. The obtained CDs were biocompatible and were found to be promising in biolabeling and bioimaging. This work has also demonstrated that inorganic ions were able to effectively promote the carbonization of carbohydrates.

Ding et al. reported the synthesis of N and S co-doped CDs by employing 1,6-hexanediamine dihydrochloride dissolved in DMSO as the only precursor. After 30 min of microwave irradiation, the CDs were obtained and purified by dialysis and freeze-drying. The nanomaterial exhibited a respectable QY of 24% and presented an emission ranging from blue to orange. The N,S-CDs were successfully employed in the detection of MnO_4^- and $Cr_2O_7^{2-}$ and showed excellent biocompatibility [199].

Jaiswal et al. developed a simple one-step microwave-mediated synthesis of CDs using biocompatible PEG as a sole source of carbon and a passivating agent. An aqueous PEG solution was irradiated for 10 min to generate amorphous CDs with an estimated average size of 3.6–5.4 nm. The obtained CDs were compliant to size separation by gel electrophoresis and possessed high photostability, which was confirmed by their ability to maintain luminescence under extended irradiation. Zhu et al. synthesized CDs by combining PEG_{200} and a saccharide (for example, glucose and fructose) in water to form a transparent solution, followed by heating in a 500 W microwave oven for 2–10 min. The solution turned from colorless to dark brown over the course of the reaction. The reaction time plays a crucial role in determining the properties and size of the CDs; in fact, longer heating times result in CDs enlarging slightly and emitting at longer wavelengths. For example, the average CD diameters were 2.75 ± 0.45 nm and 3.65 ± 0.6 nm for heating times of 5 and 10 min, respectively. Without the addition of PEG, besides the same color change, the nanomaterial obtained presents a weak and irregular PL.

In order to enhance the PL properties of the CDs, their doping with boron and nitrogen was achieved by employing urea and boric acid in combination with citric acid. The microwave irradiation of this mixture led to CDs with a mean diameter of 2 nm and a QY between 15 and 30%. Their strong luminescence was exploited for the investigation of energy transfer with photosynthetic pigments. The experiments reveal that the emission of the CDs was quenched by the pigments, meaning, that an energy transfer process between the two species was involved. This phenomenon allows the increase of the spectrum range in which the photosynthetic pigment can absorb light, enhancing their photocatalytic activity [200].

Very recently, Prato and coworkers prepared and characterized a redox library of amino-doped CDs with tunable oxidation/reduction properties starting from commercially available quinones, arginine, and ethylene diamine, highlighting their potential applicability as photocatalysts. These CDs were prepared by microwave irradiation (240°C, 26 bars, and 200 W for 180 s) of an aqueous solution of the precursors, followed by dialysis. In all cases, after the hydrothermal treatment, the color of the reaction mixture turned dark brown as a result of the formation of CDs. Benzoquinone-, naphthoquinone-, and anthraquinone-based carbon nanodots exhibited interesting electrochemistry with oxidation potentials between +1.48 V and +0.98 V vs. SCE and reducing potentials in the range −1.52 V and −2.05 V vs. SCE.

By extending this microwave-assisted multi-component synthetic approach, the Prato group prepared the first example of chiral CDs (CNDs-R or CNDs-S) by using arginine, as the core precursor, and (R,R) (1R,2R)-1,2-Diaminocyclohexane—or (S,S) (1S,2S)-1,2-diaminocyclohexane—1,2-cyclohexanediamine (CHDA) as the chiral surface precursors (Figure 6.15) [201]. These particles, with a mean particle size around 3 nm, are highly soluble in water and display a mirror-image profile both in the UV-vis and in the infrared regions, as detected by electronic and vibrational circular dichroism, respectively. The origin of chirality was ascribed to the presence of numerous cyclohexanediamine moieties around the carbon-based amorphous core. The authors [202] used the chiral nanodots as templates for the preparation of porphyrin-based supramolecular assemblies, thus opening the way for developing a variety of new chiral composite materials and applications.

6.7.1.2.4 Ultrasonication Methods

The ultrasonication method is a process in which ultrasonic waves produce alternating expansion and compression in a reaction solution, resulting in the growth and implosive collapse of bubbles irradiated with the waves. The mechanism causes high-speed interparticle collisions, which can change the morphology, composition, and reactivity of the particles. When integrated with carbonization, the energy of the ultrasonic waves generates intermediates that can be further carbonized to generate very small CDs. Li et al. described a simple synthesis of CDs from glucose or active carbon by using an ultrasonic treatment method. Such monodispersed water-soluble fluorescent CDs could emit bright and colorful PL covering the entire visible-to-NIR spectral range. Notably, the NIR emission of CDs could be obtained by NIR excitation. Furthermore, the CDs had excellent up-conversion fluorescence properties.

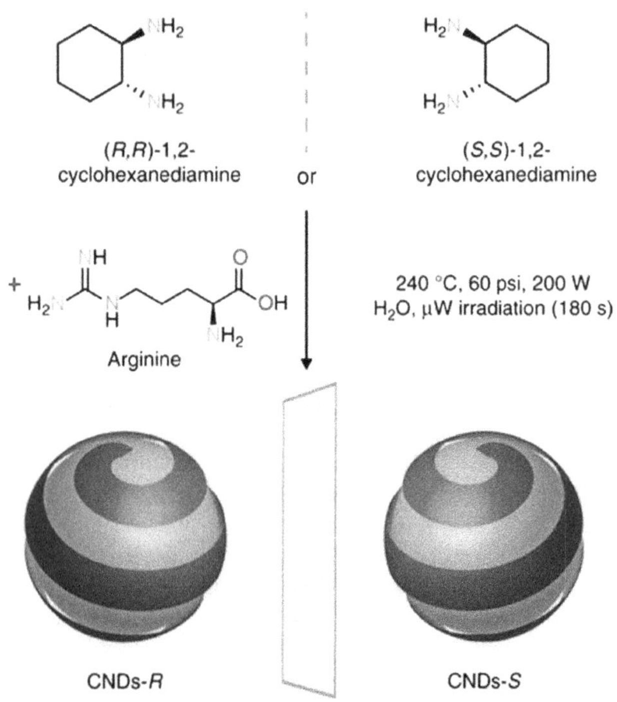

FIGURE 6.15 Design and synthesis of chiral carbon nanodots. Chiral CNDs were synthesized starting from (*R,R*)- or (*S,S*)-1,2-cyclohexanediamine and arginine, under hydrothermal microwave-assisted conditions (240°C, 70–110 psi, 200 W for 180 s).

Source: Figure adapted from ref. [201] with permission from Nature Publishing Group. Copyright 2018.

6.7.2 Chemical Composition and Structure of Carbon Dots

C, H, and O are the three main elements present in CDs, in varying ratios. The introduction of heteroatoms has been studied to tune the conduction/valence band position, which confers additional functions. For example, the quantum yield (QY) of CDs could be significantly improved by incorporating nitrogen, while CDs with a wide bandgap could be synthesized by incorporating sulfur. Furthermore, P-doped CDs showed green fluorescence, which could be utilized as an imaging signal with a low background. Other heteroatoms, such as Cl and B, could also be incorporated into CDs by changing the synthetic methods or starting materials.

Along with the elemental composition, the morphology of CDs may also be affected by both the preparation methods and the nature of the precursors. For instance, the CDs prepared by "top-down" approaches are composed of nanocrystalline cores with predominantly graphitic or turbostratic carbon (sp^2 carbon) or graphene and graphene oxide sheets fused by diamond-like sp^3-hybridized insertions. Hu et al. reported that the selected-area electron-diffraction (SAED) experiments on CDs with a size of about 3 nm prepared by laser ablation with surface modification revealed a ring pattern, with the ratio of the squares of the ring radius of 3: 8:11:16:19. This implies a diamond-like structure, with the rings respectively corresponding to the (111), (220), (311), (400), and (331) planes of diamond. This feature is retained also in the case where PEG200N is not employed as the passivating ligand. The lattice spacing observed was 0.2–0.23 nm and is, in fact, quite close to the (100) facet of graphite. The lattice fringes of the diffraction planes of diamond-like and graphitic carbon lie very close to one another, thus rendering unambiguous assignment difficult without other corroborating evidence. Additionally, Ray et al. found that the CDs prepared from oxidizing candle soot had 0.208 nm lattice spacing, which suggests sp^3 diamond-like carbon or sp^2 graphitic carbon [130]. By ^{13}C NMR analysis, Tian et al. confirmed the presence of sp^2 carbon with signals in the $\delta = 90–180$ ppm range, while the absence of signals in the $\delta = 8–80$ ppm confirms the absence of any detectable aliphatic moieties. Furthermore, FTIR measurements also confirmed the presence of C = C aromatic ring stretches. Therefore, the authors concluded that these CDs consisted of a nanocrystalline core of graphitic sp^2 carbon atoms functionalized with peripheral carboxylic/carbonyl moieties. One-step thermal decomposition reactions of citrate salts produced CDs with a size of 7 nm, whose XRD patterns were indicative of disordered carbon alongside the respective passivation agent. The XRD pattern of CDs made from octadecylammonium citrate shows two superimposed broad reflections: one centered at 4.3 Å, and a sharper peak at 4.14 Å, which are indicative of disordered carbon and densely packed alkyl groups arising from the octadecyl chains, respectively. The XRD pattern of CDs prepared by the supported method displayed a sharp, low-intensity reflection centered on d002 = 3.3 Å, which was very close to the graphite (002) lattice spacing. However, the XRD pattern of the hydrophilic CDs (prepared by controlled carbonization of sucrose) showed an (002) interlayer spacing of 4.2 Å, which is larger than that of bulk graphite (3.3 Å), indicating poor crystallization. The nanocrystalline core may also contain superficial carboxyl moieties, which impart excellent water solubility and suitable chemically reactive groups for further functionalization and surface passivation with various organic, polymeric, inorganic, or biological materials to CDs. Upon surface passivation, the fluorescence properties of CDs are enhanced. Surface functionalization also modifies their physical properties, like their solubility in aqueous and non-aqueous solvents.

Unless otherwise modified, oxidized CDs generally feature carboxylic moieties on the surface, with overall oxygen contents ranging from 5 to 50 weight (wt) %, depending upon the experimental conditions used.

Over the last few years, comprehensive research has been carried out to clarify the exact structures of the CDs prepared by "bottom-up" methods. In general, the morphology of such CDs consists of a complex mixture of crystalline or graphitic-like carbogenic cores, amorphous polymeric-like compounds, and even small molecular-like fluorophores. Moreover, the actual degrees of carbonization, size, and morphology of the CDs depend on the kind of bottom-up method (thermal/hydrothermal/solvothermal, microwave, or ultrasonication) and on the reaction conditions (i.e., the nature of the precursors, the solvents, the time, the temperature, and the presence of doping heteroatoms). Currently, citric acid (CA) is the most common source for the synthesis of highly luminescent CDs, especially in combination with other doping reagents, such as nitrogen-containing compounds. Overall, while the harsh pyrolytic conditions result in the production of CDs with a graphene-like substructure, the mild hydro/solvothermal procedures often lead to the synthesis of molecular fluorophores and amorphous CDs.

In 2012, Dong et al. demonstrated that a moderate or harsh thermal decomposition of citric acid resulted in the production of two different CDs with either an incomplete or a complete graphene-like structure, respectively. In brief, after moderate pyrolysis (30 min, 200°C), the citric acid can be partially carbonized to form nanosheets (graphene quantum dot (GQDs)) containing abundant small but uniform sp^2 clusters. The GQDs show a strong and excitation-independent photoluminescence. By heating the same reaction mixture for a longer time (120 min at 200°C), full pyrolysis occurred, forming larger nanosheets (i.e., graphene oxide (GO)). The GO contained abundant small sp^2 clusters isolated within the sp3 C–O matrix. These sp^2 clusters should be non-uniform in size and poorly passivated, resulting in a weak and excitation-dependent PL activity.

A similar study conducted by Wang et al. on the decomposition of citric acid confirms that by increasing the pyrolysis temperature and time, larger particles will be constructed which possess low luminescence. Only at relatively lower temperatures (180 and 200°C) and shorter times are sufficient quantities of highly luminescent, uniformly sized CDs formed, which therefore exhibit a strong excitation-independent photoluminescence. The authors suggest that in the first instance, the reaction proceeds toward the nucleation of some molecules of citric acid, producing highly fluorescent materials, which further evolve through cross-linking and stacking, forming extended amorphous and crystalline carbon domains.

Mild pyrolysis (180°C, 30 min) has been applied also to the synthesis of heteroatom-doped CDs, revealing the presence of molecular fluorophores; under more severe conditions (up to 400°C for 1 h or 320°C for 100 h), a carbogenic-heteroatom-doped core was observed. Specifically, the reaction between citric acid and ethanol amine was carried out at different temperatures of 180, 230, 300, and 400°C. Under mild conditions, no CNPs were detected, notwithstanding the highly fluorescent nature of the final solution. NMR and ESI-MS analyses reveal the molecular nature of the solution, and some molecular fluorophores were also identified. By increasing the reaction temperature, the formation of small spherical nanoparticles and progressive decrease of the QY were observed. The data suggest that the fluorophores produced at a low temperature are used as building blocks for the synthesis of CDs at a higher temperature.

Besides pyrolysis, also mild hydrothermal/microwave procedures have been used for the synthesis of heteroatom-doped CDs. For example, Song et al. demonstrated that the hydrothermal treatment of citric acid and ethylene diamine at low temperatures produces a mixture containing carbon cores, oligomers, and molecular fluorophores. The authors identified 1,2,3,5-tetrahydro-5-oxo imidazo[1,2-a]pyridine-7-carboxylic acid (IPCA), a bright-blue fluorophore (Scheme 6.1a) [202], which was found to exist individually or bonded to the carbon core and thus to strongly affect the luminescence properties

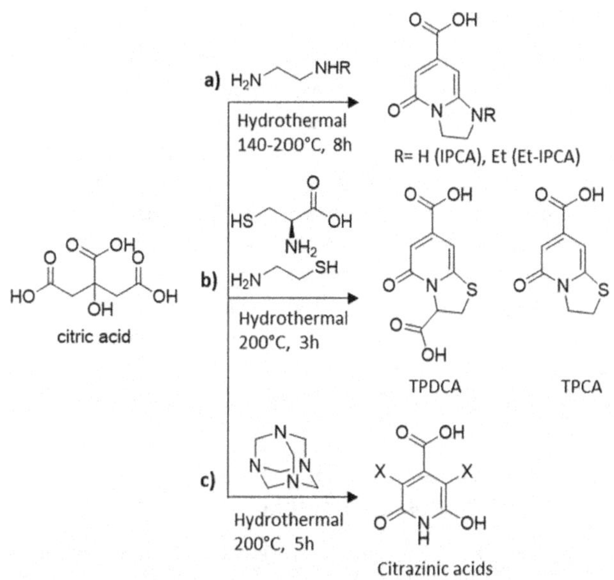

SCHEME 6.1 Molecular fluorophores identified in the synthesis of CA-based CDs using different amino-containing precursors: (a) ethylene diamine, (b) cysteine and cysteamine, and (c) hexamethylenetetramine.

of the nanoparticles. IPCA was then used in hydrothermal synthesis at two different temperatures, confirming how the temperature influences the degree of graphitization. From these experimental findings, the authors hypothesized the presence of a chemical equilibrium between IPCA and carbon cores with polymer clusters acting as a transition state. Accordingly, the synthetic outcomes could be affected by many factors, such as the reagent ratio, initial pH, and temperature. For the latter, they demonstrated that molecules/oligomers were dominant in the CDs prepared at lower temperatures, while the carbon cores prevailed in the CDs prepared at high temperatures.

Since then, many molecular fluorophores have been detected in the solution during the synthesis of CA-derived CDs. TPCA and TPDCA organic fluorophores (Scheme 6.1b) were the main ingredients and the fluorescence origins of N,S-CDs synthesized by hydrothermal treatment of CA with l-cysteine or cysteamine at low temperatures (200°C) for 3 h.

Fluorescent derivatives of citrazinic acid (Scheme 6.1c) were also identified, which are likely to constitute molecular species either free or bonded to the carbonized nanoparticles, in the CD material formed by hydrothermal treatments of CA with hexamethylenetetramine at 200°C for 5 h. The authors further compared the optical properties of different CD species, demonstrating the significant differences between samples predominantly composed of the carbon core and those containing molecular derivatives of citrazinic acids.

Many other recent contributions further describe the separation and characterization of different fluorophore molecules arising from the synthesis of CDs, leading to a deeper understanding of the existing relationship between the structural composition and the optical properties of the CDs, as clearly described in the following section.

6.7.3 Optical Properties

6.7.3.1 Absorbance

CDs typically show strong optical absorption in the UV region, with a tail extending out into the visible range.

Most of the CDs, such as those prepared by laser-passivation, electrochemical oxidation, or microwave/ultrasonic method, have an absorption band around 260–320 nm. The several shoulder peaks in UV absorption spectra are generally attributed to the π–π^* transitions of aromatic rings and C = C double bonds or to the n–π^* transitions of C = O bonds or other sub-fluorophore groups. However, the absorbance of CDs was found to increase to a longer wavelength (350–550 nm) after surface passivation with 4,7,10-trioxa-1,13-tridecanediamine (TTDDA).

6.7.3.2 Photoluminescence: Origin of Photoluminescence

One of the most fascinating behaviors of CDs, from a fundamental viewpoint of application, is their photoluminescence (PL). Although the exact mechanism which generates the light absorption and emission for CDs is still an open issue, the more reasonable hypotheses attribute it to the morphology and to the chemical/physical properties of the CDs. In summary, these are the three possible origins of PL:

1. The first is the quantum confinement effect, which is determined by the degree of π conjugation and by the size of the carbon core. This type of PL, which arises from a band-edge recombination, is commonly observed in the homologous "metal-based" quantum dots and confers to the carbon-based nanoparticles a size-dependent, excitation-independent, and a very narrow emission band.
2. The second type of emission is generated by the surface states, which are determined by surface defects, functional groups, and surface passivation of the carbogenic core. In this case, the superficial defects trap the photoexcited electrons and/or holes in the bandgap, thus generating PL with lower energy. The resulting PL is a combination of the first two types of mechanisms, leading to a luminescence with an ill-defined behavior and strongly dependent on the synthetic procedure used.
3. The third is the molecule state type, which is associated with the presence of fluorophores in the CDs. In this case, neither quantum confinement nor surface defect effects exist, and the luminescence is solely a consequence of the superposition of several "molecular"-type emissions. PL is therefore size-independent and excitation-dependent and exhibits a very broad emission band.

The photoluminescence properties of the carbon dots are therefore strictly correlated with their intrinsic structure and, consequently, to the synthetic procedure used. Despite the difficulties in determining the actual origin of luminescence and in further classifying the CDs based on their exact morphology, in general, the first two PL mechanisms are invoked for "graphitic-like" CDs synthetized via both top-down or harsh bottom-up approaches (i.e., pyrolysis), while the third for "amorphous-like" CDs prepared through soft hydro/solvothermal bottom-up treatments. Herein, recent studies on the PL properties of CDs will be discussed.

Based on the origin of PL described earlier, the PL activity of graphitic-like CDs can be easily tuned by modifying both the core size and the nature of the functional groups.

In 2010, Li et al. presented clear evidence for luminescence arising from quantum-confinement effects and size-dependent optical properties of CDs prepared by an alkali-assisted electrochemical method starting from a graphite honeycomb. The PL behavior was also retained after the plasma treatment for the removal of surface oxygen. Theoretical calculations performed on the CDs reveal that the HOMO–LUMO gap depends on the size of the graphene fragments. As the size increases, the gap energy decreases gradually, reaching the visible spectral range with CDs of 14–22 Å diameter, which agrees well with the visible emission of CDs with diameters of <3 nm. Thus, they deduced that the strong emission of CDs comes from the quantum-sized graphite structure instead of the carbon–oxygen surface.

Few years later, in 2012, by comparing carbon nanoparticles with different dimensions obtained by one-step hydrothermal treatment of orange juice followed by size separation via centrifugation, Mohapatra et al. confirmed the redshift in the emission wavelength of CDs with increasing size. As the size of CDs increases, the nature and content of sp^2-hybridized sites and the bandgap from the quantum confinement effect would be affected. In particular, the authors pointed out that excitation-dependent photoluminescence could be caused by surface states, excitons of carbon, emissive traps, aromatic conjugation structures, and free zigzag sites.

Zhang and coworkers, in 2016, prepared different-sized CDs via gel electrophoresis of the crude nanoparticles prepared through a photo-Fenton reaction of graphene oxide. They demonstrate that the PL of CDs depends on both the nanoparticle size, according to the quantum confinement effect, and the peripheral carboxylic groups. More importantly, it was revealed that for small-sized CDs, the surface status effect prevails on the PL with the contribution of the carbon skeleton, which appears only when exciting the nanomaterial at longer wavelengths. However, for the large-sized CDs, the effect of the graphitic core is dominant over their PL, leading to an emission wavelength which increases with size (minor energy gap). The latter phenomenon can only be explained with the quantum confinement effect.

An additional extensive analysis of the contribution on the PL of the carbon core of the CDs was reported by Zhu et al., who demonstrated the role of the aromatic carbon domain in achieving the blue fluorescence of the carbon nanoparticles. In more detail, in a perfect graphene core with few surface groups, the bandgap between the conjugated π-domains is the intrinsic PL center. Other important contributions to the photoluminescence of the carbon nanoparticles may derive from their surface states: the surface chemical groups and the hybridization structure of the edge groups. Carboxyl and amide groups are responsible for the green emission of the carbon nanoparticles, while the hydroxyl groups guarantee a blue photoluminescence. These results were proved by different factors; first of all, long exposure to the UV light results in an enhanced PL due to the oxidation of the hydroxyl groups to carboxyl groups. Converting the hydroxyl groups in amide groups results in an enhanced PL, and if these CDs are reduced, a strong blue luminescence is observed. These results confirmed the great complexity of the photoluminescence origin of the CDs and that different factors may contribute to it.

Considering the effect on the PL of the superficial CD decorations, many other studies have appeared in the last few years. As reported by Sun et al., the PEG_{1500N} passivation of CDs formed by laser ablation of graphite powder and cement led to an emission spectrum spanning from purple to red, which further spreads to the NIR region, with the excitation wavelength progressively increasing from 400 nm on the left in 20 nm increments. Upon surface passivation with organic or polymeric materials, such as poly(propionyl ethyleneimine-co-ethyleneimine) (PPEI-EI) attached to the CD surface, surface defects are stabilized, and strong fluorescence emissions, both in a solution-like suspension and in solid state, were detected. The emissions of such passivated CDs covered a broad range of the visible region and extended into the NIR region. It should be noted that the surface passivation agents used were not emissive in the visible and NIR regions, and thus, any fluorescence emissions observed must have originated from the surface-passivated CDs. The tunable emission properties of CDs are clearly demonstrated. From the fluorescence spectra of PPEI-EI-passivated CDs, it is evident that the emissions are broad and excitation wavelength–dependent. The tunable emissions of the surface-passivated CDs could be a result of varied fluorescence characteristics of particles of different sizes of the CDs and the distribution of different emissive sites on the surface of the CDs.

More recently, Ding and coworkers, using urea and p-phenylenediamines as precursors, prepared equal-sized CDs from blue to red with excitation-independent luminescence emission spectra. The observed color changes were found to depend on the degree of superficial oxidation structures rather than the particle size. In more detail, the observed redshift in their emission peaks from 440 to 625 nm was ascribed to a gradual reduction in their bandgaps with the increasing incorporation of oxygen species into their surface structures (Figure 6.16).

Moreover, pH-dependent PL emission was also reported, and this phenomenon can be reasonably explained by surface states, as Qu et al. have discussed. Functional groups, such as N–H and O–H, on the surface of CDs can form intramolecular and intermolecular hydrogen bonds, which endow the CDs with different surface states. pH changes could cause deprotonation or protonation of functional groups, inducing variation of surface states and fluorescence. Jia et al. reported that CDs prepared from direct heating of ascorbic acid solution show a practically linear dependence on the pH of the solution in the range of 4.0 to 8.0. The fluorescence intensity decreased by as much as 90% from acidic to alkaline pH. The shift in the pH caused the deprotonation of the carboxyl groups on the surface of the CDs, leading to electrostatic doping/charging of the CDs and Fermi level shift. A similar effect could also be triggered by solvent polarity, as Gao et al. observed, by changing the solvent from water to ethylene glycol. This may be due to the change of surface states and the decrease of non-irradiative transitions. It is worth noting that some CDs exhibit fluorescence that is independent of the excitation wavelength and pH.

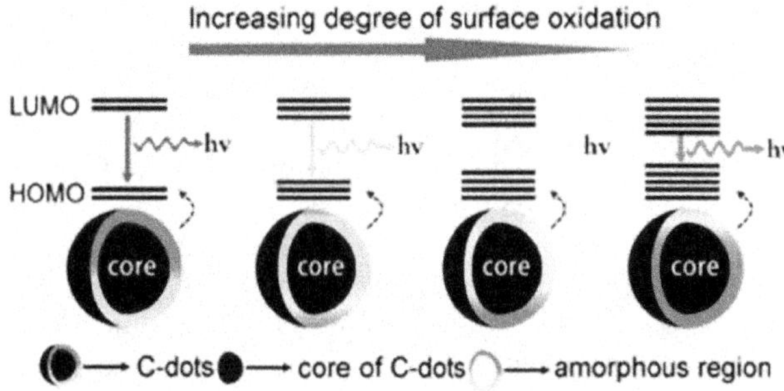

FIGURE 6.16 Model for the tunable PL of CDs with different degrees of oxidation.

Source: Figure adapted from ref. H. Ding, S.-B. Yu, J.-S. Wei, and H.-M. Xiong, Full-Color Light-Emitting Carbon Dots with a Surface-State-Controlled Luminescence Mechanism, ACS Nano, 2016, 10, 484–491.

Regarding the third molecular state effect of the PL on the CDs, an unequivocal demonstration was given in 2015 by Song et al., who were able to isolate and characterize the molecular fluorophore IPCA (5-oxo-1,2,3,5-tetrahydro-imidazo[1,2-α] pyridine-7-carboxylic acid), demonstrating that its absorption and emission spectra were identical to one of the synthetized CDs. The resulting fluorophore was found to be the main emitting species in these CDs.

Other recent research studies describe a great variety of organic fluorophores responsible for the optical properties of CDs. Worthy of mention is the study conducted by Schneider et al. on CDs derived from the soft hydrothermal treatment of citric acid in the presence of three different amino compounds.

Other important considerations regarding the role of molecular fluorophores in determining the final PL properties of the nanomaterials have been pointed out by Zhang *et al.* They demonstrated that the optical properties of CDs synthesized from citric acid and cysteine are regulated by the presence of the fluorophores TPDCA (5-oxo-3,5-dihydro-2*H*-thiazolo [3,2-*α*] pyridine-3,7-dicarboxylic acid) and TPCA (5-oxo-3,5-dihydro-2*H*-thiazolo [3,2-*α*] pyridine-7-carboxylic acid). Both the molecular fluorophores and the CDs show the same UV-vis absorption, excitation and emission, QY, fluorescent lifetime, excitation-independent emission, pH-dependent fluorescence, and photobleaching. In addition, the authors were able to isolate and characterize TPCA and TPDCA from the CD solution, confirming that the PL mechanism is governed by the molecular state.

Fu *et al.* further investigated the origin of the luminescence of CDs obtained from citric acid and ethylene diamine. The authors were able to reproduce the optical behavior of such CDs by employing simple polyaromatic hydrocarbons (PAHs) like pyrene, anthracene, and perylene. Tuning the concentration of these three compounds, they were able to reproduce most of the optical properties of the CDs. From these results, they assert that CDs likewise predominantly comprise small PAHs embedded in a matrix consisting of sp^3-hybridized carbon. Defect states and surface chemical functionalities also participate in defining the optical properties of the materials but will only play a minor role.

Based on this topic, Hinterberger et al. produced CDs from citric acid and cysteine under different hydrothermal conditions, and then they purified the mixture by silica gel chromatography. This system allowed the separation of three different fractions, the first one rich in fluorophore molecules (5-oxo-3,5-dihydro-2H-thiazolo [3,2-α] pyridine-7-carboxylic acid) (TPDCA), the second one less photoluminescent composed of fluorophores bound on the CD surface, and the last one composed of CDs without fluorophores. The analyses revealed that, under mild condition, the solution is mainly composed of fluorophores and possesses a high QY (72%). With harsher conditions, a drop in the QY was observed as the fluorophores were destroyed and embodied in the structure of the CDs. This study demonstrated the complexity and the heterogeneity of the solutions of CDs and how their luminescence properties could be tuned by employing different synthetic protocols.

An additional very recent hypothesis on the origin of the PL behavior of the CDs and the specific role played by the different components was made. They suggested that the PL of CDs is the result of a cooperative effect between the graphitic carbon core, the defect states, and the molecular fluorophore. The authors used citric acid and amino group–containing molecules as precursors to prepare CDs having luminescent pyridine derivatives along with a carbogenic core, which were separated by a dialysis treatment. The PL behavior of the molecules agreed with the one of the original CD solutions, with, however, a higher QY and a less-evident excitation-dependent behavior.

Combining these outcomes with an accurate optical study, the authors proposed a hypothetical PL mechanism in which fluorophores, defect states, and the carbon core play a different role. UV irradiation of the fluorophores generates excited electrons from the π orbitals to the π^* orbitals. Some of the excited electrons in the π^* orbitals may recombine with the holes in the π orbitals directly, emitting the PL signal centered at 420–440 nm, which can be referred to as the intrinsic emission, like the band-edge emission observed in QDs. The other excited electrons in the π orbitals may be trapped by the defect states of energies lower than in the π^* orbitals before they are finally recombining with the holes in the π orbitals. Meanwhile, some electrons may be excited and trapped directly by the defect states and relax through either radiative or non-radiative ways. Therefore, when the excitation wavelength is in the range of 280–380 nm, the CD produced both intrinsic and defect PL signals. When the excitation wavelength is longer than 380 nm, that is, at a lower energy, which is less than needed for the π–π^* transition, the electrons can only be excited to the defect states. The graphitic core, in this hypothesis, acts as a quencher of the radiative relaxation pathway of both defect and intrinsic states through a fluorescence resonance energy transfer (FRET) effect, thus lowering the QY.

In conclusion, while the PL spectra depend on both molecular fluorophores and defect states, the magnitude of QY is mainly affected by the graphitic core of the CDs.

Overall, even if this latter PL mechanism is satisfactory from an intuitive level, many other issues (such as the role of the carbon core size and the structural morphologies of the CD, that is, amorphous or crystalline) were not effectively addressed. Therefore, there is a lack of a real understanding of the mechanisms of fluorescence of these nanosystems to date.

6.7.3.2.1 Photostability

The ability to maintain stable fluorescence emission intensity after a long continuous excitation is called *photostability*. Wei et al. demonstrated that CDs have an excellent photostability when synthesized from glucose and various amino acids. After 60 min of excitation, the PL intensity of all the CDs preserved 90% of the initial intensity. PL of the CDs was much more stable than that of fluorescein isothiocyanate (FITC) dye, CdTe QDs, and previously reported polymer nanoparticles or dye-doped silica.

Ge et al. prepared red-emissive CDs using polythiophene phenylpropionic acid as a precursor, and their photostability was investigated. Fixed-cell images of the CDs labeled HeLa cells showed intense red fluorescence, after 120 min of irradiation. By contrast, the ones of FITC decay very rapidly after 10 min, confirming the higher photostability of the CDs *in vitro*.

The diversity and uncontrollable nature of the surface defects on the CDs reduce the radiative recombination, limiting their QY and their application in several fields. In order to improve the luminescence of CDs, great effort has been made through physical and chemical methods. Wang et al. reported CDs with a PL QY of 55–60% after column chromatography purification of the CD mixture with 16–20% PL QY. To enhance the QY of CDs, diverse designs have been developed, including surface passivation, element doping, and inorganic salt doping. Passivation is the common strategy to improve the QY of CDs due to its facile process ability and high efficiency. Most of the time, it implies oxidation or reduction of the CD surface and subsequent capping with organic polymers or diamine compounds. Zheng et al. reported that original CDs prepared with graphite oxide as a precursor were reduced by $NaBH_4$, and the QY of the reduced-state CDs increased greatly from 2 to 24%; meanwhile, the maximum emission wavelength shifted from 520 to 450 nm at an excitation wavelength of 360 nm (Figure 6.17).

To stabilize and maximize fluorescence, CDs are usually doped with inorganic salts or with organic precursors containing different elements. Nitrogen is the most widely used doping element, leading, in most of the cases, to higher QY. Jiang et al. prepared CDs with high QY (44.9%) from amino acids via a microwave method. Nitrogen and sulfur co-doped CDs via a hydrothermal method with extremely high QY (73%) have been prepared. In this method, L-cysteine was used as a precursor for doping of the CDs. Sulfur is also employed as a doping agent to increase the PL properties of the CDs; based on this topic, Xu et al. synthesized S-doped CDs with significant fluorescence QY (67%) via a hydrothermal method. Moreover, some other methods have been developed to improve the QY of CDs. For example, Sun et al. developed CDs doped with Zn to achieve high QY. An aqueous suspension of CDs and $Zn(CH_3COO)_2$ was hydrolyzed with NaOH, and then $Zn(OH)_2$ was converted to ZnO by thermal annealing; the QY of the ZnO-doped CDs in aqueous solution was around 45%. After precipitation with Na_2S, the QY of the ZnS-doped CDs was consistently higher than 50%. Sun et al. speculated that the combination of organic and inorganic passivation agents might provide another form of surface passivation or enhance the surface passivation effect. Under the two-photon excitation at 800 nm, these doped CDs emitted bright luminescence in the visible region, suggesting promising potential for imaging applications.

6.7.3.2.2 Up-Conversion Photoluminescence

In addition to normal fluorescence, a new and interesting phenomenon has been discovered recently: up-conversion fluorescence emission. Up-conversion fluorescence is anti-Stokes behavior, in that a longer excitation wavelength produces a shorter emission wavelength. As shown by Sun et al., CDs were strongly emissive in the visible region under irradiation by an argon-ion laser (458 nm) or a femtosecond pulsed laser for two-photon excitation in the NIR range (800 nm). The authors show that the one- and two-photon luminescence images for the same scanning area of CDs are well matched. The representative two-photon luminescence spectrum shows that such CDs have up-conversion photoluminescence (UCPL) properties. The results from further bioimaging experiments in vitro also showed the UCPL properties of CDs.

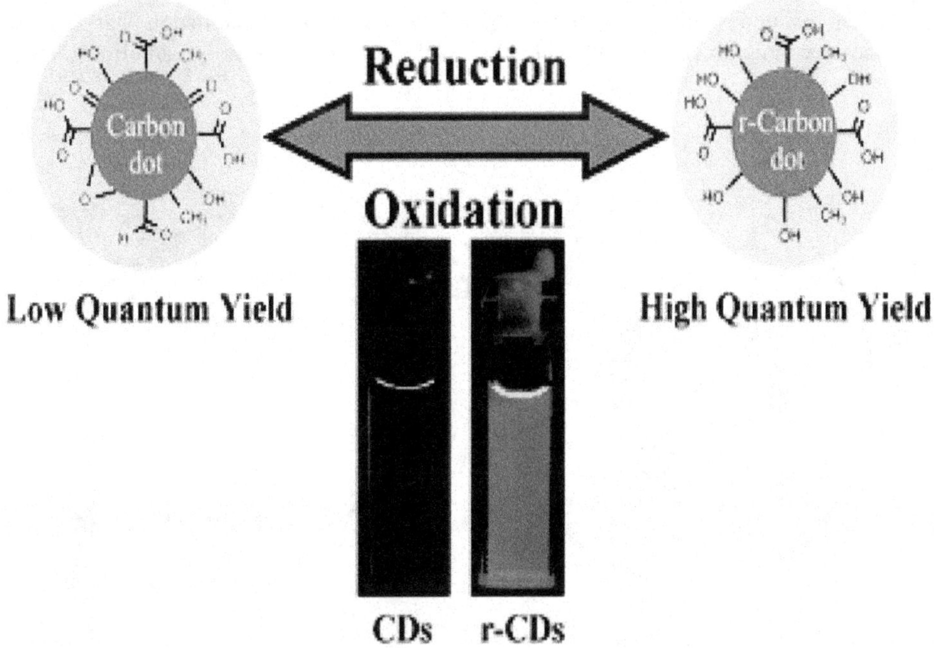

FIGURE 6.17 Graphical representation of the synthesis of reduced-state CDs (r-CDs) with blue luminescence from original CDs. Inset: photographs of aqueous solutions of the CDs (CDs) (left) and the r-CDs (right) obtained under UV light (360 nm).

Source: **Figure reproduced from H. Zheng, Q. Wang, Y. Long, H. Zhang, X. Huang, and R. Zhu, Chem. Commun., 2011, 47, 10650. With permission from Royal Society of Chemistry. Copyright 2011.**

Recently, Jiang et al. reported that CDs emitted strong UCPL under excitation with a femtosecond pulsed laser (λ = 800 nm), and this has been demonstrated to be a two-photon excitation process.

Stan et al. studied the up-conversion fluorescence of N-doped CDs in the wavelength range of 750–960 nm. Interestingly, distinct from the down-conversion case, up-conversion fluorescence showed excitation wavelength–independent and solvent polarity–dependent emission. Moreover, such up-conversion fluorescence can be easily observed by the naked eye. Shen et al. fabricated CDs surface-passivated with PEG by a one-pot hydrothermal reaction. The PL quantum yield of the CDs at an excitation wavelength of 360 nm was about 28%. The CDs possessed the up-conversion PL properties and emitted blue PL in the fluorescence microscopy images both under the ultraviolet and 808 nm laser.

To further confirm this and explain how UCPL comes from the CDs, an energy-level structural model was established, in which the UCPL spectrum could be regarded as an anti-Stokes transition. The energy levels of π and σ orbitals were provided by the carbene ground-state multiplicity, which is related to the energy difference (δ_E) between the π and σ orbitals. The energy between the excitation light and the emission light in the up-conversion process was close to 1.1 eV (Hoffmann determined δ_E should be below 1.5 eV). When a bunch of low-energy photons excites the electrons in the π orbital, the π electrons would be excited to a high-energy state, such as the LUMO, and then fall back to a low-energy state. Thus, a UCPL is emitted if the electrons transition back to the σ orbital. The electrons in the σ orbital can also be excited, and they only can emit normal PL. This explains why the difference between up-conversion excitation and emission light is a constant energy related to the energy difference of the π and σ orbitals.

The UCPL of CDs opens new opportunities for cell imaging with two-photon luminescence microscopy, as well as highly efficient catalyst design, for application in bioscience and energy technology.

6.7.3.2.3 Chemiluminescence

Chemiluminescence (CL) refers to a phenomenon whereby during a chemical reaction, a substance can absorb chemical energy to turn into an excited state and then go back to the ground state by light irradiation. The CL properties of CDs were first discovered when the CDs coexisted with some oxidants, such as potassium permanganate ($KMnO_4$) and cerium (iv). During this process, the CDs with surface energy traps serve as electron acceptors for the electron donator $O_2^{\bullet-}$ and strong CL emitter. The electron paramagnetic resonance (EPR) reveals that oxidants, such as $KMnO_4$ and cerium (iv), can inject holes into the CDs. This process increases the population of the holes in the CDs and accelerates the electron–hole annihilation, resulting in energy release in the form of CL emission. This is the first CL route accounting for the CL (CL1). The other important route (CL2) is the Mn(ii)* excited state, which returns to the ground state with CL emission at 650 nm (Figure 6.18). Moreover, CL intensity was dependent on the concentration of the CDs in a certain range. It was also found that increasing the temperature had a positive effect on the CL due to the thermal equilibrium of the electron distribution in the CDs (Figure 6.18). It is interesting to note that for this system, the CL properties can be designed by changing their surface groups.

Recently, CDs obtained from citric acid and melamine were employed to enhance the CL reaction of $K_2Cr_2O_7$ with $NaHSO_3$. The nanomaterial acts as both an energy acceptor and luminophore in the CL reaction, inducing an amplification of the signal. This effect was exploited for the determination of iodide, since this ion can interact strongly with the potassium species, leading to an enhancement of the signal [203].

A novel CL phenomenon was also observed for the CDs in a strong alkaline solution (NaOH or KOH). The

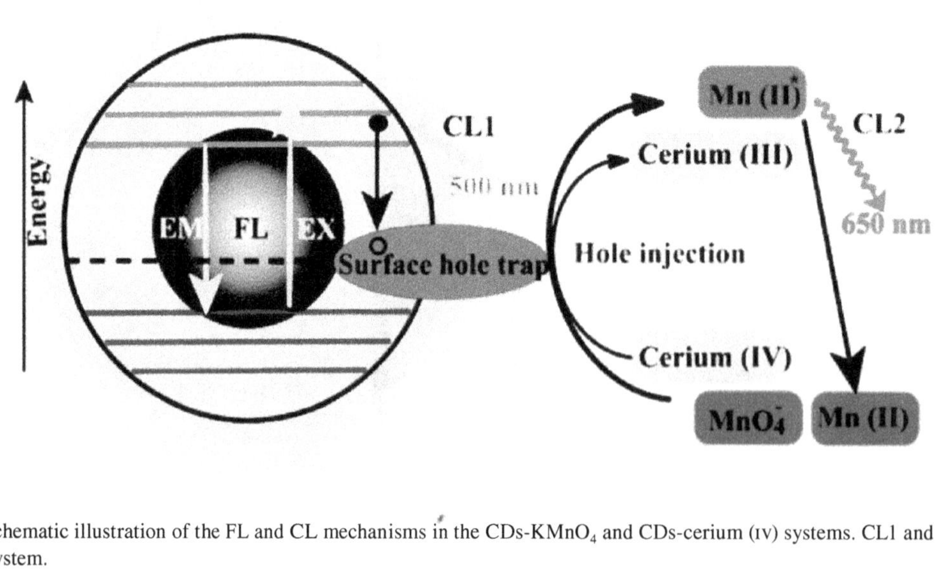

FIGURE 6.18 Schematic illustration of the FL and CL mechanisms in the CDs-$KMnO_4$ and CDs-cerium (iv) systems. CL1 and CL2 represent two CL routes in the system.

Source: Figure reproduced from Z. Lin, W. Xue, H. Chen, and J.-M. Lin, "Classical oxidant induced chemiluminescence of fluorescent carbon dots," *Chem. Commun.*, **2012, 48, 1051–1053, with permission from Royal Society of Chemistry. Copyright 2012.**

CDs exhibited excellent electron donor ability toward dissolved oxygen to form the superoxide anion radical ($O_2^{\bullet-}$) in a solution of NaOH. These results provided direct evidence for the excellent electron-donating ability of CDs. Radiative recombination of the injected electrons by "chemical reduction" of the CDs and thermally excited generated holes was suggested to account for the CL behavior in strong alkaline solutions. The dual role of CDs as an electron donor and acceptor offers great potential in optronics and catalysis.

6.7.3.2.4 Electrochemiluminescence

Differently from fluorescence and CL, electrochemiluminescence (ECL) happens when the substances produced in an electrochemical reaction are excited via electron injection and then emit light to return back to the ground state. The ECL emission of CDs (2.0 nm) produced by Zheng et al. from the electrochemical oxidation of graphite was observed as the potential was cycled between +1.8 and −1.5 V. The suggested ECL mechanism involves the formation of excited-state CDs (R*) by electron-transfer annihilation of negatively charged ($R^{\bullet-}$) and positively charged ($R^{\bullet+}$) species (the ET1 route in Figure 6.19). $R^{\bullet+}$ is the more stable of the two species, as indicated by the greater intensity of the cathodic ECL (Figure 6.19a). Interestingly, when produced by microwave synthesis, 3 nm PEG_{200}-functionalized CDs also exhibited ECL behavior, but the $R^{\bullet-}$ species was found to be more stable in this case. The presence of peroxydisulfate ($S_2O_8^{2-}$) enhanced the ECL (the ET2 route in Figure 6.19b) in the cathodic potential range and produced a stable and sensitive (as no other coreactants tested elicited an ECL enhancement) ECL response, thus suggesting the application of CDs for ECL sensing. More recently, Kumar et al. employed P-doped CDs in the fabrication of a solid-state ECL platform for the detection of Cu^{2+}. They observed that the ECL intensity of the phosphorous-doped CDs is way higher compared to that of the undoped ones. Moreover, if Cu^{2+} is added to the solution, the intensity could be further enhanced, thus increasing the detection limit for this particular ion [204].

6.7.4 Biological Properties and Applications

Carbon dots exhibit many biological applications due to their low toxicity, biocompatibility, and biodegradation. Recent advancements of CDs in the medical or pharmaceutical field include their application in bioimaging detection, drug carrier development, gene transfer, diagnosis, cancer therapy, and so on. However, some studies have reported that many factors, including CD synthesis methods, the size, the shape, and the functional groups on the surface of CDs, could affect the efficiency of CDs, causing hazardous effects on human health. Therefore, *in vitro* and *in vivo* toxicity studies of CDs are the new challenge to understand the mechanism of these nanoparticles and confirm their safety [205].

6.7.4.1 In Vitro and In Vivo Toxicity Studies

Although *in vivo* toxicity studies of CDs remain a critical issue, the low cytotoxicity of these nanoparticles could be the main reason for scarcity of studies in animal models. Wang et al. evaluated the genotoxicity, the acute toxicity, and the subacute toxicity of CDs fabricated from raw soot by nitric acid treatment and PEG passivation. The results [202] showed no genotoxic or toxic effects in the mice model used. In another study, Tao et al. investigated the *in vivo* toxicity effect of CDs following intravenous administration (20 mg kg^{-1}) in mice. The experiments were carried out for three months without showing toxic effects in the treated mice.

In recent years, zebrafish embryos have attracted widespread attention as strategies for the toxicological evaluation of CDs due to their homology to the human genome, their short generation time, and their optical transparency, which allows in real time the bioimaging detection of CDs. In a study by Tathagata et al., the authors reported the nontoxic effects of CDs from curcumin using the zebrafish model. The nonaqueous curcumin was transformed into a highly hydrophilic CD after hydrothermal synthesis. Multicolor fluorescence, high photostability, and low cytotoxicity were reported in fibroblast cells NIH-3T3, human lung adenocarcinoma cells A549,

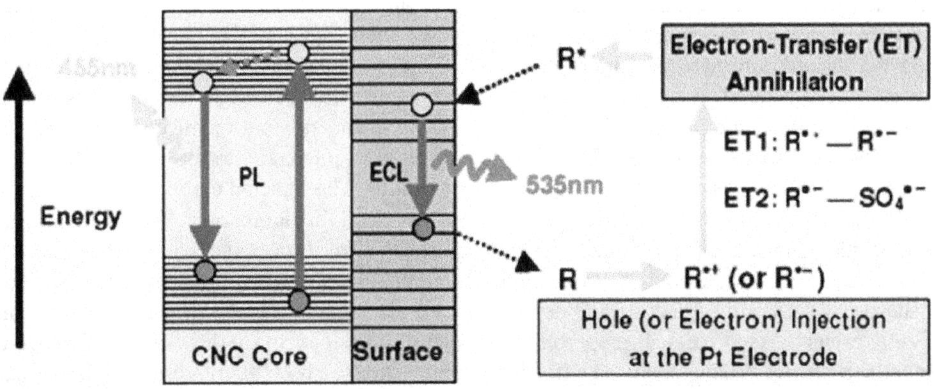

FIGURE 6.19 The ECL and PL mechanisms in CDs.

Source: **Figure reproduced from L. Zheng, Y. Chi, Y. Dong, J. Lin, and B. Wang, "Electrochemiluminescence of Water-Soluble Carbon Nanocrystals Released Electrochemically from Graphite,"** *J. Am. Chem. Soc.*, **2009, 131, 4564–4565, with permission from the American Chemical Society. Copyright 2009.**

and human colorectal adenocarcinoma HCT-15. Meanwhile, bioimaging, biocompatibility, and toxicity studies were performed using zebrafish embryo toxicity (ZET) tests. Further experiments demonstrated that fruit-based CDs from kiwi and avocado did not show sub-lethal signs of toxicity in a zebrafish model, demonstrating the low toxicity of this type of CD produced from natural sources.

On the other hand, many recent reviews have described several studies on the cytotoxic effect of CDs against different cell line models, including breast adenocarcinoma SKBR3, mouse embryonic fibroblast NIH-3T3, human renal epithelial cells 293T, normal breast epithelial cells MCF-10A, normal human liver cells HL-7702 (L-02), normal human skin fibroblasts NSFbs, human lung adenocarcinoma cells A549, human colorectal adenocarcinoma HCT-15, and others. To date, several of these cytotoxic studies have shown that CDs did not alter cell viability. Therefore, according to various researchers, the immense variety of synthesized CDs with different physicochemical properties is the next challenge in exploring the *in vitro* and *in vivo* toxicity of CDs. In fact, CD toxicity can be reduced by surface engineering techniques that use surface passivation molecules or biocompatible polymers at a minimum concentration. This approach could guarantee the combination of CDs with therapeutic agents, resulting in an excellent biological effect.

6.7.4.2 Bioimaging Detection

Real-time observation is one of the main topics of CD study, which allows the elucidation of the translocation of molecules, the interaction with targets, and the response to extracellular signals. Based on structural diversities, CDs have multiple advantages over semiconductor quantum dots (QDs), including comparable optical properties and photochemical stability. In addition, CDs are known for their tunable photoluminescence (PL) and multicolor PL properties. Indeed, these properties make CDs very desirable as alternatives to semiconductor QDs for application in bioimaging, both *in vitro* and *in vivo*.

It has already been reported that CDs mainly enter into the cells by endocytosis and are concentrated in the cytoplasm. In fact, there are few reports which show that CDs enter into the cell nucleus. Fluorescent CDs were used for cellular imaging for the first time by Cao et al. The authors used PPEI-EI passivated CDs for two-photon luminescence microscopy in human breast cancer MCF-7 cells. The cells incubated with CDs exhibited a bright luminescence in both the cell membrane and cytoplasm regions. The results indicate that the ability of the cells to take up CDs depends on the temperature.

Synthesis methods of CDs are an essential way to prepare multifunctional CDs with imaging ability. Bhunia et al. synthesized a series of fluorescent CDs from several carbohydrates, including sucrose, glucosamine, glucose, and dextrans of different molecular weights, ascorbic acid, and cellulose. The synthesized nanoparticles were then incubated with HeLa cells for 3–6 h. The CDs showed very low binding properties to the cells due to their low surface charge and small size. Moreover, the particles emitted different fluorescence spectra based on their size, suggesting that few CDs are capable of penetrating into the cell membrane and a few just help in staining the cells and cell nuclei. Thus, the surface functionalization and size of CDs play a major role for applications in bioimaging.

Several studies have indicated that surface modification of CDs is another crucial factor related to the multicolor PL properties of these nanoparticles. Bhunia et al. conducted an *in vitro* study synthesizing various CDs with different fluorescence. The target recognition was realized by surface modification of CDs with folic acid, which indicated that the fluorescence properties of these nanoparticles are stable to chemical modification. In another study by Tang et al., the authors modified CDs with doxorubicin and folic acid for specific cancer cell recognition, drug transport, and fluorescence imaging analysis.

On the other hand, some research groups discovered that CDs are able to exhibit multicolor emissions. The research group [202] synthesized fluorescent CDs that are biocompatible and suitable for bioimaging of exosomes. CD-loaded exosomes emitted blue, green, red, and violet fluorescence upon excitation at 350, 490, 550, and 630 nm, respectively. A clearly noticeable dotted appearance of CD-loaded exosomes can be observed, suggesting that these CDs can be utilized to probe exosomes for biological applications.

Other evidence indicates that changes in solvents and the adjustment of raw material proportions used in the preparation of CDs have allowed modifications in the emission wavelength of these nanoparticles. In fact, Xiong et al. acquired various colors (λ_{em} ranged from 443 to 745 nm) emitted by CDs, adjusting the type of solvent (ethanol, sulfuric acid, formamide, and N,N-dimethylformamide) and the proportions of raw materials (o-phenylenediamine and l-glutamic) used in the CD synthesis.

The fluorescence of CDs could be preserved for 60 h. Therefore, these nanoparticles could be suitable for long-term observation when performing *in vivo* bioimaging studies. Although the emission in the NIR region is relatively weak, CDs have great potential for *in vivo* fluorescence tracking studies because of the biological transparency window in the NIR region, which affords maximum penetration *in vivo*. Indeed, developing CDs with effective emissions in the visible and NIR regions has been described.

Yang et al. were the first to explore the utility of CDs as contrast agents in live mice. They obtained CDs and ZnS-doped CDs from chemical processing of raw nanomaterials by laser ablation. After PEG_{1500N} modifications, they were used for *in vivo* optical imaging of mice. CDs or ZnS-doped CDs solutions were injected into the mice body with various injection methods. The injected carbon dots in mice diffused relatively slowly, and the fluorescence faded at 24 h post-injection.

CDs were intravenously injected into mice for whole-body circulation. The abdomen was shaved for fluorescence detection of the dots trapped in organs during the circulation, but only emissions from the bladder area were observed. The images also show fluorescence of the dissected kidneys and liver. It was also observed that the injected CDs were removed from the body via the urine excretion pathway.

Furthermore, it has been noticed that blue- and green-emitting CDs are not suitable for *in vivo* imaging because the short-light excitation wavelength could harm living cells and biological systems. Hence, one of the great challenges of *in vivo* bioimaging studies is to achieve efficient and safe red-light-emitting CDs. In studies by Liu et al., the authors obtained efficient red emissive nitrogen CDs with a good excitation-independent emission, high quantum yield (QY) (10.83% in water and 31.54% in ethanol), good biocompatibility, and water dispersibility. Nitrogen-doped conjugated CDs were injected into nude mice and the fluorescence images were observed after 0.5, 1.0, 1.5, 3.0, and 20 h. As seen in Figure 6.20, the images indicate that red-emitting CDs exhibit strong penetrability and rapid excretion from the body of mice.

More recently, other studies by Li et al. reported the development of new CD-based materials with a second near-infrared emission (NIR-II). The designed watermelon-derived CDs exhibited high QY, great photothermal efficiency, and biocompatibility. The CDs were administrated by hypodermic injection in BALB/c mice, and the *in vivo* bioimaging was conducted using a NIR-II imaging apparatus (Figure 6.21). Interestingly, fluorescence signals indicated the rapid renal excretion of CDs, which was associated with the particle size.

In another *in vivo* bioimaging study, Kang et al. validated the use of zebrafish embryos as a model for bioimaging studies. The distribution of designed CDs from glucose was successfully observed in zebrafish embryos, indicating the selective accumulation of these nanoparticles in the eye and yolk sac. Furthermore, these CDs showed low toxicity and high biocompatibility in the zebrafish model.

Tathagata et al. obtained similar results evaluating the biolabeling potential of surface-passivated CDs from curcumin in zebrafish embryos. This biological model showed fluorescence in green, blue, and red, indicating the uptake of CDs through the chorionic membrane.

6.7.4.3 Biosensing

In addition to their superior biocompatibility, CDs possess the ability to serve as either excellent electron donors or electron acceptors. By monitoring the changes in their fluorescence intensity under external physical or chemical stimuli, CDs were used to detect substances such as DNA, PO_4^{3-}, thrombin, nitrite, glucose, biothiol, Cr^{3+}, Fe^{3+}, Ag^+, Hg^{2+}, Cu^{2+}, Cd^{2+}, and pH. The surface functional groups on CDs indicate distinctive affinities to different target ions, which results in the quenching of PL intensity through an electron or energy transfer process and high selectivity to other ions.

The detection of heavy metals is of importance because of their hazardous effect on the environment and human health. One of the first attempts of utilizing CDs in sensing is the selective detection of Hg^{2+} in aqueous solutions and live cells.

Based on the quenching effect of Hg^{2+} on the fluorescence of CDs, Yan et al. adopted the Hg^{2+}-CDs system for selective detection of Hg^{2+} in aqueous solution as well as in live cells. The authors reported the synthesis of two types of CDs using citric acid with N-(b-aminoethyl)-g-aminopropyl (CDs-1) and 1,2-ethyldiamine (CDs-2) that possess a high QY of 55.4 and 65.5%, respectively. The study of the effective and selective quenching of fluorescence emissions of CDs-1 and CDs-2 by Hg^{2+} demonstrated that both CDs acted as selective and sensitive fluorescent probes for the detection of traces of Hg^{2+} in both aqueous solutions and live cells. Upon the addition of 20 mM of Hg^{2+}, the fluorescence intensity of CDs-1 was rapidly quenched by 55%, while that of CDs-2 was quenched by 80%, and both remained stable after 1 h of observation. This confirms the feasibility of using CDs-1 and CDs-2 as chemical-sensing probes for Hg^{2+}. The selectivity of CDs-1 and CDs-2 toward Hg^{2+} was then assessed by comparing the

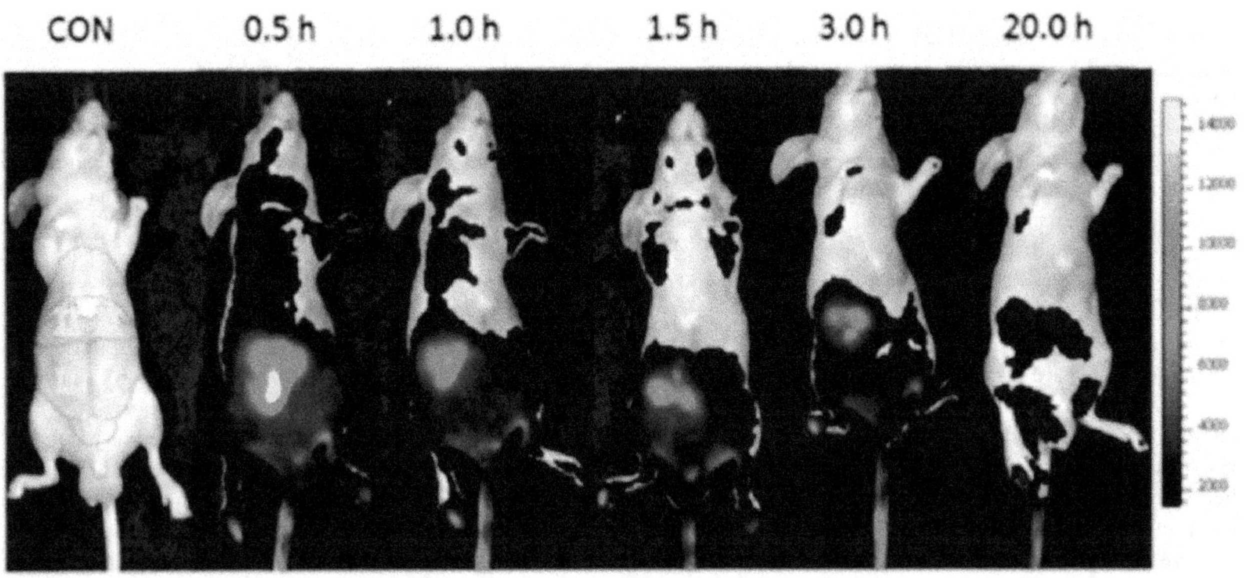

FIGURE 6.20 Real-time *in vivo* imaging of nude mice with intravenous injection of 100 μL of PBS solution of CDs-50 at different time points. (I, thoracic region; II, area of liver; III, area of small intestine; IV, area of large intestine; V, bladder region).

Source: **Figure reproduced from J. J. Liu, D. Li, K. Zhang, M. Yang, H. Sun, and B. Yang, "One-Step Hydrothermal Synthesis of Nitrogen-Doped Conjugated Carbonized Polymer Dots with 31% Efficient Red Emission for *In Vivo* Imaging," *Small*, 2018, 12, 1703919. With permission from Wiley. Copyright 2018.**

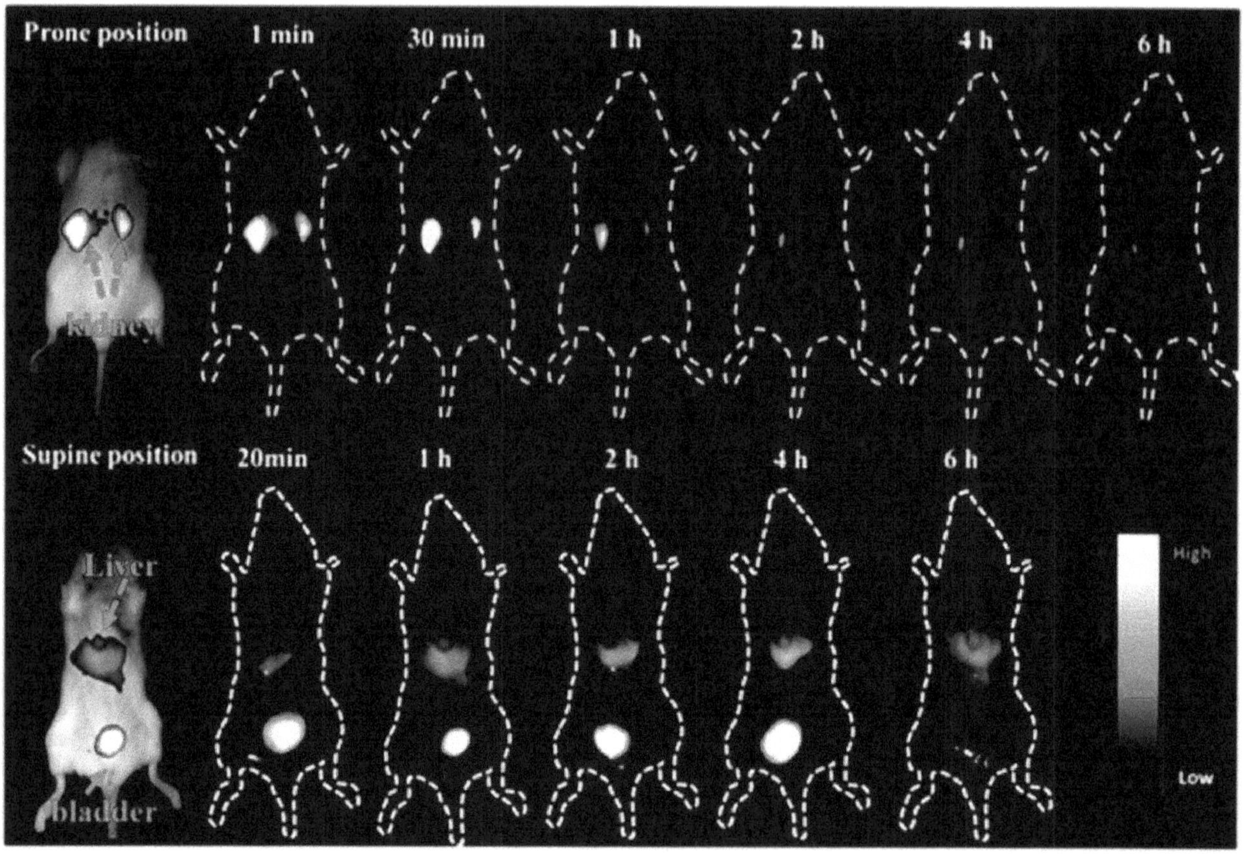

FIGURE 6.21 Time-dependent bioimaging of mouse treated with CDs (20 μg g^{-1}) through the tail vein.

Source: **Figure reproduced from Y. Li, G. Bai, S. Zeng, and J. Hao, "Theranostic Carbon Dots with Innovative NIR-II Emission for** *in Vivo* **Renal-Excreted Optical Imaging and Photothermal Therapy,"** *ACS Appl. Mater. Interfaces*, **2019, 11, 4737–4744. With permission from American Chemical Society. Copyright 2019.**

extent of fluorescence quenching of CDs-1 and CDs-2 through the addition of 20 mM of different metal ions. Among all metal ions tested, Hg^{2+} quenched the fluorescence of both CDs-1 and CDs-2 to the largest extent. However, the fluorescence was reversible and recovered by adding ethylenediamine tetraacetic acid (EDTA). Furthermore, successful attempts were made in detecting Hg^{2+} in cultured cells.

Qu et al. reported a preparative route toward distinctive fluorescent CDs from dopamine (DA). The CDs exhibited excellent PL properties, and they were used for multicolor bioimaging and as a new kind of sensor for label-free detection of dopamine (DA) and Fe^{3+} with high sensitivity and selectivity. The method depends on Fe^{3+}-induced oxidation of the hydroquinone groups on the surfaces of CDs to the quinone species, which can quench the fluorescence of the CDs and DA due to their competition with CDs to react with Fe^{3+}. It offers a favorable protocol for rapid detection of Fe^{3+} and DA. Moreover, this sensing platform exhibits high sensitivity and selectivity toward Fe^{3+} and DA versus other metal ions and the other DA analogues and offers the advantages of cost-efficiency, simplicity, and environmental friendliness.

Dong et al. designed branched poly(ethylenimine)-functionalized CDs (BPEI-CDs) as a fluorescence sensor for copper ion (Cu^{2+}) detection. On account of the inner filter effect, in that the excitation and emission wavelengths of the CDs were absorbed by the cupric amine complex formed on the surface, a quenching phenomenon would happen. Under the optimum experimental conditions, the CDs show good sensitivity and selectivity toward Cu^{2+}, and the limit of detection and the linear response range were determined to be 6 nM and 10–1100 nM, respectively.

More interestingly, a tunable ratiometric pH sensor was developed for the quantitative measurements of the intracellular pH of cells based on CDs. The amino-coated CDs were functionalized with pH-sensitive fluorescein isothiocyanate (FITC) and pH-insensitive Rhodamine B isothiocyanate (RBITC), resulting in the dual-emission probe upon single excitation. The pH sensor exhibited low cytotoxicity, good cell permeability, and excellent reversibility between pH 5 and 9. Thus, real-time quantitative determination of intracellular pH of intact HeLa cells and the pH fluctuations associated with oxidative stress was successfully performed.

On the other hand, the π–π stacking interactions between CDs and DNA can also be used as a binding strategy for the detection of DNA [269]. The fluorescence from the dye-labeled single-stranded DNA probe is quenched after adsorption onto the CD surface via π–π interactions. When the target DNA matches the dye-labeled DNA to form double-stranded DNA, the fluorescence is recovered. This strategy is also employed for the determination of metal ions such as Hg^{2+} and Ag^{+} through T–Hg^{2+}–T and C–Ag^{+}–C base pairs, respectively.

Apart from utilizing the fluorescence of CDs as an analytical signal, recent studies have revealed that CDs exhibit good chemiluminescence (CL) and electrochemiluminescence (ECL). For example, Wang et al. developed a paper-based DNA biosensor by using CDs as CL signals and nanoporous gold (NPG) as a signal amplification agent. First, they constructed microfluidic paper-based analytical devices (μPADs). Then, the captured DNA (S1) with thiol groups was immobilized onto the μPADs. Besides, in the presence of target DNA (S2), the signal DNA (S3) could fix on the surface of μPADs by hybridization with S2. Finally, by injecting with $KMnO_4$, CL reaction was triggered, and the concentration of target DNA S2 could be easily measured in the luminescence analyzer (Figure 6.22).

Wu et al. constructed an assay for cancer cell detection by using modified CDs as ECL sensors and graphene as a signal amplification agent (Figure 6.23). The sensors were developed as follows: first, the electrode was modified with amino-functionalized graphene that was covalently grafting poly(allyl amine hydrochloride) (PAH) onto graphene. Then, the CDs@Ag composite was introduced onto the surface of the electrode. After the thiol-containing amino acid cysteine was linked to the C-dot@Ag surface, folic acid was further conjugated with cysteine via a carbodiimide-mediated wet-chemistry approach between the carboxylic acid end groups on folic acid and the amine groups on cysteine. Each modifying process played a unique and important role in the sensitivity/selectivity of the sensor: (1) The metal shell on CDs accelerated the electron transfer between CDs@Ag and graphene. (2) Folic acid could specifically target folate receptors with high affinity, which enabled them to act as a bridge between the electrode and the

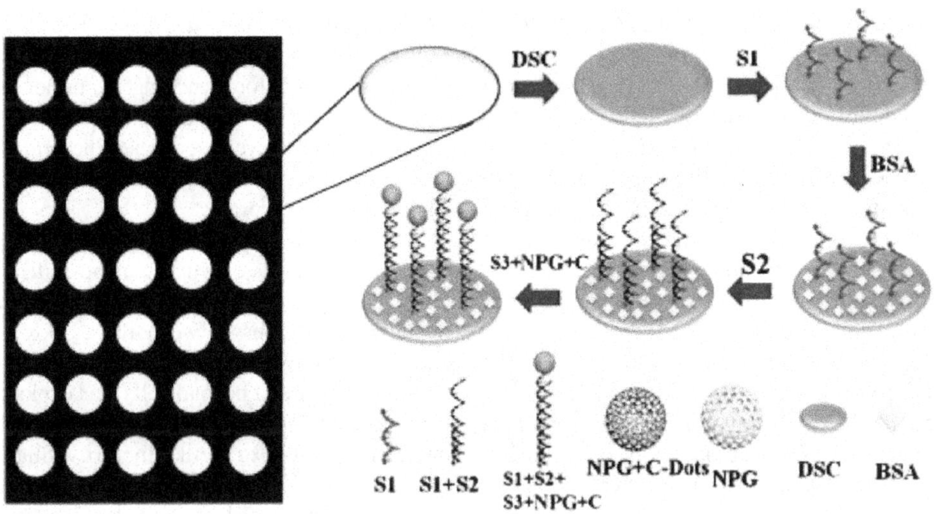

FIGURE 6.22 The CD-based CL sensor for the detection of DNA.

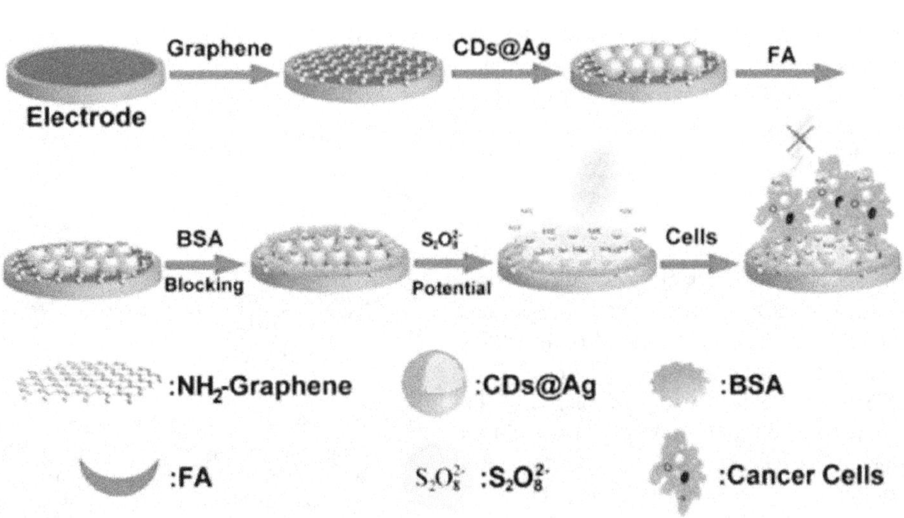

FIGURE 6.23 The CD-based ECL platform for the detection of cancer cells.

cancer cells. (3) The graphene conjugation could facilitate electron transfer due to its good conductivity and large surface area. Due to the specificity and affinity of folic acid, the fabricated electrode could selectively recognize the surface of human cervical cancer cells (HeLa) and human breast cancer cells (MCF-7) by targeting the folate receptor (FR). The presence of cancer cells caused a remarkable decrease in the ECL signal, which originated from the blocking of the CDs@Ag nanocomposite surface and preventing them from coming into contact with the ECL coreactant $N_2S_2O_8$. The detection limit was calculated to be 10 cells per mL at 3σ.

On the other hand, it is known that plant part–derived CDs can be used as biosensors to detect various bioactive molecules, including proteins, nucleic acids, enzymes, amino acids, vitamins, bacteria, thiols group, drugs, metal ions, and biological samples [206]. Based on chromium (Cr) toxicity, Roshni et al. used CDs from ground nuts (N-CDs) to detect Cr^{6+}. N-CDs showed a selective activity toward Cr^{6+} with a detection limit (LOD) of 0.1 mg L^{-1}. The methodology was carried out in the presence of Cr^{3+} and glutathione as a reducing medium for the conversion of Cr^{4+} to Cr^{3+}, which is considered one of the least-toxic micronutrients for humans.

In another study, Monte-Filho et al. used CDs derived from onion juice and lemon for the detection of riboflavin (vitamin B2). The selectivity of the CDs for the detection of riboflavin was tested with diverse substances, indicating that CDs were selective for riboflavin. Moreover, the CDs exhibited a good linear relationship between the fluorescence resonance energy transfer and the riboflavin concentration, suggesting the development of an analytical method for the determination of riboflavin in multivitamin and mineral supplements.

Ahmadian-Fard-Fini et al. were able to detect *E. coli* by using a fluorescence sensor of CDs derived from grapefruit extracts and lemon. Fluorescence signals from various concentrations of *E. coli*–labeled CDs were observed. Furthermore, the authors were able to measure unknown concentrations of *E. coli*.

6.7.4.4 Drug Carrier Development

CDs are excellent drug delivery systems (DDSs) due to their simple fabrication techniques, particle size, biocompatibility, lower cytotoxicity, and sustained drug release. CDs overcome the problems of conventional drug carriers; in fact, multicolor fluorescence CDs are considered excellent drug carriers because of their modified functional groups, maximum drug-loading capacity, and low cytotoxicity.

The most widely investigated DDSs are based on AuNPs, but their toxicity limits their applications in clinical therapy. Therefore, CDs serve as good alternatives to AuNPs since different functionalizations could result in many possibilities for conjugation with drug molecules in combination with targeting agents, expanding the drug choices for delivery. Tang et al. reported a Förster resonance energy transfer (FRET)–based CD drug delivery system that could perform real-time monitoring of drug release (Figure 6.24). The authors used the fluorescent drug molecule doxorubicin (DOX). The DOX adsorbed onto the surface of CDs via π–π stacking. Then FRET occurred between the CDs and DOX, which resulted in a decrease of the FL of CDs and an increase of the FL of DOX. With the release of DOX from the surface of CDs, FRET between CDs and DOX was weakened while the FL of CDs increased, which could be used to monitor the release of DOX.

The obtained system showed excellent targeted delivery and drug release efficiency toward cancer cells in acidic pH environments. At pH 7.4, the fluorescence barely increases over the course of 72 h, exhibiting a very low value of total release (<10% fluorescence intensity of the original CDs-FA-DOX conjugates); this indicates a negligible DOX release under the neutral conditions. A substantial increase of the drug release rate is observed for acidic solutions, in which the release rate in pH 5.0 solution is higher than that in pH 6.0 solution. In addition, compared with those of free DOX molecules, which complete release within ≈10 h, the release accumulation profiles for both pH 5.0 and 6.0 solutions show sustained release over a long period (>72 h). The percentages of accumulated release in the pH 5.0 solutions are 55%, 72%, and 78% after 24, 48, and 72 h, respectively.

This enhanced drug release rate at low pHs is particularly advantageous for cancer treatment. The slow DOX release in neutral environments can minimize the extracellular loss of drug molecules before reaching the tumor targets, as well as potential damage to normal cells. However, most of the DOX can persistently be released when the drug delivery capsules are internalized by tumor cells at low pHs (4.5–6.0), leading to enhanced cancer therapy.

More recently, the author's group developed CDs with a carboxyl-rich surface which can be utilized as a trackable drug delivery. The CDs are conjugated with doxo, via electrostatic interactions between the carboxyl groups of CDs and the amine group of doxo molecules. The pH difference between cancer and normal cells was exploited as the triggering mechanism for doxo release. The CDs maintained a stable interaction with doxo at alkaline pH with a slow-release profile, compared to a fast-release profile when the medium was acidified to levels of the extracellular space of the tumor and

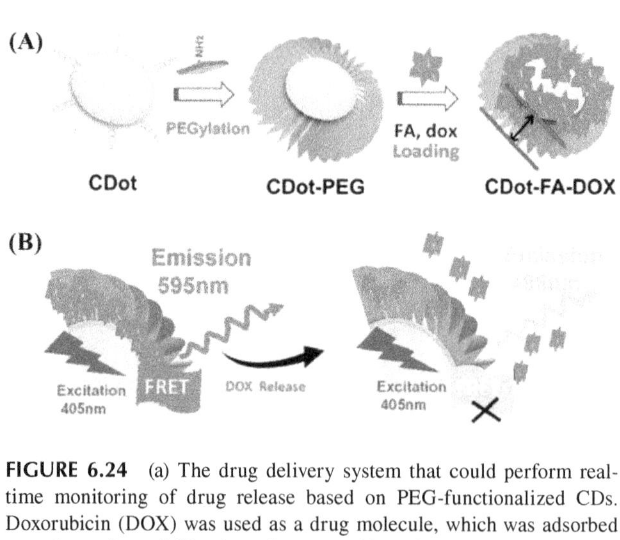

FIGURE 6.24 (a) The drug delivery system that could perform real-time monitoring of drug release based on PEG-functionalized CDs. Doxorubicin (DOX) was used as a drug molecule, which was adsorbed onto the surface of CDs through π–π stacking. (b) Proposed mechanism of real-time monitoring of DOX release based on the FRET process between DOX and CDs.

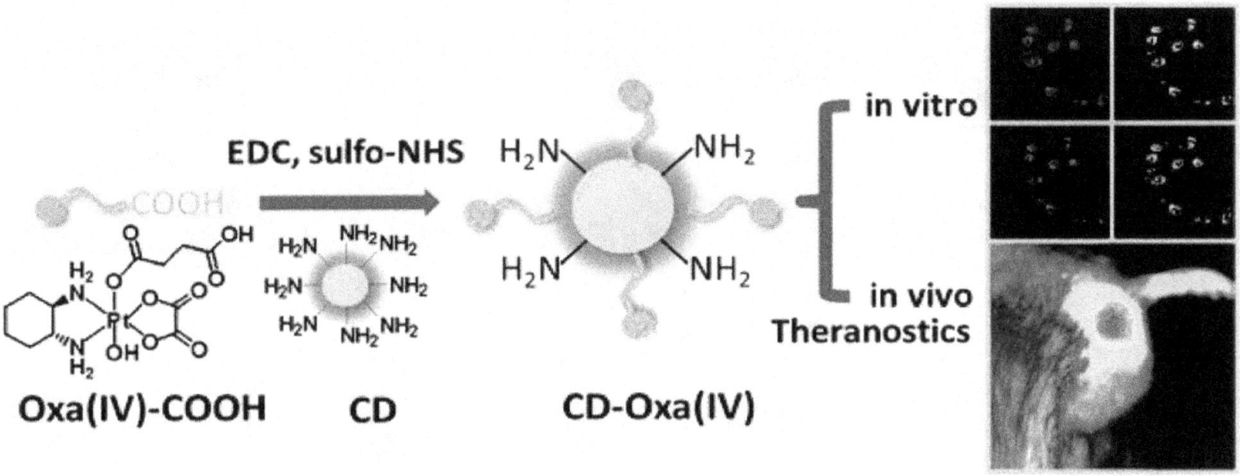

FIGURE 6.25 Synthetic scheme for CDs-oxa (CD-oxa) and its applications in bioimaging and theranostics.

in subcellular compartments. Subsequently, the cell viability of breast (MDA-MB-231) and colon (LoVo and DLD-1) cancer cell lines treated with CD-loaded doxo (Cdoxo) exhibited better cytotoxicity than free doxo in MDA-MB-231 and DLD-1 cells. An *in vivo* study followed over a period of approximately two months did not show any symptoms of stress or clinical illness. The body weight of the mice increased during the observational period. Cdoxo-treated mice demonstrate that the tumor volume was reduced compared to the tumors of mice treated with free doxo.

In view of the future use of a fully biocompatible drug delivery nanosystem, we further optimize the hydrothermal synthesis of CDs to avoid the formation of harmful chemical compounds, starting from fructose (F-CDs), glucose (G-CDs), and ascorbic acid (A-CDs), without any passivating or doping additives. Interestingly, the cytotoxicity of the CDs was affected by the choice of the starting materials: CDs synthesized from fructose were found to be toxic (due to the presence of toxic furanic compounds/frameworks formed during the hydrothermal degradation of the fructose precursor), while high biocompatibility was observed starting from glucose or ascorbic acid. Finally, the CD drug loading capabilities were evaluated by studying their interactions with DOX as a model. The study revealed the importance of the graphitic core domains, rather than the surface functional groups, in achieving high CDs–DOX affinities F-CDs > G-CDs ≫ A-CDs. With the more suitable glucose-derived CDs, up to 28% w/w of DOX loading.

Similarly, a theragnostic nanomedicine (CDs-oxa) was synthesized by a condensation reaction between the amino groups on the surface of fluorescent CDs and the carboxyl group of the oxaliplatin derivative oxa (iv)–COOH. The CDs-oxa was taken up by cancer cells through endocytosis, and the drug was released upon the reduction of oxa (iv)–COOH to oxaliplatin(ii) because of the highly reducing environment in cancer cells. It was also demonstrated that the distribution of the CDs-oxa can be closely tracked by monitoring the fluorescence signal of the CDs, thereby offering great help in the customization of the injection time and dosage of the medicine (Figure 6.25).

In an attempt to enhance the loading capacity of CDs, Mewada et al. tested the drug-carrying and folic acid–mediated delivering capacities of highly fluorescent swarming CDs. Folic acid on the CD surface was used as a navigational molecule due to its association with different types of cancer cells. The drug loading capacity for DOX was estimated to be 86%, and the release of DOX from the DOX-loaded CDs followed first-order release kinetics. Furthermore, due to the targeting ability of the folic acid molecule, CDs loaded with DOX showed greater cytotoxicity to cancer cells than free DOX.

Similarly, other researchers have also used CDs loaded with DOX. Wang et al. reported that DOX-conjugated beer CDs (DOX-BCDs) exerted a prolonged drug release profile toward MCF-7 cells. The analysis of the results confirmed the internalization of DOX-BCDs by cells and showed that DOX-BCD induced a greater cytotoxic effect than single DOX treatment. On the other hand, Zeng et al. developed green-emitting CDs by conjugating the amine moiety of DOX and native carboxyl groups present on the surface of CDs via non-covalent bonding. *In vitro* and *in vivo* studies indicated that these CDs are stable cancer drug delivery systems. Furthermore, DOX–CD conjugates showed low toxicity and selectivity toward cancer cells.

According to the different studies reported, functional groups on the surface of the CDs render them potential nontoxic candidates in targeted drug delivery. Furthermore, their fluorescence properties allow a simultaneous analysis of drug distribution and their therapeutic functions.

6.7.4.5 Gene Transfer

Gene therapy is a promising alternative for the treatment of many pathological disorders. This experimental technique requires an efficient and safe carrier for the delivery of biocompatible therapeutic loads with fluorescence properties. In this context, the properties of CDs make them efficient

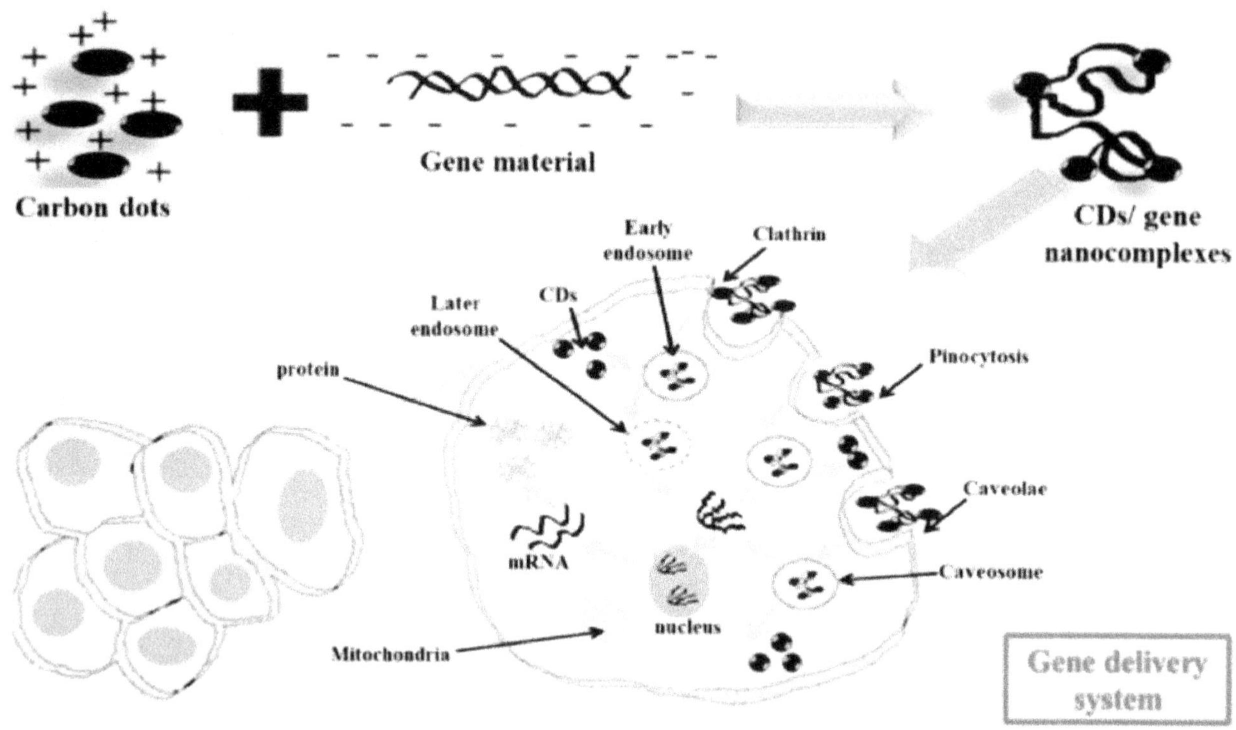

FIGURE 6.26 General mechanisms of gene delivery *via* CDs: here, CDs bind gene materials *via* electrostatic interactions, enter the cells *via* endocytosis, and release the payloads into the nucleus.

Source: **Figure reproduced from ref. [208] with permission from BMC. Copyright 2019.**

emerging carriers for cellular uptake monitoring and gene delivery. Gene therapy includes the use of pDNA, mRNA, and noncoding RNAs, which can be internalized by endocytosis [207] (Figure 6.26) [208].

In a study by Liu et al., the authors utilized polyethylenimine (PEI)–passivated CDs as transfection agents. The fluorescence properties of CDs allowed the observation of the plasmid DNA distribution during transfection, providing detailed information on the physiological function of plasmid DNA. Kim et al. also performed a DNA transfection and monitored the trafficking of cellular plasmids. The authors compared the gene delivery ability of plasmid DNA (pDNA), PEI-functionalized CDs (PEI-CDs), and PEI-functionalized gold colloids (PEI-AU). Quantitative analysis of the cellular uptake and dissociation of pDNA from the nanoassembly indicated that the fluorescence intensity of PEI-CD remained stronger compared to that of PEI-AU at the onset of cellular uptake. However, the authors reported that both the carrier systems could provide a highly intriguing method to monitor the dissociation of polyplex inside of the cytoplasm.

Recently, Zhang et al. developed hyaluronic acid (HA)/PEI–functionalized CDs (HP-CDs) for gene therapy in cancer cells. The HP-CDs showed an excellent gene condensation capacity, low toxicity, and biocompatibility. The HP-CDs were internalized into cancer cells via HA receptor–mediated endocytosis, indicating high transfection efficiency.

Additionally, Chen et al. studied the impact of gene therapy on mesenchymal stem cells (EMSCs) using different CDs derived from porphyra polysaccharide. The CDs were loaded with a combination of transcription factors Ascl1 and Brn2 (CDs-pDNA NPs). The results revealed an efficient neuronal differentiation of the EMSCs with CDs-pDNA NPs compared with the retinoic acid–containing induction medium. Another study by Ghafary et al. synthesized a nanocarrier using CDs conjugated with a chimeric peptide MPG-2H1 and DNA loading (CDs-MPG-2H1) to obtain two different color emissions (red and green). The nanocomplexes increased the gene internalization in the cells, showing that this carrier has a high potential for increasing nuclear internalization.

It is known that siRNA delivery is one of the best strategies for treating incurable diseases due to its efficiency of intracellular delivery. In this context, Dong et al. studied poly(l-lactide)-polyethylene glycol (PLA)-CDs and PEG-CDs as nanocomplexes for simultaneous gene delivery and intracellular miRNA bioimaging. The results showed that CDs conjugated with PLA or PEG provide a nanocomposite with low cytotoxicity and stable photoluminescence. Furthermore, using the HeLa cell line as a model, the authors reported that carriers exhibited an effective miRNA delivery. Moreover, Wu et al. investigated the effect of folate-conjugated reducible PEI-passivated CD for lung cancer treatment. The nanocomplexes were loaded with two types of siRNA (EGFR and cyclin B1). The results indicated that the carriers were accumulated into cancer cells and induced the silencing of the targeted gene.

6.7.4.6 Diagnosis and Clinical Prognosis

Imaging analysis has an important role in diagnosis and prognosis of certain pathologies. In this sense, the use of fluorescent nanoparticles as imaging probes is one of the best strategies. Notably, studies on the favorable properties of CDs have shown widespread research interest owing to their practical application in the fields of cell imaging and drug delivery.

Based on the ability of CDs to absorb NIR light, Wu et al. first conducted photoacoustic (PA) imaging of sentinel lymph nodes (SLN) *in vivo* by using CDs passivated by macromolecules. Observable signal enhancement of the SLN was exceptionally rapid within 2 min after injection of the agent. This nanoprobe exhibited strong optical absorption in the NIR region, a small size, and rapid lymphatic transport, offering valuable potential for faster resection of SLN, and may lower complications caused by using dyes or low-resolution imaging techniques.

The CDs can be used for photodynamic therapy (PDT). PDT is an approved therapeutic treatment for certain types of cancers. In the presence of oxygen and light, photosensitizers (PSs) can transfer the absorbed photon energy to surrounding oxygen molecules to form reactive oxygen species (ROS), such as singlet oxygen ($^1O_2$) and free radicals, resulting in cell death and tissue destruction. Huang et al. designed a PS-conjugated C-dot system featuring FRET for both enhanced fluorescence imaging and PDT therapy. Chlorin e6 (Ce6) was selected as the PS, which emitted bright-red fluorescence at 668 nm upon excitation at 430 nm due to the efficient FRET process with carbon dots. The feasibility of the system for fluorescence imaging–guided PDT was investigated in nude mice. After intravenous injection, the fluorescence from Ce6 became visible in tumor sites at 2–4 h post-injection and reached a plateau at 4–8 h post-injection, and thus the suitable time point to implement PDT was selected at 8 h (Figure 6.27).

In addition to phototherapy, CDs can be used for radiotherapy. Kleinauskas et al. developed PEG-CDs coated with a silver shell (C–Ag–PEG CDs) which could be used as radiosensitizers in DU145 cells. When irradiated with low-energy X-rays, electrons were ejected from the C–Ag–PEG CDs, which in turn generates free radicals and damages the cancer cells surrounding the CDs, reducing the damage of normal cells and increasing therapeutic selectivity.

Diagnosis of infectious diseases caused by microorganisms such as viruses, fungi, parasites, or bacteria is another area of CD applications due to their photodynamic effects that induce antimicrobial photodynamic inactivation (PDI). The mechanism of action of PDI treatment is based on nonspecific oxidative damage to the cell membrane and biomolecules (nucleic acids, proteins, and lipids), decreasing resistance by target microorganisms. ROS formation in PDI treatment is through excitation of photosensitizers with an appropriate wavelength. In this context, CDs are considered excellent photosensitizers for PDI treatment by photoinduced production of ROS, which depends on the functional groups on the surface, the optical properties, and the photoexcited state of CDs [209].

Several studies have demonstrated that EDA-CDs under visible/natural light could effectively inhibit *E. coli* cells. The antibacterial activity of these CDs was attributed to the photodynamic effects of these nanoparticles. Likewise, Li et al. reported that synthesized CDs by an electrochemical method with vitamin C show a broad-spectrum antibacterial activity against *Bacillus* sp, *E. coli*, ampicillin-resistant *E. coli*, *S. aureus*, and *B. subtilis*. Furthermore, the authors observed that these CDs also showed an antifungal effect against *R. solani* and *P. grisea*. In another reported study, Priyadarshini et al. demonstrated the antifungal potential of CDs and their derived conjugates against *C. albicans*.

Although few studies have reported the use of CDs in antiviral treatment, Huang et al. found that CDs synthesized from benzoxazine (BZM-CDs) inhibited the infection of Japanese encephalitis, Zika, and dengue viruses. The results indicated that BZM-CDs could directly bind to the surface of the virion and inhibit cell–virus interaction. Łoczechin et al. also found an antiviral effect of seven different CDs to human coronavirus HCoV-229E infection. The mechanism of action of these CDs revealed the inhibition of HCoV-229E by interactions of the functional groups of the CDs with HCoV-229E receptors. In general, these results could help replace the use of conventional antivirals with less-inhibitory activity.

According to previously published reports, CDs could be a useful tool for the treatment and diagnosis of diseases.

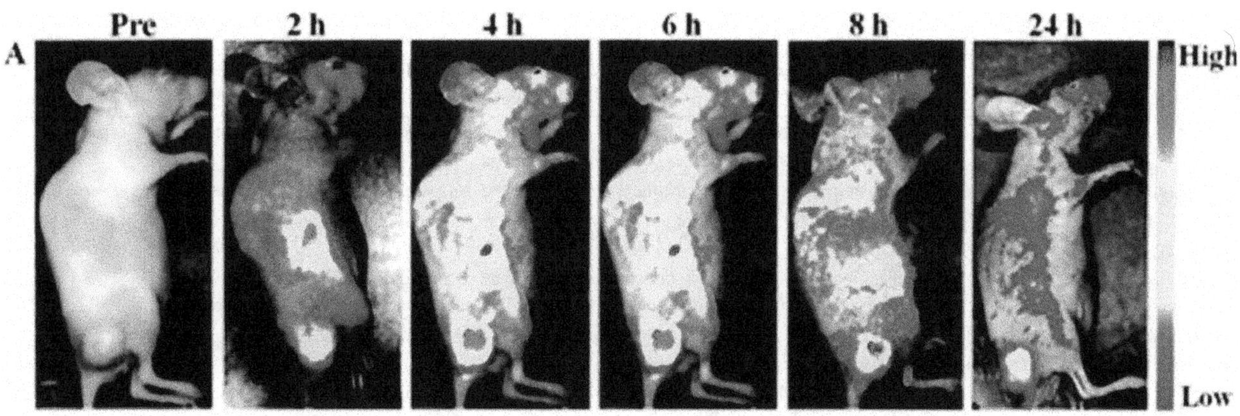

FIGURE 6.27 Real-time *in vivo* NIR fluorescence images after intravenous injection of CDs-Ce6 in nude mice at different time points.

6.7.5 Theranostic Approach in Cancer Treatment

In cancer treatment, chemotherapy, radiation, and surgery have certain limitations, because one treatment pathway cannot address all types of cancer. Tumor theranostics focuses on developing new structures that are biocompatible and biodegradable and able to perform efficient target therapy. Currently, several types of theranostic nanoparticles have been developed for treating cancer; however, not all are efficient and safe. In this respect, carbon dots are considered potential candidates for developing tumor theranostic due to the physicochemical and optical properties described earlier. Indeed, compared with other existing theranostic agents, such as metal–organic framework (MOF)–based nanomedicine, lipidosomes, and polyester micelles, CDs possess a series of advantages that include low cytotoxicity, biocompatibility, and stable photoluminescence. Consequently, CDs have been recognized as effective tumor theranostic agents for *in vivo* imaging and tumor therapy (Table 6.3) [210].

6.7.5.1 Photodynamic Therapy (PDT) and Photothermal Therapy (PTT)

The study and development of CDs for PDT and PTT have increased in recent years. As previously described, through PDT, CDs can destroy cancer cells by reactive oxygen species, which were produced from surrounding oxygen under the excitation of light with the corresponding wavelength [218]. In addition, PDT offers low toxicity and minimal invasiveness. Therefore, this therapy has gained a lot of significance because it acts on multidrug-resistant cancers and could replace conventional chemotherapy. In a study by Xie et al., the authors synthetized porphyrin-containing carbon dots, which showed intrinsic photodynamic capacity upon photoirradiation. Furthermore, the porphyrin-CDs exhibited high cellular uptake, potent cytotoxicity, good photostability, and biocompatibility. On the other hand, Zhou et al. prepared CDs from fresh tender ginger juice with good biocompatibility. The CDs showed selective cytotoxic activity toward HepG2 cells through high ROS production. However, these CDs were also cytotoxic to the normal liver cell (FL83B) and normal mammary epithelial cell (MCF-10A) lines. Another study by He et al. indicated that using a one-pot hydrothermal method to synthesize diketopyrrolopyrrole (DPP)–based fluorescent CDs with DPP and chitosan as precursors, the DPP-CDs could not only generate singlet oxygen ($^1O_2$) but also had excellent hydrophilic properties and biocompatibility. Moreover, the DPP-CDs inhibited tumor growth *in vitro* and *in vivo* with laser irradiation (540 nm).

From a theranostic point of view, photothermal therapy (PTT) is also known as hyperthermia or thermal ablation therapy. PTT, which is used as a diagnostic and treatment strategy, uses electromagnetic radiation in the infrared (IR) region to convert the absorbed energy into heat and provides high-specificity analysis and minimal invasiveness. Carbon dots are considered attractive as photothermal agents because they contain many π electrons and behave similarly to the free electrons of metallic nanomaterials. In a study by Zheng et al., the researchers synthesized multifunctional theranostic CDs (named CyCD) via a solvothermal process. CDs exhibited an excellent PTT efficiency, and the *in vitro* studies revealed that the viabilities of CT26 and HepG2 cell lines were decreased in the presence of CyCDs. Another study by Nurunnabi et al. indicated that carboxylated photoluminescent graphene nanodots (cGDs) activated by NIR laser irradiation form electron clouds to produce heat (>50°C) and decrease cell viability by ~70% of MDA-MB 231 cancer cells by thermal ablation. Bao X. et al. showed that after an *in vivo* injection of CDs, PTT significantly inhibited the growth of tumor and prolonged the life of mice. On the other side, some *in vitro* studies have demonstrated that chemotherapy combined with PTT is better at killing cancer cells than monotherapy.

Although there are some advantages of PDT and PTT in cancer treatment, there are still some difficulties in their practical application. For instance, the hypoxic environment in tumors limits the therapeutic efficacy of PDT, and the use of PTT damages the normal tissue around the tumor [210,219]. Therefore, many major challenges must be overcome.

6.7.5.2 Receptor-Mediated Therapy

Tumor-targeted CDs can specifically bind to receptors overexpressed on the cancer cell membrane [210]. Indeed, the

TABLE 6.3
Some Theragnostic Agents Based on CDs*a*

Complexes–CDs	Biological Activity	Ref.
CDs from HA	Preservation of the HA functionality, which has high specific affinity for CD44 receptors overexpressed on the surfaces of many cancer cells.	[211]
FA/DOX-CDs	The system facilitates the real-time monitoring of the drug release based on the fluorescence signal.	[211]
CDs-DOX loaded into PEG chitosan nanogels	High therapeutic efficacy through the synergistic effect of combined chemophotothermal treatments.	[212]
CDs-$MnFe_2O_4$/DOX-4 carboxyl phenylboronic acid	Acts as a cancer cell–specific targeting ligand. Effective fluorescent markers in an in vivo experiment. Moreover, it also showed the controlled release of DOX at low pH values.	[213]
CDs-DOX/biodegradable charged polyester vectors (BCPVs)/siRNA	The heat generated enhanced the anticancer activity of the nanocomplexes, which triggered the release of DOX from complexes.	[214]
CDs-PEGFA/ZnPc or R780 iodide or Ce6	The targeting of ZnPc/CDs-PEGFA was evaluated by monitoring the blue and red fluorescence of CDs. The PDT on the HeLa cells was also demonstrated	[215–217]

Note: *HA*, hyaluronic acid; *FA*, folic acid; *ZnPc*, zinc phthalocyanine.

receptor-mediated therapy of CDs is important for drug delivery [210]. Jianping Li et al. showed that hyaluronic acid (HA)–modified carbon dots (HA-CDs) obtained by hydrothermal treatment with branch-poly(ethylene mine) and citric acid specifically bind to CD44, which is overexpressed in several cancer cells. Furthermore, in this study, the antitumor effect of HA-CDs was observed in diverse tumor models, which gives it a good application prospect for targeted cancer therapy [211].

Although several studies are focusing on receptor-based tumor therapy, accumulating evidence suggests that this strategy has several important limitations because some receptors are present in both cancer cells and normal cells. In addition, different types of cancer cells may not be targeted using the same ligand [210,220].

6.8 Bright Future in the Fabrication of Portable Kits in Analytical Systems

Due to simple operation and high diversity of electroanalytical sensors, these types of sensors are expected to be the future generation of analytical systems. Therefore, many scientists and researchers have focused on designing and fabricating electroanalytical sensors with good selectivity and high sensitivity for different types of compounds, such as drugs, food, and environmental pollutants.

The coupling of mediators with highly inclined species to a particular species with conductive nanomaterials can create a highly sensitive and good selective electrochemical tool for trace-level analysis of drugs, food, and environmental pollutant compounds. This coupling has resolved selectivity and sensitivity problems of simple electrochemical sensors. In addition, the ability for simultaneous determination of drugs or food additives with one electrochemical sensor is another advantage of electrochemically modified sensors. Recently, many electrochemical sensors have been suggested for fast and simultaneous determination of drugs and environmental or food additive samples with nano-molar detection limit.

In addition, the diversity of working electrode in voltammetric and amperometric sensors is another factor contributing to the fabrication of different types of electroanalytical sensors. Gold, silver, Pt, carbon paste, glassy carbon, pencil graphite, boron-doped diamond, and carbon paper electrodes are commonly applied electrodes which have been suggested for fabrication of electroanalytical sensors. The selection of a suitable electrode for fabrication of portable kits is an important challenge in the fabrication of electroanalytical sensors. Although gold and silver electrodes have high electrical conductivity and showed better limit of detection in fabrication of electroanalytical sensors, they are not suitable for the design and fabrication of portable kits, as they are very expensive and modification of them is very hard.

Carbon-based electrodes such as pencil graphite, glassy carbon, and carbon paste electrodes with low cost and easy modification process have been considered for fabrication of highly selective and sensitive electroanalytical sensors for analysis of food, pharmaceutical, and environmental compounds. Thus, it can be concluded that, compared to other analytical techniques, electroanalytical sensors with more advantages will be used in the coming years as a unique and practical strategy for measuring a wide range of compounds. Therefore, in the present review section, it was attempted to introduce the different types of electrochemical sensors, and their analytical processes, and to review recent researches on the application of electroanalytical sensors for analysis of food, pharmaceutical, and environmental compounds. Additionally, the advantages and disadvantages of different types of electrochemical sensors for analysis of real samples and their selectivity regarding the assessment of pharmaceutical, food, and environmental compounds were also discussed in this section. Finally, this section aimed to provide readers with comprehensive information on the potential of various electrochemical sensors and their preparation.

We described the mechanism and different examples of DNA and enzymatic and electrocatalytic methods for electroanalytical determination of drug, food, and environmental compounds.

6.8.1 DNA-Based Electrochemical Sensors

Scheme 6.2 shows a biosensor diagram. As illustrated in Scheme 6.2, there are different types of biosensors with a wide range of application. The DNA sensors are one of the different types of analytical biosensors in which DNA is used as a biological recognition element. If DNA is selected as a biological recognition element and electrochemical strategy is used as transducer, then the suggested sensor is named DNA electrochemical biosensor. There are two general types of DNA electrochemical biosensors applied as analytical tool for determination of pharmaceutical, food, and environmental compounds: (1) analyte–DNA interaction type of biosensors and (2) nucleic acid hybridization biosensors.

6.8.1.1 Analyte-DNA Interaction Type of Biosensors

There are three different procedures for interaction between DNA and analytes regarding fabrication of analyte–DNA biosensors, as presented in Scheme 6.3.

In the electrostatic type of DNA biosensors, the interaction occurs between different charges of analyte and DNA structure. The phosphate group of DNA with negative charge is suitable for interaction with positive cations and could be useful as an analytical approach. This type of analyte–DNA biosensor is suitable for determination of cations, such as Mg^{2+}. There are two major and minor grooves in the DNA structure. These positions are useful for interaction of analyte with DNA. In the third approach, the intercalation of analyte and DNA is used as an analytical approach for determination of drugs and biological compounds. The intercalation of analyte and DNA is a very important and better approach compared to other approaches in analyte–DNA interaction mechanism. There are four bases in DNA structure, including adenine (A), guanine (G), thymine (T), and cytosine (C), among which guanine and adenine bases are electroactive and can be oxidized in the electrochemical systems. Oxidation signals of guanine and adenine have been used as analytical strategy for the

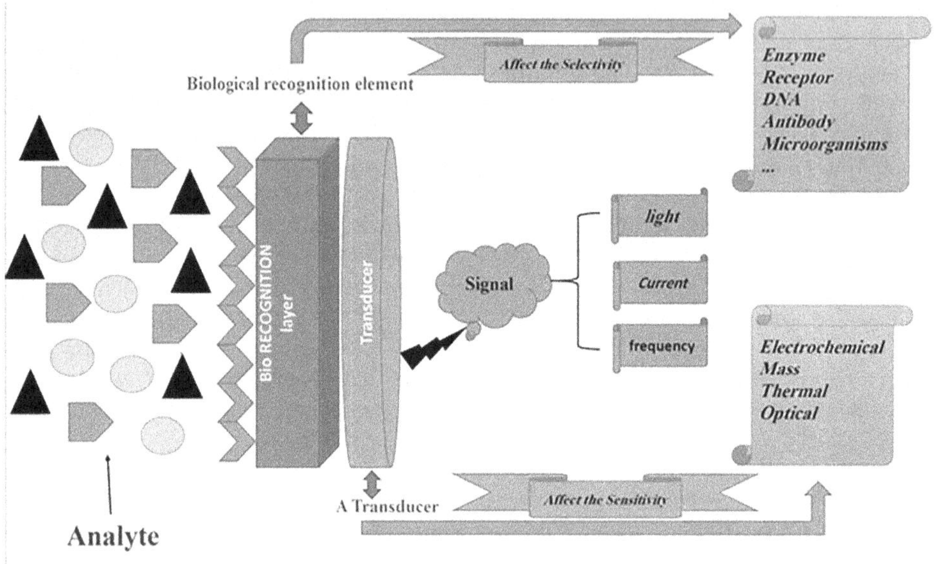

SCHEME 6.2 The overall structure of biosensor.

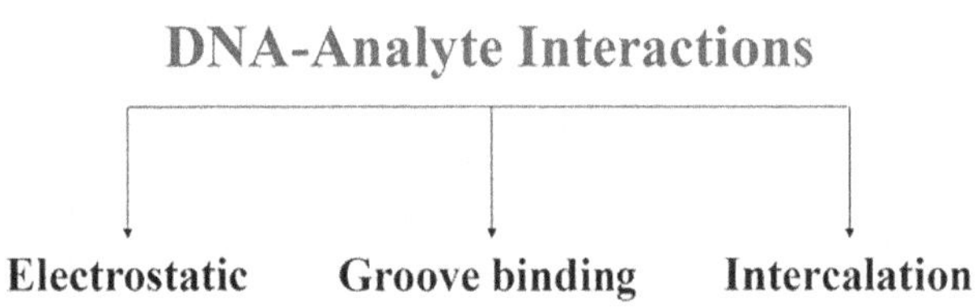

SCHEME 6.3 The different types of DNA–analyte interaction.

determination of many different analytes, especially anticancer drugs. If analyte can be intercalated in DNA structure, oxidation signals of guanine, adenine, or two bases decrease; this decrease in the current is directly related to analyte concentration. For example, Jahandari et al., in their study, reported the intercalation of Temodal with ds-DNA using a DNA biosensor as a high-performance analytical approach for the determination of this anticancer drug. The DNA biosensor was amplified with Au nanoparticles to improve the conductivity of the sensor. Figure 6.28 shows the minor groove and intercalation interaction diagram obtained by docking investigation in this study [221].

It has been shown that the intercalation between guanine base and Temodal decreased the oxidation signal of anticancer drug and created a high-performance strategy for determination of Temodal in pharmaceutical samples. In another report, and following our research group's work, a pencil graphite electrode amplified with polypyrrole and nitrogen-doped reduced graphene was modified with ds-DNA (salmon sperm) to fabricate a biosensor for determination of epirubicin anticancer drug. The use of polypyrrole and nitrogen-doped reduced graphene is essential for improving the electrical conductivity of sensors and increasing the active surface area of the sensor contributing in loading high amounts of ds-DNA at the surface of the electrode. The electrochemical impedance spectroscopy signals of unmodified

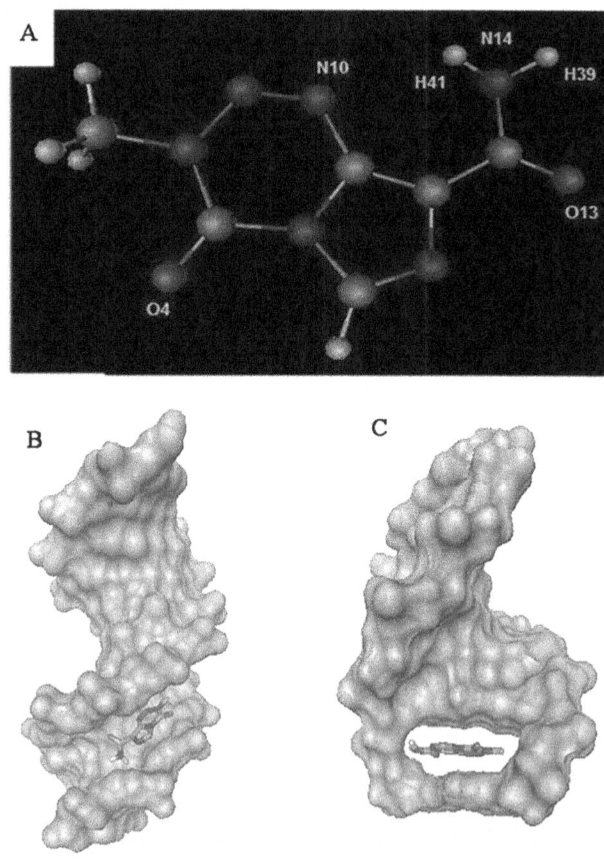

FIGURE 6.28 (a) Atomic numbering scheme of Temodal; (b) Temodal DNA minor groove interaction; and (c) Temodal DNA intercalation.

pencil graphite electrode, pencil graphite electrode modified with polypyrrole, and pencil graphite electrode modified with polypyrrole and nitrogen-doped reduced graphene are presented in Figure 6.29A [221]. It has been found that modification of electrode with conductive materials helps in improving sensitivity of sensors and reducing value of charge transfer resistance of fabricated biosensors. On the other hand, the AFM image, relative to unmodified and modified electrode, is presented in Figure 6.29B. The XPS analysis results are illustrated in Figure 6.29C, confirming the presence of two mediators at the surface of the fabricated biosensors. The amplification step is very important in the fabrication of DNA biosensors due to the response of biosensors and the association of limit of detection of systems with this step. Table 6.4 [221] shows a summary of the studies in which analyte–DNA biosensors have been used for the determination of pharmaceutical, food, and environmental compounds.

On the other hand, UV-vis spectroscopy and gel electrophoresis are two important methods which could be used for confirming DNA–analyte interaction.

6.8.1.2 Nucleic Acid Hybridization

This type of DNA biosensors works based on hybridization of immobilized probes to the sequence-specific target DNA. A specific signal relative to redox reaction such as $[Fe(CN)_6]^{-3/-4}$ before and after hybridization is selected as electroanalytical approach for the determination of target DNA. To improve electroanalytical signal, the electrode surface is usually modified with conductive mediators, such as nanomaterials. An SH group and aliphatic structure are coupled to the end of ss-DNA to provide an easy condition in the hybridization process (Scheme 6.4) [221].

This type of electrode is usually suggested for the detection of cancer. Usually, the complementary of a cancer sequence is used as a probe at the surface of the electrochemical biosensor. In the solution containing cancer sequence, their hybridization can change the redox signal of the electrochemical probe and is used as an electroanalytical approach for the detection of cancer. For example, Feng et al. reported the application of a nucleic acid hybridization DNA biosensor using methylene blue as an electroactive indicator for the detection of colorectal cancer. They used 5′-GGGCACTCTTGCCTACGCCATCAGCTCCAACTACC ACAAGTTTT-3′ as probe DNA at surface of electrode.

The 5′-AAAACTTGTGGTAGTTGGAGCTGATGGCGTA GGCAAGAGTGCCC-3′ was detected as a target probe relative to colorectal cancer using changes in methylene blue signal. Authors used nanoporous CeO_2/chitosan composite film for improving sensitivity and electrical conductivity of sensor.

6.8.2 Enzymatic Biosensors

In enzymatic biosensors, the enzyme molecule is used as a recognition element in the detection process. Selective reaction between an enzyme and an analyte helps in the fabrication of highly selective electrochemical biosensors (Scheme 6.5) [221].

The concentration of an analyte in enzymatic biosensor can be detected by impedimetric, voltammetric, potentiometric, and amperometric techniques, among which amperometric enzymatic biosensors are usually offered for real-time analysis. Immobilization of enzyme at the surface of an electrode is the main step in the fabrication of enzymatic biosensors. Reproducibility and sensitivity of enzymatic sensors depend on this stage of sensor construction. There are five approaches for modification of electrode surface with enzyme: (1) encapsulation, (2) physical adsorption, (3) cross-linking, (4) entrapment, and (5) covalent binding (see Scheme 6.6) [229]. In covalent binding strategy, the enzyme must react with a functional group at the surface of the electrode.

This type of immobilization is very useful, with high stability for fabrication of portable enzymatic biosensors. Different types of interaction, such as hydrogen bridges, van der Waals forces, ionic interactions, as well as hydrophilic and hydrophobic ones, have been suggested for physical adsorption strategy. This is an unstable procedure for fabrication of enzymatic biosensors, and previous findings have shown low reproducibility in case of applying this procedure. Polymeric films are a suitable strategy for modification of molecules of enzymes in the fabrication of enzymatic biosensors. In encapsulation strategy, semipermeable polymeric microspheres are the main source for encapsulation of enzyme molecule and modification of electrode surface. In case of entrapment of enzymatic biosensors, the enzyme molecules are entrapped in a complex matrix, such as conductive polymers. Affinity of analyte to the enzyme is an important factor in selectivity and sensitivity response of enzymatic biosensor that could be determined by the Michaelis–Menten equation. The Michaelis–Menten equation arises from the general equation for an enzymatic reaction: E + S ↔ ES ↔ E + P, where *E* is the enzyme, *S* is the substrate, *ES* is the enzyme–substrate complex, and *P* is the product. Thus, the enzyme combines with the substrate in order to form the ES complex, which, in turn, converts to product while preserving the enzyme. The rate of the forward reaction from E + S to ES may be termed k_1, and the reverse reaction as k_{-1}. Likewise, for the reaction from the ES complex to E and P, the forward reaction rate is k_2, and the reverse is k_{-2}. Therefore, the ES complex may dissolve back into the enzyme and substrate or move forward to form the product.

At initial reaction time, when t ≈ 0, little product formation occurs; therefore, the backward reaction rate of k_{-2} may be neglected. The new reaction becomes:

$$E + S \leftrightarrow ES \rightarrow E + P$$

Assuming steady state, the following rate equations may be written as:

Rate of formation of ES = $k_1[E][S]$
Rate of breakdown of ES = $(k_{-1} + k_2)$ [ES]

And set equal to each other (note that the brackets represent concentrations). Therefore:

$$k1[E][S] = (k - 1 + k2)[ES]$$

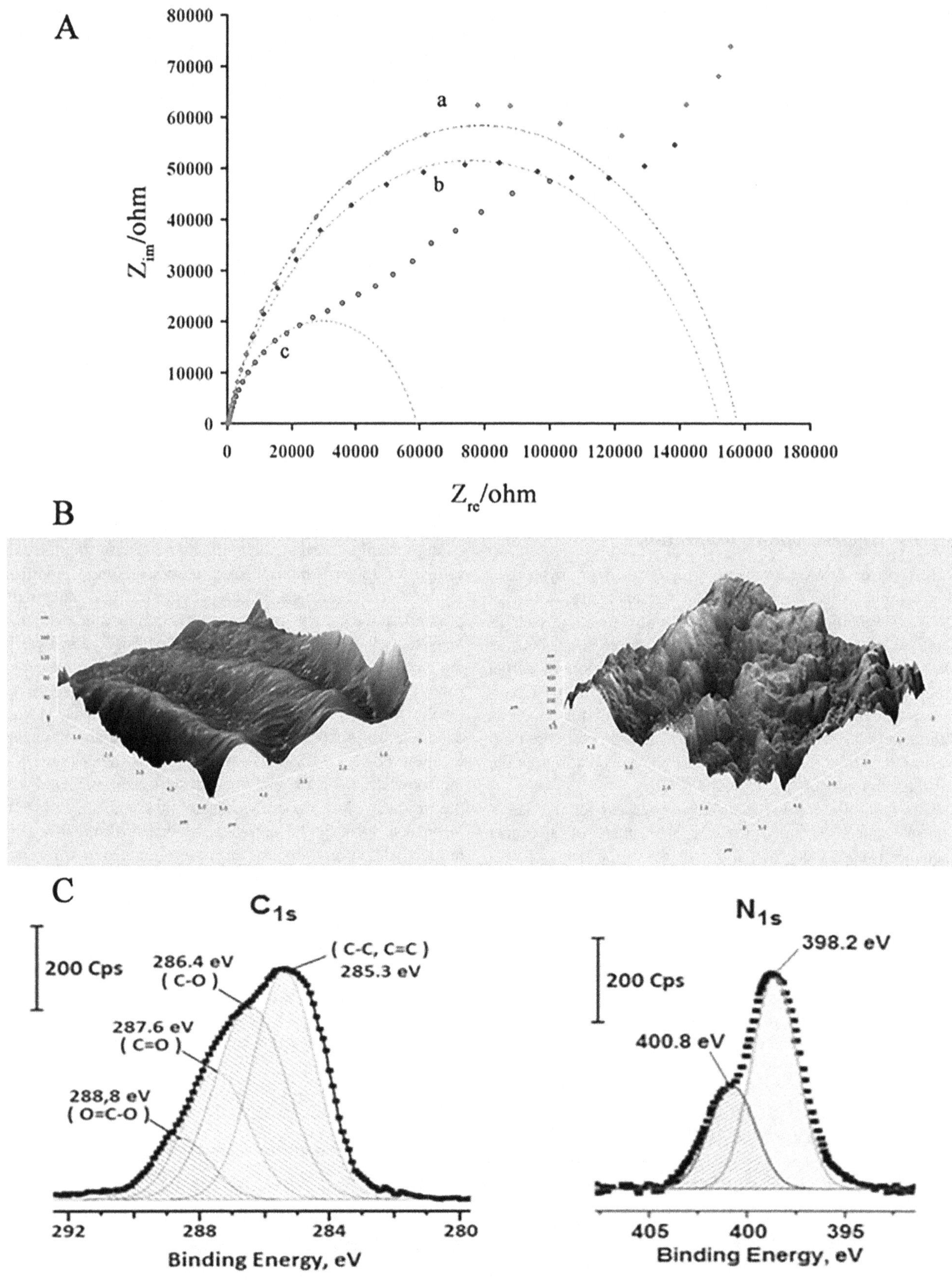

FIGURE 6.29 (A) Nyquist plots of (a) unmodified electrode, (b) PP/PGE, and (c) PP/NrG/PGE in the presence of 1.0 mM $[Fe(CN)_6]^{3+/4-}$ in 0.1 M KCl. (B) AFM images of (a) unmodified PGE and (b) PP/NrG/PGE. (C) XPS spectra of PP/NrG.

Source: **Figure reproduced from A. Khodadadi, E. Faghih-Mirzaei, H. Karimi-Maleh, A. Abbaspourrad, S. Agarwal, V. K. Gupta, Sens. Actuators B 2019, 284, 568–574. Reproduced with copyright permission of Elsevier.**

TABLE 6.4
The Electrochemical Biosensors Based on Analyte–DNA

Electrode	Type of Interaction	Analyte	Ref.
Carbon paste electrode	Not reported	Arsenic trioxide	[222]
Gold electrode	Electrostatic interactions	Ruthenium(III) hexaamine	[223]
Glassy carbon	Intercalation	Mitoxantrone	[224]
Pencil graphite electrode	Intercalation	Didanosine	[225]
Pencil graphite electrode	Intercalation	Ciprofloxacin	[226]
Pencil graphite electrode	Intercalation	6-mercaptopurine	[227]
Pencil graphite electrode	Intercalation	Epirubicin	[228]

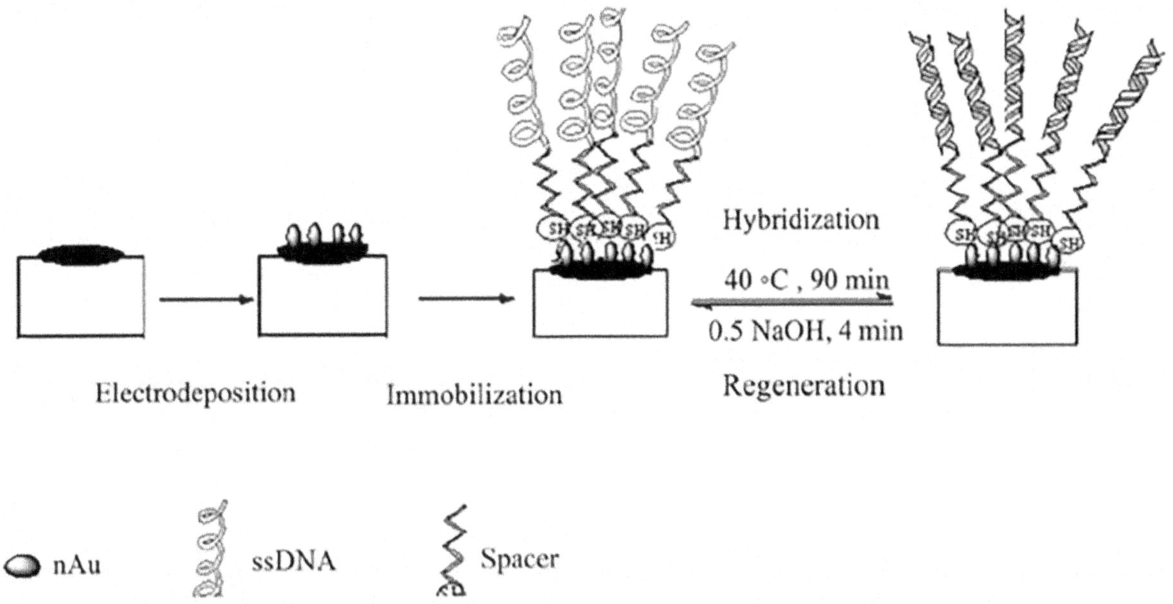

SCHEME 6.4 A typical procedure for nucleic acids hybridization biosensors.

Source: Figure reproduced from A. A. Ensafi, M. Taei, H. Rahmani, T. Khayamian, Electrochim. Acta 2011, 56, 8176–8183. Reproduced with copyright permission of Elsevier.

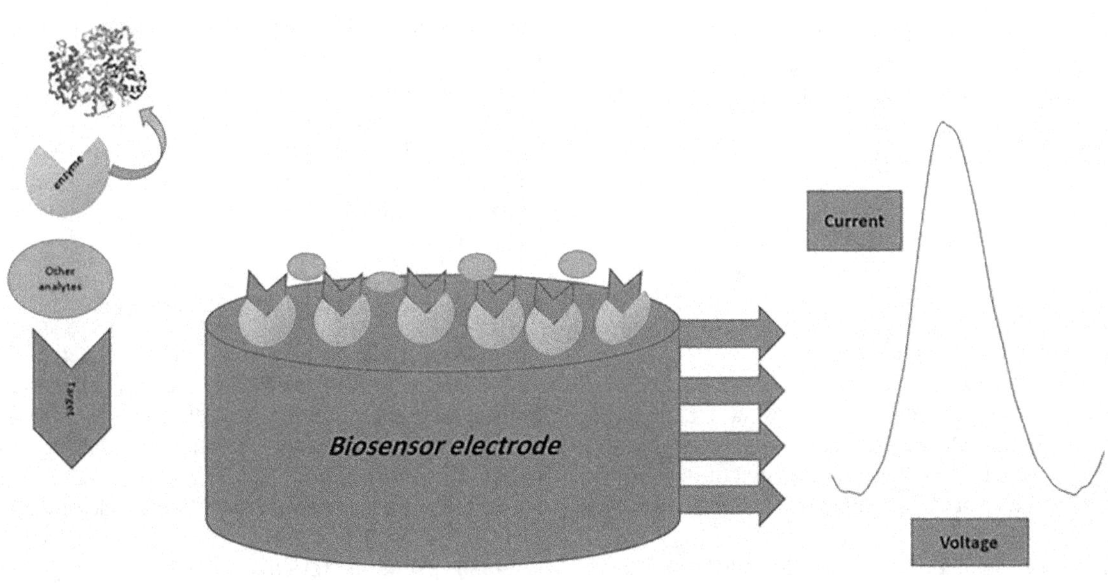

SCHEME 6.5 A typical procedure for enzymatic biosensors.

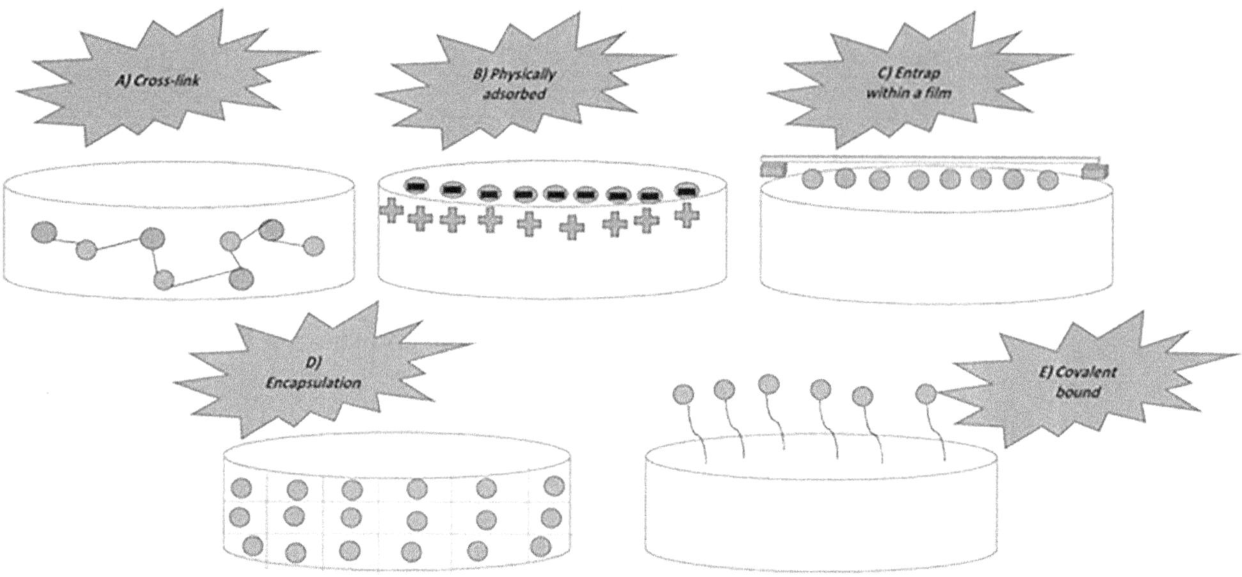

SCHEME 6.6 (a) Immobilization of enzyme by cross-linking strategy. (b) Immobilization of enzyme by physical adsorption strategy. (c) Immobilization of enzyme by entrapped-within-film strategy. (d) Immobilization of enzyme by encapsulation strategy. (e) Immobilization of enzyme by covalent binding strategy.

Rearranging terms:

$$[E][S]/[ES]=(k\text{-}1+k2)/k1$$

The fraction [E][S]/[ES] has been coined K_m, or the Michaelis constant.

According to Michaelis–Menten's kinetics equations, at low concentrations of substrate [S], the concentration is almost negligible in the denominator as KM >> [S], so the equation is essentially

$$V_0=V_{max}[S]/KM$$

which resembles a first-order reaction.

At high substrate concentrations, [S] >> KM, and thus the term [S]/([S] + KM) becomes essentially one, and the initial velocity approached Vmax, which resembles zero-order reaction.

The Michaelis–Menten equation is:

$$V_0=Vmax\left(\frac{[Substrate]}{[Substrate]+K_m}\right)$$

In this equation:

V_0 is the initial velocity of the reaction.

V_{max} is the maximal rate of the reaction.

[Substrate] is the concentration of the substrate.

Km is the Michaelis–Menten constant, which is enzyme–substrate affinity, which shows the concentration of the substrate when the reaction velocity is equal to one-half of the maximal velocity for the reaction.

It can also be thought of as a measure of how well a substrate complexes with a given enzyme, otherwise known as its binding affinity. An equation with a low K_m value indicates a large binding affinity, as the reaction will approach V_{max} more rapidly. An equation with a high K_m indicates that the enzyme does not bind as efficiently with the substrate, and V_{max} will only be reached if the substrate concentration is high enough to saturate the enzyme.

There are many electrochemical enzymatic biosensors introduced by electrochemists for the determination of different biological samples. Glucose enzymatic biosensor is an important type of enzymatic biosensors considered in many scientific reports. In all the reported papers, glucose oxidase was stabilized at the surface of the sensor. Diverse approaches for stabilization of enzyme at working electrodes and different types of nanomaterials used for improving conductivity of biosensors led to the development of new types of glucose enzymatic biosensors, as reported in the literature. For example, Umar et al. reported the application of a glucose enzymatic biosensor using immobilized glucose oxidase at the surface of flower-shaped copper oxide nanostructures as substrate, along with conductive mediator, which resulted in good electrical signal for electro-oxidation of glucose at suggested biosensors (Figure 6.30).

6.8.3 Electrocatalytic-Based Sensors

In an electrocatalytic mechanism (EC') (Scheme 6.7) [221], one mediator with reversible or quasi-reversible behavior is immobilized at the surface of an electrode and interacts with analyte. An increase in the oxidation or reduction of the signal of the mediator after interaction with analyte is an analytical factor for its determination. Due to selective interaction between mediator and analyte, this type of electrochemical sensors is useful for selective analysis of food, pharmaceutical, and compounds.

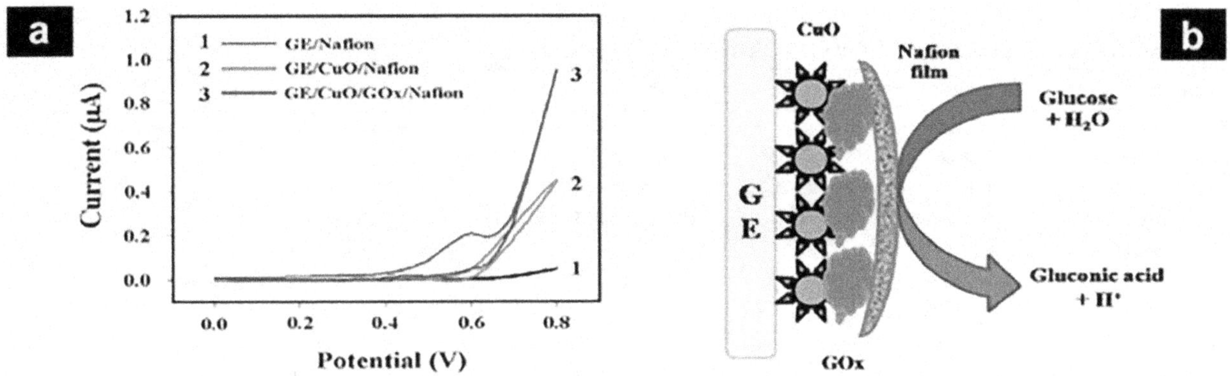

FIGURE 6.30 (a) CV sweep curves for the glassy electrode/Nafion (black line;1), GE/CuO/Nafion (red-line;2), and GE/CuO/GOx/Nafion (blue-line;3) in 0.01 M PBS (pH 7.4) at scan rate of 100 mV/s; (b) schematic of glucose detection via electrochemical method by using CuO nanostructures–modified gold electrode.

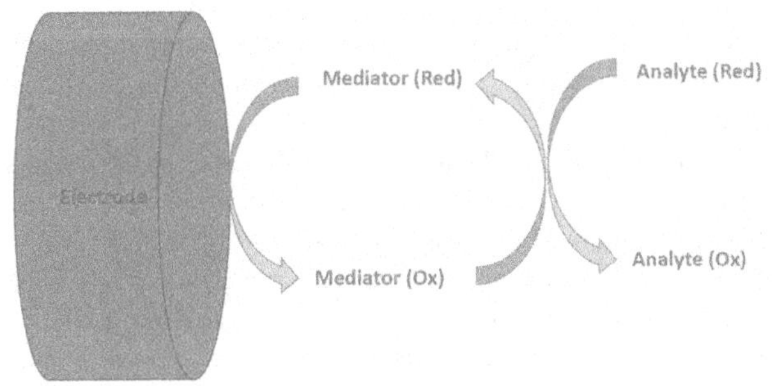

SCHEME 6.7 A simple diagrams for EC′mechanism.

Blood sugar test kit is one of the important examples of portable electrocatalytic-based sensors. Organic ligands (catechol-based structures) and inorganic complexes, such as ferrocene derivatives, are the main types of electrocatalytic mediators used for the fabrication of this type of electrochemical sensors.

For example, Ensafi and Karimi introduced ferrocenedicarboxylic acid as a suitable mediator for the modification of carbon paste electrodes in the presence of multi-walled carbon nanotubes as other conductive mediator.

Fabricated sensor was used for the electrocatalytic determination of 6-thioguanine anticancer drug. As can be seen in [221], the ferrocenedicarboxylic acid showed quasi-reversible signal in the absence of the drug. After the addition of 6-thioguanine and at surface of electrode modified with mediator, the oxidation signal of ferrocenedicarboxylic acid increased, and the reduction signal of the mediator was removed. This change in signals confirms an electrocatalytic mechanism for the determination of 6-thioguanine. The presence of MWCNTs helped in the conductivity of systems and improved the limit of detection for trace-level analysis of 6-thioguanine in this case.

On the other hand, electrocatalytic systems are a powerful and suitable strategy for simultaneous determination of electroactive compounds. In the solution containing two analytes with similar oxidation potential, the interaction of the mediator with one of them can decrease the oxidation potential of one analyte, and this point helps to separate two oxidation signals. As an example, we fabricated an electrocatalytic system for simultaneous determination of glutathione and piroxicam. At the surface of bare electrodes, the oxidation signals of glutathione and piroxicam showed to overlap together. In this work, N-(4-hydroxyphenyl)-3,5-dinitrobenzamide has been used as an electro-catalyst that interacts with glutathione. In this condition, the oxidation potential of glutathione shifted to negative value, and the oxidation potential of piroxicam remained at the same potential. This modification helps in the simultaneous determination of glutathione and piroxicam.

Many scientific reports used this type of strategy for the fabrication of an electroanalytical sensor for the determination of food, pharmaceutical, and biological samples (see Table 6.5).

6.9 Conclusions and Future Perspectives

Combining CNMs and enzymes requires a diverse skill set that is rare to find and represents a multidisciplinary research area that bears many technical and scientific challenges. However, a growing number of scientists are trying to innovate in this exciting field. The focus of this chapter has been to provide a concise overview from which it is evident how most studies have been focused on CNTs and, more recently, on graphene-based materials and CNDs, for applications in biosensing and biofuel cells. Nonetheless, CNMs offer far more benefits, and the multivarious members of the nanocarbon family still present today a valuable innovation opportunity that is worth exploring. Among other aspects that deserve further examination is their environmental fate, especially how biodegradation and photodegradation processes can improve the efficiency of CNM degradation.

Further research potential can be found in the development of computational methods to enhance enzymatic performance and robustness [240], including machine learning for enzyme engineering [241], potentially coupled to directed evolution approaches [242]. The range of enzymatic activity can be further expanded through the incorporation of unnatural amino

TABLE 6.5

Electrocatalytic-Based Sensors for the Determination of Electroactive Materials

Electrode	Electrocatalyst	Conductive Mediator	Analyte	Ref.
Glassy carbon	Alizarine red S	–	Hydroxylamine	[230]
Glassy carbon	Hematoxylin	MWCNTs	Hydrazine	[231]
Carbon paste	Isoproterenol	MWCNTs	Cysteamine	[232]
Carbon paste	Rutin	Acetylene black	Glutathione	[233]
Glassy carbon	Pyrogallol red	–	Hydrazine	[234]
Carbon paste	Catechol derivative	ZnO/CNTs	Glutathione and amoxicillin	[235]
Glassy carbon	Chlorogenic acid	–	Hydrazine	[236]
Carbon paste	Ferrocene derivative	Zinc oxide nanoparticles	Captopril	[237]
Carbon paste	Acetylferrocene	NiO nanoparticles	Glutathione	[238]
Carbon paste	Acetylferrocene	CdO nanoparticles	Hydroxylamine	[239]

acids [243], thanks to the emergence of robust methods for their genetic encoding [244]. Higher levels of complexity for the development of next-generation devices can be attained with the incorporation of multienzymatic cascade reactions [245], also in confined environments [246], in an attempt to mimic, or go even beyond, the mesmerizing performance of biochemical cascades in living organisms. To this end, advancing electrochemical techniques for the characterization of enzymes at the electrode interface will be key [247], especially to leverage the unique electronic properties of CNMs and their application to further enhancing enzymatic activity. In particular, an attractive area is the development of wearable, flexible bioelectronics for the harvesting of bioenergy and its use in self-powered biosensing for health monitoring [248].

In this chapter, ENFET with CNT nanocomposite as sensing layer has been fabricated and characterized for cholesterol detection. Due to the use of K/PPy/CNT nanocomposite, the sensor has shown high dynamic range, low detection limit, good stability, good response time, and good sensitivity of approximately Nernstian limit. Also, the fabricated device has been found to be repeatable and reproducible, with almost zero interference.

The unique physicochemical properties of carbon nanomaterials allow them to incorporate targeting ligands, chemotherapeutic drugs, and many other therapeutic agents, making them suitable for certain imaging and therapeutic applications. This urges us to establish closer interdisciplinary connections between nanotechnology, biology, and medicine in order to develop more powerful and useful tools for biologists and clinicians. Although carbon dots are considered multifunctional and low-toxicity or non-toxic nanoparticles, there are some problems associated with their use, including synthesis methods and control over their size and surface properties, which could cause interferences in their biological applications. Nevertheless, the strong optical absorption of carbon dots allows for photothermal and photodynamic therapies that harness the absorbed photons for selective destruction of malign microorganisms and tumors through targeted drug delivery and diagnostic imaging. With the many new avenues and opportunities offered by the unique properties of CDs, we envisage the future of such nanomaterials with an optimistic outlook. In this chapter, we have provided a comprehensive coverage of recent progress in biological imaging and nanomedicinal therapy using a variety of CDs. The CD synthesis, the resulting optical properties, and the recent knowledge related to the structural–luminescence relationship have also been discussed.

The number and application of these types of analytical systems is increasing rapidly and will become an integral part of human life in the coming years. According to our research group's works in electroanalytical systems, this type of analytical systems has shown many advantages for analytical determination of food, pharmaceutical, and environmental compounds, such as easy operation, portability, low cost, and fast response. It seems that, with the increase in the capacities of this field, there will be many analytical kits working on electrochemical methods in the coming years. Many companies have invested in these types of analytics systems, and indeed, tremendous progress will be observed in the future. This chapter showed that DNA–analyte interaction and, especially, intercalation reaction is a very useful strategy for the determination of anticancer drugs. Anticancer drugs deactivate the guanine and adenine bases and change the oxidation bases signals that can be used for analytical determination of drugs. On the other hand, enzymatic biosensors can be used as selective analytical tools due to the selective reaction between enzyme and analyte. In the final step, we discussed about electrocatalytic systems as sensitive and selective systems for determination of food, drug, and environmental compounds. The interaction between electroactive mediators at the surface of electrodes with analytes can help in the fabrication of a selective analytical system.

Overall, there is potential for the future clinical usage of CD nanomaterials. With the multifunctionality of these materials, and taking advantage of their low cost and low environmental impacts, high water solubility, biocompatibility, low toxicity, good cell permeability, excellent sensitivity of fluorescent imaging, and easy conjugation with therapeutics, future developments should enable the development of versatile theranostic applications for the treatment of cancer and other diseases in the near future.

7

CNMs-Based Developed Biosensors for Rapid Technologies Detection of Antiviral Infection and the Management Coronavirus Biomarkers

7.1 Background

The rapid spread of severe acute respiratory syndrome coronavirus-2 (SARS-CoV-2) around the world has ravaged both global health and economy. This unprecedented situation has thus garnered attention globally. This further necessitated the deployment of an effective strategy for rapid and patient-compliant identification and isolation of patients tested positive for SARS-CoV-2. Following this, several companies and institutions across the globe are striving hard to develop real-time methods, like biosensors for the detection of various viral components, including antibodies, antigens, ribonucleic acid (RNA), or the whole virus.

Carbon-based nanomaterials such as graphene and nanodiamonds have demonstrated impressive physical and chemical properties, such as remarkable strength, corrosion resistance, and excellent electrical and thermal conductivity, and stability. Because of these unique characteristics, carbon nanomaterials are explored in a wide range of fields, including the diagnosis and treatment of viruses.

Currently, there is no approved therapeutics for dengue virus (DENV) infection, even though it can cause fatal complications. Understanding DENV infection and its propagation process in host cells is necessary to develop specific antiviral therapeutics. Here we developed a graphene oxide–based fluorescent system (graphene oxide–based viral RNA analysis system, or GOViRA) that enables sensitive and quantitative real-time monitoring of the intracellular viral RNA level in living cells. The GOViRA system consists of a fluorescent dye–labeled peptide nucleic acid (PNA) with a complementary sequence to the DENV genome and a dextran-coated reduced graphene oxide nanocolloid (DRGON). Through a cell-based high-throughput screening of FDA-approved small-molecule drugs, we identified ulipristal, a selective progesterone receptor modulator (SPRM), as a potent inhibitor against DENV infection. The anti-DENV activity of ulipristal was confirmed both *in vitro* and *in vivo*. Moreover, we suggest that the mode of action of ulipristal is mediated by inhibiting viral entry into the host cells.

Dengue virus (DENV) is a member of the Flavivirus genus, which includes the Zika virus (ZIKV), Japanese encephalitis virus (JEV), yellow fever virus (YFV), West Nile virus (WNV), and tick-borne virus (TBEV)) [1].

3D manufacturing has significantly helped in combating the coronavirus disease (COVID-19) pandemic by facilitating the development of products with novel designs within a short duration [2]. Desktop 3D printers represent the low-cost and most accessible 3D manufacturing technique. These printers are typically based on melted thermoplastics and fused deposition modeling. Thermoplastic polymers (TPs) are the most commonly used polymers in additive manufacturing techniques, owing to their low melting temperatures and low cost. Among all TPs, PLA has gained considerable attention in medical applications owing to its biodegradability and biocompatibility. PLA degrades through hydrolysis to lactic acid, depending on the degree of water contact, autocatalytic behavior, temperature, and pH. However, certain drawbacks of PLA, such as poor thermal stability, low heat-distortion temperature, and brittleness, have limited its use in the production of medical devices. Additionally, medical devices based on PLA are ineffective in preventing virus transmission, specifically in nosocomial environments. The electrical and thermal conductivity, as well as the antiviral and antibacterial properties, of PLA can be improved using different additives, such as carbon and metal nanoparticles (NPs) and cellulose. Among nanomaterials, graphene displays significant potential in the biomedical field, owing to its robust antibacterial properties and pro-differentiating effects on eukaryotic cells. Additionally, graphene, even in small amounts, can reinforce the thermal, optical, and mechanical properties of 3D-printed structures to reduce the toxicity of these structures and the cost of production [2].

DENV, the most widespread arthropod-borne virus, is a serious human pathogen and one of the major concerns in the global public health because it causes over 300 million infection cases annually. DENV infection causes clinical symptoms that range from subclinical mild dengue fever to severe dengue, such as dengue hemorrhage fever (DHF) and dengue shock syndrome (DSS), accompanied by severe bleeding, organ impairment, and plasma leakage, which can lead to death [2]. Tridimensional (3D) manufacturing has played a pivotal role in fighting the coronavirus disease (COVID-19) pandemic with innovatively designed products developed through the collaboration between health professionals, engineers, and creatives [2]. Unfortunately, there is no approved drug or specific therapy for DENV infection up to now. The discovery of novel medications against DENV is required to resolve DENV-induced public health issues.

Effective treatments for coronavirus disease 2019 (COVID-19) are urgently needed to control this current pandemic

DOI: 10.1201/9781032635989-7

caused by severe acute respiratory syndrome coronavirus-2 (SARS-CoV-2). Replication of SARS-CoV-2 depends on the viral RNA–dependent RNA polymerase (RdRp), which is the likely target of the investigational nucleotide analogue remdesivir (RDV). RDV shows broad-spectrum antiviral activity against RNA viruses, and previous studies with RdRps from Ebola virus and Middle East respiratory syndrome coronavirus (MERS-CoV) have revealed that delayed chain termination is RDV's plausible mechanism of action. Here we expressed and purified active SARS-CoV-2 RdRp composed of the nonstructural proteins nsp8 and nsp12. Enzyme kinetics indicated that this RdRp efficiently incorporates the active triphosphate form of RDV (RDV-TP) into RNA. Incorporation of RDV-TP at position *i* caused termination of RNA synthesis at position i + 3. Almost-identical results have been obtained with SARS-CoV, MERS-CoV, and SARS-CoV-2 RdRps. A unique property of RDV-TP is its high selectivity over incorporation of its natural nucleotide counterpart ATP. In this regard, the triphosphate forms of 2'-C-methylated compounds, including sofosbuvir, approved for the management of hepatitis C virus infection, and the broad-acting antivirals favipiravir and ribavirin, exhibited significant deficits. The results collectively provide a unifying, refined mechanism of RDV-mediated RNA synthesis inhibition in coronaviruses and define this nucleotide analogue as a direct-acting antiviral.

The conventional methods of developing antiviral agents require massive resources, including time, money, and labor. Due to these limitations, tropical diseases are often neglected and disregarded by the pharmaceutical industry. Drug repurposing (or "drug repositioning"), finding effective agents from approved drugs, has appeared as an efficient way of identifying potential medications [3]. To identify the efficacy of antiviral drug candidates on virus-infected cells, a variety of in vitro assay systems have received much attention: viral infectivity assays (focus-forming assay (FFA), plaque assay, and yield reduction assay), methods measuring the viral genome and proteins (quantitative reverse transcription-PCR (qRT-PCR) and immunostaining), and methods using a gene-modified virus (reporter virus particles (RVP) and virus-like particles (VLP)). However, these *in vitro* assay systems have shown several limitations, including low reproducibility, high costs, labor-intensive process, and/or viral genetic modifications. Because of these limitations, they are not suitable for repurposing drugs through high-throughput screening. Therefore, new assays that enable a sensitive cell-level analysis of viral infection using native virus with an unmodified genome are in demand.

DENV has a single-stranded RNA genome that encodes three structural (C, prM/M, and E) proteins and seven nonstructural (NS1, NS2A, NS2B, NS3, NS4A, NS4B, and NS5) proteins. When mammalian cells are inoculated with DENV, membrane fusion occurs due to the acidic environment of the endosome, and genomic RNA is released into the cytoplasm sequentially. After the release of the RNA, a single open reading frame (ORF) is translated into viral polyproteins, and a replication complex is assembled on the cytoplasmic side of the endoplasmic reticulum (ER) membrane. Then, NS5 protein, the RNA-dependent RNA polymerase (RdRp), produces numerous copies of viral genomic RNA in the cytoplasm of the host cell, and the produced viral RNA is translated into the viral polypeptides. The immature DENV particles are transported through the trans-Golgi network (TGN), where they are converted into infectious form and are released from the host cell. The number of viral RNA copies in the cytoplasm directly reflects any change that occurred in the viral infection or proliferation process. Therefore, monitoring the change in the intracellular viral RNA level is an efficient method to analyze DENV infection.

DNA sequence detection is important for disease diagnosis, drug discovery, and bacterial identification. To date, various DNA sequence detection techniques have been developed, such as fluorescence, electrochemical, surface plasmon resonance, etc. However, these approaches are time-consuming, contain labels, and are complex to implement. Recently, a field-effect transistor, based on carbon nanotube (CNTFET), has been developed for this purpose because of their advantage potential in terms of miniaturization, high sensitivity, being label-free, high bio-compatibility, and rapid response time. This device is used to convert a small potential change at the gate surface into a detectable electric/voltage signal. The CNTFETs are fabricated by depositing SWCNTs on platinum or gold electrodes, which serve as source and drain, connected via the nanotubes channel, and the doped Si substrate serves as the gate. CNTFETs are a promising candidate for DNA sensor applications because of their numerous advantages. Star et al. reported on carbon nanotubes network field-effect transistors (NTNFETs) to detect DNA hybridization. The probe DNA sequences were immobilized on CNTs via non-covalent attachment. They found that DNA hybridization with complementary DNA sequence takes place on the device surface, resulting in the reduction of the NTNFETs conductance. CNTFET was fabricated by CNTs grown on 500 mm thick silicon oxide substrate and contacted by two electrodes labeled as source and drain. The probe DNA sequences were immobilized onto the CNTFET by covalent attachment method. The results showed that the DNA sensor based on CNTFET can determine the DNA target at concentrations as low as 1 pg mL^{-1}.

In this chapter, we propose and demonstrate a carbon nanotube (CNT) field-effect transistor (FET)–based biosensor for selective detection of severe acute respiratory syndrome coronavirus-2 (SARS-CoV-2). CNTFETs were fabricated on a flexible Kapton substrate, and the sensor was fabricated by immobilizing the reverse sequence of the RNA-dependent RNA polymerase gene of SARS-CoV-2 onto the CNT channel. The biosensors were tested for the synthetic positive and control target sequences. The biosensor showed a selective sensing response to the positive target sequence with a limit of detection of 10 fM.

7.1.1 Azvudine (FNC): A Promising Clinical Candidate for COVID-19 Treatment

A very recent work published in *Advanced Science* by the authors [4] reveals that 2′-deoxy-2′-β-fluoro-4′-azidocytidine (Azvudine, FNC), a clinical candidate originally developed for HIV treatment, has entered clinical trial in China for evaluating its efficacy and safety (ChiCTR2000029853), showing promise for treating novel coronavirus disease 2019 (COVID-19) [5]. This work suggests that nucleoside-based antivirus agents could be repurposed for COVID-19 treatment. Globally, on August 2, 2023, there have been 768,983,095 confirmed cases of COVID-19, including 6,953,743 deaths, reported to WHO. As of July 31, 2023, a total of 13,492,159,872 vaccine doses have been administered.

Since the breakout of severe acute respiratory syndrome coronavirus-2 (SARS-COV-2) in December 2019, SARS-COV-2 has spread rapidly. As of August 30, 2020, over 23 million cases have been confirmed worldwide, and more than 0.8 million deaths have been reported. Because of the lack of effective treatment, the fatal cases are increasing globally, particularly in the USA. Therefore, the developments of effective vaccines and drugs have been highly pursued for COVID-19 prevention and treatment. To date, some drugs and clinical drug candidates are currently undergoing clinical assessment for treating COVID-19 [6]. Remdesivir, originally developed by Gilead Sciences for treating Ebola virus disease, shows effectiveness in inhibiting the activity of SARS-COV-2 and has received approval in some countries for emergency use in patients with severe COVID-19 [7]. However, rationed supply, side effects, and unsatisfactory phase III clinical results limit the clinical use of remdesivir. In addition, the increasing SARS-COV-2 mutated strains G, GH, and GR have posed new challenges for COVID-19 treatment [8]. Thus, it is urgent to develop safe and effective drugs for treating COVID-19.

SARS-COV-2, a positive-sense single-stranded RNA virus, utilizes nucleosides and nucleotides for RNA synthesis (Figure 7.1a) [4]. Inside the host cells, nucleoside analogs mimic natural nucleosides and are transformed into corresponding active nucleoside triphosphates through kinase catalysis, which are then embedded in virus RNA during RNA synthesis and then block the addition of nucleotides to the 3′-hydroxy group, finally terminating RNA chain synthesis and virus replication (Figure 7.1b). Besides, nucleoside-based antiviral agents also inhibit DNA- and RNA-dependent polymerases crucial for viral replication. Therefore, the widely used nucleoside-based antiviral drugs in the clinic may have potential for COVID-19 treatment.

FNC, a novel nucleoside-based broad-spectrum antivirus clinical candidate recently developed in the laboratory for HIV infection treatment and prevention [9], is the first dual-targeting nucleoside-based agent that inhibits nucleoside reverse transcriptase and restores expression of cytidine deaminase APOBEC3G (A3G) in HIV-1 patients–derived CD4+ T cells. The 2′-fluoro group enhances its acidic stability and greatly affects the electronic properties and conformational shape of nucleosides, thus dramatically improving the activities, while modifications at the 4′-position, such as the introduction of an azido group, make the nucleosides adopt an unnatural 3′-C-endo conformation, making the compounds active against HIV and multidrug-resistant HIV strains. FNC has exhibited desirable pharmacokinetics, excellent efficacy,

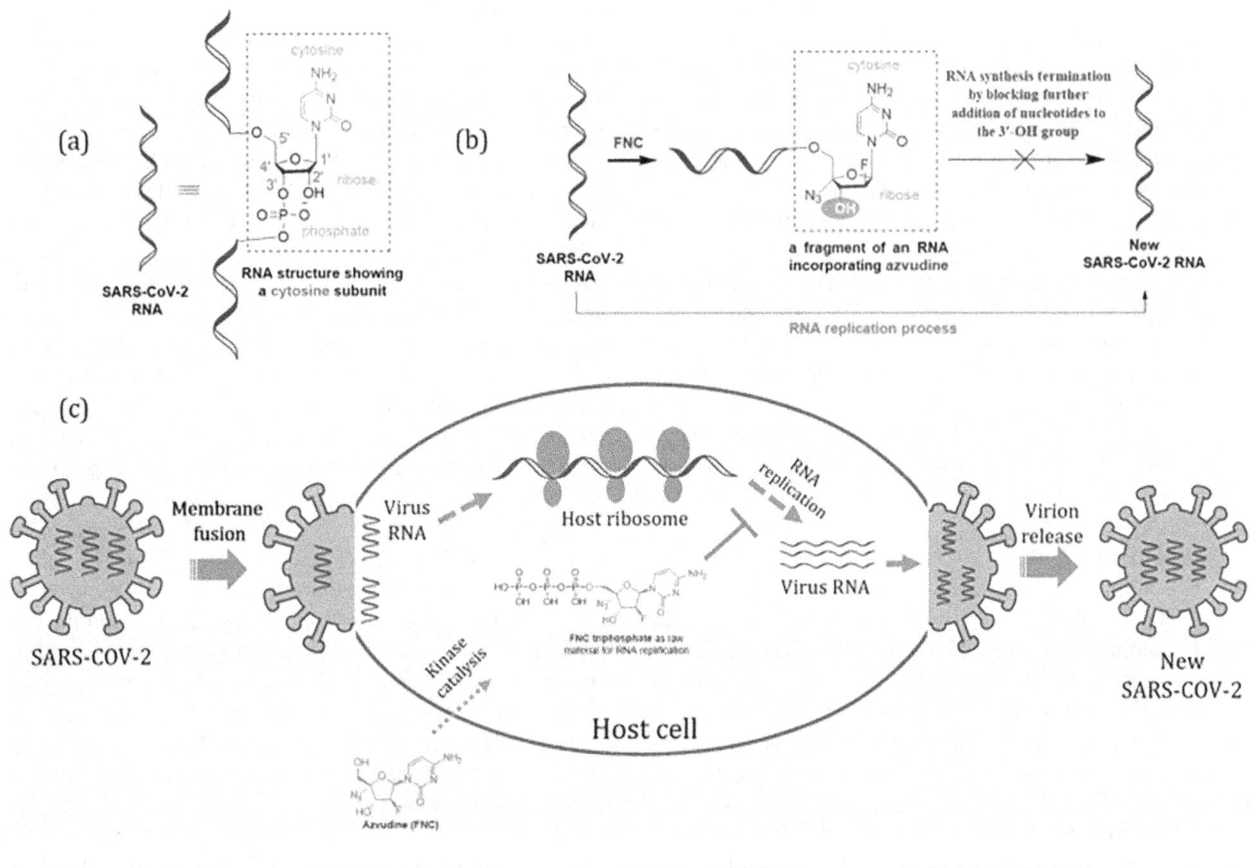

FIGURE 7.1 Nucleoside-based anti-HIV clinical candidate azvudine (FNC) for COVID-19 treatment: (a) SARS-COV-2 RNA structure showing a cytosine subunit; (b) a diagram showing the RNA replication process of SARS-COV-2 blocked by FNC; (c) proposed mechanisms of FNC for inhibiting the activity of SARS-COV-2 [4].

and safety in the phase I and II clinical trials (GQ-FNC-2014–2, GQ-FNC-201, and NCT04109183) for treating HIV infection. On March 17, 2020, a phase III clinical trial of FNC was initiated to evaluate the efficacy and safety in HIV-infected treatment naive patients (NCT04303598). On August 12, 2020, the listing application of FNC for HIV treatment was given priority in the review process (CXHS2000016/CXHS2000017). Based on the previous findings, it has been speculated that FNC could be repurposed for COVID-19 treatment, even for patients infected by mutated SARS-COV-2.

To evaluate the efficacy and safety of FNC in patients with mild and common COVID-19, we recently conducted a randomized, open-label, controlled clinical trial of FNC tablets in China (ChiCTR2000029853) [5]. In this pilot study, 20 patients were randomly assigned to receive FNC or standard antiviral treatment. It has been found that FNC could shorten the nucleic acid negative conversion (NANC) time. In the FNC group, the mean times of the first NANC is 2.60 d, while for the control group, this value is 5.60 d. The NANC rate is 100% after treatment for 4 d in the FNC group, significantly higher than that (73% after 28 d treatment) in the hydroxychloroquine treatment group. FNC is also efficacious in patients who have received other treatment regimens and could help patients recover faster. Besides, FNC is well tolerated without drug-related adverse events in the FNC group. We speculate that FNC triphosphate could be embedded during RNA synthesis of SARS-COV-2 and inhibits related polymerases, finally leading to RNA replication termination (Figure 7.1c). Overall, FNC is a safe and efficacious nucleoside-based drug candidate for treating mild and common COVID-19 and also shows promise for curing severe COVID-19. Clinical trials with larger sample size are warranted to further investigate the efficacy and safety of FNC for COVID-19 treatment. The data also suggest that repurposing existing broad-spectrum antivirus agents is a viable and promising strategy for COVID-19 treatment.

Evidence is mounting that some people can continue to pass on SARS-CoV-2 for much longer than the few days often suggested by public health agencies. A series of studies shows that many people with COVID-19 remain infectious well into the second week after they first experience symptoms. "The facts of how long people are infectious for have not really changed," says infectious disease specialist Amy Barczak, whose research suggests that one-quarter of people who have caught the Omicron variant of SARS-CoV-2 could still be infectious after eight days. "There is not data to support five days or anything shorter than ten days."

China's drug regulator granted conditional approval on Monday (July 2022) for an HIV drug to be used to treat COVID-19. The drug, azvudine, developed by Chinese drugmaker Genuine Biotech, is the first oral antiviral for the disease made in China. In an announcement, the company said that 40% of people with COVID-19 who were given azvudine for a week in a phase III clinical trial showed "improved clinical symptoms," compared with 11% of those given a placebo. Detailed data from the trial, including whether the treatment reduced the risk of hospitalization or death, have not been released. Another Chinese-made oral antiviral, VV116, is in the final stages of development, and another dozen are in various stages of development.

Most antivirals target two SARS-CoV-2 proteins that are essential for replication, a polymerase and a protease. Azvudine tricks the virus's polymerase into incorporating the drug into its RNA, which stops the virus from replicating [4].

In China and globally, the demand for COVID-19 therapies is enormous, says Sheng Ding, a pharmaceutical chemist at Tsinghua University in Beijing. Until the azvudine authorization, China had approved only one oral antiviral to treat the disease, Paxlovid, developed by Pfizer in New York City. It is highly effective—it reduces the risk of hospitalization and death by nearly 89%—but supplies in China are limited. "The market will have room for several more drugs that may not outperform Paxlovid, but allow more people to access effective therapies," adds Ding.

Another Chinese-made oral antiviral, VV116 (VV116 is a chemically modified version of the antiviral remdesivir with oral bioavailability and potent activity against SARS-CoV-2), is in the final stages of development, and another dozen are in various stages of development.

7.2 Viral Infection and Nanomaterials

The eradication of viral infections is an ongoing challenge in the medical field, due not only to the problem of spreading but also to the virus's ability to escape therapy by genetic mutations. The lack of targeted antiviral therapeutics as well as the constant emergence of new viruses make the search for antiviral agents a challenging and extremely needed research task. As part of a global strategy to prevent epidemics, some severe emerging pathogens with great epidemic potential have been identified by the World Health Organization (WHO), including, next to Ebola virus disease, the highly pathogenic human coronavirus (HCoV) infections. While circulating HCoVs (HCoV-229E, HCoV-OC43, HCoV-NL63, and HKU1) cause relatively mild common cold–like respiratory tract infections, severe acute respiratory syndrome coronavirus (SARS-CoV) and Middle East respiratory syndrome coronavirus (MERS-CoV) lead to pneumonia, requiring hospitalization and intensive care. A total of 2,266 laboratory-confirmed cases of MERS-CoV, including 804 associated deaths, have been declared to the WHO until now, with a high case fatality rate (35%). As the virus is circulating in animals and humans, it may undergo further adaptation and cause a pandemic. Therefore, therapeutic options are urgently needed.

The current treatments for MERS-CoV are extrapolated from SARS-CoV and H1N1 influenza outbreaks. These include different combinations of small molecules with broad antiviral activity (e.g., ribavirin, corticosteroids, and interferons (IFN)) and monoclonal and polyclonal antibody therapies. The membrane-anchored glycoprotein S has lately been found to be essential for the interaction between MERS-CoV and the host cell, and the development of MERS-CoV entry/fusion inhibitors targeting the S1 subunit is nowadays considered as a viable antiviral strategy.

Recently, nanoscale materials have emerged as promising and efficient platforms to modulate the viral infection cycle. Given that attachment of viruses into host cells is favored by multivalent interactions, the multivalent character of nanostructures with their high surface-area-to-volume ratio, allowing the attachment of several ligands, makes them well adapted to interfere with viral attachment and blocking viral entry into cells.

The rapid spread of severe acute respiratory syndrome coronavirus-2 (SARS-CoV-2) around the world has ravaged both global health and the economy. This unprecedented situation has thus garnered attention globally. This further necessitated the deployment of an effective strategy for rapid and patient-compliant identification and isolation of patients tested positive for SARS-CoV-2. Following this, several companies and institutions across the globe are striving hard to develop real-time methods, like biosensors for the detection of various viral components, including antibodies, antigens, ribonucleic acid (RNA), or the whole virus.

The COVID-19 outbreak came to light in December 2019, when the Chinese Center for Disease Control and Prevention (CDC) reported a new coronavirus strain which had great potential for transmission between humans [10].

Subsequently, the etiological agent of COVID-19 was confirmed to be the severe acute respiratory syndrome coronavirus-2 (SARS-CoV-2), a recently discovered strain of the Coronaviridae family that phylogenetically resembles the zoonotic SARS-CoV that previously emerged in 2020 [11]. Global molecular assay statistics state that as of February 1, 2021, there were more than 100 million subjects from over 210 countries confirmed to be infected with SARS-CoV-2 infection. Furthermore, over 2 million patients have succumbed to death from the infection, thereby posing a great peril to human physical and mental health, considerably affecting the quality of life (QoL) of people across the globe [10].

The SARs-CoV-2 infection has become one of the most serious threats to human health and society. This outbreak highlights the urgent need for developing effective and efficient detection and treatment methods. Currently, viruses are detected via antigen or antibody detection assays (ELISA, immunofluorescence, immunoperoxidase), hemagglutination testing, nucleic acid recognition (polymerase chain reaction), and genomic sequencing. Most of these conventional methods are time-consuming, labor-intensive, and costly (Table 7.1). Fast, accurate, and cost-efficient techniques, such as nanomaterial-based methods, are required for rapid and large-scale pathogenic detection. In recent years, we have witnessed great development of nanomaterials that have shown promise in meeting the needs of biomedical applications [12]. *Nanomaterials* are a material from which at least one dimension has the scale of 1–100 nm. They are unique in that they have extremely small sizes, huge surface-area-to-volume ratios, tunable optical emissions, strong mechanical properties, and superparamagnetism. Because of their small size, nanomaterials can easily interact with extracellular and intracellular biological substances, enabling the development of novel medicine (i.e., nanomedicine). Their unique optical, magnetic, and electric properties allow the development of relevant devices for disease diagnosis and medical imaging. There are over 28 Food and Drug Administration (FDA)– or European Medicines Agency (EMA)–approved nanomedicines so far, and above 60 other nanoparticle technologies that are still pending FDA/EMA approval. Common nanomedicines include Epaxal (Crucell) for hepatitis A vaccination and Inflexal V (Crucell) for influenza vaccine; both nanoparticle vaccines are liposome-based, making them highly efficient for penetrating tissues and cells to induce protective immune responses against virus. Interestingly, Alnylam developed and marketed Patisiran/ONPATTRO (ONPATTRO is a prescription medicine for adults that treats the polyneuropathy caused by an illness called hereditary ATTR (hATTR) amyloidosis). Hereditary transthyretin amyloidosis (hATTR) with polyneuropathy (formerly known as familial amyloid polyneuropathy) is a rare disease due to mutations in the gene encoding transthyretin (TTR) and characterized by multisystem extracellular deposition of amyloid, leading to dysfunction of different organs and tissues, and siRNA-delivering lipid-based nanoparticle intended for silencing gene-induced expression of transthyretin, associated with hereditary transthyretin amyloidosis.

Not surprisingly, their success in the aforementioned applications has caught the attention of the infectious disease field. For example, recent development of RNA vaccines against SARs-CoV-2 virus involves the use of lipid nanoparticles [13].

TABLE 7.1

Comparison of Traditional Virus Detection Techniques and Carbon Nanoparticle Detectors.

Detection Methods	Detection Time (Excluding Antigen/ Protein/DNA Preparation)	Detection Accuracy	Cost of Device
Enzyme-linked immunosorbent assay (ELISA)	Moderately fast (3 h to 6 h).	Extremely high sensitivity and good selectivity for specific antibodies in sera.	Inexpensive platform. However, antibody and antigen proteins are costly.
Hemagglutination assays	Relatively slow (4 h to 2 days).	High sensitivity and good selectivity for red cell agglutination.	Inexpensive platform. However, antibody and antigen proteins are costly.
PCR and genomic sequencing	Relatively fast processes, depending on the DNA fragment length. However, specific primers may take time to be synthesized.	Highly accurate detection of DNA sequences.	Machine is costly. However, repeated use of machine is enabled over long term. Primers have relatively low cost.
Carbon-based quantum dots	Extremely fast (1 min to 5 min).	Moderate sensitivity and selectivity.	Relatively inexpensive platform.
Carbon nanotubes	Relatively fast (5 min to 1.5 h).	High sensitivity and good selectivity.	Inexpensive platform. Immobilized antibody and antigen proteins are costly.
Graphene	Relatively fast (30 min to 2 h).	Moderate sensitivity and selectivity.	Relatively inexpensive platform.

TABLE 7.2

Comparison of Synthesis, Properties, and Viral Applications of Various Carbon Nanomaterials

Carbon Nanomaterials	Synthesis Techniques	Properties	Viral Applications	Reference
Carbon-based quantum dots (CDots)	Chemical ablation, laser ablation, electrochemical carbonization, microwave ray irradiation, and hydrothermal/solvothermal treatment	Excellent water solubility, good luminescence signals, chemical inertness, high resistance to photobleaching, low toxicity, good electronic properties	Treatment and detection	[15]
Carbon nanotubes	Carbon arc discharge technique, laser ablation technique, and chemical vapor deposition (CVD) technique	Exceptional strength, flexibility, resistance to fracture, and good electrical properties	Detection and prevention	[16]
Graphene and derivatives	Exfoliation and cleavage of natural graphite, CVD, plasma-enhanced CVD (PE-CVD), electric arc discharge, micromechanical exfoliation of graphite, epitaxial growth at electrical insulating surfaces, opening up CNTs, and reduction of GO using various solutions	Large surface area, high electrical conductivity, high thermal conductivity, exceptional mechanical stiffness, and adaptiveness to chemical modification	Treatment and detection	[17]
Nanodiamonds	Detonation events, high-energy ball milling of pressurized high-temperature diamond microcrystals, plasma-assisted CVD, laser ablation, ion irradiation using graphite, and ultrasound cavitation	Disperse uniformly and stably in water, high stability, high strength, good thermal conductivity, high refractive index, and enhanced resistivity	Treatment	[18]
Fullerenes	Electrical arc vaporization, combustion, laser ablation of graphite, and pyrolysis	Superconductivity, ferromagnetism, anti-HIV bioactivity, and optical limiting effects	Treatment and detection	[19]

In general, the roles of nanomaterials in medicine are roughly classified into three groups (detection, prevention, and treatment). The usage of nanomaterials is to facilitate fast detection with high sensitivity and selectivity, prevention of virus attachment or recognition, and eradication of virus before their contact with human beings through physical, chemical, and biological properties of nanomaterials.

Carbon-based nanomaterials comprise of fullerenes, nanodiamonds, carbon nanotubes, graphene and its derivatives, and carbon-based quantum dots (CDots). They own impressive mechanical, thermal, electrical, optical, and chemical properties (Table 7.2). For example, they have broad-range one-photon property (single-photon adsorption), good biocompatibility, and ease for functionalization. Carbon-based nanomaterials also contain an intrinsic two-photon fluorescence property in the long-wavelength region (near-infrared II); this property permits them to be used for deep-tissue optical imaging. Furthermore, their high conductivity, chemical stability, and fast electron-transfer rate make them exceedingly fit for biosensing applications [14]. This chapter highlights the recent development of carbon-based nanomaterials and discusses their potential and encouraging diagnostic and therapeutic applications against infectious diseases (Figure 7.2). The goal is to provide an alternative thinking about the management of infectious diseases from the field of nanotechnology.

The SARS-CoV-2 infection has been shown to spread quickly through respiratory droplets that are produced during sneezing and coughing. Subsequently, the virus anchors to the host receptors, following which it invades the cells via endocytosis or membrane fusion. The primary structural proteins that make up the coronavirus consist of the envelope (E), membrane (M), spike (S) proteins, and nucleocapsid (N). The ACE2 receptors, predominantly expressed in the pulmonary epithelium, facilitate the binding of the S protein to the host cells. Successively, the two-step protease cleavage marks the activation of the S protein, which brings about irreversible conformational changes that eventually facilitate the combination of the host and viral cell membranes with the release of viral contents into the host cell. After the viral RNA reaches the nucleus, it replicates and generates negative-strand RNA from a single-strand positive RNA template using RNA polymerase. This negative-strand RNA also helps make new positive-strand RNAs that serve as blueprints for synthesizing new viral proteins. Concurrently, while the viral mRNA is employed in the biosynthesis of new viral proteins, new viral particles are created and released into the other cells [20] (Figures 7.3–7.5 and Table 7.3).

Growing bodies of evidence have suggested the mode of transmission of SARS-CoV-2 through several routes, which is primarily attributed to the expression of human angiotensin-converting enzyme-2 (hACE2) in a multitude of cell types, including alveolar, endothelial, vascular, hepatic, and gastrointestinal cells. Furthermore, as the hACE2 gene is imperative in routine functions, the entire human race is prone to SARS-CoV-2 infection [21].

7.3 Graphene Oxide-Based Fluorescent Nanosensor to Identify Antiviral Agents via a Drug Repurposing Screen

Although assays for analyzing pathogens have been developed in recent years [29,30], robust imaging systems that enable quantitative analysis of intracellular viral genomes in live

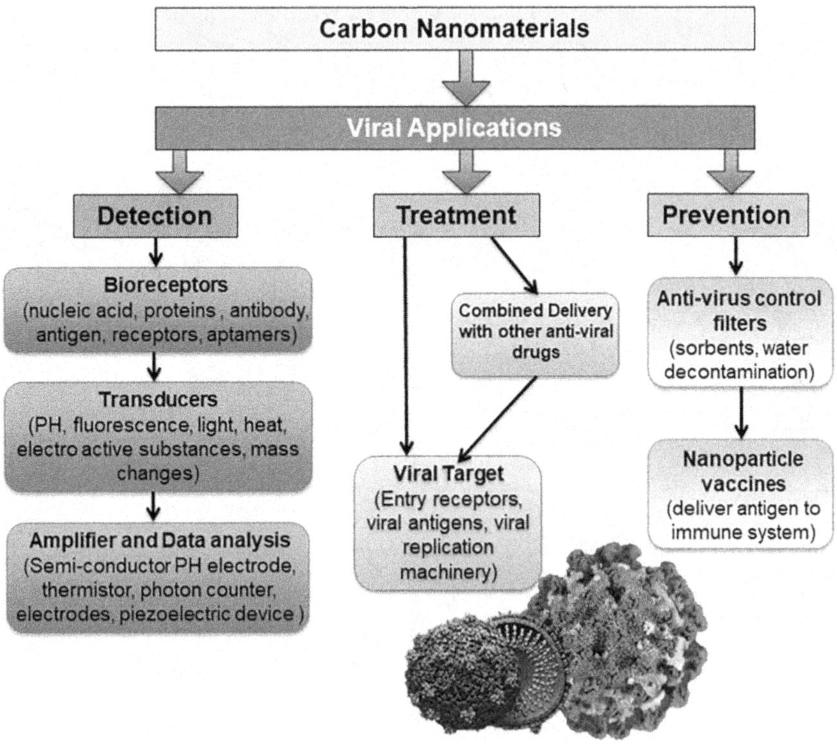

FIGURE 7.2 Carbon nanomaterials for virus management.

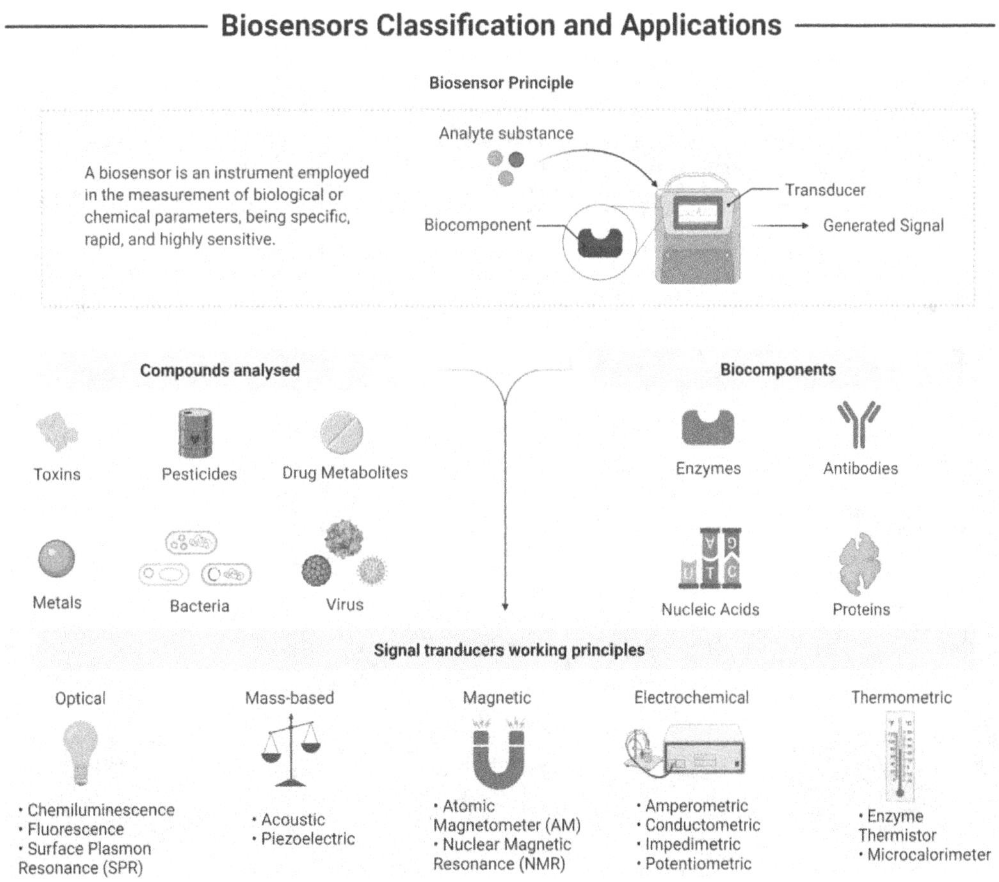

FIGURE 7.3 Classification and applications of various biosensors.

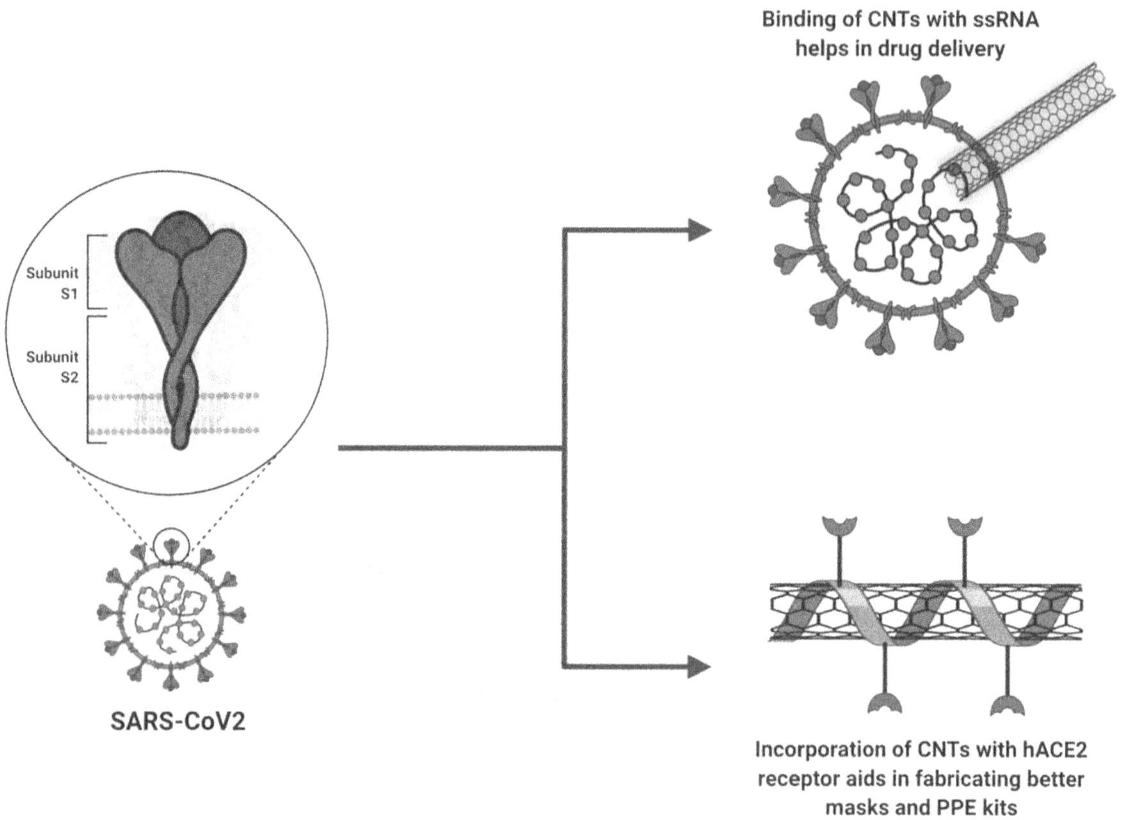

FIGURE 7.4 Models of using CNTs for the prevention and treatment of SARS-CoV- 2 infection.

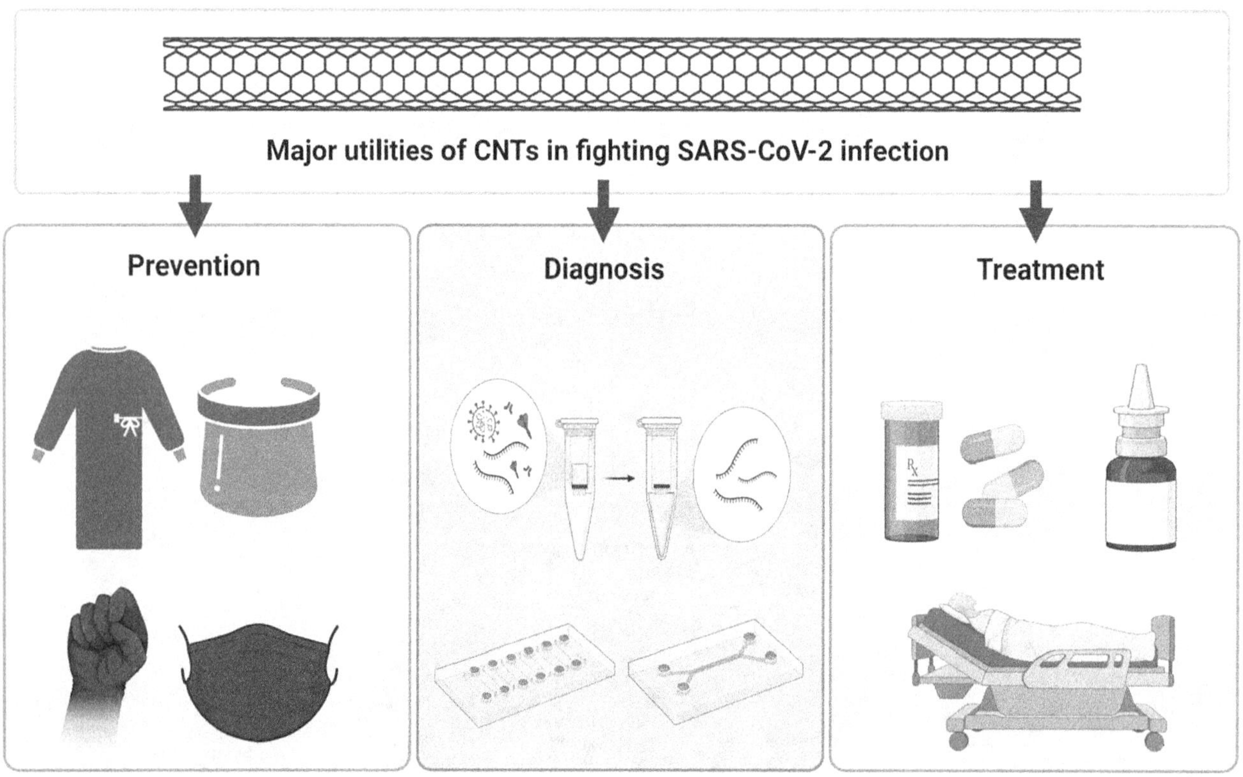

FIGURE 7.5 Future prospects of CNTs in the prevention, diagnosis, and treatment of SARS-CoV-2 infection.

TABLE 7.3
Different Types of Biosensors and Their Respective Recognition Elements for the Detection of SARS-CoV-2

Types of Biosensors	Recognition Element	References
Piezoelectric immunosensor	Spike protein S1	[22]
Thermal biosensor	RNA-dependent RNA polymerase	[23]
Optical biosensors (plasmon-enhanced fluorescence)	Fluorescently labeled antibodies attached to AuNPs	[24]
Field-effect transistor biosensors (BIO-FETs)	SpAb-PBASE/graphene-FET	[25]
Plasmonic photothermal (PPT) and localized surface plasmon resonance (LSPR)	SARS-CoV-2 nucleic acid	[26]
Colorimetric biosensors	RNA sequence of SARS-CoV-2	[27]
Surface-enhanced Raman scattering biosensors (SERS)	Spike protein receptor-binding domain (RBD) by the ACE-2 protein	[28]

cells remain challenging. It has been demonstrated that the newly developed sensitive biosensor GOViRA, using PNA and DRGON, can be used for quantitative and qualitative analysis of the intracellular DENV genome. The GOViRA system enables facile distinction between infected and non-infected cells and easily distinguishes DENV infection from other flaviviruses.

The treatment with compounds that interfere with the DENV life cycle causes a low level of intracellular DENV genome. Since it leads to a quantifiable reduction in fluorescence signal, the GOViRA system can be efficiently used for anti-DENV drug screening. High-throughput screening with FDA-approved drugs has been performed and successfully identified a new drug candidate for DENV named ulipristal. The inhibitory kinetics study revealed that ulipristal inhibits viral entry into the host cell. Based on several reports depicting the successful clinical usage of viral entry inhibitors, it could also be suggested that ulipristal has high potential as a promising antiviral candidate for clinical use. Because the way that ulipristal mediates entry inhibition and the type of interaction that is formed with a virus or host were not fully elucidated, the precise mode of action needs to be characterized.

Herein, a real-time DENV infection analysis system (graphene oxide–based viral RNA analysis system, abbreviated as GOViRA) has been designed [31] using a fluorescent dye–labeled peptide nucleic acid (PNA) and a dextran-coated reduced graphene oxide nanocolloid (DRGON) that can directly monitor and quantify intracellular viral RNA in living cells (Figure 7.6). Graphene oxide (GO)–based nanomaterials have been actively used in developing a wide range of sensors because of their physicochemical properties. In this strategy, DRGON acts as both a delivery carrier and a quencher of the dye-labeled PNA probe. When the dye-labeled PNA is adsorbed onto DRGON by the π–π interaction and hydrogen bonding, the fluorescence of the dye is effectively quenched through fluorescence resonance energy transfer (FRET). The introduction of the target viral genome induces the detachment of the PNA probe that has the complementary sequence to the viral genome and leads to the recovery of the fluorescence signal because of the high affinity and specificity of PNA to viral RNA. Therefore, when the mammalian cells are infected with DENV, several copies of viral RNA, the target of the GOViRA system, are replicated in the cytosol, and the dye-labeled PNA is hybridized with the viral RNA, resulting in the release of the PNA probe from DRGON. The observation of DENV infection with the GOViRA platform does not require terminal processing of the cells (e.g., fixation and lysis). These advantages offer real-time visualization and the analysis of DENV infection in live cells.

Moreover, it has been demonstrated that the GOViRA platform is suitable for antiviral discovery screening. The GOViRA system can discover drug candidates associated with both viral and host pathways related to the viral life cycle. Since the GOViRA platform does not require viral genome engineering, it offers great strength in targeting the complete life cycle of the native virus. To address the urgent need for anti-DENV agents, a cell-based screening of the Food and Drug Administration (FDA)–approved drugs has been conducted. Through the screening, we successfully identified a novel class of a small-molecule anti-DENV compound, ulipristal, which is previously known as a selective progesterone receptor modulator (SPRM). Used for emergency contraception or the treatment of uterine fibroids, ulipristal has never been reported to have an antiviral activity against any kind of virus. After a series of evaluations, it has been confirmed that ulipristal not only has an anti-DENV activity both *in vitro* and *in vivo* but also inhibits DENV entry into the host cell.

7.3.1 Validation of the GOViRA System in Living Cells

For the development of the GOViRA (Figure 7.6), fluorescence quenching and recovery tests were performed using the prepared DRGON and vPNA probe [31]. The fluorescence intensity was quenched down to 1% compared to the initial value when 1.2 μg of DRGON were added to 20 pmol of Cy5-labeled vPNA, and it maintained its fluorescence intensity for 24 h in the presence of serum [31]. The recovery of the fluorescence was measured using a chemically synthesized single-stranded RNA with the target sequence. The quenched fluorescence of vPNA was recovered when the target RNA was added. To examine the selectivity of the GOViRA system, Cy5-labeled scPNA was prepared with a randomly scrambled, mismatching sequence [31]. No fluorescence signal was observed from

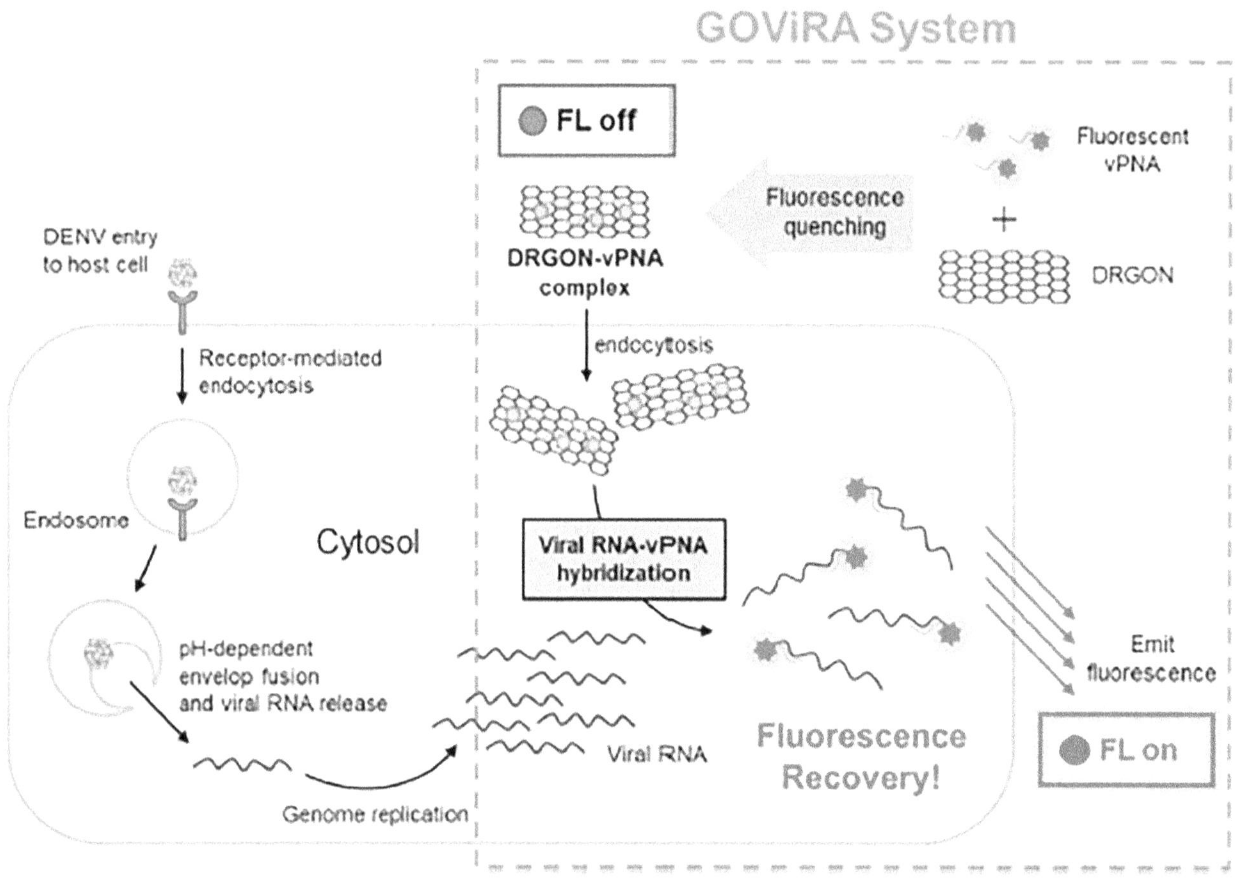

FIGURE 7.6 The strategy for real-time DENV genome monitoring GOViRA platform.

the scPNA-DRGON complex in the presence of the target RNA. Additionally, when a scrambled sequence of RNA was mixed with the vPNA-DRGON complex, there was no notable observation of fluorescence recovery as well [31]. These results indicate that the GOViRA system is highly stable and works only in a sequence-specific manner.

To investigate the ability of the GOViRA system to visualize DENV infection in live cells, we inoculated Vero E6 cells with DENV serotype 2 for 48 h and then treated them with PNA-DRGON complexes consisting of vPNA or scPNA for the next 5 h. For relative quantification, a PNA probe complementary to β-actin was conjugated with Cy3 to be used as an internal control [31]. As the intracellular viral genome was replicated after the inoculation, DENV-infected Vero E6 cells displayed a distinct fluorescence signal in the cytoplasm after the addition of the vPNA-DRGON complex, whereas that of the non-infected cells showed no fluorescence signal. In contrast, the treatment of the DENV-infected cells with the scPNA-DRGON complex did not lead to any signs of a fluorescence response (Figure 7.7a and b), indicating a high target specificity for the GOViRA system in living cells. When the z-sectioned image in the same plane was investigated, the Cy5 signals from the vPNA probe (labeled in red) were mostly observed in the cytoplasmic area (Figure 7.7d). Additionally, to verify the reliability of the GOViRA system, the number of viral RNA copies in the cytoplasm was quantified by qRT-PCR under the same experimental conditions. A high amount of viral genome was detected only in the DENV-infected cells (Figure 7.7c), which was highly correlative to the results analyzed from the fluorescence signal. Furthermore, the quantified fluorescence signal corresponding to β-actin remained constant, indicating that the β-actin is a suitable internal control [31].

DENV exists as multiple serotypes [2], which exhibit partially conserved sequences. When the sequence of vPNA was designed, the conserved region in all four serotypes was set as a target. To verify the capability of monitoring DENV infection for all four serotypes, the inoculation of DENV serotypes 1, 2, 3, or 4 was followed by vPNA-DRGON treatment. Regardless of the serotype, the DENV-infected groups showed a notable fluorescence signal in response to the vPNA-DRGON treatment, whereas those infected with other flaviviruses did not [31]. These results indicate that the GOViRA system possesses a great specificity against DENV regardless of the serotype, suggesting that this system could also be used to distinguish the infection of DENV from other flaviviruses.

To determine the capacity of the GOViRA system measuring the dynamic changes in intracellular viral RNA expression levels and monitoring the progress of the viral infection, the changes in the fluorescence intensity over time have been monitored. Vero E6 cells inoculated with DENV were treated with the PNA-DRGON complex at a series of time intervals from 12 to 72 h post-infection (p.i.) [31]. As shown in reference [31], the

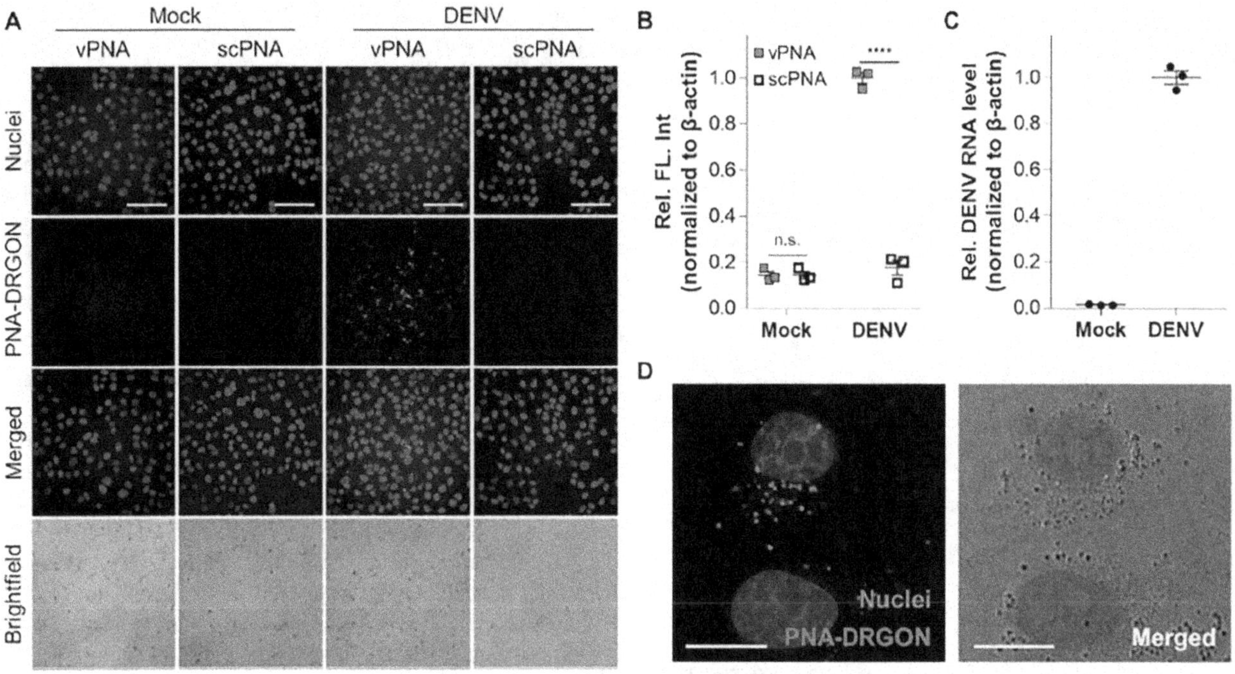

FIGURE 7.7 Qualitative and quantitative detection of the intracellular DENV genome through the GOViRA system in non-infected and DENV-infected Vero E6 cells: (a) Fluorescence images of non-infected and DENV-infected Vero E6 cells were taken after 5 h of PNA–DRGON complex treatment. PNA–DRGON complex was introduced at 48 h p.i. that includes Cy5-labeled vPNA or scPNA. Scale bar: 25 μm. (Red, Cy5 signals from PNA probe; blue, Hoechst signals from nuclei). (b) Quantitative analysis of Cy5 signals from PNA–DRGON complexes treated in non-infected and DENV-infected Vero E6 cells. The relative intensity of each signal was normalized to the β-actin signal as an internal control. Values represent mean ± SEM ($n = 3$). Statistical significance was determined by Student's *t*-test (n.s., not significant; $^{****}P \leq 0.0001$). (c) qRT-PCR analysis for the expression of the DENV genome in Vero E6 cells. Values represent mean ± SEM ($n = 3$). (d) Fluorescence images of DENV-infected Vero E6 cells were taken after 5 h of vPNA–DRGON complex treatment with DeltaVision microscope. Scale bar: 15 μm. (Red, Cy5 signals from PNA probe; blue, Hoechst signals from nuclei).

fluorescence signal from the cells showed a time-dependent increase, with a high linear correlation ($R^2 = 0.9997$) to the result from the qRT-PCR analysis [31]. Next, Vero E6 cells were inoculated with DENV at various multiplicities of infection (MOI) from 0.25 to 2, and the cells were monitored by live-cell microscopy. The quantified fluorescence signal increased in an MOI-dependent manner (Figure 7.8b). Such data suggest that the GOViRA platform facilitates not only real-time visualization of DENV infection but also quantitative analysis of intracellular viral RNA in living cells.

7.3.2 High-Throughput Screening of Approved Drugs to Identify Compounds with Anti-DENV Activity

Because the GOViRA platform with living cells was successfully demonstrated, we then tried to verify whether the GOViRA platform is suitable for high-throughput screening. To determine its systemic reliability as a high-throughput screening assay, we used Z′-factor as a statistical parameter. The Z′-factor of the GOViRA platform was calculated to be 0.87 from 20 negative and 20 positive controls (Figure 7.8c), which can be suggested as evidence of an excellent assay for high-throughput screening. To further verify whether the GOViRA system is capable of the quantitative analysis of antiviral activity, the system to investigate the cellular effect caused by a model representative antiviral compound has been utilized. The introduction of the ribavirin induced a serial decrease in the fluorescence signal dose-dependently (Figure 7.8d), indicating that the GOViRA system is suitable as a fluorescence-based quantitative antiviral assay.

Using the GOViRA system, a cell-based screening on a library of ~550 FDA-approved drugs has been conducted to find therapeutic candidates with anti-DENV activity. Vero E6 cell monolayers were treated with 10 μM of each drug in the library or with the vehicle (DMSO) for an hour before infection. Then, DENV and the PNA–DRGON complex were sequentially introduced (Figure 7.8a). Based on the screening results that considered both antiviral activity and cell viability (Figure 7.8e), ulipristal has been chosen as a potent antiviral candidate because it showed fluorescence signal decrease by <25% and minimal effects on cell viability [31].

7.3.3 Ulipristal Inhibits DENV Infection *In Vitro*

Standard assays were done to check the antiviral effect and cytotoxicity of ulipristal *in vitro*. The activity of ulipristal against DENV was evaluated by both FFA and qRT-PCR. For the FFA, Vero E6 cells were infected with DENV in the presence of various concentrations of ulipristal. The anti-DENV

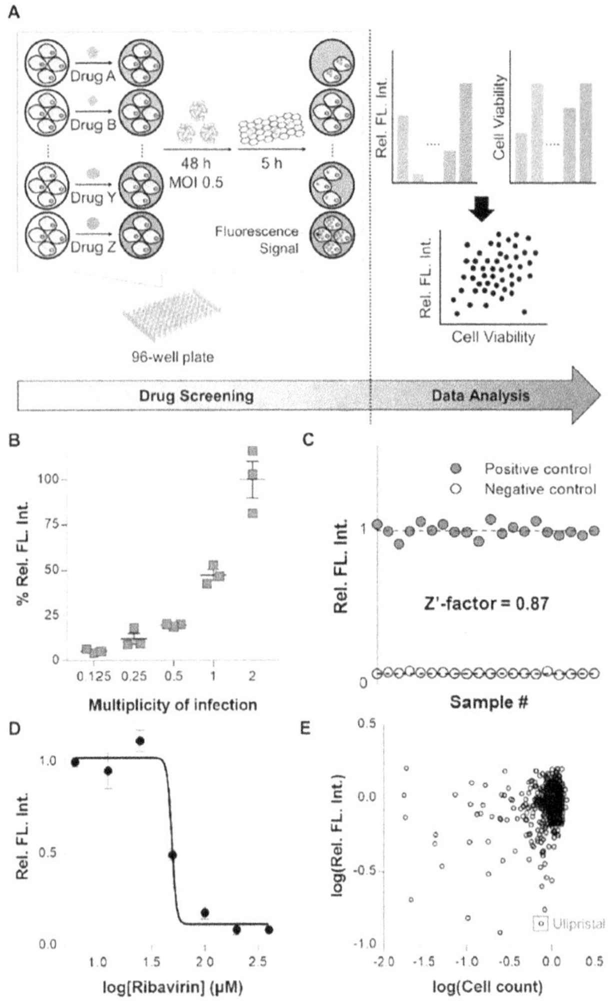

FIGURE 7.8 The application of the GOViRA platform to high-throughput DENV inhibitor screening: (a) Schematic illustration of the GOViRA system–based high-throughput screening timeline. (b) Relative quantification of the fluorescence signal with the increasing MOI. Values represent mean ± SEM (n = 3). (c) The Z′-factor was calculated for the high-throughput screening from 20 replicates of each control. (d) DENV infection assay against ribavirin with the GOViRA system. DENV-infected Vero E6 cells were treated with ribavirin concentrations ranging from 6.25 μM to 400 μM. After 48 h, the PNA–DRGON complex was treated, and DENV activity was determined. An estimated EC_{50} value against DENV serotype 2 for ribavirin was 49.2 ± 0.2 μM. Values represent mean ± SEM (n = 3). (e) A screen for anti-DENV agents was conducted. Cell viability and corresponding fluorescence intensity value for each drug are plotted.

activity was assessed by immunostaining with antibodies specific to the DENV E protein. As the number of foci decreased in a dose-dependent manner, FFA demonstrated that the compound does have an antiviral effect against DENV in the Vero E6 cells, and the half-effective concentration (EC_{50}) was 8.3 ± 0.1 μM [31]. The relative expression level of viral RNA confirmed that ulipristal was active against DENV and correlated with the FFA [31]. The cytotoxicity of the compound in the Vero E6 cells was determined by the CCK-8 assay. Ulipristal showed no impact on cell viability in the Vero E6 cells [31].

The antiviral activity of ulipristal using Huh7 (liver carcinoma cell line) and A549 (lung carcinoma cell line) cell lines has been further validated as hosts for the DENV infection. Both cell monolayers were analyzed with qRT-PCR to observe the relative DENV RNA level. The ulipristal treatment inhibited the DENV infection in both cell lines dose-dependently. Moreover, the fluorescence signal of the viral E protein from immunostaining also was reduced by the ulipristal treatment. The results [31] indicated that ulipristal effectively inhibits DENV infection *in vitro*.

7.3.4 Anti-DENV Effect of Ulipristal in Murine DENV Model

To confirm the antiviral activity of ulipristal in an *in vivo* DENV infection, this compound was evaluated in a murine DENV infection model. The DENV strain we used (KBPV-VR-29) has been reported as a mouse-adapted virus strain [32]. For the study, AG129 mice, deficient in the interferon (IFN)-α/β and γ receptors, were infected with the DENV by intraperitoneal injection at an exposure dose of 1 × 10^7 FFU, which shows lethality approximately within ~10 days. One hour after the infection, the animals were treated with ulipristal or vehicle over 14 days, and survival was monitored during that period. Ulipristal was given at a dose of 15 mg/kg every day through intraperitoneal injection. The dose was determined based on the reported rodent toxicity study and the results from the *in vitro* drug validation. It has been attempted to select a dose that would prevent toxicity but could achieve enough plasma concentration to observe an antiviral effect.

To examine whether ulipristal treatment can relieve the symptoms in the murine DENV model, the individual mouse was weighed and visually monitored for morbidity daily. Compared to the ulipristal-treated group, the control group exhibited a huge weight loss and disease symptoms, including ruffled fur, hunched posture, and decreased mobility. Ulipristal treatment in the infected mice also resulted in a statistically significant survival benefit (P = 0.0007) shown in the survival plot. Next, the systemic and local antiviral effect of ulipristal has been verified. On day 3 p.i., the ulipristal-treated group showed a significantly reduced viremia in the blood compared to that of the control group. To assess the local therapeutic effect, the viral RNA expression level in five representative organs (spleen, lung, liver, small intestine, and large intestine) and the tissue morphology was investigated. The viral RNA load in each organ of the ulipristal-administered mice was significantly decreased consistent with the viremia in the blood, although the differences between the viral RNA loads in the small intestine of the vehicle and ulipristal-treated groups were not statistically significant.

To further determine the histological differences, representative tissue samples from each group were examined. Hematoxylin and eosin (H&E)–stained sections of the spleen and liver from each group were analyzed. As shown in the uninfected control group, a normal spleen shows a distinguishable white-pulp and red-pulp structure, which is severely ruptured after the virus infection (DENV-infected, vehicle-treated group). It was observed that such a boundary loss was decreased in the ulipristal-treated group, indicating that the administration of ulipristal may relieve the virus infection–associated spleen damage. Moreover, several notable changes were also observed in the liver tissues as well. Pathological features of DENV infection include nuclear pleomorphism of hepatocytes, dilatation of sinusoids, and focal necrosis (labeled with black arrows). Compared to the control group, a significant reduction of such symptoms was observed in the ulipristal-treated group. Taken together, the overall data indicate that ulipristal may contribute to reducing the symptoms of DENV infection, resulting in a significant survival benefit *in vivo*.

In the murine DENV model, it has been reported that the viremia is very low on day 1 p.i., which gradually increases and reaches its peak level on day 3. Based on the viremia profile, the drug may function as an entry inhibitor by effectively blocking the initial process of infection. It is also suggested that serial treatment of ulipristal may prevent reinfection of newly produced DENV and relieve symptoms.

7.3.5 Mode of Action of Ulipristal Is Mediated by Inhibiting Viral Entry

A time-of-addition experiment was performed to determine which time point of the viral infection stage is affected by the administration of ulipristal. Because ulipristal is widely known as an SPRM compound, a cell line without PR expression has been chosen to exclude the influence of PR signaling on the time-of-addition experiment. PR expression was observed in three groups of A549 cells: no treatment (NT), vehicle treatment, and ulipristal treatment group. After 24 h of incubation, the RNA expression level of each group was analyzed. There was no PR expression in the NT group [31]. Additionally, the vehicle or ulipristal treatment did not influence the levels of PR expression in the A549 cells. Therefore, the mode of action of ulipristal has been examined using the A549 cell line.

A549 cells were treated with ulipristal in three different conditions: treatment before the infection (pre-treatment), treatment along with the infection (co-treatment), and treatment after the infection (post-treatment) [31]. The antiviral effect by the administration of the drug was observed in the pre-treatment and co-treatment groups. However, a less-inhibitory effect was observed when ulipristal was added after virus inoculation. Furthermore, the degree of inhibitory effect was decreased as the ulipristal administration was delayed [31]. Taken together, the inhibitory kinetics of ulipristal suggests that ulipristal inhibits viral infection at the entry stage of the DENV life cycle and acts as an endocytic inhibitor.

Ulipristal is an FDA-approved drug that has oral bioavailability and high tolerability [33]. This makes ulipristal a promising therapeutic candidate for DENV infection. It has recently been reported by the European Medicines Agency (EMA) that ulipristal may cause drug-induced liver injury (DILI) [34]. However, the hepatic safety of ulipristal was reported by a clinical development with over 1,800 patients in 2018 [35], and the mechanism of the DILI remains unsatisfactorily explained [34]. Therefore, not only further investigations on the mechanism of the DILI but also the risk–benefit assessment of ulipristal should be considered for clinical uses.

The development of novel antiviral treatments against numerous viral diseases is in high global demand. However, the difficulty of conventional antiviral drug development includes not only the expensive, laborious, and time-consuming process but also the uncertainty of success. The drug repurposing strategy with high-throughput screening could provide several advantages to overcome such issues. It has been one of the biggest obstacles of this approach that the simulated condition for the *in vitro* screening system could not perfectly mimic the complex and dynamic responses of the living organism in the presence of the drug. To address this challenge, the live cell-based GOViRA system can effectively identify the efficacy when the target viral disease is exposed to the compound within the context of a live cell, which is a more advanced feature compared to the conventional assay systems.

7.4 Carbon Nanomaterial and Its Derivatives as Nanobiosensors versus COVID-19

Tridimensional (3D) manufacturing has played a pivotal role in fighting the coronavirus disease (COVID-19) pandemic with innovatively designed products developed through the collaboration between health professionals, engineers, and creative. Examples of 3D-printed solutions established during the pandemic include valves for non-invasive ventilation respiratory supports, face shields, door handles, and COVID-19 lattice test swabs [36]. To achieve the best fit, the protective equipment has been produced using additive manufacturing combined after surface scanning of health workers' bodies; 3D printing comprises techniques of stereolithography, selective laser sintering, and fused deposition modeling. Undoubtedly, desktop 3D printers based on fused deposition modeling and melted thermoplastics are the most accessible and low-cost additive manufacturing technique.

Thermoplastic polymers (TP) are the most frequently utilized materials in additive manufacturing due to their low cost and low melting temperatures. TP includes acrylonitrile butadiene styrene (ABS), polylactic acid (PLA), polycarbonate (PC), and polyether ether ketone (PEEK).

Among these, PLA has generated significant interest for medical applications for its biocompatibility and biodegradability. PLA is the most used plastic in 3D printing since it melts easily compared to many fossil-based plastics, and thus, it is easier to print and is better-suited for parts with complex or fine details. PLA is also one of the most environmentally friendly 3D printing materials and, therefore, a promising biopolymer for medical research, capable of substituting conventional petroleum-based polymers due to recyclability and compostability. PLA degrades via hydrolysis to lactic acid, depending on pH, temperature, autocatalytic behavior, and degree of water contact.

In addition, PLA can be processed with various additive manufacturing methods [37]. Some drawbacks limit its use in medical device production, such as brittleness, poor thermal stability, low elongation at break and impact strength, and low heat-distortion temperature.

To improve PLA thermal and electrical conductivity and mechanical strength, additives such as cellulose, metals, and carbon nanoparticles have been experimented.

Among nanomaterials, graphene is a promising technology in the biomedical field due to several advantages. Graphene, a widely studied bidimensional carbon nanomaterial, and its derivatives possess pro-differentiating effects on eukaryotic cells (such as stimulation of bone/muscle tissue growth on 3D scaffolds [38]) and antibacterial properties even toward antibiotic-resistant species. Graphene has indeed high interaction with the microbial surface and can exert both a bacteriostatic and bactericidal effect, according to the damages that hydrophobic areas induce in bacterial outer membrane.

Graphene-family materials are also capable of reinforcing mechanical, optical, and thermal properties of 3D-printed constructs even in a small amount. These improvements, of great importance to produce many medical devices, can therefore be obtained at extremely low costs with low toxicity, making it an easy-to-implement strategy.

Several uses of graphene have been proposed during COVID-19 emergency: graphene field-effect transistor has been proposed for the development of a severe acute respiratory syndrome coronavirus-2 (SARS-CoV-2) diagnostic device [39], but also sensors and wearables [40].

COVID-19 is an infectious disease caused by the severe acute respiratory syndrome coronavirus-2 (SARS-CoV-2). COVID-19 was first reported in Wuhan, China, in December 2019 and spread rapidly across the world [41]. On March 11, 2020, the World Health Organization (WHO) declared the global spread of the novel coronavirus a pandemic and alerted the world to prepare for widespread community transmission [42]. Unfortunately, the transmission rate of SARS-CoV-2 is greater than that of the coronavirus for the severe acute respiratory syndrome (SARS) and the Middle East respiratory syndrome (MERS) in 2002 and 2012, respectively. COVID-19 was the leading cause of death in 2020, owing to the highly contagious and pathogenic coronavirus SARS-CoV-2. Although various vaccines have been developed and administered in various countries, the pandemic is still ongoing due to the emergence of multiple SARS-CoV-2 variants, particularly the Delta variant, which is much more transmissible. Up to July 31, 2021, there have been more than 197,252,280 confirmed COVID-19 cases globally, with 4,210,452 associated deaths [43].

The SARS-CoV-2 virus rapidly multiplies in the body tissues and triggers the immune system. The symptoms of COVID-19 may appear 2–14 days after exposure to the virus, ranging from mild fever to severe symptoms, requiring hospitalization, such as difficulty breathing or shortness of breath. To date, several biomarkers can be used for the detection of SARS-CoV-2: viral nucleic acid (single-stranded ribonucleic acid, RNA), viral protein antigen (spike (S) or nucleocapsid (N)), and antibodies (IgM, IgG, or IgA) [44]. In general, diagnostic tests for COVID-19 fall into two main categories: viral tests that detect viral nucleic acid and protein antigens, and serological tests that detect anti-SARS-CoV-2 immunoglobulins. The viral nucleic acid and antigen detection tests are used to assess the early stages of active infection, while the antibody tests provide evidence of the previous infection (recovery phase) [45].

Real-time reverse-transcription polymerase chain reaction (RT-PCR) targeting the SARS-CoV-2 RNA is the reference standard diagnostic test for COVID-19. The method is based on the reverse transcription of the viral RNA into complementary DNA (cDNA), followed by isothermally amplifying the specific regions of cDNA, and detection by quantitative RT-PCR. Although the RT-PCR test has high true positive and true negative detection rates, it is laborious, which leads to a long turnaround time from sample collection to test results. The lengthy RNA isolation step (which takes approximately 2–4 h) requires highly trained manpower. RT-PCR testing becomes challenging if there are reagent shortages and a large number of samples. PCR tests are therefore not suitable for remote or resource-limited settings. Moreover, false negatives may arise if the sample is collected before the onset of symptoms or due to inadvertent contamination of reagent or specimen.

To address these limitations, rapid diagnostic tests based on antigen or antibody detection in respiratory samples (e.g., sputum, saliva, and throat swab) or blood can provide timely detection at or near the point of care (POC), without the need for sophisticated laboratory facilities. These rapid tests have numerous benefits over the laboratory test, including rapidity of results (within 30 min), lower cost, ease of operation, and suitability for large-scale screening outside the laboratory without the need for specialist operators [46]. Rapid antigen test is useful for early detection of active infection with a high viral load of SARS-CoV-2. The viral antigen usually appears within a few days after the onset of symptoms, before the production of antibodies. A rapid antibody test is more suitable during the convalescent phase of the disease. The prevalence of antibodies in the human blood serum of individuals suspected of being infected with SARS-CoV-2 may take several days or weeks to develop after exposure to the virus. Immunoglobulin M (IgM) will be produced after three to six days of infection, and immunoglobulin G (IgG) will be detectable after eight days of infection. The Board Decision on Additional Support for Country Responses to COVID-19 has approved 47 and 48 types of rapid SARS-CoV-2 antibody and antigen diagnostic tests, respectively, for home use. However, although these rapid POC tests have high true negative rates, the true positive rates are lower than the RT-PCR test [47]. The WHO acceptable minimum true positive and true negative rates are 80% and 97%, respectively.

The coronavirus disease (2019) pandemic, caused by the rapid outbreak of severe acute respiratory syndrome coronavirus-2 (SARS-CoV-2), has claimed millions of lives worldwide. Scientists have developed various pharmaceutical and nonpharmaceutical measures to combat this pandemic. Among these, the development of effective vaccines, therapeutics, and fast and reliable diagnostic kits could aid immensely in managing the crisis. Nanotechnology has played a vital role during the pandemic. CNT-FET enables digital detection of the SARS-CoV-2 S1 antigens in saliva samples. Researchers utilized RNA hybridization as the initial signal generator, and the liquid-gated CNT network FET was used as the signal transducer. To develop this biosensor, commercially available SARS-CoV-2 S1 antigen has been used to analyze the electrical output of the CNT-FET biosensor. This technology can efficiently distinguish SARS-CoV-2 from other coronaviruses that contain SARS-CoV-1 S1 or MERS-CoV S1 antigen. Additionally, it has proved to be highly sensitive and can rapidly detect COVID-19 infection using saliva samples.

Biosensors, which satisfy the WHO's ASSURED criteria—affordable, sensitive, specific, user-friendly, rapid and robust, equipment-free, and deliverable to end users—are potential alternatives to the rapid POC antigen and antibody tests. A *biosensor* is an analytical device consisting of a biological element (e.g., nucleic acids, enzymes, antibodies, whole cells, or receptors) combined with a transducer for the detection of an analyte. The biological element binds the analyte of interest to the biosensor, and the transducer measures the interaction between the analyte and recognition element and converts the output to a measurable signal proportional to the analyte concentration. With the integration of a suitable microfluidic platform and necessary mechanical enclosure, a biosensor can be translated into a POC system, where sample collection and testing can be performed in the same device [48].

A variety of biosensors has been developed for real-time diagnosis of COVID-19, including surface plasmon resonance (SPR)–based biosensors, electrochemical biosensors, and field-effect transistor (FET)–based biosensors. These biosensors have been successfully tested in proof-of-concept studies. However, none of the sensors have been translated into a POC device for commercial use yet. In this chapter, we review the most recently developed SPR-based, electrochemical, and FET-based biosensors for SARS-CoV-2 detection. We explain how these sensors work, and discuss their advantages and limitations. Finally, we propose strategies to enhance the sensing performance of these biosensors to meet the WHO minimum requirement for true positive and negative detection rates.

With the evidence of recent pandemics and viral outbreaks, the viruses are considered a great peril to the health and well-being of humans, owing to the ravage that they cause on both health and the global economy alike. Additionally, the higher prevalence of these outbreaks can be attributed to the current improper detection tools employed for the detection of these infectious agents. Therefore, this demands a detection or diagnostic tool that is robust, rapid, selective, and accurate in its biosensing properties. *Biosensors* can be defined as analytical instruments that can assess very low concentrations of an analyte in biological samples (like the human serum, blood, tears, saliva, etc.). Compared to conventional qualitative and quantitative test kits, these biosensors are highly accurate, specific, and sensitive to the directed target. Generally, these biosensors comprise a biological element, like a microorganism, cell organelle, cellular receptor, enzyme, antibodies, nucleic acids, proteins, or any other such biological element that could potentially generate signals (like thermal, electrical, or optical signals). These signals are produced on the interaction of these biological elements with a tested element and a transducer, which further aids in converting these signals into a quantifiable electrical parameter. These measurement methods usually encompass special features for identifying and measuring these target analytes, owing to the utilization of distinct biological components. Several biosensors are currently being developed for a plethora of clinical and pharmaceutical applications. These utilities range from the early diagnosis and treatment of chronic disorders like diabetes and cancer to acute diseases like pathogen infestation. However, their pharmaceutical applications include drug discovery, assessment and measurement of drug metabolites, and drug activity. A more recent application of the same also provides the assessment of drugs in various biological samples and the preliminary diagnosis of disease by rapid and real-time tests.

In recent years, several novel biosensors have been employed in the detection of RNA viruses. The most prominent ones include aptamer-based biosensors, antigen Au/Ag-based electrochemical biosensors, CRISPR-Cas9-based paper strips, nucleic acid–based biosensors, optical biosensors, and surface plasmon resonance biosensors, to name a few. These biosensors could be potential instruments in providing a rapid, more accurate, compact, and much promising diagnostic tool in light of the World Health Organization's (WHO) test-test-test theme. Furthermore, the newer technologies, like aptamer-based bio-nanogate, DhITACT-TR chip-based biosensors, graphene field-effect transistor (FET)–based biosensors, nucleic acid hybridization, rapid-cum-portable RNA extraction preps, and surface plasmon–based (like quartz-crystal microbalance [QCM], surface-enhanced Raman scattering [SERS], and surface plasmon resonance [SPR] technologies) innovations could promote rapid, highly sensitive, and efficient solutions for better diagnosis and biosensing for COVID-19 or any further unprecedented outbreaks.

Although numerous biosensors have been developed and commercialized for regular use, they pose several downsides. These shortcomings have been studied to be eliminated by employing nanotechnology-based interventions that perform real-time direct detection of specific molecular targets. Thus, various nanomaterials, like carbon nanotubes (CNTs), quantum dots (QDs), gold (Au), and other metallic nanoparticles, are being complemented with several biosensors, owing to their characteristic features (physical, chemical, mechanical, electrical, magnetic, etc.), to accentuate the biosensing capability.

7.5 Smart Nanomaterials for Biosensing Technologies and Their Consequences

Metal and its oxides, carbon-based nanomaterials, transition metal dichalcogenide, quantum dots, polymer-based nanocomposites, and other nanomaterials are among the latest smart nanomaterials which are being widely used for biosensing applications for combating against SARS-CoV-2 infection (for various nanoparticles for combating against SARS-CoV-2, see Figure 7.9) [49]. The unique properties of these nanomaterials and their composites, such as small size, signal generation, quenching, and signal amplification, are significant for biosensors fabrication. Moreover, nanomaterials' surface, size, and shape equip biosensors with an enhanced limit of detection (LOD), sensitivity, and selectivity. Furthermore, the primary mechanism of biosensors fabricated from nano-based materials for advanced POCT (point-of-care tests) diagnostic techniques to detect the SARS-CoV-2 virus is demonstrated in Figure 7.10, proving nanomaterials can play a vital role for biosensing application for SARS-CoV-2 detection.

7.5.1 Metal and Its Oxides-Based Nanoparticles

Among the different types of metal nanoparticles, the biosensing of virus infections is majorly done by gold nanoparticles. They show excellent biocompatibility and enhanced loading capacity of bioanalyte and electrocatalytic properties. Moreover, significant

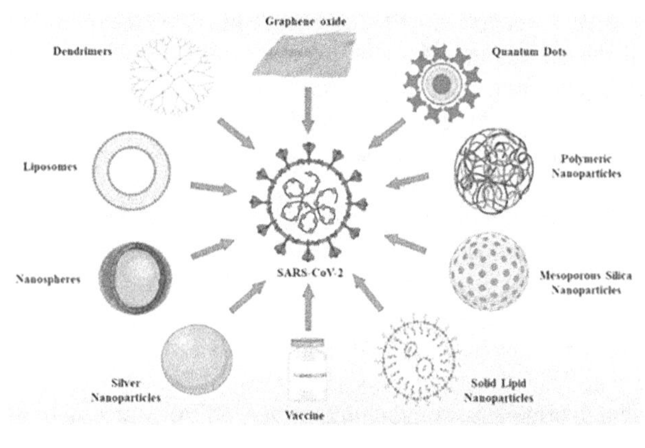

FIGURE 7.9 Various nanoparticles that are widely used for combating SARS-CoV-2 infection.

Source: [49].

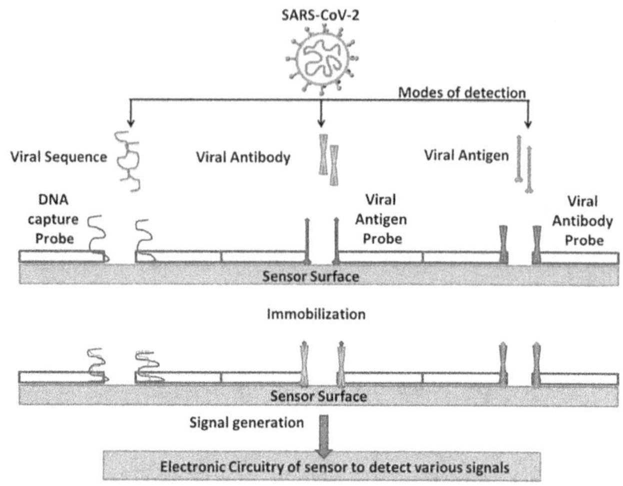

FIGURE 7.10 Schematic representation of the basic mechanism of nanomaterial-based biosensors for POCT of SARS-CoV-2 infection.

Source: [49].

work was done using gold nanoparticles to detect human samples, which detected the antigen within 30 min, and the obtained results were in complete agreement with WHO guidelines. Another work reported by Chen et al. using polystyrene nanoparticles doped with lanthanide to detect the anti-SARS-CoV-2 IgG in human serum gave very rapid detection within 10 min; the proposed mechanism of diagnosis obtained results that were comparable to the results obtained from the RT-PCR technique, making it a validated method for clinical purposes [50].

Similarly, different metal oxides are used to detect various analytes by the fabrication of sensors and biosensors. Further, silicon (Si)– and indium oxide–based nanowires are used as novel biosensing tools due to broaden the scope of detection compared to more simple optical methods, possibly due to the wide bandgap. Rashed et al. reported the fabrication of resistive immunosensors for SARS-CoV-2 antibody using gold (Au)–based electrodes, as Au nanoparticles are a safe choice, and when combined with various detection platforms, according to the need for analysis, by utilization as electrochemical sensors or biosensors, they are highly selective, specific, and sensitive. However, the efficiency of sensors gets affected not only by the properties of the substrate but also by the reproducibility of the deposited layer. Similarly, Bajo et al. analyzed the Au chip–based sensor by manipulating the unique properties of the Si substrate, functioning in three different operating modes: a sensor temperature, an electrical heater, and an electrochemical sensor for nucleic acids detection.

7.5.2 Transition Metal Dichalcogenides-Based Nanomaterials

Transition metal dichalcogenides (TMDCs) are known for their promising optical, electronic, mechanical, and magnetic properties [51]. Recently, they have emerged as excellent materials for biosensing due to the large bandgaps and better signal strength. Among the family of TMDCs, such as molybdenum diselenide ($MoSe_2$), molybdenum disulfide (MoS_2), tungsten diselenide (WSe_2), and tungsten disulfide (WS_2), MoS_2 gives unique properties, such as fast electron transfer rate, superior conductivity, and feasibility. They play a role in diverse applications, as it owns biocompatibility and stability. One study based on the use of FET-based TMDC WSe_2 acted as a promising biosensor for the ultrafast *in vitro* detection of SARS-CoV-2. Thus, a combination of efficient fabrication methods with the unique properties of MoS_2 provides exciting opportunities for multiple applications in electronic, optical, and electrochemical biosensors.

7.5.3 Quantum Dots-Based Nanomaterials

Quantum dots are tiny semiconductor nanocrystals and can convert light spectrum into various colors. They show excellent fluorescence, quantum confinement, and tunable band energy. The size of quantum dots ranges from 1 to 10 nm compared with tunable plasmonic nanoparticles (10–300 nm). Hence, for molecular imaging, quantum dots are proved as a novel fluorescent probe because quantum dots have received great attention for fighting against viral infection. Further, Łoczechin et al. investigated carbon-based quantum dots and identified them as an efficient virus-inactivation agent, with 50% efficiency. Another research showed that the graphitic carbon nitride–cadmium sulfide quantum dot nanocomposites could determine coronavirus-2 receptor–binding domain [52]. Moreover, carbon quantum dots have also proved to be predominant imaging probes (chemosensors and biosensors) for detecting microbes and viral molecules. Additionally, they can be used to label the virus's envelope, and novel fluorescent-based quantum dots may assist in developing several advanced diagnostic methods.

7.5.4 Polymer-Based Nanomaterials

Polymer-based nanomaterials are widely used for infectious disease diagnosis, and it is still evolving with time in the field of diagnostics. In the field of label-free sensing, molecularly imprinted polymers (MIPs) have gained much attention. MIPs are synthetic receptors synthesized with molecular recognition cavities complementary to the target molecule. They are ultrasensitive because of selectivity, thermal and mechanical stability, and electrical properties. According to previous research reports, it was found that MIPs have been used to detect many types of viruses, such as influenza virus, human immunodeficiency virus, hepatitis A and B virus, adenovirus, picornavirus, dengue virus, etc. For example, Raziq et al. developed the first-time electrochemical sensor to detect SARS-CoV-2 nucleoprotein from nasopharyngeal samples of COVID patients with an 11 fM LOD; the advantage of this diagnostic technique is its speed of the process of detection, along with detecting vital biomarkers [53]. Thus, MIP-based sensors are the future of upcoming sensor technology, as these sensors will be cost-effective, environmental-friendly, rapid, sensitive, selective, and specific.

7.5.5 Nanomaterial-Based Screen-Printed Electrode

To enhance electroanalytical performances and sensitivity, screen-printed electrodes (SPE) are easily modified with nanomaterials, such as graphene, carbon black, and Au nanoparticles. According to research, screen-printed graphene electrodes (SPGE) show superior electrochemical properties because of a higher electron transfer rate and a larger electrochemical surface area than other electrode-based materials. Further, a carbon-based three-electrode biosensor was developed to detect the SARS-CoV-2 virus. In another study, Au nanoparticle–based biosensing was done using SARS-CoV-2 monoclonal antibodies on the screen-printed electrodes to detect the SARS-CoV-2 virus from human saliva samples, and the obtained results from the device demonstrated LOD of 90 fM and 10–30 s response times. Further, another work was also conducted in which paper substrates were used for detecting the SARS-CoV-2 virus from the nasopharyngeal fluid samples, and it represented a LOD of 0.25 fg/mL [54].

7.6 Strategies to Enhance the Biosensor Performance

The accuracy of the reviewed biosensors in detecting negative samples is short of the WHO minimum of 97%. This can be improved by choosing biorecognition elements that are highly selective in binding with the target analytes; hence, cross-reactivity with unrelated molecules can be avoided to reduce false positives. Moreover, the true positive rate (ranging from 46.2% to 100%) of the biosensors do not all meet the WHO minimum of 80%. This can be improved by increasing the surface area of the sensor site using surface modification techniques to enhance the sensor sensitivity to a low concentration of bioanalytes. These enhancement strategies for COVID-19 biosensor performance are elaborated in the following sections.

7.6.1 Potential Biorecognition Elements

In general, the detection technique used in biosensors can be classified as labelled or label-free. Labelled biosensors commonly rely on specific labels, such as enzymes (e.g., horseradish peroxidase [HRP], alkaline phosphatase [ALP]), fluorescent molecules, or electroactive compounds, to detect analytes. The label helps in signal amplification and increase sensing selectivity, but at the same time, it increases the overall sensor cost and response time. On the other hand, label-free biosensors rely on biorecognition elements to directly detect different types of analyte targets ranging from proteins to DNA and viruses. There is a wide range of biorecognition elements—such as enzyme, antibody, nucleic acid, aptamers, molecularly imprinted polymers—with unique characteristics for the interaction with a specific target of interest [55].

In COVID-19 biosensors, antibodies and nucleic acid probes are the most common biorecognition elements used for recognizing SARS-CoV-2 biomarkers (e.g., viral proteins, human immunoglobulins, or viral RNA) through the formation of antigen–antibody immunocomplex and single-stranded-DNA/oligonucleotide complementary strands complexes, respectively.

In general, monoclonal antibodies are preferred for assay involving binding of a specific antigen. These antibodies are specific to a single epitope of a target molecule, but a slight change in conformation may lead to a dramatically reduced binding capacity. However, an alternative approach known as antibody phage display can be employed, where the monoclonal antibodies can be engineered to improve binding affinity with specific viral markers [56]. The conventional method of producing monoclonal antibodies requires expensive experimentation with animals and labor-intensive procedures. Besides high cost, the antibodies have a limited lifespan and are susceptible to high temperature.

Alternatively, high-affinity and high-specificity aptamers have emerged as a substitute to monoclonal antibodies as biorecognition elements in biosensing. Aptamers are artificial single-stranded RNA or DNA oligonucleotides that can be chemically synthesized by an in vitro selection process called systematic evolution of ligands by exponential enrichment (SELEX). Similar to antibodies, aptamers can bind specifically to the target based on structural recognition. Furthermore, aptamers offer many advantages over antibodies, including smaller size, long shelf life, and stable to changes in pH, temperature, and ionic strength. Compared to antibodies, aptamers have a much lower molecular weight (6–30 KDa, 2 nm) than antibodies (150–180 kDa, 15 nm), which allows them to bind with a wide range of potential targets, such as ions, small molecules, viruses, and proteins [57]. Aptamers also have high thermal stability (up to 95°C), and they are suitable for repeated use as they can be regenerated easily after denaturation. In particular, when used as a biorecognition element in FET biosensors, the smaller size and compact structure of the aptamers allow the binding event to take place within the Debye length, thus overcoming the Debye length limitation. The bound targets are located closer to the sensor surface, and therefore, stronger electrical signal is transduced from the binding event.

Phosphorodiamidate morpholino oligomers (PMO) are uncharged analogues of nucleic acids. Compared to natural nucleic acid probes, the PMO probe offers better stability and higher binding strength, owing to its neutral character. RNA and DNA probes are negatively charged in physiological conditions due to their phosphate groups on the nucleic acid backbone. Therefore, electrostatic repulsion exists between the highly negative charged probe and target sequence, which decreases the hybridization efficiency. Hence, RNA and DNA probes require high-ionic-strength conditions to shield their intermolecular repulsive force for hybridizations. However, PMO probes have no net charge and they are insensitive to the ionic strength of the buffer, so they can retain their excellent binding affinity to target nucleic acid under the condition of low or high ionic strength.

7.6.2 Potential Nanomaterials for Sensor Surface Modification

With the rapid development of nanotechnology in the past few years, various nanomaterials, such as gold nanoparticles, graphene, and carbon nanotubes, have been widely used in the design of biosensors as transduction substrates to enhance sensing performance. Nanomaterial characteristics, such as nanoscale size, larger surface area, and higher conductivity, aid in signal amplification. Besides that, the inherent large surface areas of nanomaterials can enhance the loading effect caused by the bioreceptor, thereby improving the sensitivity and stability of the biosensor.

In SPR-based sensors, metal nanoparticles (e.g., gold nanoparticles) have been commonly incorporated on the sensor surface. As nanoparticles possess unique physical, electronic, and chemical properties, large surface area, and high free surface energy, biomolecules (e.g., antibody) are strongly adsorbed onto the surface. This improved the SPR detection limit from the nM range to the pM range. The sensitivity improvement by nanomaterials also depends on the type of structures, such as nanoshells, nanospheres, nanorods, and nanowires. Compared to other shapes, high-aspect-ratio nanorods (NRs) offer a higher sensitivity to refractive index changes [58]. When NRs are used in a sandwich assay format, concentrations in the fM range can be detected. In another strategy, dual nanomaterials (e.g., NRs and quasi-spherical nanoparticles [qsNPs]) have yielded attomolar range (aM) detection, which is about a tenfold enhancement in sensitivity compared to sensor employing a single type of nanoparticles.

In addition, two-dimensional materials, such as graphene, are widely used in SPR, FET, and electrochemical-based biosensors. The high surface-area-to-volume ratio and carbon-based ring structures of graphene enhance the adsorption of biorecognition elements onto the sensor surface [59]. Adding graphene-based materials on the gold film of SPR sensors allows detection down to fg/mL of mass change [60]. Graphene and reduced graphene oxide possess excellent electronic properties, which allow them to be used as sensor surface material in FET and electrochemical sensors. Due to the excellent electronic and adsorption properties of these materials, the LOD of the FET biosensor reported in [59] is 1 fM and 10 fM for the detection of the Japanese encephalitis and avian influenza virus, respectively. However, graphene yields a small current on–off ratio in FETs, which limits its sensitivity. A large on–off ratio is required to reduce static leakage current for the sensor. To achieve this, two-dimensional semiconducting transition metal dichalcogenides (TMDCs) (e.g., molybdenum disulfide [MoS_2] nanoflakes, tungsten disulfide [WS_2] nanosheets) and black phosphorus (BP) can be explored. TMDCs have a larger bandgap than graphene and excellent characteristics, such as large surface area and high electron transfer. BP has adjustable bandgap value and high carrier mobility [61].

7.7 Emerging Nanomaterials-Based Biosensor for SARS-CoV-2 Detection

Severe acute respiratory syndrome coronavirus-2 (SARS-CoV-2) is a primary cause of the COVID-19 pandemic. To date, various detection approaches are already present, and many other techniques are also being developed for the rapid and real-time detection of COVID-19 infection in the wake of this pandemic. Hence, this featured review will provide an overview of COVID-19, its biomarkers, current diagnostic techniques, and emerging smart nanomaterials-based biosensing approaches; apart from this, it will also extend some light on future perspectives of biosensing technologies for SARS-CoV-2 diagnosis.

Severe acute respiratory syndrome coronavirus-2 (SARS-CoV-2) is a large coronavirus family; currently, the major cause of global pandemic threats to public health and this virus belongs to the Coronaviridae family [62]. Family Coronaviridae of coronavirus contains a single non-segmented, single-stranded ribonucleic acid (ssRNA) genome of vertebrates. Further, the World Health Organization (WHO), after detection of rare ribonucleic acid (RNA) sequences of SARS-CoV-2, confirmed that the infection is caused by the SARS-CoV-2 virus. Apart from this, it is well-known that the RNA virus can be detected through real-time polymerase chain reaction (RT-PCR) techniques based on nucleic acid amplification test, which possesses some very promising characteristics, like low detection limits and higher sensitivity, but the major drawback of this technique is its bit longer time for detection, which needs to be figured out for developing rapid diagnostic technique. Further, looking at the current pandemic scenario, researchers have extensively worked on many aspects of the RT-PCR technique to make it highly specific toward the SARS-CoV-2 virus by determining its specific targets.

According to current trends in research and development, the latest growth in nanobiotechnology gave rise to excellent diagnostic and therapeutic approaches, and advancements in biosensing techniques due to the utilization of nanomaterials as a matrix for fabricating biosensors provide them higher sensitivity, specificity, and selectivity, owing to unique properties of these nanomaterials, namely, high adsorption capacity, high surface area, high reactivity, and quantum size, which have drawn much attention toward utilization of nanomaterials for fabricating advanced biosensors. Additionally, the shape and size of nanomaterials can easily be engineered by surface modification or immobilization via covalent and non-covalent bonding with various biological species (enzymes, antibodies, etc.), which in turn help them for biosensing applications, as it offers nanomaterials high selectivity, high sensitivity, and lower detection limit toward the sample analytes [50]. Thus, a biosensor fabricated from smart nanomaterial makes the detection simple, effective, real-time, and economical, getting much attention nowadays as a rapid and effective technique for the

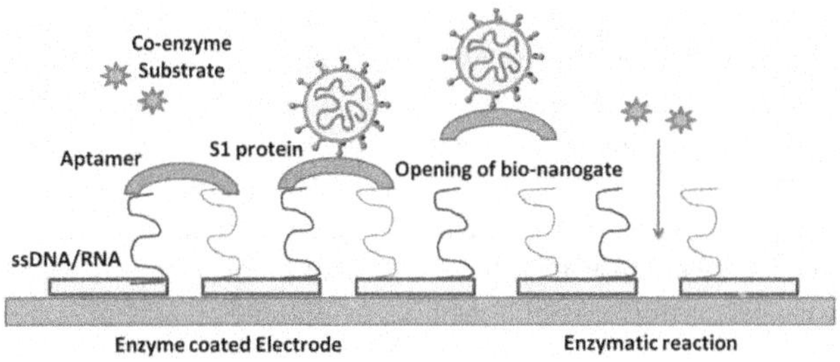

FIGURE 7.11 The basic working mechanism of bionanogate bifunctional aptamer–based biosensors for SARS-CoV-2 diagnosis.

Source: [64].

real-time quantitative and qualitative diagnosis of infectious diseases [63]. Therefore, biosensors have added advantages for identifying RNA viruses, by utilizing aptamer-conjugated nanoparticles (for working mechanism, see Figure 7.11), Au-Ag-based nanoparticles, CRISPR-Cas9-based paper strip, and surface plasmon resonance electrochemical biosensors, which serve as an efficient tool for more promising and portable diagnosis of SARS-CoV-2 [64]. Hence, this featured review intends to highlight the different smart and emerging nanomaterials used to detect SARS-CoV-2. Additionally, current diagnostic strategies, biomarkers, and future perspectives are discussed to illuminate this topic.

7.7.1 Carbon Nanotubes-Based Nanomaterials

Carbon nanotubes (CNTs) are hexagonal arrangements of carbon atoms that have a diameter of 1 nm and length ranging from 1 to 100 µm. There are two types: single-walled nanotubes (SWCNTs) and multi-walled nanotubes (MWCNTs). Notably, the structure of SWCNTs is similar to those of graphite, whose chemical bonding is constituted entirely of sp^2 bonds. This bonding structure has even higher strength than the sp^3 bonds found in diamond and provides CNTs with their exceptional strength, flexibility, and resistance to fracture. In addition, CNTs exhibit excellent electrical properties. They behave as metals or semiconductors, depending on tube diameter and the chirality.

CNTs are synthesized by three major techniques, including the carbon arc discharge technique, laser ablation technique, and the chemical vapor deposition (CVD) technique. Notably, etching agents, such as CO_2 and H_2O, are necessary components for aerosol synthesis of CNTs. It was reported that adding small amounts of CO_2 and H_2O vapor into the reactor could extend the length of synthesized CNTs. Methods affected by these etching agents include Fe particle's vapor nucleation and thermal decomposition of ferrocene vapor. In another study, laser ablation synthesis by a double-pulse Nd:YAG (neodymium-doped yttrium aluminum garnet) laser is a solid-state laser in which Nd:YAG is used as a laser medium. These lasers have many different ways performed at optimal wavelengths of 355 or 1,064 nm to synthesize CNTs.

Carbon nanotubes (CNTs) are rolled cylindrical structures made from graphene sheets with few nanometers; they show outstanding mechanical, electronic, and thermal properties [49, 65], making them a suitable choice for the development of biosensors. L. Pinals et al. developed a rapid identification system using a near-infrared mechanism by utilizing CNTs to detect the SARS-CoV-2 spike protein [66]. Another work by Aasi et al. evaluated single-walled CNTs decorated with metals for adsorption of H_2O_2 for designing inhibition surfaces to inactivate virus. Additionally, due to the metallic properties exhibited by CNTs, CNT-based sensors demonstrate excellent potential for overcoming the drawbacks of carrier migration in graphene-based sensors. Furthermore, the incorporation of metallic nanoparticles or small aromatic molecules (by covalent functionalization) in CNT-based sensors helps enhance the stability and reproducibility of sensors.

7.7.2 Graphene and Its Derivatives

Graphene is composed of a single layer of sp^2-hybridized carbon atoms arranged in a honeycomb structure with the C–C bond exhibiting a length of 0.142 nm. It is considered as a wonder material due to its impressive physical properties, such as large surface area, high electrical conductivity, high thermal conductivity, and exceptional mechanical stiffness. Graphene derivatives are graphene with chemical modification, which are to meet the needs of specific interests. Graphene oxide (GO) is one of the most studied derivatives that contain carbon–oxygen bonds, such as hydroxyl, carbonyl, and carboxyl groups. Different from graphene, GO is highly hydrophilic and more important for biomedical applications.

Graphene may be synthesized by various methods, including exfoliation, along with cleavage of natural graphite, CVD, plasma-enhanced CVD (PE-CVD), electric arc discharge, micro-mechanical exfoliation of graphite, epitaxial growth at electrical insulating surfaces, opening up CNTs and reduction of GO using various solutions. For plasma-enhanced chemical vapor deposition, methane is an effective H_2 source for high-quality graphene synthesis and saturates the nucleation density when the plasma power is above 120 W.

GO is synthesized by the oxidation of graphite via the addition of various chemicals, such as potassium chlorate plus nitric acid (Brodie and Staudenmaier method) or potassium permanganate plus sulfuric acid (Hummers method). A study showed that GO could be synthesized from natural flake graphite using the Hummers method (liquid oxidation, followed by chemical reduction, with NH_3H_2O aqueous solution and hydrazine hydrate).

Graphene is an excellent nanomaterial and shows properties like thermal conductivity, chemical stability, strength, flexibility, etc. It also provides good support for immobilizing ligands due to modifiable functional groups in its 2D plane [67]. Seo et al. fabricated a FET-based biosensor using a coating of graphene sheet for detection using specific antibodies.

Similarly, another study based on field-effect Au-decorated graphene nanosensors is developed to quickly identify the SARS-CoV-2 virus using clinical throat swab samples [68]. Zhang et al. fabricated an immunosensor using the combination of graphene–FET with antigen–antibody interaction that can give real-time detection by interacting with SARS-CoV-2 spike protein [69]. Further, it has been investigated from the current research that graphene and its derivatives are identified as essential materials because of their high conductivity and good biocompatibility, which makes them a better candidate for advanced biosensing applications for POCT.

Graphene and its derivatives were found as promising materials to help deal with the daily challenges posed by COVID-19 and related future diseases. Graphene is the thinnest two-dimensional (2D) atomic material that has emerged as a revolutionary material due to its high specific surface area and superior mechanical, electrical, optical, and thermal properties. Due to its unique properties, graphene has been applied in many applications, including sensors, biomedical aids, and membranes [70]. On top of that, graphene is acknowledged as having superior antibacterial and antiviral properties due to the movement of electron toward bacteria, which induces cytoplasmic efflux, decreases metabolism, affects lipid membrane, causes oxidative stress, produces reactive oxygen species (ROS), and finally, destroys the bacteria [71]. It is claimed that lipid bilayer of feline coronavirus is adsorbed on the surface of graphene via hydrogen bonding and electrostatic interactions. Of all the graphene derivatives, graphene oxide (GO) is the most negatively charged material which has higher affinity for positively charged viruses. Eventually, the binding of graphene destroyed the viral membrane and confirmed the effectiveness of graphene against viruses [71]. Coronavirus disease-2019 (COVID-19) has been a world pandemic since December 2019 caused by the severe acute respiratory syndrome coronavirus-2 (SARS-CoV-2) (Figure 7.12) [72].

Motivated by various properties of CNTs, research toward applying carbon nanotubes for biomedical applications has been progressing rapidly. CNT-based sensors have been developed to detect biological species, including proteins and DNA. Relying on their optical properties, SWNTs can be utilized as optical tags or contrast agents for various biological imaging techniques [73]. Many authors have shown that properly functionalized CNTs are able to enter cells without toxicity, shuttling various biological molecular cargoes into cells. The latest study has shown the promise of using CNTs for *in vivo* cancer treatment in a mouse model. However, despite these exciting findings, researchers have reported the negative sides of CNTs, showing that non-functionalized nanotubes are toxic to cells and animals [74]. The biodistribution and long-term fate of CNTs have been explored by us and several different groups, with different results obtained using different methods

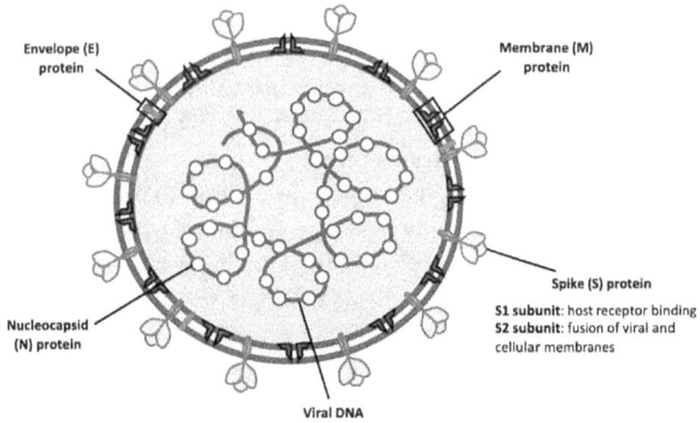

FIGURE 7.12 Illustrations of SARS-CoV-2.

and materials. These controversial findings require clarification in order to avoid confusion to the public of CNTs, showing that non-functionalized nanotubes are toxic to cells and animals [74,75]. The biodistribution and long-term fate of CNTs have been explored by us and several different groups, with different results obtained using different methods and materials. These controversial findings require clarification in order to avoid confusion to the public.

7.7.2.1 SPR/LSPR Biosensor for COVID-19

Surface plasmon resonance (SPR) and localized surface plasmon resonance (LSPR) biosensor technologies have been explored for detecting the SARS-CoV-2 virus. Recent reports on these types of sensors show promising sensitivity with fast and reliable detection. In one of the recent works, a two-dimensional heterostructure, $PtSe_2$/graphene, was attached to the gold film of the SPR sensor—the sensor configuration is shown in Figure 7.13a. The sensing region comprises three different ligand–analyte modes: (1) the monoclonal antibodies (mAbs) as ligand and the SARS-CoV-2 virus spike RBD as analyte, (2) the virus spike RBD as ligand and the virus anti-spike protein (IgM, IgG) as the analyte, and (3) the specific RNA probe as ligand and the virus single-stranded RNA as analyte [76]. The sensor employed BK_7-type prism glass, which generates stronger surface plasmon waves at the metal-dielectric interface. The heterostructure ($PtSe_2$/graphene) provided an increased surface area for better adsorption of the target analyte and hence enhanced sensitivity of the sensor. Graphene's high conductivity, large surface area, and chemical stability improved interaction between the target analyte and the ligand. It was observed that the sensitivity tend to increase by $(1 + 0.55) \times L$ times for an increase of L number of graphene layers [76]. Using multiple graphene layers is promising in detecting different analytes, such as virus spike RBD, antibodies (IgG or IgM), and viral RNA with a detection sensitivity of 183.33° RIU^{-1}, 153.85° RIU^{-1}, and 140.35° RIU^{-1} in SPR angle, respectively.

SPRi-based biosensors for detecting SARS-CoV-2 have also been developed. These sensors follow the principles of SPR and have been utilized to study binding kinetics between biomolecular species in the past. SPRi assay was used for quantitative measurement of IgG, IgM, and IgA antibodies binding to the RBD spike protein in serum sample [77]. RBD is an ideal target for blocking and neutralization therapies. This is because viral infection occurs when the S protein on SARS-CoV-2 recognizes and binds to the ACE2 receptor on the human host cell through its RBD. Hence, this assay is ideally suited for monitoring the concentration of anti-RBD antibodies of both COVID-19 patients and healthy people who are vaccinated against SARS-CoV-2.

Qiu and coworkers [78] demonstrated photothermal-assisted plasmonic sensing (PTAPS) for SARS-CoV-2 detection. Their biosensing device, as shown in Figure 7.13b, utilizes LSPR for the detection of unamplified SARS-CoV-2 [78]. Two-dimensional gold nano-islands (AuNI) played the roles of nanoabsorber, nanoheater, and nanotransducer. In this dual-functional system, AuNI functionalized with cDNA receptors were used to detect SARS-CoV-2 RNA through nucleic

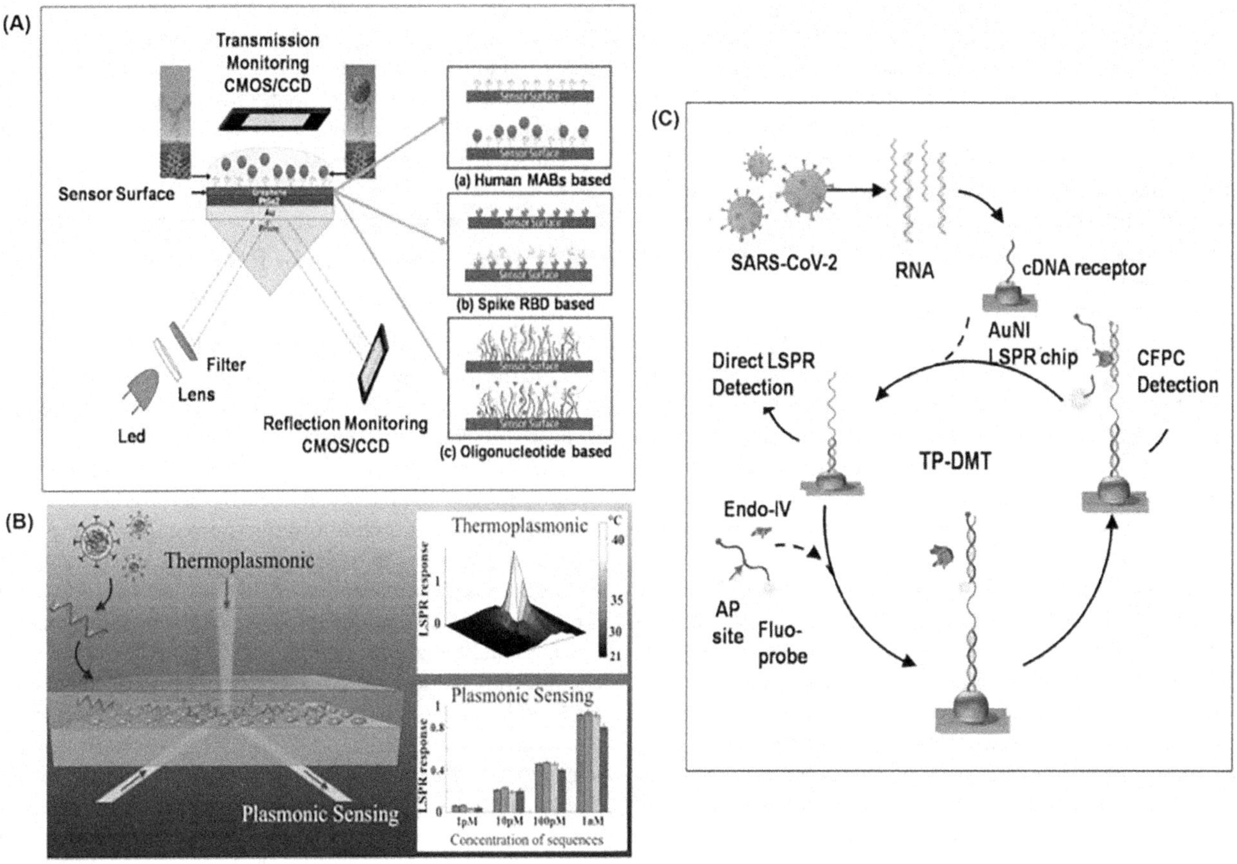

FIGURE 7.13 SPR and LSPR biosensor for SARS-CoV-2 detection: (a) Graphene-based multiple-layer coated (Bk_7/Au/$PtSe_2$/Graphene) SPR biosensor [76]. (b) Dual-functional PPT-enhanced LSPR biosensing system [78]. (c) Thermoplasmonic-assisted dual-mode transducing (TP-DMT) biosensing system [79].

acid hybridization. The entire AuNI sensing surfaces functionalized with a sufficient amount of thiol-cDNA receptor increased sensitivity and inhibit non-specific binding. Non-radiative decay of the resonantly excited LSPs produces heat that is localized near the AuNI. This plasmonic photothermal (PPT) effect aids the in situ hybridization of the RdRp-COVID sequence and its cDNA for SARS-CoV-2 detection. With the use of localized PPT heating, false positive is minimized, as the imperfectly matched sequences have difficulty remaining attached to the probe. This LSPR sensor has a detection limit of 0.22 ± 0.08 pM but is highly specific in discriminating the SARS-CoV-2 sequence from similar RdRp-SARS sequence.

Qiu et al. [79] extended the previous PTAPS method by introducing a novel concept of thermoplasmonic-assisted dual-mode transducing (TP-DMT), as shown in Figure 7.13c. This dual-mode system combines (1) an amplification-free direct viral RNA detection and (2) an amplification-based cyclic fluorescence probe cleavage (CFPC) detection to provide self-validating biosensing readout for quantifying the SARS-CoV-2 sequences within 30 min. The first LSPR signal was based on the hybridization between the target viral sequences and the functionalized thiol-DNA receptors. The amount of captured sequence is directly proportional to the virus concentration in the sample, and the limit of detection (LOD) was as low as 0.1 ± 0.04 pM. In the CFPC detection, endonuclease IV (site-specific nuclease) was utilized to cleave the apurinic/apyrimidinic (AP) site–modified fluorescent probe from the target viral sequence under local PPT heating. The released fluorescent probe was used to quantify the concentration of the virus, which improved the LOD to 0.275 ± 0.051 femtomolar (fM). This dual-mode sensing method employed two interdependent yet different tests on the AuNI chip and provides two sensitive readouts of viral sequence to yield remarkably low limits of detection in pM and fM, respectively. When the final readout of the direct viral hybridization detection exhibited a weak response, the CFPC method was used for verification, and it could even detect a trace amount of virus in the sample.

7.7.2.2 Advantages and Limitations

The SPR-based biosensors we have reviewed for SARS-CoV-2 detection have good sensitivity and reusability. However, they lack selectivity, and the refractive indexes of the biosensors are also affected by temperature, non-specific or specific adsorption on the sensor surface, and changes in buffer concentrations. Hence, the sensor surface needs to be modified with a ligand (e.g., antibody, DNA probe) to selectively capture the target analyte.

On the other hand, SPR-based biosensors allow the integration of nanostructures or nanoparticles to enhance detection sensitivity [80]. The extent of improvement depends strongly on the shape of the nanostructure and the type of metal used. As mentioned in the previous section, two-dimensional heterostructure [76] and AuNIs [78,79] attached to the gold film in the sensor exhibited maximum sensitivity of 200° RIU^{-1} and detection of sample analytes at an ultra-low concentration in the range of pM and fM, respectively. SPR-based sensors allow the tailoring of the sensing medium to improve sensor performance and sensitivity by using multi-layers for the medium or altering the medium thickness.

However, plasmonic virus detection from clinical specimens is still limited due to surface fouling of the receptor surface and interference of non-specific bindings. Surface fouling limits the application of plasmonic biosensors by blocking recognition element immobilization and specific binding. It can be prevented by selecting the appropriate sample dilution ratio or the design of ultra-low fouling surfaces with anti-fouling strategies using polymer-based surface chemistry or zwitterionic technology.

Biosensors with good reusability are highly desirable because it lowers the cost per test. The solvent environment is a key parameter that determines the binding of antibody–antigen. The reversible non-covalent interaction between antibody and antigen can be disrupted by high salt concentration, extreme pH, and detergents. Hence, chemical regeneration is the most widely used approach to regenerate the sensor by chemically altering the solvent environment with a regeneration solution (e.g., acid/base, detergent, glycine, or urea). SPR sensor could be chemically regenerated for SARS-CoV-2 detection.

7.7.3 Nanodiamonds

Nanodiamonds (NDs) are monocrystalline forms of diamond with a particle size below 100 nm. They consist of a diamond core and amorphous carbon layers. In the core, there are sp^3 C–C bonds, while the surface of NDs is covered by sp^2 C–C bonds. The most unique feature of NDs is the existence of various oxygenic functional groups on the surface; thus, NDs can disperse uniformly and stably in water. Other unique properties of NDs are high stability, high strength, good thermal conductivity, high refractive index, and enhanced resistivity [18]. In the last decade, researchers also discovered fluorescent NDs by generating point defects in the diamond structure (i.e., color centers). For example, Vlasov et al. generated a silicon vacancy in the 1.6 nm NDs to provide the stable fluorescence emission.

NDs are mainly synthesized by detonation events. However, there are also other synthesis methods, such as high-energy ball milling of pressurized high-temperature diamond microcrystals, plasma-assisted CVD, laser ablation, ion irradiation using graphite, and ultrasound cavitation. Detonation events of explosives (60/40 ratio of TNT/hexogen) in a steel chamber of 1.6 m^3 have led to the synthesis of black-powdered product containing NDs and other substances like graphite and amorphous carbon. Structural characterization by various techniques, such as X-ray diffraction spectroscopy, energy-dispersive spectroscopy, transmission electron microscopy at high resolutions, Fourier transform infrared spectroscopy, Raman spectroscopy, and differential scanning calorimetry, are critical for determining the efficiency of ND synthesis. Another study used high-energy Kr ion irradiation (350 ± 50 MeV Kr ions) of fine-grained polycrystalline using an Argonne tandem linear accelerator system (ATLAS) and acid dissolution to produce NDs at room temperature.

7.8 Carbon Nanotubes in Protection and Biosensing Applications

At the outset, the specific properties of the carbon nanotubes (CNTs), like the chemical, electrical, mechanical, and thermal characteristics, open new horizons for scientific development in nearly all fields of science. In the field of biosensors, the clinical and pharmaceutical utility of the CNTs is significant, as they play an essential part in the development of biosensors, primarily for the detection of target molecules when present in trace quantities within biological fluids. This characteristic of CNTs is attributed to their higher surface-area-to-volume ratio, low density, fine pore size, flexibility, high mechanical strength, and the ability to transmit the generated physical or chemical interactions. These CNTs are also resistant to most acids and bases, resistant to respiratory droplets, able to create reactive oxygen species (ROS), and biologically compatible with various drugs [81]. The CNTs also comprise covalent bonds (sp^2 + sp^3 hybrid phases), accounting for exceptional electrical conductivity. The single-walled carbon nanotubes (SWCNTs) and multi-walled carbon nanotubes (MWCNTs) are studied to be folded graphene sheets with lengths ranging from ~50 to 1,000 nm and diameters of ~5–20 nm. These factors thus deem SWCNTs as a favorable nanoparticle for detecting, filtering, and the inactivation of biological agents. Their use has been employed in diagnosis, viral protein detection, and drug delivery modalities for fighting viruses like influenza, SARS-CoV-1, SARS-CoV-2, and HIV [81].

The CNTs functionalized with antibodies have been created to detect a plentitude of viral proteins. Recent studies have also claimed the utility of a specific RNA lyase–coupled acidified CNTs with a photothermal conversion effect as a probable inhibitor for SARS-CoV-2 [81]. Yang et al. demonstrated the acid sensitivity of coronaviruses toward acidic and higher-temperature environments (above 56°C for more than 30 min). Thus, CNTs fabricated by acidizing, followed by conjugating a special RNA lyase to exploit the capacity of photothermal conversion, may prove to be a potential toolkit in the illumination and inhibition of SARS-CoV-2 [283].

Further studies by Yeh et al. fabricated a size-adjustable micromachine on the multi-walled carbon nanotubes (MWCNTs) for the label-free detection and quantification of the avian influenza virus. This intratubular spacing between the MWCNTs was tailored between 17 nm and 325 nm for allowing size-based viral entrapment [82]. A study conducted by Wasik et al. manufactured and demonstrated the utility of a chemiresistive biosensor in the detection of dengue virus based on a heparin-functionalized SWCNT network. Additionally, as the SARS-CoV-2 spike (S) protein experiences a conformational shift around its receptor-binding domain on interaction with heparin, which directs the utility of these heparin-functionalized CNTs in developing potent SARS-CoV-2 therapies.

Furthermore, the CNT-based filters were stated to be practical in removing pathogens. A study conducted by Vecitis et al. has demonstrated the utility of MWCNT as an anodic filter for the inactivation and removal of the bacteria (*E. coli*) and virus (bacteriophage MS2). Moreover, Németh et al. have inspected the removal of the MS2 bacteriophages from contaminated water using the inorganic nanoparticle–conjugated MWCNT hybrid membranes. These studies unraveled that the Cu_2O nanoparticle-coated MWCNT was highly efficient and removed the bacteria and viruses with ≥99.99% efficiency. Another study by Viswanathan et al. demonstrated the extrapolation of the MWCNTs as aerosol filters. The filtration quality of the MWCNT-coated cellulose fiber filters outperformed that of the cellulose filters. In a clinical setting, this salient feature could be employed in a multitude of ways, including limiting the virus transmission and bioaerosol sampling to characterize the community-wide transmission [81].

In addition, the SWCNTs have been studied for manufacturing fabrics with breathable protective layers. Bui et al. created a composite material with the vertically SWCNTs implanted in the parylene-N polymer. This SWCNT–polymer composite is an ultrabreathable and protective membrane due to a better water flow rate in the nanotube cores. Additionally, their distinct inner diameters and by size exclusion principle, the SWCNTs provide a significant level of defense from biothreats. Moreover, the nanoparticles could be coated as a layer on the protective garments to trap the pathogenic microbes. Thus, the CNTs can be coated on personal protective equipment (PPEs) to decrease the spread of the SARS-CoV-2 infection [81]. A UV irradiation has reportedly inactivated the coronaviruses at 254 nm and thermal treatment at 56°C for 30 mins, which facilitates achieving a state of photodynamic hyperthermia. However, owing to the exceptional nIR absorption behavior and photothermal conversion efficiency of the CNTs, they experience a rapid increment in temperatures greater than 51°C, which aids in achieving the state of photodynamic hyperthermia. These outstanding features could have profound applicability in both sterilizations of the infected protective equipment and PPEs functionalized with CNTs, as well as several theranostic applications [81].

Additionally, Lee et al. have developed a CNT face mask filter that demonstrates strong uniform hydrophobicity, high durability, high thermal conductivity, while exhibiting excellent barrier and antiviral effects against the COVID-19 virus. Their exceptional barrier and filter functions can be attributed to the uniformity, strength, and durability of the CNTs. They also investigated that the pore size of the CNT network is smaller than the average size of a SARS-CoV-2, thereby filtering it without impeding the breathability that was found equivalent to a conventional polypropylene filter. The simplistic processability, feasibility, and light weight of the aerosol-synthesized CNT filters underscore its practicality, especially in fighting against the COVID-19 pandemic [83].

Furthermore, owing to the powerful oxidizing nature of hydrogen peroxide (H_2O_2), several living beings produce it for a multitude of reasons, including cellular signaling, self-defense mechanism, or killing of pathogens. This has also extrapolated the utility of H_2O_2 in the cleaning and the disinfection of microbial pathogens. According to the density functional theory (DFT), the adsorption energy of a single H_2O_2 molecule onto the pristine SWCNT estimates to 0.25 eV, implying its modest interaction. Thus, for developing a filter with a long shelf life in a clinical setting, it is imperative to ensure the retainability of the H_2O_2 and the virus on the CNT filter. Thus, due to their catalytic activity, the transition metal atom-conjugated SWCNTs aid in eliminating the virus and improve the association between the target molecule and the biosensing material [81].

From a biosensing perspective, Zhang et al. investigated the molecular mechanics simulations to examine the molecular interactions between the carbon nanoparticles (CNPs) and an RNA fragment of the SARS-CoV-2. Their study unraveled that the interaction affinity between the CNPs and the SARS-CoV-2 RNA fragment increased in the order of fullerenes < graphene < CNTs. Additionally, these quantitative structure–activity relationships (QSAR) models on their interaction energies of the nanoparticles with the RNA fragment demonstrated robustness and high goodness of fit. These observations were further researched for its practical applications in different studies, which have been explored by various researchers.

Firstly, Pinals et al. demonstrated the utility of single-walled carbon nanotubes (SWCNTs) in the quantitative and qualitative analysis of a multitude of biological analytes. Furthermore, the SWCNTs inherently possess near-infrared (nIR) fluorescence. They could be functionalized with a plethora of sensing moieties or functional groups, facilitating the production of stable biological sensors with quick readouts of the alterations in the fluorescence readings. In contrast to the other traditional methods, these SWCNTs do not photobleach, thereby allowing for long-term applications. In addition, the biomolecules absorb and scatter the SWCNT nIR emission to a small extent, resulting in a readout that could pass through optically occluded patient samples, eradicating the want for sample purification and processing, substantially limiting the amount of conventional testing modalities. Moreover, SWCNTs are also easy to incorporate into portable form factors after immobilization on hydrogels or papers and subsequent detection of the SWCNT nIR signal by a Raspberry Pi system, which is a form factor similar to the smartphone.

Concurrently, Thanihaichelvan et al. demonstrated a CNT field-effect transistor (FET)–based biosensor for the selective detection of SARS-CoV-2. The sensors were made by immobilizing the reverse sequence of the RNA-dependent RNA polymerase gene of the SARS-CoV-2 onto the CNT channel on a flexible Kapton substrate. They were then evaluated for synthetic positive and control targets. The biosensor responded selectively to the positive target sequence, with a limit of detection (LOD) of 10 fM, demonstrating its potential utility in SARS-CoV-2 diagnostic kits [84].

However, the biosensors fabricated by Shao et al. detected the existence of SARS-CoV-2 in nasopharyngeal samples, by employing a high-purity semiconducting SWCNT-based field-effect transistor (FET) embellished with specialized binding chemistry. The biosensors were then conjugated with the anti-SARS-CoV-2 spike (S)-protein antibody (SAb) and anti-nucleocapsid protein antibody. This has facilitated the SWCNT-FET sensors to recognize the spike (S)–antigen (SAg) and the nucleocapsid (N)–antigen (NAg) in the calibration samples, with a LOD of 0.55 fg/mL for Sag and 0.016 fg/mL for Nag. Moreover, the Sab-functionalized FET sensors also demonstrated decent sensing performance in demarcating the negative clinical samples from positive ones, validating its utility as an economical COVID-19 antigen diagnostic device with high analytical specificity and sensitivity [85].

Additionally, Baloch et al. examined the affinity of SWCNTs with the B-domain of the S1 subunit of the S-protein based on Lennard–Jones potentials. The adsorption of the SWCNTs on the B domain surface triggered an alteration in the inner hydrogen bonds, solvent-accessible surface, and the tertiary structure, which aids in preventing ACE2 from interacting with the S-protein. Additionally, a reduction in the mean square displacement of the B-domain was observed post–SWCNT adsorption, owing to the enhancement of its hydrophobic-hydrophilic characteristics. The interaction of the SWCNTs on the B-domain was measured using the 2-acetamido-2-deoxy-β-d-glucopyranose group, which elucidated the modification in the affinity of the S1 subunit, proving as a potential barrier for viral replication. Thus, these SWCNT-based interactions can be used for drug delivery systems, following adequate *in vitro* and *in vivo* investigations.

Furthermore, Jeong et al. developed a modular technique using the "capture" ssDNA sequence–coupled CNTs for the high-yield extraction of ss-nucleic acids. These ssDNA–nanotube conjugates can be employed to isolate the SARS-CoV-2 from the liquid phase with minimal chemical reagents for the quantitative RT-PCR (RT-qPCR) detection. This nanotube-based extraction approach yields 100% of target SARS-CoV-2 RNA from the phosphate-buffered saline compared to the conventional commercial silica-column kit that yields only ~20%. These CNTs also facilitate the extraction of nucleic acids directly from the human saliva with nearly comparable efficacy as the commercially available DNA/RNA extraction kits, obviating the necessity for additional purification of the biofluids. The use of CNTs in the extraction of viral nucleic acids allows for high-yield and high-sensitivity identification of the SARS-CoV-2 nucleic acids, relying less on chemicals that are subject to change by constraints in the supply chains.

In the context of alleviating the symptoms associated with COVID-19, the CNTs may demonstrate limitations due to the toxicity issues post their intranasal administration. Upon exposure to the lungs, the CNTs tend to activate the lower respiratory tract macrophage, which paves the way for pulmonary fibrosis and collagen creation in the lesions. These changes are brought about by the instantaneous internalization of the CNTs by the lung epithelial cells via attachment to the epidermal growth factor receptor (EGFR). However, these downsides of CNT administration could be brought about by the surface functionalization of these CNTs by conjugating biomolecules like polymers or proteins, which substantially decrease their cytotoxicity on the lung tissue. In addition, the functionalization of the CNTs by conjugating hyaluronic acid moieties considerably increases their interactions with the bronchial cells. It averts the inflammatory cascade, as the alveolar macrophages do not engulf them. Further shreds of evidence have also demonstrated that the surface functionalization of CNTs using cellular ligands significantly increases the uptake of these nanoparticles. This also aids in the release of the drugs at the intended tissue by means of endocytic absorption, but without incurring damages to the plasmatic membrane. Recent studies also increased the specificity of the SWCNTs to target only receptors on the lung tissue post their functionalization with the anti-CTLA-4 antibodies. The CNTs conjugated with antiretroviral drugs were also found to be potent in inhibiting the reverse transcriptase enzyme activity in the lymphocytes of patients who tested positive with HIV. These insights may be of paramount importance in the diagnosis, treatment, and theranostics of SARS-CoV-2 infection, as the CNTs could facilitate the targeted and effective delivery of the drugs to the intended site of action. Although the CNTs could potentially lower the immune cell infiltration and, subsequently, the inflammatory cascade, they may not be recommended for use in the treatment regimen.

7.9 Carbon-Based Nanomaterials for the Management of Virus

7.9.1 Detection

A biosensor typically contains biological active components that are incorporated into equipment that enables the conversion of biochemical signals into measurable signals. Specifically, there are (1) a bioreceptor (e.g., antibody, aptamer, nucleic acid), enabling in the selectivity and specificity of the equipment; (2) a transducer (e.g., electrode, fluorophore), promoting the physical or chemical changes after sensing of analytes; and (3) a signal-processing unit (signal output). Since the biomarker may sometimes be found at very low concentrations, the sensibility, reproducibility, and stability of transducers are critically important. Due to the unique properties described earlier, carbon-based nanomaterials are perfect candidates for developing transducing components. Here, depending on the signals generated by the transducers, we group their applications in virus detection into three sub-groups.

7.9.1.1 Optical Biosensors

The optical sensors work by detecting changes in light emission during target–detector interaction. CDs, or carbon nanoparticles (CNPs), exhibit optical specifications with respect to fluorescence, chemiluminescence, electrochemiluminescence, phosphorescence, up-conversion of photoluminescence, and photo-stimulated electron transfer activity. Achadu et al. developed a fluoroimmunoassay system for detecting influenza virus (H1N1 and H_3N_2), composing of magnetic-derivatized plasmonic molybdenum trioxide quantum dots (MP-MoO_3 QDs) and fluorescent graphitic carbon nitride quantum dots (gCNQDs) [86]. Both nanomaterials were coated with specific antibody against influenza. Under the presence of the virus, a core-satellite immunocomplex was formed between Ab-MP-MoO_3 QDs and Ab-gCNQDs. The MP-MoO_3 QDs steadily generated plasmonic-induced elevation of the gCNQDs fluorescence upon escalating concentrations of influenza virus. This whole device produced a detection time of 10 min and detection limit of 0.25 pg/mL and 0.9 pg/mL for influenza virus A/New Caledonia (20/99/IVR/116) (H1N1) in de-ionized water and human serum, respectively. Furthermore, clinically isolated influenza virus A/Yokohama (110/2009) (H_3N_2) was sensed within the detection range of approximately 45–25,000 PFU/mL. In another case, Shojaei et al. developed a complex fluorometric immunoassay which consisted of anti–Citrus tristeza virus (CTV) antibody–conjugated cadmium-telluride QDs (QD-Ab) and 25 nm CNPs coated with the coat protein of CTV (CP-CNPs). When QD-Ab and CP-CNPs were mixed, the QD fluorescence was quenched by the CNPs. While in the presence of the target (i.e., CTV) in the samples, the CP-CNPs were displaced by free CPs, leading to the recovery of fluorescence intensity of the QDs. Such a system provided a detection limit of 220 ng/mL of CTV.

CNT-based optical biosensors typically rely on either the quenching activity of CNTs over conventional organic quenchers or the near-infrared photoluminescence from semiconducting SWCNTs. Tian et al. devised a biosensor for H5N1 (highly pathogenic* avian influenza [HPAI] A[H5N1] virus). Influenza A virus subtype is a subtype of the influenza A virus which can cause illness in humans and many other species that occurs mainly in birds. It is highly contagious among birds and can be deadly, especially in domestic poultry. Detection is based on the quenching effect of CNTs. Briefly, they synthesized a fluorescence resonance energy transfer system using QDs and CNTs. QDs modified with ssDNA acted as the fluorescence donor. Initially, the fluorescence of QDs was quenched by CNTs due to their complexation. Upon the recognition of the target DNA, this complexation was weakened, which restored the QD fluorescence. Harvey et al. designed SWCNT-based RNA optical sensors for detecting intact HIV in serum (characterized by wavelength shifts) within minutes. SWCNTs were modified with the DNA oligonucleotide sequence (GT)15-(T)15 DNA, which would hybridize to the polyadenylation elements of HIV RNAs. Sodium dodecyl sulfate (SDS) was used to disrupt the virus, denature the viral protein, and liberate the RNA genome. The denatured proteins interacted with the CNTs upon hybridization, leading to a greatly enhanced blueshift.

Similar principles have been explored on graphene and its derivatives as well. Kim et al. developed a biosensor using reduced GO (rGO) that can serve as an effective distance-dependent fluorescence quencher. They hybridized a single-strand aptamer possessing a fluorophore at 5′-end and a Black Hole Quencher-1 (BHQ1) on 3′-end with a complementary oligomer consisting of BHQ1-modified 5′-end. The aptamer targeted interferon-gamma (IFN-γ) specifically here. The whole complexes were anchored to rGO through two BHQ1. The presence of IFN-γ induced the complexation between single-strand aptamer, which displaced the double-stranded structure into two individual strands. Thus, two denatured strands, as well as the fluorophore, became close to the rGO surface. This quenched the fluorophore, resulting in an "off" signal. This sensor allowed the specific detection of IFN-γ at the concentration range of 0.1 ng/mL–10 μg/mL in buffer and human serum. Alternatively, Zhang et al. designed silver nanoclusters (AgNCs)/GO-based fluorescence sensor for detecting HIV genomic DNA via hybridization chain reaction (HCR). In this case, GO conducts adsorption for capturing the hairpin probes along with the selective fluorescence quencher. There are two partially complementary DNA probes, hairpin probe 1 (H1) and hairpin probe 2 (H2) as well. After adding of $AgNO_3$ and $NaBH_4$, the AgNCs were produced at the H1 and H2 probe terminals. Without HIV DNA, HCR could not be triggered. The hairpin probe shielded AgNCs attached to the GO surface that quenched fluorescence of the AgNCs. In the presence of target, H1 and H2 assembly happened via HCR, producing a long chain of H1/H2 complexes. Consequently, the HCR product (AgNCs nanowires) could not adsorb at GO surfaces and produced a strong fluorescent signal, depending on the target's concentration.

Different from the preceding three materials, NDs are mainly used for labeling and tracking. Pham et al. modified fluorescent NDs with the viral protein rA27 (a recombinant envelope protein of vaccinia virus). This allowed the targeting of glycosaminoglycans (GAGs) on cell membrane. The small size and fluorescent properties of NDs permitted the understanding of the virus–host interactions during the infectious stage. Trinh et al. complexed fluorescent NDs and bacteriophages through streptavidin and biotin interaction. NDs served as the fluorophores to visualize the interaction between phages and bacteria.

7.9.1.2 Electrochemical Biosensors

Electrochemical biosensors conduct sensing of analytes by determining electrical responses generated from electrochemical reactions between analytes and functional electrode surfaces within the sensor. The concentrations of analytes tend to linearly correlate with sensor responses for practical applications. Electrochemical biosensors are extremely sensitive, possess high signal-to-noise-ratios, and provide rapid response times. Carbon-based materials have a diverse application potential. They also are chemically inert and affordable to be used as electrode substances for electrochemical biosensors.

Carolina et al. established CNT screen-printed electrodes (CNT-SPE) immunosensor for the detection of non-structural protein 1 (NS1) from dengue virus. This sensor was made by dispersing carboxylated CNTs in carbon ink to prepare an SPE and then covalently immobilizing anti-NS1 antibodies at the CNT surface. In the measurement, the sensors were incubated with the NS1 samples and then with anti-NS1 that was labeled with horseradish peroxidase (anti-NS1-HRP). The electrochemical response was achieved by the peroxidase-catalyzed reaction of hydrogen peroxide and anti-NS1 coupling, and was accordingly resolved by chronoamperometry. Palomar et al. modified a gold electrode with a CNT/gold nanoparticles nanocomposite [87]. Dengue toxin was detected by gold nanoparticles, which immobilized dengue antibody by covalent bonding. Ferri/ferrocyanide [Fe(II/III)] ion was utilized as the signal reporter. After recognition of the dengue antibody and the toxin, the electrode's surface would be blocked, drastically reducing the Fe (II/III) redox current. Thus, detecting the sensitive change of the ferrocene-labeled probe electrochemical signals would enable transduction of the target hybridization activity.

Similar to CNTs, graphene can be used to achieve electrochemical detection too. Muain et al. immobilized hepatitis B virus core antigen (HBcAg) on gold nanoparticle–decorated rGO (rGO-en-AuNPs) nanocomposite. The biosensor can be used to detect anti-HBcAg in the electrolyte solution by the impedance method. Briefly, the electrolyte solution consists of 5 mm potassium hexacyanoferrate [$K_3Fe(CN)_6$] that acts as the redox probe and 0.1 M potassium chloride (KCl) that acts as the support electrolyte. The electrochemical response demonstrated that the electron transfer resistance was linearly related to the concentration of anti-HBcAg, ranging from 3.91 ng/mL to 125.00 ng/mL, and the lowest detection limit was 3.80 ng/mL at 3 σ/m. Huang et al. developed an electrochemical biosensor with a sandwich-type immunoassay for avian influenza virus H7 (AIV H7). The device consists of gold electrodes coated with gold nanoparticles and graphene nanocomposites (AuNPs-G). It is worth noting that the surface of gold nanoparticles was further modified by incorporating H7 monoclonal antibody (MAbs). Another component of this system is silver nanoparticle–graphene (AgNPs-G) whose surface was immobilized with H7-polyclonal antibodies (PAbs). In the detection, AIV H7, the hemagglutinin (HA) and neuraminidase (NA) genes of H7 avian influenza virus (AIV) isolated between 1994 and 2002 from live bird markets (LBM), was bound to MAbs-AuNPs-G-electrodes first. Then, PAb-AgNPs-G was added to form the sandwich structure. Finally, gold electrodes with the complexes were placed in the KCl solution with a platinum wire auxiliary electrode (counter electrode) and a saturated calomel reference electrode (SCE). Linear sweep voltammetry (LSV) was conducted for recording the stripping currents needed for AIV H7 detection.

7.9.1.3 *Field-Effect Transistor (FET) Biosensors*

Field-effect transistors are a form of semiconductor apparatus that works by current flowing from source to drain electrodes. The semiconductor channel that lies between the source and drain is modulated by the electric field generated by a gate electrode's voltage. Specifications of electrical FET biosensors may be implemented by changing the different adhesive biomolecules within the system. Both CNTs and graphene are commonly used for producing FET-based biosensors.

Mandal et al. developed a device consisting of a rectangle-shaped block of semiconducting CNT spanning a pair of Au source/drain electrodes (100 μm wide). There was no gate electrode in this device. CNT was coated with the M13-pIII antibodies that specifically bind with the pIII coat protein of M13 bacteriophage. Under the presence of M13, the specific antibody–virus (M13-pIII antibody) binding and the source–drain current decreased significantly (>20%). This device allowed the selective detection of 550 M13 viruses. Fu et al. developed the chemiresistor DNA sensors using semiconducting SWCNTs (sc-SWCNTs) and nitrogen-doped multi-walled carbon nanotubes (N-MWCNTs) for avian influenza virus (AIV) subtype H5N1. In these sensors, long CNTs (>5 μm) are positioned between the Cr/Au interdigital electrodes to allow a single CNT to be connected to the electrodes. The CNTs were functionalized with DNA probe sequences that have been non-covalently bound to the sidewalls. These chemical resistance DNA sensors can accurately detect the H5N1 complementary DNA target sequence of avian influenza virus at a concentration of 2 pM–2 nM. The working mechanism is attributed to the electrical conductivity change either to the electron doping by DNA bound to the CNT sidewall or to the change in Schottky barrier on CNT/metallic-lead interface. Besides phase and influenza virus, CNT-based FET biosensors are also used for dengue virus detection. For instance, Waski et al. constructed an SWCNT-based heparin (viral receptor analog)–modified chemical resistance to detect the whole dengue virus. The biosensor consisted of an SWCNT network chemical resistor that is functionalized with heparin instead of using an antibody, which serves as a biomolecule for viral recognition. The SWCNT network chemical resistance sensor was fabricated on the patterned interdigital gold electrode by the self-assembly method. Heparin was covalently attached on the SWCNT surface. The virus would bind to heparin and cause the increase of resistance of the electrodes. This chip-based biosensor had a detection limit of ~8 virus/chip. It was sensitive to detect the presence of dengue virus, but unfortunately not influenza H1N1.

Similar to CNTs, graphene can be used to build FET biosensors as well. Afsahi et al. built a FET biosensor using single-layer graphene for Zika virus detection [88]. Graphene was then functionalized by the target, anti-Zika NS1 mouse mAb 6B1 antigens. The C-response sensorgram (capacitance of biosensor toward the liquid) was used to monitor the binding of the virus and the biosensor. Jin et al. used a similar strategy to develop a FET biosensor for the detection of inactivated Ebola virus [89]. An equine antibody targeting the virus glycoprotein was immobilized on reduced graphene oxide–modified FET surface. Different from Afsahi's work, [88] this work measured the shift of Dirac voltage during the binding of Ebola virus and the antibody.

The current coronavirus pandemic (SARS-CoV-2) has been posing a serious threat to global public health. Reliable laboratory diagnosis of this virus is the first step toward effective preventive intervention. Seo et al. demonstrated that graphene and its derivatives could be used to make biosensors for detection of COVID-19 (Figure 7.14) [90]. Their device consisted of anti-SARS-CoV-2 spike protein antibodies immobilized on graphene sheets that recognized SARS-CoV-2 spike protein. FET sensor utilized PBS buffer as the electrolyte to modulate an effective gating effect. This biosensor detected the SARS-CoV-2 based on alterations in channel surface potential and the consequential effects on the electrical response. The device exhibited the detection limit of 16 pfu/mL in culture medium and 2.42×10^2 copies/mL in clinical samples.

7.9.2 Diagnosis of SARS-CoV-2

The diagnosis of the COVID-19 infection is primarily carried out by identification of the SARS-CoV-2 viral genetic material. The generally preferred targets for gene-based analysis of the SARS-CoV-2 include the testing for spike (S) glycoprotein, envelope (E) protein gene, nucleocapsid (N) protein gene, non-structural RNA-dependent RNA polymerase gene, and the open reading frame of the 1a/bc ORF1 a/b genes. However, in the molecular testing methods, the E and ORF1a/b genes

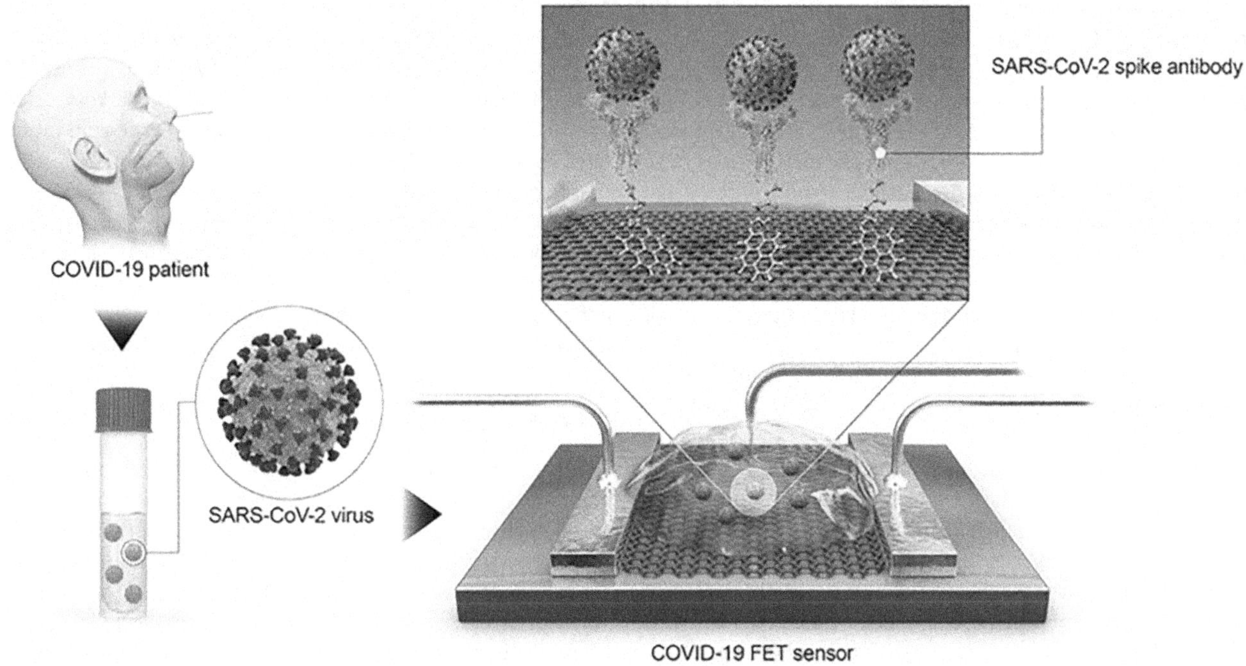

FIGURE 7.14 FET biosensor for the detection of SARS-CoV-2 in human nasopharyngeal swab specimens.

Source: [90].

are the most commonly employed genes for detecting SARS-CoV-2 infections.

The current testing regimen is broadly classified into two types, viz., serological and molecular testing. However, nucleic acid amplification tests (NAAT) like real-time reverse-transcription-based polymerase chain reaction (RT-PCR) are considered to be the gold standard for the diagnosis of a multitude of samples from nasopharyngeal swabs to bronchoalveolar lavage.

Although for geographies with profound community-level transmission and limited laboratory resources, RT-PCR for detecting SARS-CoV-2 is deemed adequate, in most cases, serological tests like the chemiluminescence immunosorbent assay (CLIA) and the enzyme-linked immunosorbent assay (ELISA) may be recommended to detect the humoral response mediated by IgA, IgG, and IgM that is characteristic of viral proteins. Additionally, the evidence of prior immune response to the virus is attributed to the cytotoxicity demonstrated by the natural killer (NK) cells and the CD8+ lymphocytes.

Ponti et al. opine that there is an interplay of several biochemical, hematological, and inflammatory indicators that exert their influence in the COVID-19 infections. They also reported that the major hematological indicators in COVID-19 include the absolute and relative (ratios) counts of the circulating neutrophils and lymphocytes in the blood. Several studies also reported clinical incidences of lymphopenia in progressing and more severe cases of COVID-19 infections in patient populations. Of the numerous biomarkers in the progression of COVID-19 infection, the most conspicuous ones include creatine kinase, D-dimer, and troponin. The evidence presented by Tersalvi et al. and Yao et al. underscores the direct relation of D-dimer levels with the severity of the COVID-19 conditions. However, Garg et al. state that the severity of the SARS-CoV-2 infection can be analyzed by measuring the elevated levels of inflammatory biomarkers like C-reactive protein (CRP), ferritin (FT), interleukin-6 (IL-6), and procalcitonin (PCT).

Nevertheless, there has not been a commercially available test kit that facilitates the evaluation of specific immune responses while eliciting a robust cellular response. Although antibodies targeted against the receptor-binding domain (RBD) of the S protein are highly specific for the SARS-CoV-2, their role against other proteins in the pathogenesis of COVID-19 still needs to be elucidated and studied further.

Furthermore, factors such as the individual, test technique, and data collection strategy can profoundly affect the test sensitivity, which may further introduce inconsistencies and errors between the tests. Additionally, a negative test report in a typical clinical setting does not rule out the possibility of COVID-19 infection, reiterating the need for additional laboratory and serological studies. In addition, the entire scientific community across the globe is working relentlessly to find a viable and economical diagnostic option for the early diagnosis of COVID-19 for people across the globe.

With the rapid community-level spread of the SARS-CoV-2 and associated morbidity and mortality, statistics have produced a great demand for rapid, highly selective, and sensitive detection methods to ensure early diagnosis and to avail treatment, primarily in cases where there are limited prevention and mitigation strategies in place.

Most diagnostic toolkits that employ antigen-based or human blood serum–based lateral-flow immunoassays usually suffer from low-sensitivity issues. In addition, the performance is improved by advanced digital systems, but at the cost of speed and the requirement for massive equipment.

Furthermore, the gold standard currently employed for detecting COVID-19 is the commonly utilized quantitative real-time polymerase chain reaction (qRT-PCR). Nevertheless, these methods are arduous, are cumbersome, require skilled labor, and might be of limited utility in distant and resource-constrained surroundings. Moreover, this method may also produce specific individual false-positive results. It could fail to meet the newer challenges (like rapid viral mutation) or the need for mass-producing methods for quicker and more direct detection of viral particles or proteins. In contrast, most biosensors work by detecting the viral internal genetic material or the viral surface proteins.

Therefore, these shortcomings limit its utility while impeding the ability to produce accurate data on the infectivity and extent of COVID-19 infection in the community or population.

In addition, the pandemic has strained the testing resources, further prompting the development of rapid point-of-care assays along with the deployment of isothermal DNA amplification. Several emerging technologies, like CRISPR gene-editing tools, also prove advantageous due to their ease of utility in lateral-flow assays. They complemented with their high sensitivity and high specificity of molecular diagnostics. Furthermore, DNA sequencing and sample pooling methodologies are required to maximize the capabilities of available biosensors and to expedite mass testing.

7.9.3 Biomarkers and Current Diagnostic Strategies

The term "biomarkers," a portmanteau of "biological markers" refers to objective indications of medical symptoms analyzed from the patient's outer look, which can be measured with high reproducibility and accuracy, which help diagnose a patient's clinical conditions or state without affecting his body [67]. Further, as per pre-existing literature data, it is evident that enormous biomarkers can be employed for SARS-CoV-2 detection, and similarly, many different biomarkers of various viruses, namely, the Middle East respiratory syndrome (MERS) and influenza virus, are known to have special types of primers and may be fully expressed by RT-PCR assays with high sensitivity toward SARS-CoV-2 detection [91]. Moreover, the four structural proteins, including matrix (M), spike (S), nucleocapsid (N), and envelope (E), are used as antigens for the diagnosis of SARS-CoV-2. Several studies reported that assembling the structure of virus M and E proteins plays a crucial role. In contrast, S and N proteins serve as necessary biomarkers that might be used to detect SARS-CoV-2, in which S-proteins play an important role in combining with receptor-binding and host cell domains that interact with angiotensin-converting enzyme 2 (ACE2) receptors [92]. However, specific antibodies are also carried out for SARS-CoV-2 detection over the patient's serological sample. According to research, the adaptive immune response of the infected patients will develop antibodies naturally to the S proteins, and then the process is known as "active immunity." As binding occurs between antibodies and S protein, the ability of a virus to infect more cells gets neutralized, and the interaction of the virus with ACE2 gets prohibited. Thus, the progression of diseases gets limited. If antibodies develop against the spike proteins, then the process is known as "passive immunity." S proteins enzyme-linked immunosorbent assay (ELISA) is one of the immunological assays used to measure the antibodies that can help detect the SARS-CoV-2 virus, which can help treat SARS-CoV-2 infections [68]. Hence, the current biomarkers detection techniques for antibody detection and nucleic acid testing have evolved well, including ELISA and RT-PCR. However, these approaches still undergo some feasible drawbacks, like a bit longer time for diagnosis. Therefore, compared to current biomarkers detection techniques, biosensors can serve as alternative tools, as they possess high accuracy, rapid response, enhanced sensitivity, portability, selectivity, non-sophisticated, and awareness of infection's critical trends and severity.

7.9.4 Treatment

Viruses rely on infecting host mammalian cells to conduct genome replication and generation of new virus particles. The infection process is a major part of the virus life cycle; therefore, viral treatments target this stage. Current replication inhibitors comprise of antiviral drugs designed to interfere with viral replication and intracellularly prevent production of new virus particles. Conversely, entry inhibitors block virus particles extracellularly to combat infection. These aim to decrease viral loads along with improving prophylactic or therapeutic end points. Carbon nanomaterials exhibit low to moderate cytotoxicity and specific antiviral actions [93]. They work by either directly interacting with the virus (also via photo-induced mechanisms) or as platforms for delivering other antiviral substances.

Huang et al. synthesized benzoxazine monomers–derived Cdots (BZM-CDs) as a broad-spectrum antiviral drug [10]. BZM-CDs could directly attach to virion surfaces and thus block the first step of virus–cell interaction. They found that BZM-CD treatment could prevent cell infection by flaviviruses (JEV, ZIKV, and DENV) and non-enveloped viruses (porcine parvovirus, PPV, and adenovirus-associated virus, AAV). Barras et al. discovered that boronic acid or amine functionalization on Cdots was critical to prevent the entry of herpes simplex virus type 1 (HSV-1). In another independent study, Aleksandra Łoczechin et al. confirmed this observation. They explored the usage of seven different CQDs made of different methods for inhibiting HCoV-229e through inhibition of human coronavirus (HCoV-229E) infections [94]. The most effective CQDs were either made from boronic acid derivatives or coated with amine groups. Another interesting report examined the antiviral activity of positively charged 2,2′-(ethylenedioxy)bis(ethylamine) (EDA)-Cdots and non-charged 3-ethoxypropylamine (EPA)-Cdots. This group studied the infection of two strains of human norovirus virus-like particles (VLPs), GI.1, and GII.4 VLPs. Both types of Cdots effectively inhibited both strains of VLPs' bindings to histo-blood group antigens (HBGA) receptors from human cells. However, the positively charged EDA-Cdots proved to be more efficient. Taken together, Cdots/CQDs execute their antiviral functions mainly through blocking the antigens on the viral particle surface. The surface charge and functional groups control the efficiency of this process. Roy et al. made use of NDs as carriers for the anti-HIV-1 drug efavirenz. This system showed excellent drug dissolution profile (approximately 5–10 ng/mL greater dissolution for ND–drug complex compared to free drug), transmigration through the blood–brain barrier in vitro (~450 ng/mL greater transmigration for ND–drug complex compared to free drug at day 2), and therapeutic efficacy (significantly reduced number of HIV-1-infected macrophages from over 8,000 pg/mL for untreated group, 2,500 pg/mL for free drug, to below 1,500 pg/mL for ND–drug complex by day 7).

Yang et al. reported a sulfonate GO system that was modified with β-cyclodextrin (CD) and curcumin. Through the tissue culture infectious dose assay and immunofluorescence assay, this functional GO provided effective inhibition of RSV infections. It works through three possible mechanisms: directly inactivating viruses, blocking viral attachment, and interfering with virus replication. Deokar et al. explored the photothermal antiviral properties of graphene by taking that sulfonated magnetic nanoparticles functionalized with rGO (SMRGO) as a hot plate surface for herpes simplex virus type 1 (HSV-1) capture and destruction under irradiation. The captured HSV-1 became non-infectious after SMRGO irradiation, and average infection percentage reduced from 65.62% without irradiation to 0% after near-infrared light irradiation.

7.9.5 Prevention

As everyone knows nowadays, the best way to prevent illness is to avoid being exposed to the virus. Before the development of the vaccines, any strategy to minimize exposure to the virus is welcomed. It has been shown that SWCNT could act as a filter to efficiently remove bacterial and viral microbes from water. The filter was a polyvinylidene fluoride (PVDF)–based microporous membrane (5 μm pore size) sheltered by a thin layer of SWCNTs. SWCNT filters had depths of 2.0 to 6.0 μm. When the water containing T model virus particle (MS2 bacteriophage) ran through the filter using a peristaltic pump, the virus could be completely removed (no remaining plague-forming units detected at filter outlet) based on size exclusion or sieving. Later, the same group further developed an anodic MWCNT micro-filter for removal of MS2 viruses. MWCNT filters were made of 5 μm PTFE membrane and MWCNTs that had diameter distribution of 17 ± 9 nm along with a length distribution of 91 ± 21 μm. The solution with the virus ran through filters under the peristaltic pump as well. However, previous work purely depended on the sieving to remove the bacteria and virus. This new system has an integrated electrolysis component. Concomitant electrolysis on the filters during filtration led to significantly elevated viral inactivation. At applied potentials of 2 and 3 V, the electrochemical MWCNT filter decreased the viral numbers in the effluent lower than the detection limit.

7.10 Rapid and Label-Free Detection of H5N1 Virus Using Carbon Nanotube Network Field-Effect Transistor

DNA hybridization–based detection techniques are widely used in genetics, medicine, and drug discovery. However, the current techniques are usually based on labels and reagents that are time-consuming and complex to implement. In this study, we report a label-free DNA sensor based on single-walled carbon nanotube field-effect transistor (SWCNTFET) for selective DNA hybridization detection of H5N1 virus. A network of single-walled carbon nanotubes (SWCNTs) acts as the conductor channel. Probe DNA sequences were adsorbed onto SWCNTs. The developed DNA sensor can effectively detect full-complementary DNA with concentration as low as 1.25 pM. The sensitivity of the DNA sensor reached approximately 0.28 nM/nA. The effect of the parameters, including DNA probe concentration, its complementary concentration, mismatched sequence, and hybridization time, on the sensor response was also studied. The potential application of the DNA sensor for medical, environmental, and epidemic detection has been investigated.

In the current section, a DNA sensor based on single-walled carbon nanotube field-effect transistor (SWCNTFET) for detecting DNA sequence hybridization has been developed. This sensor has advantages, such as label-free, simple, convenient, and inexpensive. In this study, complementary detection mechanism using SWCNTFET has been proposed. The effect of the parameters, including probe DNA concentration, its complementary concentration, mismatched sequence, and hybridization time, on the sensor response was also studied. The results of the studies showed the potential application for other kinds of DNA biosensors in the future.

7.10.1 DNA Hybridization Detection Using SWCNTFET

Hybridization signal was measured using a Keithley semiconductor parameter analyzer, model 4200-SCS. Measurements were performed by immersing the SWCNTFETs in a measuring cell filled with 2 mL of buffer solution. Sample concentration was adjusted by adding defined volumes of the target DNA sequences. For each concentration, the SWCNTFETs were immersed for 1 h at 37°C, rinsed with distilled water, dried with nitrogen, and then electrically characterized. By applying a bias to the gate voltage, the I_{ds}–V_{gs} characteristics of the SWCNTFET sensor were monitored. The schematic of SWCNTFET is shown in Figure 7.15.

7.10.2 Electrical Characterization of SWCNTFET Based on the DNA Sensor

The transfer characteristics of bare SWCNTFET immobilized with probe DNA sequence and hybridized with the target DNA sequence has been studied by measuring three times the dependence of the source–drain current I_d on the back gate voltage V_{gs} at fixed bias voltage V_{ds} of 1 V at room temperature. For bare SWCNTFET, the source–drain current I_d decreased significantly with increasing back gate voltage V_{gs}. The studies suggested that the device operates as a field-effect transistor with a p-channel; the transport through the semiconductor CNT is dominated by holes. When SWCNTFET immobilized the probe DNA sequence, channel current was significantly reduced compared with that of the bare sensor. Subsequently, the electrical current was further reduced when the probe DNA sequences were hybridized with its complementary sequences.

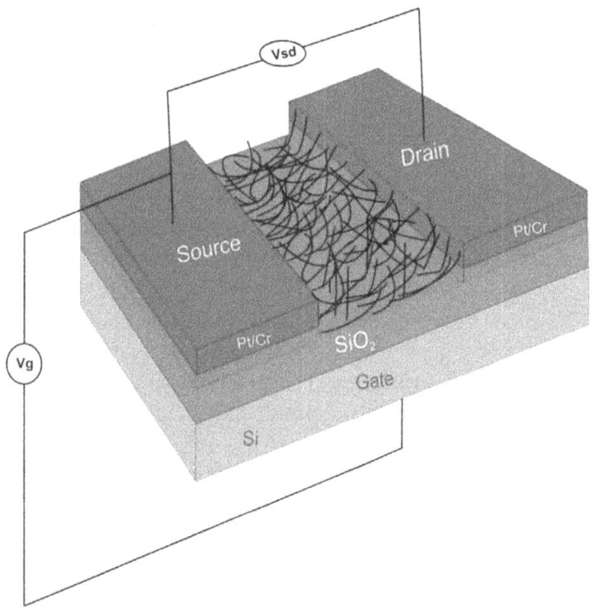

FIGURE 7.15 Schematic of the SWCNTFET. The distance between the source and the drain is 50 μm.

To date, the mechanism of DNA hybridization detection using CNTFETs device is still under argument. Thus, DNA hybridization can be detected by electrical conductance change because of the modulation of energy-level alignment between SWNTs and Au electrodes. It has been suggested that the DNA hybridization detection mechanism of SWCNTFET is based on specific interaction between the DNA probe and its complementary sequences. Given that the phosphate groups of the DNA molecules are negatively charged, two DNA sequences were bound and formed a double helix that produces a high density of negative charges on the sensor surface when hybridization happens, providing an electrostatic gating effect on SWCNTFET and resulting in the change of channel current. In other words, threshold voltage V_T would be changed, leading to a change in drain current I_d. DNA hybridization can be detected from the difference of V_T or I_d. In another suggestion, the binding between the probe DNA sequence and its complementary sequence creates a change in free energy that can generate stress on the sensor surface.

7.10.3 Effect of the Target DNA Concentration on the Electrical Sensor Response

The functionalized SWCNTFET was used to determine different target DNA concentrations. For each concentration, the SWCNTFETs were immersed in PBS solution containing the target DNA sequences for 1 h at 37°C, rinsed thoroughly with DI water, dried with nitrogen, and then electrically characterized by measuring the I–V characteristics. A maximum channel current was observed at the target DNA concentration of 1 pM. When the target DNA concentration increased, the channel current of the device decreased dramatically. According to measurement data, the average electrical current decrease was approximately 16% for each target DNA concentration. The sensitivity of the sensor was 0.28 nM/nA. The performance of the different DNA sensors with this work has been compared, and the results are shown in [95].

7.10.4 Effect of the Probe DNA Concentration on the Electrical Sensor Response

Previous studies indicated that the probe DNA concentration significantly affects the DNA hybridization efficiency. Thus, the effect of the probe DNA concentration on electrical sensor response was also investigated in this study. For this purpose, probe DNA concentration was studied in the range of 1 μM–20 μM under standard reaction conditional with 10 nM perfectly matched target DNA. The experiment was performed under the same conditions of immobilization time, solution concentration, and ion strength. Channel current is inversely proportional to probe concentration. The current decreased with increasing probe concentration. It has been found that the signal decreased to 10 nA when the probe DNA concentration increased to 20 μM. However, as the probe concentration continues to increase, hybridization efficiency is low (data not shown). This result can be attributed to the repulsive electrostatic or steric interaction between the bases of the DNA sequences.

7.10.5 Effect of the Mismatched DNA on the Electrical Sensor Response

Mismatch detection was the first trial step for sensor selectivity investigation. In this study [95], two different mismatched sequences were used. The hybridization signals of the mismatched sequences were compared with those of fully complementary sequences. A decreasing, much stronger signal of DNA hybridization containing one- and three-base mismatched DNA strands was clearly found compared with the system containing fully matched DNA strands. It has been found that if the fully targeted DNA was replaced by mismatched base C (cytosine) instead of a G (guanine) at the 7th position of the DNA molecule and three bases C (cytosine) instead of a G (guanine) at the 7th position and CC instead of AA at the 12th and 13th positions close to the 5′ end of the DNA molecule, the I_d current was decreased in the range of 20% and 25%, respectively. From these results, we could deduce that the DNA sensor has sufficient high sensitivity to detect a single base pair mismatched DNA at certain positions within the sequence.

7.10.6 Effect of Hybridization Time on the Electrical Sensor Response

The dependence of the electrical sensor response on the hybridization time at target DNA concentration of 2 nM, $V_{gs} = -8$ V, and $V_{ds} = 1$ V has been investigated. The I_d current decreased linearly upon exposure to the complementary sequence when hybridization time was increased up to 60 min. The signal slowly decreased and reached saturation value until maximum hybridization was obtained. In the experiment [95], the optimal hybridization time for the sensor was 140 min, which was selected as representative in the following experiments.

7.10.7 Stability of SWCNTFET-Based DNA Sensor

The stability of SWCNTFET was also investigated in this study. Eleven sensors were fabricated under the same conditions. The shift in drain current I_{ds} of the 11 sensors in response to the hybridization of 20 nM of target DNA is indicated. The average value of the drain current *Ids* was 64.45 nA, corresponding to the relative standard deviation (RSD) of 29.69%.

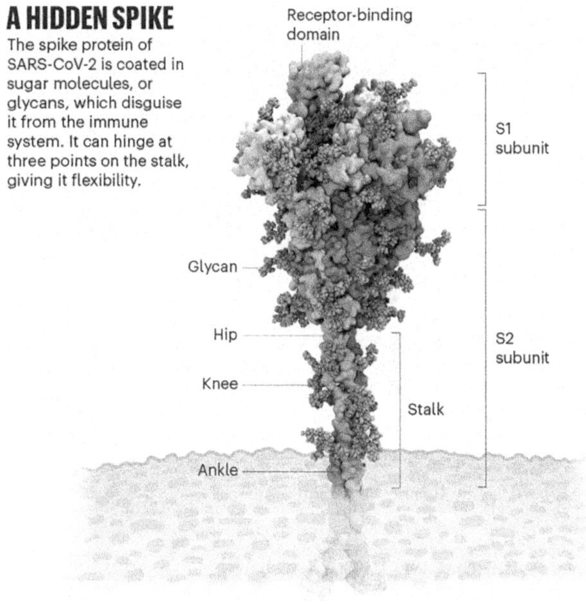

FIGURE 7.16 Spike protein of SARS-CoV-2.

7.11 How the Coronavirus Infects Our Cells

The coronavirus sports a luxurious sugar coat. “It’s striking,” thought Rommie Amaro, staring at her computer simulation of one of the trademark spike proteins of SARS-CoV-2, which stick out from the virus’s surface. It was swathed in sugar molecules, known as glycans. “When you see it with all the glycans, it’s almost unrecognizable,” says Amaro, a computational biophysical chemist at the University of California, San Diego.

Many viruses have glycans covering their outer proteins, camouflaging them from the human immune system like a wolf in sheep’s clothing. But last year, Amaro’s laboratory group and collaborators created the most detailed visualization yet of this coat, based on structural and genetic data and rendered atom-by-atom by a supercomputer. On March 22, 2020, she posted the simulation to Twitter. Within an hour, one researcher asked in a comment: What was the naked, uncoated loop sticking out of the top of the protein?

Amaro had no idea. But ten minutes later, structural biologist Jason McLellan at the University of Texas at Austin chimed in: the uncoated loop was a receptor binding domain (RBD), one of three sections of the spike that bind to receptors on human cells (see “a hidden spike”).

In Amaro’s simulation, when the RBD lifted up above the glycan cloud, two glycans swooped in to lock it into place, like a kickstand on a bicycle. When Amaro mutated the glycans in the computer model, the RBD collapsed. McLellan’s team built a way to try the same experiment in the lab, and by June 2020, the collaborators had reported that mutating the two glycans reduced the ability of the spike protein to bind to a human cell receptor—a role that no one has previously recognized in coronaviruses, McLellan says. It is possible that snipping out those two sugars could reduce the virus’s infectivity, says Amaro, although researchers do not yet have a way to do this.

Since the start of the COVID-19 pandemic, scientists have been developing a detailed understanding of how SARS-CoV-2 infects cells. By picking apart the infection process, they hope to find better ways to interrupt it through improved treatments and vaccines and learn why the latest strains, such as the Delta variant, are more transmissible.

What has emerged from 19 months of work, backed by decades of coronavirus research, is a blow-by-blow account of how SARS-CoV-2 invades human cells (see “life cycle of the pandemic coronavirus”). Scientists have discovered key adaptations that help the virus grab on to human cells with surprising strength and then hide itself once inside. Later, as it leaves cells, SARS-CoV-2 executes a crucial processing step to prepare its particles for infecting even more human cells. These are some of the tools that have enabled the virus to spread so quickly and claim millions of lives. “That’s why it’s so difficult to control,” says Wendy Barclay, a virologist at Imperial College London.

That allows the spikes to flop around, sway, and rotate, which could make it easier for them to scan the cell surface and for multiple spikes to bind to a human cell. There are no similar experimental data for other coronaviruses, but because spike protein sequences are highly evolutionarily conserved, it is fair to assume the trait is shared, says Beck.

Early in the pandemic, researchers confirmed that the RBDs of SARS-CoV-2 spike proteins attach to a familiar protein called the ACE2 receptor, which adorns the outside of most human throat and lung cells. This receptor is also the docking point for SARS-CoV, the virus that causes severe acute respiratory syndrome (SARS). But compared with SARS-CoV, SARS-CoV-2 binds to ACE2.

The spike protein of SARS-CoV-2 (Figure 7.16) is coated in sugar molecules, or glycans, which disguise it from the immune system. It can hinge at three points on the stalk, giving it flexibility.

7.11.1 Viral Entry Up Close

Virus and host cell membranes fuse after the TMPRSS2 enzyme cuts a SARS-CoV-2 spike protein. This exposes hydrophobic amino acids in the spike that rapidly embed themselves into the nearest membrane—that of the host cell, as shown in Figure 7.17.

7.11.2 Restricted Entry

Once the viral spikes bind to ACE2, other proteins on the host cell’s surface initiate a process that leads to the merging of viral and cell membranes.

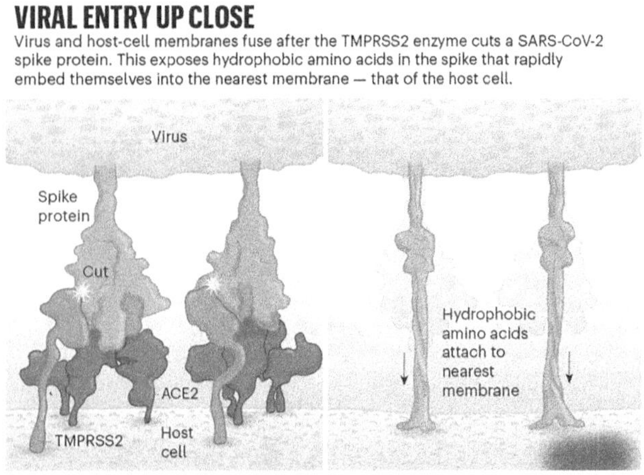

FIGURE 7.17 Viral entry up close.

The virus that causes SARS, SARS-CoV, uses either of two host protease enzymes to break in: TMPRSS2 (pronounced "tempress two") or cathepsin L. TMPRSS2 is the faster route in, but SARS-CoV often enters instead through an endosome—a lipid-surrounded bubble—which relies on cathepsin L. When virions enter cells by this route, however, antiviral proteins can trap them.

SARS-CoV-2 differs from SARS-CoV because it efficiently uses TMPRSS2, an enzyme found in high amounts on the outside of respiratory cells.

The discovery also points to protease inhibitors as a promising therapeutic option to prevent a virus from using TMPRSS2, cathepsin L, or other proteases to enter host cells. One TMPRSS2 inhibitor, camostat mesylate, which is approved in Japan to treat pancreatitis, blocked viral entry into lung cells, but the drug did not improve patients' outcomes in an initial clinical trial [96].

"From my perspective, we should have such protease inhibitors as broad antivirals available to fight new disease outbreaks and prevent future pandemics at the very beginning," says Stefan Pöhlmann, director of the Infection Biology Unit at the German Primate Center in Göttingen, who has led research on ACE2 binding and the TMPRSS2 pathway.

7.11.3 Deadly Competition

The next steps of infection are murkier. "There are a lot more black boxes once you are inside the cell," says chemist Janet Iwasa at the University of Utah in Salt Lake City, who is developing an annotated animation of the viral life cycle. "There's more uncertainty, and competing hypotheses."

After the virus shoots its RNA genome into the cell, ribosomes in the cytoplasm translate two sections of viral RNA into long strings of amino acids, which are then snipped into 16 proteins, including many involved in RNA synthesis. Later, more RNAs are generated that code for a total of 26 known viral proteins, including structural ones used to make new virus particles, such as the spike, and other accessory proteins. In this way, the virus begins churning out copies of its own messenger RNA. But it needs the cell's machinery to translate those mRNAs into proteins.

Coronaviruses take over that machinery in many ways. Virologist Noam Stern-Ginossar and her team at the Weizmann Institute of Science in Rehovot, Israel, zoomed in on three mechanisms by which SARS-CoV-2 suppresses the translation of host mRNA in favor of its own. None are exclusive to this virus, but the combination, speed, and magnitude of the effects seem unique, says Stern-Ginossar.

First, the virus eliminates the competition: viral protein Nspl, one of the first proteins translated when the virus arrives, recruits host proteins to systematically chop up all cellular mRNAs that do not have a viral tag. When Stern-Ginossar's team put that same tag on the end of a host mRNA, the mRNA was not chopped up [97].

Second, infection reduces overall protein translation in the cell by 70%. Nspl is again the main culprit, this time physically blocking the entry channel of ribosomes so mRNA cannot get inside, according to work from two research teams. The little translation capacity that remains is dedicated to viral RNAs, says Stern-Ginossar.

Finally, the virus shuts down the cell's alarm system. This happens in numerous ways, but Stern-Ginossar's team identified one clear mechanism for SARS-CoV-2: the virus prevents cellular mRNA from getting out of the nucleus, including instructions for proteins meant to alert the immune system to infection. A second team confirmed this finding and again pointed to Nspl: the protein seems to jam up exit channels in the nucleus so nothing can escape.

Because gene transcripts cannot get out of the nucleus, the infected cells do not release many interferons—these are signaling proteins that alert the immune system to the presence of a virus. SARS-Cov-2 is particularly efficient at shutting down this alarm system: compared with other respiratory viruses, including SARS-CoV and respiratory syncytial virus, SARS-CoV-2 infection induces significantly lower levels of interferons. And this June, researchers reported mutations in the Alpha variant that seem to enable it to subdue interferon production even more efficiently.

"It's clear that SARS-CoV-2 is a very fast virus that has a unique ability to prevent our immune system from recognizing and combating infection in the first stages," says Stern-Ginossar. By the time the immune system does realize there is a virus, there is so much of it that immune-response proteins sometimes flood the bloodstream at a faster rate than normal—which can cause damage. Doctors saw early in the pandemic that some people with COVID-19 who become very ill are harmed by an overactive immune response to SARS-CoV-2, as well as by the virus itself. Some proven treatments work by dampening down this immune response.

7.11.4 Renovation Station

Once the virus has taken over host translation, it starts a home makeover, extensively remodeling the interior and exterior of the cell to its needs.

First, some of the newly made viral spike proteins travel to the surface of the cell and poke out of the host cell membrane. There, they activate a host calcium ion channel, which expels a fatty coating onto the outside of the cell—the same coating found on cells that naturally fuse together, such as muscle cells. At this point, the infected cell fuses to neighboring cells expressing ACE2, developing into massive individual respiratory cells filled with up to 20 nuclei.

On the inside of the cell, even more change is occurring. Like other coronaviruses, SARS-CoV-2 transforms the long thin endoplasmic reticulum (ER), a network of flat membranes involved in protein synthesis and transport, into double-membrane spheres.

7.11.5 "There Are a Lot More Black Boxes Once You Are Inside the Cell"

As if the ER were blowing bubbles. These double-membrane vesicles (DMVs) might provide a safe place for viral RNA to be replicated and translated, shielding it from innate immune sensors in the cell, but that hypothesis is still being investigated.

Proteins involved in making DMVs could be good drug targets, because they seem to be necessary for viral replication. For instance, a host protein, TMEM41B, is needed to mobilize cholesterol and other lipids to expand the ER membranes so that all the virus parts will fit inside. "When you take TMEM41B out, it has a major impact on infection," says Vineet Menachery, a coronavirus researcher at the University of Texas Medical Branch in Galveston who was involved in the research. The coronavirus transmembrane protein Nsp3 could also be a target: it creates a crown-like pore in the walls of the DMVs to shuttle out newly made viral RNA.

Most viruses that have an outer wrapping, known as an envelope, form this feature by assembly directly at the edge of the cell, co-opting some of the cell's own plasma membrane on their way out. But newly made coronavirus proteins take a different path.

For years, evidence has suggested that coronaviruses are transported out of the cell through the Golgi complex, an organelle that works like a post office, packaging molecules in membranes and sending them off to other parts of the cell. There, the virus forms a lipid envelope from the Golgi complex's membrane; newly formed virions are then carried inside Golgi vesicles to the cell surface, where they are spat out of the cell, says virologist and cell biologist Carolyn Machamer at Johns Hopkins University in Baltimore, Maryland, who has studied coronaviruses for 30 years.

Leaving a cell through either the Golgi or lysosomes is slow and inefficient compared with budding out of a plasma membrane, so scientists do not know why SARS-CoV-2 does it. Machamer suspects that the lipid composition of a Golgi- or lysosome-derived envelope is somehow more beneficial to the virus than one from the plasma membrane. "If we understood this part a little bit better, there would be great opportunities for novel antiviral therapeutics," she says.

On the way out of the cell, one more event makes this virus into an infectious juggernaut: a quick snip at a site of five amino acids prepares the virus to strike its next target.

Where other coronaviruses have a single arginine amino acid at the junction of the S1 and S2 subunits of the spike, SARS-CoV-2 has a line of five amino acids: proline, arginine, arginine, alanine, and arginine. "Because the site was unusual, we focused on it, and it turned out that, yes, the site is essential for invasion of lung cells," says Pöhlmann. In May 2020, he and his colleagues reported that a host cell protein called furin recognizes and clips that string of amino acids—and the cut is "essential" for the virus to enter human lung cells efficiently.

It is not the first time that researchers have identified a furin cleavage site on a virus; highly pathogenic avian influenza viruses also have it, says Barclay. When a colleague sent Barclay a strain of SARS-CoV-2 in culture that had spontaneously lost the furin cleavage site, her team found that ferrets infected with this strain shed viral particles in lower amounts than did those infected with the pandemic strain and did not transmit the infection to nearby animals.

7.11.6 "We Would Hypothesize That This Is the Virus Getting Even Better at Transmitting"

In a host cell membrane, says Gallagher, if spikes are not pre-clipped by furin—and they are not always—they bypass TMPRSS2 and enter through the slower endosomal pathway, if at all.

Two coronavirus variants, Alpha and Delta, have altered furin cleavage sites. In the Alpha variant, the initial proline amino acid is changed to a histidine (P681H); in the Delta variant, it is changed to an arginine (P681R). Both changes make the sequence less acidic, and the more basic the string of amino acids, the more effectively furin recognizes and cuts it, says Barclay. "We would hypothesize that this is the virus getting even better at transmitting."

More furin cuts mean more spike proteins primed to enter human cells. In SARS-CoV, less than 10% of spike proteins are primed, says Menachery, whose lab group has been quantifying the primed spike proteins but is yet to publish this work. In SARS-CoV-2, that percentage rises to 50%. In the Alpha variant, it is more than 50%. In the highly transmissible Delta variant, the group has found, greater than 75% of spikes are primed to infect a human cell.

7.11.7 Known Unknowns

The scientific community is still scratching the surface of its understanding of SARS-CoV-2. Key unknowns include the number of ACE2 receptors needed to bind to each spike protein, when exactly the S2 site is cleaved by TMPRSS2, and the number of spikes needed for virus–cell membrane fusion, says McLellan—and that is just for entry. In April 2020, a team at the University of California, San Francisco, identified at least 332 interactions between SARS-CoV-2 and human proteins [98].

It is not easy to keep pace with the quickly mutating virus. Most mutations so far are associated with how effectively the virus spreads, not with how much the virus damages the host, experts agree. This month, a study reported that the Delta variant grew more rapidly and at higher levels inside people's lungs and throats than did earlier versions of the virus.

But it is not yet certain how Delta's mutations have supercharged the variant in this way, says Stern-Ginossar. "This is something many labs are trying to figure out."

7.12 Life Cycle of the Pandemic Coronavirus

A simplified account of how SARS-CoV-2 enters and exits cells is represented in Figure 7.18.

Fused cell structures (syncytia) seen in cells expressing the SARS-CoV-2 spike protein (green). Nuclei are in blue and the cell skeleton is in red (Figure 7.19).

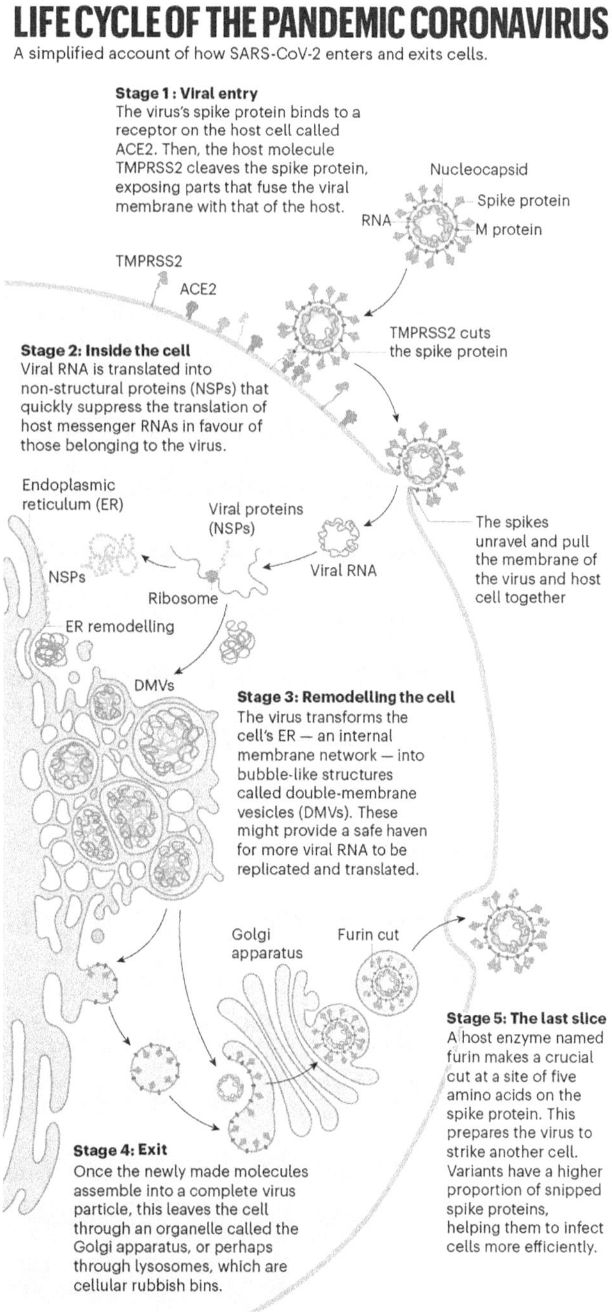

FIGURE 7.18 Stages of life cycle of the pandemic coronavirus.

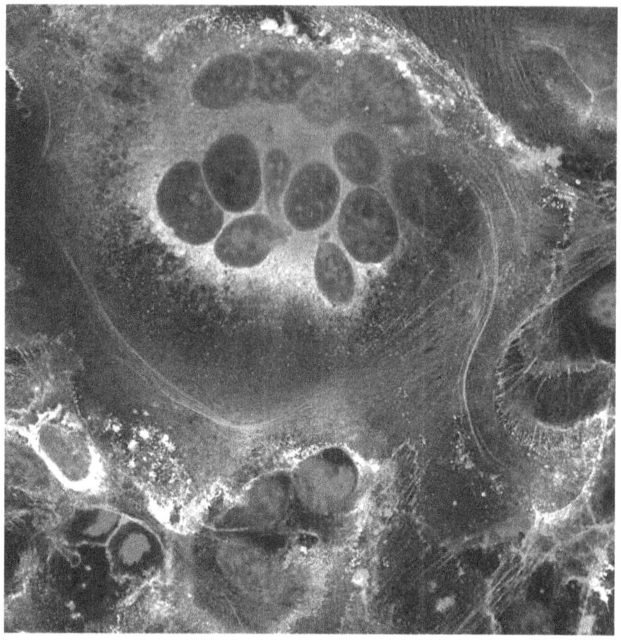

FIGURE 7.19 SARS-CoV-2 spike protein in the cell.

7.13 Latest Developed Biosensors for COVID-19

The World Health Organization (WHO) announced on March 11, 2020, that the SARS-CoV-2 epidemic was a pandemic and a global health emergency [99]. It is well-known that there have been three human pathogenic coronavirus outbreaks in the 21st century that triggered transmission and posed immense challenges to global public health and economic growth. The three virus outbreaks were SARS-CoV in 2003, MERS-CoV in 2012, and the new SARS-CoV-2 in December 2019 [100]. Phylogenetic data analysis suggests that SARS-CoV-2 is further away from the SARS-CoV (79%) and MERS-CoV (50%) strains. As a result, the world increasingly needs diagnostic tools with the capability of identifying the infected individuals, for example, the source of infection.

Electrochemical biosensors are advantageous for sensing biomolecules because of their ability to detect biomarkers with accuracy, specificity, and high sensitivity. Previously, electrochemical biosensors have been successfully used in medical diagnostics for the detection of viruses such as MERS-CoV, hepatitis C virus (HCV), human influenza A virus H9N2, and avian influenza virus (AIV) H5N1. Recently, Shao et al. developed a SARS-CoV-2 S antigen detection device based on a carbon nanotube field-effect transistor (CNT-FET) functionalized with anti-SARS-CoV-2 spike antibody with a detection range of 5.5 fg/mL to 5.5 pg/mL [101]. The real-time polymerase chain reaction (RT-PCR) rigorously used for the diagnosis of SARS-CoV-2. RT-PCR is excellent in terms of sensitivity and selectivity but can only be performed in well-equipped laboratory-based hospitals, requires costly chemicals, enzymes, spacious machinery, and up to 1–2 days. In order to detect SARS-CoV-2 quickly with high accuracy, a simple, sensitive, and low-cost biosensor is needed.

Compared to time staking laboratory tests, a biosensor with fast response and high accuracy in the form of a point-of-care device would be an excellent aid for the early diagnosis of SARS-CoV-2 infection. As shown in Figure 7.20a, generally, a biosensor comprises of biosensing elements, such as nucleic acids, enzymes, or antibodies that can interact with the target analyte in the form of biological or chemical sample, a transducer that can convert the changes in the biosensing element to an electrical signal, and an amplifier and necessary electronic system to process the electrical signal to digitize the output. The COVID-19 outbreak has spurred the development of various types of biosensors with different biosensing platforms that can be used for the diagnosis of COVID-19.

SARS-CoV-2 contains four structural proteins: spike (S), membrane (M), envelope (E), and nucleocapsid (N) proteins, as shown in Figure 7.20b. The S protein is composed of two subunits, S1 and S2, which are responsible for the attachment, fusion, and entry of the virus. The S1 subunit contains a receptor-binding domain (RBD) that recognizes host cell receptors and human angiotensin-converting enzyme 2 (ACE2). The S2 subunit facilitates membrane fusion for virus entry. N proteins bind to the viral RNA genome to form the nucleocapsid. M proteins release nutrients at the transmembrane and form the viral envelope. E proteins are small polypeptides that are responsible for the assembly and release of the virus. The SARS-CoV-2 viral RNA genome consists of open reading frames (ORFs) genes, which encode a total of 16 non-structural proteins (e.g., ORF1ab gene) and at least four structural proteins (e.g., S gene, E gene, M gene, N gene). For SARS-CoV-2 detection, three types of diagnostic tests—nasopharyngeal swab, throat swab, blood and saliva samples—have been widely used based on (1) virus detection: hybridization between sequence complementary (capture probe) to the target RNA genome; (2) antigen protein detection: interaction of monoclonal antigen-specific antibody and virus antigen protein; and (iii) antibody detection: interaction of recombinant antigen and target-neutralizing antibody. As described in the following sections, the current development of biosensors employs these approaches to target SARS-CoV-2 RNA genome (ORF1ab gene, RNA-dependent RNA polymerase (RdRP) gene, S gene, N gene) [76, 78, 79, 102], specific antigen protein (S protein [S1 subunit/RBD], N protein) [103], and neutralizing antibody (IgM, IgG) [76, 77].

7.14 CNT-FET-Based Biosensor for Rapid Detection of SARS-CoV-2 (COVID-19)

As of today, the COVID-19 pandemic is a global challenge, and scientists are working on therapeutics, vaccines, and fast diagnostic techniques. Since therapeutics are delayed and vaccines are underway, fast diagnostic techniques could help control the spread and open the borders without affecting the economy. Rapid detection techniques have been developed and commercialized using antibody and antigen sensors. However, the

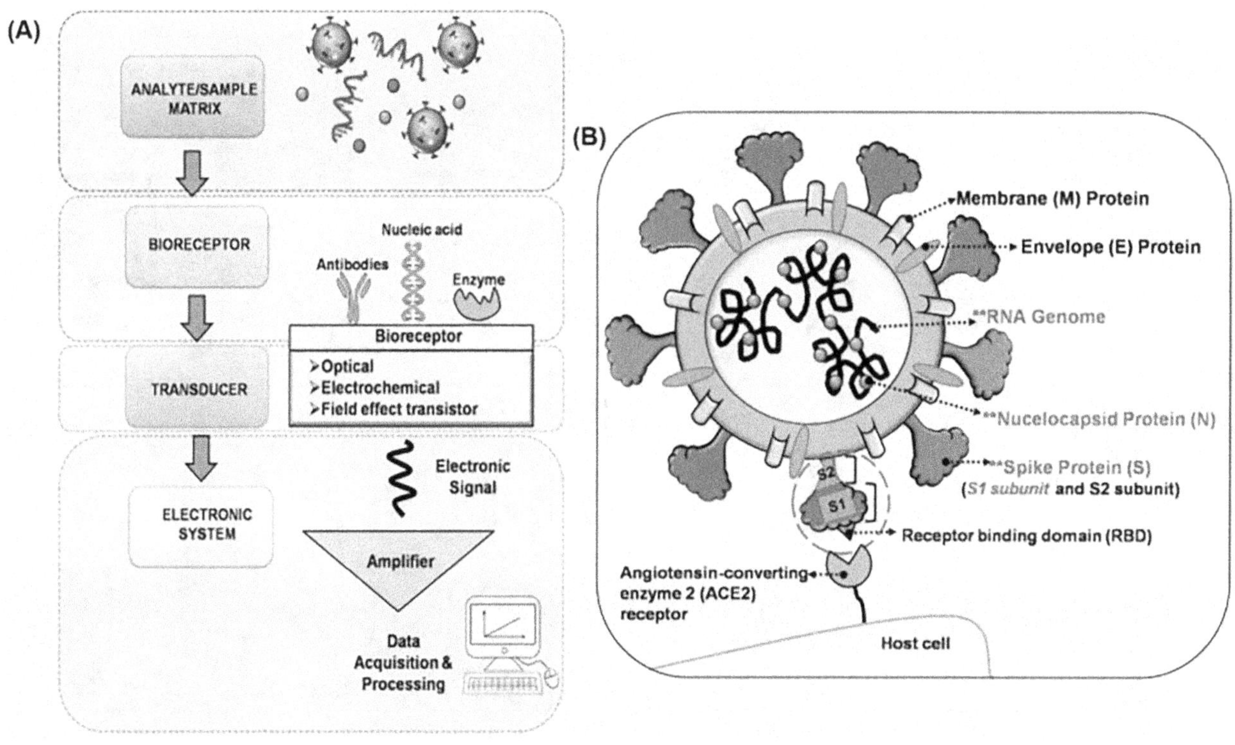

FIGURE 7.20 (a) Schematic diagram of a biosensor. (b) Structure and function of SARS-CoV-2 virus. The main four viral surface proteins are spike (S), envelope (E), membrane (M), and nucleocapsid (N). S protein contains the receptor-binding domain (RBD) that recognizes the host cell receptor, that is, the human angiotensin-converting enzyme 2 (ACE2). E protein contributes to the assembly and morphogenesis of virions. M protein, which is embedded in a lipid bilayer, is responsible for the release of nutrients at the transmembrane and forms the viral envelope. N protein binds to the RNA genome to form the nucleocapsid. Note: **Preferred target analyte used for current COVID-19 biosensor development.

antibody test is not a reliable test for detecting SARS-CoV-2. As per WHO, real-time polymerase chain reaction (qPCR) is the recommended test for detecting SARS-CoV-2. However, expensive equipment, trained personnel, and longer processing time make qPCR a non-effective method for point-of-care application. Longer time taken for qPCR test is due to longer amplification step before detecting the positive sequence. The time taken for the amplification step can be saved by employing a highly sensitive and selective detection mechanism instead of the optical labeling method used in qPCR test. CNT network FETs are known as one of the best platforms for electronic biosensors that can selectively detect metal ions and biomolecules, including hormones, viruses, and whole cells. Recently, a graphene FET–based biosensor is reported using a specific antibody against SARS-CoV-2 spike protein as the primary sensing element for detecting SARS-CoV-2.

In this work, a carbon nanotube (CNT) field-effect transistor (FET)–based biosensor has been proposed and demonstrated for selective detection of severe acute respiratory syndrome coronavirus-2 (SARS-CoV-2). CNTFETs were fabricated on a flexible Kapton substrate, and the sensor was fabricated by immobilizing the reverse sequence of the RNA-dependent RNA polymerase gene of SARS-CoV-2 onto the CNT channel. The biosensors were tested for the synthetic positive and control target sequences. The biosensor showed a selective sensing response to the positive target sequence with a limit of detection of 10 fM. The promising results from the study [104] suggest that the CNTFET-based biosensors can be used as a diagnostic tool for the detection of SARS-CoV-2.

In this work, a proof-of-concept electronic biosensor has been reported for rapid detection of SARS-CoV-2 based on liquid-gated CNT network FETs. The sensors were successfully fabricated, and selective detection of SARS-CoV-2 was demonstrated.

Attachments of carbon-based two-dimensional materials and nanotubes (CNTs) on the surface of FET biosensors have been explored to enhance the detection of the target analyte. CNTs and graphene-based FETs have shown high sensitivity in detecting small concentrations of target analyte.

Recently, a FET biosensor was developed by depositing SARS-CoV-2 spike protein and anti-nucleocapsid protein antibodies–functionalized single-walled carbon nanotube (SWCNT) on the sensor surface to detect complimentary SARS-CoV-2 antigens (Figure 7.21A) [105]. Based on 28 positive samples, the SWCNT-based FET biosensor exhibited a true positive rate of 82.1% and 53.6% for detecting spike protein and nucleocapsid protein, respectively. Based on ten negative samples, the true negative rate was 70% for both proteins. Overall, the SWCNT-based FET sensor exhibited excellent sensitivity with a LOD of 0.55 fg mL^{-1} and 0.016 fg mL^{-1} in detecting spike protein and nucleocapsid protein, respectively [105]. The sensor has the potential to be used as a rapid SARS-CoV-2 antigen test using clinical nasopharyngeal samples, without pre-processing, in less than 5 min.

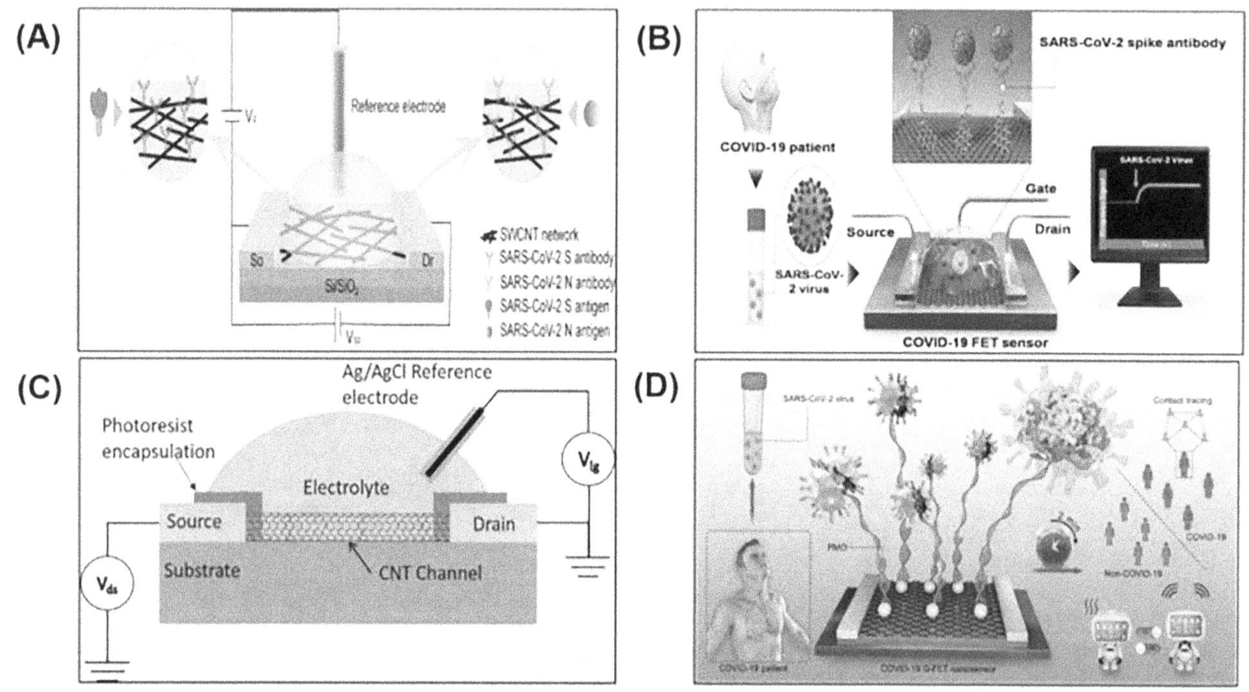

FIGURE 7.21 Field-effect transistor biosensor for COVID-19 detection: (a) SWCNT-based FET biosensor. (b) Graphene-based FET biosensor. (c) CNT-based FET fabricated on a flexible Kapton substrate. (d) PMO-functionalized graphene–FET biosensor.

(a) Reprinted with permission from Seo, G.; Lee, G.; Kim, M. J.; Baek, S.-H.; Choi, M.; Ku, K. B.; Lee, C.-S.; Jun, S.; Park, D.; Kim, H.G. "Rapid detection of COVID-19 causative virus (SARS-CoV-2) in human nasopharyngeal swab specimens using field-effect transistor-based biosensor." ACS Nano 2020, 14, 5,135–5,142. Copyright 2020, American Chemical Society.

In another approach, SARS-CoV-2 spike protein antibodies were functionalized on graphene sheets, which were then deposited on the sensor surface. This graphene-based FET biosensor is depicted in Figure 7.21B. The sensor was able to detect the SARS-CoV-2 spike antigen protein down to fg mL^{-1} in phosphate-buffered saline samples or clinical transport medium and with a LOD of 2.42×10^2 copies mL^{-1} in clinical samples, at a response rate between 0 and 400 s.

However, for viral detection of SARS-CoV-2, the RNA probe is required to detect the presence of complementary nucleic acid sequences (target sequences). To fulfill this need, recently, a liquid-gated CNT network FET was fabricated on a flexible Kapton film [104], as shown in Figure 7.21c. The sensor was able to selectively detect a portion of the SARS-CoV-2 RNA through hybridization. Here, the reverse sequence of the RNA-dependent RNA polymerase gene of SARS-CoV-2 was immobilized onto the CNT sidewalls. RNA hybridization was used as the primary signal generator, and the liquid-gated CNT network FET was used as the signal transducer. The biosensor showed a selective sensing response to the target sequence with a LOD of 10 fM.

In another remarkable FET biosensor, gold nanoparticles (AuNP)–decorated graphene sheets and phosphorodiamidate morpholino oligos (PMO) probes were employed on the sensor surface for ultrasensitive and rapid SARS-CoV-2 detection (Figure 7.21D) [106]. The PMO probe is usually 25 bases in length, and they bind to complementary sequences of RNA or single-stranded DNA according to standard nucleic acid base pairing. The PMO enabled direct detection of SARS-CoV-2 RNA through the hybridization between the PMO probe and SARS-CoV-2 RdRp without the need for further PCR amplification. For clinical readiness, a FET biosensor needs to have good reusability. For SARS-CoV-2 RdRp detection, this sensor can be chemically regenerated for reuse by denaturing the PMO–RNA duplex with 8.3 M urea solution for 5 min. The high surface-area-to-volume ratio of AuNP, high conductivity of graphene, and high density of neutral PMO immobilization provided more responsive testing than using charged oligonucleotide capture probe (e.g., single-stranded DNA probe) [106] for RNA detection. The sensor accuracy was analyzed with a receiver operating characteristic (ROC) curve, and it achieved an AUC of 0.995.

This research section describes the development of a new CNT-FET-based biosensor for reliable, fast detection of SARS-CoV-2 S1 antigen with high selectivity and sensitivity. Here, we present a highly sensitive electrical immunosensor for the detection of SARS-CoV-2 S1 antigen using single-walled carbon nanotubes (SWCNTs) deposited on the surface of SiO_2 between the S-D channels. The developed biosensor is based on the field-effect transistor (FET) technology, and its fabrication involves the immobilization of antibodies between the S-D sensing areas. The newly developed CNT-FET immunosensor can detect SARS-CoV-2 S1 antigen, based on the change in source–drain current (IDS), and the antigen-binding effect is characterized by a change in electrical signal (Scheme 7.1). The basic advantages of the FET-based biosensor are easy fabrication, fast sensing response, and ease of use, because the dynamic real-time response can be acquired with low-cost digital readers that can be calibrated for different applications. Certainly, at central hospitals and testing centers, advanced and traditional equipment can analyze and diagnose SARS-CoV-2 infection with high accuracy and precision. In pandemic circumstances, CNT-FET-based biosensors could be helpful as potential detection devices for tracing SARS-CoV-2 infection at the mass level.

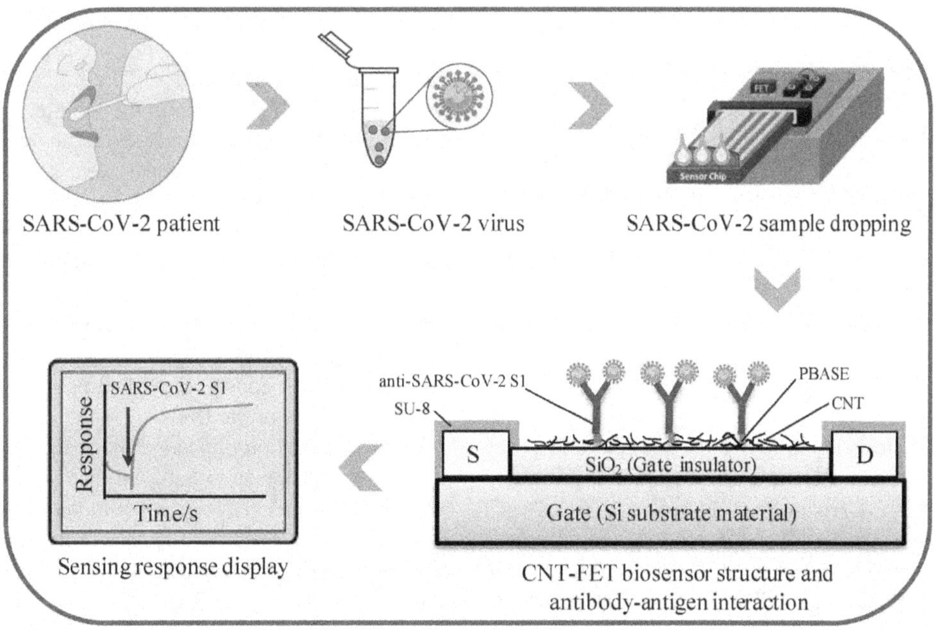

SCHEME 7.1 Schematic diagram of CNT-FET biosensor and SARS-CoV-2 S1 testing steps. SWCNT as a sensing nanomaterial and anti-SARS-CoV-2 S1 immobilized on the CNT via PBASE (linker). The CNT-FET biosensor senses the SARS-CoV-2 spike protein based on the corresponding effects on the electrical signal properties.

7.14.1 CNTFET and Sensor Fabrication

Carbon nanotube field-effect transistors on flexible Kapton substrates with encapsulated electrodes were fabricated as reported earlier. Around 99% semiconducting CNTs with an average diameter of 1.5 nm were used to fabricate the CNT network. The CNT thin films on the Kapton substrate were deposited by a simple solution process technique. The CNT suspension was made by sonicating a tweezer tip amount of CNT buckypaper. Then the Kapton substrate was functionalized with a monolayer of 2-mercaptopyridine using polydimethylsiloxane (PDMS) (Sylgard 184) stamping method. The functionalized Kapton film was immersed into the CNT suspension for 20 min. The CNT-deposited Kapton surface was cleaned by immersing it into absolute ethanol for 10 min and dried in nitrogen. The CNTs in the unwanted area were removed by plasma cleaning at 600 mTorr pressures and 10 SCCM flow of 99.99% oxygen gas. The electrodes were then deposited using successive evaporation of 5 nm Cr and 50 nm Au after defining the electrodes using photolithography. The electrodes were encapsulated using AZ1518 photoresist to avoid gate leakage and hard-baked at 200°C for 10 min [107]. The probe sequences were immobilized onto the CNT sidewalls, as described in refs [108], using pyrenebutanoicacid, succinimidyl ester as the molecular linker.

All the sequences used in this section were purchased from Integrated DNA Technologies, USA. The probe sequence that was immobilized onto the CNT sidewalls is the reverse sequence of the RNA-dependent RNA polymerase gene of the SARS-CoV-2. Before functionalization, the probe suspension in 20 mM Tris buffer was annealed at 70°C in an electric oven (BioBase).

A CNTFET-based biosensor has been fabricated to selectively detect a portion of the SARS-CoV-2 RNA. The positive target sequence was the RNA-dependent RNA polymerase gene (RdRP) of the SARS-CoV-2, as reported previously. The probe for selective detection used was the reverse sequence of the positive target sequence with an amino modification at the 5′ end for immobilization purpose. The negative control sequence was the RNA-dependent RNA polymerase gene of the SARS virus. The negative sequence has four mismatches with the reverse sequence of the RNA-dependent RNA polymerase gene of the SARS-CoV-2. The control sequence has been chosen to differentiate the closely related RNA sequence of the severe acute respiratory syndrome (SARS) viral RNA from the RNA of SARS-CoV-2.

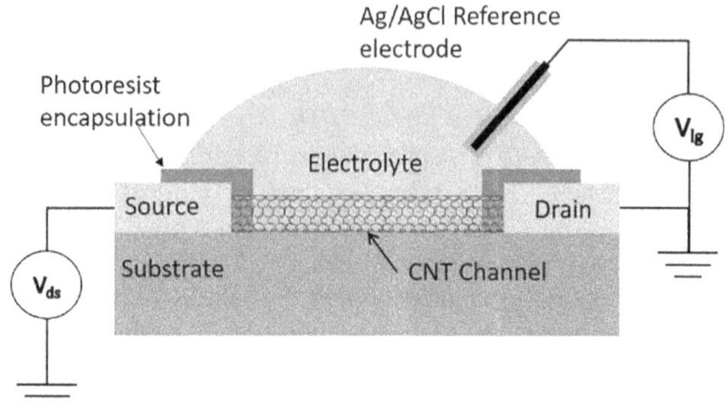

FIGURE 7.22 Schematic of the CNTFET fabricated on a flexible Kapton substrate with encapsulated electrodes with external electrical circuit for FET and sensor measurements.

Source: [104].

TABLE 7.4

Sequences of Probes and Positive and Negative Targets Used in This Study

	Sequence of the Primers and Probes
Probe	Amine-5′-GCATC TCCTG ATGAG GTTCC ACCTG-3
Positive target sequence (SARS-CoV-2 RdRP)	CAGGT GGAAC CTCAT CAGGA GATGC
Control target sequence	C CAGGT GGAAC ATCAT CCGGT GATGC

7.14.2 CNTFET and Sensor Measurements

The transfer characteristic curves of the pristine and probe immobilized CNTFETs were measured under liquid-gated conditions using 2 mM Tris buffer solution, and an Ag/AgCl standard electrode as the gate. The schematic of the fabricated device, along with the measurement setup, is illustrated in Figure 7.22. A well made up of PDMS was mounted onto the channel to hold the electrolyte and target solution in the channel area. A computer-interfaced Kiethley 2602 source measure unit was used for electrical measurements. The device current (I_{ds}) was measured by sweeping the gate voltage (V_{lg}) from −0.5 V to 1 V with a step size of 0.02 V. The sensor measurements were done by continuously monitoring Ids with a sample time interval of 1 S. The sensors were tested for both positive and negative target sequence, as given in Table 7.4 [104]. Both positive and control sequence solutions were prepared by dissolving the purchased sequences in 2 mM tris buffer.

The target sequences were prepared with different concentrations in 2 mM Tris buffer. The initial stock solution was prepared at 10 μM, as given in the suppliers' information, and diluted further to obtain target sequences with concentrations of 10 pM. The target sequences were added into the PDMS well by monitoring the current Ids with an interval of 1 S. The response of the biosensors for both positive and control targets has been investigated. The addition of positive target shows a clear concentration depended on the drop in the device current. The drop in the device current could be attributed to the change of band realignments and electrostatic gating at the metallic–semiconductor carbon nanotube junction due to the hybridization of the DNA.

The concentration-dependent normalized current response is studied. The deviation between the response of the positive and control sequences is prominent, and this could be a clear indication of the selective response of the tested biosensor. As discussed earlier, the control sequence is selected to differentiate SARS-COV-2 and SARS virus. Hence, we can say that the relatively higher response of the biosensor for the control sequence at concentration of 1 nM is due to the aggregation of the negative sequence within the electrical double layer of the CNT channel.

7.14.3 Immobilization of the Probe Sequence

The CNTFETs were electrically tested to ensure the immobilization of the probe sequence. The transfer characteristic curves of the pristine and probe-immobilized CNTFETs have been investigated. The pristine CNTFET showed ambipolar characteristics with a positive threshold voltage (V_{th}) which indicate the hole-dominated electrical conduction at a gate bias of 0 V. A clear positive shift in threshold voltage is observed after immobilization of probe sequence. This is consistent with our previous works and ensures the tethering of probes on the sidewalls of CNTs. The Debye length of the 2 mM tris buffer solution used was about 10 nm. The length of the probe sequence is also about 10 nm, and any changes in the probe sequence will be in the vicinity of the CNT channel.

7.14.4 Basic Structure of the CNT-FET Device and Optical Microscopy (OM)/SEM Imaging

The basic structure of the field-effect transistor (FET) is shown in Figure 7.23a. The complete fabricated CNT-FET device

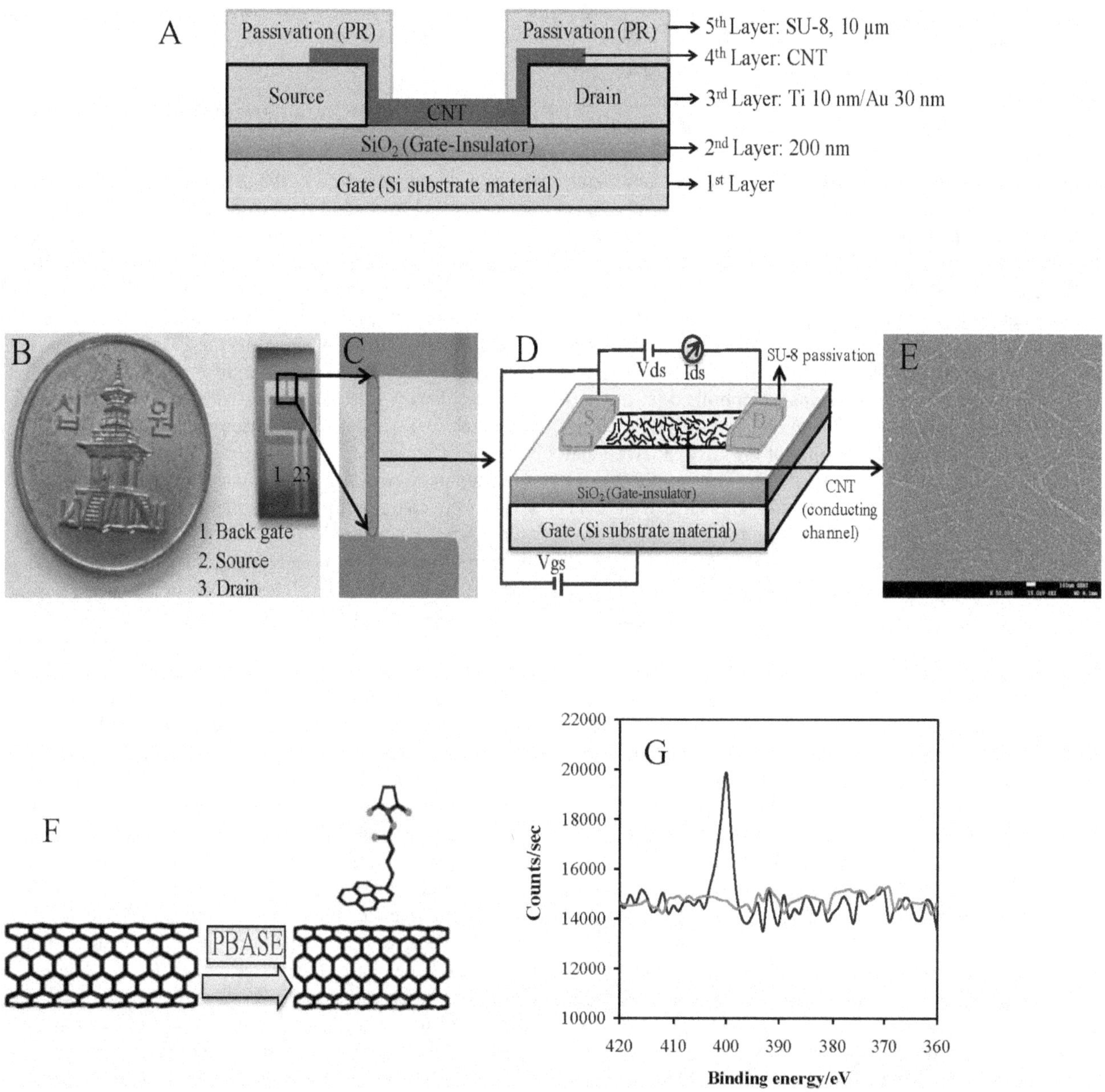

FIGURE 7.23 (a) Schematic representation of CNT-FET device illustrating structural components and thickness of fabricated nanomaterial. The CNT network makes contact with metal electrodes (source–drain). An SU-8 photoresist on the source–drain electrodes is used to prevent leakage of gate current. (b) Optical image of single-die CNT-FET device from wafer. (c) Optical microscope image of CNT-FET device showing source–drain electrodes. (d) Schematic structure of FET circuit diagram and CNT network situated between source–drain electrodes on conductive substrate. (e) SEM image of deposited CNT network on surface. (f) Surface functionalization of CNT-FET by 2 mM PBASE (linker). (g) XPS spectra of CNT-FET surface before (red line) and after PBASE treatment (blue line). Change in N1s peak at 400.2 eV assigned for PBASE successfully modified the CNT surface.

after a single die is shown in Figure 7.23b. Optical microscopy (OM) was used to identify the locations of nanotubes bridging source–drain (S-D) electrode pairs in order to determine the fabrication process (Figure 7.23c). Inkjet printing was used to deposit CNTs, random network on the SiO_2 surface between the S-D of the device. The schematic structure of the FET circuit diagram along with the CNT semiconductive network situated between S-D electrodes on the substrate is shown in Figure 7.23d. The deposited CNT network characterized by SEM imaging is shown in Figure 7.23e.

7.14.5 Characterization of CNT-FET Surface

The basic mechanism of PBASE functionalization with CNT surface is shown in Figure 7.23f. To confirm the CNT-FET biosensor surface modification and the presence of PBASE on the surface of the device, X-ray photoelectron spectroscopy (XPS) was employed. The peak height of XPS difference spectra can be used to confirm the absence or presence of functionalized PBASE on the CNT surface by analyzing the N1s peak at 400.2 eV. As seen in Figure 7.23g, the bare surface did not show any peak increase at 400.2 eV, and after PBASE modification of the device, the N1s peak appeared at 400.2 eV. The binding energy values after N substitution were assigned in the range of 400.2 to 401.8 eV. These XPS results clearly suggest successful functionalization, since the only source of nitrogen atoms in functionalized CNT is the PBASE molecule. The PBASE was immobilized on the surface of the carbon nanostructure by π–π non-covalent stacking between the six-membered ring of the CNT sidewall and the pyrene group of PBASE, while the succinimidyl ester group of the PBASE facing upward on the surface of CNT can react with an amine group of the target antibody and forms an amide bond.

7.14.6 SEM Characterization of Patterned CNT

The morphology of CNT from scanning electron microscopy (SEM) is investigated. SEM images show the microstructure of the unaligned CNT needle-like fine network. On a nanometer scale with open pores, the CNTs formed an interconnected and well-entangled porous network. Aligned CNT bundles with varying diameters are shown by scanning electron microscopy, averaging approximately 30 μm to confirm the immobilization pattern of anti-SARS-CoV-2 S1 on the PBASE-modified CNT-FET between the S-D channel areas of the biosensor. On the dry surface of anti-SARS-CoV-2 S1 immobilized area, AuNPs-SARS-CoV-2 S1-conjugated antigen solution was applied, and AuNPs-conjugated SARS-CoV-2 S1 antigen was bound with the immobilized anti-SARS-CoV-2 S1 between the S-D channel area. For the sphere-like structure that proves the presence of AuNPs-conjugated SARS-CoV-2 S1 antigen, the AuNP sizes are in the range of 19.3 to 23 nm. The increased size of AuNPs was due to the binding of the highly glycosylated SARS-CoV-2 S1 antigen. These findings suggest that the SARS-CoV-2 S1 antibody was successfully immobilized on the biosensing area, and the formation of the antibody–antigen complex localized by AuNPs is studied.

7.14.7 Study of Anti-SARS-CoV-2 S1 Specificity by Western Blot

To confirm the specificity of anti-SARS-CoV-2 S1 with target SARS-CoV-2 S1 antigen, a Western blotting experiment was performed. Western blot data of SARS-CoV-2 S1, SARS-CoV-1 S1, and MERS-CoV S1 antigens at a concentration of 1 μg/mL (lanes 1, 2, and 3). A single distinct band recognizes the 77 kDa SARS-CoV-2 surface spike glycoprotein S1 antigen (lane 1). The increased molecular size was observed due to the high glycosylation of the S1 protein. The nonspecific SARS-CoV-1 S1 and MERS-CoV S1 antigens did not show binding with the anti-SARS-CoV-2 S1 (lanes 2 and 3). The results indicate that the used anti-SARS-CoV-2 S1 was specific for the SARS-CoV-2 S1 antigen.

7.14.8 Electrical Characterization of the Biosensor

Before any treatment, the transfer property of the CNT-FET device was characterized as the best fit for a p-type CNT-FET device, acting as a conductor with semiconductor properties. Oxygen and water molecules adsorbed on the CNT surface withdraw electrons from the CNT, which results in the p-type operation. Due to variations in the amount of SWCNT deposition on the individual chips, small variations in IDS can be observed. The transistor output of the individual chips, however, is very similar because the differences in SWCNT distribution density across are relatively small and reasonably comparable. The CNT-FET biosensor was electrically characterized after each functionalization step in dry conditions at room temperature. The semiconductor properties of the biosensor were characterized before the treatment (i.e., only CNT on the surface), after CNT surface modification by PBASE, and after antibody immobilization. No gate current leakage was observed, with almost zero IDS, suggesting a superior p-type transistor compared to previous reports.

SARS-CoV-2 S1 (1 μL of 100 μg/mL) antibody diluted in 0.01 × PBS was then exposed to the PBASE-modified CNT surface. After anti-SARS-CoV-2 S1 immobilization, the surface was washed and dried in N_2 gas blow, and the IDS of the CNT-FET biosensor was measured; a depleted drain current indicated that the antibody was successfully immobilized on the biosensor surface. Antibody immobilization leads to a 10–50% decrease in ON-state current because of enhanced electron dispersion from crowded and more complex chemical environments along the CNT-FET source–drain channel area. In each of these steps, the mobility of the CNT-FET device generally decreases by a small amount, as there are additional sources of dispersion of the charge carrier. Garcia-Aljaro et al. reported that the decrease in IDS of the biosensor, that is, the increase in resistance, is due to the accumulation of negative charge from the immobilized antibodies on the biosensor. Based on the same modification and attachment chemistry, changes in IDS versus VGS induced by the functionalization process were consistent with previously reported findings. The mechanism of source–drain current (IDS) decrease in carbon nanotube transistors may arise from the electrostatic gating effect and the Schottky barrier effect. On the dry surface of the CNT-FET biosensor, 1 μL of SARS CoV-2 S1 antigen was dropped on the immobilized anti-SARS CoV-2 S1, and IDS of the CNT-FET biosensor was measured; a depleted drain current indicated that the SARS CoV-2 S1 antigen solution strongly binds with immobilized anti-SARS CoV-2 S1 on the biosensor surface.

7.14.9 Determination of Response Time, Detection Limit, and Detection Range of CNT-FET Biosensor

The CNT-FET biosensor response time, limit of detection, and detection range were characterized by loading of target antigen (SARS-CoV-2 S1) at serially increased concentrations. The anti-SARS-CoV-2 S1 immobilized CNT-FET biosensor was used in systematic electrical signal measurements. First, at 10 s, 0.8 μL of 10 mM (AA) buffer solution at pH 6.0 was dropped on the sensor to equilibrate the source–drain current (IDS). After achieving a stable IDS signal, continuously increasing SARS-CoV-2 S1 antigen concentrations (0.8 μL each drop) were loaded. The real-time response with increasing concentration of SARS-CoV-2 S1 antigen added every 50 s was recorded after achieving saturation of the observed IDS. Each concentration of the SARS-CoV-2 S1 antigen generated a characteristic spike and saturation, seen in all tested antigen concentrations.

A calibration curve was investigated as a function of SARS-CoV-2 S1 antigen concentrations against normalized sensor response (ΔI/Io). These results indicate that the CNT-FET biosensor detection lies in the range of 0.1 to 5,000 fg/mL. The calibration curve indicates that the sensing response starts becoming saturated from 100 fg/mL of SARS-CoV-2 S1 antigen concentration; however, little increase in IDS was observed above a 100 fg/mL concentration. The limit of detection (LOD) was determined in the only linear portion of the curve based on the dose-dependent sensor response. The LOD of the biosensor was 4.12 fg/mL in 10 mM (AA) buffer solution of pH 6.0. The sensitivity of the CNT-FET biosensor (immunochemical method) is non-linear at increasing SARS-CoV-2 S1 antigen concentration; probably, the immobilized antibody number on the CNT surface is limited.

Recently, Seo et al. [109] fabricated a graphene-based FET biosensor for instant detection of SARS-CoV-2 spike S1 protein using monoclonal antibody immobilized, which had a LOD of 1 fg/mL. The variation in LOD values of graphene and CNT-FET was due to the varying amount of semiconducting graphene and CNT in the device fabrication. Table 7.5 presents the data on SARS-CoV-2 detection by various biosensors reported in recent years. The summarized parameters collected from the relevant publications, as shown in Table 7.5, include the analyzed biomarker target, LOD, measurement range, time required for final result generation, and compared with the results of this study on detection of SARS-CoV-2 S1. Our biosensor is highly sensitive compared with the other reported biosensors. The sensitivity and time response of the biosensor vary with the number of immobilized detecting antibodies on the semiconducting CNT layer. The dimension and width of the S-D may be other parameters that are responsible for the sensitivity of the biosensor [109].

7.14.10 Physiochemical Properties of the SARS-CoV-2, SARS-CoV-1, and MERS-CoV Spike Proteins

The SARS-CoV-2 S1 antigen is positively charged (*pI* = 8.27) [115], and the SARS-CoV-2 S antigen is negatively charged (*pI* = 6.24) at neutral pH [101]. Table 7.6 summarizes the physicochemical properties of the SARS-CoV-2, SARS-CoV-1, and MERS-CoV spike proteins. The SARS-CoV-2 S1, SARS-CoV-1 S1, and MERS-CoV S1 antigens carry a net charge of +5, −8, and −7, respectively, at pH 7.0 (Table 7.6) [114]. Based on these data, it was concluded that the SARS-CoV-2 S1 antigen carries more positive charge than the other two antigens at neutral pH. The SARS-CoV-2 S1 antigen was prepared in 10 mM AA buffer at pH 6.0. At this acidic pH, the antigen was more protonated and carried a net charge of +13. This increased positive charge (+13) on the antigen strongly binds with the SARS-CoV-2 S1 antibody and generates a strong IDS response.

TABLE 7.5

Performance Comparison of Previously Developed Biosensor for SARS-CoV-2 Target Biomarker, Detection Method, LOD, Detection Range, and Time Required to Generate Final Test Result

Biomarker	Detection Method	LOD	Detection Range	Detection Time	Ref.
SARS-CoV-2 spike protein (S)	CNT-FET	5.5 fg/mL	5.5 fg/mL to 5.5 pg/mL	2 min	[101]
SARS-CoV-2 spike protein (S1)	Graphene-FET	1 fg/mL	1 fg/mL to 10 pg/mL	5–8 min	[109]
SARS-CoV-2 nucleic acid/ SARS-CoV-2 thiol-cDNA	Optical LSPR	0.22 pM	0.10 pm to 1.0 μM	15–20 min	[110]
SARS-CoV-2 spike RBD	SWCNT intrinsically near-infrared (nIR) fluorescence	12.6 nM	Not determined	5 s	[111]
SARS-CoV-2 spike protein (S)	Graphite electrode functionalized with AuNPs-cys	229 fg/mL	1 pg/mL to 1 ng/mL	6.5 min	[112]
SARS-CoV-2 spike protein (S)	Tungsten diselenide (WSe_2) based-FET	25 fg/μL	25 fg/μL to 10 ng/μL	2 min	[113]
SARS-CoV-2 spike protein (S1)	CNT-FET	4.12 fg/mL	0.1 fg/mL to 5.0 pg/mL	2–3 min	[114]

TABLE 7.6

Molecular Weight (Mw), Net Charge, Isoelectric Point (pI), and Comparative Physiochemical Properties of Spike Protein of SARS-CoV-2, SARS-CoV-1, and MERS-CoV

Properties	SARS-CoV-2	SARS-CoV-1	MERS-CoV
Spike (S) protein, UniProt ID	P0DTC2	P59594	A0A140AYZ5
Spike protein sequence length	1,273	1,255	1,353
Molecular weight (kDa)	141.1	139.1	149.4
Spike (S1/S2) protein cleavage site	R685/S686	R667/S668	R751/S752
Spike protein net charge	−7	−16	−17
S1 subunit net charge	+5	8	−7
S2 subunit net charge	−12	−8	−10
S protein isoelectric point (pI)	6.24	5.56	5.73
S1 subunit isoelectric point (pI)	8.27	5.67	5.98
S2 subunit isoelectric point (pI)	5.25	5.45	5.46
RBD sequence length	Sequence 333–526	Sequence 306–527	Sequence 367–606
RBD net charge	+2	+4	−3

Note: Summarized values are predicted by online ProtParam tool [114]. ProtParam tool does not consider post-translational modification in the physiochemical parameter calculations. These estimated values should be followed with caution.

7.14.11 Selectivity Study of the CNT-FET Biosensor

Practically, a biosensor should not only be sensitive but also selective to a specific antigen. Selectivity is an important parameter in immunosensor applications because of the complex composition of biomolecules. Therefore, to confirm the selectivity of the CNT-FET biosensor, a control set of specific (SARS-CoV-2 S1) and non-specific (SARS-CoV-1 S1 and MERS-CoV S1) antigens was tested under identical experimental conditions. Figure 7.24a shows the normalized biosensor response of the tested antigens prepared in 10 mM AA buffer at pH 6.0. First, after running the test, at time 10 s, the 10 mM AA buffer was dropped to stabilize the IDS of the CNT-FET biosensor. After IDS stabilization up to 50 s, the MERS-CoV S1 antigen was loaded on the biosensor. After saturation of the IDS signal, the SARS-CoV-1 S1 antigen was again dropped (Figure 7.24a). These negative control experiments provide strong evidence that the no signal response of the CNT-FET biosensor reflects a highly selective response against non-specific antigens that reveals a non-specific binding. Immobilized anti-SARS-CoV-2 S1 recognized the target antigen, not the two tested non-specific antigens (Figure 7.24B). SARS-CoV-2 S1 antibodies binding with specific antigens produced far greater changes in the IDS signal than did the non-specific antigens. For particular antigen–antibody pairs, the CNT surface showed high electron transport properties compared to the non-specific pairs. These findings show a reduced normalized biosensor response by 8 to 9.5% compared with specific antigen–antibody pairs.

Saliva samples with and without SARS-CoV-2 S1 antigen were tested. There was no significant change in IDS after dropping of non-fortified saliva on the biosensor (Figure 7.24c). Saliva without SARS-CoV-2 S1 antigen showed a negligible response and did not show binding with immobilized anti-SARS-CoV-2 S1. However, saliva with SARS-CoV-2 S1 antigen showed a strong binding response with immobilized anti-SARS-CoV-2 S1. The concentration-dependent SARS-CoV-2 S1–fortified saliva was tested to see the biosensor response. As shown in Figure 7.24d, the sensor response was dependent on the SARS-CoV-2 S1 concentration present in the fortified saliva. The sensor response was almost saturated at 4,000–5,000 fg/mL SARS-CoV-2 S1–fortified saliva. These results indicated that the sensor response data is very similar, as discussed before.

7.14.12 Reproducibility and Reusability Study of the CNT-FET Biosensor

Furthermore, the reproducibility tests of each biosensor are needed to characterize the parameters for practical applications. Because reproducibility is one of the key factors that affect the practical application of electrochemical immunosensors, the reproducibility, therefore, of fabricated CNT-FET biosensors from three batches (1, 2, and 3) was tested under identical experimental condition by the SARS-CoV-2 S1 antigen dropping experiment (Figure 7.25a). The obtained results demonstrate that all tested CNT-FET biosensors fabricated in all three batches exhibited very similar SARS-CoV-2 S1 antigen responses. The relative standard deviation (RSD) was estimated to be 2.65% based on the generated electrical signal of the 12 replicates of SARS-CoV-2 S1–fortified saliva (Figure 7.25a). Thus, these results indicate that fabricated CNT-FET biosensors have stable and good reproducibility for antigen recognition.

For the reusability experiment of CNT-FET biosensor, SARS-CoV-2 S1 –tested biosensor was washed five times with 0.01 × PBST to clean the bound SARS-CoV-2 S1 antigen with anti-SARS-CoV-2 S1 and dried with N_2 gas blow. The MERS-CoV S1, SARS-CoV-1 S1, and SARS-CoV-2 S1 antigens were tested, and the observed sensor response shows that after one use, still the fabricated material was stable and not damaged in the washing process. The normalized sensor response drop of SARS-CoV-2 S1 was 0.068; however, in the reused biosensor, the normalized sensor response was 0.062 (Figure 7.24a and 7.25b). Based on the comparison of normalized sensor response (Figure 7.24a and 7.25b), it was concluded that the sensitivity

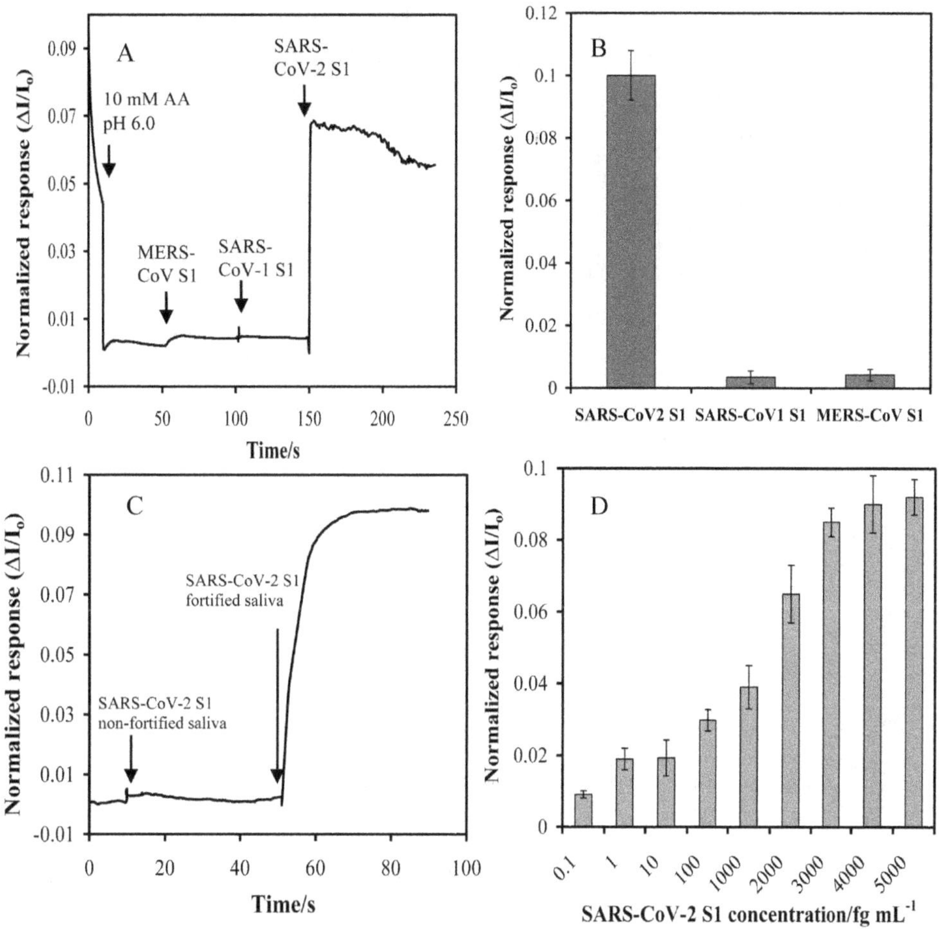

FIGURE 7.24 (a) Real-time biosensor response for selectivity test of target SARS-CoV-2 S1 and non-target SARS-CoV-1 S1 and MERS-CoV S1 antigens. Antigen concentration was 100 fg/mL, prepared in 10 mM AA buffer at pH 6.0. (b) Normalized response ($\Delta I/I_o$) of target SARS-CoV-2 S1 and non-target SARS-CoV-2 S1 and MERS-CoV S1 antigens. Error bars represent the standard deviation of three biosensor replicates. Each experiment was repeated a minimum of three times, and typical results are shown. (c) Normalized real-time biosensor response ($\Delta I/I_o$) versus time characteristics after SARS-CoV-2 S1 non-fortified and fortified saliva dropping. The used antigen concentration in fortified saliva was 100 fg/mL. (d) Normalized real-time biosensor response ($\Delta I/I_o$) versus SARS-CoV-2 S1 antigen (0.1, 1, 10, 100, 1,000, 2,000, 3,000, 4,000, and 5,000 fg/mL) fortified saliva. Error bars represent the standard deviation of three biosensor replicates. Each experiment was repeated a minimum of three times, and typical results are shown.

of the biosensor was decreased by 8.82% (Figure 7.25b). With less than 10% of sensor response decrease, the regeneration step was working quite well for the developed system. The biosensor reusability response depends on the retained CNT-FET fabricated materials, and the biosensor offers 91.18% retained or higher sensing response.

7.14.13 Advantages and Limitations

Overall, the FET-based sensor provides fast detection and low LOD and does not require additional procedures for labelling during sample preparation. It is low-cost, small in size, and simple to operate. Nevertheless, the device sensitivity could be further improved, especially at a high concentration of sample analyte, as the total number of antibodies anchored on the surface is limited by the small sensor size. Non-specific interaction and screening effect could also diminish response and sensitivity. To prevent non-specific binding, a blocking reagent (e.g., BSA or polyethylene glycol) is required to block the un-reacted active sites, or a covalent coupling (e.g., amide bond) is required to attach the antibody to the sensor [116].

The Debye length problem remains an entrenched obstacle [117]. A layer of ions in the electrolyte above the sensor surface effectively "shields" or "screens" the analytes from the charge carriers in the semiconductor channel. The thickness of this layer is called the Debye length [116]. As shown in Figure 7.26a, the Debye length under physiological conditions (in 10 mM phosphate buffer saline (PBS) solution) is close to 0.7 nm, which is smaller than the size of antibody receptor molecules immobilized on the sensor surface, which are generally 10–15 nm in size [117]. It is difficult to detect analyte-binding that is beyond the Debye length in the physiological environment. There have been attempts to address this problem by using short antibody fragments (e.g., nanobody receptor) or aptamers (Figure 7.26B), which enable the analyte to bind closer to the sensor surface and achieve a detection limit down to the sub-picomolar range without the loss of selectivity.

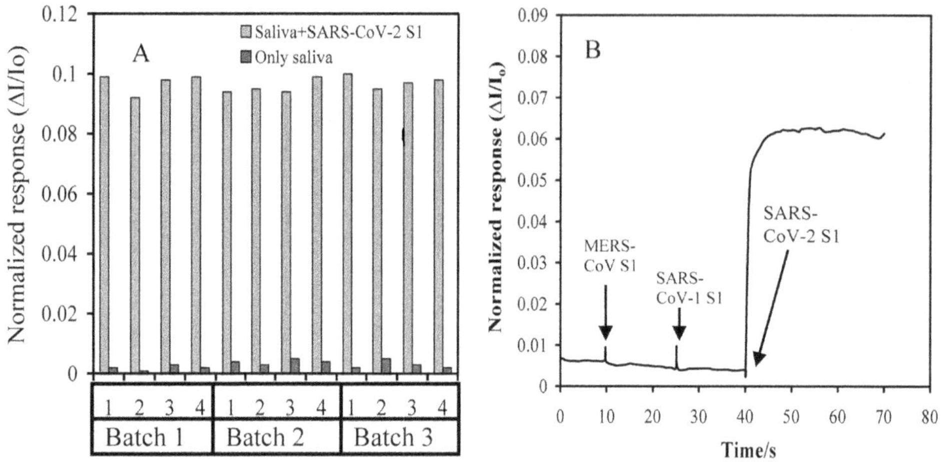

FIGURE 7.25 (a) CNT-FET reproducibility test of 24 CNT-FET biosensors from three batches: 12 CNT-FET used for SARS-CoV-2 S1–fortified saliva and 12 CNT-FET used for only saliva test. Fixed drain–source voltage (Vds = 0.5 V) and Vg = −1.5 V were applied in the electrical signal measurements. (b) Normalized real-time biosensor response ($\Delta I/I_0$) versus time characteristics after 0.01 × PBST washing and drying (reused CNT-FET biosensor). Target SARS-CoV-2 S1 and non-target SARS-CoV-1 S1 and MERS-CoV S1 antigens were tested. Each antigen's 100 fg/mL were prepared in 10 mM AA buffer of pH 6.0.

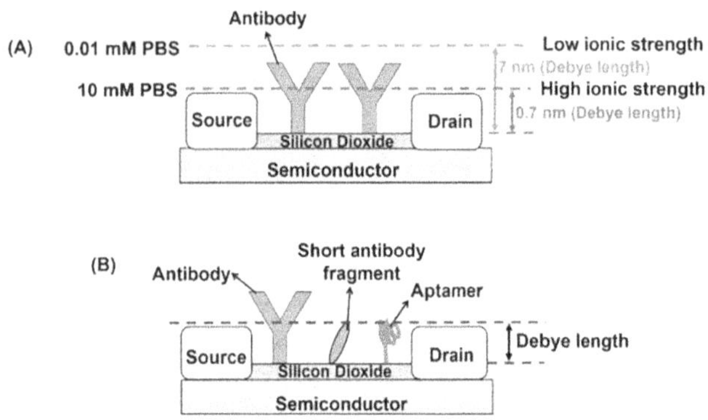

FIGURE 7.26 (A) The Debye length increases with the reduction of buffer ionic strength. (B) Short antibody fragments or aptamers could be used to bring the analyte-binding closer to the sensor surface and within the Debye length.

The Debye length is proportional to the reciprocal of the ionic strength. To increase the Debye length, the electrolyte ionic strength can be lowered by diluting the sample, but this, in turn, dilutes the analyte concentration and may cause a change in protein structure, resulting in the loss of protein activity and binding affinity as well. For example, in [118], the 10 mM PBS buffer was diluted to 0.01 mM, which increased the Debye length from 0.7 nm to 7 nm, comparable to the size of the positive-charged spike protein S1 subunit antibody (7–10 nm). However, dilution makes it difficult to detect low-abundance analytes [119].

7.15 Functional Carbon Quantum Dots as Medical Countermeasures to Human Coronavirus

Carbon-based quantum dots comprising of graphene quantum dots (GQDs) and carbon quantum dots (CQDs, C-dots, or CDs) have sizes that are lower than 10 nm. Different from the bulk carbon, carbon-based quantum dots have excellent water solubility and good luminescence signals. Compared with traditional semiconductor quantum dots and organic dyes, they are better in terms of chemical inertness, high resistance to photobleaching, and low toxicity. The last but not the least, carbon-based quantum dots have good electronic properties as either electron donors or acceptors. All these make them suitable in applications in biomedicine, catalysis, optronics, and sensors.

Carbon-based quantum dots can be prepared or synthesized via "top-down" and "bottom-up" approaches, including chemical ablation, laser ablation, electrochemical carbonization, microwave ray irradiation, and hydrothermal/solvothermal treatment [15]. Keys in this synthesis process are to avoid carbonaceous aggregation, to achieve size control and uniformity, and to enable surface modification. For example, we synthesized 15 nm GQDs with the green emission (497 nm) from Vulcan CX-72 carbon black by being refluxed with concentrated nitric acid. Synthesized GQDs contained plenty of carboxyl and hydroxyl groups on the surface. In another study, the hydrothermal approach (Hummer's method) was used to make 5 nm GQDs with blue emission (430 nm).

Therapeutic options for the highly pathogenic human coronavirus (HCoV) infections are urgently needed. Anticoronavirus therapy is, however, challenging, as coronaviruses are biologically diverse and rapidly mutating. In this work, the antiviral activity of seven different carbon quantum dots (CQDs) for the treatment of human coronavirus HCoV-229E infections was investigated. The first generation of antiviral CQDs was derived from hydrothermal carbonization of ethylenediamine/citric acid as carbon precursors and postmodified with boronic acid ligands. These nanostructures showed a concentration-dependent virus inactivation with an estimated EC_{50} of 52 ± 8 μg mL^{-1}. CQDs derived from 4-aminophenylboronic acid without any further modification resulted in the second generation of anti-HCoV nanomaterials with an EC_{50} lowered to 5.2 ± 0.7 μg mL^{-1}. The underlying mechanism of action of these CQDs was revealed to be inhibition of HCoV-229E entry that could be due to interaction of the functional groups of the CQDs with HCoV-229E entry receptors; surprisingly, an equally large inhibition activity was observed [120] at the viral replication step.

In this section, we investigate the potential of functional carbon quantum dots (CQDs) as inhibitors of host cells infection by HCoV-229E coronavirus (Figure 7.27). CQDs with an average diameter below 10 nm and excellent water dispersion are highly attractive for nanomedical applications due to a lack of visible signs of toxicity in animals. They can be synthesized quickly via several different inexpensive and simple methods, and their excellent optical properties offer in vivo tracking possibilities. It was recently demonstrated that CQDs are suitable scaffolds to interfere with the entry of viruses into cells. Boronic acid–modified CQDs were able to inhibit, for example, HIV-1 entry by suppressing syncytium formation. Some of us have shown lately the potential of CQDs functionalized with boronic acid and amine moieties to interfere with the entry of herpes simplex virus type 1 [12]. Han and coworkers reported the potential of CQDs as viral inhibitors by activation of type I interferon responses.

This unique study reveals that boronic acid functions can be responsible for anti-HCoV activity. CQDs derived from citric acid/ethylenediamine and further conjugated by "click" chemistry with boronic acid functions display an effective 50% inhibition concentration EC_{50} = 52 ± 8 μg mL^{-1}. Likewise, CQDs derived from 4-aminophenylboronic acid and phenylboronic acid without any further modification exhibit antiviral behavior with a decreased effective EC_{50} down to 5.2 ± 0.7 μg mL^{-1}. The underlying mechanism of action of these CQDs was revealed to be the CQDs' interaction with the HCoV-229E S protein. Surprisingly, an equally large inhibition activity was observed at the viral replication step.

7.15.1 First Generation of CQD Inhibitors of Host Cell Infections by HCoV-229E Coronavirus: Boronic Acid-Modified CQDs

7.15.1.1 Formation and Characterization

7.15.1.1.1 Carbon Quantum Dots Formed from Ethylenediamine/Citric Acid

Boronic acid derivatives have been proposed as low-toxicity agents for inhibiting the entry of various viruses. To test if such concepts can be extrapolated to human coronavirus HCoV-229E infections, boronic acid functional groups were chemically integrated onto CQDs-1 formed through hydrothermal carbonization of ethylenediamine/citric acid (Figure 7.28a) [120]. The approach consists of sealing the organic precursors in a Teflon-lined autoclave chamber and performing the formation of CQDs at elevated temperature under reduced pressure for 5 h. The pH value of the resulting CQDs suspensions was found to be 7.2 ± 0.2 (*n* = 5). To remove larger precipitates, the as-obtained CQDs suspension was first centrifuged and then dialyzed against water for 24 h, with a final yield of CQDs of 40%. CQDs-1 exhibits a spherical shape with an average diameter of 4.5 ± 0.2 nm (Figure 7.28b). XPS analysis (Table 7.7) [120] indicates the presence of C, O, and N. The C1s high-resolution XPS spectrum of CQDs-1 depicts three different carbon features: the graphitic C = C at 283.4 eV, 284.9 eV (C–H), and 286.4 eV (C–O, C–N) (Figure 7.28c). Analysis of the N_{1s} high-resolution XPS shows the presence of surface NH_2 groups (399.9 eV) (Figure 7.28d). The Raman spectrum of the CQD-1 (Figure 7.28e) displays the characteristic G band at 1,570 cm^{-1} related to in-plane vibration of sp^2 carbon, and the D band at 1,350 cm^{-1} attributed to disorder and defects. The ratio of the intensity of these bands (I_D/I_G), used to express the extent of sp^2/sp^3 hybridization of carbon atoms, is found to be 0.93 ± 0.15 for all particles. XRD patterns indicate their crystalline nature with a broad diffraction peak centered at 25.5° corresponding

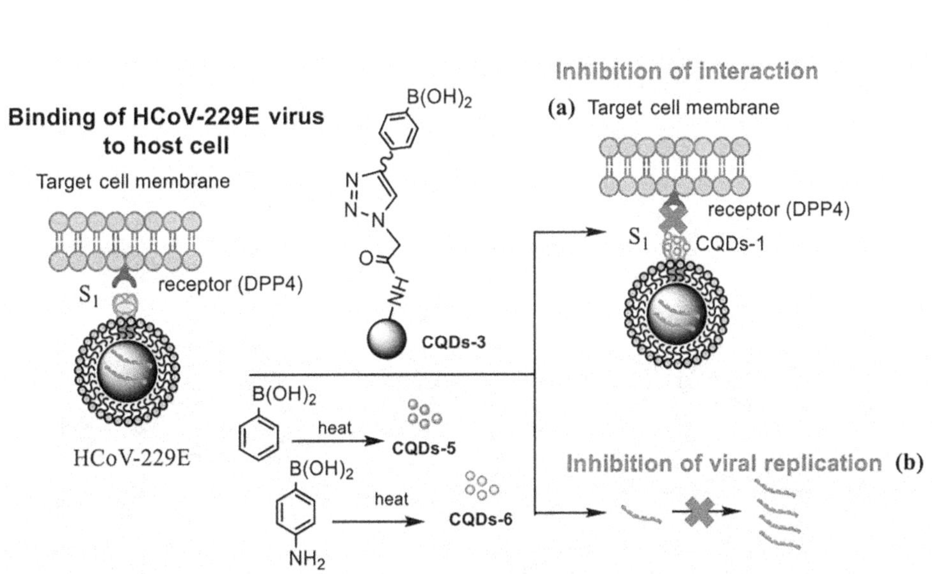

FIGURE 7.27 Influence of CQDs, prepared by hydrothermal carbonization, on binding of HCoV-229E virus to cells: (a) inhibition of protein S receptor interaction, and (b) inhibition of viral RNA genome replication.

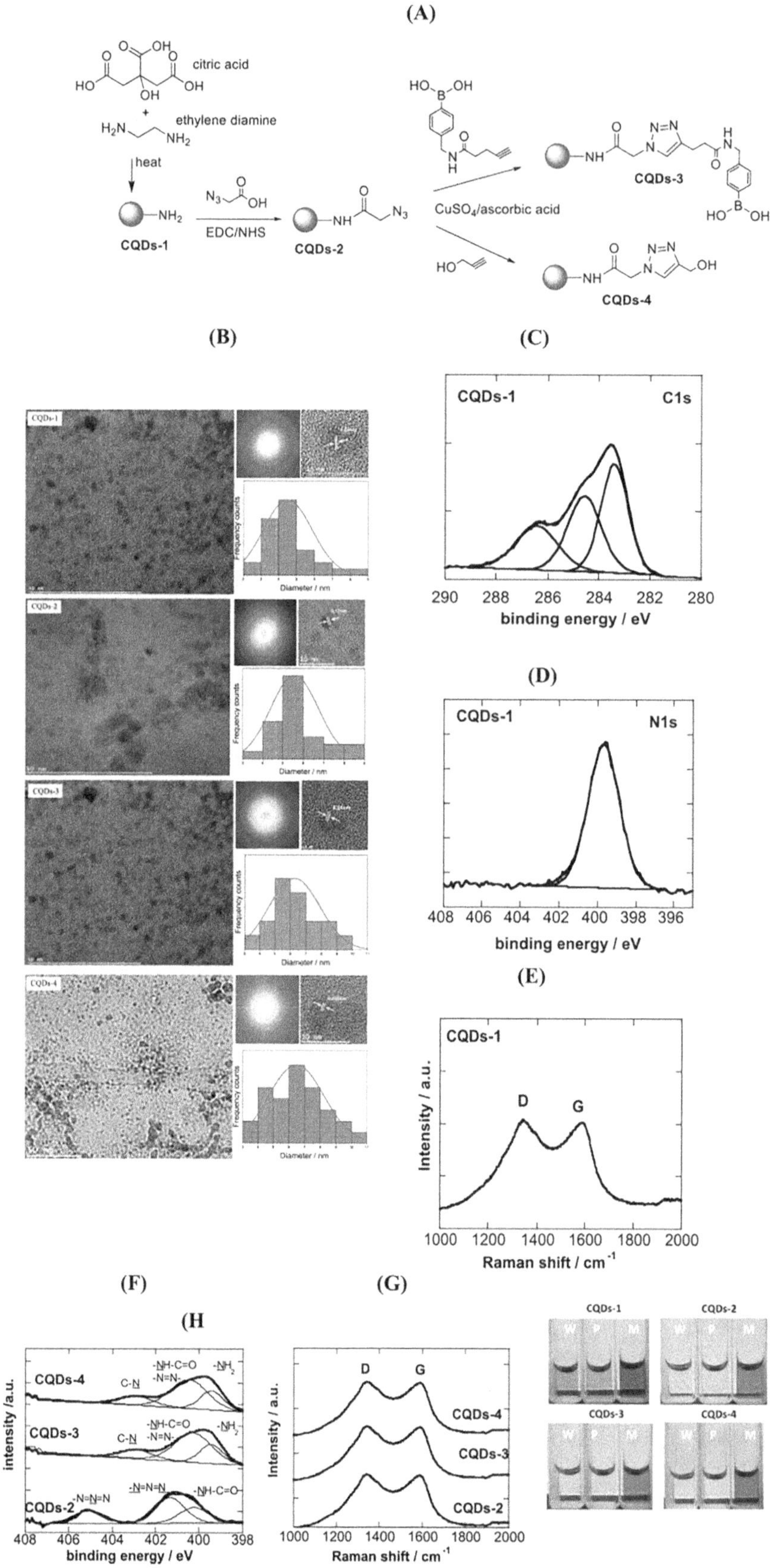

FIGURE 7.28 (a) Schematic representation of the synthesis of CQDs-1–4; (b) TEM, magnified TEM, HR-TEM images, and size distribution histograms of CQDs-1–4; (c) C1s high-resolution XPS spectrum of CQDs-1; (d) N_{1s} high-resolution XPS spectrum of CQDs-1; (e) Raman spectrum of CQDs-1; (f) N_{1s} high-resolution XPS spectra of CQDs-2–4; (g) Raman spectrum of CQDs-2–4; and (h) photographs of CQDs-1–4 suspensions (1 mg mL^{-1}) after 1 month in water (W), PBS (0.01 M, P), and Dulbecco's Modified Eagle's medium (M) [120].

TABLE 7.7
Physicochemical Characteristics of the CQDs

CQDs	ζ (mV)[a]	Size (nm)	Hydrodynamic Size (nm)[b]	PDI	C_{1s}[c] (at. %)	O_{1s} (at. %)	N_{1s} (at. %)	B_{1s} (at. %)
CQDs-1	−9.9 ± 3.4	4.5 ± 0.2	11 ± 0.1	0.22 ± 0.11	72.6	12.5	14.9	
CQDs-2	−7.9 ± 2.7	5.5 ± 0.3	12 ± 0.1	0.23 ± 0.11	68.8	13.9	17.3	
CQDs-3	−15.9 ± 4.3	6.3 ± 0.4	12 ± 0.25	0.15 ± 0.10	67.9	7.3	20.3	4.5
CQDs-4	−15.9 ± 1.3	6.5 ± 0.4	11 ± 0.19	0.13 ± 0.10	68.5	13.6	17.9	

[a] ζ, zeta potential; *PDI*, polydispersity index.
[b] The hydrodynamic size was recorded at 37°C.
[c] XPS was used to determine the atomic percentage of the elements, respectively.

to an interlayer spacing of 0.35 nm. This is larger than the spacing between (100) planes in bulk graphite (0.23 nm) due to the incorporation of functional groups along the edges of the CQDs. The UV-vis of CQDs-1 reveals an absorption maximum at ~242 nm attributed to π–π* transition of C = C and a band at 344 nm due to n–π* transition of C = O and C = N bonds. The fluorescence quantum yield (QY) is 0.33 as compared to that of quinine sulfate used as reference (QY, 0.54 in 0.12 M H_2SO_4). A wavelength-dependent fluorescence emission is observed, whereupon increasing the excitation wavelength, the emission gradually shifts to the red region with an increase in fluorescence intensity. The phenomenon of excitation-dependent emission is typical for such nanostructures. The zeta potential and hydrodynamic size of the CQDs-1 are summarized in Table 7.7.

7.15.1.1.2 Functionalization of CQDs-1

The formation of CQDs-3 is based on a two-step chemical process. In the first step, azido-functionalized CQDs-2 is prepared by coupling 2-azido acetic acid moieties to CQDs-1. The N_{1s} signal of CQDs-2 shows signals at 405.2 (–N = N^+ = N–) and 401.6 eV (N = N^+ = N–) in a 1:2 ratio, as theoretically expected (Figure 7.28f). The azide functions in CQDs-2 quantitatively react with alkyne functions, as indicated by the absence of the azide band at 405.2 eV in the relevant spectra of CQDs-3 and CQDs-4 (Figure 7.28f). The band at 399.2 eV (–NH_2) most likely results from partial hydrolysis of surface-linked 2-azido acetic ester function. CQDs-4 was synthesized as a control to check whether the triazole function acts as a passive linker or not. The morphologies of CQDs-3 and CQDs-4 are comparable to that of CQDs-1, with an average diameter of 6.25 ± 0.17 nm (Figure 7.28b) and diffraction peak centered at 25.3° for CQDs-3 and an average diameter of 6.50 ± 0.40 nm (Figure 7.28b), and diffraction peak centered at 25.4° for CQDs-4. The Raman spectra of the CQDs-2–4 (Figure7.28g) are similar to that of CQDs-1, displaying the characteristic G and D bands with ID/IG = 0.93 ± 0.15 for all particles. The colloidal stability of CQDs-1–4 in water, phosphate buffer (PBS, 10 mM), and Dulbecco's modified Eagle's medium (M) was, in addition, examined. All the particles had good long-term colloidal stability, as seen from the photographs in Figure 7.28h.

7.15.1.2 Cytotoxicity Assay

The cell toxicity of CQDs-1, CQDs-3, and CQDs-4 was established on Huh-7 cell lines after 8 h (time points corresponding to HCoV-229E infections) and 24 h incubation. The CQDs toxicity was evaluated using cell viability assessment by the resazurin assay, based on the conversion of nonfluorescent dye to a fluorescent molecule by mitochondrial and cytoplasmatic enzymes. All CQDs are nontoxic to Huh-7 cells even at the highest concentration (100 μg mL^{-1}) investigated when incubated for 8 and 24 h. Neither the presence of boronic acid nor triazole units had a negative effect on cell toxicity.

The uptake mechanism proved to be the same for all the nanostructures. Taking the example of CQDs-3 (which later proves to have antiviral activity), Huh-7 cells were fixed after 1 h incubation at 4 and 37°C, and then nuclei were stained with Hoechst 33342, a fluorescent dye for labeling DNA in fluorescence microcopy. The green fluorescence, which is attributed to the CQDs-3, is homogeneously distributed in the cytoplasm after 1 h when incubated at 37°C, which confirms the internalization of CQDs-3 inside the cells. The reduction of green fluorescence, observed in the cytoplasm after 1 h incubation at 4°C, suggests that the active internalization mechanism may be partially blocked, and a small portion of CQDs was internalized by passive penetration.

The endocytosis of CQDs-3 was, in addition, quantitatively evaluated using flow cytometry by treating Huh-7 cells with 100 μg mL^{-1} of CQDs-3 for 1 h at 4°C and for 1, 3, and 6 h at 37°C. The excitation fluorescence of CQDs-3 at 488 nm allowed the analysis of CQDs intracellularly. A progressive shift in the cell population toward higher fluorescence values was observed with a subsequent increase of time incubation due to the time-dependent cellular uptake likely through endocytosis. Lower fluorescence intensity was observed upon incubation at 4°C for 1 h, where the active uptake process is blocked. The low percentage of green cells (0.8%) observed after 1 h at 4°C suggests that only a very low quantity of CQDs-3 penetrates via passive uptake.

7.15.1.3 Antiviral Assay of First Generation of Antiviral CQDs

The antiviral activity of CQDs-1, CQDs-3, and CQDs-4 was evaluated on Huh-7 cell monolayers infected with HCoV-229E-Luc (Figure 7.29a). The addition of CQDs-1 after 1 h infection and further incubation for 6 h at 37°C shows no inhibition of infection. This contrasts to CQDs-3, where a concentration-dependent virus inactivation is observed with an estimated EC_{50} = 52 ± 8 μg mL^{-1} (Figure7.29b). The addition of mannose to CQDs-3 results in a complete loss of antiviral activity of the latter at low particle concentrations, with some antiviral

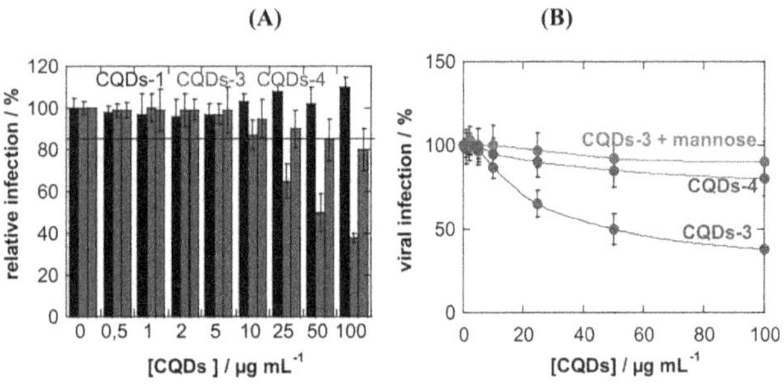

FIGURE 7.29 Viral infection inhibition in the presence of CQDs: (a) Viral inhibition using CQDs at various concentrations. Huh-7 cells (1.5×10^4 cells/well) were inoculated with HCoV-229E-Luc for 1 h (in atmosphere with 5% CO_2 at 37°C) in the presence or absence of different CQDs in medium without FBS for 1 h. Afterward, the inoculum was removed and replaced by DMEM with FBS for 6 h. Cells were lysed, and luciferase activity was quantified. The results are expressed as percentage of infection normalized to the control without CQDs, which is expressed as 100% infection. Data are means of two independent experiments with each treatment performed in triplicate. (B) Determination of EC_{50} for CQDs-3 and CQDs-4, and effect of viral inhibition using CQDs-3 after incubation with mannose (2:1) overnight at 4°C.

activity above 50 µg mL^{-1} CQDs. These data reveal two important findings. First, it highlights that boronic acid functions, where the mode of action is the selective and reversible formation of tetravalent complexes with cis-diols, and thus, glycan units are interacting with HCoV-229E. CQDs-3 is, in this context, speculated to be pseudolectins, targeting the S protein of HCoV-229E via a lectin–carbohydrate binding mechanism, similar to that of the oligomannose-specific lectin Griffithsin. Thus, the presence of mannose blocks the antiviral activity in favor of this mechanistic behavior. The presence of some antiviral activity of the mannose-saturated CQDs-3 might be due to the presence of the triazole function on the particles' surface. Indeed, the control particles CQDs-4, bearing no boronic acid function but a triazole ring, display some antiviral activity, even though largely decreased when compared to CQDs-3.

7.15.2 Second Generation of CQD Inhibitors of Host Cell Infections by HCoV-229E Coronavirus

7.15.2.1 Formation and Characterization of CQDs-5–7

With the aim to validate if boronic acid functions can be formed directly on CQDs, hydrothermal carbonization of phenylboronic acid and 4-aminophenylboronic acid was performed, resulting in CQDs-5 and CQDs-6, respectively. As control, hydrothermal carbonization of aniline and polyethylene glycol (PEG_{600}), both lacking boronic acid functions, was conducted. Unfortunately, several attempts to prepare CQDs from aniline as a starting material failed. Dulbecco's modified Eagle medium (DMEM) is a widely used basal medium for supporting the growth of many different mammalian cells. Cells successfully cultured in DMEM include primary fibroblasts, neurons, glial cells, HUVECs, and smooth muscle cells, as well as cell lines such as HeLa, 293, Cos-7, and PC-12.

The TEM images of CQDs-5–7 have been studied. CQDs-5 have an average diameter of 9.2 ± 0.3 nm, somehow larger than CQDs-6 with an average size of 7.6 ± 0.2 nm (Table 7.8). The particles formed from PEG (CQDs-7) display a spherical shape, with an average diameter of 8.0 ± 0.2 nm.

The XRD diffractograms display broad diffraction peaks centered at 21.3° for CQDs-5, 22.6° for CQDs-6, and 22.1° for CQDs-7, corresponding to an interlayer spacing of 0.42 nm (CQDs-5), 0.40 nm (CQDs-6), and 0.39 nm (CQDs-7). The UV-vis absorption spectra of the CQDs are depicted. The absorption shoulders at 250–300 nm correspond to a typical absorption of an aromatic π system, in accordance with the literature data [121]. The CQDs exhibit different fluorescence quantum yields (QY) of 0.03 (CQDs-5), 0.05 (CQDs-6), and 0.09 (CQDs-7). The wavelength-dependent fluorescence emission properties of the CQDs are comparable. The zeta potential and hydrodynamic size of CQDs-5–7 are summarized in Table 7.8. Raman spectra of the CQDs-5–7 are comparable to that of CQDs-1, displaying the characteristic G and D band with ID/IG = 0.93 ± 0.15 for all particles.

The chemical composition of the particles was thus further assessed using X-ray photoelectron spectroscopy and ^{11}B NMR. The XPS survey spectra of different CQDs (Table 7.8) indicate the presence of C_{1s}, O_{1s}, N_{1s}, and B_{1s} in agreement with the chemical composition of the particles. Deconvolution of the C1s XPS spectrum of CQDs-5 reveals bands located at 284.3 eV (C = C, sp^2), 285.1 eV (C–H, C–B), and a small contribution centered at 287.0 eV (C = O). The boron content is lower; this indicates that some of the phenylboronic acid groups were carbonized under the experimental conditions. The low B content might also indicate doping rather than the presence of boronic acid function. CQDs-6 particles depict bands at 284.3 eV (C = C, sp^2), 285.2 eV (C–H, C–B), 287.3 eV (C = O), and a band at 290.3 eV due to O–C = O functions. In the case of CQDs-7, the C1s XPS spectrum comprises three different carbon features: the graphitic C = C at 283.4 eV,

TABLE 7.8
Physicochemical Characteristics of the CQDs-5–7

CQDs	ζ (mV)[a]	Size (nm)	Hydrodynamic Size (nm)[b]	PDI	C1s[c] (at. %)	O_{1s} (at. %)	N_{1s} (at. %)	B_{1s} (at. %)
CQDs-5	−20.0 ± 5.5	7.6 ± 0.2	13 ± 1.8	0.14 ± 0.09	77.4	21.7		0.9
CQDs-6	−41.2 ± 1.0	9.2 ± 0.3	12 ± 0.2	0.11 ± 0.06	69.4	21.5	7.4	1.7
CQDs-7	−39.2 ± 1.5	8.0 ± 0.2	13 ± 3.1	0.28 ± 0.34	60.8	39.2		

[a] ζ, zeta potential; *PDI*, polydispersity index.
[b] The hydrodynamic size was recorded at 37°C.
[c] XPS was used to determine the atomic percentage of the elements, respectively.

284.9 eV (C–H), and 286.4 eV (C–O, C–N). Analysis of the N1s high-resolution spectrum of CQDs-5 reveals the presence of surface NH_2 groups.

The FTIR spectra of CQDs-5–7 exhibit a distinct band at 3,465 cm^{-1} attributed to the stretching vibration of –OH groups and bands at around 2,874 and 2,924 cm^{-1} due to CH_2 stretching bands. The sharp band at 1,618 cm^{-1} is assigned to graphitic C = C, and the C–H deformation mode is seen at 1 460 cm^{-1}. The C = O band at ~1,780–1,650 cm^{-1} is also visible in all cases. In the case of CQDs-6, the band at 1,090 cm^{-1} might be due to C–B stretching modes. This band is less defined in the case of CQDs-5, which might underline doping rather than the presence of boronic acid functions. The FTIR spectrum of CQDs-7 displays the C–O–C bands of the PEG units at 1,043 cm^{-1}.

CQDs-5–7 exhibited a negative zeta potential in water (pH 7.4) at room temperature and showed excellent long-term stability even in biological medium, such as Dulbecco's modified Eagle's medium (DMEM).

The cytotoxicity of CQDs-5–7 is comparable to that of CQDs discussed, with CQDs-6 being slightly more toxic at concentrations >25 μg mL^{-1} after 24 h incubation. This might be due to the presence of NH_2 groups on these particles. The uptake mechanism of these particles was comparable and is exemplified using CQDs-6. Because of low intrinsic fluorescence of CQDs-6 particles, they were labeled with fluorescein-NHS.

7.15.2.2 Antiviral Assay of the Second Generation of CQDs-5–7

The addition of CQDs-7 after 1 h infection and further incubation for 6 h at 37°C showed no inhibition of infection, indicating that these particles are not interfering with HCoV-229E-Luc entry or replication. CQDs-5 and CQDs-6 display a concentration-dependent virus inactivation. The dose–response curve reveals that the effective concentration to achieve 50% inhibition (EC_{50}) against HCoV-229E-Luc infection is 5.2 ± 0.7 μg mL^{-1} for CQDs-6 and 11.6 ± 1.1 μg mL^{-1} for CQDs-5. Surprisingly, the addition of mannose did not result in a loss of the antiviral activity, as observed previously for CQDs-3.

Performing ^{11}B NMR analysis of CQDs-5 and CQDs-6 and comparing the obtained spectra to those of the respective starting materials, 4-aminophenylboronic acid and phenyl boronic acid, reveal large differences in chemical composition. 4-aminophenylboronic acid and phenyl boronic both exhibit a strong signal at around 29 ppm, in accordance with literature data for -$B(OH)_2$ functions. The small signal at about 20 ppm arises most likely from residual $B(OR)_3$ often used in boronic acid synthesis. The ^{11}B NMR spectra of CQDs-5 and CQDs-6 display, however, peaks at 13 ppm (CQDs-5) and a band at 10 ppm, with a shoulder at 12 ppm for CQDs-6. This means that boron was incorporated through doping rather than surface functionalization during the hydrothermal reaction. Indeed, one-pot solvothermal synthesis using aminophenylboronic acid precursor was reported by Wang et al. to result in N and B co-doped CQDs. They indeed reported the presence of 0.7 at. % B by XPS, comparable to the amount obtained here (Table 7.8).

7.15.3 Mechanism of Action

The mechanism of action of CQDs-3 and CQDs-6 on viral infection has been further investigated [120] by performing a time-of-addition assay. CQDs (at 10 μg mL^{-1}) were added at different time points during infection. As expected, a strong inhibition of infection was observed when CQDs were added after 1 h inoculation. Moreover, the inhibition activity of CQDs was stronger when the nanoparticles were added during the entry step, that is, 30 min before and after inoculation and during inoculation. The results agree with the hypothesis of an interaction of CQDs with HCoV-229E S protein, or an interaction of CQDs with entry factors. Surprisingly, a strong inhibitory activity of CQDs was also observed when they were added after 5.5 h after the entry step, the replication step. The inhibition is not significantly different for the entry step as compared to the replication step. This suggests that, in addition to its major effect on HCoV-229E entry, CQDs can also affect the genomic replication of this virus. This could potentially be explained by an interaction between the CQDs and a cell surface protein, leading to signal transduction affecting viral replication, or by an interaction with cytosolic proteins as CQDs are internalized.

To determine if CQDs interact directly with viral particles, HCoV-229E-Luc was incubated with CQDs at 10 μg mL^{-1} for 30 min at 37°C before inoculation. The inoculum was diluted ten times, leading to a final concentration of CQDs of 1 μg mL^{-1}, and infection assay was performed. In parallel, Huh-7 cells were inoculated with HCoV-229E-Luc in the presence of CQDs at 1 or 10 μg mL^{-1}. The inoculum titers were kept constant in the different conditions. The results [121] showed that the preincubation of the virus with CQDs at high concentration does not impair HCoV-229E infection, meaning, that CQDs do not interact with the particles before infection. Taken together, our results are in favor of an interaction of CQDs with cellular factors, which may explain their antiviral effects at different steps of infection.

7.16 3D-Printed Graphene Polylactic Acid Devices Resistant to SARS-CoV-2

Graphene-family materials are capable of reinforcing mechanical, optical, and thermal properties of 3D-printed constructs. In particular, graphene can adsorb near-infrared light with high efficiency. Here it has been demonstrated that the addition of graphene nanoplatelets to PLA filaments (PLA-G) allows the creation of 3D-printed devices that can be sterilized by near-infrared light exposure at power density analog to sunlight. This method has been used to kill SARS-CoV-2 viral particles on the surface of 3D-printed PLA-G by 3 min of exposure. 3D-printed PLA-G is highly biocompatible and can represent the ideal material for the production of sterilizable personal protective equipment and daily life objects intended for multiple users.

Additive manufacturing has played a crucial role in the COVID-19 global emergency, allowing for rapid production of medical devices, indispensable tools for hospitals, or personal protective equipment. However, medical devices, especially in nosocomial environments, represent high-touch surfaces prone to viral infection, and currently used filaments for 3D printing cannot inhibit transmission of virus.

Recently, it has been demonstrated that graphene can inhibit the infectivity of SARS-CoV-2 if embedded in textiles and that graphene oxide can trap and induce precipitation of viral particles in solution. An interaction between graphene and SARS-CoV-2 surface proteins has also been recently demonstrated [122].

One of the most noteworthy features of graphene is its strong interaction with light: a single layer of graphene (<0.5 nm of thickness) can absorb 2.3% of incident visible light [123]. This property is essential for photothermal therapies (PTT) as well as wound healing, muscle repair, and angiogenesis, for regenerative medicine. NIR absorbers like graphene are used for the hyperthermic killing of cancer cells and microbial species due to hyperthermic effects. Furthermore, graphene and its derivatives are easily added to thermoplastic polymers for 3D printing, making this technology easily implementable in laboratories.

Graphene-family materials are capable of reinforcing mechanical, optical, and thermal properties of 3D-printed constructs [2]. In particular, graphene can adsorb near-infrared light with high efficiency. Here we demonstrate that the addition of graphene nanoplatelets to PLA filaments (PLA-G) allows the creation of 3D-printed devices that can be sterilized by near-infrared light exposure at power density analog to sunlight. This method has been used to kill SARS-CoV-2 viral particles on the surface of 3D-printed PLA-G by 3 min of exposure. 3D-printed PLA-G is highly biocompatible and can represent the ideal material for the production of sterilizable personal protective equipment and daily life objects intended for multiple users (Scheme 7.2) [2].

Given these advantages, in this work chapter [2], the feasibility of adding graphene nanoparticles to PLA filaments (PLA-G) has been investigated for the creation of sterilizable objects intended for healthcare applications. PLA-G filaments containing graphene in a range from 0.5% up to 5% have been tested for (1) mechanical strength, (2) near-infrared adsorption and thermal properties, and (3) anti-SARS-CoV-2 properties. All the concentrations had high biocompatibility when eukaryotic cells have been grown on PLA-G surfaces. Using NIR light with power intensity analog to sunlight, we demonstrate the feasibility of using PLA-G for protective equipment production. Besides the intrinsic graphene inhibition of SARS-CoV-2 attachment, viral particles that might come in contact with PLA-G can be easily killed by sunlight, offering an economic and environmentally sustainable method for surface sterilization. This nanotechnology-based system can greatly impact the production of face masks, surgical instruments, and daily objects in healthcare or other working or public environments, such as schools or public transport.

7.16.1 PLA-G Filaments and 3D Printing

PLA filaments containing G+ (Directa Plus) with different amounts of G+ flakes (0%, 0.5%, 2%, 5%) have been used. G+ was produced according to a proprietary patented technology involving three steps: expansion, exfoliation, and drying. In Table 7.9, the main features of G+ are summarized. Full characterization of this nanomaterial is reported elsewhere. The structure of 3D-printed scaffolds was designed using modeled 3D computer graphics and computer-aided design (CAD) software Rhinoceros (Robert McNeel & Associates). Ultimaker S3 3D printer was used to produce 3D-printed structures using a nozzle extruded at temperature of 180°C and printing velocity of 20 mm/s. The nozzle diameter was 400 μm, and the thickness of a single layer was set to 200 μm. Shapes printed for different tests are presented in Table 7.10 and Figure 7.30 [124].

The COVID-19 pandemic has prompted the use of PLA (polylactic acid), a biodegradable hydrolyzable aliphatic semicrystalline polyester produced through the direct condensation reaction of its monomer, lactic acid, as the oligomer, and followed by a ring-opening polymerization of the cyclic lactide

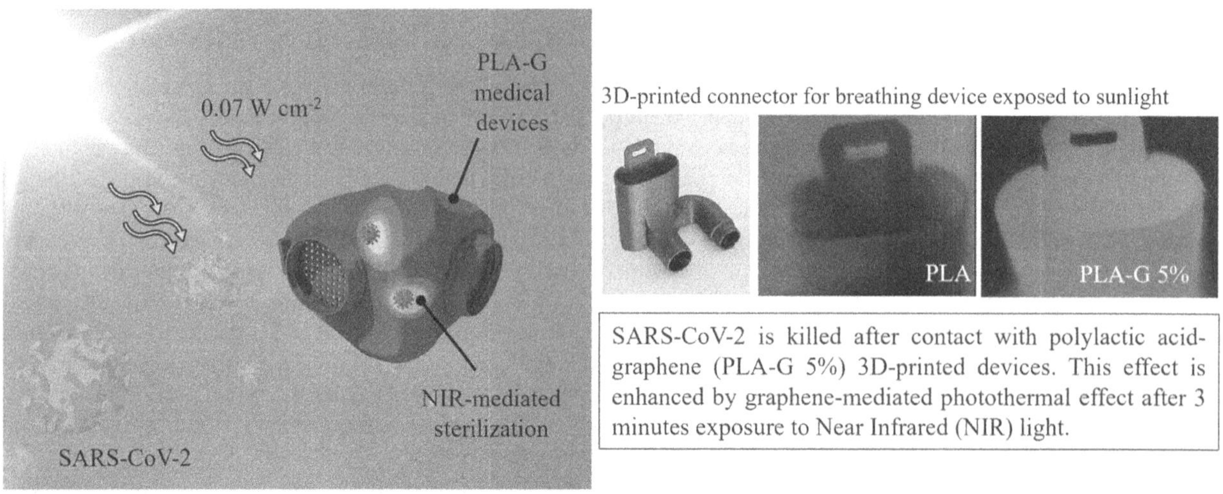

SCHEME 7.2 3D-printed graphene polylactic acid devices resistant to SARS-CoV-2.

Source: [2].

TABLE 7.9
Characterization of G+ Nanoplatelets

	G
ID/IG (Raman spectroscopy)	0.127
Thickness (atomic force microscopy)	4–6 layers
Lateral dimension (atomic force microscopy)	3 μm

TABLE 7.10
3D-Printed Structures

Shape	Test
Cylinder	Compression test
Dog bone	Tensile test
Disc	SEM, cell viability, SARS-CoV-2, NIR
Connectors to breathing devices (Cavallo *et al.*, 2020)	NIR

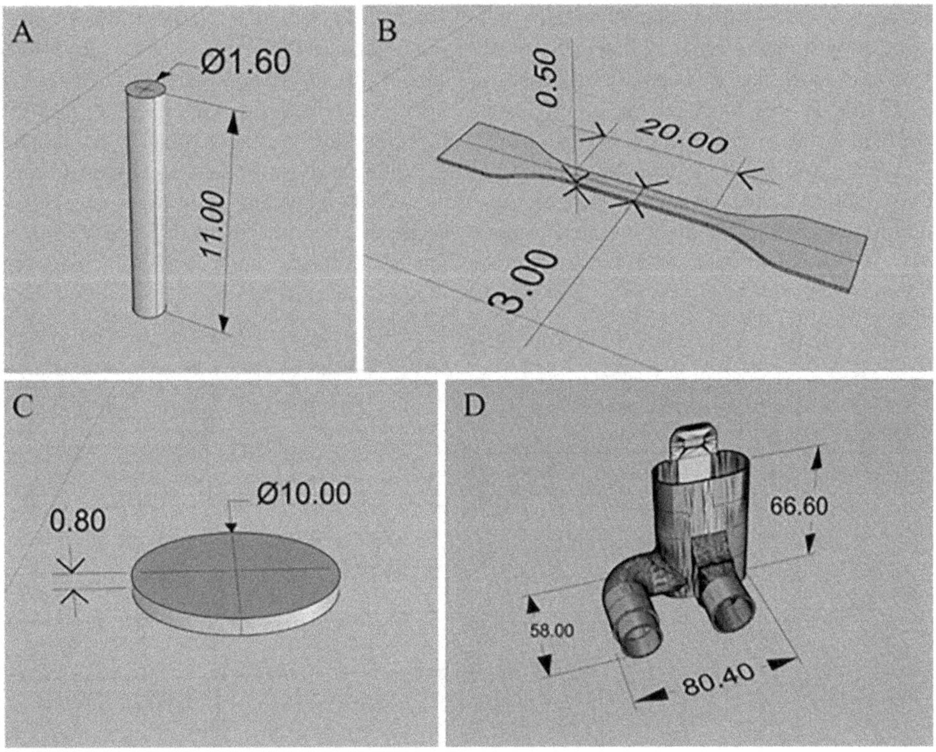

FIGURE 7.30 3D-printed structure models: 3D renders using Rhinoceros software of (a) cylinder, (b) dog bone, (c) discs, and (d) connector for breathing device used for experiments.

dimer, and other thermoplastic-based printing filaments to produce PPE (personal protective equipment), which refers to specialized garments or accessories, such as clothing, helmets, gloves, and so forth, that fulfil a protective function against various hazards, mechanical or chemical, when worn by workers; medical devices; and daily life objects. PLA filaments' composition can be modified with carbon nanomaterials, such as bidimensional graphene, to improve the performance of 3D-printed medical devices. Indeed, the bare PLA filaments can lack the strength to produce fully functioning engineering parts, restricting the adoption of 3D technology [125].

SEM images of 3D-printed structures made of PLA or PLA-G with different graphene nanoplatelets concentrations (0.5%, 2%, or 5%) are shown. Graphene nanoplatelets used in this study have an average lateral dimension of 3 μm and a layer number comprised between 4 and 6 layers, as presented in Table 7.9. The structures have been produced with a deposition speed of 20 mm/s and nozzle diameter of 0.4 mm using the Ultimaker S3 3D printer. Since the presence of graphene can alter the printing process and, consequently, the diameter of filaments, quantification of this parameter obtained from SEM has been performed. Overall, the presence of G nanoplatelets in the PLA filaments does not alter the printed structure significantly, as shown by SEM. Nanoscale roughness has been quantified from AFM imaging with an evident increase of surface roughness as graphene percentage goes from 0.5% to 5%. The increase of amount of G changes PLA viscosity and melting point, causing faster polymer solidification and a slower polymer relaxation after 3D printing [126]. This thermodynamic behavior, during post-printing solidification, increases the local roughness of the surfaces as the graphene concentration increases.

PLA and PLA-G have very similar hydrophobicity, as measured by contact angle experiments. Data reported in the literature report contact angles for PLA and graphene between 70° and 90°. This value can change due to several factors, like the specific polymer preparation, the number of graphene layers, temperature, humidity, etc.

In Table 7.11, the results of tensile tests of 3D-printed dog bones of PLA with or without graphene are shown. In Table 7.12, the results of compression tests on PLA and PLA-G cylinders are shown. The addition of G in the filaments increases the tensile and compression elastic modules up to 35% in compression and 20% in elongation using G at 5% in PLA-G (Table 7.11). The elongation at break increases up to 17.5%, the max stress in tension increases up to 13%, and the yield stress up to 24%.

The mechanical properties of medical devices that are put under physical stress, like ventilator valves or connectors for breathing devices, are exceptionally important. Indeed, the device must be sufficiently strong to retain its integrity under conditions of normal wear and tear. Biocompatibility assessment is fundamental for devices intended for in vivo use. Biocompatibility of PLA and PLA-G was evaluated on VERO, C2C12, and A549 cells plated on 3D-printed supports after 24 h of growth. Cell viability assays did not show any significant cell growth inhibition even at the highest concentration of G tested (PLA-G 5%). As highlighted from representative images of C2C12 cells grown on PLA-G 5% reported, cells were attached and grew easily on supports. Biocompatibility is maintained in these cells even after several days of growth have been investigated, quantified by luminescence and normalized to control samples. No significant differences have been observed.

To assess the ability of PLA-G to capture SARS-CoV-2, a solution of SARS-CoV-2 containing ~105 viral particles/mL was let to interact with PLA and PLA-G supports (discs) for 2 h at 37°C. Following incubation, contaminated discs were harvested, and the plastic surface exposed to the SARS-CoV-2-containing solution washed. Discs and washing solution were recovered in 5 mL of sterile fresh medium, and an aliquot of this suspension was used to infect VERO cells to measure viral infectivity (Figure 7.31a). VERO cells are derived from the kidney of an African green monkey and are one of the more commonly used mammalian continuous cell lines in microbiology and molecular and cell biology research. Representative images of infected VERO cells are shown in Figure 7.31b: exposure of SARS-CoV-2-containing solution,

TABLE 7.11

Results of Mechanical Characterization after Tensile Tests of PLA and PLA-G Samples

	Stress Max (Mpa)	% break	E (Gpa)
PLA	69	4.00%	2.9
PLA-G 0.5%	73	4.50%	3
PLA-G 2%	74	4.60%	3.2
PLA-G 5%	78	4.70%	3.5

TABLE 7.12

Results of Mechanical Characterization after Compression Tests of PLA and PLA-G Samples

	Yield Stress (Mpa)	E (Gpa)
PLA	76	2.6 ± 0.2
PLA-G 0.5%	80	2.6 ± 0.2
PLA-G 2%	94	3.2 ± 0.26
	96	3.5 ± 0.28

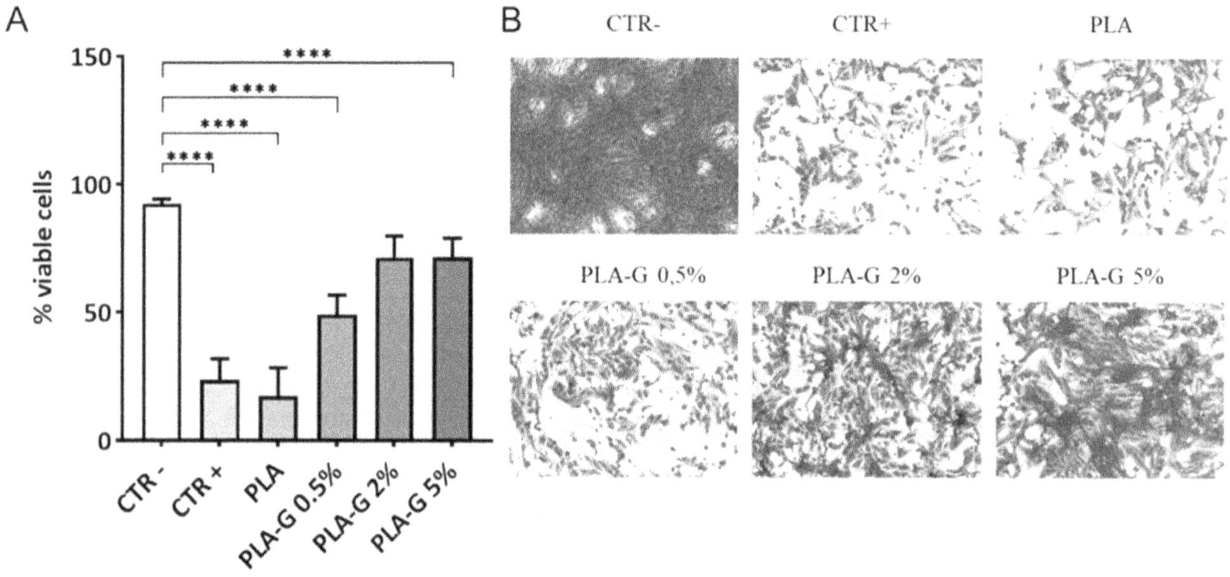

FIGURE 7.31 Graphene-functionalized PLA reduced infectivity of SARS-CoV-2. PLA- and PLA-G- (0.5%, 2.0%, and 5%) functionalized PLA were incubated with a suspension of SARS-CoV-2 at the final concentration of ~10^5 viral particles/mL, for 2 h at 37°C, to assess the ability to capture SARS-CoV-2 and subsequently reduce infectivity in VERO cells. Three days post-infection with solution recovered from surfaces, VERO cells were fixed and stained with crystal violet. Images were acquired using Cytation instrument an analyzed with ImageJ software, and data were expressed as mean ± SD and analyzed by one-way ANOVA comparison tests, followed by Tukey's correction. Asterisks indicate p <0,001 (a). Representative images were obtained after crystal violet staining of VERO cells for each sample (b).

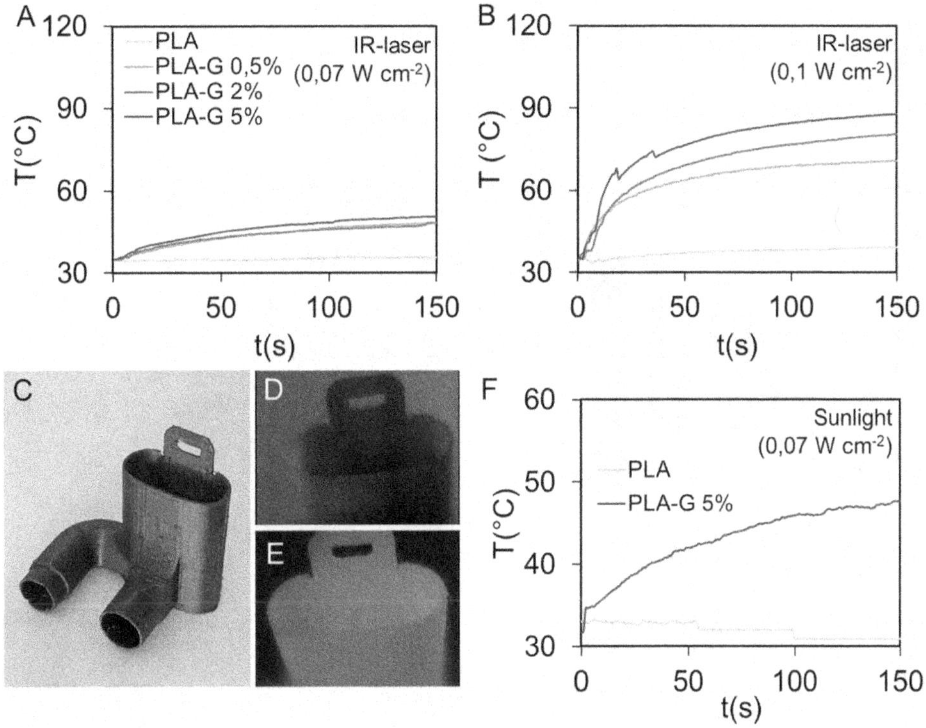

FIGURE 7.32 Effects of exposure of PLA or PLA-G to 808 nm laser light at (a) 0.07 W cm^{-2}, (b) 0.1 W cm^{-2}. (c) 3D-printed connector for breathing device. Thermal images of 3D-printed connector for breathing device in (d) PLA and (e) PLA-G-5% exposed for 150 s to sunlight (about 0.07 W cm^{-2}), and the (f) relative temperatures obtained by the thermal camera.

even at the lowest concentration of graphene tested (PLA-G 0.5%), significantly reduced viral infectivity. Reduction in viral infectivity was proportional to the concentration of G in the PLA filaments, reaching a maximum with PLA-G 5%, supporting previous findings indicating the ability of G to bind and "trap" viral particles. However, it cannot exclude a detrimental effect of G on viruses' envelopes and consequent destabilization of the versions.

Graphene absorbs infrared light and has photocatalytic effects [127]. Since IR light occupies the largest proportion in the solar spectrum, we tested whether the graphene in the filaments could represent an easy and low-cost method to promote the adsorption of IR light by 3D-printed constructs and consequently sterilize surfaces [127]. The photothermal catalytic disinfection experiment has been carried out with less than 808 nm lasers light; the average temperature of the 3D structures has been monitored by a thermal camera. In Figure 7.32, the results of temperature monitoring after exposure for 3 min of PLA and PLA-G samples are reported. In Figure 7.32a, the illumination of samples with a NIR light having a power density of 0,07 W cm^{-2}, which corresponds to the measured average exposure of sunlight, causes an increase of temperature up to 50°C, with no marked differences between samples. On the contrary, when using the average power density of summer light (i.e. 0,1 W cm^{-2}), PLA temperature does not significantly increases, whereas samples containing graphene nanoplatelets substantially increase in temperature, reaching, after 3 min, 60°C, 70°C, and 80°C for PLA-G 0.5%, PLA-G 2%, and PLA-G 5%, respectively.

Figure 7.32c shows a 3D-printed connector for a breathing device made of PLA or PLA-G. These connectors have been irradiated with an average power density of 0.07 W cm^{-2}, and results obtained with thermal imaging are shown in Figure 7.32d and Figure 7.32e. Temperatures of devices during irradiation are shown in Figure 7.32f, where it is demonstrated that PLA-G 5% temperature increases up to 50°C using a power intensity analog to sunlight.

To mimic sunlight effects, a suspension of SARS-CoV-2 was incubated on the discs for 2 h, and the surfaces were exposed to NIR light. The increase of temperature correlated with a significant drop in infectivity compared to physiological body temperature (BT in Figure 7.33a). At 0.07 W cm^{-2} and 0.1 W cm^{-2}, the further increase of temperature (≈55° and ≈85°C, respectively) was able to reduce SARS-CoV-2 infectivity, maintaining cell viability up to values of the not-infected cells. The killing efficiency for PLA-G 5% surfaces toward SARS CoV-2 is reported in Figure 7.33b, ranging from 55.9% at BT to 91.4% at 0.1 W cm^{-2}, which corresponds to 85°C. Since SARS-CoV-2 is extremely sensitive to high temperature, the method which has been developed can be used to easily clean and efficiently sterilize the surfaces using power density as sunlight exposure.

7.17 Conclusion and Perspective

Nowadays, smart and emerging nano-based materials play a crucial role in biomedical sciences, owing to the unique

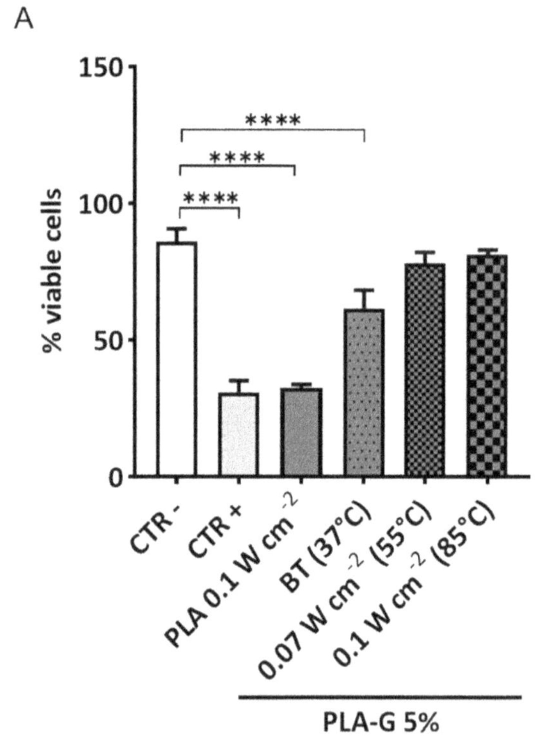

B

	% SARS-CoV-2 killed
PLA 0.1 W cm^{-2} (85°C)	2,9
PLA-G 5% BT (37°C)	55,9
PLA-G 5% 0.07 W cm^{-2} (55°C)	85,8
PLA-G 5% 0.1 W cm^{-2} (85°C)	91,4

FIGURE 7.33 Effects of exposure to different NIR light of PLA and PLA-G-5% surfaces incubated with SARS-CoV-2 solutions. PLA and PLA-G 5% were incubated with a suspension of SARS-CoV-2 at the final concentration of ~10^5 viral particles/mL and exposed to different NIR light conditions (37°C, 55°C, 85°C) for 2 h. Three days post-infection with solution recovered from surfaces, VERO cells were fixed and stained with crystal violet. Data are expressed as mean ± SD after analysis with ImageJ and analyzed by one-way ANOVA* comparison tests, followed by Tukey's correction. Asterisks indicate p <0.001 (a). The ability to kill SARS-CoV-2 was quantified and significantly improved after NIR treatment, as shown from the values in the table (b). *Note:* *Analysis of variance (ANOVA) is a statistical formula used to compare variances across the means (or average) of different groups.

properties of nanomaterials, such as high adsorption capacity, high surface area, and high reactivity. This featured review attempts to explore the various biomarkers, indicators for SARS-CoV-2 detection, and smart nanomaterials for biosensing technologies and their consequences. Moreover, this work will also give a gist of the biological properties of SARS-CoV-2 that will enable researchers to develop novel diagnostic strategies to combat this pandemic and upcoming pandemics due to other mutating viruses/bacteria/fungus. 3D-printed graphene devices can kill SARS-CoV-2 with sunlight (Scheme 7.3).

This chapter is one of a kind, mainly focusing upon smart and emerging nanomaterials as biosensors for detecting SARS-CoV-2. Here in this work, we have also discussed the use of current biomarkers and indicators of the SARS-CoV-2 virus. However, from the established studies, it has been reported that, for the early and rapid diagnosis of SARS-CoV-2 infection, biosensors can serve as an analytical and powerful device that will offer more awareness of critical trends and conditions severity. Thus, this review will, in detail, provide an up-to-date literature review of smart and emerging nanomaterials as a biosensor in SARS-CoV-2 detection during this prevailing pandemic.

The viral infection cycle produces important biological and structural changes in the host cell, resulting in cell damage. The possibility to interfere with viral attachment to cells as well as viral replication to reduce viral infection and spreading is an appropriate antiviral approach. We presented here the antiviral performance of seven different CQDs, with their main features summarized in Table 7.13. Three of these CQDs (CQDs-3, 5, 6) were shown to interfere significantly with HCoV-229E-Luc infection in a concentration-dependent manner, while CQDs-4 showed a very moderate antiviral activity. The estimated EC_{50} value decreased considerably from CQDs-3, boronic acid–modified quantum dots, derived from ethylenediamine/citric acid as carbon precursors (EC_{50} = 52 ± 8 μg mL^{-1}) to 5.2 ± 0.7 μg mL^{-1} in the case of CQDs-6. While the presence of boronic acid functions proved to be vital for covering CQDs-3 with antiviral activity, CQDs-5 and CQDS-6 did not carry a substantial amount of boronic acid functions, as revealed by ^{11}B NMR. (The ^{11}B NMR spectrum shows a single broad resonance at δ = −34.7 ppm, which is characteristic for a four-coordinate boron center attached to two phosphorus atoms and validated by mannose addition experiments.) These findings reveal the complex nature of identifying viral inhibitors for human coronaviruses, such as HCoV-229E-Luc. Mechanistic studies suggest that the particles are acting at the early state of virus infection through the inhibition of entry that could be due to inhibition of protein S-receptor interaction with the host cell membrane. All different particles interfere in addition with the viral replication step, something less common. These results are extremely encouraging to replace currently used antiviral agents, such a ribavirin and IFN, known to

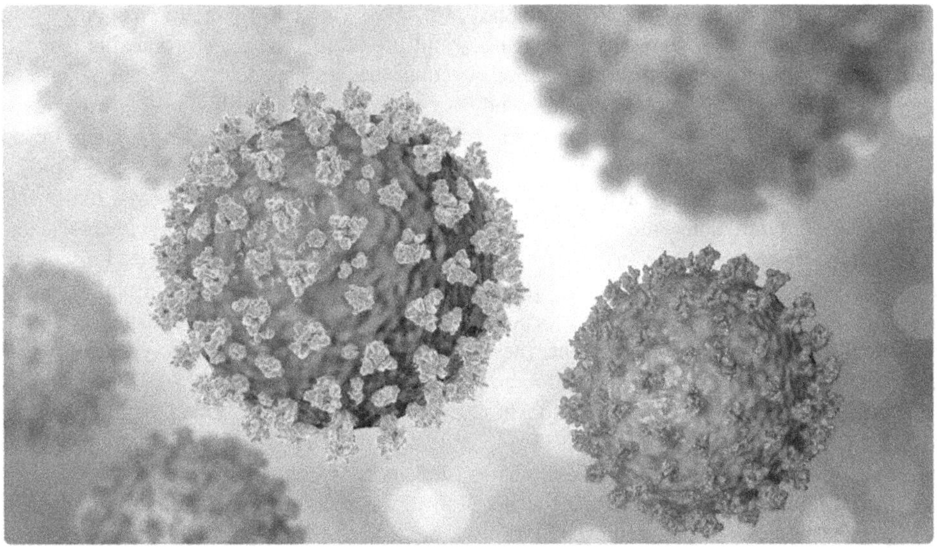

SCHEME 7.3 3D-printed graphene polylactic acid devices resistant to SARS-CoV-2.

TABLE 7.13
Summary of the Main Features of CQDs-1–7

CQDs	Size (nm)	Charge	Functions	Antiviral	EC_{50}/µg mL^{-1}
CQDs-1	4.5 ± 0.2	−9.9	NH2, COO−	–	
CQDs-2	5.5 ± 0.3	−7.9	N_3	–	
CQDs-3	6.3 ± 0.4	−15.9	Triazole, R–B$(OH)_2$	++	52 ± 8
CQDs-4	6.5 ± 0.4	−15.9	Triazole, OH	+	n.d.
CQDs-5	7.6 ± 0.2	−20.0	R–B$(OH)_2$	+++	11.6 ± 1.1
CQDs-6	9.2 ± 0.3	−41.2	R–B$(OH)_2$, NH_2	++++	5.2 ± 0.7
CQDs-7	8.0 ± 0.3	−39.2	PEG	–	

have major side effects, such as confusion, short-term memory loss, deficits in executive functions, as well as extrapyramidal effects. Further experimental confirmations are required if this approach can be extrapolated to other coronaviruses, notably to the clinically relevant MERS-CoV, to validate the potential of these nanostructures as alternative anti-MERS therapeutics and approaches to confront this severe and life-threatening disease. Also, how such particles work *in vivo* has to be shown in the future.

As we are observing, infective diseases continue to provoke global risk to public health. Despite the development of biology and electronic devices in the past 50 years, our capabilities to cope with the pandemic, including large-scale and fast detection and the development of vaccines, are obviously insufficient. There is a great need for multidisciplinary collaboration to prepare the humankind for any future outbreak.

Materials science is one of the fast-developing fields and offers numerous potentials for revolutionizing the medical industry. As we discussed in this chapter, carbon nanomaterials, one representative new type of materials, are highly promising for virus management. They ease diagnostic processes via various platforms by conducting direct real-time sensing of biomolecule targets. They block the entrance of virus to the cells to prevent infection. They can also be used to remove the virus from the water.

Although it does not seem to be far away before we bring carbon-based sensors/medicine/purifier from bench to our real life, there are a few things to notice in the following process. The immobilization methods of nanomaterials and the incorporated biological components should be standardized to improve precision during virus detection/targeting. The protocols reported in most of the articles are individually developed. The lifetime of the biosensor/medicine/purifier may be considerable. Another important consideration is the clearance of carbon nanomaterials. Although Singh et al. revealed that functionalized SWNT linked with ^{111}Indium are excreted as intact nanotubes by renal excretion, CDots and CNTs may accumulate in the reticuloendothelial system (RES), which could prevent renal uptake.

With the global burden of SARS-CoV-2-infected patients increasing by the day, the urge for rapid and convenient testing methods has never been more. Compared to the conventional sensing methods, nanomaterial-conjugated or nanomaterial-based biosensors offer a superior level of selectivity, sensitivity, reliability, robustness, reproducibility, and repeatability of the samples, all being economical in the first place, as it may be required for the mass populations. Additionally, with the increasing importance of nanotechnology-based biosensing platforms in clinical practice, studies demonstrating the applicability and utility in diagnosing RNA viruses have increased substantially. Based on these conclusions, it can be made concrete that these nanotechnology-based biosensors will surely play an indispensable role in the efficient and convenient diagnosis of the SARS-CoV-2 infection. Additionally, their utility can also be extrapolated to detect various other respiratory and systemic RNA viruses, with sufficient calibration and modifications based on the biological fluid used for testing purposes. With further research and development, these biosensors could present a realistic view of the several nanomaterials and interface-based nanotechnological approaches for detecting SARS-CoV-2 in various biological fluids. These biomedical gadgets being both reliable and economically feasible are projected to give rapid, convenient, and easy-to-use toolkits for masses across the globe. Additionally, clubbing it with interventions like the Internet of Things (IoT) and artificial intelligence (AI) can efficiently track, control, and forecast the spread of the COVID-19 pandemic and any other such unforeseen outbreaks.

The recently developed SPR-based, electrochemical- and FET-based, biosensors for SARS-CoV-2 detection we have reviewed are promising alternatives to currently available point-of-care (POC) tests. However, in addition to the limitations we have highlighted, none of the sensors met the WHO minimum requirement for true positive and true negative detection rates. Some of the sensors met the former requirement, but none met the latter requirement. The detection accuracies (particularly the true negative/false positive rate) need to be significantly improved before the sensors could be translated into POC devices for commercial use. The biorecognition elements and sensor surface modification materials we have suggested could be explored to improve the true negative and true positive rate, respectively.

A proof-of-concept electronic detection technique for selectively diagnosing SARS-COV-2 has been demonstrated. RNA hybridization was used as the primary signal generator, and liquid-gated CNT network FET was used as the signal transducer. The sensors produced a promising sensing signal at 10 fM concentrations of the positive target sequences at real-time sensing conditions. The proposed CNTFET-based biosensor can be developed as a reliable, fast, and cheap alternative for existing diagnostic techniques.

A very sensitive, selective, and quantifiable CNT-FET-based antibody–functionalized biosensor for SARS-CoV-2 S1 antigen detection has been designed and successfully developed in buffer solution and not in real samples. The biosensor was fabricated and operated under the p-type channel depletion principle. The source–drain metal electrodes were passivated by SU-8 photoresist to diminish direct contact with applied antigen samples and prevent a short circuit of the electrical components. The device showed excellent semiconductor properties. The quick response of the antigen drop confirms that source–drain semiconducting channels were quite sensitive to the transfer of electrons during antigen–antibody interaction. The CNT surface of the biosensor was modified by PBASE linker molecules, and anti-SARS-CoV-2 S1 were immobilized on the PBASE layer. The biosensing responses were rapid (minutes) and produced reliable, reproducible results. Antigen-specific concentration-dependent sensing response over a broad range of concentrations (0.1 to 5,000 fg/mL) was shown in the calibration experiments. The CNT-FET biosensor is highly sensitive and able to discriminate SARS-CoV-2 S1, SARS-CoV-1 S1, and MERS-CoV S1 antigens, indicating good selectivity to SARS-CoV-2 S1. The experimental data indicate that the biosensor can be a good, low-cost biosensor for rapidly testing people for SARS-CoV-2 infection that is easy to handle. Thus, the developed biosensor is inexpensive, simple, versatile, and easy to use and can be a prototype for SARS-CoV-2 S1 antigen detection and diagnosis of SARS-CoV-2 infection.

In the context of the pandemic challenges facing humanity today, the 3D printing production of protective equipment and more, in general, any surface that can readily warrant viral inactivation, is of paramount importance. Traditionally, chemical disinfectants are the most widely used method to kill harmful pathogens, though the release of by-products toxic for human health and the environment is a cause of major concern [127]. Nanotechnology has offered several approaches to cope with the COVID-19 emergency, as initially hypothesized in several papers [128]. Here we propose to exploit the photocatalytic properties of graphene nanoparticles embedded in the widely used biocompatible 3D-printable PLA. The most important feature which differentiates graphene from many nanomaterials besides its mechanical and optical properties is the interaction between graphene and different kinds of microorganisms [129]. The use of 3 min of NIR (808 nm) with a power density of 0.1 W cm^{-2} allows killing SARS-CoV-2 deposited on surfaces using a light with intensity analog to sunlight. These results allow for extensive use of graphene PLA filaments, considering that exposure to sunlight can be a method to sterilize the surfaces of 3D-printed objects. We also demonstrate that the mechanical behavior of the material is improved while the biocompatibility is retained toward eukaryotic cell lines. The World Health Organization highlighted the need for the prioritization of personal protective equipment supplies for frontline healthcare workers, and PLA-G-based objects could represent the game changer against pandemic spreading. Furthermore, NIR-mediated sterilization could represent a sustainable method to recycle medical devices and lower the impact on the environment. The applications of PLA-G-based devices go beyond the nosocomial settings: with its high biocompatibility and mechanical resistance, PLA-G can become building materials for high-touch surfaces, such as handles and buttons, in public transport. Furthermore, 3D-printed SARS-CoV-2 can be used to produce long-term wearable prosthetic devices. Indeed, the improvement of mechanical properties and the possibility to sterilize the surface by NIR could cope with the necessity, in the emergency setting, to reduce plaster and cast making. Indeed, given the hospital overflow together with the risk of transmission, protocols during pandemics could envisage the use of medical data files to send 3D-printed prosthetics to the patient directly at home [130]. Any PLA-G-printed medical device could indeed be ordered remotely to reduce the hospitalizations and could be easily self-removed by the patient. Finally, 3D-printed air filters [131,132] made of PLA-G could be particularly useful for the possibility to use NIR light sterilization daily to maintain SARS-CoV-2-free air.

The most commonly relied upon COVID-19 sensing techniques, ELISA, PCR, and RT-PCR, are reliable but require expansive instrumentation, training, and time for diagnosis. PCR is predominantly used to detect specific organisms, such as viruses. PCR is a very powerful technique as it can identify the residual fragments of a virus even after the disease disappears, and so it has enabled rapid analysis to diagnose diseases in humans. RT-PCR is a laboratory-based investigation process which produces copies of specific DNA/RNA sequences for investigation. Enzymes belonging to RT are manipulated and used to vary a specific sequence of RNA to a matching piece of DNA. After producing numerous pieces of DNA in large quantities through DNA polymerase, it can identify a specific mRNA sequence which makes up a gene. RT-PCR can help to efficiently diagnose a disease and monitor an infection. So in standard PCR analysis, a DNA template is amplified and a thermocycler is used, but in RT-PCR, RNA is utilized as a template and is reverse-transcribed into complementary DNA. PCR is typically employed for viruses that have DNA for amplification [133]. Similarly, SARS-CoV-2 has only RNA, and it can be detected through RT-PCR. Figure 7.34 [133] shows the structure of and components present in SARS-CoV-2.

Electrochemical detection is among the significant, low-cost, and high-performance sensing techniques [134,135] which can effectively detect changes in the current, voltage, or charge generated from surface interactions with a working electrode and analyte. The aforementioned detection techniques [133,134] suffer from certain demerits, such as the need for trained and qualified personnel and also more demand for expensive chemical reagents. Importantly, traditional techniques are not suited for large-scale diagnosis in quick time frames. Although these techniques exhibit great sensitivity, sometimes they provide false positive or negative test results. It is noteworthy to mention that the sensitivity and the limit of detection (LOD) are respective to the COVID-19 viral dose and infective virus dose, which becomes an issue for sensing platforms. For RT-PCR testing of nasal samples, standard COVID-19 detection techniques provide an average LOD of 100 copies of viral RNA per mL [136]. Having said that, more than 10,000-fold, the LOD can be achieved through electrochemical-based detection techniques (Figure 7.35) [133].

In conclusion, a label-free DNA sensor based on SWCNTFET has been developed for the selective detection of DNA hybridization. The DNA sensor used in this study contains a random network of SWCNTs that covered a large surface area of interdigitated electrode. The effect of the parameters, including target DNA, probe DNA concentration, and hybridization time, on the sensor response was studied. The results in the reference showed the SWCNTFET-based DNA sensor is a promising candidate for the development of biosensors for medical, forensic, and environmental purposes.

Finally, the cost is also critical. The research field has aimed to produce accessible, precise, real-time, portable, and recyclable devices to detect viruses. The development of next-generation carbon-based nanomaterials for virus treatment devices must also be safe, cheap, and efficacious to treat the infection. In conclusion, carbon-based nanotechnology is positioned to provide a better life.

In summary, this chapter proposes that a graphene oxide–based viral RNA analysis system (GOViRA) platform can be helpful to study the DENV life cycle and to develop antiviral drugs. A biosensor using PNA and DRGON that can quantitatively analyze the intracellular DENV genome level in live

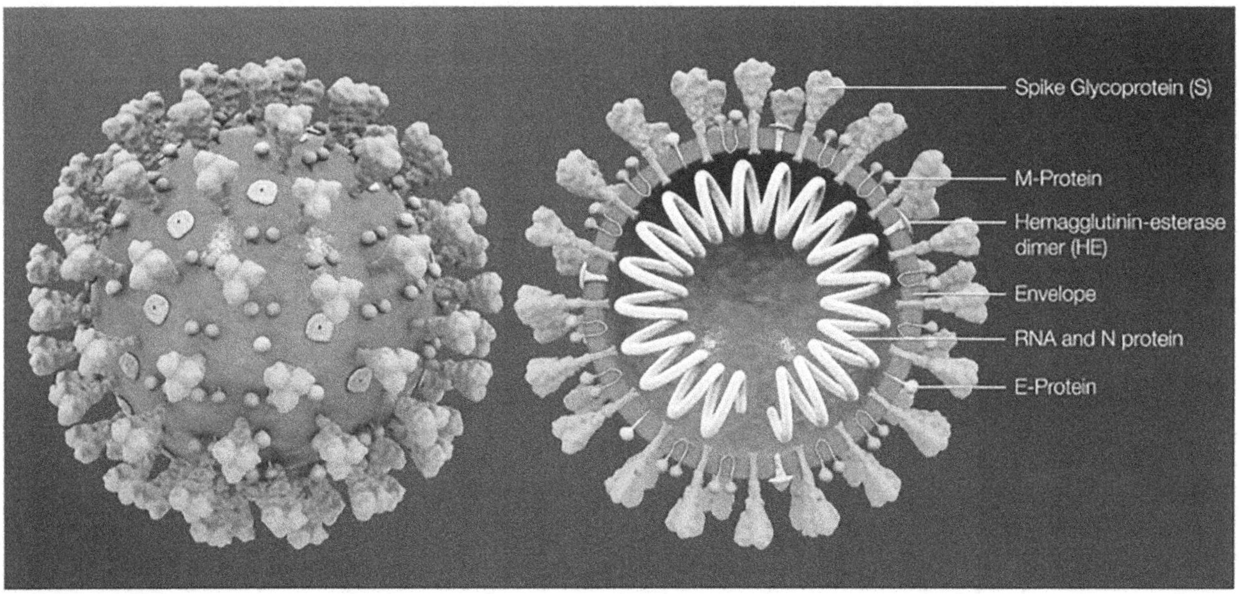

FIGURE 7.34 Structure and components of SARS-CoV-2.

Source: [133].

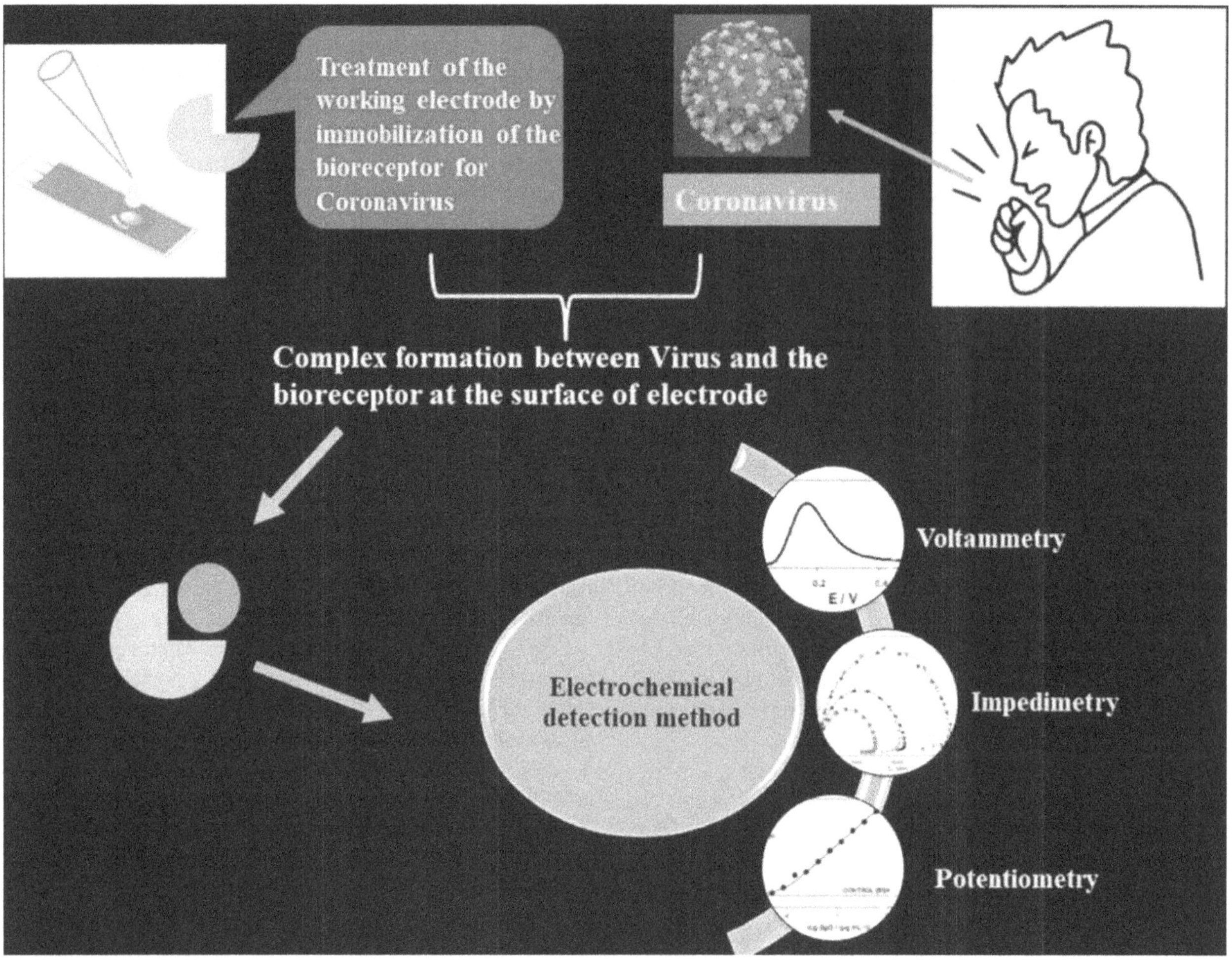

FIGURE 7.35 Schematic of an electrochemical COVID-19 detection technique using voltametric, impedimetric, and potentiometric sensors.

Source: [133].

cells has been developed. In addition, anti-DENV drug repurposing through high-throughput screening was facilitated by the GOViRA platform. Through this process, ulipristal was identified as a new entry inhibitor against DENV infection having an anti-DENV activity in cells and a murine model. The repurposing of ulipristal in DENV treatment may provide great potential in clinical use. To do so, further study on the precise mode of action of ulipristal and evaluation in a non-human primate DENV infection model are necessary. The successful identification of a novel anti-DENV agent suggests that this approach can facilitate repurposing antiviral therapeutics for other various viral infections. We anticipate that the GOViRA system can accelerate the discovery of effective antiviral drug candidates at the initial stage of the drug discovery process.

8

Insights on Carbon-Based Nanomaterials as Smart Nanosystems Platform for Cancer Theranostics Sustainable Technology

8.1 Background

Carbon nanotubes (CNTs), one of the most promising carbon-related nanomaterials, have already achieved much success in the biomedical field. Due to their excellent optical property, thermal and electronic conductivity, easy functionalization ability, and high drug loading capacity, CNTs can be applied in a multifunctional way for cancer treatment and diagnosis.

The nanoplatform offers an exciting opportunity to gain targeting strategies and multifunctionality. The advent of nanotechnology, in particular, the development of smart nanomaterials, has transformed cancer diagnosis and treatment. The large surface area of nanoparticles is enough to encapsulate many molecules and the ability to functionalize with various biosubstrates, such as DNA, RNA, aptamers, and antibodies, which helps in theranostic action. Comparatively, biologically derived nanomaterials perceive advantages over nanomaterials produced by conventional methods in terms of economy, ease of production, and reduced toxicity.

The unregulated proliferation of cells that damage healthy organs and tissues is known as cancer. Cancer cells develop traits, including self-sufficiency in proliferation factors, infinite cell expansion capability, and susceptibility to signals that inhibit rapid cell growth or induce cell death in normal cells as a result of numerous mutations and excessive growth and division. *Cancer* is a broad denomination that refers to a range of disorders distinguished by uncontrollable neurogenesis. Currently, there are more than 200 known forms of cancer; all these have their terminology depending on the nature of the organ from where cancer originated. Numerous medicines are present in the trial phase. Nanostructures have provided important development in the recent decade, owing to one's enormous possibility in biological devices. Carbon nanotubes (CNTs), quantum dots, and dendrimers are nanotechnology with distinctive features which could be used for cancer detection, laser therapy, as well as medicinal administration. These are thought to be amongst the foremost potential nanotechnology since they can monitor malignant cells as well as transport medications or tiny medicinal compounds to patients.

Despite the exciting breakthroughs in medical technology, cancer still accounts for one of the principal triggers of death, and conventional therapeutic modalities often fail to attain an effective cure. Recently, nanobiotechnology has made huge advancement in cancer therapy with gigantic application potential because of their ability in achieving precise and controlled drug release, elevating drug solubility and reducing adverse effects.

Cancer is one of the deadest diseases that cause increasing mortality rates over the past decades [1]. This malignant illness is often characterized by an uncontrolled growth of cancer cells, which proliferates in an unlimited manner and invasively spreads to other organs and tissues throughout the body, disturbing the physiological function of normal cells and severely threating people's health and affecting their quality of life [2]. Though the rapid development of treatment strategies like surgery, chemotherapy, radiotherapy, endocrine therapy, immunotherapy, phototherapy, and gene therapy has greatly improved the current situation of cancer therapy and prolonged the patients' survival time, these therapeutic modalities still face many challenges that hinder their broad application, especially for metastatic cancer treatment [3]. For instance, surgery stalls cancer progression at the cost of significant pain and disfigurement of patients who have solid tumor [4]. Chemotherapy and radiotherapy lack specificity toward cancer cells, which can result in many unavoidable side effects, and are able to promote drug resistance [5]. Nanobiotechnology has emerged as a novel treatment opportunity against cancer in recent decades. The employment of nano-based drug delivery systems (DDS) opened a new avenue to integrate multiple anticancer agents in one platform for more efficacious therapeutic outcome with reduced side effects and enhanced targeting ability [6]. Due to their unique potential for passive targeting through enhanced permeability and retention (EPR), high surface area for drug loading and modification, and prolonged plasma half-life, nanomedicine possesses numerous benefits over conventional therapeutic modalities [7]. In this field, many nanocarriers, like liposomes, micelles, reconstituted high-density lipoprotein (rHDL), metallic NPs, hybrid NPs, nanogel, nanoemulsion, black phosphorus, carbon-related nanomaterials, and other inorganic nanomaterials, have been extensively explored in anticancer drug delivery both clinically and pre-clinically [8]. Among various nanocarriers, carbon nanotubes (CNTs) have arisen many researchers' interest due to their multifunctional application possibilities in both cancer treatment and diagnosis. CNTs possess tiny tubular shapes comprising carbon atoms which are ordered to form a honeycomb nanostructure with exceptional physicochemical properties [9]. Generally, CNTs can be classified into either single-walled carbon nanotubes (SWNTs) or multi-walled carbon nanotubes (MWNTs) according to the sheet number of carbon atoms, both playing a critical role in cancer research with different properties.

An innovation in nanomedicine has guided the improved outcomes for cancer diagnosis and therapy. However, the

DOI: 10.1201/9781032635989-8

frequent use of nanomaterials remains challenging due to specific limitations, like non-targeted distribution, causing low signal-to-noise ratio for diagnostics, complex fabrication, reduced biocompatibility, decreased photostability, and systemic toxicity of nanomaterials within the body. Thus, better nanomaterial systems with controlled physicochemical and biological properties form the need of the hour. In this context, smart nanomaterials serve as promising solution, as they can be activated under specific exogenous or endogenous stimuli, such as pH, temperature, enzymes, or a particular biological molecule. The properties of smart nanomaterials make them ideal candidates for various applications, like biosensors, controlled drug release, and treatment of various diseases. Recently, smart nanomaterial–based cancer theranostic approaches have been developed, and they are displaying better selectivity and sensitivity with reduced side effects in comparison to conventional methods. In cancer therapy, smart nanomaterials system only activates in response to tumor microenvironment (TME) and remains in deactivated state in normal cells, which further reduces the side effects and systemic toxicities. Cancer is one of the deadliest diseases, and despite global efforts, the number of cancer patients are increasing continuously. Anticancer approaches, including chemotherapy, radiotherapy, and tumor surgical resection, which are developed with time, could not attain complete cure of the disease. Moreover, traditional anticancer treatments are responsible for the compromised lifestyle of the patient, and they have significant side effects. The presence of biological barriers like genetic mutations, endothelial cell barriers, and blood–brain barriers (BBB) is the main reason for the unavailability of proper diagnostic and treatment against cancer. The pharmaceutical barriers like limited biodistribution, perfusion, toxicity, permeability, inefficacy, and penetration are the main difficulties in the translation of any anticancer approach into clinical platform. Further, most of the recent anticancer approaches target any rapidly dividing cells, irrespective of whether the target is tumorous or not. Thus, it is necessary to develop effective anticancer approaches for accurate diagnosis and treatment that can overcome the previously cited limitations to provide an optimistic solution.

The alarming increase in new cancer cases worldwide concerns people's lives and physical well-being. Despite advancements in science and technology and drug discovery methods, cancer is still the second leading cause of death worldwide, after cardiovascular diseases. The global survey, including the individual medical data of 37.5 million cancer patients diagnosed between 2000 and 2014, shows that overall, cancer survival rates are improving, including those for cancers with high malignancies. Cancer is responsible for about one in six deaths worldwide. Global Cancer Statistics 2020: GLOBOCAN estimates of incidence and mortality worldwide for 36 cancers in 185 countries (https://doi.org/10.3322/caac.21492) implies that 19.3 million new cancer cases will be responsible for approximately 10 million deaths [10]. It turns out that low- and middle-income countries account for over 70% of cancer-related fatalities globally. Five main dietary and lifestyle disorders, including tobacco use, high body mass index, inadequate intake of fruits and vegetables, inactivity, and high alcohol consumption, are responsible for one-third of cancer-related fatalities. The complex, multifaceted origin makes cancer treatment more difficult. Additionally, many cancer treatments fail because of the development of multidrug-resistant cells. Consequently, a single line of treatment cannot apply to all patients. Recurrence is frequently possible because cancer may become resistant to therapies that formerly cured it successfully [11].

Effective and personalized treatment plans incorporating cancer diagnostic and therapeutic approaches are required to achieve excellent clinical results. Afterward, monoclonal antibody–based therapy has been explored by utilizing tumor-specific antigens (TSAs) and tumor-associated antigens (TAAs). Antibody–drug conjugates (ADCs) are biopharmaceutical drugs designed for targeted cancer therapy and sparing healthy cells. This approach has also paved the way from the bench side to the bedside in a majestic way. Despite the substantial progress of these techniques, the aforementioned techniques have their own advantages and disadvantages. To address this, researchers and scientists have worked on several methods and techniques, including organic chemistry, supramolecular chemistry, nanotechnology, oncology, and pharmacology [12]. Nanotheranostics harnesses the capabilities of nanotechnology; due to their small size and leaky tumor vascularization, nanosystems can preferentially aggregate in tumor cells and exhibit enhanced therapeutic efficacy and diagnostic capability. Additionally, these nanoparticles (NPs) can be redirected and reoriented in a variety of ways while carrying the medicines on them. The emerging area of nanotechnology brings the concept of nanotherapeutics, and this technique has proven very promising in cancer treatment. *Nanotechnology* has been considered as the engineering of the molecule at the nanoscale level, which endows high drug loading capabilities due to high external surface area. Moreover, owing to the small size, which is comparable with the biological system, nanomaterials actively interact with cellular components of the cell and show promising application in both *in vivo* and *in vitro* biomedical applications.

It is apparent that overcoming cancer is a battle against complexities and intricacies due to mutations, the metastatic nature of cancer cells, a lack of early detection techniques, and the inability of the scientific community to solve many cancer-related problems. However, the recent developments in nanotechnology can be a key to unlock the secrets of cancer diagnosis and treatment strategies [13]. Nanotechnology is one of the emerging multidisciplinary areas dealing with physics, biochemistry, material science, chemistry, biology, medicine, informatics, and engineering. The nanomaterials are typically between 0.1 and 100 nm in size, and they exhibit extraordinary capabilities due to higher surface-area-to-volume ratio, and they find applications in food science, agriculture, marine science, environmental chemistry, veterinary medicine, medicine detection, and several other industries [14].

The use of nanotechnology-based approaches and nanomaterials in oncology can lead to early diagnosis, targeted drug delivery, drug development, and efficient anticancer therapies. For example, gold nanoparticles (AuNPs) have extensively been employed as drug delivery vehicle for breast and prostate cancers [15]. Gold nanoparticles are considered due to their reliable properties, like capacity to absorb/scatter light and converting optical energy into heat. On the other hand, recently investigated nanotoxicity of different types of nanomaterials may promote off-target reactions and bioaccumulation of metal-based nanoparticles, limiting full potential of nanomaterials in oncology. However, there are still opportunities for future investigations in terms of nanotherapy's sensitivity to tumor microenvironment, which could result in improved palliative care in addition to diagnosis and therapy.

The field of theranostic nanosystems is promising and extensive, and it warrants further research for the discovery of effective theranostic NPs, which enable a more personalized approach to nanomedicine. To this, NPs can be coated with hydrophilic materials, such as folate, polyethylene glycol (PEG), hyaluronic acid, transferrin, aptamers, and antibodies, which make NPs hydrophilic, which, in turn, increase the period of drugs, targeting efficiency by specific recognition, and enhance their penetration and accumulation in tumors. Numerous NPs also act as imaging agents due to the unique physicochemical properties of nanomaterials, along with improved transport. Hence, they need not be loaded with an additional imaging agent. For instance, the use of iron oxide in magnetic resonance imaging (MRI) allows diagnosis and therapy to be carried out concurrently rather than before or after therapy. The unique properties of noble metal Au and Ag nanoparticles show unique tunable optical properties because of their surface plasmon resonance (SPR) and have a strong penetrating ability, which makes them appropriate for theranostic applications [16]. Thus, as theranostic agents, nanomaterials provide a unique advantage, including passive or active accumulation in tumor tissues and monitoring all activities within one formulation, ultimately reducing the patient's inconvenience and potential adverse effects on the human body. The challenge associated with nanomaterials is their toxic properties, which should be addressed before their administration in clinical applications.

This chapter describes the documented literature on the recent progress of nanotechnology-based theranostic systems that have been extensively employed to support numerous clinical and preclinical cancer treatments, as given in Scheme 8.1 [17]. This provides an overview of nanomaterials used for cancer theranostics platforms, along with a brief introduction to nanomaterial synthesis and its types, and attempts were also made to summarize the comprehensive novel nanotheranostic systems that have the potential for simultaneous cancer diagnosis and treatment in clinical translations, followed by future perspectives and challenges. We conclude this chapter with a retrospective outlook of this important field and identify potential implications of this field's paradigm in healthcare. With continued innovation and serious attention to the key challenges, it is expected that this important field will play a pivotal role in cancer diagnosis and treatment in clinical translations. We believe the summary of recent developments for the use of carbon-based nanomaterials in cancer theranostics will provide a comprehensive understanding of the applications of NPs in biomedical research investigations and clinical uses.

8.1.1 Insights on Functionalized Carbon Nanotubes for Cancer Theranostics

CNTs are nanometer-size tubular substances possessing axial concord, which gives the key qualities which could be used in diagnostics and therapy. CNTs possess the ability to transport

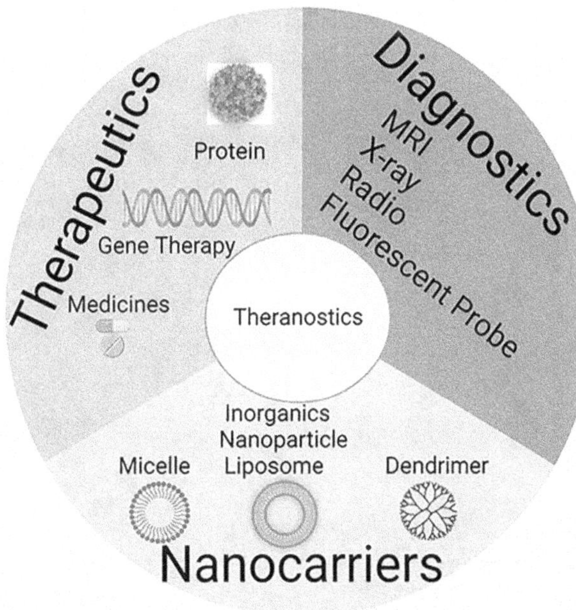

SCHEME 8.1 Recent progress of nanotechnology-based theranostic systems.

Source: [17].

medications to specific sites. Along with the remarkable progress in the production of nanoscale materials technologies, it is equally critical to understand the toxic effects of nanomaterials. CNTs have been utilized in almost all cancer therapy techniques in recent years, encompassing medication administration, lymph-specific treatments, thermal treatments, photodynamic therapy, and gene therapy. Inside this overview, we will look at the ways they have been integrated into diagnostics and therapy. Chemical conjugation is a critical part of the studies in both schemes, as is emphasized in this chapter. It is attempted to categorize the studies by cancer type and to introduce novel therapeutic strategies developed for cancer diagnosis and treatment. The focus is primarily on the biomedical aspects of the methodologies, as well as the cancer cells' subsequent biological responses to the procedures.

Owing to their unique physiochemical features, CNTs are extensively studied in cancer theranostics, with versatile application potentials. For instance, the strong absorption of CNTs in near-infrared (NIR) regions enables their application in photothermal therapy (PTT). CNTs can transform the laser energy to acoustic signals and exhibit great resonant Raman scattering and photoluminescence in NIR region, which are all beneficial to their utilization in cancer imaging [18]. Besides, it has been reported that only a tiny amount of nanodrugs can be successfully delivered into solid tumors because of the biological obstacles and complicated tumor microenvironment (TME) that hinder their deep penetration. Excitingly, numerous reports have demonstrated that CNTs can be taken up by various cell types due to their needle-like architecture, which promotes their tumor penetration as ideal vehicles for anticancer targeted drug delivery. Moreover, CNTs can carry therapeutic agents to many intracellular targets, like nucleus, mitochondria, and cytoplasm, or target the TME components to disturb tumor cells' living condition, both of which can result in an enhanced antitumor effect (Scheme 8.2) [19].

Taken together, owing to their outstanding physicochemical characteristics, ultrahigh surface for conjugation and drug loading, thermal conductivity, optical property, and tumor penetration ability, CNTs are becoming rising stars in many biomedical fields, including drug delivery, genetic engineering, imaging, and biosensing, to treat and diagnose a variety of cancers (Figure 8.1) [20].

Of course, every coin has two sides; the distinctive structures of CNTs increase their hydrophobicity in water and leave them with inherent cytotoxicity [21]. Therefore, elevating hydrophilicity and reducing cytotoxicity through functionalizing CNTs

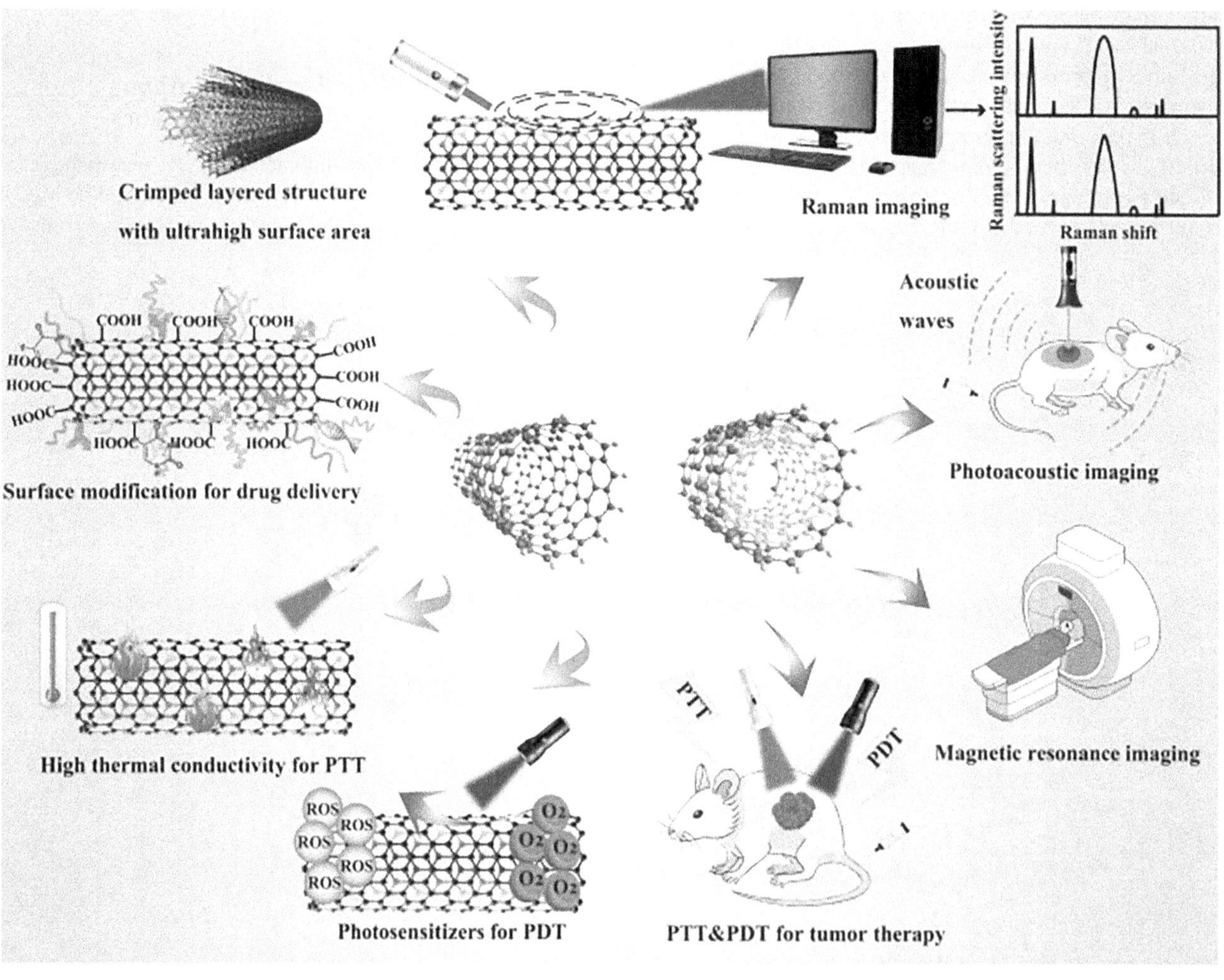

FIGURE 8.1 Schematic overview of the diverse applications of CNTs in cancer theranostics.

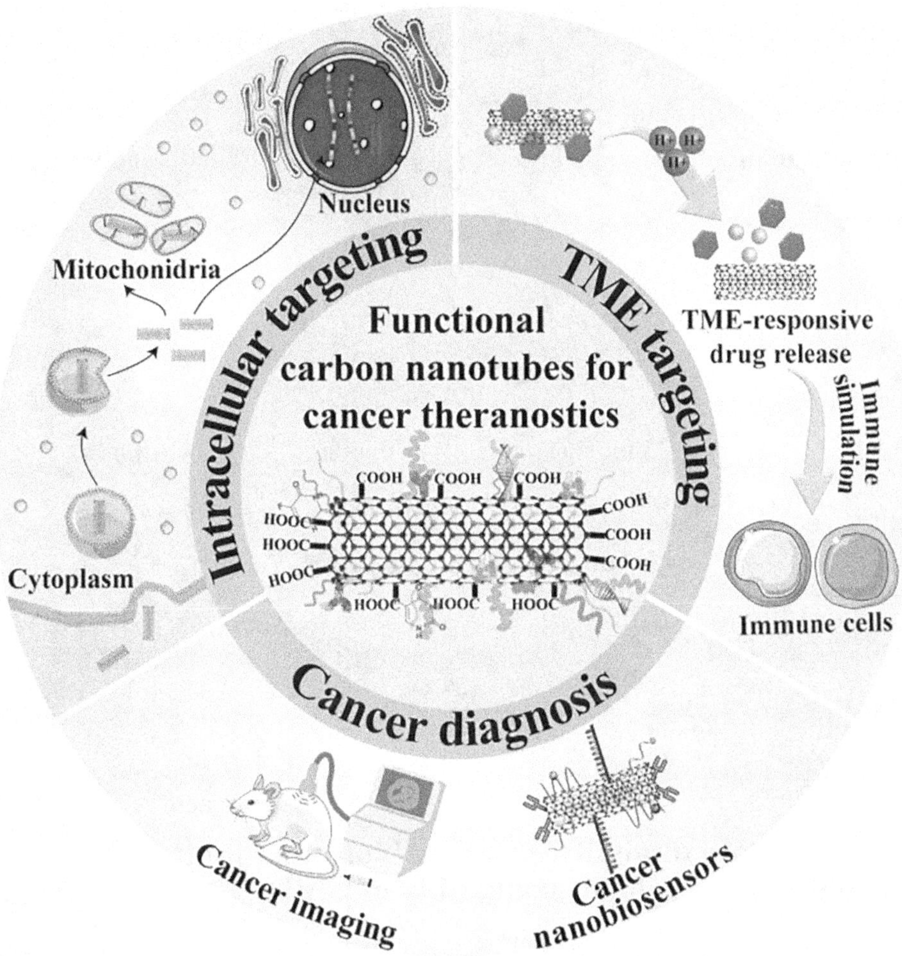

SCHEME 8.2 Functional carbon nanotubes for cancer theranostics

Source: [19].

with different chemical groups or biomolecules are of great significance to improve their safety and the effectiveness for broad application in cancer therapy [22]. Thus, this chapter highlights the update on the progress of CNTs as promising drug delivery vehicles in cancer treatment. Different strategies used for their functionalization, as well as their key roles in targeting various intracellular spots and TME constituents, will be introduced. In addition, the recent advances of their application in cancer diagnosis will be outlined in detail. Therefore, compared to the previous reviews that summarized CNTs, the novelty of this chapter is that we systemically introduce the theranostic applications of CNTs against many cancer types from the aspect of various therapeutic targets and emphasize the combination therapeutic modalities based on the physiochemical features of CNTs by using the fresh reported literatures [23].

8.2 Functionalization Methods of Carbon Nanotubes

CNTs are initially insoluble and less-dispersible substances; their inherent limitations, such as poor solubility, agglomeration, and toxicity, severely hinder their wide applications. Hence, improving their natural properties through surface modification is of great necessity to acquire enhanced solubility, better biocompatibility, deeper penetration, and decreased cytotoxicity in biological systems. Typically, there are two functionalization methods to modify CNTs; one is covalent, and the other is non-covalent. *Covalent modification* of CNTs, such as oxidation and carboxylation, offers a stable platform for drug delivery, while *non-covalent functionalization* through van der Waals interactions, π–π interactions, and hydrophobic interactions causes minimal damage to the surface of CNTs [24]. A lot of bioactive molecules, such as antibodies and aptamers, various polymers, and surfactants, have been adopted to non-covalently functionalize CNTs to achieve increased biocompatibility and reduced toxicity (Figure 8.2) [25]. Moreover, the biodegradability of raw CNTs is low because their hydrophobic interaction prevents enzymes from approaching it; however, their biodegradability can be improved through functionalization, which increases their solubility and produces defect sites to provide preferred binding sites for enzymes and promote enzymatic degradation. For instance, defective sites on the carbon walls and ends of

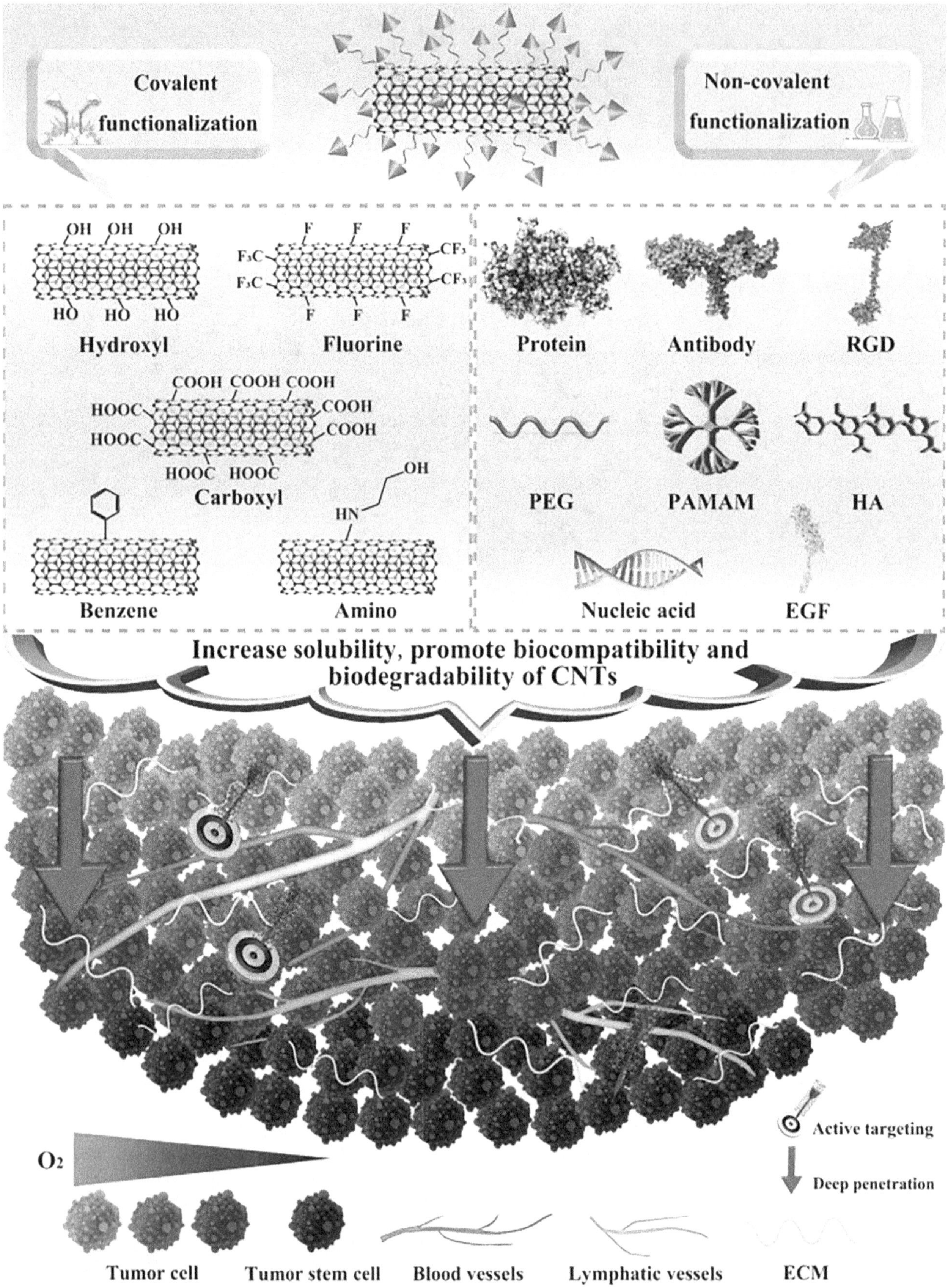

FIGURE 8.2 Schematic demonstration of different functionalization methods of CNTs. CNTs can be functionalized in covalent and non-covalent ways through various chemical groups, ligands, and polymers to improve their solubility, biocompatibility, and biodegradability for active drug targeting and deep tumor penetration [19].

TABLE 8.1

Summary of the Functionalization of CNTs through Various Molecules

Type of CNTs	Functionalized Molecules	Effectiveness	Tumor Model	Biocompatibility Test	Refs.
SWNTs	PEG	Increase solubility, prevent particle aggregation, decrease side effect of the whole DDS	Gastric cancer	Show decreased toxicity toward normal tissue	[26]
Both SWNTs and MWNTs	PEI	Improve solubility, homogeneity, and dispersity; reduce particle size; increase positive charge to interact with siRNA	Cervical cancer	N/A	[27]
SWNTs	Hyaluronic acid	Enhance serum stability and target CD44-overexpressing cancer cells; overcome multidrug resistance	Ovarian cancer	Show no cytotoxicity toward normal tissue with no body weight drop in mice	[28]
MWNTs	Chitosan	Increase water solubility and cell-penetrating ability; decrease toxicity	Breast cancer	Show low cytotoxicity	[29]
MWNTs	PLGA	Improve dispersity, reduce toxicity, provide attachment sites for drugs, and tune temporal release	Osteosarcoma	Show low cytotoxicity in normal cells	[30]
SWNTs	CD33 mAB	Recognize and specifically target GNM-CD33+ cells	Glioblastoma	N/A	[31]
SWNTs	IGF1R mAB and HER2 mAB	Enable multi-component to target IGF1R and HER2 surface receptors	Breast cancer	Exhibit negligible in vitro toxicity in normal cells	[32]
SWNTs	RGD peptide	Target $\alpha_v\beta_3$-expressing cancer cells	Malignant melanoma	Induce little toxicity in vitro	[33]
SWNTs	EGF receptor	Achieve active targeting ability and enhance the uptake of drugs	Head and neck squamous carcinoma	Show negligible toxicity in vitro and in vivo	[34]

carboxylated or nitrogen-doped MWNTs are more likely to bind to horseradish peroxidase (HRP), thus facilitating their enzymatic degradation. Hence, the following sections mainly focus on the modifications of CNTs through various functionalized molecules. Different functionalization methods of CNTs are summarized in Table 8.1.

8.2.1 Functionalization Using Polymer

Polyethylene glycol (PEG), a widely used polymer, was approved for pharmaceutical application by FDA and has been utilized as an adjuvant material in drug delivery for many years due to its versatility and safety. Therefore, PEG functionalization is a favorable choice to elevate the physiochemical characteristics of CNTs to achieve enhanced solubility and biocompatibility. To this aim, Taghavi et al. developed PEGylated SWNTs to carry DOX and Bcl-xL-specific short hairpin RNA (shRNA) for gastric cancer treatment, which exhibited an enhanced cancer cell death through the synergistic therapeutic effect of DOX and shRNA [26]. To achieve the active targeting purpose, the constructed PEGylated SWNTs were covalently linked to the nucleolin ligand AS1411 aptamer. PEG modification increased the solubility of SWNTs as well as prevented aggregation of particles and decreased the side effect of this DDS. According to the data of in vitro experiments, this combinational strategy through shRNA-based gene silence and chemotherapeutic agent DOX displayed excellent tumoricidal efficacy. In addition to PEG, polyethylenimine (PEI) is another widely used polymer that is suitable for gene delivery. As a polycation, PEI can incorporate with CNTs to reinforce the combining ability of CNTs with nucleic acid by π-stacking and electrical reaction. Huang et al. modified both SWNTs and MWNTs with PEI by amination to obtain PEI-NH-SWNTs and PEI-NH-MWNTs [27]. As a result of PEI functionalization, both functionalized CNTs were capable of dispersing better in aqueous solution than SWNTs and MWNTs alone. Besides, CNTs modified with PEI could interact with siRNAs by electrical reaction due to CNTs' positive charge on their surface, successfully delivering siRNAs into cells and resulting in higher transfection and gene silence efficiency. Hyaluronic acid (HA) is a linear macromolecular mucopolysaccharide with excellent biodegradability and biocompatibility, and it is composed of alternatingly linked two saccharide units of N-acetylglucosamine and glucuronic acid. CD44 receptor, the main binding receptor of HA, is usually overexpressed in many tumor types. Therefore, HA is a promising material which can not only endow various nanoplatforms with active targeting ability to tumor tissue but also enhance the biocompatibility of the whole DDS without additional toxicity during antitumor therapy. Bhirde et al. designed a CNT-based DDS by self-assemble method to actively deliver anticancer drug DOX to tumor site through the interaction between cholic acid–derivatized HA (CAHA) wrapped around semiconducting single-walled carbon nanotube (sSWNT) and CD44 receptors expressed on tumor cells [28]. According to the confocal video imaging results, DOX contained in this DDS could be effectively taken up by both drug-sensitive ovarian cancer cells OVCAR8 and resistant OVCAR8 (OVCAR8/ADR). In contrast, free DOX could only be taken up by drug-sensitive OVCAR8, but not by OVCAR8/ADR, demonstrating that CD44-targeted DDS was able to circumvent drug resistance during antitumor therapy and enhance the accumulation of drug in cancer cells. Other polymers like chitosan and polylactic-co-glycolic acid (PLGA) can also be adopted to modify CNTs [29, 30]. Chitosan is a bioactive polymer derived from natural polysaccharides chitin, while PLGA is a synthetic polymer that has been approved by the FDA for medical application due to its great biodegradability and low toxicity. Both modifications can greatly improve the inner properties of CNTs to achieve a better anticancer therapeutic efficacy.

8.2.2 Functionalization Using Antibody

Monoclonal antibodies (mAbs) are artificial proteins with similar functions, like human antibodies, and were firstly applied as antagonists of oncogenic receptor tyrosine kinases. Nowadays, mAbs have been regarded as one of the promising substance for antitumor targeted therapy. Several receptors, like cluster of differentiation-133 (CD133), human endothelial receptor 2 (HER2), and insulin-like growth factor 1 receptor (IGF1R), often show an overexpression on numerous types of cancer cells and cancer stem cells (CSCs). Therefore, conjugating monoclonal antibody on CNTs opens a new era for antitumor treatment. CD133 is a common biomarker to detect CSCs, and it serves as a prognostic indicator to guide tumor progression, remission, and patient survival. Thus, the application of CD133 monoclonal antibody (anti-CD133) can obviously enhance the targeting ability to CSC. Wang et al. combined SWNTs with anti-CD133-conjugated chitosan, forming anti-CD133-CS/SWNTs for glioblastoma (GBM) treatment [31]. *In vitro* experiment showed that this nanosystem exhibited excellent targeting ability to GBM-CD133+ cells and could effectively eliminate cancer cells upon NIR irradiation without damaging surrounding tissues. Besides, the combination of monoclonal antibody with PTT displayed good inhibitory effects on tumor invasion through preventing the self-regrowth of GBM-CD133+ cells *in vitro*. Integrated molecular targeting is another approach that can be combined with CNTs during antitumor therapy. IGF1R and HER2 are two surface markers that both overexpress in various cancer types, exhibiting great research values. Shao et al. designed a nanosystem consisting of SWNTs, IGF1R monoclonal antibody (anti-IGF1R), and HER2 monoclonal antibody (anti-HER2), which could target IGF1R and HER2 in tumor cells [32]. *In vitro* experiments based on breast cancer cell lines showed that antibody-modified SWNTs could internalize into cancer cells more effectively through the interaction between specific antibodies and their corresponding antigens. In addition, the integration of PTT with the aforementioned mAB therapy could significantly destroy the breast cancer cells *in vitro*, indicating that antibody-functionalized SWNTs, combined with their intrinsic optical properties, could provide an effective way for anticancer treatment.

8.2.3 Functionalization Using RGD Peptide

Arginylglycylaspartic acid (RGD) is a small peptide that serves as an ideal ligand for most integrin types expressed on various cancer cells. Thus, combining RGD peptide onto the surface of CNTs can improve the active targeting ability of the DDS as well. Integrin $\alpha v\beta 3$, a common form of integrin, is overexpressed on many cancer cells and contributes a lot to tumor progression. Koh et al. constructed RGD peptide–modified, carboxylic acid–functionalized SWNTs with the encapsulation of the topoisomerase I inhibitor camptothecin (CPT) (CPT@f-CNT-RGD) to treat malignant melanoma [33]. According to the results of cell viability assay, 3D-cultured cells model, and Western blot assay, the human malignant melanoma cell A375 incubated with CPT@f-CNT-RGD exhibited the lowest cell viability and expressed the highest level of apoptosis-related proteins, such as caspase-3 and Bax. In addition, *in vivo* distribution studies showed that CPT@f-CNT-RGD could localize in tumor sites to a great extent, confirming the excellent targeting effects of this nano-DDS.

8.2.4 Functionalization Using Epidermal Growth Factor

Epidermal growth factor (EGF) is the ligand of EGF receptor (EGFR) overexpressed on the surface of various tumor cells. Therefore, combining CNTs with EGF endows CNTs with tumor-targeting ability and can be regarded as another method to improve therapeutic efficacy of anticancer treatment. Cisplatin is a classic anticancer drug with broad spectrum to treat many cancer types. Bhirde et al. conjugated both cisplatin and EGF to the surface of oxidized SWNTs, which endowed the nanosystem with active targeting ability through the interaction between EGF and EGFR overexpressed on tumor cells for enhanced antitumor efficacy of cisplatin [34]. *In vitro* and *in vivo* studies based on head and neck squamous carcinoma model showed that EGF/cisplatin/CNTs exhibited the best active targeting ability and the strongest cytotoxicity to tumor cells, which could inhibit the tumor growth to the greatest extent compared to other groups without EGF modification, further demonstrating that the active targeting ability of the whole DDS could be enormously improved with the existence of EGF, while the potential adverse effects due to the lack of specificity could be accordingly avoided.

8.3 Tumor Microenvironment (TME) and Opportunities

Cancer consists of a complex environment with heterogenous cells involved in dissimilar, unpredictable, and mutually interactive patterns of growth. The major hallmarks of cancer are defined as sustaining proliferative signals, inducing angiogenesis, resisting cell death, evading growth suppressors, enabling replicative immortality, activating invasion, and metastasis. Cancer controls the various hallmarks by governing the energy metabolism alterations, genome instabilities, and inflammation by employing the normal cells to recruit and sustain the microenvironment required for the propagation of cancer.

The TME refers to the exterior of malignant/benign cell's surrounding components comprising of extracellular matrix, blood vessels, fibroblasts, signaling molecules, secreted factors, tumor vasculature, and lymphatics. Additionally, the TME is created by the interaction between the malignant and non-transformed cells. Other than the malignant cells, cancer also consists of other cells which get corrupted from the transformed cells. TME is created by the interaction between the malignant and non-transformed cells. Functionally, malignant cells invade the local tissues during carcinogenesis by releasing pro-tumorigenic factors, which are responsible for the formation of TME, characterized by angiogenesis and hypoxia. Further, proliferation and progression of tumor are controlled by the subsequently reprogrammed TME, such as redox potential alteration, nutrient and oxygen uptake (hypoxia conditions) changes, and blood flow alteration in the due time course. Parallelly, at all stages of carcinogenesis, non-malignant cells of TME have tumor-promoting and dynamic functions.

The significant abnormalities in TME, like altered redox potential, hyperthermia, acidic pH, and upregulated expression of selected proteins, and enzymes have drawn the interest of employing stimulus-responsive nanomaterials in cancer diagnosis and therapy. This approach enables the synthesis of nanomaterial, which responds to endogenous and/or exogenous stimuli like pH, temperature, magnetism, light, and enzymes to improve drug targeting and internalization. Thus, nanotechnology finds application as a stimulus-responsive nanomaterial which (1) inhibits tumor growth by enabling tumor or TME targeting, (2) facilitates the accumulation of drugs in altered TME, and (3) improves therapeutic ability.

The mild acidic nature of TME is one of the key characteristic, and an alteration in tissue pH indicates the pathological progression. Lactate (metabolite of aggravate aerobic glycolysis) accumulation is the major reason of acidic pH in TME, which is popularly termed as "Warburg's effect." Various other factors governed by programmed oncogenes, like Na^+/H^+ exchange, carbonic anhydrase-9, and mono-carboxylate transporters, also maintain the acidic environment, with the extracellular and intracellular pH at 6.0–7.0 and 6.0–6.5, respectively. This mild acidic nature has been successfully employed in cancer theranostics, like stimuli-responsive drug release, accurate diagnosis of tumor state, and micro-metastasis tracking. Higher rate of glycolysis places high nutritional demand, leading to increased glucose uptake into the cancer cells. This has enabled the utilization of glucose metabolism for targeting the TME with the help of metabolic programmer nanosensors [35]. Additionally, lipid is also found as an important component in cancer progression, and involvement of lipid in cell-to-cell interaction in TME has also been demonstrated. However, lipid-based targeting of nanotherapeutics is not fully developed and considered as a future of targeted nanomedicine in the treatment of cancer.

The high nutritional requirements give rise to several redox conditions. Therefore, cancer cells are under high oxidative stress due to excessive production of hydroxyl radicals ($OH^\bullet$), superoxide anion radical ($O_2^\bullet$), and hydrogen peroxide (H_2O_2). These reactive oxygen species (ROS) produced from various metabolic pathways occur in peroxisomes, mitochondria, and endoplasmic reticulum of the cells. To counteract the enhanced oxidative stress, cancer cells overexpress the antioxidant system, like glutathione (GSH), glutathione peroxidase, and superoxide dismutase (SOD). As a result, the intratumoral glutathione level in tumor cytoplasm rises to $2–10\times^{-3}$ M, which is 100–1,000 times higher concentrations than the blood and extracellular fluid. Overall, the oxidation/reduction potential of TME remains relatively high, and several nanotherapies can harness on this dysregulated microenvironment to develop diagnostics and therapeutics.

Additionally, the tumor cells undergo excessive proliferation, due to which they consume high amount of oxygen and nutrients, leading to a hypoxic condition. Although dense neovasculature construction is present, the supply of oxygen and nutrient remains insufficient, in addition to the leaky characteristics of the neovasculate systems. Hypoxic areas of tumor are very less prone to chemotherapeutic drugs due to limited drug delivery by circulation. Therefore, an abundant oxygen supply to tumor site enhances the efficacy of chemotherapeutic drugs. Thus, efforts have been made to promote the hypoxic-responsive nanomaterials which follow the oxygenation strategy. Matrix metalloproteinase (MMP) enzymes are proteolytic enzymes governing the tumor cells' behavior, like proliferation, invasion, metastasis, and apoptosis. Thus, overexpression of MMP within TME serves as a specific biomarker for designing enzyme-responsive imaging nanoprobes. Similarly, caspase is a protease enzyme which regulates cell death and thus serves as an important biomarker to follow the apoptosis process. Synthesis of caspase-responsive nanoprobes to monitor the apoptosis in TME to evaluate the therapeutic efficacy of anticancer drugs has been reported.

From the discussion, it is evident that "intelligent/smart materials" or "stimuli-responsive materials" can be prepared, that undergoes essential changes/transformations (physical, chemical, or biological) with minor environmental fluctuations for better diagnostic and therapeutic effects. The response might be reversible or irreversible, depending on the nanomaterial's ability to regain the initial state [36]. Such materials are influenced by (1) internal stimulus (any biological component functions as a stimulation to which the material immediately responds, such as temperature, pH, redox potential, glucose/antibody concentrations, or lysosomal/other enzymes) and (2) external stimulus (magnetic field, electric field, ultrasound, or light needed to activate the responsiveness of materials).

8.4 Carbon Nanotubes for Tumor Microenvironment Targeting

A number of researches have clearly revealed the critical role of TME in tumorigenesis. TME is composed of a complicated system involving various cell types, including endothelial cells, pericytes, immune cells, CSCs, cancer-associated fibroblasts (CAFs), and the dense extracellular matrix (ECM). TME-constituting cells have a dynamic interplay with the cancer cells, serving as the soil for tumor initiation, development, invasion, migration, and therapy response. Therefore, TME exhibits great research and clinical importance in cancer therapy. Recent decades have witnessed the huge progress of employment of nanotechnology in cancer therapy. Except for the tumor cells, nano-based DDSs can be designed as demand to accurately target TME elements and remodel the TME for tumor regression increases [37]. Owing to their unique properties, multifunctional CNT-based nano-DDSs have shown outstanding ability in targeting the components of TME [38]. Thus, this section highlights the recent applications of CNTs in TME-based cancer therapy—various strategies, including

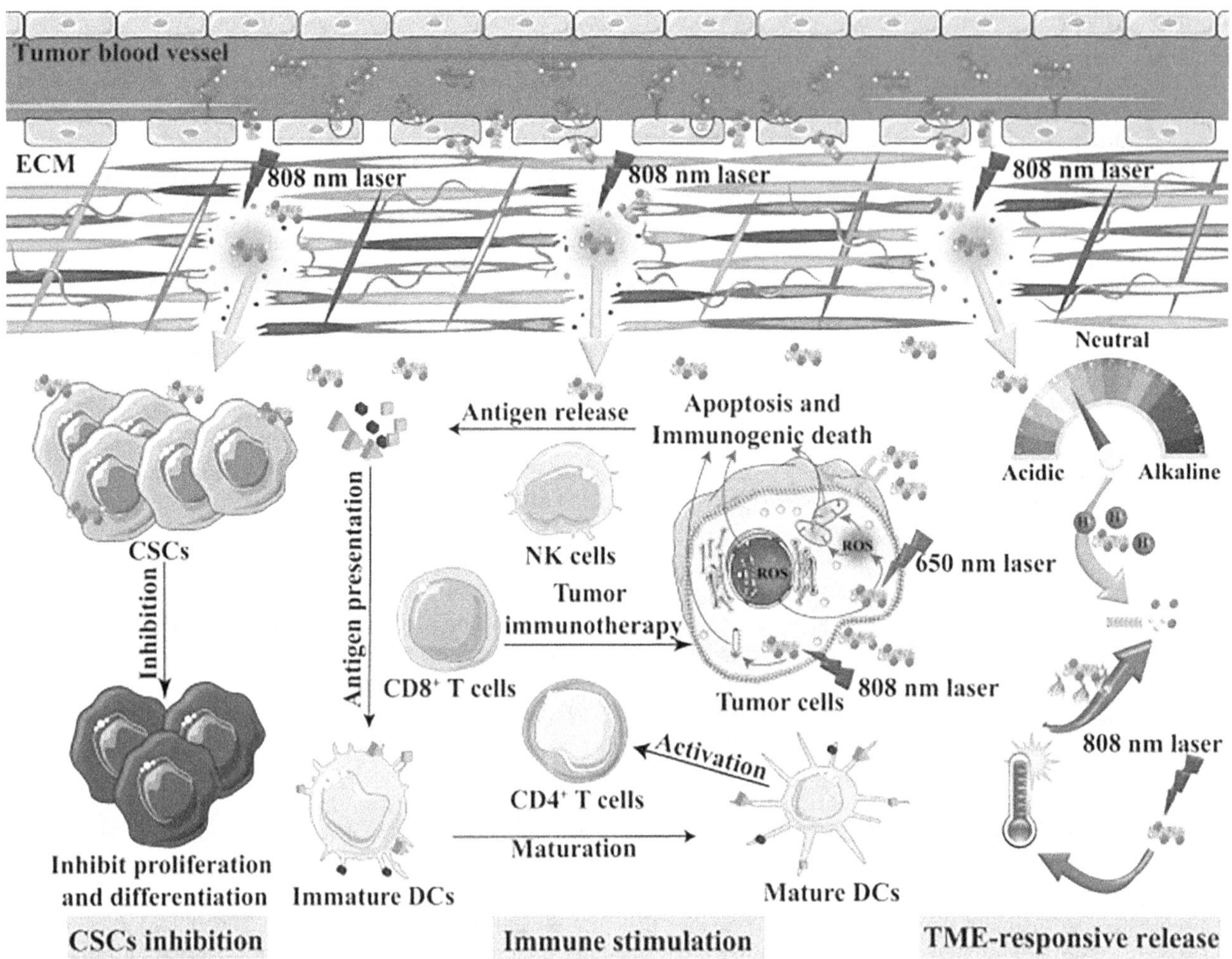

FIGURE 8.3 Schematic graph of CNT-based DDS in TME targeting.

ECM remodeling, tumor vasculature targeting, immune stimulation, CSCs inhibitory, and TME-responsive drug release, will be outlined (Figure 8.3).

8.4.1 Extracellular Matrix Remodeling

ECM is commonly defined as the non-cellular constituents of three-dimensional macromolecular scaffold that supplies biochemical and structural support for its cellular constituents. Fundamentally, ECM is a dense environment mainly composed of collagen, proteoglycans, laminin, and fibronectin. This diverse composition of ECM endows it with distinct biophysicochemical properties to regulate various cellular processes within the TME [39]. Besides, several studies have demonstrated that ECM is the first barrier before tumor migration, metastasis, and proliferation, and its dysregulation can accelerate tumor progression. Thus, understanding the interplay between tumor cells and ECM, as well as investigating potential therapeutic strategies through targeting ECM components, will open a new era for anticancer therapy.

Collagen is considered as the basis of ECM structure and is the most abundant protein discovered in human tissue. As tumor cells are usually embedded in a dense ECM comprising cross-linked collagen, hyaluronic acid, and different proteins, the rich matrix composition of these substances impedes the deep penetration of therapeutic agents to tumor cells, thus greatly limiting their therapeutic efficacy. Therefore, reduction of collagen density and tumor stiffening resulting from the abnormal organization of ECM are possible approaches to enhance the penetration and accumulation of drug at tumor sites. Marangon et al. studied the effects of local hyperthermia produced by MWNTs on epidermoid carcinoma microenvironment to explore the relationship between tumor stiffness evolution and tumor progression. Physical strategies using hyperthermia or photothermia represent as an alternative strategy to ablate the components of ECM. In their study, two conditions of heating, including mild hyperthermia (43°C for 15 min) and thermal ablation (52°C for 3 min), were generated by light-exposed MWNTs through tuning NIR irradiation power to explore the effects of nanomaterial-mediated heating on ECM remodeling. According to their observation, the irradiated tumors showed an obvious softening, accompanied with volume decrease over the days after PTT, compared to the non-irradiated group. In addition, with the imaging of second-harmonic generation (SHG) microscopy and two-photon excitation fluorescence (TPEF) microscopy, MWNTs-mediated

PTT was shown to induce the destruction of collagen and cell damage, indicating that nanohyperthermia was an alternative approach to decrease tumor stiffening and remodel the dense ECM for better drug penetration.

8.4.2 Cancer Stem Cell Inhibition

CSCs are a subpopulation of cancer cells which are characterized by highly tumorigenic and are intrinsically drug-resistant. They are able to self-renew and differentiate into diverse tumor cell types. Accumulating researches have evidenced the key role of CSCs in modulating TME, which involves different stages of tumorigenesis, including tumor growth, metastasis, and recurrence. In addition, a growing evidence demonstrated that CSCs are capable of withstanding classical therapeutic modalities, like chemotherapy and radiotherapy, through various mechanisms, such as elevated expression of drug transporters, enhanced DNA repair ability, and maintenance of a slow dividing state, which result in the development of drug resistance [40]. Besides, owing to their good tumorigenic and survival abilities, a group of CSCs can probably survive under conventional cancer treatment strategies and are able to seed new tumors in the second generation, leading to the quick relapse of cancer. Therefore, CSCs are regarded as potential target spots within the TME for cancer therapy. As CNTs are able to integrate molecular targeting and PTT in one platform, CNTs-based therapeutic strategies are thus promising methods to destroy CSCs as well as induce their apoptosis through hyperthermia.

Osteosarcoma stem cells (OSCs) are a kind of CSCs that are very closely related to the metastasis and recurrence of osteosarcoma. Transforming growth factor β type I (TGFβ1) is an important cytokine that contributes to the progression and carcinogenesis of osteosarcoma. Zhang et al. revealed that TGFβ1 signaling acted in a pivotal role in maintaining the OSCs population, and the high level of TGFβ1 in the osteosarcoma microenvironment induced the differentiation of osteosarcoma cells into OSCs. Therefore, inhibition of TGFβ1 signaling was a possible solution to alter OSCs state and reduce their population. Interestingly, an investigation by Miao et al. found that both raw SWNTs and carboxyl-modified SWNTs could specifically inhibit TGFβ1-induced differentiation of osteosarcoma cells, prevent the alteration of OSC phenotypes, and attenuate the viability of OSCs under osteosarcoma microenvironment-mimetic conditions. In addition, carboxyl-SWNTs were found to specifically bind to TGFβ1-induced activation of TGFβ type I receptor (TGFβR1) and suppress its downstream signaling, which drove OSCs formation and maintenance. All these observations indicated the unexpected biological effect of CNTs themselves to modulate OSCs, offering rational references for the CSCs-targeted therapy through the further application of CNTs-mediated treatment (Figure 8.4).

8.4.3 Tumor Vasculature Targeting

Tumor vasculature targeting is an important therapeutic strategy for cancer treatment because tumor blood vessels can secrete a high level of pro-angiogenic factors that cause the formation of abnormal vascular networks to give rise to poorly perfused tumors. Besides, tumor cells are able to produce a large number of hydrogen ions, lactate, and pyruvate through anaerobic glycolysis, thus creating an acidic microenvironment. These abnormalities of tumor vasculature build an intricate TME featured by hypoxia, acidity, and high IFP, which facilitate tumor progression, immunosuppression, and drug resistance. Therefore, anti-angiogenesis or tumor vasculature normalization is a potential approach to prevent their growth and metastasis, exhibiting great research and clinical prospects in cancer treatment.

Compared to other carbon nanomaterials, CNTs, especially MWNTs, possess a better anti-angiogenic properties and can be applied as excellent inhibitors of blood vessel growth for tumor angiogenesis targeting. Recent studies have also reported many cases on the application of CNT-based drug carriers against angiogenesis. For instance, Das et al. designed an injectable nanocarrier that combined f-CNTs with pH- and thermo-responsive polymer after rational modification [41]. Then, curcumin and DOX were loaded in this nanocarrier to obtain a synergistic antitumor effect. This nanocarrier achieved multidrug delivery with more than 90% drug encapsulation efficiency and a sustained drug release over 30 h under the stimulation of TME. Owing to the optical property of CNTs, a mild PTT effect could be simultaneously realized. Moreover, an outstanding antiangiogenic potential of this drug-loaded nanocarrier was firstly demonstrated *ex-ovo* by chorioallantoic membrane assay. *In vivo* results obtained from hepatocellular carcinoma (HCC)–bearing mice evidenced that these CNTs-involved carriers displayed an obvious effect on the reduction of MMP-9, which is closely related to cancer progression, implicating the potential of this nanocarrier in combinational cancer treatment for anti-angiogenesis. Cheng et al. conjugated SWNTs with three different agents, including the anti-angiogenesis drug thalidomide, cRGD peptide, and a fluorescent marker rhodamine. They proved that f-SWNTs could target angiogenic sites and effectively inhibit angiogenesis in transparent zebrafish embryos and mammalian cells. In addition to chemical drugs, radiotherapy substances can also be attached to SWNTs and produce anti-angiogenesis effects. Ruggiero et al. modified SWNTs with radiometal-ion chelates and the tumor neovascular-targeting antibody E4G10. Through the guide of E4G10 antibody toward tumor angiogenic vessels, radionuclide cargoes were specifically delivered to the tumor vasculature, after which the vessel image of the colon adenocarcinoma tumor model was acquired by performing PET radioimmunoimaging. Their study provided an alternative approach for tumor vessel targeting by combining SWNTs-based platform with radiotherapy and imaging.

Similar to SWNTs, MWNTs can also be functionalized to load different therapeutic agents to realize multiple effects for tumor vasculature targeting. αvβ3 is integrin that regulates cell attachment, spreading, and migration against cancer cell proliferation and metastasis. Targeting of αvβ3 integrins expressed on tumor tissue and neovasculature using fluorescent small molecules and nanoparticles has been studied. The nanoparticles remained within the vasculature for prolonged period, which allows thorough interrogation of αvβ3 integrin receptor expression within the blood vessels. Integrin αvβ3 has been extensively investigated as a potential target for cancer

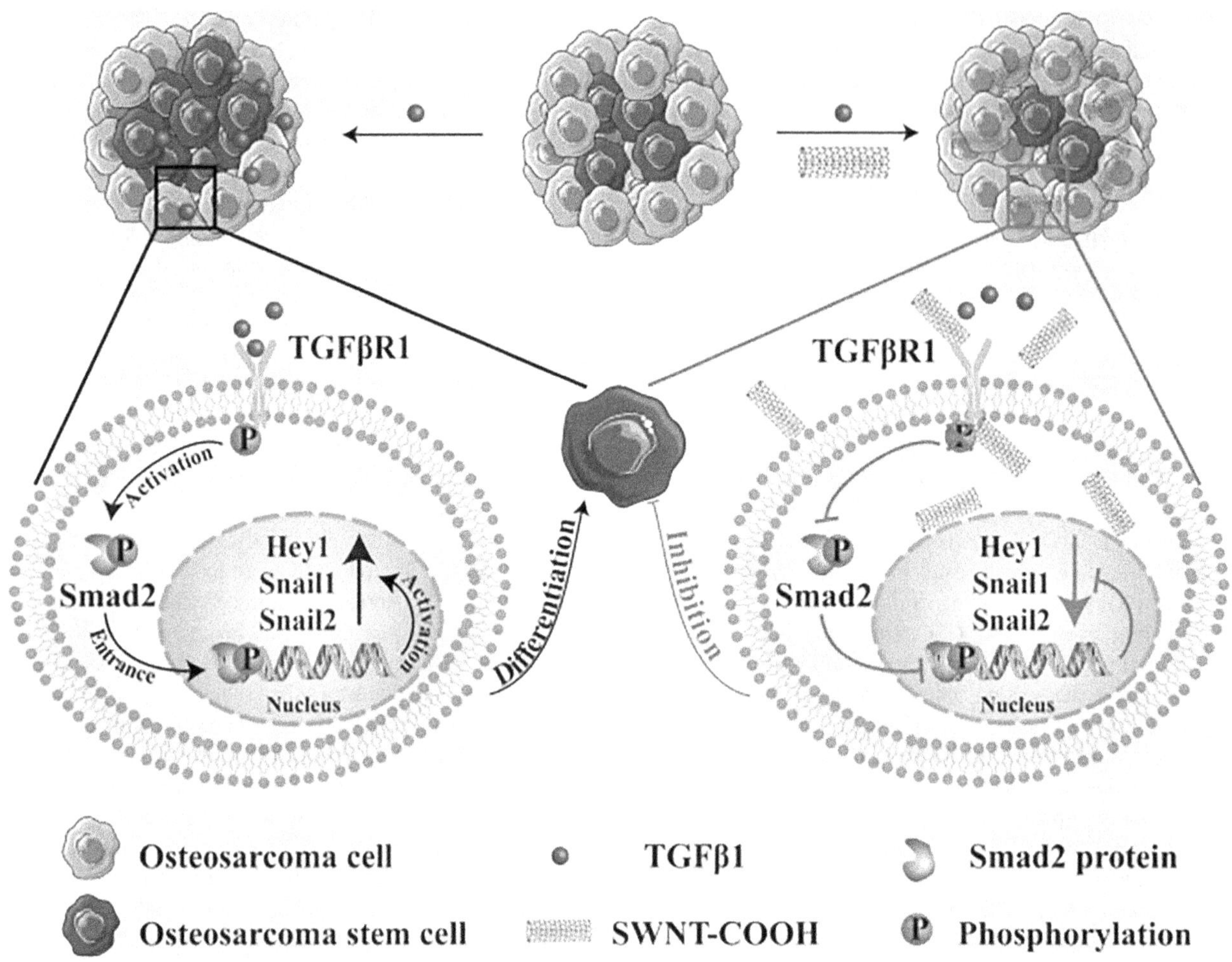

FIGURE 8.4 Schematic illustration of the working mechanism and therapeutic effects of SWNT-COOH on OSCs targeting.

treatment due to its close relationship with angiogenesis. RGD peptides were reported to specifically bind with integrin $\alpha v\beta 3$ and thereby could be employed as targeting ligand for $\alpha v\beta 3$-anchored delivery. $\alpha v\beta 3$ and $\alpha v\beta 5$ are coordinated cell adhesion and movement of diverse cell types. In the previous work, a co-delivery system based on MWNTs with dual-targeting ability was designed to aim at angiogenesis for lung cancer treatment. iRGD peptide and candesartan were linked to PEI-modified MWNTs, which was then assembled with plasmid angiotensin II type 2 receptor (pAT2) through electrostatic interaction to form the final nanocomposites. Owing to the intracellular penetration ability of MWNTs, candesartan and pAT2 were successfully delivered into cytoplasm to achieve synergistic anti-angiogenic effects in A549 lung cancer cell. A549 cells are lung carcinoma epithelial cells that constitute a cell line. A549 is one of the commonly used cell lines for a wide range of research applications, which also exhibited a significant suppression of tumor growth in A549 xenograft nude mice.

8.4.4 CNTs for Immunotherapy

As is described previously, TME is a very complicated environment composed of parenchymal cancerous cells and stromal non-cancerous components. Immune cells, the most abundant cell types in TME, act a significant part in TME-based targeted therapy. These immune cells dynamically interact with other components in TME and endow TME with immunosuppressive properties. Thus, targeting specific immune cells or modulating the immunosuppressive environment of TME present great significance in cancer immunotherapy. Owing to the feasible modification possibility of CNTs, a number of immunomodulators can be either directly connected on the surface of CNTs through functionalization or encapsulated into their inner structure for efficient delivery. In addition, it was reported that the systematic immune activity could be elevated by s.c. injection of water-soluble MWNTs in HCC tumor-bearing mice, which subsequently activated the complement system, activated the phagocytosis of macrophages, and facilitated the production of inflammatory cytokines, indicating the promising application prospect of CNTs in cancer immunotherapy. By using a combination of light energy, CNTs can also be applied as useful tools in phototherapy to effectively kill cancer cells; the released tumor-associated antigens (TAAs) and damaged-associated molecular patterns (DAMPs), through the induced immunogenic cell death (ICD) in target tumors, can stimulate systemic immune response for enhanced immunotherapy effect. Therefore, CNT-mediated DDS displays a great research potential for precise immunotherapy.

Carbon nanotubes (CNTs), as advanced nanotechnology with specific properties and structures, have presented practical drug delivery properties. Ginsenoside Rg3 is a component of puffed ginseng and demonstrates anticancer activities. To explore the effect of CNT-loaded Rg3 (Rg3-CNT) on the PD-1/PD-L1 signaling and the development of triple-negative breast cancer (TNBC), ginsenoside Rg3 enhances the anticancer effect of 5-FU in colon cancer cells via the PI3K/AKT pathway. Recently, Luo et al. designed a nanosystem composed of MWNTs-loaded ginsenoside Rg3 (Rg3-CNT) for triple-negative breast cancer (TNBC) treatment, which firstly demonstrated the new function of Rg3-CNT in elevating the therapeutic efficacy of Rg3 against TNBC through the inhibition of PD-1/PD-L1 axis, providing a potential strategy for TNBC treatment through immunotherapy. Programmed cell death protein 1 (PD-1) plays a vital role in inhibiting immune responses and promoting self-tolerance through modulating the activity of T cells, activating apoptosis of antigen-specific T cells, and inhibiting apoptosis of regulatory T cells. Programmed cell death ligand 1 (PD-L1) is a transmembrane protein that is considered to be a co-inhibitory factor of the immune response; it can combine with PD-1 to reduce the proliferation of PD-1 positive cells, inhibit their cytokine secretion, and induce apoptosis. PD-L1 also plays an important role in various malignancies, where it can attenuate the host immune response to tumor cells. Based on these perspectives, PD-1/PD-L1 axis is responsible for cancer immune escape and makes a huge effect on cancer therapy. In their study, Rg3-CNT was found to reduce PD-L1 expression and PD-L1 upregulation induced by IFN-γ in TNBC cells; meanwhile, PD-1 expression and PD-1/PD-L1 signaling were also suppressed, which remarkably inhibited the TNBC cell growth *in vivo*. Luo's investigation offered new insights in revealing the correlation between Rg3-CNT and PD-1/PD-L1 signaling, indicating that the application of Rg3-CNT might be an alternative approach for TNBC immunotherapy. Another update study by Jin et al. showed that intratumoral delivery of immunoadjuvant CpG through CNTs could enhance the uptake of CpG in colon cancer cells, which remarkably inhibited primary tumor growth and liver metastasis [42]. Cytosine-phosphorothioate-guanine oligodeoxynucleotides (CpG ODN) have shown significant potential for treatment of a wide variety of diseases, including cancer. CpG ODN can be used either as a standalone molecule or as an adjuvant to alternative therapies. Stimulation of toll-like receptor-9 (TLR9) by CpG oligodeoxynucleotides (CpG) has been shown to counteract the immunosuppressive microenvironment and to inhibit tumor growth in glioma models. Since TLR9 is located intracellularly, it has been hypothesized that methods that enhance its internalization may also potentiate its immunostimulatory response. *In vitro* results obtained from HCT116 human colon cancer cells demonstrated that CNTs-CpG complex could result in significant inhibitory effects on cancer cell growth, invasion, and migration, implying the promising application potential of this nanocomplex for colon cancer immunotherapy. Besides, various f-CNTs were reported to deliver vaccines like ovalbumin (OVA) or siRNA to protect them from degradation for enhanced immunotherapy effects, which shows great research interest and clinical value to treat many cancers [43].

8.4.5 Tumor Microenvironment-Responsive Drug Release

The conventional DDS based on EPR effect and receptor-mediated endocytosis often faces many limitations due to the biological complexity of TME where tumor cells live. However, the hypoxic and acid features of TME with high levels of GSH and H_2O_2 enable the development of multistage TME-responsive drug release strategy. Triggered by various stimuli factors within TME, the carried drugs can be sequentially released in a controlled or sustained profile to realize multiple therapeutic effects and deep tumor penetration. In addition, the reaction with these sensitive factors can alleviate tumor hypoxia and acidity, which creates a suitable environment for better therapeutic outcome. Therefore, the ongoing section highlights the recent examples about smart drug delivery systems based on CNTs for TME-responsive drug release.

Yang et al. designed a kind of oxidized MWNTs with a large inner diameter to encapsulate anticancer drug cisplatin in their inner structure and to load DOX on the external surface. PEG and folic acid were also employed to block the release of cisplatin from the inner MWNTs. Consequently, the carried cargos showed a pH-sensitive release profile under pH 6.5, which mimicked the weak acidic TME, indicating the TME-responsive potential of this MWNTs-based nanosystem. Moreover, the antitumor efficacy tested on MCF-7 breast cancer cells showed that a more pronounced cytotoxicity was observed in the pH 6.5 conditions than that in pH 7.4, confirming the best tumor-killing effect of this nanosystem in acidic TME. Wang et al. constructed MWNTs-based nanosystem for MRI-guided and TME-responsive phototherapy. A uniform MnO_2 layer and photosensitizer Ce6 were modified on MWNTs for enhanced phototherapy. MnO_2 could decompose H_2O_2 in the TME to produce $^1O_2$ for promoting the photothermal effect generated by MWNTs, relieving tumor hypoxia, and facilitating Ce6-mediated PDT. In addition, MnO_2 was able to rapidly deplete GSH in the acidic TME through redox reaction to reduce Mn^{4+} into Mn^{2+} ions, which augmented ROS-mediated cell death via chemodynamic therapy and accelerated Ce6 release, meanwhile acting as a contrast agent for T1-MRI. Altogether, this multifunctional MWNTs-based platform offered a promising strategy to achieve synergistic cancer theranostics due to its TME-sensitive properties. Another case by Qin et al. showed that CNTs-based nanoplatforms could also be encapsulated into a type of thermo-/pH sensitive nanogel to achieve NIR-triggered, TME-responsive drug release. The loaded DOX in this nanosystem showed a faster release rate at a higher temperature of 40°C than 25°C; meanwhile, more DOX was released from this nanosystem at pH 5.0 than pH 7.4, which indicated that the combinational effects of photothermal effect mediated by CNTs upon NIR irradiation and acidic environment of TME were able to facilitate the release of DOX under dual stimuli.

8.5 Stimuli-Responsive Intelligent Nanomaterial in Cancer Theranostics

Intelligent or smart nanomaterials can be classified into various categories, depending on the response to specific stimulus or a group of stimuli, and their properties can be governed in a controlled manner by external or internal factors, like temperature, pH, electric or magnetic fields, biomolecules, and stress. Figure 8.5 [44] exemplifies classification of smart nanomaterials depending on their specific responses, with suitable examples.

8.5.1 Bio-Responsive Intelligent Nanomaterials

Bio-responsive nanomaterials are designed especially for biomedical applications in response to specific stimuli, like biological signal and pathological abnormalities. Thus, in recent years, it has shown great achievement in the development of novel precise medicines for various diseases. Generally, these

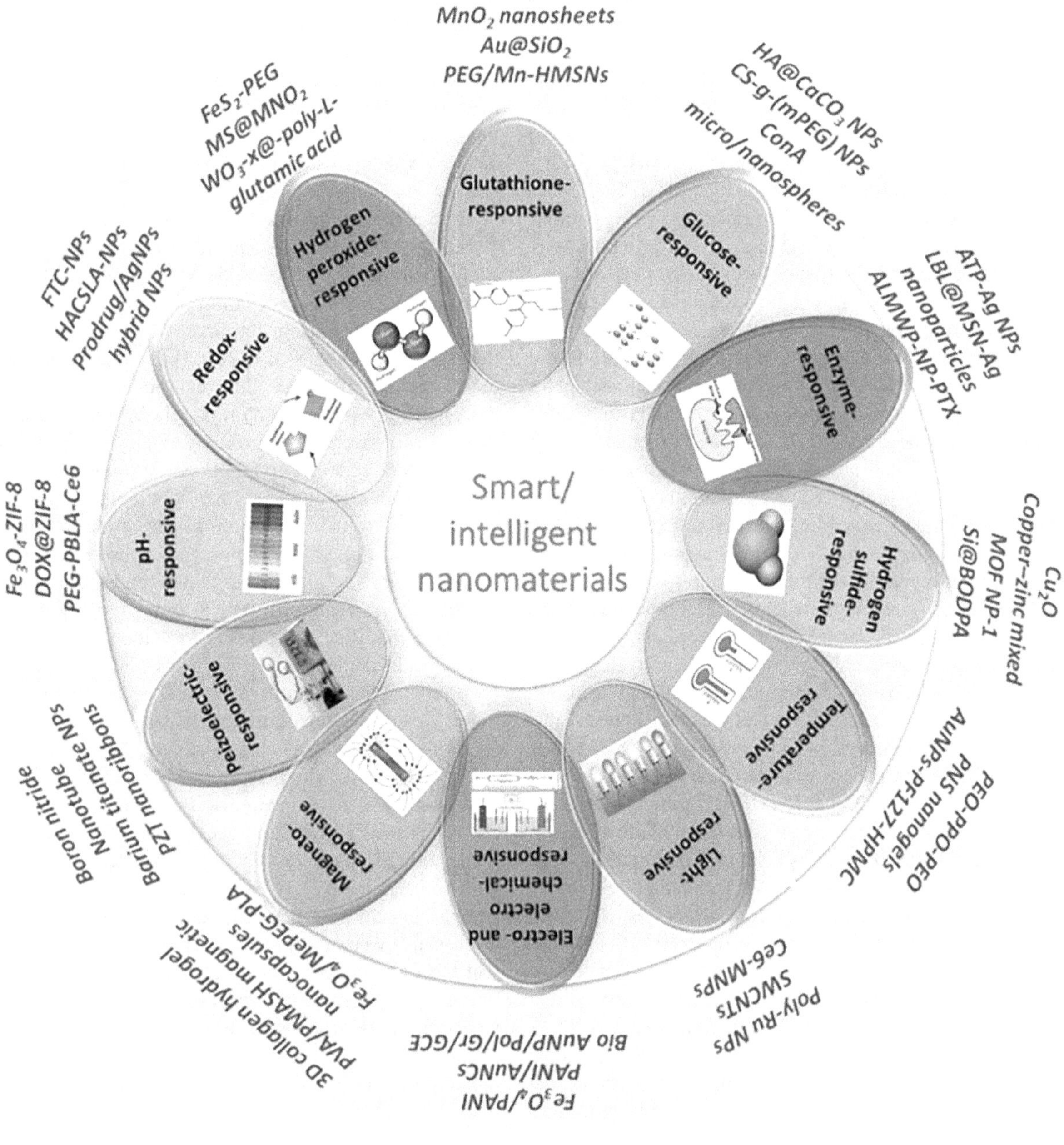

FIGURE 8.5 Schematic representation of intelligent nanomaterials classification based on the specific stimulus and relevant examples.

Source: [44].

theranostic smart nanomaterials are in an "OFF" state in normal condition, whereas in disease condition, it switches "ON" under specific stimuli, like enzymes, glucose, H_2O_2, H_2S, or glutathione. Thus, intelligent nanomaterials provide high sensitivity and selectivity with low side effects. The roles of different bio-responsive nanomaterials in cancer theranostics are discussed in the following and summarized in [44].

8.6 Progress of Smart Nanoparticles-Based Theranostics

Theranostics is a unique concept that integrates therapy and diagnosis in a single system to achieve an accurate cancer diagnosis. It has been recognized as a potential breakthrough in resolving the problems with conventional oncotherapy.

Nanoparticles are ideal candidates as carriers for theranostic agents due to their exceptional physicochemical characteristics, such as nanoscale sizes, functional properties, active or passive tumor targeting, specific cellular uptake, and excellent optical properties, that perfectly meet the needs of phototherapy and imaging at the same time. Metals and biological materials have significantly advanced cancer therapy and personalized medicine with the advancement of nanotechnology and medical technology. Theranostics has advanced significantly with the advancement of nanotechnology and is currently in the "bench-to-bedside" transition phase. In this review, we summarize recent progress on nanotechnology-based theranostics, that is, nanotheranostics, that has significantly surpassed conventional therapies and has provided new therapeutic strategies, as well as "cocktail" theranostics (mixing various treatment modalities), as shown in Figure 8.6.

8.6.1 Applications of Targeted Nanotheranostics in Cancer Therapy

Chemotherapeutic medications suffer from several problems, including significant side effects and poor therapeutic efficacy. Nanomedicines help improve the biodistribution and target accumulation of chemotherapy drugs, which allows them to better balance the effectiveness and toxicity of the treatment. Many nanomedicines have been investigated throughout the years, including liposomes, polymer–drug conjugates, and polymeric assemblies, to enhance tumor-targeted drug delivery. These nanomedicines use passive targeting, active targeting, and triggered release techniques. Recently, nanoscale biomaterial-based technologies have resolved several complicated and challenging issues in science and technology.

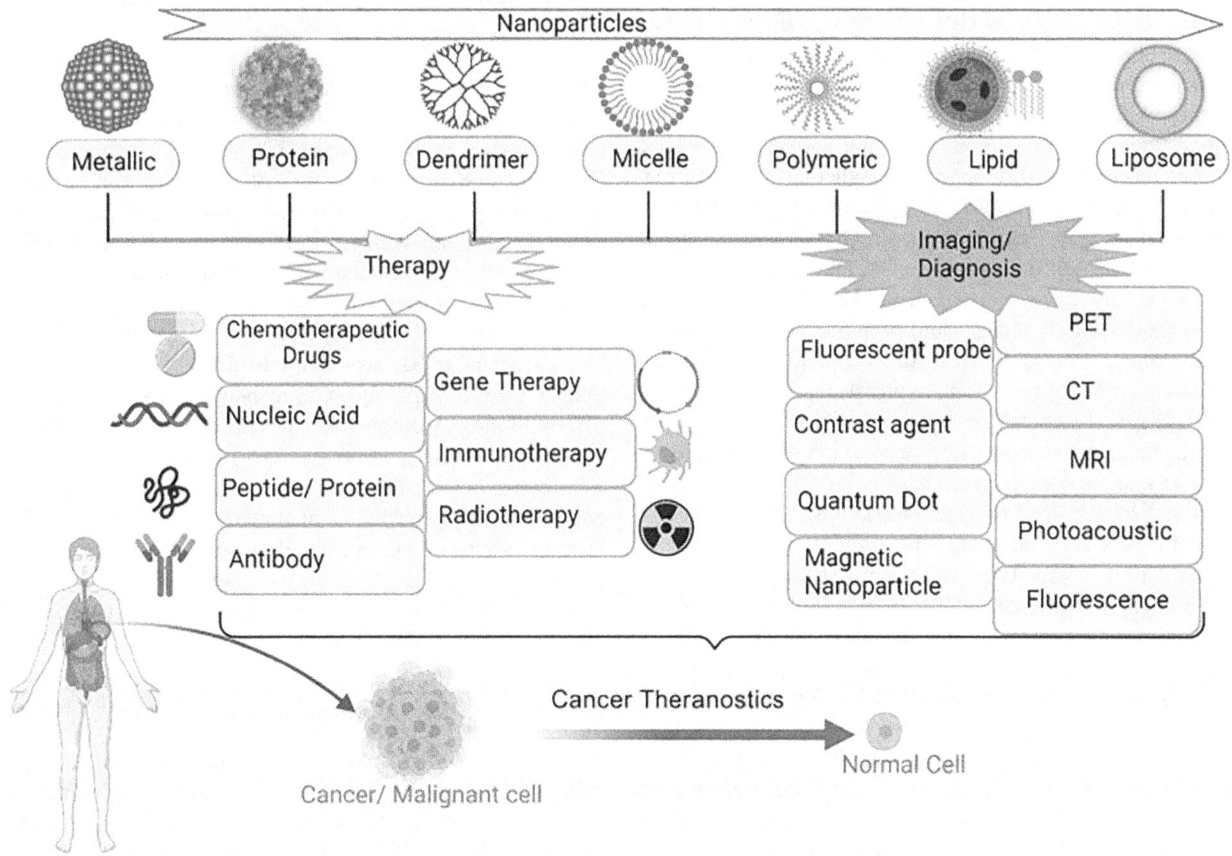

FIGURE 8.6 Nanotheranostic platform for simultaneous therapy and diagnosis. Comprehensive smart nanoplatforms from organic, inorganic, and carbon-based nanoparticles for cancer theranostics. *PET*, positron emission tomography; *CT*, computer tomography; *MRI*, magnetic resonance imaging.

Source: [17].

Nevertheless, they also opened a new window in biomedical research focusing on personalized medicine. Nanoparticles are one of the greatest scientific breakthroughs because they have unique properties, including a high specific surface area and physicochemical features, like optical, magnetic, electronic, catalytic, and antibacterial qualities. To combat the negative effects of cancer treatment, it is crucial to transport therapeutic medication molecules to the targeted tumor site. To enable site-specific cancer therapy, numerous efforts have been made over the past 20 years to develop drug delivery systems based on nanomaterials. Theranostics integrates therapy and diagnostics in one system, which helps in developing an improved understanding of the treatment for its side effects and benefits and captures an image while dispensing therapeutic medications at a precise dosage.

An overview of recent advancements in targeted nano-based cancer treatments is provided in this review chapter, along with a variety of diagnostic probes and therapeutic medications. Moreover, syntheses and applications of inorganic nanoparticles, carbon nanoparticles, micelles, protein conjugates, linear and branching polymers, and dendrimers in theranostics are also covered. The use of theranostics in imaging methods like computed tomography, magnetic resonance imaging, single-photon emission computed tomography, and fluorescence/optical imaging for *in vivo* imaging was also highlighted. About a dozen nanomedicines based on polymeric micelles are currently undergoing clinical trials for various cancers. The latter is desirable for delivering chemotherapeutic drugs with low water solubility. Integrating therapy with non-invasive imaging is extremely valuable for understanding the *in vivo* fate, pharmacokinetics, target site accumulation, and therapeutic efficacy of nanomedicines. By selecting patients in advance who are most likely to respond to nanotherapy, this information can be utilized to evaluate the suitability of nanotherapeutic treatments based on nanomedicine. The fundamental ideas of nanoparticle-based tumor targeting and clinical and preclinical cancer treatments from chemotherapy to radiotherapy and to photodynamic therapy, and from photothermal therapy to gene therapy, are outlined in this chapter, along with the advantages of utilizing imaging to preselect patients and tailor nanomedicine therapies.

Being heterogeneous by nature, cancer is a complicated disease. Despite notable advancements in the development of new drugs and conventional treatment modalities, still the success rates of cancer survival remain undermined. Drug resistance and cancer heterogeneity are the main obstacles that reduce a drug's efficacy. A patient-centric or individualized approach is required for a poor medication response for a better therapeutic result. Nanotheranostics has become a promising way to handle such complex problems which amalgamates therapy and diagnosis.

These advanced nanocarriers are capable of drug targeting while enabling diagnostic attributes like imaging. Recent studies indicate that a cancer nanotheranostics platform provides improved pharmacology of the drugs, leading to low toxicity compared to conventional approaches. Passive or active, the targeting of drugs by nanoparticle-based drug delivery systems (NDDSs) achieves a better distribution of the drug to the tumor sites, which shows a great advantage in cancer therapy. A nanoparticle-based theranostic agent is rendered more attractive for personalized therapy because it integrates the three perspectives—diagnosis, drug delivery, and treatment response monitoring—in a single platform. Nanotheranostics, in combination with the targeted drug, could provide great potential for an individualized therapeutic paradigm for cancer. In addition, NDDSs could also combine distinct therapeutic modalities into a single feasible platform to offer synergistic effects, and also to reverse the development of drug resistance. Lipid-based nanoparticles, polymers, dendrimer-based nanoparticles, metal nanoparticles (noble metals, such as gold and silver), semiconductor nanoparticles, carbon nanotubes, metal oxide nanoparticles, metal–organic frameworks (MOFs), and up-converting nanoparticles (UCNPs) are NDDSs which are available for cancer therapy. Cancer nanotheranostics aims to utilize nanotechnology to combine cancer therapy and imaging. Engineering nanomaterials can greatly enhance the effectiveness and specificity of therapy for cancers to interact with cancer cells at the molecular level [45]. The greatest therapeutic challenge for targeted therapy is posed by metastasis, drug-resistant cancers, and cancer stem cells. Nanoparticles, adult stem cells, or T cells in immunotherapy can appropriately be developed as drug delivery systems to achieve a targeted therapy.

8.7 Physical and Chemical Properties-Responsive Nanomaterials

The application of nanomaterials for the identification and treatment of cancer by harnessing the inherent properties of nanomaterials holds a promising milieu in nanomedicine. Cancer nano-diagnostics and nanotherapeutics can be implemented using various physical and chemical properties intrinsic/extrinsic to cancer microenvironment or the nanomaterials. The incorporation of nanomaterials may enhance the effectiveness of the chemotherapeutic, may delay the development of chemoresistance, and may be able to overcome the systemic and intracellular barriers through differential properties of temperature, electricity, photo-responsiveness, piezoelectric, pH, and redox. Moreover, the physicochemical properties of nanomaterials are fine-tunable toward various applications with enhanced efficiency [13,46]. In addition, the physical and chemical properties of nanomaterials can be controlled exogenously or endogenously. However, the physical- and/or chemical-responsive nanomaterials are popular due to their non-invasive nature, simplicity of operation, and good controllability to achieve high spatiotemporal resolution.

8.7.1 Thermo-Responsive Nanomaterials

Thermoregulation is a major homeostatic system in all organisms, and it may be used for therapeutic benefits. When the vertebrates are treated at temperatures above the physiological temperature (37°C), which is popularly termed as "hyperthermia," it is indicated that there will be an increase in the oxygenation states of the cancers. It is also indicated that hyperthermia stimulated the heat-inducing factor I (HIF-I) and its downstream molecules of vascular endothelial growth factor (VEGF) and pyruvate dehydrogenase kinase I (PDK I), leading to enhanced perfusion and oxygenation. Thereby, the combination of radiotherapy and the conventional treatment of cancer with heat treatment improved the efficiency of such treatments, especially in multicentric randomized trials for high-risk soft-tissue sarcomas.

Cancer ablation is mostly used as an adjunct treatment, with radiotherapy or chemotherapy displaying an impact on the tumor vascular perfusion, immune function and immunogenicity, cytokine activity, lymphocyte trafficking, metabolism, and gene expression. Traditionally, heat is applied locally, regionally, or systematically either through the local insertion of a needle or using external machines transmitting high energy waves. Nowadays, the magnetic nanoparticles consisting of iron nanoparticles are frequently used as thermal-responsive nanomaterials. The usage in the form of nanofluids with external application of the magnetic field is predicted to generate enough heat postulated to produce adequate sensitivity and specificity to achieve clinical diagnostics and treatments effectively. Moreover, the superparamagnetic nanoparticles (SPIONs) conjugated with radionuclides, such as ^{223}Ra (radium-223), Technetium-99 (^{99}Tc), yttrium-90 (^{90}Y), lutetium-177 (^{177}Lu), ^{111}In (índium-111), ^{59}Fe (iron-59), and 18F-2-fluoro-2-deoxyglucose (^{18}FDG), have substantially grown for biomedical applications. Apart from inorganic nanomaterials, polymers, self-assembly amphiphilic micelles, core–shell nanoparticles, and lipids are commonly used in the thermo-responsive treatment of cancers. Polymeric nanomaterials can be made highly thermo-responsive for local radiotherapy by varying the hydrophilic/hydrophobic moieties ratio, for example, poly(N-isopoprylacrylamide) (pNIPAAm) labeled with L-tyrosinamide or diethyltriaminepenta acetic acid, and the delivery of docetaxel loaded in biodegradable thermosensitive copolymer poly(N-isopropylacrylamide-co-acrylamide)-b-poly(DL-lactide) can be increased for the chemotherapeutic effects. Among various polymeric systems used, pNIPAAm, pluronics, and poly(hydroxypropyl methacrylamide-lactate) (p(HPMAm-Lacn)) are frequently used in clinical trials.

Moreover, externally applied sources, such as laser, can induce change in the temperature above lower critical solution temperature, which can change the phase of nanomaterial to release the contents. The release of the active drug is through the conversion of gel phase to crystalline liquid phase, modification of interaction between the hydrophobic and hydrophilic regions, and temperature-mediated chain modification. The nanomaterials may have high stability at physiological pH; however, they may quickly release the cargo locally in hyperthermia conditions. The nanomaterials provide better biodistribution profiles as they release drugs in high concentrations regionally and reduce systemic toxicity. Moreover, recent trends like the MRI-guided thermometry as shown in Figure 8.7a have added more value to the present thermo-responsive nanomaterials.

8.7.2 Photo-Responsive Nanomaterials

An external stimulus such as ultraviolet light or visible light can also provide precise spatiotemporal drug release at the site of interest. Some nanomaterials have inherent photo-based imaging capabilities, and others, such as polymeric nanomaterials, respond to differential photo-absorbing potentials as nanocarriers to the fluorescent dyes or photosensitizers. The photo-responsive materials respond to ultraviolet light, visible light, or near-infrared light. The near-infrared is perceived to produce minimal toxicity and enhance penetration. The resulting effect can be photothermal, photodynamic, or photoconversion mechanism, to give a phototoxic effect as a chemotherapeutic. Photothermal (nano)materials, such as near-infrared-absorbing dyes like Prussian blue, copper sulfite, bismuth sulfide, and AuNPs, can convert the incoming radiation to heat, which can be externally controlled to produce local effects. An agglomerate of cyclic arginine-glycine-aspartic acid conjugated 1,2-distearoyl-sn-glycero-3-phosphoethanolamine-N-[amino(poly(ethylene glycol))] (DSPE-PEG), 1,2-dipalmintoyl-sn-glycero-3-phosphatidylcholine (DPPC), cholesterol, photosensitizer, and polyamidoamine (PAMAM) dendrimers were grafted with cisplatin prodrug (CIS). The photosensitizer was present in the outermost layer of the dendrimer, which encapsulated a liposome containing the chemotherapeutic. Upon near-infrared irradiation at 808 nm, the photosensitizer elevated the temperature above physiological, releasing the Cis-liposome (~8.6 nm) to achieve deeper penetration, site targeting, and long circulation abilities. A similar strategy has been utilized to target mitochondria [47]. Interestingly, phase-changing materials such as 1-tetradecanol transition from solid to liquid to release the drug at the targeted site, most frequently introduced with photothermal nanomaterials such as Bi2S3 (Figure 8.7B) [48].

In contrast to PTT, PDT utilizes the hypoxia-cleavable moieties to convert light energy into ROS, and in some cases, this leads to increase in the hypoxia conditions of the cancers. Generically, a photosensitizer is encapsulated within the nanomaterials and linked to an active drug, which, upon exposure to optimum wavelength of light, induces the ROS moieties upgradation to cleave the linker, releasing the active drug.

On the other hand, some materials, such as 2-nitrobenzyl, coumarin, azobenzene, or 7-nitroindoli, have the ability for photolysis through photocleaving, photo-switchable, or photo-reductive properties [49]. When such up-conversion materials are included with the nanomaterials and the active drug, they can release the active material in a controllable fashion by converting light from longer wavelength to shorter wavelength (for example, near infrared to ultraviolet), sometimes targeted with suitable surface moieties. The frequently used up-conversion materials display excellent stability against photochemical degradation, which photoconverts by hydrophobic to hydrophilic conversions, by changing the effective surface charges, or by changing conformations. For example, MSNs were capped with azobenzene and DOX and surface-conjugated with the transactivator of transcription peptide (to enhance membrane permeability) and silanol group. Upon irradiation of laser at 990 nm, the azobenzene emitted ultraviolet and visible light to switch azo from trans to cis isomer, which leads to rotation-inversions movement and release of drug DOX. This photoconvertible nanosystem displayed ~80% drug release efficiency as compared to ~5% in the absence of photolysis. Working on a similar line, more recently, a small targeting molecule, CFMQ (near-infrared photodynamic therapy agent),

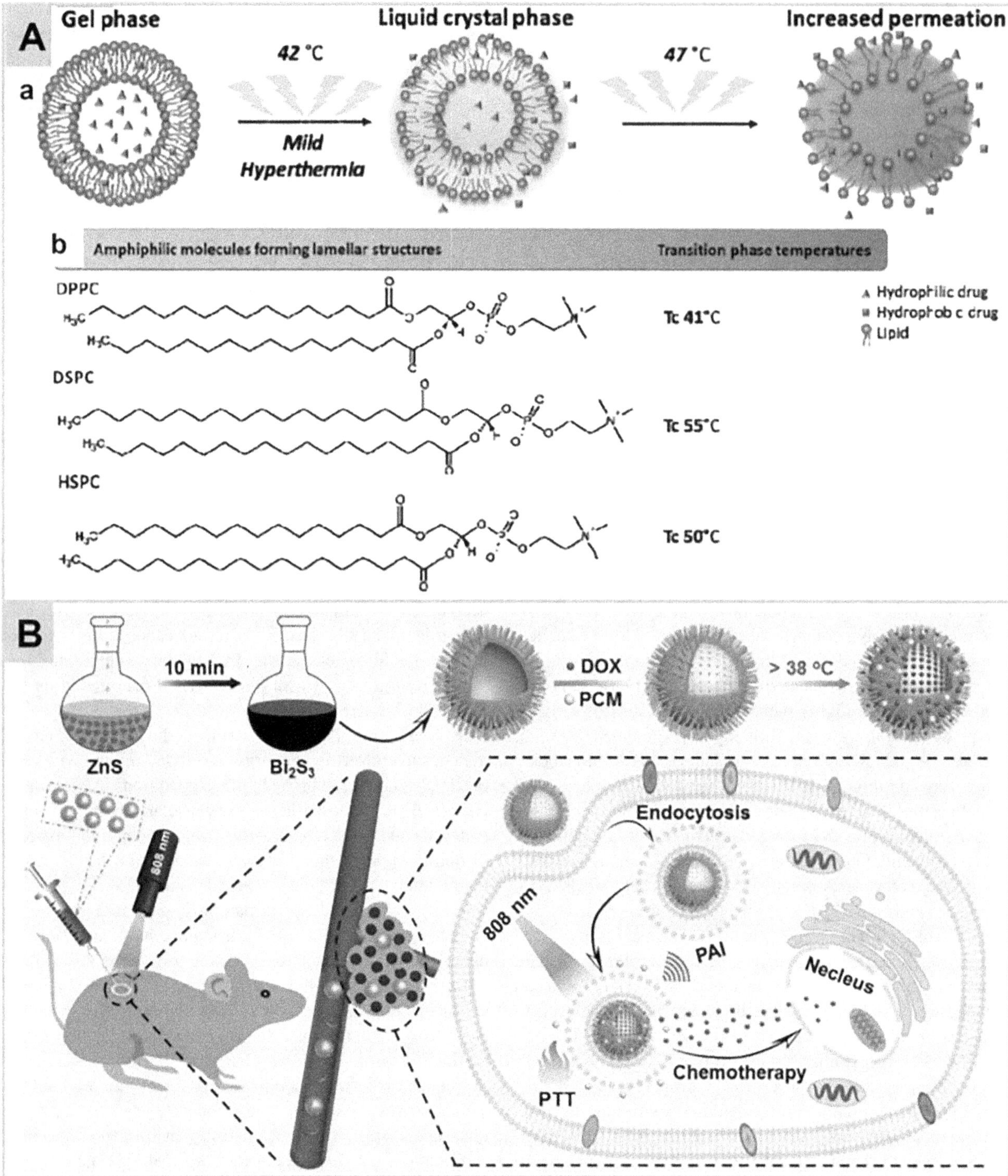

FIGURE 8.7 Mechanism of drug release from thermosensitive liposomes: (a) Schematic illustration of the mechanism of phase transition of the lipids that form the liposome bilayer. The increase of the temperature above the transition phase temperature (47°C) leads to higher bilayer permeability, and consequently, the drug release is favored. (b) Amphiphilic molecules forming lamellar structures and their transition phase temperatures. Tc: Phase transition temperature (panel A). A representation of the usage of hallow nanomaterials conjugated with phase-changing materials for photolytic release of doxorubicin. The photothermal agent (Bi_2S_3 nanomaterials) was synthesized using the polyol route, displaying a photoconversion efficiency of 26.8%. The photothermal agent was encapsulated with doxorubicin and coated with 1-tetradecanol acting as a gatekeeper until melting temperature of 38°C was attained for the photothermal-responsive drug release to be activated (panel B) [48].

was tagged with chitosan-coated poly(lactic-co-glycolic) acid nanoparticles encapsulating chemotherapeutic temozololomide to effectively treat glioblastoma multiforms [50].

8.7.3 Electro- and Electrochemical-Responsive Nanomaterials

The membrane potential (Vm) of cells is developed due to the electric selectivity of the transport ions and channels for the permeability of selected molecules. It modulates important biophysical properties of the cell, such as proliferation, migration, cytoskeleton reorganization, direction sensing, and differentiation. In the case of cancer cells, the membrane potential is dysregulated due to enhanced proliferation. In cancer, it is shown that membrane potential undergoes hyperpolarization before entering M phase, and the levels are highly correlated with the sarcoma cell cycle progressions acting as an effective bioelectric regulator. Moreover, the electric charges may act as a driving force for the cancerous cells to metastasize via Ca^{2+}. Preceding that, in vivo studies have demonstrated that membrane depolarization may lead to cancer transformation, manifested as increased proliferation, changes in morphology, and abnormal angiogenesis. More specifically, intracellular Na^+ levels are found to be high in cancers, whereas K^+ concentrations remain stable. Additionally, in order to maintain cancer stem cells (CSCs) to sustain the cancerous nature, hyperpolarization of the membrane potential is found essential. Therefore, the dysregulation of the electrochemical potential developed across the cancerous cells acts as an important indicator of cancer progression and an important biomarker. In this regard, there is a. general suggestion that ether-a-go-go ion channel may serve as a biomarker for cancer, which is cell-cycle dependent.

The conventional methods for measuring membrane depolarization include Western blotting, flow cytometry, and enzyme-linked immunosorbent assay for cancer diagnostics or therapeutics. However, the usage of smart nanomaterials for cancer diagnostic and therapeutics based on electro- or electrochemical properties is frequent in the field of diagnostics. Electrochemical nanobiosensors are applied for rapid cancer biomarkers, cancer screenings, and cancer management.

Basically, electrochemical nanomaterials consist of a biometric element (aptamers, lignins, or antibodies), an electrochemical sensor, a transducer, and a signal processor. The interaction between the biometric element and the cells is detected through sensors which are transformed into meaningful signals by the transducer. Different cancers possess different biomarkers, which are expressed in Table 16.2. In this direction, harnessing the ligand–receptor affinity, an aptamer, AS1411, to nucleolin has been developed. Targeted cancer therapy has become one of the most important medical methods because of the spreading and metastatic nature of cancer. Based on the introduction of AS1411 and its four-chain structure, research progress in cancer detection and drug delivery systems by modifying AS1411 aptamers based on graphene, mesoporous silica, silver, and gold has been reviewed. The application of AS1411 in cancer treatment and drug delivery and the use of AS1411 as a targeting agent for the detection of cancer markers, such as nucleoli, are summarized from three aspects of active targeting, passive targeting, and targeted nucleic acid aptamers. Although AS1411 has been withdrawn from clinical trials, research surrounding its structural optimization is still very popular. Further progress has been made in the modification of nanoparticles loaded with TCM extracts by AS1411. The progress in cancer drug delivery based on AS1411-oriented nanomaterials is shown in Scheme 8.3[51].

A platform consisting of ionic liquid–hydroxyapatite nanorod–gold nanoparticles nanocomposite was created and tagged with the aptamer. In the presence of MCF-7 cells, the aptamer was released and replaced to decrease the current in proportion to increasing concentration of the cancer cells, resulting in the detection range of $10^{-1} \times 10^6$ cells/mL, with detection limit of 8 ± 2 cells/mL. Additionally, an indium tin oxide electrode modified with iron phthalocyanine and Ag-$ZnIn_2S_4$ quantum dots was prepared to generate electric signals under the influence of near-infrared. The HA was tagged, which reacted with the A549 cells to reduce the electric signal, displaying a linear range of 2×10^2–4.5×10^6 cells/mL and a detection limit of 15 cells/mL. It was shown that conjugating aptamers on the nano-coated electrode provided good specificity and stability, which also help detect HeLa cells as low as 5 cells/mL (Figure 8.8A) [52]. An increasing concentration of HeLa cells reacts with aptamer and leads to decreased photocurrent (Figure 8.8B-a), and this decrease in photocurrent exhibited linear correlation with increased concentration of HeLa cells (Figure 8.8B-b). The aptamers are also tagged to the cells to improve detection. For example, the EpCAM aptamer modified with polyadenine at the 3'OH end was tagged to the cells. The modified aptamer was conjugated with the gold electrode to give a linear range of 10–10^3 cells/mL and detection limit as low as 3 cells/mL. Interestingly, an electronic transfer peptide YYYYC possessing excellent electroactivity and functionality of hydrate-mimicking peptides has also been designed. In studies, YYYYC was conjugated to myelopeptide-4, which is derived from bone marrow and fixed on electrode through collagen and measured through electrochemical impedance

TABLE 8.2

Different Types of Cancers and Their Respective Biomarkers Overexpressed on Their Surfaces During Metastatic Transformations

Cancer Type	Biomarkers	Refs
Breast cancer	Transmembrane glucoprotein mucin 1 (MUC1), nucleoli, epidermal growth factor receptor (EGFR), CD44	[54]
Lung cancer	Transferrin receptors, E-Cadherins, CD44, carcinoembryonic antigen, sialic acid, nucleoli	[55]
Cervical cancer	Nucleoli, CEM, PTK7, carcinoembryonic antigen	[56]
Liver cancer	Alpha-fetoprotein, MUC1, folic acid (FA) receptors, EpCAM, CD44, CD90, CD133/2, OV-6	[57]
Leukemia	ASCP receptors, p-glycoprotein, CD44, PTK-7	[58]
Gastric and colorectal cancer	M2-PK, ESM1, CTHRC1, and AZGP1, CA72-4, CA125, alpha-fetoprotein, sialic acid, mannosyl groups, folic acid receptors	[59]

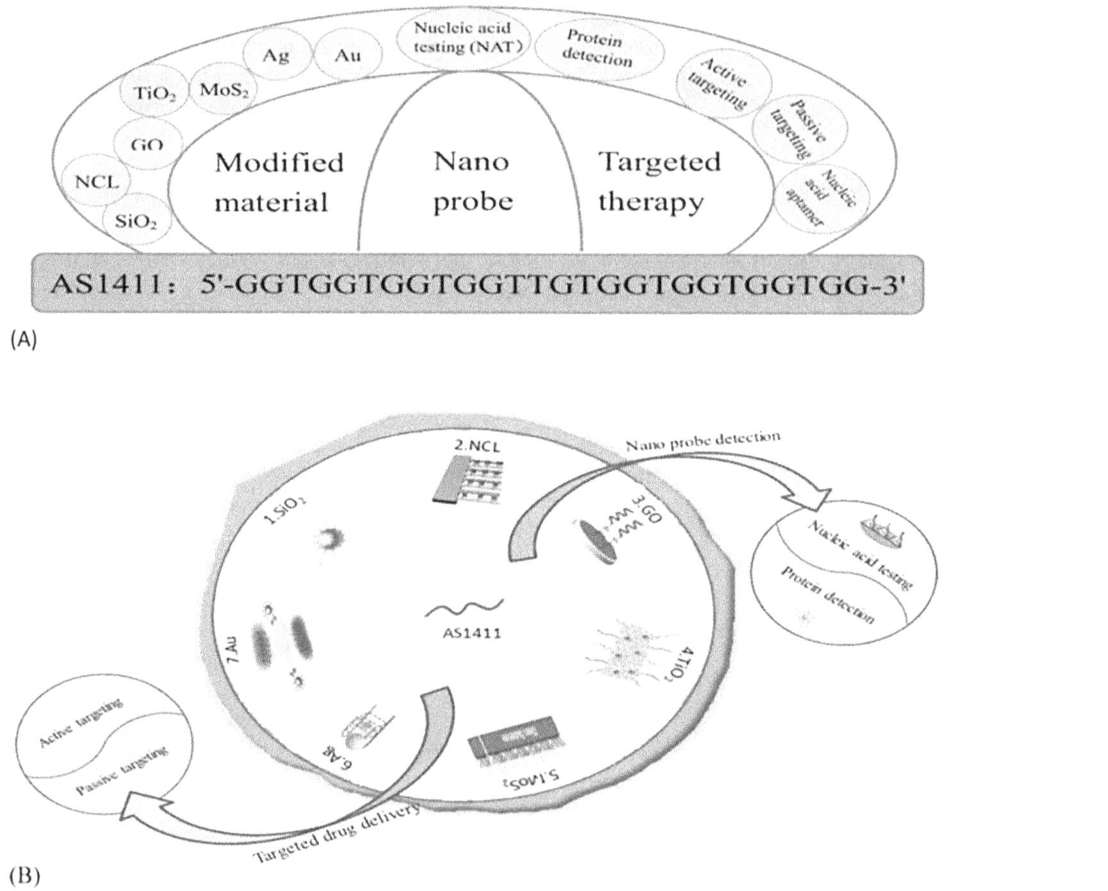

SCHEME 8.3 (a) The modified material of AS1411 and its general application in biomedical targeted therapy and nanoprobe. (b) Schematic diagram of AS1411-modified nanomaterials and their application in biochemistry.

Source: [51].

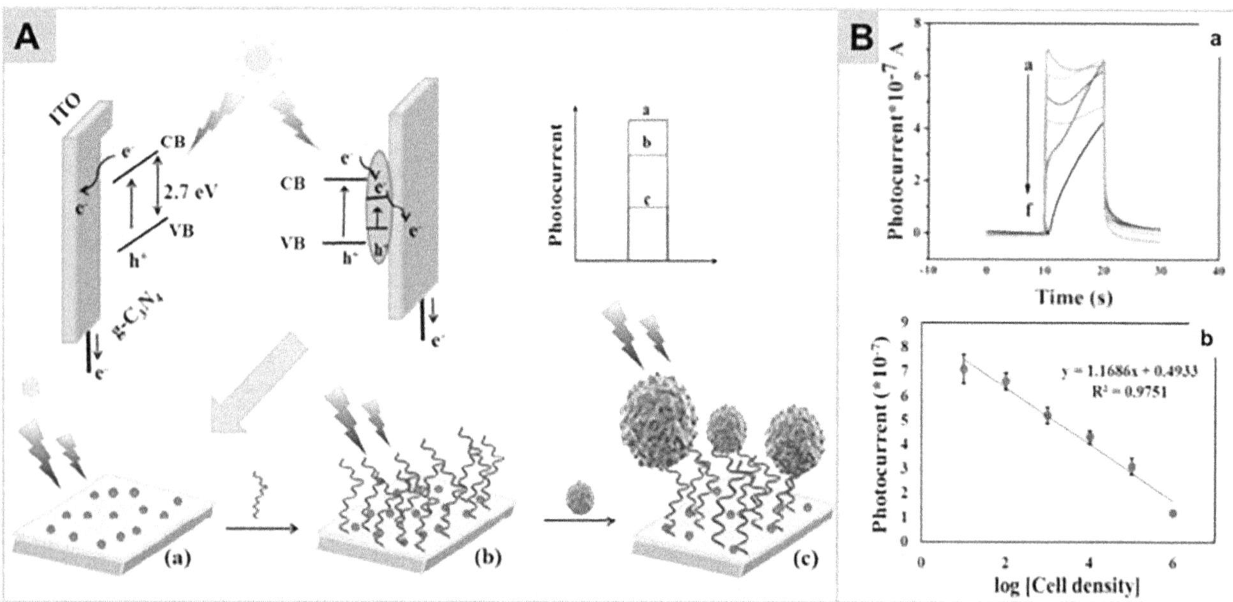

FIGURE 8.8 Panel A: PEC cytosensor fabrication process and its corresponding photocurrents. Panel B-a: Photocurrent responses of ITO/C3N4-AgI/aptamer after incubating with various concentrations of the HeLa cells: (a) 10, (b) 1×10^2, (c) 1×10^3, (d) 1×10^4, (e) 1×10^5, (f) 1×10^6 in PBS (0.1 M, pH 7.4). Panel B-b: Calibration curve of the cytosensor for HeLa cells detection. Corresponding data points and error bars are related to the average and standard deviations from four individual experiments.

Source: [52].

spectroscopy. Additionally, electrochemical nanosensors were utilized to detect the cancer stem cell, which predominantly expresses the cell surface markers CD44, CD90, CD133/2, and OV-6 through their antibodies of gold electrodes. Molecular frameworks (Cr-MOF) were also popularly utilized for the detection of CT26 colorectal cancers [53].

8.7.4 Magneto-Responsive Nanomaterials

Magnetic nanoparticles are multifunctional nanomaterials for multimodal theranostic applications. Nanomaterials are popularly used due to their unique physicochemical properties, facile synthesis, possibility of multiple functionalities, biocompatibility, biodegradability, and controlled toxicity. For example, size-dependent hyperthermia and theranostics have been researched. The surface charge of the nanoparticles can be used to bind with nucleic acid or increase the circulation time, while spherical or hollow-shaped nanomaterials are used for drug delivery. Cube-shaped nanomaterials, meanwhile, are used for guided chemo-photothermal therapy [60]. Due to these properties, nanomaterials are extensively used in biosensing, MRI, gene therapy, magnetic hyperthermia, PDT, and photothermal ablation. The approval of various iron-based drugs by the Food and Drug Administration (FDA), such as Combidex®, Endorem®, Feraheme®, Feridex, Ferumoxytol®, Gastromark®, Lumiren®, and Radiogardase®, for iron deficiency, iron replacement therapy, lymph node metastasis imaging, and magnetic resonance imaging contrast agent are in use. The European Union (EU) also approved Nanotherm® for the treatment of glioblastoma multiform, which proves the immense potential of magnetic nanoparticles. More commonly, magnetic iron oxide (frequently maghemite γ-Fe_2O_3 or magnetite Fe_2O_3), nickel, cobalt, Prussian blue, or gadolinium remains the most extensively researched nanomaterials. The functionalization usually provides colloidal stability and allows for stearic or electrostatic binding with the active therapeutic drug, targeting moieties, or the imaging probe, and tuning important properties of pharmacokinetics, systemic toxicity, clearance, cellular interactions, and non-specific protein absorptions [13, 46, 61].

The nanomaterials may obtain a shell–core structure consisting of magnetic nanomaterials forming the core and a polymeric material establishing the shell, such as chitosan-PEG-PEI-coated iron oxide nanoformulations encapsulated with chlortoxin (CTX) and green fluorescent encoded DNA (NP:DNA-CTX). Likewise, magnetic mesoporous silica nanoparticles (M-MSNs) were targeted to the HepG2 cells–bearing mice, where the MSNs were externally directed using the electromotive force (EMF) and/or alternating current magnetic force (ACMF), which, in combination, was found to be most effective. MSN were used to deliver chemo-radionuclides, such as cisplatin, with neutron-activated holmium-166 for non-small-cell lung cancer. The application of the magnetic field enhanced the radionuclides concentration.

8.7.5 Piezoelectric Responsive Nanomaterials

It is well-known that the stimulation of a mild electric signal proves toxic to cancer cells and inhibits their proliferation. However, its application is limited because of drawback, like unintended stimulation of healthy cells due to electric signal. Therefore, delivery of electric cues to targeted cancer site will be appreciated [62]. In order to overcome the limitation, "ultrasound-stimulated piezoelectric nanoparticle activation" came in existence, which is able to generate electricity upon exposure of mechanical deformation and serves as a promising tool in targeted stimulation of cells and tissues. Mechanical stimulation, such as ultrasound, can be used for the activation of piezonanotransducers. A report revealed that a biocompatible piezoelectric barium titanate nanoparticle (BTNPs), in combination with ultrasound, triggers the stimulation of various cell types. BTNPs have several advantages, like high piezoelectric coefficient (d33~30 pm/V), biocompatibility, excellent optical properties, and ability for morphology control. The barium titanate nanoplatform conjugated with anti-HER2 antibody has been demonstrated to target the HER2 positive cancer cells. Thereby, the anti-proliferative effect of the synthesized nanoparticles reduces cell proliferation by inducing cell cycle arrest in G0/G1 phase.

In a similar way as low-intensity electric field, piezoelectric system stimulation inhibits cell proliferation due to the upregulation of gene-encoding Kir3.2 inward rectifier potassium channels, causing disturbance in Ca^{2+} homeostasis and mitotic spindle organization. BTNPs functionalized with transferrin receptor antibody have been used for the dual-targeting purpose of the blood–brain barrier and glioblastoma cells. Ultrasound-mediated stimulation of BTNPs significantly reduces the proliferation of glioblastoma cells with lowered Ki-67 expression. In combination with a sub-toxic dose of temozolomide, BTNPs increase the sensitivity of chemotherapy with anti-proliferative and pro-apoptotic effect. Racca et al. exhibited the cytotoxic effect of zinc oxide (ZnO) nanocrystals in combination with high-energy ultrasound shock waves; however, the role of the piezoelectric effect remains unclear in the study [63].

Recently, ultrasound in the presence of piezoelectric tetragonal barium trioxide ($BaTiO_3$) has been demonstrated to act as a microscopic pressure resource and generate ROS for piezocatalytic tumor therapy. Ultrasonic vibration enables the separation of holes and electrons due to piezoelectricity and leads to the establishment of an electric field, and the generation of hydroxyl and superoxide radicals in situ downregulates the Ki-67 proliferative marker, leading to tumor eradication. The Ki-67 proliferation marker rest and breast cancer treatment plays a role in predicting chemotherapy response and prognosis. Both *in vitro* and *in vivo* result indicated that exposure of nanoparticle-embedded hydrogel causes ultrasound-induced cytotoxicity and piezocatalytic tumor eradication (Figure 8.9a–e), in addition to *in vivo* biosafety. Yet adoption of this technology in clinical practice is still in its infancy, as several open issues must be addressed, including piezoelectric property measurement, control of the ultrasound dose delivered *in vitro*, modelling and measurement of the piezo effects, knowledge of triggered bioeffects, biocompatibility studies, therapy targeting, and control of the ultrasound dose delivered *in vivo*.

8.7.6 Photochromism- and Electrochromic-Responsive Nanomaterials

Photochromism is a phenomena in which the color of a substance changes when it is exposed to photon energy [64]. Carbon-based nanomaterials functionalized with

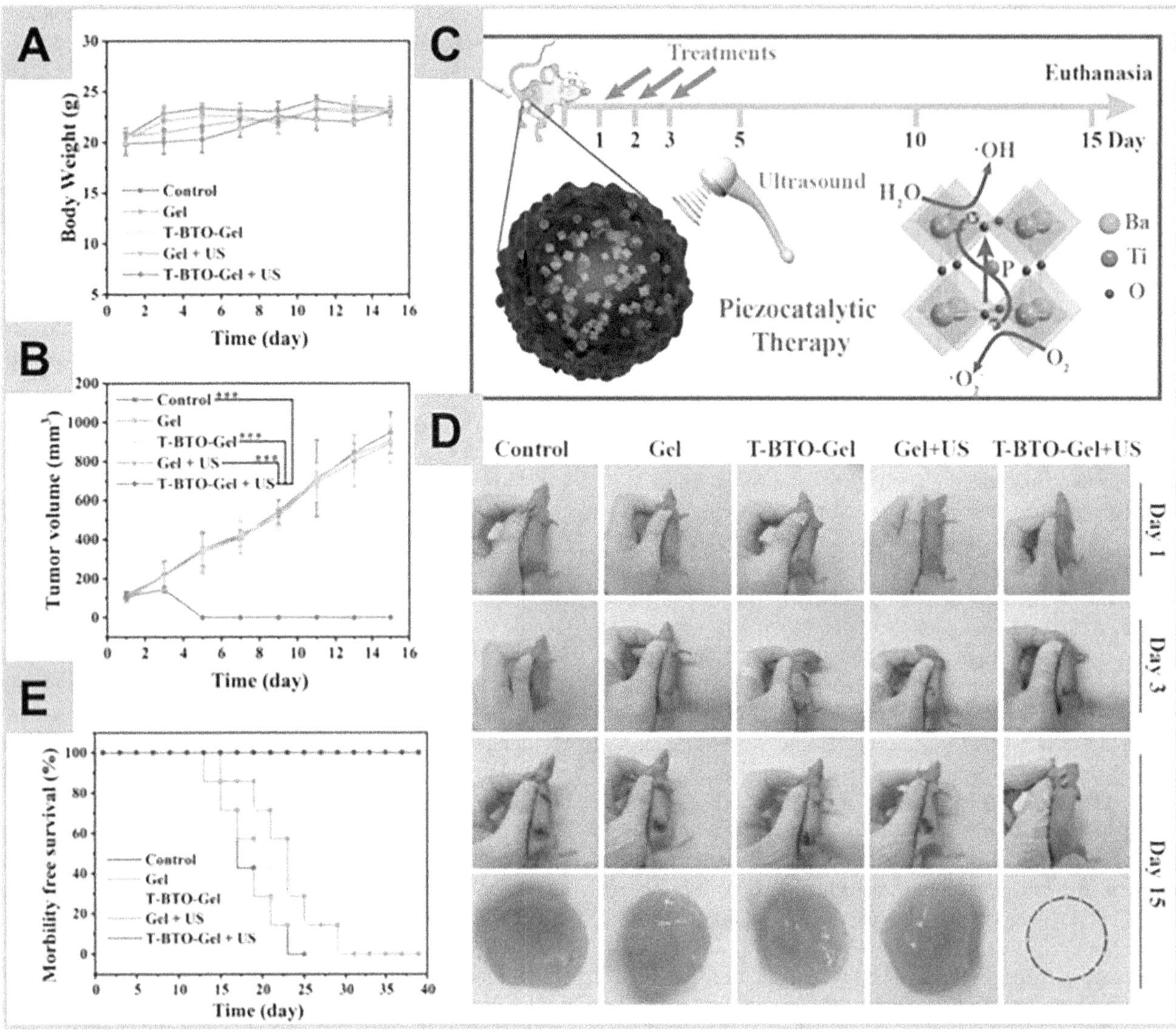

FIGURE 8.9 In vivo piezocatalytic therapy on tumor regression under US irradiation. Time-dependent body weight curves (panel A) and time-dependent tumor growth curves of tumor-bearing mice after different treatments, including control group, gel group, T-BTO-gel group, gel + US group, and T-BTO-gel + US groups (*$p<0.05$, **$p<0.01$, ***$p<0.001$) (panel B). Schematic illustration of piezocatalytic therapy in vivo (panel C). Digital photos of 4T1-tumor- bearing mice and their tumor regions after various treatments at different intervals (panel D). Survival curves of tumor-bearing mice after treatment (panel E).

photochromic moieties confer the property of photochromism to respond against a specific wavelength of light. *Spiropyran* is a well-reported photochromic molecule which can be easily interconverted between merocyanine (open-ring, colored, polar, and hydrophilic) and spiropyran (closed-ring, colorless, nonpolar, and hydrophobic) form upon specific light irradiation. Spiropyran-conjugated reduced graphene oxide (r-GO) has been demonstrated to retain its photochromic behaviour and can be utilized in the detection and therapy of tumor cells both *in vitro* and *in vivo*. Complex can be converted to merocyanine form upon irradiating with ultraviolet light and can be detected by fluorescent microscopy. Synthesized complex is capable as anticancer drug carrier, is non-toxic, as well as exhibits fluorescent property. Another study has also reported about spiropyran-conjugated graphene oxide for imaging of tumor cells. Composite showed the reversible change in color upon irradiation with light, thus confirming the photochromic property. In this direction, other photochromic molecules, like diarylethene, have been shown to be encapsulated into the same nanoparticles with conjugated polymer.

Like photochromism, the electrochromic effect is recognized to change their optical properties (light/dark) when exposed to change in electric potential and voltage change. Several polymers, inorganic and organic materials, exhibit an electrochromic property, including metal oxides, viologens, organic polymers, and polyaniline composite. Interestingly, cathodic coloring under negative potentials and bleaching states under positive potentials were discovered in inorganic materials (WO_3, TiO_2, V_2O_5 films, etc.). It is mostly due to charge-balancing ions (H^+, Li^+, Na^+, and K^+ ions) and electron insertion/extraction processes (reduction/oxidation). Dicationic 1,1,4,4-tetraarylbutadiene, 1^{2+} has been shown as an H_2S-responsive electrochromic material which can be used for PDT in mice. Different fluorescences (580, 700, or 830 nm) of fluorophores within 1^{2+}-SPNs are efficiently quenched by EM 1^{2+} with a strong absorption (500–850 nm), while selective conversion into colorless diene2 by H_2S-mediated two-electron reduction significantly recovers fluorescence, allowing for non-invasive imaging of hepatic and tumor H_2S in mice in real time.

Additionally, an electrochromic system composed of photovoltaic cells, plastic antibodies, and plasmonic nanomaterials (AuNPs) has been designed for color response detection of carcinoembryonic antigen (CEA) [65]. It has been observed that, when one of the photovoltaic cell's electrodes was modified with plastic antibodies, it was responsible for generating power for the electrochemical device and functioned in a concentration-dependent way. This energy passed through an electrochromic cell, which turned it into a colored event; because the intensity of the created color was power-dependent, the color observed was concentration-dependent, allowing visual detection. The plasmonic nanoparticles were investigated as an extra component in this system that might improve the photovoltaic cell's performance and contribute to higher sensitivity, as seen by better color detection. In terms of application, the hybrid device was able to respond to CEA in concentrations ranging from 0.1 to 10 g/mL, which is a critical range for disease screening, diagnosis, and progression. Introduction of plasmonic AuNPs boosted the sensitivity of the developed system. Simple visual inspection of the color gradient gave semi-quantitative data, but the color coordinates could be employed to obtain quantitative data.

8.7.7 pH-Responsive Nanomaterials

Cancers exhibit a slightly acidic pH (6.5), which may act as discerning factor from the normal cells. Due to the vulnerability of the acid–base haemostasis, the cancer may propagate to other pathological conditions, such as ischemia, inflammatory diseases, infections, or rheumatoid arthritis. The solid tumor will further proliferate, resulting in increased H^+ concentrations and production of lactate, owing to the aerobic glycolysis, leading to an acidic pH vs. normal cell of 7.4. It is imperative to consider the intracellular components present in different pH (for example, ~5.5 for endosomes and ~5.0 for lysosomes), which requires intricate designing of the delivery systems to release the cargo in the cytoplasm. Nanoparticles are more popularly used, harnessing the differential pH property of the cancers that can resist the non-specific interactions and the uptake by non-targeted cells or the immune system. More specifically, intelligent pH-responsive nanocarriers can increase the concentration of the chemotherapeutics, resulting in higher therapeutic effects.

Some pH-responsive nanomaterials are activated by the charge reversal of the surface moieties by the acidic environment exhibited by the cancer microenvironment. Metal organic framework with high DOX loading with redox responsive release has been investigated [66]. The traditionally used pH biosensors suffered from photobleaching and autofluorescence in the background, which affected the resolution of the images. Through expansion, the pH can invoke changes in the protonation or the deprotonation states of the functional groups, leading to changes in the hydrophobicity, conformation, or electrostasis altered to release the cargo from the nanomaterials. Apart from these, the temperature and the ionic states of the solutions are also used to alter the states. In such kind of application, polymeric micelles, polymerosomes, or hydrogels are more frequently used.

More commonly, in the direct cleavage of the bonds, the active drug or the fluorophore is linked to an inert nanomaterial through a linker which is susceptible to variable pH. In this aspect, the upconverting nanomaterials (UCNs) are appreciated due to the ability to function via anti-stokes emission, converting excitation in near-infrared to emission in the visible spectrum, minimizing the fluorescence background or tissue-induced scattering problems and increased photostability. In one such study, NaYF4:Yb^{3+} UCNs were conjugated to pH-sensitive dye pHrodo™ red though biocompatible aminosilane, which was seen to exhibit sensing in the dynamic range of 7.2–2.5 pH when tested on the HeLa cells. The pHrodo™ red fluorescence increases with decreased pH, imaged in confocal microscopy at 980 nm excitation. Similarly, charge reversal upon encountering cancerous cells' membranes (pH = 6.8) and, subsequently, the release of the DOX from the deblock co-polymer monomethoxyl poly(ethylene glycol)-b-poly(allyl ethylene phosphate) in the endosomes (pH = 5.0) formed a dual pH-sensitive therapeutic strategy (Figure 8.10A-C) [67].

Alternatively, the expansile nanoparticles swell or shrink in response to the differential protonation/deprotonation states, leading to transitions of the hydrophilic groups to hydrophobic groups. The expansion or swelling of the polymerosomes (poly-(L-glutamic acid)-block-poly(L-lysine) pointed to fenestrated nanostructures to release the drug or imaging agent. In case of nanomaterial swelling, it is imperative to control the swelling/contraction ratio for obtaining controlled release of the active material. On the other hand, gatekeeping strategies include caging the cargo materials, which opens to release the contents upon pH changes. MSNs, due to their ability to manipulate the pore volumes, large surface area, and lower cytotoxicity, are the most reasonably popular nanomaterials used with bio-orthogonal gatekeepers such as β-cyclodextrin or hydrazone bonds.

However, certain nanomaterials inherently degrade or dissemble into pieces completely by a single stimulus, the ranges of which have the spatial and temporal controls of release of the cargo. Polymeric nanomaterials such as poly(lactic acid) or polylactide-co-glycolide (PLGA) have ester bonds which undergo hydrolysis at a lower pH to release the cargoes, while co-block polymers containing boronic acid moieties possess altered solubility in the acidic environment. Surprisingly, aggregation of the nanomaterials into discrete and ordered nanostructures in response to pH has also been harnessed for drug delivery, more often involving a change in phase. Aggregation-based methods generally deliver the non-toxic nanomaterials through enhanced permeation and retention (EPR) effect to the cancers, also leading to decrease in the background signals with diagnosis. For example, magnetic resonance (MR) molecule-masked amphiphilic peptides were used to assemble the nanofibers, wherein the magnetic resonance units intracellularly increased the T1 relaxation time for three-dimensional

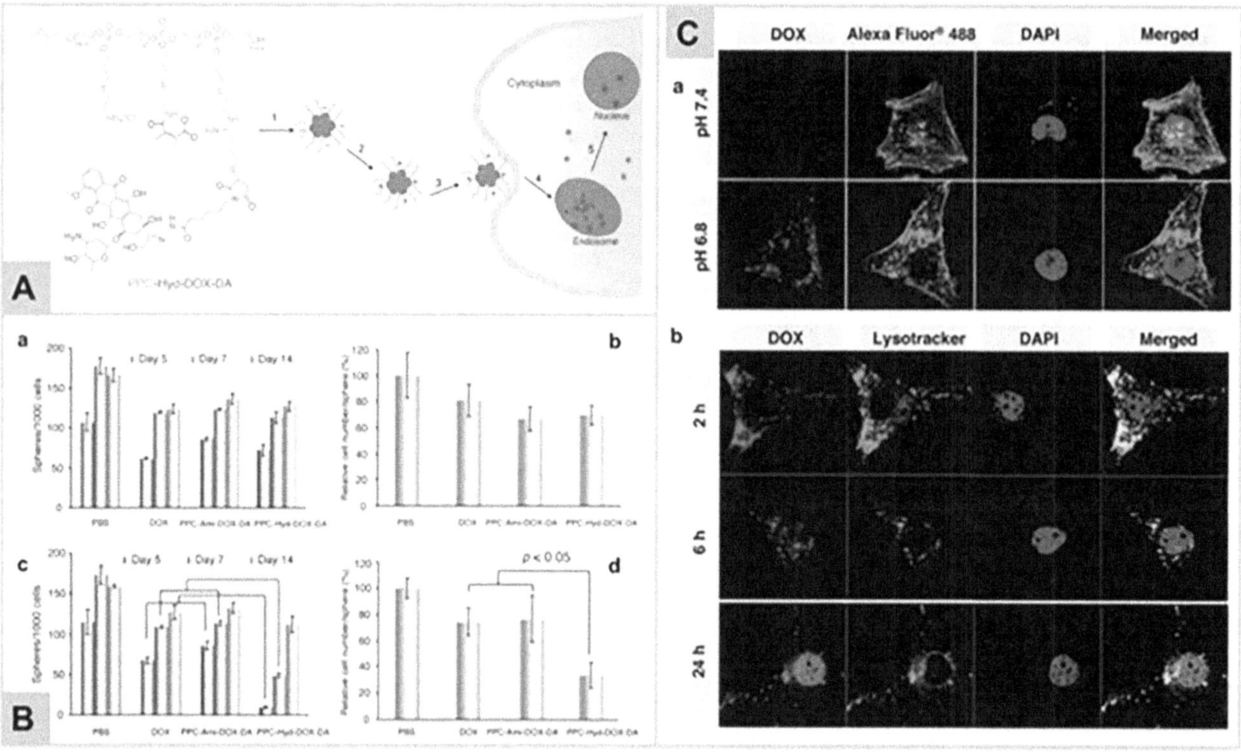

FIGURE 8.10 Chemical structure of the dual pH-responsive polymer doxorubicin (DOX) conjugate (PPC-Hyd-DOX-DA) and schematic illustration of its pH-triggered cellular internalization and intracellular drug release (panel A). Time-dependent sphere formation of SK-3rd cells after incubation with various formulations (a and c) and the relative cell numbers/sphere measured at 14 days (b and d). Cells were first incubated with the formulations in culture media for 2 h at pH 7.4 (a and b) or 6.8 (c and d), and then the media were replaced with fresh media and further incubated at pH 7.4. $p<0.005$. PBS control was set as 100%. The dose of DOX or its equivalent was 2 µg/mL (panel B). (a) Cellular uptake of PPC-Hyd-DOX-DA NPs (red) at pH 6.8 or 7.4 after incubation with MDA-MB-231 cells for 1 h. DAPI (40, 6-diamidino-2 phenylindole, blue) and Alexa Fluor488 phalloidin (green) were used to stain cell nuclei and F-actin, respectively. (b) Subcellular distribution of PPC-Hyd-DOX-DA NPs (red) at pH 6.8. DAPI (blue) and LysoTracker green were used to stain the cell nuclei and acidic organelles. Cells were imaged using a 60 water-immersion objective (panel C). [67].

magnetic resonance mapping of tissue-engineered scaffolds. Alternative to aggregation, a morphological switch operates by changing the shape of the nanomaterials in response to the pH of the local environment, changing the pharmacological properties of the material. For example, in poly(butadiene) m – poly(l-lysine)n (m – n = 107 – 200, 107 – 100, and 60 – 50), the micelle structures at physiological pH were swollen due to charge–charge repulsions to transit to helix-like nanostructures, releasing the cargo.

8.7.8 Redox-Responsive Nanomaterials

ROS includes OH•, O_2•, and H_2O_2, which play an important role in the body for key cell signalling pathways (redox signalling), cellular differentiation, and proliferation. However, the production of ROS is elevated in tumor cells because of increased metabolic rate, gene mutation, and relative hypoxia. Moreover, in the mitochondria, the energy cycle is mostly directed toward aerobic glycolysis and pyruvate oxidation, which is popularly termed as "Warburg's effect," which can increase the ROS production. The elevated ROS leads to several pathological conditions, as well as the propagation of cancer. More specifically, ROS has an effect on the calcium channels by releasing calcium from the cellular reserves and affecting the kinases (such as protein kinase C) for the proliferation of cancer cells. Interestingly, it is observed that cancer-associated fibroblasts (CAFs) are involved in a two-way cross-talk with the ROS in the tumor microenvironment to increment H_2O_2 level.

Moreover, ROS may affect the activity of histone regulators, such as histone deacetylases or DNA methyltransferases, known to oxidise the guanine residues; the rate of oxidation is increased to 35–50% in transformed cells. The ROS may also impair the MDR of the cancer cells. The differing ROS and the GSH concentrations can provide an altered redox condition in cancerous cells. Generally, in cancer cells, the GSH produced is about 2×10^{-3}–10×10^{-3} M, while it is ~1,000-fold lower extracellularly (2×10^{-3}–20×10^{-6} M), wherein the ROS provides excellent selectivity for the release of the cargo. Contrarily, the antioxidant transcription factors such as Nrf2 are found to be important for maintaining tumorigenesis. Therefore, ROS behaves as double-edged swords, which are regulated to be useful in some therapies through apoptosis [68], autophagosomes, necroptosis, or ferroptosis.

Chen et al. synthesized the nanocarrier comprised of ROS-responsive poly(β-amino ester) (PBAEROS) by introducing thioketal groups in the monomer structure. It can be used as a nanocarrier to facilitate the controlled release of DOX and near-infrared photosensitizer IR780 to achieve the synergistic combined anticancer effect of PTT/PDT and chemotherapy. Further, nanoparticles were loaded with marine sulfated polysaccharide, known as poly(β-amino ester) PPID nanoparticles, which have the capacity to respond to ROS and release DOX in a regulated way. Upon irradiation with 808 nm laser, temperature elevation has been observed in response to poly(β-amino ester) nanoparticles and induces high ROS generation, displaying their high PTT/PDT therapy efficiency. It was shown that poly(β-amino ester) nanoparticles increased the cellular uptake of the IR780 and DOX in hepatoma cells, and that they also significantly decreased cell growth following laser irradiation, showing the synergistic anticancer effects. ROS-responsive liposome nanocarrier was also demonstrated for their synergistic antitumor effect in breast cancer cells, with no cardiotoxicity or side effects to normal cells, as shown in Figure 8.11a, b [69].

The nanomaterials conjugated with redox-responsive functional groups may degrade the nanoprotective shield, undergoing structural and functional changes to provide superior cancer-targeted ability and reduced toxic side effects. In general, the redox-responsive functional groups include sulphur-containing, selenium-containing, tellurium-containing, and arylboronic ester linkages. It has been observed that the nanomaterials containing the ROS-sensitive linkages underwent a phase transition to degradation, amphiphilic transitions, and changes in the solubility, and fracture of the nanomaterials to release the contents.

Under ROS conditions, hydrophobic monoselenide groups are oxidized to hydrophilic selenones, causing ROS-responsive nanoparticles to disassemble and the loading drug to be released at specified targeted site [70]. Ma et al. demonstrated the amphiphilic triblock copolymer composed of two PEG moieties attached to both terminals of polyselenide moiety. In aqueous solution, it tends to form block copolymer aggregates and have enhanced oxidation-responsiveness. It dissociates under a mild oxidation condition, that is, 0.1% H_2O_2 v/v, due to high sensitivity of selenide group.

To enhance the stability and avoid the premature delivery of drugs, hydrophobic drugs covalently attached to the polymer have been explored. Epalrestat and DOX were co-delivered at tumor-targeted site using redox-sensitive polymer micelles composed of tocopherol polyethylene glycol succinate conjugated with vitamin B6, which acts as cancer targeted moiety. Synthesized prodrug micelles disrupt in redox tumor environment of MDA MB 231 and 4T1 cell lines and release both drugs in ratiometric manner. The synergistic combined effect of drugs induces cell cycle arrest, apoptosis, and alteration to mitochondrial membrane potential in cancer cells, as well as down-regulates the expression of CD44 receptor, which is the main factor for cancer metastasis. Both drugs show the prolonged circulation half-life and tumor bioavailability with developed approach. Moreover, *in vivo* study clarifies the reduced cardiotoxicity effect of DOX, and thus, nanoencapsulation proves to be the new opportunities in combined chemotherapy.

MSN offers great advantage as a redox-sensitive delivery system due to the presence of abundant Si–OH group on the surface, large surface area, and high biocompatibility. Zhang et al. demonstrated the redox-responsive disulfide-bridged and DOX-embedded silica nanoparticles for desirable gene/drug codelivery. To facilitate gene delivery, a nanoparticle has been functionalized with polycation, comprised of one β-cyclodextrin core and two ethanolamine-functionalized poly(glycidyl methacrylate) arms. Another study also reported the redox-responsive, β-cyclodextrin-gated silica nanoparticles containing DOX and conjugated with azobenzene/galactose-grafted polymer (GAP) for the treatment of HepG2 cells. Azobenzene/galactose-grafted polymer acts not only as a sealing gatekeeper to prevent leakage but also as a targeting moiety to target the asialoglycoprotein receptor (ASGPR) present on HepG2 cells. Controlled and stimuli-responsive drugs can be achieved by the exposure of ultraviolet radiation, followed by exposure to endogenous GSH (Table 8.3) [44].

8.8 Synthesis of Nanomaterials

The various techniques used to synthesize nanomaterials can be broadly categorized as bottom-up and top-down, as shown in Figure 8.12.

8.8.1 Bottom-Up Approach

This method is called a constructive approach for synthesizing nanomaterials. Common bottom-up approaches are sol–gel, spinning, chemical vapor deposition (CVD), pyrolysis, and biosynthesis.

8.8.1.1 Chemical Vapor Deposition Technique (CVD)

In the chemical vapor deposition method, a thin film is deposited onto a substrate via the chemical reaction of the gaseous substrate. This reaction is generally carried out at ambient temperature. A thin film is formed by the chemical reaction which occurs when a heated substrate comes into contact with the precursor gas. This method can obtain a uniform, pure, rigid, and robust film with good reproducibility. One of the major disadvantages of this technique is the requirement of special equipment and gaseous by-products, which are sometimes highly toxic [84].

8.8.1.2 Solvothermal and Hydrothermal Methods

Solvothermal and hydrothermal methods are popular conventional approaches for synthesizing nanomaterials, such as nanowires, nanorods, nanosheets, and nanospheres. In the solvothermal process, the reaction is carried out in a closed, sealed vessel whose pressure should be greater than the solvent's boiling point. In the hydrothermal process, instead of solvent, water is used. The microwave-assisted hydrothermal approach combines the merit of microwave and hydrothermal methods. In this approach, temperature affects the morphology of the nanomaterials.

8.8.1.3 Sol-Gel Method

The sol–gel method is one of the most widely used wet chemical approaches for synthesizing nanomaterials, owing to its simplicity, economic viability, and environmental benignity. As

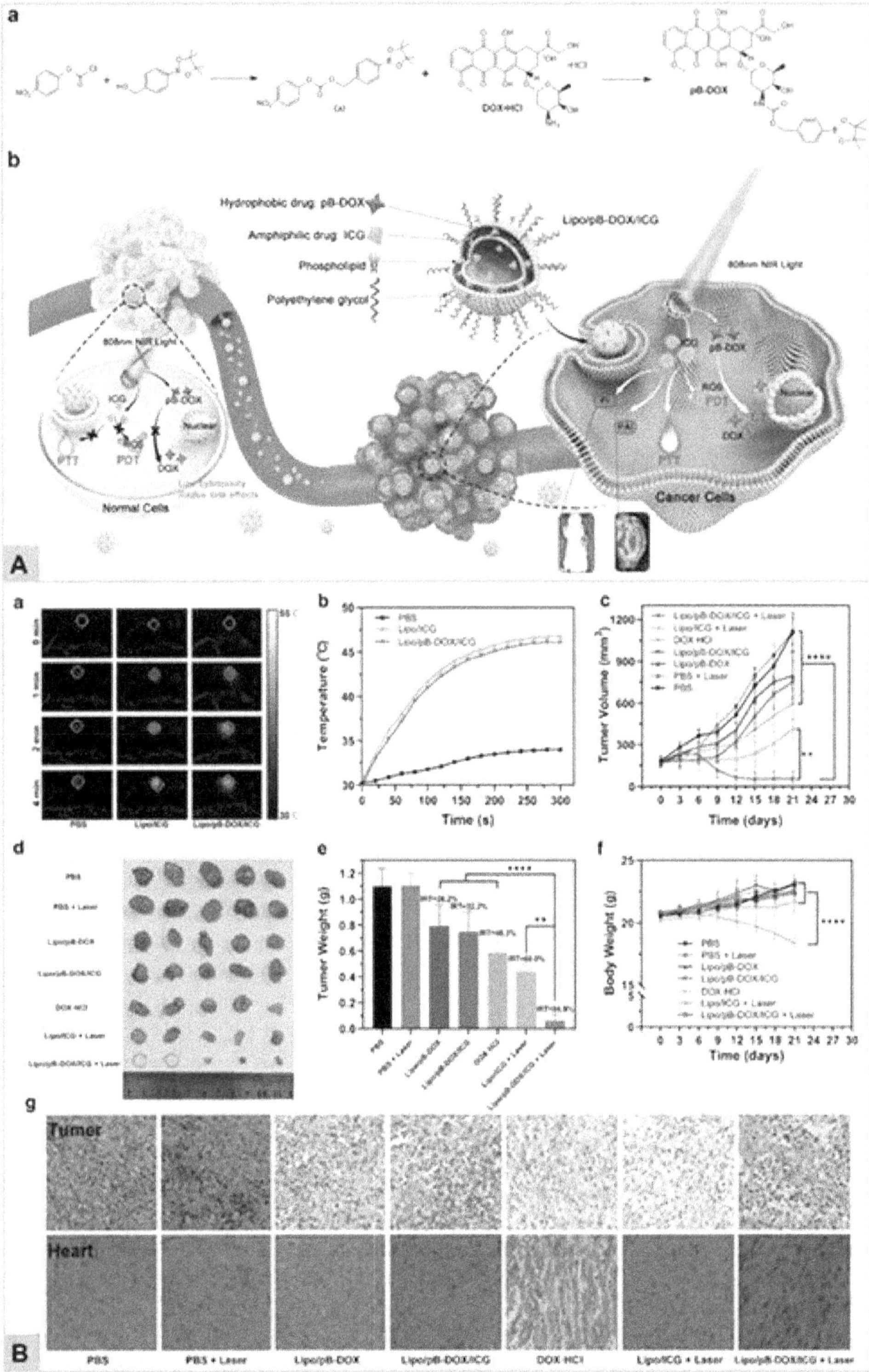

FIGURE 8.11 (a) Synthesis of pB-DOX. (b) Schematic illustration of lipo/pB-DOX/ICG-combined photodynamic therapy with ROS-responsive chemotherapy to synergistically treat cancer cells (panel A). The ICG-generated ROS would exert photodynamic therapy by inducing cell necrosis or apoptosis and selectively cleave the boronate moiety of pB-DOX under 808 nm laser irradiation, triggering DOX release for chemotherapy. ICG could generate localized hyperthermia by absorbing NIR for PTT. Lipo/pB-DOX/ICG offers FI and PAI approaches for visualizing its dynamic distribution within the whole body. With low endogenous ROS levels and without light irradiation, normal tissues could be free from damage (panel A). (a) Thermal images of MDA-MB-231-tumor-bearing mice from different treating groups (PBS+laser, lipo/ICG+laser, and lipo/pB-DOX/ICG+laser) under 808 nm laser irradiation for different irradiation periods. (b) Temperature change curves at the tumor sites of different treatment groups during 808 nm laser irradiation. (c) Tumor volume curves of different groups after various treatments, including PBS, PBS+laser, DOX·HCl, lipo/pB-DOX, lipo/ICG+laser, lipo/pB-DOX/ICG, and lipo/pB-DOX/ICG+laser. (d) Photographs of tumor tissues removed from groups treated with different formulations after 21 d. The red circles indicate disappeared tumors. (e) Tumor weights of each group at the end of experiment and IRT. (f) Body weight curves of MDA-MB-231 tumor-bearing mice for each group. (g) Representative histological images of tumor and heart samples from the treated mice (panel B) [69]

TABLE 8.3

List of Nanomaterials Activated by Thermal Differences, Photo-, Electro-, Redox-, Photochromic-, Wlectrochromic-, and pH-Responsive Nanomaterials and Their Reactivities

Nanomaterials Used	Physical or Chemical Effect Displayed	Reactivity	Refs.
Pluronic F-127 (polyoxyethylene-propylene co-polymer)	Thermosensitive	High hydrophilicity, low toxicity; used frequently for high lipophilic chemotherapeutics	[71]
Poly(N-isopropylacrylamide-co-acrylamide)-b-poly(DL-lactide)	Thermosensitive	Inhibited 80% growth of gastric cancers	[71]
1,2-Distearoyl-sn-glycero-3-phosphoethanolamine (DPPH-2) liposomes	Thermosensitive	Plasma half-life of gemcitabine increased from 0.07 to 2.59 h	[72]
Gold nanoparticle coated by polyethylene glycol (AurolyseTM)	Thermo-responsive	Laser-irradiated ablation of prostate tissue with no toxicity observed	[73]
Mitoxantrone and SB-431542 loaded reduced graphene oxide	Photo-responsive	Near-infrared irradiation destroys primary tumor and inhibits metastasis in 4T1 in vivo tumor model	[74]
Phthalocyanine chloride disulfonic acid (AlP) and camptothecin prodrug nanoparticles	Photo-responsive	660 nm light irradiation induces 1O2 generation, which disrupts the nanosystem and suppresses tumor growth and metastasis	[75]
PEG-methotrexate and indocyanine green–loaded bismuth sulfide nanoparticles	Photo-responsive/ redox-responsive	Nanosystem shows cellular internalization, proapoptotic behavior, and cellular cytotoxicity upon near-infrared and redox responses	[76]
Keratin-coated gold nanoparticles	Photo-responsive	Excellent biocompatibility, efficient cellular uptake, and localized photothermal heating capabilities observed	[77]
Nanoparticle composed of polylactic-co-glycolic acid (PLGA) wrapped with bovine serum albumin shell functionalized with acidity-triggered rational membrane (ATRAM) peptide	pH-responsive	ATRAM facilitates the internalization of nanosystem in acidic tumor environment and releases therapeutic cargo with no cytotoxic effect on healthy cells	[78]
Endosomolytic polymer nanoparticles loaded with 3pRNA	pH-responsive	Intratumoral delivery of NPs inhibited CT26 tumor growth and enhanced the therapeutic efficacy of anti-PD-1 immune checkpoint blockade and caused 30% complete response rate and generation of immunological memory that protected against tumor reoccurrence	[79]
Clustered iron oxide core within the polymer PPy-polyethylene glycol	Magneto-responsive	Nanosystem generates heat in response to an alternating current magnetic field, and its exposure destroys the tumor cells and protects against tumor reoccurrence without any significant toxicity effect	[80]
Trastuzumab- doxorubicin PVA/PMA_{SH} magnetic nanocapsules	Magneto-responsive	Magnetic targeting optimizes intratumoral distribution and utilization to inhibit the tumor growth	[81]
Oleic acid–, chitosan-, and 5-FLU-conjugated iron oxide nanoparticle (Fe_3O_4@OA-CS-5-FLU-NPs)	ROS-responsive	Induces cytotoxicity and morphological deformation with inhibition in colony formation of A549 and HeLa cells	[82]
Doxorubicin modified with a phenylboronic acid ester group and an amphiphilic polymer (DSPE-PEG) modified with internalized RGD (DSPE-PEG-iRGD)	ROS-responsive	Targeted delivery shows synergistic combined effect of photodynamic therapy and chemotherapy	[83]

Source: [44].

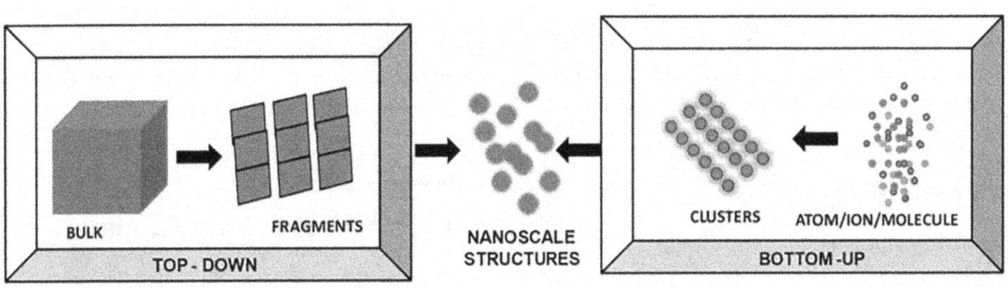

FIGURE 8.12 Synthesis of nanomaterials: top-down and bottom-up approaches.

the name suggests, in this method, there is the dissolution of a precursor in a solvent system, which is transformed into the sol, and the sol is finally converted into gel through the process of condensation, hydrolysis, gel aging, etc. Metal oxides and chlorides are the conventional precursors for this method. During the condensation process, hydroxo (M–OH–M) or oxo (M–O–M) bridges synthesize metal–hydroxo or metal–oxo clusters in the solution. The material's structure, characteristics, and porosity change due to ongoing polycondensation. Aging results in a reduction in porosity and an increase in the spacing between colloidal particles and formation of a gel. After the aging process, the gel is dried, which removes water and organic solvents from it, followed by calcination to get nanoparticles.

8.8.1.4 Pyrolysis

In industry, *pyrolysis* is a well-used technology for the large-scale synthesis of nanomaterials. Herein, the precursor is fed into the furnace at high pressure through a small orifice and burned in the flame at a high temperature, involving the thermal decomposition of materials in an inert atmosphere. This method is simple, efficient, and economically viable with a high yield.

8.8.1.5 Biosynthesis

This is a greener approach for synthesizing nontoxic and biodegradable nanoparticles. Instead of using conventional chemicals for bioreduction and capping, the biosynthesis method produces NPs using bacteria, plant extracts, fungi, and other microorganisms together with the precursors. Because of their distinctive and improved features, biosynthesized NPs are used in various applications, including drug carriers for targeted delivery, cancer treatment, gene therapy, DNA analysis, antibacterial agents, biosensors, separation science, and magnetic resonance imaging (MRI).

8.8.1.6 Reverse Micelle Method

The reverse micelle method is an intriguing wet chemical method that can be used to synthesize nanomaterials with the desired shape and size. In this process, reverse micelles are formed from at least three components; two are immiscible, and the third is a surfactant with amphiphilic properties. Aqueous systems with nanometer dimensions are used to carry out specific reactions in order to develop materials with controlled size and shape. For controlling the size of the nanomaterial, the reverse micelles' size plays a crucial role. In this method, the reverse micelle acts as a nanoreactor, leading to an enhanced reaction rate and uniform distribution of NPs. The advantage of this approach over other approaches lies in the improved control of particle size, shapes, uniformity, and dispersibility.

8.8.2 Top-Down Method

In contrast to bottom-up approaches, top-down approaches reduce bulk materials to nanoscale particles. As a result, this method is also known as a destructive method for nanoparticle synthesis. Some of the common synthetic methods for this approach include lithography, mechanical milling, laser ablation, sputtering, and thermal decomposition.

8.8.2.1 Lithography

A focused electron beam is used to synthesize nanomaterials. This approach is broadly classified into two main categories: masked lithography and maskless lithography. Generally, lithography is used in microfabrication to pattern part of a thin film using the bulk substrate.

8.8.2.2 Mechanical Milling

Among the various top-down approaches, mechanical milling is a physical method for synthesizing various nanoparticles. Milling aims to reduce the particle size and blend the particle in an inert atmosphere. Plastic deformation determines the particle shape and fracture and reduces particle size, and cold welding, which increases particle size, is the influencing factor in mechanical milling. This method is simple, is low cost, and can produce various nanoparticle sizes.

8.8.2.3 Laser Ablation

This is a common method for fabricating a wide range of nanomaterials, including semiconductors, metal NPs, nanowires, composites, ceramic carbon nanotubes, etc., from various solvents. In this approach, a laser beam is irradiated on a metal solution. Due to the high laser energy, the precursor vaporizes, followed by nucleation and growth of a plasma plume, which leads to the synthesis of nanoparticles. This technique is considered a green process as it obviates the need to stabilize and reduce agents for the NP synthesis.

8.8.2.4 Sputtering

In this process, high-energy particles bombard the solid surface, which leads to the production of NPs. It is a very effective technique for producing a thin film. Sputtering is usually a deposition of a thin layer of materials onto a particular surface by ejecting atoms from that material and condensing ejected atoms onto the surface when a high-vacuum environment is applied [85]. Sputtering can be carried out in a number of ways, including radio frequency diodes, magnetrons, and DC diodes. Sputtering is often carried out in an evacuated chamber that is then filled with sputtering gas. Free electrons collide with the gas due to a high voltage supplied to the cathode target, creating gas ions. Atoms are ejected off the cathode target's surface due to the positively charged ions' rapid acceleration in the electric field as they approach the target. The thickness of the layer, temperature, duration of annealing, substrate type, etc. determine the shape and size of the synthesized film over the substrate.

8.9 Classification of Nanomaterials

Nanoparticles can be classified according to their physical and chemical properties. Generally, NPs can be classified into organic, inorganic, and carbon-origin nanoparticles.

8.9.1 Organic Nanoparticles

Organic nanoparticles are synthesized utilizing natural or synthetic organic molecule templates, as shown in Figure 8.13. There are many different types of organic NPs in nature, including protein aggregates, lipid bodies, milk emulsions, and more complex structures like viruses, to mention a few [86]. Common names for organic nanoparticles or polymers include dendrimers, micelles, chitosan, silk fibroin, liposomes, and ferritin. These nanoparticles are biodegradable and nontoxic, and some are like micelles and liposomes, which have hollow centers, so they are also called "nanocapsules." The high stability of organic NPs in biological fluids and during storage makes them an ideal choice for stimuli-responsive materials triggered by electromagnetic radiation, like heat and light [86]. Biopolymer nanoparticles offer several advantages, including the ease of their preparation, higher colloidal stability, improved dispersibility, and surface reactivity, making them a perfect candidate for drug administration.

8.9.2 Inorganic Nanoparticles

Inorganic nanoparticles are biocompatible, hydrophilic-toxic, and highly stable. Some common examples of inorganic nanoparticles include quantum dots and metal and metal oxide nanoparticles. These inorganic NPs are highly efficient for diagnosis and imaging due to their unique electrical, chemical, and magnetic properties.

8.9.2.1 Metal-Based NPs

Metal nanoparticles are currently being used for biological applications. This covers a broad range of substances, including elemental metals, such as cadmium (Cd), cobalt (Co), aluminum (Al), iron (Fe), copper (Cu), gold (Au), silver (Ag), lead (Pb), and zinc (Zn), as well as metal oxides and metal salts. Silver nanoparticles (AgNPs) and gold nanoparticles (AuNPs) show optical plasmonic behavior that leads to enhancement in the electromagnetic field due to collective oscillation of the electrons and accordingly enhances the radiative properties for cancer theranostics applications. Moreover, iron nanoparticles are exclusively used for magnetic resonance imaging (MRI) applications.

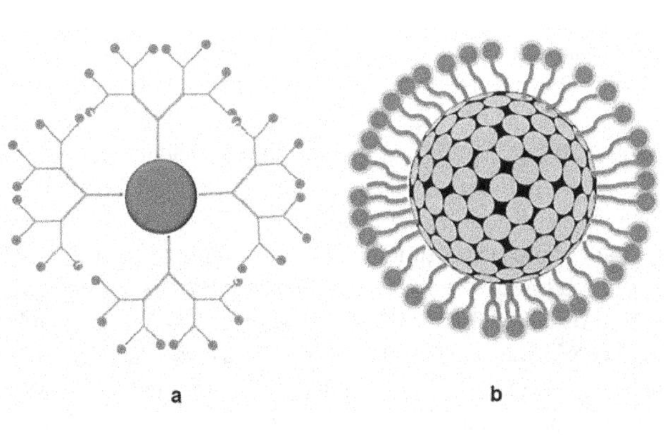

a b

FIGURE 8.13 Organic nanoparticles: (a) dendrimer and (b) liposome.

8.9.2.2 Metal Oxide NPs

Metal oxide NPs are well-known for their anticancer activity and enhanced radiosensitization ability. In order to modify the properties of their respective metal-based nanoparticles, metal oxide nanoparticles are synthesized. For example, in the presence of oxygen at room temperature, iron (Fe) nanoparticles instantly oxidize to iron oxide (Fe_2O_3), increasing their reactivity compared to iron NPs. It has also been proven that ZnO NPs are most effective in targeting certain cancer cells. The genotoxic ZnO NPs offer a promising platform for designing more potent anticancer agents for therapeutic use. The surface modification of metal oxides can be performed with carboxylate, oleic acid, and polyethylene glycol to deliver various therapeutic agents. Surface modifications of these NPs make them more biocompatible, reactive, and biodegradable by improving properties such as cytotoxicity, hydrophilicity, large pore volume, high surface area, and pore size. These modifications lead to an enhancement in therapeutic efficacy. Metal oxides such as aluminum oxide (Al_2O_3), iron oxide (Fe_2O_3), cerium oxide (CeO_2), and zinc oxide (ZnO) are attracting particular interest due to their enormous potential in anticancer therapy [68]. Particularly CeO_2, by virtue of its redox-modulatory enzyme-like activities, is envisaged as a promising candidate in nanomedicine. The ability of cerium nanoparticles to mimic various redox activities, allowing them to scavenge reactive oxygen species, such as catalase, superoxide dismutase, peroxidase, phosphotriesterase, phosphatase, and oxidase, makes it a potential candidate for cancer theranostics.

8.9.3 Carbon-Based NPs

Carbon-based nanomaterials are extensively used in biomedical applications, particularly for cancer theranostics, thanks to their unique physicochemical properties and inert nature, which enhances their ability to deliver drugs to the cell without any adverse effects. The feasibility of surface functionalization with organic and biological molecules makes them some of the most promising materials capable of targeted drug delivery. Carbon nanomaterials show strong absorption in the near-infrared region (NIR), which is helpful for photothermal tumor ablation. Furthermore, these materials are capable of releasing heat in a radio frequency field, which can be utilized to kill cancer cells by heating them. As a result, they can be applied to photodynamic and photothermal therapies. Carbon-based nanomaterials can be classified into activated carbon, fullerenes, graphene, carbon nanotubes (CNTs), carbon nanofibers, carbon black, etc., as shown in Figure 8.14.

8.9.3.1 Activated Carbon

Activated carbon (AC) is an amorphous form of carbon and is produced from a range of carbonaceous sources, such as bamboo, wood, coconut shells, and coal, by the process of carbonization and activation. AC is economically viable and biofriendly, making it an ideal candidate as a carrier for tumor therapeutic agents.

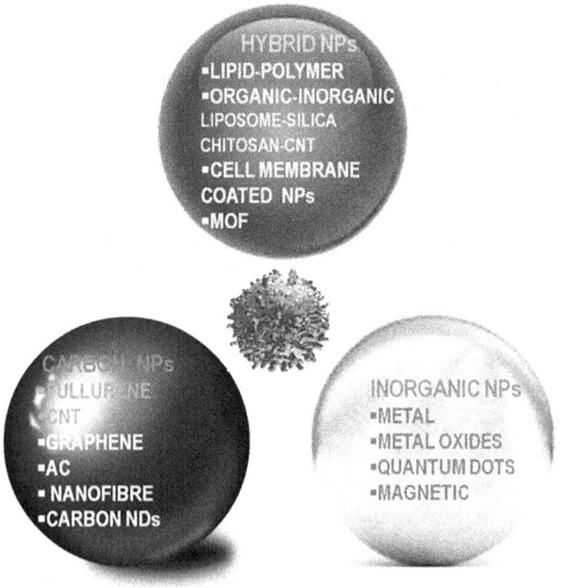

FIGURE 8.14 Different types of nanoparticles for cancer theranostics.

8.9.3.2 Graphene

Graphene is a carbon allotrope and comes under two-dimensional materials. Graphene possesses extraordinary physicochemical properties, including ultrahigh carrier mobility, excellent electrical conductivity, superior thermal conductivity, large specific surface area, high optical transmittance, and good biocompatibility. Due to the preceding properties, graphene has been widely used as an excellent drug delivery system, in fluorescence imaging, and in cancer theranostics.

8.9.3.3 Carbon Nanotubes

Carbon nanotubes (CNTs) are novel-type synthetic nanomaterials a few nanometers in diameter with distinct hollow and cylindrical structures. CNTs are formed by rolling graphene sheets. CNTs possess extraordinary chemical, electronic, mechanical, and optical properties. The functionalization of CNTs with other biological systems makes them ideal for biocompatible drug delivery strategies for targeting and eliminating specific tumor cells.

8.9.3.4 Fullerene

A *fullerene* is also an allotrope of carbon. In a fullerene, carbon atoms are held together by sp^2 hybridization and belong to the carbon nanomaterials family. The distinct cage-like structure and electron-deficient nature impart fascinating properties, making fullerenes a promising focus of various research areas, including cancer theranostics.

8.9.3.5 Carbon Nanodots

Carbon nanodots (CNDs) are zero-dimensional nanoparticles having a size of less than 10 nm. CNDs are fluorescent materials and exhibit unique characteristics, such as high water solubility, chemical inertness, low toxicity, ease of functionalization, and good biocompatibility. CNDs are fascinating carbon-based materials and have received much attention in bioimaging, optical sensing, anticancer, photocatalysis, lasers, drug delivery, and optoelectronics.

8.10 Recent Trends of Nanomaterials in Cancer Theranostics

Due to their low cost, simple synthesis, and minimal toxicity, bioinspired nanoparticles surpass traditionally synthesized nanoparticles by mimicking nature. This chapter provides a comprehensive overview of cancer theranostics using a variety of bioinspired materials, which include lipid nanoparticles, protein-based nanoparticles, liposomes, inorganic nanoparticles, viral nanoparticles, chitosan, and silk fibroin. Because of their dimensions in the range of 1–100 nm, nanocarriers possess greater and more effective interactions with cancerous cells and are greatly explored for biomedical applications.

Due to their distinct physicochemical characteristics, bionanoparticles have received a lot of attention recently. Viral NPs, protein NPs, apoferritin, aptamers, solid–lipid NPs, etc. [87] appear to be the most promising members of the cauldron. Recent trends in cancer theranostics are displayed in Figure 8.15.

However, it has been shown that biosynthesized multifunctional nanoparticles encapsulating therapeutic and imaging agents possess theranostic activity. The following approaches can synthesize a bioinspired theranostic agent: (1) screening of plant extracts; (2) standardizing a variety of physicochemical parameters for biosynthesis; (3) inclusion of therapeutic and imaging agents; (4) characterization of nanocarriers to determine their properties.

The hybridization of gold NPs with quantum dots (QDs) can produce multifunctional nanohybrids with superior imaging and anticancer properties. Chen et al. created ZnO QDs conjugated to gold nanoparticles containing the anticancer drug camptothecin [88]. AuNPs convert absorbed light energy into localized heat responsible for tumor cells' destruction via photothermal therapy. Nanocarriers, with and without drug loading, exhibited similar cytotoxicity toward HeLa cells. On the contrary, hybridization of the paramagnetic Gd ion and CuInS/ZnS QDs could enable dual fluorescence/magnetic resonance–mediated imaging.

Yang et al. synthesized Gd-doped ZnS QDs without Cd in lipid vesicles with enhanced fluorescence and improved colloidal stability. Similarly, to avoid fluorescence quenching of QDs, superparamagnetic Fe_3O_4 was separated from fluorescent graphene–CdTe QDs by a SiO_2 shell. 5-fluorouracil could be loaded into this bifunctional cytocompatible model, which would be effective against hepatoma cells. Overall, the hybridization of QDs with different types of inorganic NPs enables their use in multimodal imaging, such as fluorescence, magnetic, and ultrasound imaging. By combining magnetic hyperthermia, photothermal therapy, and photodynamic therapy, synergistic cancer therapy could also be achieved.

8.10.1 Organic Nanoparticles in Cancer Theranostics

In the past decade, there have been significant increases in the application of nanotechnology to detect and treat numerous diseases, including cancer. Nanotechnology helps improve the biodistribution and target accumulation of chemotherapy drugs, allowing them to balance better the efficacy and toxicity of the treatment. In response to the various limitations in conventional therapeutic strategies and to improve tumor-targeted drug delivery, various nanomedicines, including liposomal nanoparticles, nonmetallic nanoparticles, viral nanoparticles, protein nanoparticles, and lipid nanoparticles, have been studied [89]. It is important to note that nanoparticles offer a small size and enhanced drug loading capacity, ease of functionalization, simple penetration capabilities, and improved retention inside the targeted tissue, which have significantly improved the diagnostics and therapeutics of various cancers. These nanomedicines use passive targeting, active targeting, and triggered release techniques. In the recent era, nanotechnology has resolved several complicated issues in the fields of science and technology. It may also open a new window in the biomedical realm focusing on personalized medicine. To combat the negative effects of cancer treatment, it is crucial to transport therapeutic medication molecules to the targeted tumor site. Numerous efforts have been made over the past 20 years to enable site-specific cancer therapy to develop drug delivery systems based on nanomaterials. Theranostics is a recently developed nanotechnology that describes a method of combining medicinal, diagnostic, and imaging methods into a single unit. Doxil is the first nanomedicine approved by the US Food and Drug Administration (FDA). About a dozen nanomedicines based on polymeric micelles are currently undergoing clinical trials for various cancers. The latter is particularly attractive for delivering chemotherapeutic drugs with low water solubility. Integrating therapy with non-invasive imaging is extremely valuable for better understanding the *in vivo* fate of nanomedicines, pharmacokinetics, target-site

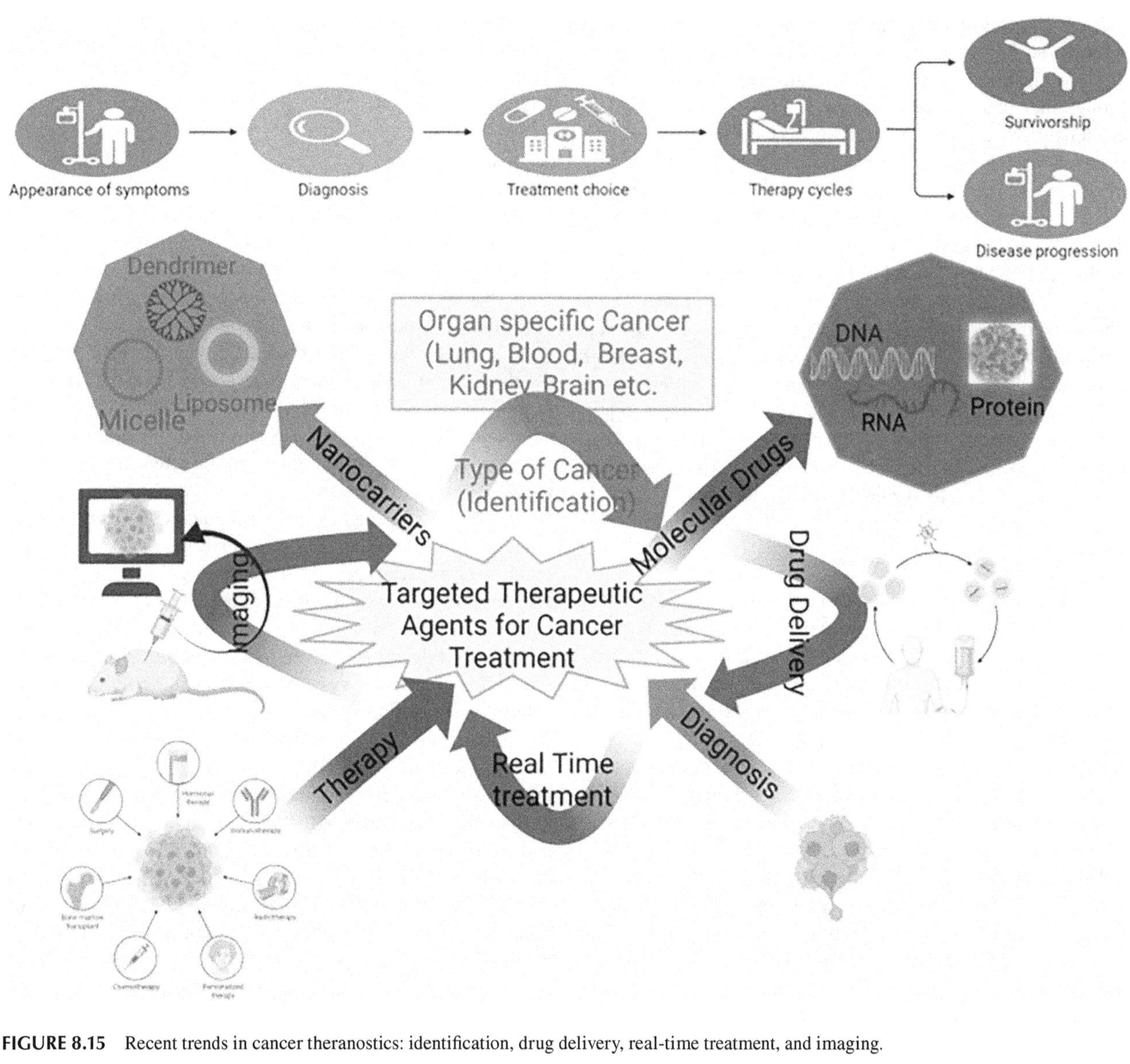

FIGURE 8.15 Recent trends in cancer theranostics: identification, drug delivery, real-time treatment, and imaging.

accumulation, and therapeutic efficacy. Furthermore, these nanomaterials' outstanding biocompatibility, biodegradability, and multifunctional uses for biosensing, bioimaging, diagnostics, and therapies have expanded their applications in a vast range of biomedical applications [90]. Following are the details of the organic cancer theranostics platform.

8.10.1.1 Liposome Nanoparticles

In cancer theranostics, liposomes, a type of biomimetic nanoparticle, are undoubtedly the most well-known and adaptable lipid-based nanoweapon for cancer theranostics. These are generally made of concentric lipid bilayers that self-assemble around an aqueous core domain. They have proved to be effective nanocarriers for the delivery of a variety of drugs by encasing hydrophilic ones inside the liposomal aqueous core domain (or on the bilayer membrane surface) and hydrophobic ones inside the liposomal bilayer. These carriers offer many advantages, including biocompatibility, biodegradability, ease of synthesis, sustained release of the therapeutics, low toxicity, and the ability to incorporate both hydrophilic and hydrophobic chemotherapeutic compounds. Additionally, the liposome surfaces can be tailored for targeted cancer therapy [91]. Liposomes can accumulate in cancerous tissues passively through the enhanced permeability and retention (EPR) effect and actively by specifically targeting a cancer cell or an angiogenic marker. Liposomal therapeutic agents with multimodality imaging make it highly impressive for individual monitoring of *in vivo* cancer and pharmacokinetics of therapeutic drugs. This platform also predicts the therapeutic efficacies of the drugs in combination with the useful information collected by imaging techniques. Numerous liposomal medications are now used in clinical trials or have received clinical approval due to their numerous benefits. Liposomes can transport small and large molecules and have also been investigated for the delivery of various diagnostic agents, such as ^{64}Cu and ^{14}C isotopes, quantum dots (QDs), gadolinium (Gd)–based contrast agents, etc. It is expected that liposomes as a theranostic tool for cancer patients will soon be applied in clinical trials.

8.10.1.2 Lipid Nanoparticles

In cancer therapy, lipid nanoparticles (LNPs) remain one of the most promising platforms for cancer theranostics because of their biocompatibility and scalability. Lipidic nanocarriers have unique benefits that set them apart from other nanoformulations. Recent investigations have shown that lipidic theranostic nanomedicines are a promising and prospective strategy for increasing the efficacy of cancer treatment to a benchmark level. LNPs can penetrate the vascular endothelial gaps of tumors and deliver chemotherapy drugs to tumor tissue. In one of the studies, it has been found that DiR'; DiIC18(7) (1,1'-Dioctadecyl-3,3,3',3'-tetramethylindotricarbocyanine iodide) is weakly fluorescent in water but highly fluorescent and quite photostable when incorporated into membranes. The sulfonate groups incorporated into this DiI analog improves water solubility. It has an extremely high extinction coefficient and short excited-state lifetimes (~1 ns) in lipid environments. Once applied to cells, the dye diffuses laterally within the plasma membrane. Dyes have the ability of enhanced tissue penetration, owing to an elongated absorption wavelength for superior antitumor activity. The size of the nanocarrier strongly depends on the targeted organ and type of imaging. For the purpose of sensitive and specific tumor detection, Zhang et al. [92] developed a fluorinated nanoemulsion. These nanoemulsions showed dramatically improved fluorescence imaging signals. Their theranostic method was extremely effective at identifying a particular type of tumor tracking the possible in vivo fate of the nanoemulsion and providing highly effective photodynamic therapy. Zheng et al. developed a nanoemulsion with a porphyrin shell that allows the encapsulation and stabilization of the oil core, resulting in a monodisperse nanostructure for imaging and phototherapy. A non-invasive and real-time monitoring of drug delivery for an orthopedic prostate tumor model was presented by Lin et al. by utilizing LNPs loaded with dye and siRNA. Liang et al. developed a theranostic nanoplatform based on a relatively smaller (<20 nm) iron oxide loaded with porphyrin-grafted lipid nanoparticles (Fe_3O_4@PGLNPs), demonstrating an excellent photodynamic effect against HT-29 cancer cells *in vitro* [93]. LNPs are exclusively used in cancer theranostics agents for curing different types of tumors due to their negligible toxicity, multifunctional potential, and functionalization flexibility, which helps them cross different physiological barriers.

8.10.1.3 Protein Nanoparticles

In cancer theranostics, scientists extensively explored protein NPs because of their natural availability and compatibility with physiology. Proteins belong to the biological molecules with distinctive properties and perspectives, making them amenable to biomedicine and materials science. Due to the amphiphilicity nature of a protein, it interacts favorably with the drug and solvent, making it an ideal choice for NP preparation. The natural origin of a protein makes it biodegradable, metabolizable, and readily susceptible to changing surfaces to facilitate drug attachment and targeted ligand attachment. Albumin has been recognized as a potential carrier for delivering imaging/anticancer medicines to tumor microenvironments after the FDA's clinical approval of Abraxane (paclitaxel bound to albumin). Patients had a better response rate with Abraxane than with conventional paclitaxel (Taxol), which increased progression-free survival with the least amount of side effects. Eventually, albumin was developed into a flexible delivery system for medications with poor water solubility, such as rapamycin (water solubility is 2.50 mg/mL). A clinical trial involving albumin-bound rapamycin ABI-009 (Nab-sirolimus) in patients with genetically confirmed Leigh or Leigh-like syndrome total bilirubin $\leq 1.5 \times$ upper limit of normal (ULN) mg/Dl (ABI-009) was conducted to treat non-hematologic cancers. There are many albumin-based NPs currently undergoing clinical studies. Human serum albumin (HSA) caps are among other intriguing possibilities, since the human liver supplies a plentiful amount of the same (35–50 mg/mL). To build effective theranostics, HSA has been investigated as a natural transporter of superparamagnetic iron oxide, organic/inorganic oxides, IR780, IR825, and chlorin e6 (Ce6). NIR probes like IR825 (a near-infrared dye), after encapsulation into nanoparticles, may be useful for cancer photothermal and photodynamic treatmeent; indocyanine green (ICG) and IR780 are becoming more popular because of their ability to penetrate relatively deep tissue and their low autofluorescence interference. A recent publication noted that IR825 and gadolinium (Gd) were encapsulated in HSA to produce HAS-Gd-IR825 complexes for dual imaging-guided photothermal treatment (PTT) to prevent lymphatic metastases after surgery. Yu et al. developed gemcitabine and pheophorbide-a (P@)–loaded human serum albumin (HSA) (P@-Gem-HSA) to create multifunctional nanoparticles for the treatment of lymphatic pancreatic ductal adenocarcinoma (PDAC) metastases, which constitutes 90% of pancreatic cancers, the fourth leading cause of cancer-related deaths in the world.

8.10.1.4 Metal–Organic Frameworks

In cancer theranostics, metal–organic frameworks (MOFs), a fascinating and intriguing class of porous hybrid coordination polymers with metal ions or ion clusters serving as nodes and organic ligands serving as linkers, have been synthesized and utilized for a variety of applications, including gas storage, catalysis, sensing, biomedical applications, and cancer theranostics, addressing the drawbacks of conventional cancer treatment or the inability of therapeutic drugs to target the tumor sites without damage to healthy tissues and organs. In order to synthesize structurally diverse MOFs (specific physical and chemical properties), metal (such as d- and f-block elements) and organic linkers (such as carboxylates and nitrogen heterocycles) can be varied, which leads to the synthesis of thousands of MOFs with distinctive characteristics. The development of nanoscale MOFs (nMOFs) presented potential applications in photodynamic therapy (PDT), drug delivery, and imaging and has led to considerable contemplation of their potential as therapeutic platforms in oncology and other fields of medicine, as shown in Figure 8.16. Their remarkable characteristics, which include easy surface functionalization, structural diversity, high surface area, enormous porosity, tunable energy gap, tailored synthesis, excellent biocompatibility, and a variety of physicochemical properties, make MOFs suitable candidates for cancer theranostics. A major reason for the failure of conventional cancer treatment is the inability of therapeutic drugs to reach the target tumor sites without damaging healthy tissues and organs. Due to their exceptional qualities, MOFs not only enhance the outcomes of conventional therapies like radiation therapy (RT) and chemotherapy but also benefit the recently developed phototherapy methods [94].

Moreover, MOFs are suitable materials for imaging-guided cancer theranostics, as they can codeliver various bioactive substances, including medications, enzymes, genes, and gases. Zn-based MOFs have also been reported as nanocarriers. Wang et al. developed a chiral Zn-based MOF using zinc ions and achiral 5,5′,5″-(1,3,5-triazine-2,4,6-triyl)tris(azanediyl)triisophthalate (TATAT) ligands for the delivery of the anticancer medication 5-fluorouracil (5-FU). The experimental results indicated high drug loading capacity and slow release of the loaded drug, with a complete delivery time of about 1 week. A multifunctional tumor-targeting MOF nanocomposite with fluorescence (FL) imaging, MRI, and controlled drug release has been reported for cancer therapy. The targeting group folic acid (FA) and 5-fluorouracil agent were decorated on the surface of 5-FU-loaded Fe-MIL-53-NH_2 as an outer layer through an amidation reaction to give Fe-MIL-53-NH_2-FA-5-FAM/5-FU. In this approach, Fe-MIL-53-NH_2 was utilized to encapsulate the drug and magnetic resonance imaging feature. NH_2-MIL-53 (Fe): molecular formula, $C_8H_6FeNO_5$; CAS no. 1291088–77–1; appearance, dark-red crystals; storage, store at room temperature or 4°C in dry state.

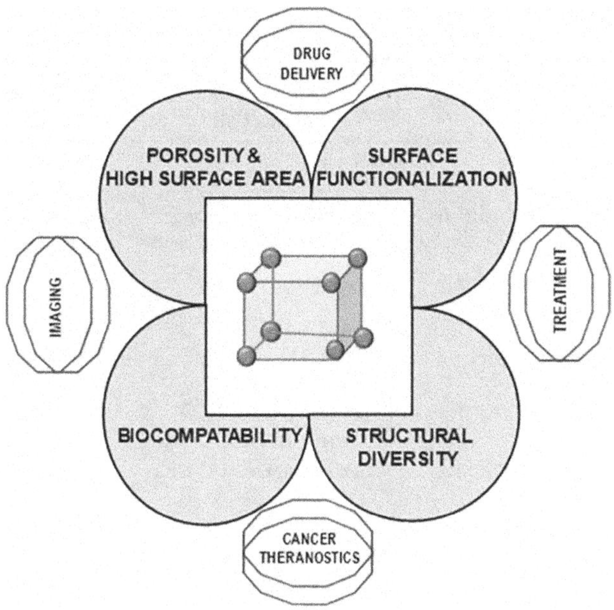

FIGURE 8.16 Schematic illustration of MOFs showing different applications for cancer diagnosis and treatment.

Liu and coworkers [95] have synthesized UiO-66-NH_2 with controlled particle sizes of 20–200 nm. Later, the MOF was modified with FA, and the fluorescence imaging agent 5-carboxyfluorescein (5-FAM) is a green fluorescent reagent used for in situ labeling of peptides, proteins, and nucleotides, known as UiO-66-NH_2-FA-5-FAM/5-FU, a multifunctional theranostic nanoplatform with FL imaging. The *in vivo* studies indicated that UiO-66-NH_2-FA-5-FAM/5-FU could be accumulated in the tumor and display more vital antitumor efficiency due to long-term drug release. In one study, Cherkasov et al. synthesized an MOF through antibodies to selectively absorb HER2/neu-positive cancer cells [96]. A biomimetic MOF, Hf-DBP-Fe, was synthesized for effective cancer therapy utilizing a synergistic combination of radiation and an immune checkpoint blockade [97]. Chen et al. synthesized folic acid–modified hafnium-based manganoporphyrin metal–organic framework nanoparticles (MnTCPP-Hf-FA MOF NPs) to enhance radiotherapy and prevent postoperative recurrence [98]. Table 8.4 shows some representative MOFs for cancer therapy.

8.10.2 Carbon-Based Nanomaterials in Cancer Theranostics

One of the most promising fields of biomedical sciences with the fastest growth is nanotechnology, which has been cleverly applied to unravel various biological challenges. In recent

TABLE 8.4
Some Common MOFs for Cancer Therapy

MOF	Active Unit	Therapeutic Method	Model	Administration Type	Ref.
Hf-DBB-Ru	Hf and Ru	Radiotherapy	Colorectal tumors in mouse models/ MC38 tumor-bearing C57BL/6 mice	Intratumoral	[99]
W18@Hf12-DBB-Ir	Hf12 (SBUs), Ir bridging ligands, W-polyoxometalates	Radiotherapy	Murine colorectal adenocarcinoma models of MC38 tumor–bearing C57BL/6 mice and CT26 tumor–bearing BALB/c mice	Intravenously	[100]
Hf-DBP-Fe	Hf, H2DBP, Fe	Radiotherapy	MC38 cells	Intraperitoneal	[97]
MnTCPP-Hf-FA MOF NPs	TCPP-Hf, Mn	Radiotherapy	B16-F10 cells, melanomatumor	Intravenous	[98]
DOX-loaded MOFs	Zr4+ metal–organic framework nanoparticles, DOX	Chemotherapy	MDA-MB-231 breast cancer cells	—	[99]
Fe-MIL-53-NH2-FA-5-FAM/5-FU	5-fluorouracil, Fe, BDC-NH_2	Chemotherapy	MGC-803 and HASMC, mice-bearing glioblastoma	Intratumoral injection	[101]
Fe_3O_4/IRMOF-3/FA	Fe_3O_4, $Zn(NO_3)_2{\cdot}6H_2O$, NH_2-H_2BDC	Chemotherapy	HeLa cells and normal NIH3T3 cells	—	[102]
Zr-UiO-66	Zr-UiO-66, DOX	Chemotherapy	BALB/c mice, breast cancer cells, and L929 fibroblasts	Intravenous injection	[103]
DOx/FA/CDs/ IRMOF-3	DOX, CDs, IRMOF-3	Chemotherapy	L929 (murine fibroblast) and human cervix adenocarcinoma (HeLa) cell lines	—	[104]
Fluorescein/ZIF-8	2-methyl imidazolate and zinc ions, fluorescein	Chemotherapy	MCF-7 cell	—	[105]
UiO-66 and UiO-67	Terephthalic acid (BDC), $ZrCl_4$, 4,4′-biphenyldicarboxylic acid (BPDC)	Chemotherapy	HSC-3 (human oral squamous carcinoma) and U-87 MG (human glioblastoma grade IV; astrocytoma)	—	[106]
Selenium-polymer@ ZIF8	2-methylimidazole, DOX@ P$Zn(NO_3)_2{\cdot}6H_2O$	Chemotherapy	MDAMB-231 cells breast carcinoma cell line (MDA-MB-231)	—	[107]
Cisplatin/doxorubicin/ NMOF	Cisplatin (14.4 wt %) and doxorubicin ZnII (p-phenyleneethynylene) (OPE) dicarboxylate linker	Chemotherapy	HeLa cells	—	[108]
Ti-TBPMOF	Ti–oxo chain (SBUs), 5,10,15,20-tetra(p-benzoato) porphyrin (TBP) ligands, Ti3+	Photodynamic therapy	CT26 tumor–bearing BALB/c mice	Intratumorally	[109]
Porphyrinic Zr-MOF	Porphyrinic Zr metal–organic framework, MnO_2, apatinib	Photodynamic therapy	4T1 cells or mouse macrophage RAW 264.7 cells	Subcutaneous and intravenous	[110]
Zr-TBB MOF	Zr, 5,10,15,20-tetra(p-benzoato) bacteriochlorin (TBB) ligands	Photodynamic therapy	Breast and colon cancers, 4T1 murine breast carcinoma cells, subcutaneous 4T1-bearing BALB/c mice, and murine colon carcinoma MC38-bearing C57Bl/6 mice	Subcutaneous	[111]
ZnP@Hf-QC	Zinc phthalocyanine, $HfCl_4$, H_2QC	Photodynamic therapy	CT26 cells, CT26 tumors on BALB/c mice, and MC38 tumors on C57BL/6 mice	Subcutaneous	[112]
MOF199	Cu(II) carboxylate Ce, benzene-1,3,5-tricarboxylate (BTC), $Cu(NO_3)_2$	Photodynamic therapy	HepG2 cells and NIH-3T3, HepG2 cells, and 3T3	Intravenous injection	[113]

years, carbon-based nanomaterials have significantly increased the detection and treatment of cancer and neurodegenerative diseases. Various research groups have concentrated on the development of carbon-based nanomaterials, such as fullerene, carbon nanotubes, graphene, and derivatives, for biomedical applications, which has opened the way for their application in the emerging field of cancer theranostics. Carbon-based nanomaterials exhibit several extraordinary properties, such as high surface area, tunable pore structure, and nonreactive and easy surface functionalization, making them suitable for their biological application, in particular, for cancer diagnosis, which, in turn, opens up a new avenue for improved therapeutic strategies [114]. In addition to this, these nanomaterials possess outstanding biocompatibility, biodegradability, and multifunctional uses for biosensing, bioimaging, diagnostics, and therapies, which have boosted their potential for biomedical applications [115].

8.10.2.1 Carbon Nanotubes

In one of the studies, carbon nanotubes (CNTs) have been shown to be a promising material for drug delivery. In this study, CNTs are loaded with ginsenoside Rg3 and fabricated Rg3-CNT, and the effect was studied on triple-negative breast cancer (TNBC). This study has established that Rg3-CNT is a potential therapeutic strategy for the immunotherapy of TNBC. M13 phage-functionalized CNT (M13-CNT) was explored for the fluorescence imaging of targeted tumors even at low concentrations. In another work, a targeted M13 virus–stabilized CNT probe was utilized for the detection of the human ovarian tumor by Ghosh et al. with a high signal-to-noise ratio. Results were compared with those with visible and NIR dyes, and it was found that the M13 virus–stabilized CNT probe can detect a tumor in the submillimeter range. A fluorescence imaging system for ovarian cancer was developed by Ceppi et al. utilizing single-walled carbon nanotubes (SWCNTs) conjugated to M13 bacteriophage, which carries a peptide-specific protein [116]. The developed system helps in intraoperative tumor debulking in real time. There was an improved survival rate in animals when treated with CNT fluorescence image surgery compared to conventional surgery. Lee and colleagues developed CNTs coupled with a platelet-derived aptamer, and the result showed a significant change in NIR fluorescence due to conformal aptamer change. Zhang et al. synthesized a nanocomposite comprising CNTs and CDs for dual-modal imaging of cancer cells. It was observed that the drug loading capabilities of CNTs depend on several factors, including the material's nature, the medium's pH, the free sites of the material, and the nature of the drug. Due to their substantial surface areas, SWCNTs have demonstrated a higher drug-loading capacity than MWCNTs. Peptides having aromatic content showed high binding affinity toward CNTs due to π–π interaction [117]. Yang et al. proved that the functionalized SWCNTs as DOX carriers are useful for treating MCF-7 cells. Results demonstrated that, when compared to CNT-COOH and CNT-PEG, SWCNT-PEG-PEI had the most substantial antitumor impact and drug delivery capacity. Fluorescence-based research and flow cytometry investigations show that SWCNT-PEG-PEI is internalized more readily, promoting the apoptosis that leads to tumor cell death due to increased dispersibility and a stronger affinity for cancer cells. CNTs are exclusively used for the pH-responsive release of cancer drugs as they are very susceptible to the acidic environment, making them a promising candidate for drug therapy [118]. Lu et al. functionalized CNTs with poly(acrylic acid) and used them for the FA for DOX drug loading. It has been found that DOX-loaded CNTs showed higher efficiency when compared to free DOX; this could be due to hydrogen bonding and π–π stacking. The developed platform serves as an efficient tool for cancer theranostics.

8.10.2.2 Carbon Dots

Owing to their small sizes, carbon dots (CDs) are particularly promising since they can target cancerous tumors with an increased permeability and retention (EPR) impact. The urinary system can readily eliminate CDs to reduce *in vivo* toxicity. Additionally, CDs have shown to be a unique platform for delivering different therapeutic agents. CDs are widely used for various applications, such as chemotherapy, photodynamic therapy (PDT), photothermal therapy (PTT), gene therapy, and radiation therapy.

The quantitative cellular accumulation of free CDs and CDs with targeting ligands on cancerous (MDAMB and A-549) and healthy (MDCK) cells showed that diseased cells were more effectively treated than healthy cells. Madin–Darby canine kidney (MDCK) cells are a model mammalian cell line used in biomedical research. MDCK cells are used for a wide variety of cell biology. The Madin–Darby canine kidney (MDCK) cell line is widely used as an epithelial cell model in studies ranging from viral infection to environmental pollutants and vaccines production.

Mesenchymal stem cell–conditioned medium promotes MDA-MB-231 cell migration and inhibits A549 cell migration by regulating insulin receptor in humans. The ligand-attached CDs that ingested cancer cells demonstrated target-selective endocytosis via receptor-mediated therapy. Additionally, the tumor's uptake of nano-sized CDs may be significantly influenced by the enhanced permeability and retention effect [119]. Photosensitizing properties of CDs have been extensively explored for NIR light triggered photodynamic therapy alone or in combination with photosensitizing agents, such as photoporphyrin, zinc phthalocyanine, etc., which are responsible for the production of reactive oxygen species (ROS) for the treatment of cancer cells [120,121].

The targeted cancer cells can be hyperthermally killed by NIR-responsive photothermal treatments, like PDT. Numerous carbon-based nanomaterials tend to absorb NIR light from the electromagnetic spectrum and transform it into heat, which thermally kills cancerous cells [122]. For example, under various excitation wavelengths, carbonized polydopamine has shown multiple fluorescence emissions along with NIR-responsive photothermal conversion and heat, which is responsible for the destruction of cancerous cells. CD-based hybrid systems are extensively explored for PDT, PTT, and pH- or NIR-responsive drug release all at once. Synergistic cancer therapy is made possible by such a multipurpose intelligent delivery system. For instance, CD nanogels with integrated PEG–chitosan have demonstrated PTT against tumor cells and dual pH- and NIR-light-responsive drug release [123]. Mauro et al. developed an efficient protocol for one-pot synthesis of N, S doped CDs having a high NIR photothermal conversion efficiency and efficient ROS production in the cancer cell. S-CD triggers more ROS generation in cancer cells when compared to a healthy cell. The NIR laser is responsible for enhancing the oxidative stress in cancer cells at a moderate power density and for opening up a range of possibilities for real biomedical applications. In another work, [124] NIR-responsive core–shell hybrid nanocomposite as a smart theranostic platform based on hyaluronic acid–PLA and hydrophobic carbon dots (HA-g-PLA/HCDs) was designed to selectively recognize cancer cells overexpressing CD44 receptors and NIR-triggered chemo-phototherapy of solid tumors.

Moreover, combining the anticancer drug with NIR-triggered photothermal treatment may utilize the potential benefits of carbon dots, which may be overcome with specific resistance to apoptosis, eliciting alternative RCD routes, such as necroptosis. Nicosia et al. developed a hybrid material CD bearing biotin and a high amount of irinotecan (CDs-PEG-BT/IT) for controlled release and imaging of MDA-MB231 and MCF-7 cancer cells and killing them by photothermal and chemotherapeutic means. The results indicate that CDs-PEG-BT/IT is a safe and potentially effective candidate as a theranostic agent in IG-PTT of breast cancer. Geng et al. have synthesized nitrogen and oxygen co-doped CDs with an excellent optical response to NIR lasers [125]. These synthesized doped CDs showed excellent therapeutic efficacy and bioimaging ability, with 100% tumor destruction, without affecting the healthy cell.

8.10.2.3 Graphene

Graphene and its derivatives have been explored for biological and biomedical applications, owing to their high surface areas, easy functionalization, and biocompatibility, which render them essential for high drug loading capability and make them potential candidates as drug carriers, in imaging, and in drug delivery systems.

Chen et al. have synthesized an rGO/PEG/ICG nanosystem which is made up of the functionalization of reduced graphene oxide (rGO) with polyethylene glycol (PEG) and indocyanine green (ICG) and later used as a dual-modality contrast agent. It was observed that the rGO/PEG/ICG nanosystem was sustained for a longer time in *in vivo* and was capable of targeting tumors. Mirrahimi et al. used GO for anchoring superparamagnetic iron oxides (SPIOs) and AuNPs adapted with phase-change material (PCM) for stimulus-based drug release. The study also reveals that the synergistic effect of all, like NIR absorbance of GO, MRI contrast of SPIOs, AuNPs for X-ray attenuation, and PCM for thermosensitive features, makes this platform ideally suited for synergistic thermo-chemotherapy in a controllable drug release. Graphene has the potential for use in PET, imaging, and dual-modality MRI/fluorescence imaging [126]. A novel platform consisting of GO with PEGylated and oxidized sodium alginate was used to load the anticancer drug paclitaxel to get a synergistic chemotherapy/PTT/PDT effect. Yang et al. bound a molecular beacon (MB) on the surface of GO, which resulted in the enhanced fluorescence quenching of cy5 when compared to the self-quenching effect [127]. The nanocomplex bound to miRNA-21, and the fluorescence response of cy5, was restored. With this technique, the fluorescence intensity was enhanced while the imaging's fluorescence background was diminished. The synthesized nanocomplexes showed excellent imaging capability for numerous tumor cells, as shown by *in vitro* and *in vivo* studies, suggesting that GO-based nanomaterials had promising potential in cancer diagnostics. Graphene was also explored for breast tumor PTT and photoacoustic imaging (PAI). In this context, polydopamine (PDA) was bound to rGO, and then the diagnostic reagent ICG was loaded for PTT. It was found that PDA improved the nanosystem's water solubility and biocompatibility, which, in turn, quenched rGO's fluorescence and improved the effectiveness of PAI. The ICG-PDA-rGO was processed with higher sensitivity and PAI ability than other control groups, according to in vivo imaging investigations. The endogenous contrast agent hemoglobin also allowed for the clear observation of the vascular tissue in tumor tissue. The aforementioned findings suggested that rGO-based nanomaterials could be employed in PAI for tumor diagnostics as well as PTT to increase the effectiveness of cancer treatment. Graphene quantum dots (GQDs) show strong absorption in the NIR-II region. Liu et al. reported 9T-GQDs as a breast, cervical, and lung cancer imaging tool utilizing phenol as a precursor [128]. The photoluminescence (PL) quantum yield of the 9T-GQDs was 16.67%, almost 1.8 times more than that of ordinary GQDs. The synthesized 9T-GQDs are able to reach the cytoplasm of the 4T1 cancer cell by penetration of the cell membrane to induce continuous fluorescence.

8.10.2.4 Fullerene

A *fullerene* is a third allotrope of carbon with fused rings of five to seven carbon atoms joined by single and double bonds to form a closed or partially closed mesh [129]. Fullerene exhibits a unique physicochemical characteristic, making it a promising candidate for several industrial and medical applications. Pristine fullerenes are insoluble in water, limiting their use in biological applications. The surface modification of fullerenes has opened up a new horizon for pharmaceutical and biomedical applications due to their water solubility after modification [207]. Furthermore, fullerenes have drawn much interest in biomedical applications due to their small diameters, large specific surface areas, and high reactivity. Many water-soluble fullerene derivatives (C_{70}, C_{80}, C_{94}) with various carbon atoms have also been studied to utilize their small sizes, shapes, and molecular topologies for various biological applications. For the cancer theranostics application, fullerenes can be functionalized to make them have distinct physicochemical characteristics, such as biocompatibility and water solubility. Additionally, the fullerene cage functions as a unique 3D scaffold and may be utilized to attach a variety of drugs to it covalently.

Fullerene is a promising nanomaterial for cancer imaging, PDT, and photo/thermoacoustic-assisted theranostics due to its intrinsic optical and thermodynamic qualities. Due to their distinctive physical–chemical characteristics, fullerenes have attracted a lot of attention in the field of cancer theranostics. Notably, fullerene can act as a potent antineoplastic agent due to its anticancer action and sensitization effect on cancer cells. Fullerene also acts as a free radical scavenger and can be employed as an antioxidant. It is interesting to note that metal atoms can also be added to fullerene to create metallofullerene, which inherits the combined properties of the carbon cages and internal metal and has promising potential for use as contrasts in magnetic resonance imaging (MRI), X-ray, radiotracers, and anticancer agents [130]. Though, with chemical modification, fullerene can be tailored for specific applications for cancer, there are some intrinsic challenges associated with fullerenes, such as intrinsic toxicity and solubility in water. In this context, various research groups tried numerous approaches, such as modification of fullerene with water-soluble functional groups (hydroxyl, carboxyl, and amino groups)/polymers or grafting of the biocompatible molecule through covalent bonding. Hence, owing to the unique advantages of biocompatible fullerene, it has been extensively explored as a potential platform for targeted drug delivery. To cure pancreatic cancer, Serda et al. created Sweet-C60 (highly water-soluble hexakis-glucosamine fullerene derivative), a novel targeted anticancer drug that mostly accumulated in the nucleus of pancreatic stellate cells (PSCs). It was observed that a glycoconjugate of fullerene could improve the cancer-targeting characteristics since the proliferation of tumors required the energy associated with glucose metabolism.

Wang et al. synthesized an amphiphilic fullerene derivative (C_{60}-Dex-NH_2) to deliver siRNA into cancerous cells to address the lysosomal degradation of RNAi. The results showed that the synthesized fullerene derivative promoted the lysosomal entrapment and caused the destruction of the lysosomal membrane by triggering controllable ROS under visible light irradiation. Through binding to the MYH9 protein, Zhou et al. created a class of C_{70} fullerene derivatives (C_{70}-EDA) modified with multiple ethylenediamine (EDA) moieties that might prevent cancer cell migration, alter intracellular MYH9 distribution, and prevent EMT. C_{70}-EDA treatment inhibited cancer cell migration and reversed the EMT process in A549 cells in vitro. Li et al. modified gadofullerene with β-alanine (GF-Ala) to develop a strategy against tumor immunity [131]. This study revealed that immunosuppressive TME (ITM) is crucial for successful immunotherapy. This strategy could induce macrophages to exert an inhibitory tumor growth to convert to tumor-supportive M1 type from M2 type. From the preceding discussion, it can be concluded that judicial modification of fullerene is required to explore the excellent biocompatibility and significant antitumor activity, which can open up the horizon of materials for the broad application prospects in cancer therapy. Table 8.5 summarizes the use of graphene and its derivatives for cancer imaging and theranostic applications.

8.10.3 Engineered Inorganic Nanoparticles in Cancer Theranostics

Due to their unique physicochemical characteristics, inorganic nanoparticles such as platinum, gold, silica, palladium, silver, iron oxides, zinc oxide, and rare earth oxides have been widely used for a number of biomedical applications, including cancer theranostics, nucleic acid delivery, bioimaging, drug administration, and biosensing [159].

Green chemistry is a promising approach that can be used for the natural design of metallic or nonmetallic nanoparticles. Many advantages are associated with this technique, including their eco-friendly setups (which ignore harmful chemicals), simplicity, robustness, time savings, and use of safe solvents, especially water. This green approach uses bioreducing agents comprising plant extracts, bacteria, algae, etc., in place of hazardous chemical catalysts. Because of these benefits, such safe, natural nanoparticles are highly desirable for cancer theranostics.

In many parts of the world, various research teams are utilizing nanoparticles of silver and gold synthesized by a biological process that can work as one of the ideal candidates for cancer theranostics applications. AuNPs and AgNPs produced through biosynthesis have the potential to be used in the *in vitro* and *in vivo* delivery of anticancer medications.

8.10.3.1 Quantum Dots in Cancer Theranostics

Over the past few decades, researchers have paid significant attention to multimodal medication delivery systems. Due to their distinct physiochemical properties, quantum dots (QDs) are among the most effective tools utilized in theranostic applications for diagnosis and therapy [160]. QDs are semiconductor crystals in the 2–10 nm nanoscale range and show emission from visible to near-infrared wavelengths along with outstanding light stability [161]. The best QDs for cell labeling and cancer biomarker detection are those with intense photoluminescence and high molar extinction coefficient values. Symmetrical broad-absorption spectra and narrow-emission spectra distinguish QDs.

High-stability protein–QD nanohybrids in biological fluids are essential for bioimaging applications. QDs can combine with proteins by either physical trapping or chemical interaction. For instance, gemcitabine-loaded human serum albumin nanoparticles have successfully had graphene QDs attached to their surfaces (NPs) [162]. Hyaluronic acid and graphene QDs–functionalized human serum albumin nanoparticles have been reported for bioimaging and targeted delivery of gemcitabine to pancreatic cancer [162]. In a different work, spray-dried single bovine serum albumin (BSA) nanospheres were used to physically encapsulate several CdTe/CdS QDs of various sizes to create multifluorescent nanospheres which can be achieved by altering the QDs' size. When the QD-BSA nanospheres comprised a high molar ratio of QD:BSA, the fluorescence emission was reduced by 4% after being continuously irradiated (at 365 nm) for 1 h. These findings demonstrated the potential of QD-BSA nanospheres for long-term fluorescence observation in biomedical research fields. Song et al. synthesized a nanocomposite of phosphorus QDs with Bi@RP-PEG-DOX and bismuthene, which showed an effective platform for photothermal and photodynamic effects and controlled release of the drug in the presence of NIR-II irradiation. Zein–ZnS QD nanohybrids could be used to deliver drugs like 5-fluorouracil. Girija Aswathy et al. examined the impact of these nanohybrids on the viability of L929 and MCF-7 cancer cells to ascertain their biocompatibility. For zein-QDs and ordinary zein nanoparticles, cell viability was found to be above 90 and 80%, respectively, which showed that they were compatible. Cell viability was considerably decreased when the cells were exposed to 5-FU-loaded zein-QDs. Furthermore, the zein–ZnS QD NPs' fluorescence emission demonstrated that they had successfully entered the cells. Shao et al. synthesized biodegradable titanium nitride quantum dots (Ti_2N QDs), which showed excellent photothermal conversion efficiency under NIR [163]. The prepared material showed excellent biocompatibility, photoacoustic effect, and efficiency of photothermal therapy (PTT). Another study indicated multistage QD nanocarriers by joining silica-coated QDs to the surface of gelatin NPs to create 100 nm nanohybrids, among other intriguing methods to improve tumor penetration. In the tumor microenvironment, the increased matrix of metalloproteinases dissolved the gelatin core after extravasations into the tumor tissue, producing incredibly tiny 10 nm QDs that effectively penetrated the tumor parenchyma. In general, utilizing proteins to hybridize QDs can be a viable method to extend their time in the body, boost

TABLE 8.5

Graphene and Its Derivative–Based Nanosystems for Cancer Imaging and Theranostics

System	Cancer Cell	Experimental Model (*In Vitro/In Vivo*)	Main Finding	Ref.
Graphene oxide	Murine lung metastasis model of breast cancer	*In vitro/in vivo*	Enhanced drug delivery efficiency in cbgLuc-MDA-MB-231 metastatic sites was demonstrated. It can serve as a useful tool for early metastasis detection and targeted delivery of therapeutics.	[132]
	B16F0 melanoma tumors using a mouse model	*In vitro/in vivo*	This work shows a nanocomposite as a theranostic nanomedicine for fluorescent imaging and combined nanomaterial-mediated photodynamic therapeutic and photothermal therapy for clinical cancer treatments.	[133]
	Bel-7402, SMMC-7721, HepG2 cell line hepatocellular carcinoma	*In vitro*	This work provides a multifunctional drug delivery system that has the ability to target hepatocarcinoma cells, is pH-responsive, and can be efficiently loaded with a number of therapeutic agents for biomedical applications.	[134]
	MCF-7 cells	*In vitro*	Photo-responsive ICG-loaded HArGO nanosheets could serve as a potential theranostic nanoplatform for image-guided and synergistic photothermal antitumor therapy.	[135]
	KB cell–bearing nude mice	*In vitro/in vivo*	This provides an effective tool to visualize intracellular low-level miRNAs and to help in understanding the role of miRNAs in cellular processes.	[136]
	PC-3 cells prostate cancer	*In vitro*	This work evaluated interactions between halogenated amino acid–tagged fluorescent NDIs and flat aromatic carbon materials.	[137]
rGO-$MnFe_2O_4$-PEG	4T1 tumor	*In vitro/in vivo*	Multimodal imaging using nanomaterials in a single platform can provide exact information, including the tumor location and size. This study also promotes the biomedical applications of nanographene-based nanocomposites.	[138]
$CoFe_2O_4$/GO cobalt ferrite/graphene oxide	Cancer cell	*iIn vitro*	The prepared material showed great potential as an effective multifunctional nanoplatform for magnetic resonance imaging and controlled drug delivery for simultaneous cancer diagnosis and chemotherapy.	[139]
GO/$ZnFe_2O_4$/UCNP graphene oxide/Zn ferrite/upconversion luminescence nanoparticles	HeLa cell	*In vitro/in vivo*	Diagnosis to therapy realized the integration of imaging and high antitumor efficiency. It provides a feasible strategy to solve the main problems in current light-triggered theranostics.	[140]
GO-CD/Fe@C graphene oxide–cyclodextrin, carbon-coated iron NPs	MDA-MB-231 breast cancer cells	*In vitro*	The material was used for potential magnetic-directed drug delivery and as a diagnostic agent. The finding highlights the multifunctional GO-CD/Fe@C nanohybrid for magnetic-sensing anticancer drug delivery to tumor cells.	[141]
MNP/GO/chitosan chitosan-grafted graphene oxide/magnetic nanoparticle	CD44-expressing breast cancer cells, MCF-7 human breast cancer, and L-929 mouse fibroblast cells	*In vitro*	This work highlighted cancer treatment for transformative theranostic technologies combining imaging with drug delivery.	[142]
Fullerene	HCT 116 colon cancer	*In vitro*	Fullerene was used for high-resolution fluorescent imaging of tumor sites in vivo and resulted in a significant regression of HCT-116 tumors.	[143]
Fullerene derivative (C_{60}-Dex-NH2)	MDA-MB-231 cells	*In vitro/in vivo*	This work presented a novel photosensitive siRNA delivery carrier, C60-Dex-NH2. The C60-Dex-NH2/siRNA complex destroyed the endolysosomal membrane via the controllable generation of ROS when exposed to visible light, which enhanced the gene-silencing efficiency of the siRNA *in vitro* and *in vivo*.	[144]
C_{70} fullerene derivatives (C_{70}-EDA)	A549 cells	*In vitro*	This work provides a precise biological target and new strategies for fullerene applications in cancer therapy.	[145]

Gadofullerene (Gd@C82) with β-alanines (GF-Ala)	RAW 264.7 cells, 4T1, and A549 cancer cell	*In vitro*	This study provides an effective immunomodulation strategy using gadofullerene nanoparticles by rebuilding ITM and synergizing immune checkpoint blockade therapy.	[131]
Fullerene modified with diadduct malonic acid, micelles	HeLa cells, S180 tumor–bearing mouse models	*In vitro/in vivo*	This study suggested the tremendous promise of DMA-C60 as a carrier material of MC and significant advantages in a combination of chemo-phototherapy of some tumors.	[146]
Fullerene modified with distearoyl-sn-glycero-3-phosphoethanolamine, polyethylene glycol, Asn-Gly-Arg (NGR)	4T1 cells (mouse breast cancer cell line)	*In vitro/in vivo*	To address the problem of traditional drug delivery, such as unexpected drug release during circulation and the sluggish release of drug in the target site, an "off–on" type of drug delivery system with precise control was developed in this study.	[147]
Fullerene with Cremophor EL micelles	Human cervical HeLa cancer cells	*In vitro*	This study reported the synthesis and anticancer photodynamic properties of two new decacationic fullerene (LC14) and red light–harvesting antenna–fullerene conjugated monoadduct (LC15) derivatives.	[148]
SWNT	KB oral epithelial carcinoma	*In vitro*	This work presents a facile approach to synthesizing water-soluble noble metal-coated SWNTs with a strong SERS effect for Raman spectroscopic imaging of biological samples. The nanocomposite can be used as an optical theranostic probe for cancer imaging and therapy.	[149]
	MCF-7 breast cancer	*In vitro/in vivo*	In this work, an aspargine–glycine–arginine peptide–modified SWCNT system was developed by a non-covalent approach and loaded with doxorubicin and MRI contrast agent gadolinium diethylenetriamine pentaacetic acid.	[150]
	Human breast cancer	*In vitro*	In the present study, the efficacy of multiscale photoacoustic microscopy was investigated to detect, map, and quantify trace amounts (ng to µg) of SWCNTs in a variety of histological tissue specimens consisting of cancer and benign tissue biopsies.	[151]
	4T1 breast cancer	*In vitro*	This work presented a new type of theranostic platform based on SWNTs coated with a shell of polydopamine, followed by polyethylene glycol.	[152]
	MDA-MB-468 breast cancer	*In vitro/in vivo*	In this work, SWNTs dispersed in sodium cholate with the biocompatibility of SWNTs dispersed in PL–PEG and established the use of bright biocompatible SWNTs as versatile in vivo NIR photoluminescence imaging agents for live animals.	[153]
MWNT	B16F10 melanoma	*In vitro/in vivo*	This study suggests the utilization of MWNTs for the codelivery of tumor-derived antigen, CpG, and αCD40 for efficient tumor eradication.	[154]
	A549 lung cancer	*In vitro/in vivo*	This work presents a dual-targeting strategy that improves the delivery performance of MWNT and opens a new avenue for RAS-related lung cancer therapy.	[155]
	MCF-7 human breast cell lines	*In vitro*	In this work, novel biomaterials utilizing water-soluble chitosan (CS), phycocyanin, MWCNTs were prepared and characterized with the potential for PDT and PTT.	[156]
MWNTs/gemcitabine (Ge)/lentinan	MCF-7 cells	*In vitro/in vivo*	Multi-walled carbon nanotubes (MWNTs)/gemcitabine (Ge)/lentinan) three-component anticancer composite was prepared and shown to be a promising candidate for cancer therapy in the combination of chemotherapy and photothermal therapy.	[157]
MWCNTs-TAM-LEN lentinan tamoxifen	MCF-7 cells	*In vitro/in vivo*	A lentinan (LEN)–functionalized multi-walled carbon nanotube (MWCNTs) drug delivery system, using tamoxifen (TAM), was developed. This system possessed good stability, water dispersibility, and extraordinary photothermal properties.	[158]

their physical stability, improve their capacity to target tumors, and lessen their toxicity.

To enable nontoxic imaging, various polysaccharide types can be used to increase the safety and biocompatibility of QDs. Chitosan toxicity can be decreased by adding Mn-doped ZnS QDs (Mn:ZnS QDs), making folic acid functionalization possible. Bwatanglang et al. integrated the targeted drug delivery properties of folic acid (FA) with the imaging properties of Mn:ZnS QDs into a unified nanodelivery system. In order to create an FACS–Mn:ZnS nanocomposite, FA–chitosan conjugate (FACS) was first synthesized and electrostatically complexed with Mn:ZnS QDs. After 24 h, neither bare Mn:ZnS QDs nor FACS–Mn:ZnS (7–500 g/mL) displayed toxicity to cancer models of breast cells (MCF-7 and MDA-MB-231) or a healthy model of breast cells (MCF-10). Only a minor decrease in viability was seen in FACS–Mn:ZnS-treated cells as compared to treatment with Mn:ZnS QDs when the QD concentration was increased from 62 to 500 g/mL. This marginal decrease in cell survival for the cells treated with FACS–Mn:ZnS may be attributed to the enhanced binding of the FA-coupled QDs to the cancer cell that expresses the folate receptor. Also, upon binding to the folate receptors expressed on the cancer cells, the FA-conjugated QDs increased the intensity of the cellular fluorescence.

Hyaluronic acid and QD pairing have been discovered to be an intriguing strategy for improved intracellular transport into liver cells, mediated by contact with CD44 receptors, permitting *in vivo* real-time observation. In another work, CdTe QD theranostic nanocapsules were coated with chondroitin sulfate, followed by loading with rapamycin and celecoxib for cancer applications. To prevent chondroitin sulfate nanocapsules from being absorbed by healthy cells unintentionally, an exterior coating of cationic gelatin-coupled QDs was applied to them. Gelatin was degraded by matrix metalloproteinases at tumor locations, releasing both medication nanocapsules and quantum dots (QDs) into cancer cells for imaging. In a related experiment, lactoferrin, an iron-binding cationic protein, was used in place of gelatin to produce an on–off effect, where the fluorescence of QDs was first quenched by energy transfer and subsequently recovered upon bond cleavage in tumor cells. As a result, QD fluorescence was used to show how nanocapsules were localized both *in vitro* and *in vivo* within breast cancers. On the basis of the studies mentioned, it is clear that combining QDs with polysaccharides can enhance their ability to target tumors by interacting with their receptors, which cancer cells tend to overexpress. This leads to an increase in the amount of QDs that accumulate at the tumor site. Table 8.6 summarizes the application of various nanomaterials in targeted cancer therapy and imaging.

8.11 Carbon Nanotubes in Cancer Treatment

CNTs have been widely investigated in targeted drug delivery for cancer therapy due to their distinguished properties. CNTs can not only serve as drug carriers to deliver various anticancer cancer agents but also function as excellent mediators in phototherapy because of their inherent optical features. The multifunctionality of CNTs enables their multiple applications in treating various cancers. Currently, many anticancer therapeutic strategies are aiming at targeting tumor cells and the environment where they survive. Targeting tumor cells can effectively destroy their parenchyma in a direct way, while targeting TME can inhibit their growth and metastasis through disturbing their living conditions, which also kills tumor cells indirectly. Therefore, the following sections will give a detailed introduction on how CNT-based nano-drug delivery systems target various therapeutic spots, including intracellular targeting spots of tumor cells and the extracellular components in TME for cancer therapy (Table 8.7)

8.11.1 Carbon Nanotubes for Intracellular Drug Delivery

Intracellular drug delivery has gained a considerable attention in cancer therapy. By this delivery strategy, anticancer agents can be delivered to particular intracellular targeting spots, which not only maximizes their therapeutic efficacy but also reduces their corresponding toxicity. The most popular intracellular targets include nucleus, cytoplasm, and mitochondria. Nucleus acts as a regulatory center for cellular genetics and plays a key role in cell metabolism, growth, and differentiation. Cytoplasm is composed of cytoplasmic matrix, endomembrane system, cytoskeleton, and inclusions, serving as the main site of cellular activity. Mitochondria are vital intracellular organelles that carry out a variety of functions and are involved in many metabolic pathways. In addition, mitochondria are responsible for the synthesis of the energy-rich molecule adenosine triphosphate (ATP), which is required for many cellular processes. Therefore, these three intracellular elements can be used as potential therapeutic targets for precise cancer treatment. Nanocarriers offer a number of advantages for intracellular drug delivery, by which therapeutic agents can be specifically transported to their sites of action with much lower drug concentration to elicit a better effect than drugs administered in the free form. CNTs are attractive carriers to deliver both biomolecule and small-molecule anticancer drugs. Through appropriate functionalization, the biological performance of CNTs can be intensively elevated with reduced toxicity, which benefits their application in anticancer drug delivery. Thus, the following sections give an introduction of the recent examples in CNT-mediated anticancer intracellular targeting via various delivery strategies (Figure 8.17).

8.11.1.1 Nucleus Targeting

The nucleus of cells serves as the regulation center to control the proliferation and metabolism of cells, manage cell cycle, and activate certain genes; therefore, the nucleus is considered as a desired therapeutic target for malignant tumor treatment. Nucleus targeting or nucleus membrane-penetrating nanoparticles are expected to provide a more effective approach in cancer therapy. Oh et al. constructed a DDS that carried DOX with PEGylated SWNTs for combined NIR-irradiated PTT and chemotherapy [199]. DOX is a widely adopted topoisomerase inhibitor in chemotherapy; however, the toxic side effects generated by DOX due to its non-specific distribution and high administration dosage significantly limit its further

TABLE 8.6

Representative Theranostic Nanomaterials and Their Applications

No.	Type of Nanomaterial	Characteristics	Application	Cancer Treatment	Technique Used	Ref.
1	Lipid-based nanoparticles	Colloidal carriers, biocompatible, biodegradable, and amphiphilic	Nanocarriers for codelivery of hydrophilic and hydrophobic drugs controlled and modified drug release, preventing drug degradation	Improving antitumor activities of several chemotherapeutic agents	ME cold dilution	[164]
2	Protein nanoparticles	Self-assembled supramolecular structures, biocompatible, biodegradable, and low immunogenicity; one of the FDA-approved drugs; easy functionalization	Cancer imaging and therapy	Metastatic breast cancer	Genetic recombination	[165]
3	Viral nanoparticles	Nanomaterials derived naturally from plant viruses, bacteriophages, and mammalian viruses; noninfectious, biocompatible, and biodegradable	Drug delivery, imaging, immunotherapy, theranostic applications, cancer vaccine, and immune modulators	Cancer immunotherapy	Computer-based technology	[166]
4	Inorganic nanoparticles	SPR effect and photothermal effect with unique properties, including optical, thermal, and electrical conductivity, potential magnetic and catalytic properties; some of the materials have issues with *in vivo* long-term circulation and potential toxicity	Drug carrier, imaging, therapy, and functional coating drugs that lead to more effective antitumor activity	Cancer imaging and therapy	Photodynamic therapy and hyperthermia	[167]
5	Bioinspired nanoparticles			Cancer theranostics	Fluorescence	[87]
6	ZnO QDs conjugated with gold NPs	Porous structure, biocompatibility, biodegradability, and unique physicochemical properties	Delivery platform, photodynamic therapy, photothermal therapy, imaging, PA imaging, radiotherapy, and phototherapy	Tumor-targeted drug delivery	Electrochemical	[168]
7	Pectin–guar gum–zinc oxide (PECGG–ZnO) nanocomposite	Porous structure, biocompatible, biodegradability, and unique physicochemical attributes	Effective drug carrier for targeted and sustained delivery of various bioactive and chemotherapeutic anticancerous drugs; specific toxicity via generation of reactive oxygen	Tumor-targeted drug delivery	Precipitation	[169]
8	Mesoporous ZnO nanofibers (ZnOnFs)	Porous structure, biocompatible, biodegradability, and unique physicochemical attributes	Effective drug carrier for targeted and sustained delivery of various bioactive and chemotherapeutic anticancerous drugs; specific toxicity via generation of reactive oxygen	Breast cancer	Electrospinning	[170]
9	Mn-doped ZnS QDs	Nonradiative decay, superior stability, such as high fluorescence intensity, long lifetime, and good resistance to photobleaching	Delivery platform, photodynamic therapy, photothermal therapy, and imaging	Chondrosarcoma	Photodynamic therapy	[171]
10	Nonmetallic nanomaterials	Cost-effective, biocompatible, easy modification protecting drug against multidrug resistance	Environmental friendliness, diminutive toxicity, and low cost, stimuli-responsive systems for the transport and delivery of materials, optical labeling or other detectable tracers, carrier, NIR fluorescent probe, and photothermal therapy	Cancer theranostics	Microemulsion	[172]
11	Paclitaxel-loaded PLGA nanoparticles	Biodegradable polymeric NPs used in medicine delivery systems and given approval by the FDA for its controlled and sustained release features	Drug carriers and drug delivery, and ease of processing	Anticancer therapy	Ultrasound imaging	[173]

(*Continued*)

TABLE 8.6 (Continued)

Representative Theranostic Nanomaterials and Their Applications

No.	Type of Nanomaterial	Characteristics	Application	Cancer Treatment	Technique Used	Ref.
12	Nanoscale metal–organic frameworks (nMOFs)	High surface areas, tunable pore size, crystallinity, thermal stability, and easy surface modification	Effective cellular uptake, focused molecular targeting, smart nanodrug delivery devices, and drug-responsive behavior; extensive therapeutic stimuli and drug release	Cancer immunotherapy	Radiotherapy–radiodynamic therapy (RT–RDT) and chemodynamic therapy (CDT)	[174]
13	Polylactide nanoconjugates	Biodegradable and biocompatible polymer and easy to modify	Suitable for usage as a nanoparticulate platform for administration of antigens and drugs	Prostate cancer therapy	Intravenous therapeutic strategy	[175]
14	DOX/ICG/BSA nanoparticles	Large surface-area-to-volume ratio, biocompatible	Effective carriers for delivering ICG to tumor tissue, drug delivery	Breast cancer therapy	Photothermal therapy	[176]
15	Dendrimer-based nanoparticles	Polymer containing repetitive unit with a symmetric, almost-spherical shape; the majority of polymers are not soluble in water; it is possible to make dendrimers water-soluble	High loading capacity for guest molecules; diagnosis using imaging techniques with low toxicity, low immunogenicity, and high permeability so that they can cross biological barriers	Cancer therapy	MRI	[177]
16	Carbon nanotubes	One-dimensional material, inert, stable, and biocompatible	Drug carriers deliver various anticancer agents; excellent mediators in phototherapy because of their inherent optical features	Cancerous cells detection and drug delivery	Photoacoustic imaging	[178]
17	Porous nanomaterials (PNMs)	Porous structure, easy modification, and protecting drug against multidrug resistance, stable, and biocompatible	Drug carrier	Cancer immunotherapy	Photothermal	[179]
18	Gold nanoparticles	One-dimensional, SPR effect, and photothermal effect; strong photostability and photoluminescence	Excellent plasmonic materials size-adjustable energy regulation; immobilization of bioreceptors, improved analyte loading, strong catalytic characteristics	Cancer therapy	Photoacoustic imaging	[180]
19	Plasmonic palladium (Pd) nanospheres coated with titanium dioxide shell	SPR effect and photothermal effect; strong photostability and photoluminescence	Immobilization of bioreceptors, improved analyte loading, strong catalytic characteristics	Cancer therapy	Photothermal technique	[181]
20	Silver nanoparticles	One-dimensional, unique physicochemical properties, including optical, thermal, and electrical conductivities, as well as their capability to combat viruses, fungi, and even bacteria	Immobilization of bioreceptors, improved analyte loading, strong catalytic characteristics	Antitumor agents	Biomedical imaging	[182]
21	Gold nanorods	One-dimensional, SPR effect and photothermal effect; high photostability and photoluminescence	Excellent plasmonic materials size, adjustable energy regulation; immobilization of bioreceptors, improved analyte loading, strong catalytic properties	Breast cancer therapy	Photothermal	[183]
22	Aptamer-based nanoparticles	Aptamers are single-stranded DNAs or RNAs; highly selective recognition ability; good reproducibility, low toxicity, high stability, low molecular weight, and compact size	Aptamers, due to structure diversity, have higher rates of tumor penetration, retention, and uniform dispersion, while the attachment process to the surface of nanomaterials is more amenable and repeatable	Cancer therapy	Cellular imaging	[184]
23	Porphyrin-based inorganic nanoparticles	Photosensitizer, tunable surface area, and biocompatibility	Photodynamic therapy, cancer treatment, and photothermal therapy as well as enhanced photodiagnosis	Cancer treatment	Photodynamic therapy	[185]
24	Gold nanoparticles/graphene oxides	SPR effect, strong NIR light absorption, and high surface area; high photostability and photoluminescence	Immobilization of bioreceptors, improved analyte loading, strong catalytic properties; drug carriers, NIR florescence probes, PA imaging photothermal therapy	Breast cancer therapy	Near-infrared (NIR) light-activatable photothermal therapy	[186]

25	Liposome-based nanoparticles	Amphiphilic and good biocompatibility; however, easily oxidized, structurally unstable	Nanocarriers for codelivery of hydrophobic and hydrophilic drugs	Cancer therapy	Chemo-immunotherapy (CIT)	[187]
26	Mesoporous MnO_2	Porous structure, easy modification, and protecting drug against multidrug resistance; stable, biocompatible	Drug carrier	Breast cancer	Photodynamic therapy	[188]
27	Fe_3O_4-based nanoparticles	Magnetic properties and biocompatibility, high surface-to-volume ratio, and easy separation methodology	MRI imaging, hyperthermia treatment, drug delivery, superparamagnetism	Targeted drug/gene delivery systems	Chemotherapy	[189]
28	Ag–Au nanostructure	SPR effect and photothermal effect	PA imaging, Raman spectroscopy imaging radiotherapy, phototherapy, immobilization of bioreceptors, improved analyte loading	Breast cancer therapy	Near-infrared photothermal therapy	[190]
29	Gold nanoparticles	SPR effect and photothermal effect; photostability and photoluminescence	Immobilization of bioreceptors, improved analyte loading, strong catalytic properties	Colorectal cancer therapy	Chemotherapy	[191]
30	Fmoc-H/Zn2+/OMHEPzEOPP nanoparticles	Photothermal conversion properties, high surface area, and biocompatible	Exceptional superparamagnetic characteristics, photothermal therapy, photodynamic therapy, and enhanced drug delivery systems (DDSs)	Cervical cancer therapy	Near-infrared nanocomposite photosensitizer	[192]
31	Persistent luminescence nanoparticles	Unique optical materials, easily doped or modified with elements, hollow or mesoporous structures, and versatile surface functionality	Optical imaging of tumors, high sensitivity, high penetration depth, fluorescence-guided surgery, photothermal therapy, photodynamic therapy, drug/gene delivery, and combined therapy	Cervical cancer therapy	Tumor imaging	[193]
32	Black quantum dots/mesoporous silica framework/Pt nanoparticles		Drug carrier, delivery platform, photodynamic and photothermal therapies	Liver cancer therapy	Self-compensation mechanisms	[194]
33	Polymeric nanoparticles	Biocompatible and easy to modify	Drug intelligent responses, functional coating	Cancer therapy	Chemotherapy	[195]
34	Cyclodextrin polymer (CDP)–based nanoparticles	Low toxicity, soluble in water, insoluble in organic solvents, and easy to modify	Potential to improve the loading capacity of nanostructured lipid carriers, solid lipid nanoparticles, and liposomes	Cancer therapy	Chemotherapy	[196]
35	mAb nanoparticles	Biocompatible, highly specific; recognize and find specific proteins on cancer cells	Used to deliver nanoparticles and improve drug targeting to cancer cells	Cancer therapy	Chemotherapy	[197]
36	Nanoemulsion (NE)	Colloidal particulate system in submicrometer-size range; these carriers are solid spheres with an amorphous, lipophilic, negatively charged surface	Drug delivery, biological or diagnostic agents, safeguard the effective content of drugs from hydrolysis and oxidation	Cancer therapy	Chemotherapy	[198]

TABLE 8.7
Application of CNT-Based DDS in Targeting Various Intracellular Therapeutic Spots and TME Components

Targeting Spot	Drug Delivery System	Therapeutic Modality	Tumor Model	Effectiveness	Biocompatibility Test	Refs.
Nucleus	PEG-SWNTs-DOX	Photothermal therapy + chemotherapy	Breast cancer	Increase delivery efficiency, promote the accumulation and localization of DOX inside the nucleus, cause effective cancer cell death	N/A	[199]
Nucleus	SWNTs carrier	Chemotherapy	Colorectal cancer	Achieve targeted therapy and controlled drug release	Show good biocompatibility	[200]
Nucleus	*f*-SWNTs–p53 plasmid complexes	Gene therapy	Breast cancer	Transport the target gene into the nucleus effectively, induce apoptosis strongly	N/A	[201]
Cytoplasm	Chim/PEI/5-FU/CNT nanoparticles	Gene therapy + chemotherapy	Gastric cancer	Achieve targeted delivery and silence the drug-resistant gene, promote the apoptosis of drug-resistant cancer cells	Show negligible in vivo toxicity, and none of the mice dead after treatment, with no statistically significant difference in body weight between the groups	[202]
Cytoplasm	MWNTs/Sor/siRNA	Gene therapy + chemotherapy	Liver cancer	Enhance the release of sorafenib and improve siRNA stability, display significant antitumor effect	N/A	[203]
Cytoplasm	SWNT-HIF-1α siRNA complexes	Gene therapy	Pancreas cancer	Transfect and induce the RNAi response, effectively suppress tumor growth	Negligible toxic effect in vitro and in vivo	[204]
Cytoplasm	oxDWNT-siRNA	Gene therapy	Prostate cancer	Release siRNA into the cytoplasm to suppress survivin protein synthesis, directly cause cancer cell apoptosis	Show good biocompatibility	[205]
Mitochondria	MWNT-Rho (PtBzt + BP)	Chemotherapy	Ovarian cancer	Increase the selectivity of platinum-based chemotherapy, minimize the side effects	N/A	[206]
Mitochondria	PEG-CNTs-ABT737	Chemotherapy	Lung cancer	Improve the mitochondrial targeting of lung cancer cells, cause cancer cell apoptosis	Show lower cytotoxicity in NHFB normal cells than A549 lung cancer cells	[207]
Mitochondria	P-D-CS-CNTs	Photothermal therapy	Bladder cancer	Enhance mitochondrial targeting, induce the ROS burst, result in mitochondrial damage and cell death	N/A	[208]
Mitochondria	PL-PEG-SWNT	Photoacoustic therapy	Breast cancer	Transform pulse laser energy into sound energy, bomb the mitochondria into dysfunction, and trigger mitochondrial outer membrane permeabilization	Show low toxicity without epidermis injury	[209]
Extracellular matrix	MWNTs	Photothermal therapy	Epidermoid carcinoma	Significantly soften tumors together with volume reduction, induce the destruction of collagen and cell damage	N/A	[210]
Cancer stem cells	SWNT-Raw and SWNT-COOH	Chemotherapy	Osteosarcoma	Specifically bind to TGFβ1-induced activation of TGFβR1 and suppress its downstream signaling, decrease the OSCs population	Exhibit no obvious toxicity to normal cells	[211]
Tumor vasculature	DOX/CD-CNT and CUR/CD-CNT	Photothermal therapy + chemotherapy	Hepatocellular carcinoma	Enhance drug entrapment efficiency and achieve sustained release of both drugs	Cause minimal damage to normal cells	[41]
Tumor vasculature	iRGD-PEI-MWNT-SS-CD/pAT2	Chemotherapy	Lung cancer	Promote the cellular uptake and transfection efficiency, inhibit angiogenesis, suppress tumor growth significantly	Not induce obvious tissue damage or inflammatory cell infiltration, not affect blood, hepatic, or kidney function in mice	[212]
PD-1/PD-L1	Rg3-CNT	Immunotherapy	Triple-negative breast cancer treatment	Inhibit PD-1/PD-L1 axis and the TNBC cell growth	N/A	[213]
Immune cells	MWNTs-DOX and MWNTs-CpG	Immunotherapy + chemotherapy + phototherapy	Melanoma	Inhibit tumor growth, enhance the number of CD4+ and CD8+ T cells, promote TAM shifting, reduce the number of Tregs in TME	Show non-toxicity to the organs (liver, spleen, kidneys, heart, and lungs) in mice	[214]

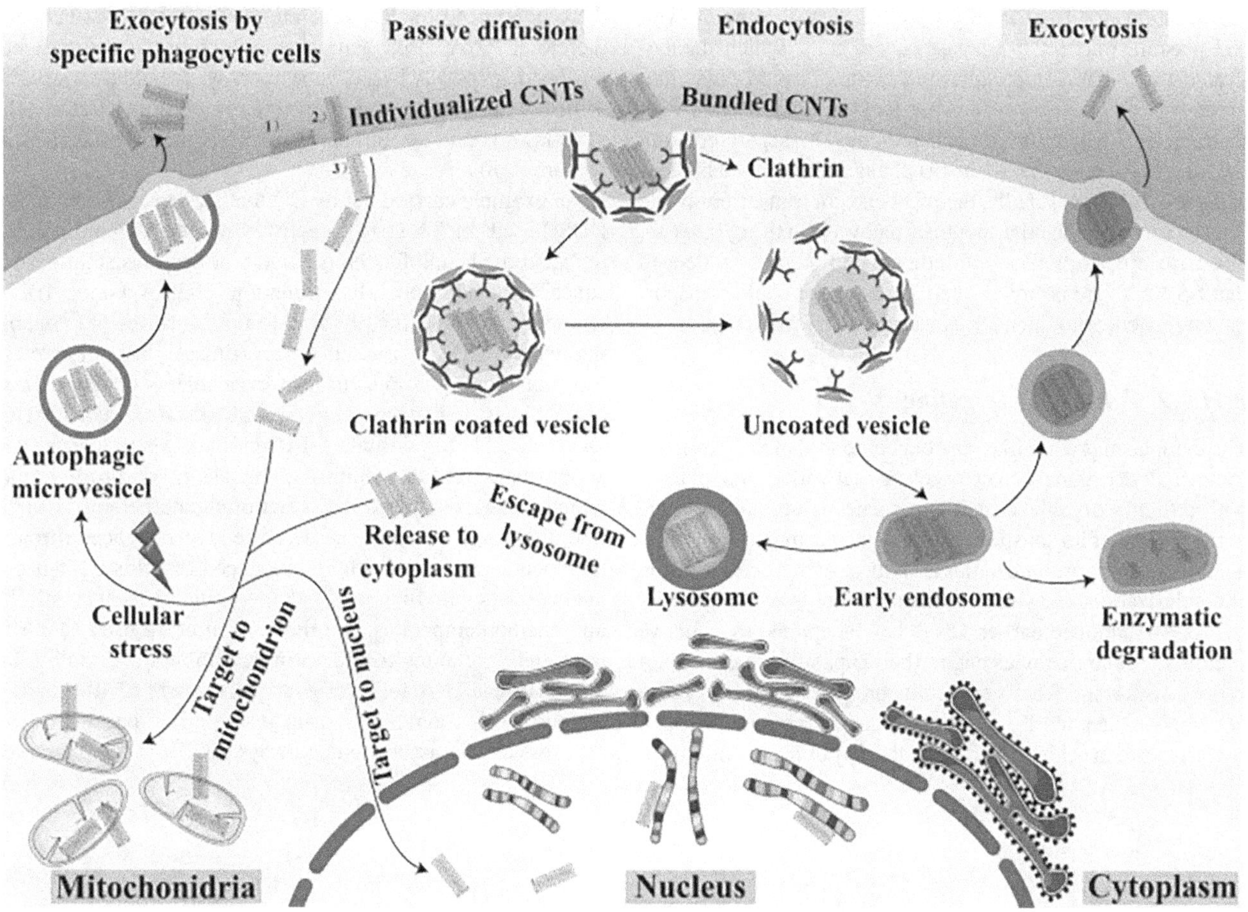

FIGURE 8.17 Schematic demonstration of intracellular targeting spots, uptake, and cellular fate of CNT-based DDS.

application. Therefore, SWNTs with high surface area provide an approach for the efficient drug delivery of DOX. In this study, the synthesized PEG-SWNTs-DOX could lead to effective breast cancer cell death in comparison to the single treatment with DOX or PTT alone. Besides, the released DOX from carrier could accumulate inside the cancer cells at high concentration to effectively localize into their nucleus, demonstrating the excellent potential of PEG-SWNTs-DOX for breast cancer treatment. Lee et al. designed a nanotube system that used SWNTs to conjugate with an EGFR inhibitor cetuximab and topoisomerase I inhibitor SN38 to realize the precise treatment of EGFR over-expressing colorectal cancer [200]. SN38 was covalently linked to SWNTs via carbamate bond that could be gradually broken up by carboxylesterase enzyme (hCE) in lysosomes; therefore, SN38 was controllably released inside the cells. In vitro results obtained from different colon cancer cell lines showed that SN38 was able to enter the nucleus after dissociation from the SWNT-carrier, while leaving the carrier in the cytoplasm, which confirmed that SWNTs were excellent vehicles for the targeted transportation of SN38 to the nucleus.

Gene therapy is an emerging area with the goal to rectify genetic disorders at the molecular level. Gene therapy mainly includes the transport of genes with plasmid DNA (pDNA) to elevate downregulated genes and change mutated genes, or through the application of small interfering RNA (siRNA), micro-RNA (miRNA), and shRNA to decrease protein expression by interference in RNA level (Figure 8.18) [215].

A satisfactory gene therapy effect is dependent on the vector that protects exogenous DNA from degradation and inactivation or avoids lysosomal degradation within the cells. Therefore, an effective delivery vehicle plays a key role in achieving successful gene therapy outcomes. CNTs, a class of non-viral gene vector, have attracted increasing attention in gene delivery. CNTs are reported to have an interaction with many biological constituents and are able to be effectively internalized in various cell types via distinct mechanisms. In addition, unlike viral vectors, non-viral vectors tend to display a better immunogenic performance, which will not cause severe immunogenic side effects to the body. The TP53 gene provides instructions for making a protein called tumor protein p53 (or p53). This protein acts as a tumor suppressor, which means that it regulates cell division by keeping cells from growing and dividing (proliferating) too fast or in an uncontrolled way. Therefore, Karmakar et al. used the oncogene suppressor protein 53 (p53) genes as the mode gene and functionalized SWNTs as the vector for breast cancer treatment [201]. p53 is an important anti-oncogenic gene which is involved in the DNA repair procedure or triggers cell suicide when DNA damage is irreparable. *In vitro* experiments verified the feasibility of transporting f-SWNTs-DNA complex with p53 plasmid into MCF-7 breast cancer cells, which demonstrated that f-SWNTs-p53 plasmid complex could enter into the cytoplasm of cancer cells via endocytosis and then arrive at their nucleus, where the p53 plasmid could be separated from the f-SWNTs vector due to the pH change between the nucleus and the cytoplasm. Finally, the p53 gene got transcription and translation to activate the apoptosis pathways in the cytoplasm. Taken together, all these aforementioned studies evidenced that f-SWNTs are promising gene vectors that could transport the target gene into the nucleus with good effectiveness.

8.11.1.2 Cytoplasm Targeting

The cytoplasm is a gel-like scaffold composed of various macromolecules, organelles, cytoskeletal networks, and cytosol with a highly organized and heterogeneous architecture due to the variety of its constituents. The cytoplasm participates in a number of important cellular activities, such as cell division and polarization, and serves as the main site for cellular activity. As is mentioned earlier, CNTs can be applied as effective vectors for gene therapies due to their capability to efficiently enter cells. Apart from gene insertion into the host genome via pDNA, silencing the pathogenic gene expression through siRNA can also achieve great gene therapy efficacy. Moreover, there is no need for RNA to integrate into the host genome; therefore, RNA-based gene therapy exhibits a better safety profile than pDNA-based gene therapy. In addition, siRNA achieves its sites of action in the cytoplasm; therefore, the cytoplasm is an essential place for RNA interference (RNAi) (Figure 8.18).

An example carried out by Chen et al. constructed a nano-DDS based on CNTs to effectively deliver chemotherapeutic agent 5-FU and for the treatment of drug-resistant gastric cancer with peritoneal dissemination [202]. Aptamer-siRNA chimera could specifically bind to the cancer cells to enable the whole DDS with active targeting ability for precise transportation of 5-FU. In vitro experiments obtained from MKN45 gastric cancer cell line revealed that this constructed DDS was able to facilitate 5-FU-resistant gastric cancer cell apoptosis as well as inhibit their invasion and proliferation, which in turn enhanced the effect of chemotherapy. In addition, the drug-resistant gene was effectively silenced through therapeutic siRNA, which all evidenced that this CNT-based nanocarrier could function as a great vehicle to deliver siRNA and chemotherapeutics. Similarly, Wen et al. used MWNTs to co-deliver the multi-target kinase inhibitor sorafenib (Sor) and EGFR siRNA for liver cancer treatment [203]. Sor is a widely applied anticancer drug in the clinic because it can suppress cancer-associated pathways. EGFR is overexpressed

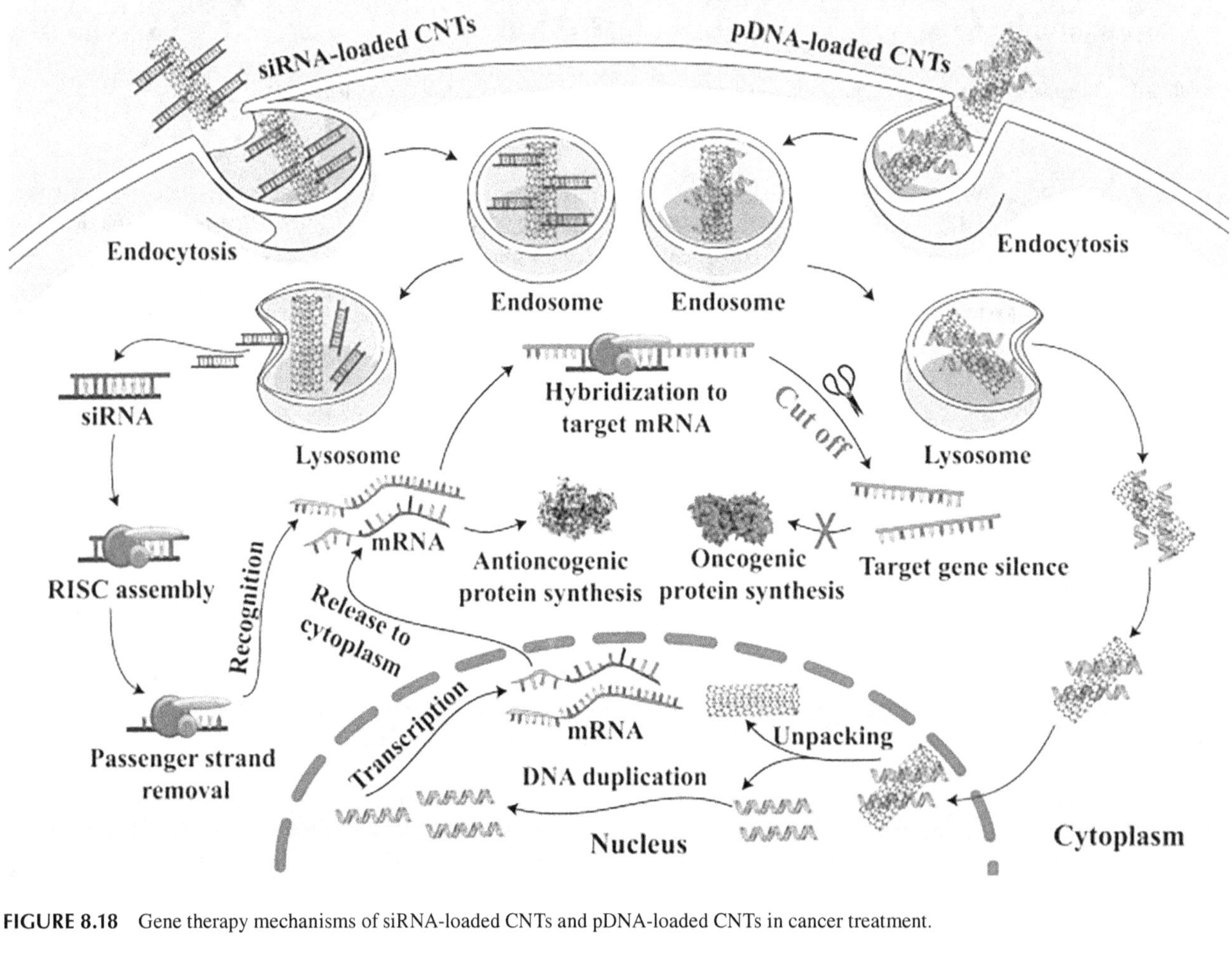

FIGURE 8.18 Gene therapy mechanisms of siRNA-loaded CNTs and pDNA-loaded CNTs in cancer treatment.

in many cancer types; therefore, specific inhibition of EGFR expression can induce cell apoptosis through reducing the activity of EGF. As a result, combinational treatment strategy of Sor and EGFR targeting through CNT-based DDS is an ideal therapeutic approach for liver cancer treatment. The obtained nanocomposite could increase the release of Sor and enhance siRNA stability by protecting it from degradation. In vitro results demonstrated that this nanocomposite could significantly inhibit the replication of liver cancer cells and induce their apoptosis compared to the control group. In vivo experimental data further evidenced that treatment with this nanocomposite could obviously decrease the tumor volume and weight in tumor-bearing mice, indicating its superior effectiveness for liver cancer treatment. Apart from the examples mentioned earlier, Bartholomeusz et al. used SWNTs to deliver hypoxia-inducible factor 1 alpha (HIF-1α) siRNA into pancreas cancer cell to inhibit the expression of HIF-1α [204]. As hypoxia is one of the most characteristic features of rapidly proliferating solid tumor, which makes them aggressive and difficult to treat, therefore, tumor hypoxia is regarded as a potential therapeutic target, and a lot of researches have already reported that HIF-1α inhibition can suppress tumor growth by reducing its activity. This nanocomplex could efficiently achieve the goal of RNAi and effectively suppress tumor growth, further demonstrating the key role of CNTs as a good siRNA delivery platform. In addition to SWNTs and MWNTs, double-walled carbon nanotubes (DWNTs), which bridge the gap between SWNTs and MWNTs, could also be applied to delivery siRNA. Neves et al. loaded survivn siRNA by polypeptide (-oly(Lys: Phe))-coated DWNTs for prostate cancer treatment [205]. Due to the nano-needle structure, DWNTs could efficiently enter mammalian cells and was able to escape from lysosomes and release siRNA into the cytoplasm to suppress survivin protein synthesis, directly causing cancer cell apoptosis. To summarize, CNT-based nano-DDS is a promising tool to carry siRNA into the cytoplasm for efficient gene therapy.

8.11.1.3 Mitochondria Targeting

Mitochondria, one of the most important organelles within the cells, are around 1 μm in diameter with variable length. Mitochondria are well-known to participate in energy metabolism, such as ATP synthesis. Besides, they are pivotal cellular organelles involved in the generation of ROS and regulation of apoptosis, autophagy, and necroptosis. Accumulating evidence have already demonstrated that mitochondrial bioenergetics, biosynthesis, and signaling play a fundamental role in tumorigenesis, and mitochondria are indispensible energy supporter for highly proliferating cancer cells; thus, mitochondria are regarded as important therapeutic targets in cancer treatment. However, the lack of efficient delivery vehicle that can load therapeutic molecules with specific targeting ability and internalization capability limits the therapeutic strategy based on mitochondrial targeting. Fortunately, CNTs are capable of being internalized by various cancer cells and can target mitochondria by mitochondrial targeting ligands, such as mitochondriotropics. In addition, CNTs possess excellent optical properties and can be applied in PTT, photoacoustic therapy (PAT), and thermoacoustic therapy (TAT) to directly destroy the mitochondria of cancer cells, thus causing obvious killing effect on cancer cells.

Chemotherapy remains to be the most widely adopted strategy to treat various cancers; however, due to their nonspecificity, indiscriminate destruction of normal cells, and the development of multidrug resistance, chemotherapy often causes undesirable side effects, and the application of chemotherapy is still limited. Benefiting from their attractive properties, CNT-based DDS have been explored and designed for the precise delivery of chemotherapy drugs to mitochondria. Platinum (IV) complexes take advantage of the exclusive conditions that occur within the tumor to carry out their cytotoxic activity. On the other hand, silk fibroin has natural properties which make it very interesting as a biomaterial: high biocompatibility, biodegradability, low immunogenicity, high cellular penetration capacity, and high reactive surface. Herein we report the preparation of silk fibroin nanoparticles (SFNs) loaded with the hydrophobic Pt(IV) complex cis,cis,trans-$[Pt(NH_3)_2Cl_2(O_2CC_6H_5)_2]$ (PtBz). Yoong et al. functionalized MWNTs with fluorescent rhodamine-110 with mitochondrial targeting ability (MWNTs-Rho) to co-encapsulate a chemopotentiator 3-bromopyruvate (BP) and platinum (IV) prodrug (PtBz), constructing a DDS called MWNT-Rho (PtBzt+BP) for cancer treatment [206]. PtBz, which were entrapped within the core of hydrophobic MWNTs, could be transformed into platinum (II) by glutathione, which turned to be hydrophilic species and could be released from MWNTs. After reaching mitochondria of the cancer cells via active targeting effect of Rho-110, platinum (II) could covalently cross-link and inhibit the transcription and replication of mitochondrial DNA (mtDNA) that encodes 13 polypeptides essential for mitochondrial function, eventually causing cell apoptosis. *In vitro* experiments showed that co-incubation of PtBz with BP exhibited significant cytotoxicity to human ovarian cancer cells. In addition, owing to the unique shape of CNTs and the lipophilic cationic nature of Rho-based dyes, MWNTs-Rho (PtBz+BP) could be effectively internalized into cells and target mitochondria, which mitigated the poor selectivity of platinum-based chemotherapy and minimized the side effect. Although targeting mitochondria is an effective method to induce cancer cell apoptosis, the limited targetability toward mitochondria impedes its clinical effectiveness for cancer treatment. ABT-737 binds to the hydrophobic groove of multiple members of the anti-apoptotic Bcl-2 protein family, including Bcl-2, Bcl-xl, and Bcl-w. This inhibits the activity of these pro-survival proteins and restores apoptotic processes in tumor cells, via activation of Bak/Bax-mediated apoptosis. To address this chapter, Kim et al. designed a ABT737-loaded PEGylated CNT-based nano DDS (PEG-CNTs-ABT737) with enhanced mitochondrial targetability toward lung cancer cells [207]. ABT737 is a small-molecule inhibitory compound that can suppress B-cell lymphoma-2 (Bcl-2) protein, which is an anti-apoptotic protein for efficacious cancer treatment. As is illustrated in Figure 8.19, PEG-CNTs-ABT737 nanodrug was able to escape from endosome and could deliver ABT737 into the mitochondria of A549 lung cancer cells, which resulted in the mitochondrial accumulation of nanodrug to cause cancer cell apoptosis (Figure 8.19).

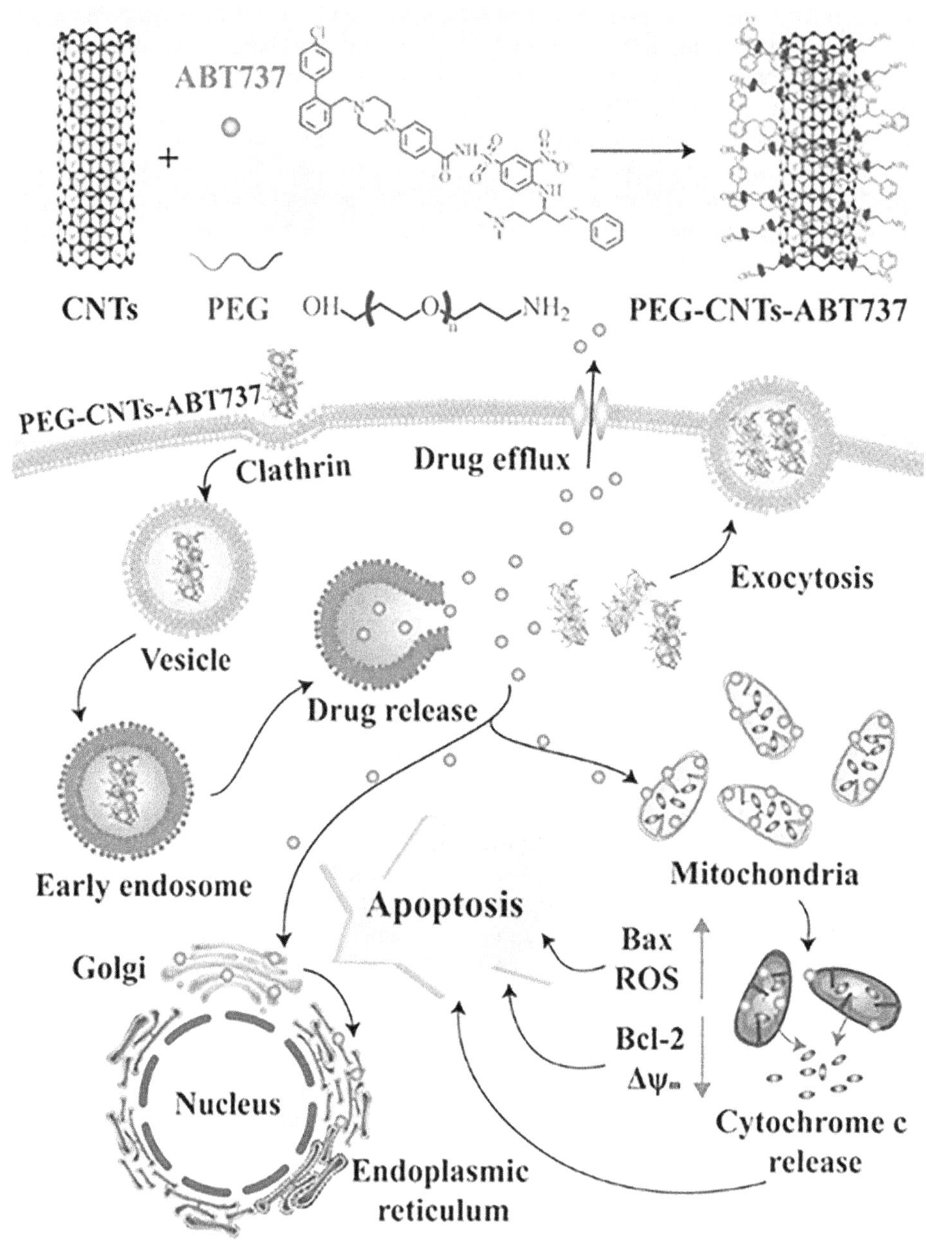

FIGURE 8.19 Schematic demonstration of the construction and working mechanism of PEG-CNTs-ABT737 nanodrug for anticancer therapy.

Apart from the application as drug carriers, CNTs can be utilized in PTT due to their superior NIR absorption efficiency. Mitochondria were reported to be sensitive to hyperthermia and can be considered as targets for PTT [216]. Wang et al. fabricated a nanosystem based on SWNTs for the PTT of bladder cancer [208]. *In vitro* experiments showed that this nanosystem could destroy the mitochondria of MB49 murine bladder cancer cells after mild hyperthermia produced by SWNTs-mediated PTT, which led to the burst of ROS from damaged mitochondria to induce cell death. Although PTT is one of the emerging therapeutic modalities with non-invasive or slightly invasive properties for cancer treatment, it can also inevitably induce partial skin damage. Therefore, photoacoustic therapy (PAT), another innovative phototherapy strategy, is adopted to selectively eliminate tumor cells without causing epidermis injury. The dose of laser and treatment model are two main differences between PTT and PAT. PTT usually irradiates the local tissue continuously with a higher laser dose, while PAT can be generated through a lower laser dose by transducing light energy into acoustic pressure [217]. For example, Zhou et al. applied PAT for mitochondria-targeting destruction by using the photoacoustic transducer property of SWNTs with the selective absorption of 1064 nm NIR pulse laser [209]. SWNTs were able to transform pulse laser energy into sound energy that could bomb the mitochondria into dysfunction and trigger mitochondrial outer membrane permeabilization

(MOMP) to cause intrinsic apoptosis. In vitro experiments showed SWNTs-based treatment accompanied with laser irradiation could induce obvious cell death in EMT6 mouse mammary tumor cells compared to the control group, confirming that the sound energy stimulated by SWNTs was able to trigger a much higher level of apoptotic cell death due to the initiation of cancer cell apoptosis through mitochondrial pathway.

8.12 Carbon Nanotubes in Cancer Diagnosis

Cancer diagnosis is a process of examining and detecting the etiologies and the related symptoms of different types of cancer through modern technologies. As a kind of inorganic nanomaterials with many unique properties, CNTs have arisen much attention in the field of cancer diagnosis. Therefore, in this section, the application of CNTs in various cancer imaging, including Raman imaging, nuclear magnetic resonance imaging, ultrasonography, photoacoustic imaging, radionuclide imaging, near-infrared fluorescence imaging, as well as their contributions to cancer nanobiosensors, will be discussed in detail (Figure 8.20). Table 8.8 [19] is a summary of all these CNT-based applications in cancer diagnosis.

8.13 CNTs in Cancer Imaging

CNTs are multifunctional bio-probes with numerous unique properties, such as strong absorbance in NIR, good resonance Raman scattering, and high modifiability. Thus, CNTs can be regarded as a kind of suitable material for cancer imaging. Recently, the application of CNTs in cancer imaging has gained increasing attention in detecting various cancer types, which shows a promising research and clinical prospective in cancer diagnosis.

8.13.1 Raman Imaging

Raman scattering is the transfer of emission wavelength of photons with light excitation. Due to the sharp electronic density of states at the van Hove singularities, CNTs exhibit numerous strong Raman peaks, including radial breathing

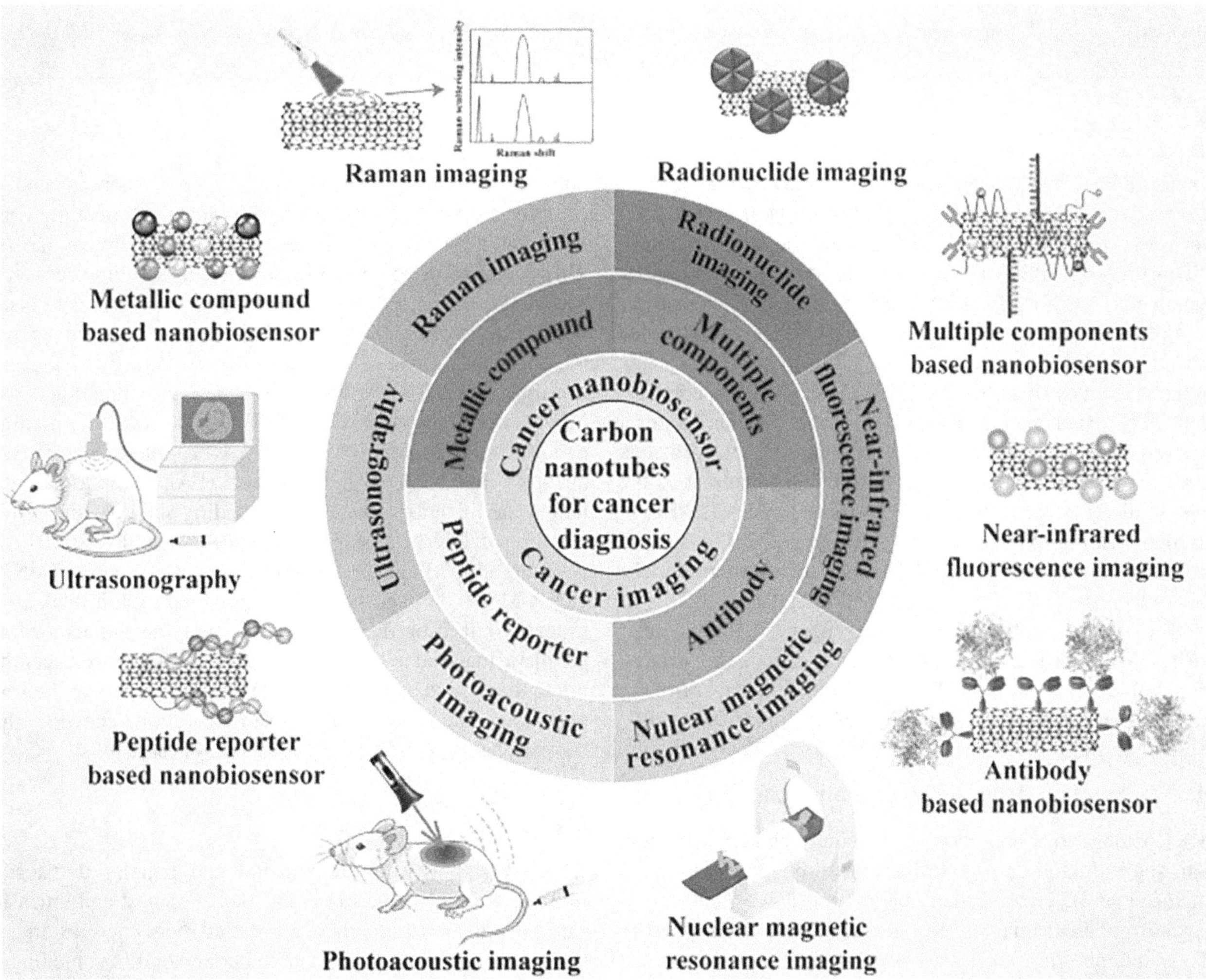

FIGURE 8.20 An overview of the contributions of CNTs to cancer diagnosis.

TABLE 8.8
Summary of the Application of CNTs in Cancer Diagnosis

Type of CNTs	Diagnostic Methods	Effect	Refs.
SWNTs	Raman imaging	Strong spots of Raman signals derived from the o-SWNTs-PEG in colon-26 cells can be obtained five days after administration.	[218]
SWNTs	Raman imaging	Possess a strong SERS effect suitable for labeling and fast Raman spectroscopic imaging of biological samples.	[219]
SWNTs	MRI	Exhibit excellent MRI function for tumor diagnosis.	[220]
MWNTs	MRI	Magnify the longitudinal proton relaxation process, possess T1-enhanced MRI effect.	[221]
MWNTs	Ultrasonography	Show high contrast in ultrasonic imaging.	[222]
MWNTs	Ultrasonography	Exhibit ultrasound signal with strong, long-lived, and high-quality properties after sonication treatment.	[223]
SWNTs	PA imaging	Shows obvious and stable PA signals.	[224]
MWNTs	PA imaging	Precisely target the tumor site in vivo; strong PA imaging effect can be obtained.	[225]
MWNTs	Radionuclide imaging	Enable easy and direct SPECT/CT imaging.	[226]
SWNTs	Radionuclide imaging	Achieve efficient tumor tissue accumulation for the subsequent radionuclide imaging.	[227]
SWNTs	NIRF imaging	Produces outstanding signal-to-noise performance and exhibits high specificity toward the in situ ovarian tumor and the implanted tumor nodules.	[228]
SWNTs	NIRF imaging	Obtain high-resolution intravital tumor vessel images through the thick skin in live mice.	[229]
MWNTs	Nanobiosensor	Obtain high biosensing ability and provide a wide linear range for detecting miR-21 with a very low detection limit in the early diagnosis of pancreatic cancer.	[230]
SWNTs	Nanobiosensor	Exhibit broad detection range, low detection limit, and high specificity to only OPN during prostate cancer detection.	[231]
MWNTs	Nanobiosensor	Achieve the simple detection of CDK1, and report the enzymatic activity of CDK1 for cancer diagnosis.	[232]
MWNTs	Nanobiosensor	Possess high selectivity and sensitivity to HPV-18 for the early, rapid, easy, and accurate diagnosis of cervical cancer.	[233]

Source: [69].

model (RBM) and tangent G-module (TGM), which can be detected by a Raman microscope. Sekiyama et al. constructed epoxide-type oxygen-doped SWNTs with the modification of PEG (o-SWNTs-PEG) as a recently developed over-thousand-nanometer (OTN) NIR fluorescent probe for the investigation of the time-dependent change in OTN-NIR fluorescence images of colon-26 cancer cells [218]. Raman microscopy was adopted to study the o-SWNTs-PEG's distribution in colon-26 cells. The experiment result showed that the Raman signals derived from this constructed nanostructure in colon-26 cells were enhanced evidently on the fifth day, in contrast to the past, indicating the suitability of applying o-SWNTs-PEG in Raman imaging. Wrapping noble metal around CNTs' surface is a common way for the enhancement of their Raman signals. For this purpose, Wang et al. modified PEGylated CNTs with gold or silver to achieve the surface-enhanced Raman scattering (SERS) effect of nanocomposites. After NIR irradiation, noble metal–modified CNTs consumed the least time to acquire the Raman images compared with single CNTs [219].

8.13.2 Nuclear Magnetic Resonance Imaging

MRI belongs to a non-invasive imaging technology without ionizing radiation damage to the human body. It can obtain the original 3D cross-section images and shows great advantages in medical imaging. Because CNTs can be applied as T2 spin dephasing contrast agents, they are common contrast agents that can be utilized to enhance nuclear magnetic resonance (MR) in the clinic, and the MR images were generally obtained through an MRI scanner. Yan et al. non-covalently combined NGR (asparagine-glycine-arginine) peptide with DOX and a type of MR contrast agent, Gd-DTPA, on CNTs. This nanosystem possessed both excellent antitumor efficacy and MRI function, exhibiting outstanding synergistic effect on tumor diagnosis and treatment [220]. Another research regarding the application of MWNTs in MRI was done by Zhang and teammates [221]. They synthesized a type of functionalized MWNTs (FA-GdN@CQDs-MWNTs/DOX) with the modification of gadolinium NPs (GdN), magnetofluorescent carbon quantum dots (CQDs), and folic acid (FA). These aforementioned modifications ensured outstanding stability and water stability of MWNTs, which are both essential for MRI. *In vitro* targeting MRI experiment result revealed that FA-GdN@CQDs-MWNTs magnified the longitudinal proton relaxation process, indicating the feasibility of applying this nanoparamagnetic material to be a T1 contrast agent. Moreover, according to the in vivo experiment, the MR signal at tumor site was positively enhanced after IV administration, showing the tumor specificity for T1-enhanced MRI of these NPs.

8.13.3 Ultrasonography

Ultrasonography is a fundamental and popular diagnostic imaging technique due to the low detection cost and intrinsic safety. Compared with other nano-based inorganic substances, CNTs are the most suitable nanomaterials for ultrasonic imaging due to the high signal produced by them during ultrasonography, and the signal could be detected by a contrast-enhanced ultrasound imager. Besides, the small size of CNTs enables them to cross the endothelial barriers and, subsequently, to become a targetable material to reach tumor regions. Saghatchi et al. designed a kind of functionalized MWNT that was modified with both magnetic Fe_3O_4 and gold NPs, obtaining mf-MWNT/AuNPs for cancer imaging and therapy [222]. According to the ultrasonic imaging effects, these NPs showed high contrast under all the employed concentrations, exhibiting the possibility to become a type of contrast agent in ultrasonography. Moreover, Delogu et al. also carried out a study on MWNTs applied in ultrasonography [223]. In their research, MWNTs were firstly modified with azomethine ylides to improve their biocompatibility. According to various experiment results, these prepared functionalized MWNTs (ox-MWNT-NH_3^+) showed the ultrasound signal with strong, long-lived, and high-quality properties after sonication treatment.

8.13.4 Photoacoustic Imaging

PA imaging is a booming imaging technique which provides in vivo pathology with new characterization methods. With irradiation by pulsed laser, the absorbed luminous energy can be converted into ultrasonic through the thermal expansion of tissues and organs and can subsequently be detected by sensors. In contrast to other tumor diagnosis methods, the application of PA technology can improve tissue penetration and spatial resolution effectively. Because CNTs possess strong NIR absorption and deep tissue penetration, it is regarded as an ideal contrast agent for PA, and the PA signal could be recorded through a photoacoustic microscopy. For example, Avti et al. directly detected, localized, and measured the content of CNTs in different tissue samples through PA technology in cell imaging, and the signals of these samples were obvious and stable because of the powerful NIR absorbance of CNTs [224]. Besides, Wang and his teammates reported a kind of RGD-modified silica-coated Au nanorods-functionalized MWNTs with active targeting ability for the in vivo PA imaging of gastric cancer [225]. They originally combined silica-coated Au nanorods (sGNRs) onto MWNTs and then attached RGD peptides to the sGNR/MWNTs nanostructure. After IV administration of this obtained RGD-conjugated sGNR/MWNTs probe, the treated mice were all diagnosed by an optoacoustic imaging system, which evidenced that this designed probe could precisely target the tumor site in vivo to obtain strong photoacoustic imaging effect.

8.13.5 Radionuclide Imaging

Radionuclide imaging is another type of imaging technology that is related to radioactive isotopes. Radiation source can form *in vivo* after the injection of radioactive chemicals, such as ^{111}In, ^{131}I, ^{64}Cu, and ^{86}Y, into the body and absorb subsequently human tissues and organs [234]. The γ-ray released by *in vivo* radioactive isotopes during their decay process can be detected by nuclear detection devices *in vitro*, and the distribution density of the radioactive isotopes *in vivo* can be simultaneously obtained. In contrast to other imaging technologies, radionuclide imaging possesses both deep tissue penetration with negligible limitation and high sensitivity [235]. With the aim to investigate the organ biodistribution of various f-MWNTs *in vivo*, Wang et al. radiolabeled MWNTs with ^{111}In to enable the *in vivo* single-photon emission computed tomography/computed tomography (SPECT/CT) imaging [226]. With this radionuclide modification, detection of the f-MWNTs *in vivo* through whole-body SPECT/CT imaging could be achieved easily and directly. ^{131}I is another important radio isotope that can be applied in radionuclide imaging. Zhao et al. firstly modified SWNTs with polydopamine (PDA) and PEG, forming a nanostructure named SWNTs@PDA-PEG [227]. The functionalization of PDA shell enabled ^{131}I to be labelled onto SWNTs@PDA-PEG for the subsequent radionuclide imaging. After administration, outstanding tumor tissue distribution of ^{131}I-labelled SWNTs@PDA-PEG was observed *in vivo* through a gamma counter.

8.13.6 Near-Infrared Fluorescence Imaging

Near-infrared fluorescence (NIRF) imaging is an exciting and fast-progressing imaging technique which can be applied in deep tissues and organs for cancer diagnosis. NIR biological window ranges from 780 to 1,700 nm, and CNTs possess obvious optical absorption and intrinsic fluorescence in this range. Therefore, CNT is a type of promising material which can be applied in NIRF imaging during cancer diagnosis, and NIRF images are commonly acquired through an in-house *in vivo* imager. In contrast to MWNTs, SWNTs are more suitable for NIR imaging due to the higher absorbing properties with stronger optical absorption, better E11 optical transitions, and less photobleaching. Ghosh et al. designed an M13-stabilized SWNTs probe which could precisely target secreted protein, acidic and rich in cysteines (SPARC)–expressing tumor nodules *in vivo* [228]. Second-window NIR light (NIR-II) was applied in this research as the fluorescence source to circumvent optical scattering and obtain deeper tissue penetration effect during NIRF imaging. According to the diagnostic result, these NIR2-emitting SWNTs probes produced outstanding signal-to-noise performance and exhibited high specificity toward in situ ovarian tumor and the implanted tumor nodules that existed on the surfaces of other peritoneal organs. Another research of adopting SWNTs to NIRF imaging was done by Welsher et al. [229]. In this research, SWNTs were firstly combined with phospholipid-PEG (PL-PEG) for the formation of a biocompatible nanosystem with negligible destruction of the integrity of WNTs' sidewall, which effectively enhanced the stability of SWNTs as well. With the application of an InGaAs camera, intravital tumor vessel images with high resolution were obtained through the thick skin of the live mice made by the aforementioned functionalized SWNTs.

8.14 CNTs in Nanobiosensors

Biosensors were studied in 1962 by Clark and his teammates for the first time to qualify the glucose concentration combining electrochemical oxygen and glucose oxidase enzyme in aqueous media. Recently, nanobiosensors have become more and more attentive mainly due to their easy application, fast response, and low cost. Nanobiosensors are an important type of biosensors that usually consist of both biological recognition elements and nanomaterials with the dimensions range from 1 to 100 nm. Therefore, the events at nanoscale level, such as the interaction between small molecules and specific receptors, can be monitored and detected by nanobiosensors sensitively. Due to the outstanding electrical conductivity, excellent electrocatalytic activity, high stability, with slow oxidation kinetics and good modifiability, CNTs are a class of suitable inorganic material for the application as nanobiosensors in cancer diagnosis [236].

8.14.1 CNTs in Combination with Metallic Compound

Some types of metallic NPs, like AuNPs and AgNPs, can be applied to modify CNTs for the construction of nanobiosensors. Rawashdeh et al. reported that AuNPs-modified MWNTs were electrochemical nanobiosensors that detect a kind of micro–ribonucleic acid named miR-21 [230]. The miR-21 derived from body fluid exhibits an important role in the early diagnosis of pancreatic cancer. However, the miR-21 existing in bloodstreams is generally at very low level during the early stage of pancreatic cancer, which brings great difficulty to cancer diagnosis. With the application of AuNPs-decorated MWNTs, the detection of miR-21 was greatly improved. According to the experiment result, this nanobiosensor was able to provide a broad linear range for detecting miR-21, with a detection limit as low as 3.68 femtomolar (fM), using the source measure unit (SMU). Thus, this nanobiosensor constructed by MWNTs possessed excellent application prospect in the early diagnosis of pancreatic cancer.

8.14.2 CNTs in Combination with Antibody

Nanoimmunosensors based on antibody are another kind of nanobiosensors for cancer diagnosis. Osteopontin (OPN) is a biomarker which can be applied to detect prostate cancer. And the OPN level is important for predicting the survival time of prostate patient. Traditionally, the measurement of OPN is usually achieved by ELISA assay; however, lack of sensitivity, high cost, and complex operation greatly hinder this detection method. Sharma et al. covalently combined OPN monoclonal antibodies onto the surface of carboxylated SWNTs, forming a nanoimmunosensor to determine OPN based on electrical detection for prostate cancer diagnosis [231]. This nanoimmunosensor exhibited high specificity to only OPN, which showed outstanding selectivity during detection. Moreover, broad detection range and low detection limit can both be achieved with this nanoimmunosensor during prostate cancer detection.

8.14.3 CNTs in Combination with Peptide Reporter

Peptide reporter–modified nanobiosensors enable implementation to quantify peptide activity sensitively and dose-dependently in complex biological environments. CDK1 (cyclin-dependent kinase 1) is a protein coding gene. Diseases associated with CDK1 include polyploidy and retinoblastoma. Among its related pathways are regulation of activated PAK-2p34 by proteasome-mediated degradation and loss of Nlp from mitotic centrosomes. CDK1 is responsible for the progression through mitosis and the coordination of G2/M transition; however, diagnostic methods for the detection and measurement of relative activities of CDK1 possess great difficulties due to the lack of sensitivity and specificity. Tilmaciu et al. designed functionalized MWNTs that were modified with a kind of fluorescent peptide reporter which was specific to CDK1 for the sensitive and fluorescence-based quantification of CDK1's activity through fluorescence imaging [232]. This nanobiosensor could not only achieve the simple detection of CDK1 but also report the enzymatic activity of CDK1 as well. Therefore, the information on kinase function in the biological environment could be subsequently provided. And this nanobiosensor exhibited a promising future for the application in cancer diagnosis, because CDK/cyclin activity could be detected in numerous cancer types and was associated with poor prognosis.

8.14.4 CNTs in Combination with Multiple Modifications

In contrast to single modification, multiple modifications to CNTs can further improve the diagnostic effects obtained from the constructed nanobiosensors. Cervical cancer severely threatens women's health, and its incidence keeps growing at a very fast rate. Human papillomaviruses (HPVs), especially HPV type 18 (HPV-18), are important factors leading to cervical cancer. Mahmoodi et al. designed an rGO-MWNTs/L-Cys-AuNPs nanocomposite through the modification of reduced graphene oxide (rGO), AuNPs, L-Cysteine (L-Cys), and single-strand DNA (ssDNA) probe to MWNTs as an electrochemical DNA biosensor to diagnose HPV-18 [233]. rGO improved the electrical conduction of this nanobiosensor; AuNPs not only increased electrical conductivity but also immobilized DNA on the electrode surface as well. In addition, L-Cys also plays an important role in immobilizing the ssDNA probes on the surface of this nanobiosensor [237]. According to their research, this nanobiosensor possessed high selectivity and sensitivity to HPV-18. Both the extracted DNA from HPV-18 patients and the synthetic DNA could be detected by this nanobiosensor in very small quantities with large detection range. Altogether, this constructed nanobiosensor could be regarded as an essential tool for the early, easy, rapid, and accurate diagnosis of HPV-18 compared with other classical detection methods.

8.15 Multi-Responsive Intelligent Nanomaterials

Designing smart systems with dual- or multi-responsiveness capabilities is highly promising to provide accurate, systemic, and site-specific drug administration. Additionally, dual- and multi- responsiveness might substantially boost the diverse usability of such systems by integrating the drug administration with other desirables, like imaging, sensing, or monitoring. Such systems do provide yet another possibility to tweak their response toward each stimulus individually, enabling medication release to be precisely controlled under cumulative effect of multiple stimuli. In these systems, multiple impulses are integrated to enable nanoformulation in milder environment, by introducing external stimulus like pH, temperature, etc., since in such systems one of these stimuli will be employed to load drug in carriers and other/s for activating the release of drug; also, the activation of drug release under external stimulus, including magnetic field, temperature, light, or ultrasonic waves; further, the release of drugs can also be initiated at targeted site. Owing to diverse TME, including as perfusion, oxygenation, vascular irregularities, and other metabolic conditions, such stimuli-responsive systems are especially developed for anticancer medication.

Yet another research conducted by Ying et al. demonstrated distillation-precipitation polymerization to develop novel redox/pH dual-stimuli responsive camptothecin (CPT) prodrug nanogels (Figure 8.21A) [238]. In aqueous phase, the as-prepared P(CPT-MAA) prodrug nanogels had a high CPT grafting rate (approaching 92.4%) and were uniform spheres. The CPT release results suggested that its release depends on pH and redox dual-responsive phenomenon. This might be due to the redox-sensitive feature of the disulfide link and the acid-sensitive property of MAA, which may further limit tumor development both *in vitro* and *in vivo*. Figure 8.21Ba–c shows the highest efficiency of nanogel prodrug in the inhibition of tumor growth among all groups, whereas Figure 8.21B-b shows decrease in body weight of mice by 22% in only CPT-treated group. Zhong et al., in their research, mentioned biocompatible triple-responsive nanocages (acid pH, temperature, and reducing agent). Under triple stimulation, the aforementioned nanocages greatly enhanced the release of drug, pharmacokinetic properties, and bioavailability of anticancer drugs, affirming the potent in vivo therapeutic effect with minimal adverse effects. You et al. developed a dual-responsive GSH and near-infrared light system for targeted cisplatin and indocyanine green delivery. Result showed that at pH of 7.4 after 72 h, a higher percentage of drug was released in acidic conditions, particularly when exposed to GSH and near-infrared irradiation (99.35%) compared to GSH alone (58.45%), near-infrared light alone (73.46%), or neither stimulus (12.35%). The previous study results, even so, were not significant at pH 5.5. In a cytotoxicity assay, cell viability was reduced to 1.95% (SGC-7901) when exposed to near-infrared light and to 1.25% in MCF-7 cells. Human gastric cancer cell line (SGC-7901) was established by Wang Long-Bao et al. in cooperation with Shanghai No. 6 People's Hospital and other institutions. SGC7901 is a human gastric cancer cell line that is commonly used in research to study gastric cancer, a type of cancer that affects the stomach. The SGC7901 cell line was originally derived from a patient with gastric adenocarcinoma.

Recent years of rapid advancement in the establishment of mono-, dual-, and multi-responsive polymeric nanoparticulate systems with tailored targeted drug delivery have limitless potential in design and chemical composition. Every mono-responsive or hybrid responsive system does have its own set of advantages and disadvantages. Despite numerous advances, there are still several barriers to transforming stimuli-responsive drug delivery devices for clinical use. The need of the hour is to create systems with improved sensitivity, biocompatibility, non-toxicity, and multi-responsive qualities. Many multi-responsive polymer systems are only proof-of-concept studies that are only examined *in vitro*. As a result, rigorous in vivo performance evaluation of multi-stimuli sensitive systems is required.

8.16 Toxicological Effects of Nanomaterials

As stated in the preceding sections, different types of nanoparticles are frequently being employed as nanomedicine and nanocarriers due to their small size and unique physicochemical properties. Properties like morphology (shape), size, surface functional groups, and dose-dependent characteristics may also contribute to nanomaterial-induced toxicity in healthy human cells, tissues, and organs.

For example, cellular uptake of nanomaterials is mainly regulated by the shape, which plays a vital role in toxicity as well as biological reactivity [239]. Studies have indicated that the needle-shaped nanomaterials are more toxic in comparison to spherical-shaped due to enhanced adhesiveness to the target cell surface, rate of internalization, and better multiple endocytic mechanism. In zebrafish embryos, Ag nanoplates possesses higher toxicity in comparison to Ag nanospheres, whereas Au nanorods cause less autophagosome accumulation in contrast to Au nanospheres. Likewise, surface-area-to-volume ratio increases exponentially with decrease in nanomaterials size, resulting in increased chemical and biological reactivity. The toxic effect of nanomaterials is mainly dominated by the interaction between the surface of nanomaterials and the cellular components. Therefore, with the same chemical composition, nanoparticles show different toxicity level, depending on the particle size and surface area [239]. Inhalation of different-size nanomaterials exhibits different levels of distribution pattern in the respiratory tract, as inhalation of AgNPs demonstrated size-dependent pulmonary inflammation. Similarly, smaller AuNPs (10 and 30 nm size) can cross the nuclear membrane and break DNA, whereas, large-sized AuNPs (60 nm size) are reported to have higher accumulation in the spleen [240].

Further, surface functionalization or coatings of nanomaterials enables in modification of their property; however, it can convert non-toxic particles into toxic ones due to enhanced bioavailability. Polyethyleneimine (PEI)–coated iron oxide nanoparticles are shown to be highly internalized in both cancer cells and macrophages and consequently display higher toxicological effects in comparison to PEG-coated iron oxide nanoparticles. This may be attributed to higher affinity of cationic nanoparticles to protein domains or negatively charged phospholipid present in cellular membrane. Therefore, it is essential to consider the impact of surface functionalization while studying the toxicity effect of nanomaterials. In the lungs, aspect ratio–based nanoparticle toxicity has also been observed. The aspect ratio of nanomaterials is directly proportional to toxicity. In this context, Li et al. demonstrated the in vivo toxic effect of MSN with different aspect ratios of 1, 1.75, and 5. With decrease in aspect ratio, absorption through organs increases, whereas excretion via urine reduces. Furthermore, toxicity of nanomaterials can be defined by its dissolution

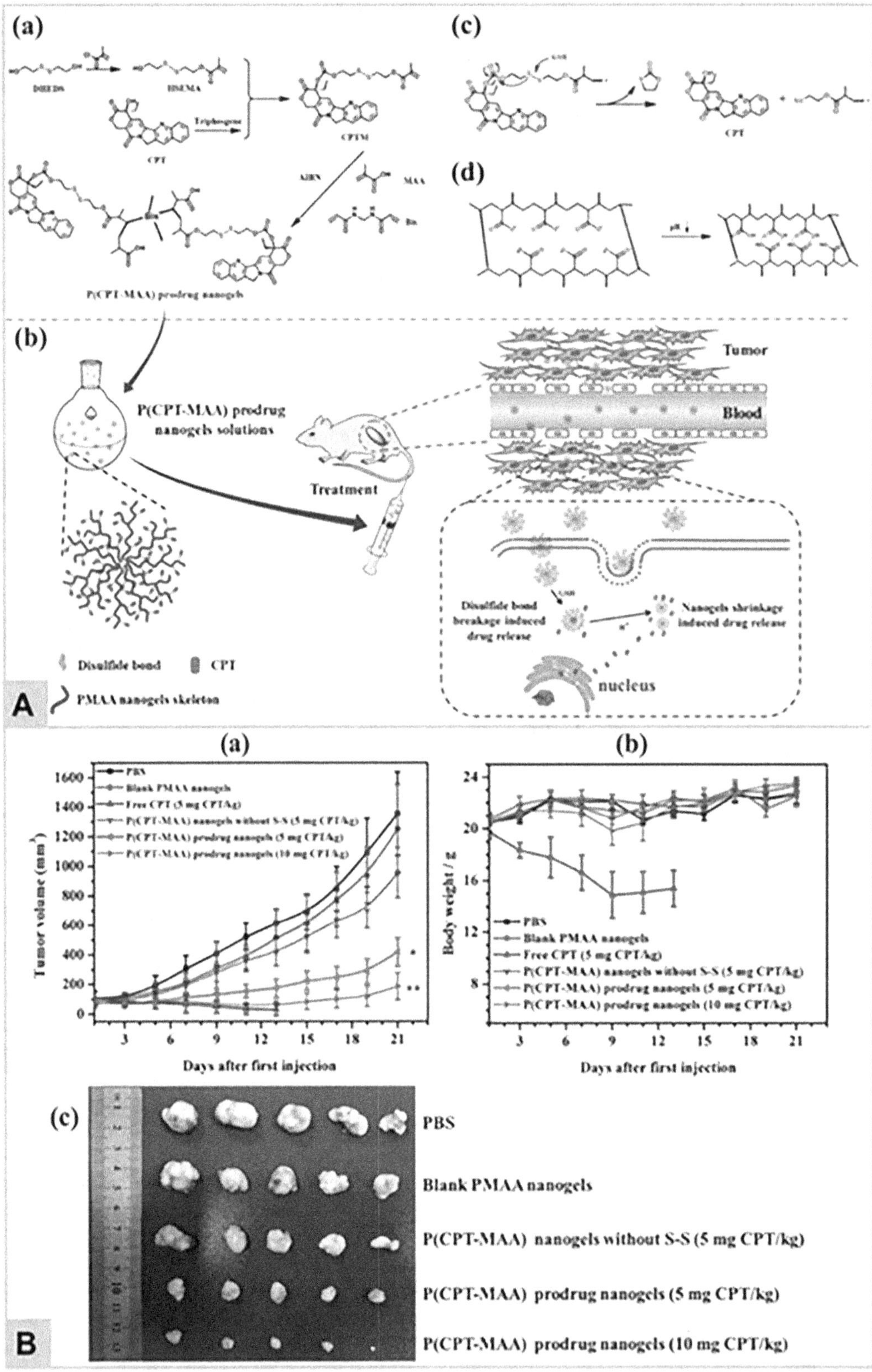

FIGURE 8.21 (a) Synthesis of the P(CPT-MAA) prodrug nanogels. (b) Schematic illustration of the pH and redox dual-responsive drug release of P(CPT-MAA) prodrug nanogels. (c) The redox-responsive drug release mechanism. (d) The pH-responsive mechanism (panel A). In vivo antitumor assays. (a) Relative tumor volume and (b) body weight of the Hep G2 tumor-bearing BALB/c nude mice administrated by the intravenous injection of PBS, blank PMAA nanogels, free CPT (5 mg CPT/kg), P(CPT-MAA) nanogels without single bond (5 mg CPT/kg), and P(CPT-MAA) prodrug nanogels (5 mg CPT/kg and 10 mg CPT/kg), respectively. (c) Photo images of the harvested tumors at 21 days post the first injection; no tumor of free CPT group obtained due to the death of all mice at 13 days. *Note:* *$p<0.05$; **$p<0.01$, compared with PBS, blank PMAA groups (panel B).

Source: [238].

ability. Depending on the surface modification, nanoparticles with similar composition may experience a different degree of dissolution.

Furthermore, the surface charge of nanomaterials is essential in governing their cellular internalization, interaction with biomolecules, or cellular organelles. Therefore, the surface charge of nanomaterials directly influences the toxic behaviour of nanomaterials. Studies have confirmed that an iron oxide nanoparticle with higher positive charge possesses more toxic effect in human hepatoma BEL-7402 cells. This might be due to high electrostatic interaction of more positively charged nanoparticles, leading to more endocytic effect. Recently, smart nanomaterials–mediated drug delivery systems have been developed for targeting brain, but very less information is available on neurotoxicity. Nevertheless, various researches suggest that neurotoxicity of nanomaterials is due to the free radical–mediated oxidative stress [241]. Interestingly, due to high surface energy, a nanomaterial tends to be agglomerated and may induce inflammatory condition in human lungs. Generally, oxides and carbon nanotubes exhibit the agglomeration-dependent toxic effect. Agglomerated carbon nanotubes are reported to induce additional toxic effects in comparison to well-dispersed carbon nanotubes. On the contrary, large AgNPs agglomerate induces less haemolytic toxic effect in comparison to smaller aggregates.

In addition to this, recent studies have demonstrated that chemically manufactured nanomaterials are more harmful to human cells than biosynthesized nanoparticles, which consist of biocompatible surface functional groups. However, certain biosynthesized nanoparticles may also be hazardous, by disintegrating into smaller fragments and bioaccumulation. ROS-mediated oxidative stress is reported as one of the most common nanoparticle-induced toxicity phenomena at cellular level. ROS generally attacks cellular proteins, nucleic acid, lipids, and key biomolecules, which lead to membrane damage, membrane depolarization, electron transfer chain impairment, and NADPH-like system activation [239]. Nanoparticles like ZnO are well reported to induce oxidative stress–mediated DNA damage and ROS-triggered apoptosis in both human and bacterial cells. Zhao et al. demonstrated ZnO nanoparticles–mediated acute toxicological effect and developmental abnormalities in zebrafish embryo [242] due to DNA damage and apoptosis induction by p53-mitochondria-caspase-mediated pathway. Besides oxidative stress, toxicity of nanomaterials can be caused by various other biochemical, physicochemical, and molecular mechanisms. Excessive Ca^{2+} production is another way of nanoparticle-induced toxicity, as it induces apoptosis via releasing cytochrome c. From the discussion, it is apparent that the full potential of nanomaterials is yet to be achieved in nanomedicine, and it can only be exploited if we can control their toxicity and develop smart nanomaterials.

8.17 Current Technological Challenges and Limitations of Effective Theranostics

Smart nanomaterials offer a robust platform for effective cancer theranostics as they can be triggered in response to specific external or endogenous stimuli, like pH, temperature, enzymes, or a particular biological molecule. Compared to traditional cancer theranostic approaches, smart nanomaterials–based approaches exhibit improved selectivity and sensitivity with fewer adverse effects. Furthermore, an additional benefit of using a theranostic device is the non-invasive, rapid, and precise identification of early chemotherapeutic responses. Overall, using theranostic platforms based on nanotechnology gives chemotherapy unmatched advantages for overcoming its long-accompanied disadvantages. Early cancer detection, tailored medication delivery, drug discovery, and effective anticancer therapy are all possible with nanotechnology-based techniques and nanomaterials in oncology. Gold nanoparticles (AuNPs) have been widely used in treating breast and prostate cancers as drug delivery systems. AuNPs are considered because of their dependable qualities, such as their ability to scatter light, absorb light, and convert optical energy into heat [243]. Though the nanomaterials have proven their anticancer activities, one of the most challenging problems in the field of nanotheranostics is system complexity, having numerous functionalities in a single nanometer particle size. Industrial scale-up production and its clinical translation are also two of the main obstacles in the field of NPs. Scientists and engineers should adopt an interdisciplinary approach to successfully absorb this field in cancer theranostic nanomedicine. With many of their intrinsic molecular properties and multifunctionality, different nanomaterials have recently become an exciting tool in cancer theranostic applications, assisting in successful therapy, diagnosis, and imaging. However, several obstacles prevent their clinical translation, including systemic toxicity of nanomaterials within the body, nontargeted distribution, complex synthesis, high cost, reduced biocompatibility, stability, and reduced photostability [180, 244]. Another major obstacle to the use of nanomaterials in cancer theranostics is the selection of models, as most of the research is in and around cell and animal models that may not be the right models to assess the anticancer efficacy of both diagnostic and therapeutic agents, as these models suffer from various degrees of different chemical and physical stresses and might not be representative of those of whole human organs. In the complex human system, it is difficult to replicate a reaction using just one model.

A single model may not mimic the complex human system; however, the possibility to link several of these models, which are capable of recapitulating the *in vivo* interaction, extracellular matrix, intercellular signaling, and *in vivo* growth, may provide a system that more closely resembles and can harness a better understanding of *in vivo* events. Biomimetic organ/tumor-on-a-chip tools and organoid model systems are possible solutions to imitate *in vivo* conditions of nanocarriers used in cancer patients [245]. First and foremost, developing a low-cost synthesis method and an easy purification procedure is vitally necessary to enable the mass production of nanomaterials. The focus on engineered nanomaterials with high hydrophilicities will open the door to anticancer drug carriers with enhanced tumor therapy efficacy and drug delivery. Last, but not the least, the focus should be directed toward delivering genetic material to the cancer cell for effective cancer theranostics. So far, the full potential of nanomaterials in cancer is not fully utilized, as nanotoxicity and bioaccumulation of NPs constrain their broader applicability.

TABLE 8.9

Some Cancer Theranostics Agents and Their Characteristics and Indications

Nanoparticles	Purpose in Cancer Treatment	Biocompatibility	Diagnostic Potential	Indications (Approved and/or in Clinical Phases)	Ref.
Liposome	Therapeutics, diagnostics, theranostics	Yes	Nanocarriers for the delivery of a variety of drugs	Under clinical trial/phase II	[246]
Lipid NPS	Therapeutics, diagnostics, theranostics	Yes	Negligible toxicity, multifunctional potential, and functionalization flexibility help them cross different physiological barriers; LNPs can deliver chemotherapeutic medications to tumor tissue by penetrating the vascular endothelial gaps of tumor	Phase I clinical trial (nct00355888) of MBP-426 was completed, with phase II started	[247]
Protein NPs	Therapeutics, diagnostics, theranostics	Yes	Natural availability and biocompatibility; physiology makes it amenable to biomedicine and materials science; amphiphilic in nature; albumin has been recognized as a potential carrier for delivering imaging/anticancer medicines to tumor microenvironments	Clinical trials completed for albumin and albumin-based NPs currently undergoing clinical studies/phase II	[248]
MOF	Therapeutics, diagnostics, theranostics, imaging	Yes	High surface areas, adjustable pore size, crystallinity, thermal stability, and easy surface modification; effective cellular uptake, focused molecular targeting, smart nanodrug delivery devices, and drug-responsive behavior	Translation to clinical settings; long-term toxicity and biosafety of NMOFs still need to be further evaluated	[249]
Carbon-based nanoparticles	Therapeutics, diagnostics, theranostics, imaging	Yes	Carbon-based nanomaterials exhibit several extraordinary properties, such as high surface area, tunable pore structure, and nonreactive and easy surface functionalization, making them suitable for biological applications	FDA has approved over 35 imaging or therapeutic nanoparticles for clinical trials; under preclinical studies and no clinical trials to date	[250]
Inorganic nanoparticles (platinum, gold, silica, palladium, silver, iron oxides, zinc oxide, and rare earth oxides)	Therapeutics, diagnostics, theranostics, imaging	Yes	Inorganic NPs have enormous potential as drug carriers, owing to the easy modification of targeting molecules, different stimuli-driven drug release, and effective delivery to target sites; inorganic NPs are investigated in preclinical and clinical studies for the detection, diagnosis, and treatment of many diseases	Currently used in clinical practice, gold nanoparticles or nanoshells (nct00356980, nct00848042), silica nanoparticles (nct02106598), and silica–gold nanoparticles (nct01270139) might hold a greater chance to speed up the translational process	[251]
Quantum dots	Therapeutics, diagnostics, theranostics, imaging	Yes	Compact size, high surface area, surface charges, and precision targeting are distinctive features; increases solubility, prolongs the period of retention, and lessens the negative effects of loaded drugs	FDA has approved a clinical trial for Cornell dot, or c-dot, for melanoma patients	[252]

QDs have generated a great deal of attention in various biological domains due to their several significant benefits over conventional dyes in bioimaging. However, these applications face numerous difficulties, including cellular toxicity brought by producing reactive oxygen species and cadmium leakage, which might threaten the patient after the treatment. For example, graphene QDs have been demonstrated to be safe and nontoxic to normal cells. However, extensive *in vivo* toxicity studies are required prior to its administration in cancer theranostics. Despite QDs' effectiveness in cancer theranostics, one of the biggest problems is the possibility of nonspecific reticuloendothelial absorption, which lowers the likelihood and effectiveness of these theranostic agents binding to the targeted cancer site.

In this chapter, we covered the development of many multifunctional platforms for cancer therapy and diagnosis, as well as diverse methods utilized to reduce the toxicity of nanomaterials through the process of hybridization with different biocompatible lipids, proteins, polymers, or nanoparticles. Table 8.9 summarizes some cancer theranostic agent characteristics, biocompatibility, and translation stages.

8.18 Global Opportunities of Smart Nanomaterials in Next-Generation Cancer Theranostics

The use of nanomaterials has shown a paradigm shift in cancer theranostics when compared to conventional approaches. Nanotechnology has revolutionized the cancer theranostics field, as the sizes of biomolecules, such as DNA, hemoglobin, proteins, and enzymes, are in accordance with the size of NPs, which leads to enhanced biomedical application, owing to their effective interactions. Owing to the unique properties of nanomaterials, a high surface-to-volume ratio leads to a broader surface area for interactions with biological molecules, resulting in increased sensitivity, enhanced selectivity, and shorter reaction times. Quantum dots (QDs), liposomes, micelles, metallic nanoparticles, dendrimers, and polymeric nanoparticles have recently been utilized for cancer therapy and imaging. Contrarily, the traditional approaches to treating cancer are ineffective and lack selectivity [253]. As these traditional procedures affect healthy and cancerous cells, opponents of health also dispute their selectivity. The most significant benefit of smart nanomaterials is their ability to overcome these constraints. Nanomedicine advancements have influenced better outcomes for cancer detection and treatment and have opened new avenues for cancer treatment. Nanomaterials have shown improved pharmacokinetics, biocompatibility, tumor targeting, and stability compared to conventional methods. However, numerous uses of nanomaterials are still challenging because of certain restraints, such as nonspecific delivery, multistep synthesis, poor bioaffinity, reduced light immovability, and toxicity of nanomaterials inside the living system. Therefore, enhanced nanomaterial moieties with well-ordered physicochemical and biological characteristics are strongly considered for cancer theranostics.

Recent advancements in smart nanomaterials–based cancer theranostic methodologies have been cultivated, and they are exposing recovering sensitivity and selectivity by condensed negative effects in contrast to traditional methods. In cancer treatment, the smart nanomaterials system reacts to the tumor microenvironment (TME) and leftovers in the neutralized form in standard cells, decreasing the side effects and overall toxicities. Nanomaterials expand drug effectiveness by enhanced sensitivity, light-absorbing capacity, drug half-life lengthening, and drug solubility enhancement, with long-standing confirming drug discharge. Additionally, smart nanomaterials can also be applied to intensify the healing, drug loading capability, and organized continuous discharge of drugs, and specific and selective biodissemination, by engineering their conformation, designing methodologies, morphology, size, and surface chemistry. Unlike traditional materials, engineered smart nanomaterials can pierce transversely biological obstacles and empower pH-, light-, and heat-based pursuit of malicious cells. Manufacturing procedures may be fine-tuned to normalize the functionality and specificity of nanomaterials by transforming the chemical configuration, shape (morphology), and size. For cancer-dealing approaches, nanomaterials can overwhelm the stability and solubility of anticancer drugs [254]. Nanomaterials also help in the treatment of persistent tissue by pointing to the cancer spots, delivery of various drugs, and falling drug conflict. Additionally, to overwhelm the cytotoxic influence of nanomaterials, novel methodologies have been projected to cultivate biocompatible nanomaterials resembling surface reformation with diverse biodegradable fragments. Extensive research studies need to be carried out for engineered hybrid NPs better suited for cancer treatment with specific binding. The size, shape, composition, and surface of the NPs impact the immune system. Though the nanomaterial approaches are more effective than traditional approaches, the clinical efficacy of this therapy is still inadequate, and further research into the safety and tolerance of these novel techniques is required. Exploiting nanomaterial characteristics to improve target specificity can achieve significant therapeutic efficacy. Though many research studies were carried out for the uses of nanomaterials in cancer theranostics, only a handful of nanomaterials have successfully translated to clinical applications. Extensive research needs to be carried out for the successful implementation of nanomaterials in clinical applications amid tumor heterogeneity, which poses one of the greatest technological challenges to theranostics.

8.19 Advantages, Challenges, and Outlooks of Nanomaterials

Employing nanomaterials for biomedical applications offers better prospects because biomolecules such as DNA, proteins, enzymes, and hemoglobin occur in the nanometer range inside the living entity. At this scale, the surface-to-volume ratio is high, and it provides large surface area for interactions with the biological molecules, leading to higher sensitivity and enhanced specificity with reduced time for reaction. In this context, quantum dots (QDs), metallic nanoparticles, liposomes, dendrimers, micelles, and polymeric nanoparticles have emerged in the recent past for cancer therapy and imaging. On the contrary, the conventional methods of cancer therapeutics have limited effectiveness and lack of selectivity. Further, poor solubility, inadequate biodistribution, lower stability, and poor metabolism pose different challenges of toxicity and inefficacy, making these methods less effective. Health critics also raise questions on selectivity of these conventional methods as they harm both healthy cells and cancer cells. Overcoming these limitations is the utmost advantage of smart nanomaterials.

Nanomaterials are promising and the best possible choice for controlled drug delivery systems, diagnostics, and imaging. It improves therapeutic efficacy by enhancing sensitivity, the capacity to absorb light, extending drug half-life, boosting drug solubility, and ensuring long-term drug release. These smart artificially engineered nanomaterials exhibit higher cellular uptake, targeted tumor site delivery with more specificity, as compared with conventional materials. Moreover, smart nanomaterials can also be extensively used to increase the therapeutic drug loading capacity, controlled sustained release of drugs, as well as selective and specific biodistribution, by engineering their composition, synthesis methods, size, morphology, and surface chemistry. Unlike conventional materials, the artificially engineered smart nanomaterials can penetrate across biological barriers and enable pH, thermal, and light-based targeting of malignant cells. Synthesis processes may be fine-tuned to regulate the functionality and specificity of nanomaterials by modifying the chemical composition, size, and shape (morphology) according to the applications. Specifically, for cancer treatment strategies, nanomaterials can overcome the limitations of solubility and stability of anticancer drugs. Furthermore, these nanomaterials prevent pharmaceuticals from being degraded by enzymes, enhance drug half-life in *in vivo* responses, and improve anticancer drug biodistribution. Nanomaterials also help in the sustained release of anticancer drug by targeting the cancer sites, delivery of multiple drugs at single platform, and reducing drug resistance.

From the preceding discussion, it is apparent that nanomaterials exhibit various advantages in biomedical industry, like biodegradability, high drug loading capacity, and release characteristics, accompanied with stimuli sensitivity. Despite their extensive use in the development of various drug delivery systems, some limitations, including toxicity, uniform size/shape of nanomaterials, and limited biocompatibility with specific cell membrane, need to be resolved. Further, to overcome the cytotoxic effect of nanomaterials, new approaches have been proposed to develop biocompatible nanomaterials, like surface modification with different biodegradable molecules. In this context, research has been conducted on different shapes (nanoflowers, nanospheres, nanowires, nanostars, and nanoprisms) of AuNPs to compare their toxicity, which clearly indicates that the toxic behaviour of nanoparticles depends on their shape and size. Functional group–dependent cytotoxic research showed that AuNPs modified with polyethylene glycol-SH exhibit no cytotoxicity when compared with polyethylene glycol and polyethylene glycol-NH_2. Further, it has also been reported that the coating of Fe_3O_4 over silica shell reduces its cytotoxic effect by minimizing the oxidative stress and altering the iron homeostasis.

Although stimuli-responsive nanomaterials provide targeted delivery to the specific site, more precise imaging in biological system is still a challenge. Currently, various imaging modalities are available, but each one has their own pros and cons. For example, fluorescence imaging lacks in tissue penetration ability and spatial resolution. On the contrary, MRI experiences high cost, has low sensitivity, and is time-consuming. Thus, for future application, stimuli-responsive nanomaterial-activated multimodality imaging should be developed for more accurate and complementary information regarding disease of patients. Further, the responsiveness of multifunctional nanomaterials also needs to be considered, as sometimes the response of one stimulus may fail, leading to the compromised efficiency of the whole system. Nowadays, research is mainly focused on the use of universal nanoparticles which are more compatible to incorporate the drug/genes at the same time or separately and allow their release spatially and temporally. Thus, theragnostic nanomaterials with multiple actions at the same time should be explored further, which leads to early diagnosis and drug/gene therapy.

In addition, biodegradability is another key factor that is important for the stability of nanomaterials in biological medium. Various biodegradable nanomaterials, like chitosan, liposomes, dendrimers, and poly(lactic-co-glycolic acid) (PLGA) micelles, are utilized to improve the therapeutic effect and decrease the side effects. In this context, poly(lactic-co-glycolic acid) microspheres–coated particles protect the cells from harsh oxidative stress conditions. Moreover, conjugating the stimuli-responsive nanomaterials with highly specific gene editing tools like zinc finger nucleases, transcription activator-like effector nucleases (TALENs), and CRISPR-cas gene editing tools can provide specific cleavage of the DNA.

Exogenous stimuli sources (light, ultrasound, temperature, magnetic fields) may damage the normal cells. However, designing a nanomaterial which utilizes the endogenous stimuli sources, such as redox potential, pH, enzymes, and glucose concentrations, can deliver safe, efficient, and intelligent nanocarriers, where more research in this area is encouraged. Although the stimuli-responsive nanomaterials are designed extensively, it is still a challenge to provide clinical efficiency due to the variability of different cancers and patient-to-patients biases, limiting the stimuli-responsive targeted drug delivery and diagnosis. The selection of the method of physical, chemical, or biological-responsive nanomaterials adopted is based on clinical applications. For example, in the treatment of cancers such as glioblastoma, a high degree of specificity and sensitivity is required, where the enzyme-responsive nanomaterials hold high applications. Moreover, toxicity to the healthy tissues may be avoided by using exogenous stimuli-responsive nanomaterials. Many state-of-art tools developed lack the efficiency to precisely measure the in vivo dynamics. Moreover, many more physical or molecular biomarkers to distinguish between cancer cells and normal cells can open avenues for the development of the chemo-diagnostics and chemo-therapeutics field. The use of nanomaterials for cancer treatment and diagnosis provides many advantages, as these materials can be functionalized and can also be easily tuned. Smart nanomaterials consist of the ability to deliver specifically in therapeutic, diagnostic, or both fields. These anticancer drugs can be delivered across traditional biological barriers in the body, such as the dense endothelial blood–brain barrier, with the help of nanocarriers.

Overall, stimuli-responsive smart nanomaterials provide great potential to improve the efficacy of cancer diagnosis and therapy. New strategies should be developed to address the challenges which significantly contribute to the designing of precise nanomedicine.

8.20 Conclusions and Future Prospect

This chapter gives a summary of the updated advances of CNTs in cancer theranostics. Recent decades have witnessed the booming progress of nanotechnology in the biomedical field. CNTs, one of the most widely investigated carbon-related nanomaterials, have gained considerable attention since their discovery. Because of their distinguished physiochemical properties and unique architecture, like extensive surface areas, rich surface modification possibilities, high drug loading capacity, and great optical features, CNTs can not only be adopted as fantastic transporters in drug delivery but also occupy an important position in phototherapy-based cancer treatment. Through optimal functionalization, the inherent limitations of CNTs, like unsatisfactory solubility, agglomeration, and toxicity toward cells, can be overcome, which improves their therapeutic performance in cancer treatment due to the enhanced biocompatibility and biodegradability, promoted tumor-penetration ability, and acquired active targeting capability. Moreover, many researches have demonstrated the multifunctional applications of CNTs in anticancer targeted drug delivery, which ranges from intracellular targeting spots to TME components, from single therapeutic modality to combinational treatment strategies, all indicating the promising future of CNTs in cancer treatment. In addition to their therapeutic applications, CNTs are also important participants in cancer diagnosis because of their peculiar characteristics. CNTs can be utilized in different cancer imaging, like PA imaging, MRI, Raman imaging, radionuclide imaging, and NIR fluorescence imaging. Besides, when combining with other diagnostic agents, CNTs are able to be employed in nanobiosensors for the early detection of various cancer types, like pancreatic cancer, prostate cancer, and cervical cancer with a high specificity. Therefore, CNTs are one of the versatile nanomaterials with broad biomedical application potential in both cancer treatment and diagnosis.

Early detection of different types of cancers, targeted drug delivery, and controlled drug release are the future of cancer treatment. The success of nanotechnology in recent times indicates that it is a promising field which can provide valuable information about the disease and future techniques for therapeutic possibilities. Moreover, designer nanomaterials with controlled toxicity have demonstrated significant influence on the pharmaceutical business, resulting in the emergence of nanomedicine. Due to nanomaterials biocompatibility, high loading capacity, and stimuli-responsive drug release properties, stimuli-responsive nanoparticles have garnered the attention of the scientific community and are widely utilized in biomedical applications, particularly in drug delivery. These qualities also offer a viable path for improving the efficacy of existing medications and accelerating the development of disease diagnostics and therapies.

The quick expansion of theranostics based on nanotechnology has impressively endorsed the uprising of diagnosis methodologies and cancer oncotherapy. The present chapter discusses the most relevant advancements in smart nanomaterials, from organic, inorganic, and carbon-based nanoparticles for cancer theranostic applications. The review article's findings are incredibly inspiring and strongly urge the exploration of nanomaterials as nanocarriers, and their physicochemical attributes can be harnessed to improve *in vivo* performances in cancer theranostics. This chapter also detailed the limitation and global opportunities for the successful implementation of nanomaterials-based cancer theranostics, which can be translated into clinical applications. One can expect that, by giving attention to the key challenges mentioned earlier, the nanomaterials-based cancer theranostic platform will bring many exciting opportunities for therapy and diagnosis to achieve accurate cancer diagnoses and address the challenges of conventional oncotherapy. Nanotechnology has demonstrated a new dimension for cancer theranostics by delivering tiny molecules for cancer detection, diagnosis, and therapy. Many different types of cancer are treated using cancer medicines that are based on the exceptional qualities of NPs. With advancement in this vital field, nanomaterials in their different forms have proved to possess enhanced drug delivery effectiveness for cancer. Perfect nanotheranostic arrangements are projected to be (1) harmless and biologically tuned, (2) greatly unwavering and effectual for drug stuffing, (3) simple to modify and prepare, and (4) targeting malignant cells and active for endocytosis.

Despite the merits mentioned, there are still many obstacles that impede the clinical application of CNT-based therapies. For instance, the safety issues of CNTs in human body have not been fully studied. Although *in vitro* experiments carried out in many cell lines have demonstrated the safety of CNTs, *in vivo* tests based on animal models are often studied in a comparatively short period. Therefore, the long-term safety of CNT-based nanomedicine in the human body still requires more investigations to confirm their application possibility in the clinical setting. Besides, several functionalization methods of CNTs are relatively complicated in terms of large-scale production; thus, controllable industrial production with good reproducibility of functionalized CNTs is another problem that hinders their clinical translation. In contrast, another kind of carbon nanomaterials, carbon quantum dots (CQDs), seems to perform better in terms of large-scale synthesis because of their relatively simple synthesis method, low cost, and environmentally friendly property. Unfortunately, CQDs also have concentration-dependent toxicity, which limits their application [255]. Therefore, in order to reduce the administration dosage to reduce toxicity, the accuracy of cancer cell targeting or TME components targeting through these carbon-based therapy should be evaluated and improved. From the aspect of diagnosis, graphene and its derivatives possess an extraordinary electronic property, which appears to be more promising in cancer biosensing [256]. However, although there are some difficulties that need to be solved, we are confident that CNTs are very promising nanotools with great research and clinical potential in cancer treatment and diagnosis. With the rapid progress in science and technology, more mature preclinical studies will be designed for CNT-based nanocarriers to provide us with more relevant data to explore their clinical possibilities.

Furthermore, the groundwork and superiority mechanism of nanoparticles are still complex. Last, the equilibrium between the reliability and efficiency of nanotheranostic settings would be reflected, though the overview of numerous agents in one theranostic stage may fetch various purposes. It is anticipated that, with the advancement in proteomics research on the mechanism of cancer origin, cancer heterogeneity, and multidrug resistance behavior, a large number of NP-based drugs can be exploited. Though extensive research has been carried out on NPs, only a few NP-based medications are presently in use, a smaller number are in clinical trials, and the majority is still in the infancy stage. An interdisciplinary approach is required to realize nanomaterials in cancer therapy. Though the application of nanomaterials is in the midst of development, this can be proved to be a new and promising platform that can bring new hope not only for the diagnosis of cancer but also for imaging, treating, and preventing cancer, owing to their small sizes, their functionalization potentiality, and the ability to introduce multiple therapeutic agents on their surfaces. This will be a paradigm shift in the way that we treat cancer. Nevertheless, the nanosystems could be too intricate for bulk-scale engineering. Since the present chapter and development efforts have placed a cumulative effect on these nanosystems, innovation in materials science integrated with biological material may accomplish more real-world presentations of nanotheranostic platforms in cancer diagnostics.

Recently, the use of stimuli-responsive nanopolymers in lab-on-a-chip systems has resulted in considerable decrease in cost, time, and reagents, as well as a reduction in the number of tests performed. However, some challenging biological in vitro hurdles remain unresolved, that is, enhancing biocompatibility, stability, and biodegradability, assuring nontoxicity, timely turns on and off, and precise control over response locations of stimuli-responsive nanoplatforms. Additionally, dual- and multi-stimuli-responsive nanomaterials (e.g., temperature/pH dual stimuli; pH/redox potential dual stimuli; pH/light/enzyme presence multi-stimuli) may pave the way for novel nanomaterials with biological applications in the long run. Thus, designing multifunctional nanoplatforms can provide new approaches and strategies for future clinical cancer nanomedicine, and they can also support in improving the efficacy of diagnosis and therapies. In summary, we have provided evidence to anticipate that stimuli-responsive nanomaterials will undoubtedly lead to effective strategies in cancer therapy and will provide a significant advantage in the biomedical area because of the rising development and ongoing innovation in science and technology.

In conclusion, the rapid advancement in theranostics based on nanotechnology has significantly acelerated the revolution in cancer oncotherapy and diagnosis. The best nanotheranostic systems should be (1) nontoxic and biocompatible, (2) very stable and effective in drug loading, (3) easy to prepare and modify, and (4) capable of tumor targeting and endocytosis. Although the majority of the nanoparticles listed do not appear to have obvious cytotoxicity, additional experiments are required to ensure safety in clinical translations. Moreover, nanoparticle preparation and quality assurance are still challenging tasks. Notably, the synthesis of organic nanomaterials is frequently laborious, with low yields. Last, but not the least, although combining several agents in a single theranostic platform may bring about a variety of activities, it is important to balance the efficiency and dependability of nanotheranostic systems. However, the nanosystem could be too complicated for large-scale synthesis. We presuppose that the revolution in clinical translation for NP-based cancer therapy with rational approaches dealing with synthetic strategies, toxicity, and cellular and physiological factors will be accomplished with nanotechnology and cancer therapy development. Laboratories are coming up with nanomedicine-based drug delivery systems with a strong emphasis on cutting-edge technological and scientific advancements that succeed on a small scale. These laboratories often are familiar with the technical problems that occur in the industry for the commercializing processes. A strong collaboration among pharmaceutical companies and academic laboratory groups must be established to bridge this gap. Nevertheless, current investigators are emphasizing these difficulties, and several initiatives are being taken to achieve more practical applications of nanotheranostic platforms in the treatment of cancer.

Abbreviations

α	the residual activity
$α_2β_2$	the tryptophan synthase
αvβ3	integrin regulates cell attachment, spreading, and migration; thyroid hormone-integrin to cancer cell proliferation and metastasis
αvβ3 and αvβ5	coordinated cell adhesion and movement of diverse cell types
β-2M	β-2 microglobulin
β-GP	β-glycerophosphate
ρ	electron density
λex	excitation wavelength
σf	flexural strength
εf	strain at failure
μPADs	microfluidic paper-based analytical devices
$∇^2ρ$	Laplacian
ΔE	binding energy
ΔG	Gibbs free energy
Δv	stretching frequencies
ΔS	entropy
0D	zero-dimensional
1D	one-dimensional
2D	two-dimensional
3D	three-dimensional space (tridimensional)
3DSG	3D sulfur-doped graphene

(A)

(A)	adenine
l-AA	L-ascorbic acid
AA	ascorbic acid
AA	all-atomistic molecular dynamics
AAAS	American Association for the Advancement of Science
AA/CGMD	all-atomistic/coarse-grained molecular dynamics
AAMD	all-atomistic molecular dynamics
AANL	
AAS	atomic absorption spectroscopy
AAV	adenovirus-associated virus
ABEI	N-(4-Amino-Butyl)-N-Ethyl-Isoluminol
Ab-gCNQDs	antibodies graphitic carbon nitride quantum dots
Ab-MP-MoO_3 QDs	antibodies plasmonic molybdenum trioxide quantum dots
ABS	acrylonitrile butadiene styrene
Abs	antibodies
ABS-75	Ankaferd blood stopper
ABTS	(2,2′-azino-bis(3-ethylbenzathiazoline-6-sulfonic acid))
AC	alternating current
AC	activated carbon
a-C	amorphous carbon
ACD	6-amino-g-cyclodextrin
a-CDs	amorphous carbon dots
A-CDs	ascorbic acid- carbon dots
ACE	angiotensin-converting enzyme
ACE2	angiotensin-converting enzyme 2
ACh	acetycholine
AChE	acetylcholinesterase
ACMF	alternating current magnetic force
ACMO	acryloyl morpholinc
ACS	American Chemical Society
ACV	acyclovir
ADCs	antibody–drug conjugates
ADFs	amino acid fullerene derivatives
ADHD	attention deficit hyperactivity disorder
ADME	absorption, distribution, metabolism, and excretion properties
ADP	adenosine diphosphate
AETP	activated endothelium targeting peptide
AEY	Auger electron yield
af-GQDs	amino-functionalized graphene quantum dots
AFM	atomic force microscope
AFP	alpha-fetoprotein
AF-SWCNTs	acid-functionalized single-walled carbon nanotubes
Ag	silver
AGA	N-acryloyl-D-glucosamine
A-GA	annealed graphene aerogel
AgNCs	silver nanoclusters
$AgNO_3$	silver nitrate
Ag NPs	silver nanoparticles
AgNPs-G	silver nanoparticle–graphene
AGNRs	armchair graphene nanoribbons
AGQDs	alkylated GQDs
aGQDs	activated graphene quantum dots
$AgVO_3$	silver vanadium trioxide
Ag_2WO_4	silver tungstate
AI	artificial intelligence
AIDS	acquired immuneodeficiency syndrome
AIM	atom in molecule
AIV	avian influenza virus
Al	aluminum metal
AL_4C_3	aluminum carbide
$AlCl_3$	aluminum trichloride
ALD	atomic layer deposition method
Al_2O_3	aluminum oxide
ALP	alkaline phosphatase

ALS amyotrophic lateral sclerosis
AM acrylamide
AM additive manufacturing
aM attomolar range
AMBER amplitude-modulated burst energy radiograph
AMP adenosine monophosphate
AMT associate in mechanical technology; associate in medical technology
a-N-CDs amorphous nitrogen-doped carbon dots
ANG angiopep-2
ANOVA analysis of variance
AP alkaline phosphatase
AP ammonium perchlorate
AP apurinic/apyrimidinic
APT atom probe tomography
Apt aptamers
APTMS 3-Aminopropyl)trimethoxysilane
AP-XPS ambient pressure X-ray photoelectron spectroscopy
Ar argon
ARES autonomous research system
Arg178 arginine residue
ARGO reduced graphene oxide–based aerogels
AS activated sludge
ASCP American Society for Clinical Pathology
ASE atomic simulation environment
ASGPR asialoglycoprotein receptor
ASNase L-asparaginase enzyme
Asp aspartic acid
ASSURED affordable, sensitive, specific, user-friendly, rapid and robust, equipment-free, and deliverable to end users
ASTM American Standard Test Method
ATCC American Type Culture Collection
AT–Fe_3O_4 magnetic attapulgite/Fe_3O_4 nanoparticles
ATLAS Argonne Tandem Linear Accelerator System
ATP adenosine triphosphate
4-ATP 4-aminothiophenol
ATP-s adenosine 5′-[γ-thio] triphosphate
ATRA atom transfer radical addition
ATRAM acidity-triggered rational membrane
Au gold
Au–GO gold nanoparticles and graphene oxide
AuNI gold nano-islands
AuNPs gold nanoparticles
AuNPs-$B(OH)_2$ gold nanoparticles with 3-mercaptophenyl boronic acid
AVL automatic vehicle locator

(B)

BA n-butyl acrylate
BAC bis(acryloyl)cystamine)
BALF bronchoalveolar lavage fluid
$BaTiO_3$ barium trioxide
BaWO4 barium tungstate
BBB blood–brain barrier
B-doping boron doping
BChE butyryl cholinesterase
BCPs bond critical points
BCPs block copolymers
BCQDs boron-doped CQDs
BDC Breast Diagnostic Center
BEAS-2B human bronchial epithelial
BEM boundary element method
BEN bendamustine
BET Brunauer-Emmett-Teller theory
BFG bovine fibrinogen
BFO bismuth ferrites ($Bi_2Fe_4O_9$)
BGA biological graphene aerogel
BGDs boron-doped graphene quantum dots
BGE butyl glycidyl ether
BGNs/Fe_3O_4 polyethylenimine-graphene-iron oxide
B-GQDs boron-doped GQDs
(B)-GQDs blue GQDs
$BH(N_3)_2$ diazidoborane
$B_3H_6N_3$ borazine
BHQ1 Black Hole Quencher-1
Bi–g-C_3N_4 bi-doped g-CN
BIO-FETs field-effect transistor biosensors
BioFETs biologically modified field-effect transistors
Bi_2MoO_6 bismuth molybdate nanoplates
BIOH biochanin
Bi_2S_3 bismuth (III) sulfide
Bi_2WO_6 bismuth tungstate
$BiVO_4$ bismuth vanadate (V)
BLM bilayer lipid membranes
B3LYP Becke, 3-parameter, Lee–Yang–Parr
BMC BioMed Central
BMCN B-doped mesoporous g-CN prepared by Badiei's group
[BMim][BF_4] 1-butyl-3-methylimidazolium tetrafluoroborate
BM-MSC bone marrow–derived mesenchymal stem cells
bMWCNTs bamboo-like multi-walled carbon nanotubes
BNCQDs CQDs co-doped with boron and nitrogen
BNNTs boron nitride nanotubes
BNSCQDs CQDs co-doped with boron, nitrogen, and sulfur
BP 3-bromopyruvate
BP buckypaper
BP black phosphorus
BPA bisphenol A
BPDC biphenyl-4,4′-dicarboxylic acid
BPEI branched polyethylenimine
BPEI-CDs branched poly(ethylenimine)-functionalized CDs
BP/PVA buckypaper/polyvinyl alcohol
$(bpy)_3^{2+}$ tris(bipyridine)
BRCA1 breast cancer gene 1

BRCA2 breast cancer gene 2
BRENDA BRaunschweig ENzyme DAtabase
BSA bovine serum albumin
B-SSCN B-doped carbon nitride microspheres using ammonia borane, cyanuric chloride
BSSE basis set superposition error
BT bentonite
(BTC) benzene-1,3,5-tricarboxylate
BTNPs barium titanate nanoparticle
BVIm 1-butyl-3-vinyl imidazolium
BZ Brillouin zone
BZM-CDs benzoxazine monomers derived Cdots

(C)

(C) cytosine
(C) covalent
C60 fullerene
CA citric acid
CA19–9 carbohydrate antigen 19–9
CA125 carcinoma antigen 125
Caco-2 colorectal adenocarcinoma cells
CAD computationally assisted design (computer-aided design software)
CADASIL cerebral autosomal-dominant arteriopathy with subcortical infarcts and leukoencephalopathy
CADD computer-aided drug design
CAFM conductive atomic force microscopy
CAFs cancer-associated fibroblasts
CAGR compound annual growth rate
CAHA cholic acid–derivatized HA
CAR carmustine
CAS catalytic active site
CB cucurbit
CB conduction band
CB chlorobenzene
CBNMs carbon-based nanomaterials
C_2C_{12} subclone from a myoblast line established from normal adult C3H mouse
CC BY-NC Creative Commons Attribution Non-Commercial License 4.0
CCG chemically converted graphene
CCl_4 carbon tetrachloride
C_6-CNTPC coumarin-6 loaded TPGS conjugated MWCNT.
CCVD catalytic chemical vapor deposition
CD β-cyclodextrin
CD circular dichroism
CD carbidopa
CD candesartan
CD133 cluster of differentiation-133
CDC Chinese Center for Disease Control and Prevention
CDK1 cyclin-dependent kinase 1
cDNA complementary DNA
CDots carbon-based quantum dots
C-dots-PPEI-EI poly(propionylethylenimine-co-ethylenimine) coated C-dots
Cdoxo CD-loaded doxo
CDP cyclodextrin polymer
Cd-QDs CdS quantum dots
CDs carbon-based quantum dots (carbon dots)
CdSe QDs cadmium and selenium quantum dots
CDT chemodynamic therapy
CdTe cadmium tellurite
CdTe QDs cadmium telluride quantum dots
CE catalytic efficiency
Ce6 chlorin e6
CEA carcinoembryonic antigen (carcino-emryogenic antigen)
C_{70}-EDA fullerene modified with multiple ethylenediamine
CEE cross-link enhanced emission
CeO_2 cerium oxide
CF carbon fiber
CF_4 tetrafluoromethane
CFE carbon fiber
cFLISA competitive fluorescence-linked immunosorbent assays
CFPC cyclic fluorescence probe cleavage
CFRP carbon fiber reinforced polymer
CFs C60-fullerenes
CFX cefotaxime
CG coarse-grained molecular dynamics
cGDs carboxylated graphene nanodots
$(C_{12}G_2)$ diglycerol monolaurate
$(C_{14}G_{12})$ diglycerol monomyristate
CGCs critical gel concentrations
CGMD coarse-grained molecular dynamics
CGN colloidal gold nanobeads
CH chitosan
CH_4 methane
C_2H_2 acetylene
$C_{10}H_{16}$ turpentine oil
CHARMM Chemistry at Harvard Macromolecular Mechanics
$C_6H_8BNO_2$ 3-Aminophenylboronic acid
CHC clonidine hydrochloride
(C_6H_4COOH) benzoic acid
CHDA 1,2-cyclohexanediamine
CHI HA–chitosan
CHI-SWNTs chitosan-SWNTs
CHIT chitosan
CHNCH2 nitrile ylide
CH_2NHCH_2 azomethine ylide
$CH_2N(H)O$ nitrone
$(C_6H_4NH_2)$ amino-phenyl
$(C_6H_4NO_2)$ nitro-phenyl
CHNNH nitrile imine
CHO Chinese hamster ovary cells
$C_{10}H_{16}O$ camphor
$C_{10}H_{18}O$ eucalyptus oil
$C_{16}H_{36}O_4Ti$ tetrabutyl titanate
$C_{39}H_{74}O_6$ coconut oil

$C_{54}H_{100}O_7$	castor oil
$C_{67}H_{127}O_8$	palm oil
ChOx	enzymecholesterol oxidase
Ci	cisplatin
CIP	ciprofloxacin
CIS	cisplatin
CIT	chemo-immunotherapy
CL	chemiluminescence
CLB	colibactin resistance protein
ClCN	Cl-doped g-CN
CLEAs	cross-linked enzyme aggregates
CLIA	chemi-luminescence immunosorbent assay
ClPCN-1–ClPCN-4	P–Cl co-doped g-CN
CLSM	controlled low-strength material analysis
CMC	critical micellar concentrations
CME	chemically modified electrodes
CME	clathrin-mediated endocytosis
CMOS	complementary metal oxide semiconductor
CMSD	Center for Molecular Spectroscopy and Dynamics
(C ≡ N)	nitriles
–C≡NC	cyano group
C_3N_3	triazine
C_6N_7	tri-s-triazine/heptazine
CNBr	cyanogen bromide
CNBS	B–S co-doped g-CN
CNDs	carbon nanodots
CNFs	carbon nanofibers
CNZCel	g-C_3N_4/ZnO/cellulose
C_2H_5OH	ethanol
$C_3N_6H_6$	melamine
CNHs	carbon nanohorns
13C NMR	nuclear magnetic resonance to determine the type and number of carbon atoms
CNMs	carbon nanomaterials
CNOs	carbon nano-onions
CNP	carbon nanoplatelets
CNPs	carbon nanoparticles
CNRs	carbon nanoribbons
CNS	central nervous system
CNSs	carbon nanostructures
CNTs	carbon nanotubes
CNT-Ch-ENFET	carbon nanotubes based ENFET for detection of cholesterol
CNT-ENFETs	carbon nanotubes based Enzyme modified field-effect transistor
CNT-FET	field-effect transistor, based on carbon nanotube
CNTs	carbon nanotubes
CNT-SPE	CNT screen-printed electrodes
CNW	carbon nanowall
CNZ	g-C_3N_4/ZnO
CO	carbon monoxide
(C-O)	carbonyl group
Co^{2+}	cobalt ions
CoB/g-C_3N_4	cobalt boride/g-C_3N_4 nanosheets
C-OC	epoxy
Co/C-dots	cobalt-doped C-dots
COD	crystallography open database
Co–g-CN	co-doped g-CN
$C_{60}(OH)_{12}$	low-hydroxylated fullerenol
COMPASS	condensed-phase optimized molecular potentials for atomistic simulation studies
COMPASS	COMPrehensive Addiction Service Systems
Con A	concanavalin A
(-CONH-)	amide
Con-R	Congo red
CO_2	carbon dioxide
Co_3O_4	cobalt (II, III) oxide
(–COOH)	carboxylic group
CoMoCAT®	cobalt-molybdenum catalytic method SWNTs
CoPc	cobalt-phthalocyanine
copo	copolymer
COVID-19	coronavirus disease 2019
CP	chlorophenols
CP-CNPs	coat protein-–carbon nanoparticles
CPDs	carbonized polymer dots
CPE	carbon paste
CpG	Cytosine-phosphorothioate-guanine
CpG ODN	Cytosine-phosphorothioate-guanine oligodeoxynucleotides
CPPs	cell-penetrating peptides
CPT	camptothecin
CPT@f-CNT-RGD	camptothecin functionalized CNT-Arginylglycylaspartic acid
CQDs	Carbon quantum dots
CQDt	carbon quantum dots
CR	Congo red
Cr	chromium
Cr	coreactant
cRGD	conjugated Arginylglycylaspartic acid
CRISPR	clustered regularly interspaced short palindromic repeats
CRISPR-Cas9	clustered regularly interspaced short palindromic repeats -associated protein 9.
CRL	Candida rugosa lipase
CRP	C-reactive protein
CS	chitosan
CS	chitosan solution
CS	citrate synthase
CSCs	cancer stem cells
CSGQDs	chitosan-GQDs
CSWCNT	carboxylated SWCNT
CT	charge-transfer
CT	computer tomography
CT	calf-thymus
CTAB	cetyltrimethyl ammonium bromide
(cTnT)	cardiac troponin T
CTV	Citrus tristeza virus
CTX	chlortoxin
Cu-CDs	copper doped carbon dots
Cu-CNB	Cu and B co-doped g-CN

CuFoam copper foam
(^{64}Cu@GNTs) $^{64}Cu^{2+}$ ions at gadolinium nanotubes
CuNCs–CNQDs copper nanoclusters@nitrogen-doped carbon quantum dots
Cu NPs Cu nanoparticles
CuPc Copper-phthalocyanine
CUR curcumin
$CuWO_4$ Copper tungsten oxide
CV cyclic voltammetry
CVD Chemical vapor deposition
CW continuous wave
Cy5 cyanine 5
l-Cys L-cysteine

(D)

DA Diels-Alder
DA Dopamine
DAMPs damaged-associated molecular patterns
DAPI 4',6-diamidino-2-phenylindole
dba dibenzylideneacetone
DBP dibenzoyl peroxides
DBP dibutyl phthalate
DC direct current
DC 1,3-dipolar cycloaddition
DCB Double cantilever beam
DCB 2-dichlorobenzene
DCC N,N′-dicyclohexylcarbodiimide
DCCA Drying Control Chemical Additives
DCDA dicyandiamide
DCDA-CNZ dicyandiamide (DCDA) to ZnO and $g\text{-}C_3N_4$ nanoparticles
DCE dichloroethane
dc-ELISA direct Enzyme-linked immunosorbent assay
DCF Dichlorofluorescein
DCFH-DA 2′,7′-dichlorofluorescein diacetate
DCM Device Communication Manager
DCMU 3, (3,4-dichlorophenyl) 1,1-Dimethyl Urea
DCPC 1,2-dicaproyl- sn-glycero-3-phosphocholine
DCs Dendritic cells
DDAO N,N-dimethyldodecylamine N-oxide
DDM Deformation-driven metallurgy
DDSs drug delivery systems
DEA diethylamine
DEAE diethylaminoethyl
DENV dengue virus
DET direct electron transfer
DETDA diethyltoluenediamine
$DexP\text{-}g\text{-}C_3N_4$ phenoxy dextran-graphite-like carbon nitride
DFT density functional theory
DFX deferoxamine mesylate
Dh hydrodynamic diameter
DHF dengue hemorrhage fever
DHODH dihydroortate dehydrogenase
DHPC 1,2-dihexanoyl-sn-glycero-3-phosphocholine
DI dielectric
DIEA Diisopropylethylamine
DILI drug-induced liver injury
DIW Direct ink writing
DL degree of labeling
DLC diamond-like carbon
DLC drug loading capacity
DLPC 1,2-dilauroyl-sn-glycero-3-phosphocholine
DLS dynamic light scattering
DMA dynamic mechanical analysis
DMA 2,3 dimethylmaleic acid
DMAEMA dimethylaminoethyl methacrylate
DMAEMA-co-NBM 2-nitrobenzyl methacrylate copolymer dimethylaminoethyl methacrylate
DMD disintegrated melt deposition
DMEM Dulbecco's Modified Eagle Medium
DMF N,N-dimethylformamide
DMFC Direct Methanol fuel cell
DMPC 1,2-dimyristoyl-sn-glycero-3-phosphocholine
DMPE 1,2-Bis(dimethylphosphino)ethane
DMPO 5,5-dimethyl-1-pyrroline N-oxide
DMSO dimethyl sulfoxide
DMVs double-membrane vesicles
DNA deoxyribonucleic acid
DNA-SWNT DNA-dispersed carbon nanotubes
DND detonation nanodiamond
DNP 2, 4-dinitrophenol
DOPC 1,2-dioleoyl-sn-glycero-3-phosphocholine
DOQ dopamine-o-quinone
DOS density of states
DOTA 1,4,7,10-tetraazacyclododecane-1,4,7,10-tetraacetic acid
DOX doxorubicin
DOX-BCDs DOX-conjugated beer CDs
DOXO doxorubicin
DP synthetic monocrystalline diamond
DPA Docosapentaenoic Acid
DPH Diphenylhexatriene (Diphenhydramine)
DPD Dissipative Particle Dynamics
DPP diketopyrrolopyrrole
DPPH-2 1,2-Distearoyl-sn-glycero-3-phosphoethanolamine
DPV Differential Pulse Voltammetry method
DRGON dextran-coated reduced graphene oxide nanocolloid
DRS diffuse reflectance spectroscopy
DSC differential scanning calorimetry
dsDNA double-stranded DNA
dsDNA/Au double-stranded DNA modified gold electrodes
DSF Differential scanning fluorimetry
DSPC 1,2-distearoyl-sn-glycero-3-phosphocholine
DSPE-PEG 1,2-distearoyl-sn-glycero-3-phosphoethanolamine-N-[amino(poly(ethylene glycol))]

DSPE-PEG-iRGD	DSPE-PEG modified with internalized Arginyl-glycyl-aspartic acid
DSS	dengue shock syndrome
DSSC	dye-sensitized solar cells
dt	diameter
DTAB	dodecyl trimethylammonium bromide
DTG	derivative thermal gravimetric
DTPA	diethylenetriamine-pentaacetic acid; N 4: 6-(carboxyl)-1,4,8. . .
DTX	docetaxel
Du145	is a human prostate cancer cell line
DV	double vacancies
DVB	diagrammatic valence bond
DW	double-walled
DWCNTs	double-walled carbon nanotubes
DWNTs	double-walled carbon nanotubes

(E)

(E)	envelope
(E)	Young's modulus
***E*a**	Arrhenius activation energy
Ea	barrier heights
EA	electron affinity
EA	Elemental analysis
EAC	Ehrlich-Lettre ascites carcinoma
E_{ads}	adsorption energy
EAE	experimental allergic encephalomyelitis
EC	Enzyme Commission
EC	electrocatalytic mechanism
EC_{50}	Half maximal effective concentration to achieve 50% inhibition
ECBs	electrochemical biosensors
ECD	electrochemical deposition
ECD	electronic circular dichroism
ECG	electrocardiogram
ECH	electroconductive hydrogel
ECL	electrochemiluminescence (electrogenerated chemiluminescence)
ECL-RET	ECL resonance energy transfer
E. coli	*Escherichia coli*
ECM	Electronic Content Management
ECT	emission computed tomography
ED	Electrochemical deposition
ED_{50}	50% median effective dose
EDA	2,2′-(ethylenedioxy)bis(ethylamine)
EDA	ethylenediamine
EDAC·HCl	1-ethyl-3-(3-dimethylaminopropyl) carbo-diimide hydrochloride
EDAX	Energy Dispersive X-Ray Analyzer
EDB-FN	extra domain-B fibronectin
EDC	1-ethyl-3-(3-dimethylaminopropyl) carbodiimide
EDC	N-(3-dimethylaminopropyl)-N′-ethylcarbodiimide hydrochloride
EDC•HCl	1-(3-dimethylaminopropyl)-3-ethylcarbodiimide hydrochloride

EDC/NHS	ethyl(dimethylaminopropyl) carbodiimide/N-hydroxy succinimide
EDC-NHS	1, 1-ethyl-3-(3-dimethylaminopropyl) carbodiimide/N-hydroxysuccinimide
EDS	Energy-dispersive X-ray spectroscopy
EDTA	ethylene diamine tetra-acetic acid
EDX	Energy Dispersive X-Ray Spectroscopy
EE2	Ethinylestradiol
EELS	electron energy loss spectroscopy
Ef	Fermi level
Ef	flexural modulus
EFTEM	energy Filtered Transmission Electron Microscopy
EG	Ethylene glycol
(E_g)	bandgap (energy gap)
EGB	Ethylene Glycol butyl ether
EGF	Epidermal growth factor
EGFR	epidermal growth factor receptor expression
EGQDs	extended graphene quantum dots
E_{HB}	hydrogen bond energies strength
EIS	electrochemical impedance spectroscopy
ELISA	enzyme-linked immunosorbent assay
ELR	extrapolation in linear region
EM	electromagnetic
E_m	energy of up-converted emission light
EMA	European Medicines Agency
EMF	electromotive force
EMFs	endohedral metallofullerenes
ENF	end-notched flexure
EMI	electromagnetic interference
EMIs	electropolymerized molecular identifiers
EMSCs	encapsulated mesenchymal stem cells
EMT	epithelial–mesenchymal transition
ENFET	enzyme-modified field-effect transistor
ENMs	engineered nanomaterials
Epa	anodic peak
EPA	Environmental Protection Agency
EPA	3-ethoxypropylamine
Epc	cathodic peak
EpCAM	epithelial cell adhesion molecule
EPD	electrophoretic deposition
Epi	epirubicin
EpiSkin™	reconstructed human epidermis model within IATA for skin corrosion and irritation (epidermis model can be used to assess skin irritation potential of chemicals)
EPO	erythropoietin
EPR	enhanced permeability and eetention effect
EPR	electron paramagnetic resonance
ER	endoplasmic reticulum
Er	reaction energies
ES	screen-printed electrode
ESD	electrospray deposition

ESF	European Science Foundation
ES GQDs	screen-printed electrode graphene quantum dots
ES GNMs	electrospun graphene-based nanomaterials
ES GNMs NF	electrospun graphene-based nanomaterials nuclear factor
ESI	Employee's State Insurance Corporation
ESNFs	electrospun nanofibres
ES PS-b-PMMA NF	electrospun mesoporous poly(styrene-block-methylmethacrylate) nanofibers
ESR	electron spin response
(ET)-1	endothelin
ETEM	environmental transmission electron microscopy
Et_2O	diethyl ether ($C_8H_{20}O_2$)
EtOAc	ethyl acetate
ETOH	ethanol (C_2H_5OH)
EU	European Union
Eu	europium
EVA	ethylene-vinyl acetate
E_x	energy of up-converted excitation light
EXAFS	extended X-ray absorption fine structure

(F)

F_2	fluorine
FA	folic acid or folate acid
FA-CHI-SWNTs	folic acid—chitosan SWNTs
FACS	fluorescence-activated cell sorting
FACS	FA–chitosan conjugate
FACS–Mn:ZnS	
FAD	flavin adenine dinucleotide
FAM	fluorescein amidites
FAU	FBR-MuSV-associated ubiquitously
FB	flurbiprofen
FBCVD	fluidized bed chemical vapor deposition
FBR	foreign body response
FBR-MuSV	Finkel-Biskis-Reilly murine sarcoma virus
FBS	fasting blood sugar
FBS	fetal bovine serum
Fc	ferrocene
FCC	phase cubic lattices
FCCCD	face-centered central composite design
FCCVD	floating catalyst chemical vapor deposition
F-CDs	fructose–carbon dots
fCNT	functionalized nanotubes
FCR	fractional change in resistance
FCVA	filtered cathodic vacuum arc
FDA	US Food and Drug Administration
18FDG	18F-2-fluoro-2-deoxyglucose
FDM	finite difference method
59Fe	iron-59
FEA	finite element analysis
$Fe(CO)_5$	iron pentacarbonyl
$Fe(C_5H_5)_2$	ferrocene
Fe–Cu@PANI	iron–copper co-doped polyaniline NPs
FEDs	field emission displays
FEL	free electron laser method
FEM	finite elements method
$Fe(NO_3)_3.9H_2O$	iron (III) nitrate nonahydrate
Fe_2O_3	iron oxide
γ-Fe_2O_3	maghemite
Fe_3O_4	magnetite
Fe_3O_4@PGLNPs	iron oxide loaded with porphyrin-grafted lipid nanoparticles
FE-SEM	field emission-scanning electron microscopy
FETs	field-effect transistors
FFA	focus-forming assay
F-GQDs	fluorinated GQDs
FIB	focused ion beam
FISPE	fullerene impregnated screen-printed electrode
FIT	fluctuation-induced tunneling
FITC	fluorescein isothiocyanate
FL	fluorescence intensity
FLG	few-layer graphene
FLU	flutamide (4-nitro-3-trifluoromethyliso butylanilide)
fM	femtomolar
FMN	flavin mononucleotide
FMN	formononetin
f-MWCNT/AgNP	functionalized multi-walled carbon nanotube/silver nanoparticle
FNC	azvudine is a nucleoside analog that inhibits HIV-1 (RdRp)
FNDs	fluorescent nanodiamonds
FNTs	fullerene C_{60} nanotubes
FO	forward osmosis
FOH-SWCNTs	SWCNTs functionalized with a hydroxyl (-OH) group
FPG	fasting plasma glucose comet assay
FR	folate receptor
FRET	fluorescence (Förster) resonance energy transfer
FRP	fiberglass-reinforced polymer
FRs	fullerenes
FS	Forcespinning® technology
FSCV	fast-scan cyclic voltammetry
FSP	friction stirs processing
FT	ferritin
FT-EXAFS	Fourier-transformed extended X-ray absorption fine structure
FT-IR	Fourier-transformed infrared spectroscopy
FTIR-ATR	FTIR-attenuated total reflection
FTO	fluorine-doped tin oxide
FTS	Fischer–Tropsch synthesis
5-FU	fluorouracil
FWHM	full width at half maximum
FWNTs	few-walled carbon nanotubes

(G)

(G) graphene
(G) guanine
GA graphene aerogels
GAGs glycosaminoglycans
GAMESS General Atomic and Molecular Electronic Structure System
GAP azobenzene/galactose-grafted polymer
GAPDH glyceraldehyde-3-phosphate dehydrogenase
GAs graphene aerogels
GBM gradient boosting model
GBM glioblastoma multiforme
GC glycated chitosan (glycol chitosan)
g-CDs graphitic carbon dots
G-CDs glucose–carbon dots
GCE glassy carbon electrode
GC-g-DMA-g-C_{60} glycol chitosan-grafted 2,3 dimethylmaleic acid–grafted C_{60}
GCMD grand canonical molecular dynamics
g-C_3N_4 graphitic carbon nitride
GCNF F-doped g-CN
gCNQDs graphitic carbon nitride quantum dots
g-C_3N_4–Zn/BiS zinc-doped g-C_3N_4 with Bi_2S_3
Gd gadolinium
GD gestational day
Gd@$C_{82}(OH)_{40}$ hydroxylated gadofullerenes
Gd^{3+} gadolinium (III)
Gd-DTPA gadolinium-diethylenetriamine pentaacetic acid
Gd-DTPA-BMA gadolinium 3-diethylenetriamine pentaacetate-bis(methylamide)
GDs graphene derivatives
GDE glycerol diglycidyl ether
GdN gadolinium NPs
Ge gemcitabine
GEM gemcitabine
GF graphene foam
GF graphite fibers
GF-Ala gadofullerene with β-alanine
GFP green fluorescent protein
GFs graphite flakes
GFs gauge factors
GGA generalized gradient approximation
(G)-GQDs green GQDs
GIT gastrointestinal tract
GLOBOCAN Global Cancer Statistics 2020
GLP good laboratory practice
Glu glutamic acid
Gly glycine
GM Göppert–Mayer
g-N-CDs graphitic nitrogen-doped carbon dots
GNDs graphene nano-dots
GNMs graphene-based nanomaterials
GNPs graphene nanoplatelets
GNRs graphene nanoribbons (graphene nanorods)
GNs graphene nanosheets
GNTs gadolinium nanotubes
GO graphene oxide
GOA graphene oxide aerogel
GOD glucose oxidase
GOF graphene of fluoro-doped
GOQDs graphene oxide quantum dots
GO-SF graphene oxide/silk fibroin
GOViRA graphene oxide–based viral RNA analysis system
GOx glucose oxidase enzyme
GOxNPs glucose oxidase nanoparticles
GPa grade point average (gigapascal)
GPAW grade projector-augmented wave
GQDs graphene quantum dots
GQD-PEG graphene quantum dots–polyethylene glycol
GQDs-PEI polyethylenimine-functionalized graphene quantum dots
GR graphene
GRAS generally regarded as safe
GRMMCs graphene-reinforced metal–matrix composites
GRMMNCs graphene-reinforced metal–matrix nanocomposites
GROMACS GROningen MAchine for Chemical Simulations
GROMOS GROningen MOlecular Simulation computer program package
GRP-R gastrin-releasing peptide receptor
GRs graphenes
GRT graphite
GSH glutathione
GSs graphene sheets

(H)

H1 hairpin probe 1
H2 hairpin probe 2
($h(v)$) photon energy
HA hyaluronic acid
HA the hemagglutinin genes of H7
HAADF-STEM high-angle annular dark field-scanning transmission electron microscopy
hACE2 human angiotensin-converting enzyme-2
HA-g-PLA/HCDs hyaluronic acid–polylactic acid and hydrophobic carbon dots
$HAuCl_4$ chloroauric acid
HB hydrogen bond
4H2B 4-hydroxy-2-butanone
HBcAg hepatitis B virus core antigen
HBEpCs human bronchial epithelial cells
HBGA histo-blood group antigens
HBMECs human brain microvascular endothelial cells
hBN hexagonal boron nitride
HBs hydrogen bonds
HCC hepatocellular carcinoma
hCE human carboxylesterase enzyme

HCl hydrochloric acid
hCG human chorionic gonadotropin
HCoV human coronavirus
HCoV-229e human coronavirus (HCoV-229E) infections
HCR hybridization chain reaction
HCV hepatitis C virus
H&E hematoxylin and eosin
HEA hydroxyethyl acrylate
HEK human neonatal epidermal keratinocytes
HeLa human cervical cancer cells
HepG2 human hepatocarcinoma cells
HER hydrogen evolution reaction
HER2 human endothelial receptor 2
HF high frequency
HFCVD hot-filament chemical vapor deposition
HfDBP hafnium/5,15-di(p-benzoato)porphyrin
HFF-QCM high-fundamental-frequency quartz crystal microbalance
HFs hydroxyl fullerenes
Hg^{2+} mercury ion
(h-GQDs) hydrophobic graphene quantum dots
HIF-I heat-inducing factor I
HIF-1α hypoxia-inducible factor 1 alpha
HiPCO high-pressure carbon monoxide
HIV human immunodeficiency virus
HKUST-1 Hong Kong University of Science and Technology
HMA (hydroxymethyl)amino-methane
HMME hematoporphyrin monomethyl ether
H_3N_2 sub-type of influenza A virus
4-HNE 4-hydroxynonenal
HNO_3 nitric acid
HNS hollow nanospheres
H_2O water
H_2O_2 hydrogen peroxide
$Ho@SiO_2$ holmium silica dioxide
Ho-HF Hoechst 33258-hyaluronate fullerene
HOMO highest occupied molecular orbital
HOPG highly ordered pyrolytic graphite
HPAI highly pathogenic avian influenza H5N1
HP-β-CD hydroxypropyl-β-cyclodextrin
HPC hydroxypropyl cellulose
HP-CDs hyaluronic acid (HA)/PEI-functionalized CDs
HPCNTs hollow-structured carbon nanotubes
HPG hyperbranched polyglycerol
H_3PO_4 phosphoric acid
HPPH (HK-peptide) functionalized and photosensitizer
HPPT 4-hydroxy-1H-pyrrolo[3,4-c] pyridine-1,3,6 (2H,5H)-trione
HPVs human papillomaviruses
HPV-18 HPV type 18
HQ hydroquinone
HR heart rate
HRP horseradish peroxidase
HR-SEM high-resolution scanning electron microscopy
HR-TEM high-resolution transmission electron micrograph
H_2S hydrogen sulfide
HSA human serum albumin
HSC-3 helicopter sea combat squadron
HS-CNTO hollow sphere and melamine
H_2SO_4 sulfuric acid
HSV-1 herpes simplex virus type 1
HSVM high-speed vibration mill
HT high temperature
HT-29 human adenocarcinoma colorectal cell line
HUGO Human Genome Organisation
HUVECs human umbilical vein endothelial cells
HY-SWCNTs hyaluronate-functionalized SWCNTs

(I)

IATA integrated approaches on testing and assessment
IBM International Business Machines Corporation
IBS Institute for Basic Science
IC_{50} concentration of a drug that reduces the activity (or binding) of another drug to an enzyme by 50%
ICD immunogenic cell death
ICG indocyanine green
ICP inductively coupled plasma
ICP-AES inductively coupled plasma atomic emission spectroscopy
ICP-MS inductively coupled plasma mass spectrometry
ICP-OES inductively coupled plasma optical emission spectroscopy
I_{DS} source–drain current
I_d device current
IDS intrusion detection system
IEC ion exchange chromatography
IECDNA-SWNT ion exchange chromatography DNA-dispersed carbon nanotubes
IEEE Institute of Electrical and Electronics Engineers
IEF isoelectric focusing electrophoresis analysis
IFE inner filter effect
IFN interferon
IFN-α interferon-alpha receptor
IFN-β interferon-beta receptor
IFN-γ interferon-gamma receptor
IFP interstitial fluid pressure
Ig gamma immunoglobulin
IgA immunoglobulin A
IGF1R insulin-like growth factor 1 receptor
IgG immunoglobulin G
IgM immunoglobulin M
IG/ID intensity ration of G-band to D-band

IITC	International Interconnect Technology Conference
IL	ionic liquid
IL-1β	interleukin-1β
IL-2	interleukin-2
IL-6	interleukin-6
IL-8	interleukin-8 from HEKs
IL-13	interleukin-13 gene
ILSS	interlaminar shear strength
IM-CNTs	isopropyl myristate–treated CNTs membrane
111In	Indium-111
IncRNA	long non-coding RNA
InGaN LED	indium gallium nitride light-emitting diode
INH	isoniazid
IoT	Internet of Things
IP	ionization potential
IPA	isopropyl alcohol
IPA	iodophenyl acetate
IPCA	international parental–child abduction system
IPCA	(5-oxo-1,2,3,5-tetrahydro-imidazo[1,2-α]pyridine-7-carboxylic acid)
IPEG	isoprenyloxy polyethylene glycol
IPR	isolated pentagon rule
IR	infrared
$IrCl(CO)(PPh_3)_2$	iridium, carbonylchlorobis (triphenylphosphine)
iRGD	integrin-binding arginine-glycine-aspartic acid
IRMOF	isoreticular metal–organic framework
ISF	skin interstitial fluid
ISFET	ion-sensitive field-effect transistor
ITM	immunosuppressive tumor microenvironment
ITO	indium tin oxide
IU	international unit
IUBMB	International Union of Biochemistry and Molecular Biology
IV	intravenous

(J)

JCPDS	Joint Committee on Powder Diffraction Standards
JEV	Japanese encephalitis virus
JP	Jicama peroxidase

(K)

K562	human leukemia cells
KCl	potassium chloride
KEGG	Kyoto Encyclopedia of Genes and Genomes
$[K_3Fe(CN)_6]$	potassium hexacyanoferrate
KMapp	Michaelis constant
KC	keratin-derived carbon
$K_2Cr_2O_7$	potassium dichromate
Kd	dissociation constant
Km	Michaelis–Menten constant
$KMnO_4$	potassium permanganate
$KNbO_3$-AuNPs@Bi_2S_3	potassium niobate-Au NPs@bismuth sulfide
KOH	potassium hydroxide
K/PPy/CNT	potassium-doped polypyrrole/carbon nanotubes
ks	electron transfer rate constant

(L)

LA	laser ablation
LASER	light amplification by stimulated emission of radiation
LbL	layer by layer
LBM	live-bird markets
LC	liquid chromatography
LCA	life cycle assessment
LC-MS	liquid chromatography–mass spectrometry
LCO	lactosylated chitosan oligosaccharide
L-CQDs	L-tryptophan-capped CQDs
L-Cys	L-cysteine
LD	linear dichroism
LDH	lactate dehydrogenase
LDL	low-density lipoprotein
LDPE	low-density polyethylene
LED	light-emitting diode
LEDs	light-discharging diodes
LEEM	low-energy electron microscopy
Le	lentinan
Leu	leucine
LFIA	lateral-flow immunochromatographic assay
LIBs	lithium-ion batteries
$LiCoO_2$	lithium–cobalt oxide cathode materials
LIG	laser-induced graphene
LiP	lignine peroxidase
L-J	Lenard–Jones (Leanard–Jones)
LLC-PK1	Lilly Laboratories cell-porcine kidney 1
LLIP	liquid–liquid interfacial precipitation
LM	liquid metallurgy
LM	light microscopy
LNPs	lipid nanoparticles
LOC	lab-on-a-chip devices
LOD	limit of detection
LOQ	limit of quantification
LP	lumbar puncture
LP	lipophilic potential
LP	lone pair
LPC	lysophosphatidylcholines
LPG	liquefied petroleum gas
L-Phe	L-phenylalanine
LRP	lipoprotein receptor–related protein
LSG	laser-scribed graphene
LSPR	localized surface plasmon resonance
LSV	linear sweep voltammetry
177Lu	lutetium-177

Luc luciferase
LUMO lowest unoccupied molecular orbital

(M)

(M) matrix
mAb monoclonal antibody
H7 MAbs H7 monoclonal antibody
MAG micro-architected graphene
MARTINI coarse-grained (CG) force field developed by Marrink for MDS
MB methylene blue
MB molecular beacon
MC Monte Carlo
MCBF-CQDs multicolor bandgap fluorescent CQDs
MCF-7 Michigan Cancer Foundation-7
MCF-10A Michigan Cancer Foundation-10A
MCGO magnetic chitosan–GO nanocomposite
MCH 6-mercaptohexanol
MCM medical countermeasure
MCN mesoporous carbon nanoparticles
MCN-PVDF mesoporous carbon nanoparticles–polyvinylidene fluoride
MCNTs magnetic CNTs
MCs mesoporous carbons
MCs multicellular spheroids
MC3T3-E1 osteoblastic cell line has been established from C57BL/6 mouse calvaria
MD molecular dynamics simulation studies
MD malate dehydrogenase
MDA-MB-231 M. D. Anderson metastatic breast 231 cells
MDCK Madin–Darby canine kidney cells
MDPI Multidisciplinary Digital Publishing Institute
MDR multidrug resistant
MECs multi-enzyme complexes
MEH-PPV poly[2-methoxy-5-(2-ethylhexyl-oxy)-p-phenyleneviny-lene]
MEH-PPV/PCBM MEH-PPV/phenyl-C_{61}-butyric acid methyl
MeOH methanol (CH_3OH)
MEP molecular electrostatic potential
MEROPS the database of proteolytic enzymes, their substrates and inhibitors
MERS Middle East respiratory syndrome
MERS-CoV Middle East respiratory syndrome coronavirus
MES 2-(N-morpholino)ethanesulfonic acid ($C_6H_{13}NO_4S$)
MF middle frequency
MF mangiferin
MFC microbial fuel cells
MFs microflowers
MHC major histocompatibility complex
MHI 2-methyl heptyl isonicotinate
MHP maximum hardness principle
MIPs molecularly imprinted polymers
miRNA micro-RNA
miRNAs micro-RNAs
ML machine learning
MLM molecular-level mixing technology
MLN mediastinal lymph node
MMA methyl methacrylate
MMCs metal–matrix composites
MMIPs-CDs@VPA magnetic microspheres vinyl phosphate–modified CDs
MMNCs metal–matrix nanocomposites
MMP mitochondrial membrane potential
MMP matrix metalloproteinase
M-MSNs magnetic mesoporous silica nanoparticles
Mn/C-dots manganese-doped C-dots
MNCO molybdenum-nickel-cobalt ternary oxide
MNi micronuclei
Mn(II)-NGQDs manganese ion (Mn^{2+})–bonded nitrogen-doped graphene quantum dots
MnP manganese peroxidase
Mn:ZnS QDs Mn-doped ZnS QDs
MO molecular orbital
MO methyl orange
MOFs metal–organic frameworks
MOF-199 Cu(II) carboxylate–based metal–organic framework
MOG myelin-oligodendrocyte glycoprotein
MOI multiplicities of infection
(MOLT-4) T lymphoblast cell line derived as the MOLT-3 cell line
MOMP mitochondrial outer membrane permeabilization
MOP myeloperoxidase enzyme
MoS_2 molybdenum disulfide
MoSe2 molybdenum diselenide
(MPa) megapascal
MPECVD microwave plasma–enhanced chemical vapor deposition
MP-MoO_3 QDs plasmonic molybdenum trioxide quantum dots
mPmPD modified poly(m-phenylenediamine)
MPO myeloperoxidase
MPS mononuclear phagocyte system
MPYLDC60-PC N-methyl-pyrrolidino[60]fullerene to polycarbonate chain
MR magnetic resonance
MRFS molecular recognition force spectroscopy
MRI magnetic resonance imaging
MROM modified rule of mixture
M–S Mott–Schottky curve
MS multiple sclerosis
MS mass spectrometry
MS2 model virus particle (bacteriophage)
MSF mesoporous silica nanochannel film
MSG-CLEA mesoporous silica gel cross-linked PAL
MS/m mho or siemens per meter
MSNs mesoporous silica nanoparticles

MSP	membrane scaffold protein
(m-) SWCNTs	metallic SWCNTs
mt	mitochondria protein
MTCN	S-doped g-CN
mtDNA	mitochondrial DNA
mTEG	monomethoxy triethylene glycol
MTT	3-(4,5-dimethylthiazol-2-yl)-2,5-diphenyl-2H-tetrazolium bromide
MTX	mitroxantrone
MTX	methotrexate
MUC1	mucin 1
Mw	molecular weight
MW	multi-walled
MW	microwave
MWCNTs	multi-walled carbon nanotubes
MWCNT-COOH	carboxylic-functionalized multi-walled carbon nanotubes
MWCNTs	multiple-walled carbon nanotubes
MWCO	molecular weight cut-off
MWI	microwave irradiation
MWNTs	multi-walled carbon nanotubes
MWNTs-PEG	MWNTs with polyethylene glycol
MWNTs-Rho	rhodamine-110 with multi-walled carbon nanotubes

(N)

N	nitrogen
(N)	nucleocapsid
N_2	nitrogen gas
NA	neuraminidase genes of H7
NAAT	nucleic acid amplification tests
$NaBH_4$	sodium borohydride
$Na_2B_4O_7$•$10H_2O$	borax
NaCl	sodium chloride
NADH	nicotinamide adenine dinucleotide (NAD) + hydrogen (H)
NADPH	nicotinamide adenine dinucleotide phosphate
NAF	Nafion
NAg	nucleocapsid (N) antigen
NaI	sodium iodine
NAMD	nanoscale molecular dynamics
NANC	nucleic acid negative conversion
NASA	National Aeronautics and Space Administration
NBE-T-CQDs	narrow-bandwidth emission T-CQDs
$NbCl_5$	niobium chloride
NBM	2-nitrobenzyl methacrylate
NBO	natural bond orbital
NBS	N-bromosuccinimide
NC	non-covalent
NC	nucleocapsid
NCs	nanocrystals
NCBI	National Center for Biotechnology Information
NCDs	nitrogen-doped carbon dots
NCF	non-covalent functionalization
N-CQDs-Tb	Terbium (III)-referenced N-doped carbon dots
NCs	nanoclusters
NCs	nanocomposites
NDDSs	nanoparticle-based drug delivery systems
N-dots	nitrogen-rich quantum dots
NDs	nanodots
NDs	nanodiamonds
Nd:YAG	neodymium-doped yttrium aluminum garnet
Nd:$Y_3A_{15}O_{12}$	neodymium-doped yttrium aluminum garnet
NE	nanoemulsion
NED	normal electron demand
NEM	nanoelectro-mechanic
NEXAFS	near-edge X-ray absorption fine structure
NF-κB	nuclear factor kappa-light-chain enhancer of activated B cells
NFs	nanofibers
N-GQDs	nitrogen-doped graphene quantum dots
(N-H)	amine group
(-NH_2)	amine unit
NHE	normal hydrogen electrode
NH_4HCO_3	ammonium bicarbonate
NH_2-SWCNTs	amino-functionalized single-walled carbon nanotubes
N_2H_4	hydrazine
$(NH_4)_6Mo_7O_{24}.4H_2O$	ammonium molybdate tetrahydrate
NHS	N-hydroxylsuccinimide
$(N_2H_4)_2S_2O_8$	ammonium persulfate
NHSS	N-hydroxysulfosuccinimide
NiFe@PCN	Ni-Fe co-doped g-CN
Ni@PCN	Ni-doped g-CN
NIPAAm	poly-N-isopropyl acrylamide
NIR	near-infrared (700–900 nm)
NIR-II	second-window NIR light
NIRF	near-infrared fluorescence imaging
NIST	National Institute of Standards and Technology
$NiTiO_3$	Nickel(II) titanate
NiTMTAA	Ni(II) tetramethyldibenzotetraaza-annulene
$NiWO_4$	nickel tungstate
NK	natural killer cells
NLC	nanostructured lipid carriers
NMDA	N-methyl D-aspartate
NMOF	nanovesicular metal–organic framework
NMP	N-methylpyrrolidone
NMR	nuclear magnetic resonance
NMRD	magnetic relaxation dispersion profiles
NMs	nanomaterials
N-MWCNTs	nitrogen-doped multi-walled carbon nanotubes
NO	nitric oxide
NO_2	nitrogen dioxide
NP3	triphosphor nitrogen
NPC	nanoporous copper
NPG	nanoporous gold

NPs nanoparticles
NPT a constant particle number, a pressure, and a temperature
NP-TFC nylon 66/para-phenylenediamine thin film composite
NPM–EG nylon 66/pPD/MWCNTs, catalyst-free in ethylene glycol
NPM–EtOH nylon 66/pPD/MWCNTs, catalyst-free in ethanol
NPM–SiG/EG nylon 66/pPD/MWCNTs, silica gel catalyzed in ethylene glycol
NPM–SiG/EG–TFC nylon 66/pPD/MWCNTs, silica gel in ethylene glycol thin film composite
NPM–SiG/EtOH nylon 66/pPD/MWCNTs, silica gel catalyzed in ethanol thin film composite
NPM–SiG/EtOH–TFC nylon 66/pPD/MWCNTs, silica gel catalyzed in ethanol
NPM–SiG/H_2O nylon 66/pPD/MWNTs, silica gel catalyzed in distilled water
NPM–SiG/H_2O–TFC nylon 66/pPD/MWNTs, silica gel in distilled water thin film composite
NPM-TFCs nylon 66/pPD/MWCNTs, catalyst thin film composite
NRAM nonvolatile random access memory
NRs nanorods
NS1 non-structural protein 1
NS1-HRP non-structural protein 1 labeled with horseradish peroxidase
NSAIDS non-steroidal anti-inflammatory drugs
NSF nephrogenic systemic fibrosis
NS-GDs nitrogen and sulfur co-doped GDs
NS-GQDs nitrogen and sulfur co-doped graphene quantum dots
NT no treatment
NTA nitrilotriacetic acid
NTCOCl COCl-functionalized CNT
NTCOOH COOH-functionalized CNT
NTNFETs carbon nanotubes network field-effect transistors
NTs nanotubes
NVP N-vinylpyrrolidone

(O)

$1O_2$ singlet oxygen
$O_2^{•-}$ superoxide anion radical
O_3 ozone
OA oxalic acid
OAPI octadecyl amine-p(Asp-API)10
OCCAM open curation of computation and metadata
O.D. optical density
ODN oligodeoxynucleotides
OECD Organisation for Economic Co-operation and Development
OELs occupational air exposure limits
OER oxygen evolution reaction
(O)-GQDs orange GQDs
(–OH) hydroxyl group
•OH hydroxyl radicals
8-OHdG 8-oxodeoxyguanosine
OLED organic light-emitting diode
OM optical microscopy
OMC ordered microporous carbon
OPE optical proximity effect
OPG osteoprotegerin
OPH organophosphate hydrolase
OPLS orthogonal projections to latent structures
OPN osteopontin
Ops opsonins
OPVs organic photovoltaics
ORF open reading frame
ORR oxygen reduction reaction
OSCs osteosarcoma stem cells
(O)-SWCNTs oxide single-walled carbon nanotubes
o-SWNTs-PEG epoxide-type oxygen-doped SWNTs with the modification of PEG
OTA ochratoxin A
OTN-NIR over-thousand-nanometer near-infrared
OVA ovalbumin
OVCAR8 ovarian cancer cells and resistant
oxCNTs oxidized multi-walled carbon nanotubes
8-oxodG 8-oxo-7,8-dihydro-20-deoxyguanosine

(P)

p53 tumor protein
PμSL projection microstereolithography
P@-Gem-HSA gemcitabine and pheophorbide-a (P@)–loaded human serum albumin
PA polyamide
PA photoacoustic
PAA polyacrylic acid
PAbs polyclonal antibodies
P(AGA) poly(acryloylglucosamine)
[P(AGA)(AA)] poly(acryloylglucosamine) (acrylic acid)
PAGE polyacrylamide gel electrophoresis
PAGenes propagatively alkylated graphene sheets
PAH poly(allyl amine hydrochloride)
PAI photoacoustic imaging
PAHs polyaromatic hydrocarbons
PAL phenylalanine ammonia lyase
PAM polyacrylamide
PAMAM polyamidoamine
PA-MWCNTs multi-walled carbon nanotube polyamide
PAN polyacrylonitrile
PANI polyaniline
PANI/MWCNT polyaniline MWCNTs
PAni/NMP polyaniline emeraldine base dissolved in N-methyl-2-pyrrolidone
PAniNT/rGOA polyaniline nanotube/reduced graphene oxide aerogel
PARP poly-ADP ribose polymerase
PAS peripheral anionic site

PAS proline, alanine, and serine
PAT photoacoustic therapy
pAT2 plasmid angiotensin II type 2 receptor
PATEI poly(amidethioesterimide)
PA-TFC polyamide-based thin-film nanocomposite
PAVE poly(acrylic acid-r-(7-(4-vinylbenzyloxy)-4-methyl coumarin)-r-ethylhexyl acrylate)
PAW projector-augmented wave
PB polyetherimide betaine
Pb^{2+} lead ions
PBAE-ROS ROS-responsive poly(β-amino ester)
PBASE 1-pyrenebutanoic acid succinimidyl ester
PBE Perdew–Burke–Ernzerhof
PBMCs peripheral blood mononuclear cells
PBS phosphate buffer solution
PBST phosphate-buffered saline solution
PBT preliminary breath test
PC polycaprolactone
PC polycarbonate
Pc petroselinum crispum
PC3 considered to be the standard prostate cancer cell lines used in therapeutic research
PCBG polymerized C_{61}-butyric acid glycidol ester
PCBM phenyl-C_{61}-butyric acid methyl ester
PCM Tomasi's polarized continuum model
PCM phase-change material
PCN P-doped g-CN
PCNNFs P-doped g-CN nanoflakes
P-CNTs purified carbon nanotubes
PCP pentachlorophenol
P(CPT-MAA) poly(camptothecin methacrylic acid)
PCR polymerase chain reaction
PCT procalcitonin
Pd palladium
PD-1 programmed cell death protein 1
PDA polydopamine
PDAC pancreatic ductal adenocarcinoma
PDDA poly(diallyl-dimethyl-ammonium-chloride)
$Pd_2(dba)_3$ palladium dibenzylideneacetone polymer
PDGF-BB platelet-derived growth factor B-chain
PDK I pyruvate dehydrogenase kinase I
PD-L1 programmed cell death ligand 1
PDMS polydimethylsiloxane
$_P$DNA plasmid DNA
$Pd(OAc)_2$ oxime carbapalladacycle
PDOS projected electronic density of states
PD phenylenediamine
PDA polydopamine
PDI photodynamic inactivation
PDI perylene diimide
PDMS polydimethylsiloxane
PDs Parkinson's diseases
PDT photodynamic therapy
PE plasma-enhanced
PEC photoelectrochemical
PE-CVD plasma-enhanced chemical vapor deposition
PEDOT poly-(3,4-ethylene dioxythiophene)
PEDOT-PSS-G poly-(3,4-ethylene dioxythiophene)/polystyrene sulfonate-functionalized graphene
PEEK polyether ether ketone
PEG polyethylene glycol
PEG-BT polyethylene glycol (PEG)–bentonite (BT)
PEG-b-PBLA poly(ethylene glycol)-block-poly(β-benzyl-L-aspartate)
PEG-CNTs polyethylene glycol carbon nanotubes
PEG-MWCNTs polyethylene glycol MWCNTs
PEI polyethylenimine
PEI polyetherimide
PEI poly(ether imide)
PEI-AU polyethylenimine–gold
PEI-GQDs polyethylenimine-functionalized GQDs
PEI-SA polyethyleneimine/sodium alginate
PEMFC proton exchange membrane fuel cell
PEO poly(ethylene oxide)
PEOX poly(2-ethyl-2-oxazoline)
PES polyethersulfone
PET positron emission tomography
PET photoinduced electron transfer
PF127 Pluronic F-127
PFA polyfluoroalkyl
PFM piezoelectric force microscopy
PGQDs pristine graphene quantum dots
P-GR-CdSe protected graphene—cadmium selenide
P-gp P-glycoprotein
PhA pheophorbide A
PHPMA-CNOs 4-hydroxyphenyl methacrylate-carbon nano-onions
p(HPMAm-Lacn poly(hydroxypropyl methacrylamide-lactate)
P3HT poly(3-hexylthiophene)
PI polyimide
PI propidium iodide; used as a marker of cell membrane permeability
pI isoelectric point
Pl-PEG phospholipid–PEG
PKA protein kinase A
pKa dissociation constant
PKU phenylketonuria
PL photoluminescence emission spectra
PL CDs photoluminescence carbon dots
PL peptide lipid
PLA polylactic acid
PLA pulsed laser ablation
PLE photoluminescence excitation spectrum
PLGA poly(lactic-*co*-glycolic acid) or polylactide-co-glycolide

PL GQDs	photoluminescence graphene quantum dots
PL-PEG	phospholipid–polyethylene glycol
PL QY	photoluminescence quantum yield (photons)
PM	powder metallurgy
PMF	potential of mean force
PMMA	polymethylmethacrylic acid
P(MAA-co-BAC)	poly(methacrylic acid-co-N,N-bis(acryloyl)cystamine
PMNs	polymorphonuclear leukocytes
PMO	phosphorodiamidate morpholino oligos
PMOA	poly(2-(2-methoxyethoxy)ethyl methacrylate-co-oligo(ethylene glycol) methacrylate-co-acrylic acid)
PmPV	poly(m-phenylenevinylene)
PMT	photomultiplier tube
pMWCNT	pristine multi-walled CNTs
P-MWNCNTs	prisitine multi-walled carbon nanotube
p-MWNTs	purified MWNTs
PNA	peptide nucleic acid
PNA-DRGON	peptide nucleic acid–dextran-coated reduced graphene oxide nanocolloid
pNIPAAm	poly(N-isopoprylacrylamide)
(P(NIPAAm-co-GMA-co-BAC)	poly(N-isopropylacrylamide-co-glycidyl methacrylate-co-N,N-bis(acryloyl)cystamine)
POC	point of care
POCT	point-of-care tests
POD	peroxidase
poMWCNTs	O_2-plasma-oxidized MWCNTs
POPC	1-palmitoyl-2-oleoyl-sn-glycero-3-phosphocholine
POSS	polyhedral oligomeric silsequioxane for superhydrophobicity
PP	polypropylene
PPAc	poly(phenyl acetylene)
PPD	paired pulse depression
pPD	para-phenylenediamine $(C_6H_4(NH_2)_2$
PPE	personal protective equipment
PPEI-EI	poly(propionyl ethyleneimine-co-ethyleneimine)
PPID	human peptidyl-prolyl cis-trans isomerase D
PPT	photothermal therapy
PPT	plasmonic photothermal
PPV	porcine parvovirus
PPy	polypyrrole
PPy-co-PAni	polypyrrole-co-polyaniline
PR	progesterone receptor
pRF-GQDs	pH-responsive fluorescent graphene quantum dots
PS	photosensitizer
PS	polystyrene
PS	photosystem
PSA	prostate-specific antigen
PS-b-PMMA NFs	poly (styrene-block-methyl methacrylate) nanofibers
PSCs	pancreatic stellate cells
PSF	polysulfone
PSF	phagolysosomal simulant fluid
PSI	post-PSII inhibitor
PS-PDMS	polystyrene-bpolydimethylsiloxane
PS-PDMS BCP	polystyrene-bpolydimethylsiloxane block copolymers
PSS	polystyrene sulfonate
PSS	polysodium 4-styrenesulfonate
PSs	photosensitizers
Pt	platinum
Pt@CNOs	platinum-decorated carbon nano-onions
PT-APS	photothermal-assisted plasmonic sensing method
PtBz	complex cis,cis,trans-$[Pt(NH_3)_2Cl_2(O_2CC_6H_5)_2]$
PTCDA	3,4,9,10-perylenetetracarboxylic dianhydride
PTC-NH$_2$	amino functionalized 3,4,9,10-perylenetetracarboxylic dianhydride
PTEN	phosphatase and tensin homologue
PTFE	polytetrafluoroethylene
PtNCs	Pt nanochains
PtNPs	Pt nanoparticles
PTT	photothermal therapy
PTX	paclitaxel
PU	polyurethane
PVA	polyvinyl alcohol
PVA/PMA$_{SH}$	poly(methacrylic acid)–grafted poly(vinyl alcohol) copolymer
PVB	polyvinyl butyral
PVD	physical vapor deposition
PVDF	polyvinylidene fluoride
PVP	poly(4-vinlypyridine)
PXM	product experience management
PZ	piezoelectric crystals
PZA	pyrazinamide
(Q)	
Qbd	quality by design
QC	2″,3′-dinitro-[1,1′:4′,1″;4″,1‴-quaterphenyl]-4,4‴-dicarboxylate
QCM	quartz crystal microbalance
QDs	quantum dots
QD-BSA	quantum dots–bovine serum albumin
QE	quantum efficiency
QM	quantum mechanics
QoL	quality of life
qPCR	real-time polymerase chain reaction
QPEIs	quaternized hyperbranched poly(ethyleneimine) derivatives
qRT-PCR	quantitative real-time polymerase chain reaction
QSAR	quantitative structure–activity relationship
qsNPs	quasi-spherical nanoparticles

QSPR quantitative structure–property relationship
QTAIM quantum theory of atoms in molecules
QY quantum yield

(R)

R^2 linear coefficient correlation
223Ra radium-223
RAFT reversible addition–fragmentation chain transfer
RAMD randomly accelerated molecular dynamics simulation
RANK receptor activator of nuclear factor-kappa B (RANK)
RANKL receptor activator of NF-κB ligand
RBD receptor-binding domain
RBM radial breathing mode or radial breathing model
R-BF-CQDs red bandgap fluorescent carbon quantum dots
RBITC Rhodamine B isothiocyanate
RBS random blood sugar
RCA rolling circle amplification
RDF radial distribution function
RDG reduced density gradient
rDNA ribosomal DNA, DNA sequence that codes for ribosomal RNA
RdRp RNA-dependent RNA polymerase gene of the SARS-CoV-2
RDV remdesivir
RDV-TP remdesivir triphosphate
RES reticuloendothelial system
RET resonance energy transfer
RF radio frequency
RF-CVD radio frequency chemical vapor deposition
RF-QDs radio frequency quantum dots
RFP red fluorescent protein
Rg3 ginsenoside
Rg3-CNT MWNTs-loaded ginsenoside Rg3
RGB red, green, and blue
RGD arginyl-glycyl-aspartic acid
RGD-CS-SWCNT-DTX arginylglycylaspartic acid–chitosan–docetaxel–SWCNT complex
RGO reduced graphene oxide
rGO/PEG/ICG reduced graphene oxide/polyethylene glycol/indocyanine green
rGQDs reduced graphene quantum dots
Rh–B Rhodamine-B
$RhCl(PPh_3)_3$ tris(triphenylphosphine)rhodium(I) chloride
Rh/3D-GA Rh-decorated three-dimensional graphene aerogel
rHDL reconstituted high-density lipoprotein
Rho rhodamine-110
RI red ink
RIU refractive index unit
RLNs infrared (NIR) objective lens/ PAL-50-NIR-L-LC07
RME receptor-mediated endocytosis
RMI relative membrane integrity
RMSD root mean square deviation
RMSF root mean square fluctuations
r-MWNTs raw multiple-walled carbon nanotubes
RNA ribonucleic acid
RNAi RNA interference
R-NBE-T-CQDs red narrow-bandwidth emission triangular CQDs
RO reverse osmosis
ROC receiver operating characteristic
ROM rule of mixture
ROMP ring-opening metathesis copolymerization
ROS reactive oxygen species
RRA relative recovered activities
RSDs relative standard deviations
RSM response surface methodology
RSV respiratory syncytial virus
RT radiation therapy
R–T resistance–temperature
RTM resin transfer molding method
RT-PCR real-time-based polymerase chain reaction
RT-qPCR quantitative RT-PCR detection
RT–RDT radiotherapy–radiodynamic therapy
$Ru(bpy)_3^{2+}$ tris (2, 2'-bipyridine) ruthenium (2+) ion
RVP reporter virus particles
Rxn reversible reaction

(S)

(S) spike glycoprotein
SA South Africa
SAb pike (S) protein antibody
SAED selected-area electron-diffraction
SAg spike (S) antigen
SAM self-assembled monolayer
SARS severe acute respiratory syndrome
SARS-CoV severe acute respiratory syndrome coronavirus
SARS-CoV-2 severe acute respiratory syndrome coronavirus-2
SARS-CoV-2 RdRps severe acute respiratory syndrome coronavirus-2 RNA–dependent RNA polymerase
SASA solvent accessible surface area
SBA-15 Santa Barbara amorphous-15
S_{BET} specific surface area calculated by the BET method
s-BLMs supported bilayer lipid membranes
SBM Solomon, Bloembergen, and Morgan theory
SBS polystyrene-polybutadiene-polystyrene
SBS short-beam shear
SCD standard current divider
SCE saturated calomel reference electrode
SCN thiocyanate
$SCN/CoFe_2O_4$ S-doped g-CN and $CoFe_2O_4$

SCRF	self-consistent reaction field
S-D	source–drain
SD	standard deviation
SD	silver dendrites
SDBS	sodium dodecyl benzene sulfate
SDS	sodium dodecyl sulfate
SDS-PAGE	sodium dodecyl sulfate-polyacrylamide gel electrophoresis
SEBS	styrene ethylene butylene styrene
SEC	size-exclusion chromatography
SECM	scanning electrochemical microscopy
SEI	solid electrolyte interface
SELEX	systematic evolution of ligands by exponential enrichment
SEM	scanning electron microscopy
SERS	surface-enhanced Raman scattering
SFNs	silk fibroin nanoparticles
SG	specific gravity
SGA	S-doped g-CN nanotubes/graphene oxide aerogel
SGC-7901	human gastric cancer cell line
S-g-C_3N_4/FTO	S-doped g-CN–modified fluorine-doped tin oxide
S-g-CN–GCE	sensor of S-doped g-CN nanoflakes–modified glassy carbon electrode
sGNRs	silica-coated gold nanorods
SGQDs	sulfur-doped graphene quantum dots
SG-SWCNTs	specific gravity–single-walled carbon nanotubes
SH	spontaneous hypertensive
SH	thiolation
SHG	second harmonic generation
SH-g CDs	thiol-terminated CDs
SH-gC-Dots	thiol-terminated C-dots prepared from glycerol
SH-MWCNTs	thiol-functionalized multi-walled carbon nanotubes
shRNA	short hairpin RNA
Si	silicon
siBraf	siRNA raised against the B-raf oncogene
SiC	silicon carbide
SiG	silica gel
siGFP	siRNA against GFP
SiNPs	silica nanoparticles
siRFP	siRNA against RFP
siRNA	small interfering RNA
SIS	polystyrene-polyisoprene-polystyrene
SLA	stereolithography
SLG	single-layer graphene
SLGQDs	single-layer graphene quantum dots
SLN	solid lipid nanoparticles
SLN	sentinel lymph nodes
$SmCl_3$	samarium chloride
152$SmCl_3$	152-samarium chloride
SMD	steered molecular dynamics
SMRGO	sulfonated magnetic nanoparticles functionalized with rGO
SMU	source measure unit
SnO	stannous oxide
SNUR- MWCNT	significant new use rules–multi-walled carbon nanotubes
SO_3^{2-}	sulfite ion
$S_2O_8^{2-}$	peroxydisulfate ion
$S_2O_8^{2-}/O_2$	peroxydisulfate/oxygen
$SOCl_2$	thionyl chloride
SOCS1	suppressor of cytokine signaling 1
SOCT	sodium octanoate
SOD	superoxide dismutase
Sor	sorafenib
SPAN	sulfonated polyaniline
SPAN-MWCNT	composites of multi-walled carbon nanotubes and sulfonated polyaniline
SPARC	secreted protein, acidic and rich in cysteines
SPE	serum protein electrophoresis
SPE	screen-printed electrodes
SPECT	single-photon emission computed tomography
SPECT/CT	single-photon emission computed tomography/computed tomography
SPGE	screen-printed graphene electrodes
SPIONs	superparamagnetic iron oxide nanoparticles
SPIOs	superparamagnetic iron oxides
SPR	surface plasmon resonance
SPRM	selective progesterone receptor modulator
SPS	spark plasma sintering
SQE	static quenching effect
SRA	specific radioactivity
SSA	specific surface area
STDEV	standard deviation of the calculated average in the simulation
ssDNA	single-stranded DNA
ssRNA	single-stranded ribonucleic acid
sSWNT	single-walled carbon nanotube
STEM	scanning transmission electron microscopy
STEM-EELS	scanning transmission electron microscopy–electron energy loss spectroscopy
STEM-HAADF	scanning transmission electron microscopy–high angle annular dark field
STM	scanning tunneling microscopy
STNNE	stretchable and transparent nanofiber-networked electrode
SUTW	super ultra-thin window
SV	single vacancies
SW	single-walled
SWBNNT	single-walled boron nitride nanotubes
$SWCNT_{COOH}$	carboxylated single-walled carbon nanotubes
SWCNTFET	single-walled carbon nanotube field-effect transistor
SWCNTs	single-walled carbon nanotubes
s-SWCNTs	semiconducting SWCNTs

SWNTs	single-walled carbon nanotubes
SWV	square wave voltammetry

(T)

T1	longitudinal
T2	transverse
(T)	thymine
TA	tannins
ta-C	tetrahedral amorphous carbon
TAAs	tumor-associated antigens
TADF	thermally activated delayed fluorescence
TALENs	transcription activator-like effector nucleases
TAM	tumor-associated macrophages
TAT	thermoacoustic therapy
TATAT	5,5′,5″-(1,3,5-triazine-2,4,6-triyl) tris(azanediyl)triisophthalate
TATB	1,3,5-triamino-2,4,6-trinitrobenzene
Taxol	paclitaxel
TB	thrombin
TB	tight binding
TBA	tetrabutyl alcoholic
TBA1	thrombin capture aptamer
TBA2	aptamer of thrombin
TBAB	tetrabutyl ammonium bromide
TBA^+ClO4^-	tetrabutylammonium perchlorate
TBB	5,10,15,20-tetra(p-benzoato) bacteriochlorin
TBEV	tick-borne virus
TBP	5,10,15,20-tetra(p-benzoato)porphyrin
TC	tetracycline
99Tc	Technetium-99
TCA	tricarboxylic acid
TCB	trichlorobenzene
1,3,5-TCB	1,s3,5-trichlorobenzene
TCE	trichloroethane
TCFs	transparent conducting films
TCM	traditional Chinese medicine
TCNEO-C60	1,2-(1′,1′,2′,2′-tetracyanomethanoxymethano) C_{60}
T-CQDs	triangular CQDs
TD-DFT	time-dependent density functional theory
TDOS	tape/disk operating system
TEA	triethylamine
TEG	tri(ethylene glycol)
TEM	transmission electron micrograph
TEY	total electron yield
Tf	transferrin
TFA	trifluoroacetic acid
TFCs	thin-film composites
TFNs	thin-film nanocomposites
TFTs	thin-film transistors
TG	thermogravimetric
Tg	transition temperature
TGA	thermogravimetric analysis
TGF-β1	transforming growth factor-β type I
TGFβR1	TGFβ type I receptor
TGM	tangent G-module
TGN	trans-Golgi network
THF	tetrahydrofuran $(CH_2)_4O$
THFF	tetrahydrofurfuryl
THP-1	acute human monocyte leukemia cell line
THPP	tetra-phenyl-porphyrin
Thr	threonine
THRI	temperature heat-resistance index
TIMs	thermal interface materials
TINKER	a complete and general package for molecular mechanics and dynamics
Ti_2N QDs	titanium nitride quantum dots
$Ti(OC_4H_9)_4$	titanium (IV) butoxide
TLC	thin-layer chromatography
TLR9	toll-like receptor-9
TM	mean residence lifetime
TMA	trimesic acid
TMA	trimethylamine
TMAC	tetramethylammonium chloride
TMA-C_{60}	tris(malonic)acid-C_{60}
TMB	3,3′,5,5′ tetramethylbenzidine
TMDCs	transition metal dichalcogenides
TMDC WSe_2	transition metal dichalcogenides tungsten diselenide
TME	tumor microenvironment
TMPRSS2	transmembrane protease, serine 2
TNBC	triple-negative breast cancer
TNBO	$TiNb_2O_7$
TNF-α	tumor necrosis factor-α
TNO	$TiNb_2O_7$
TNT	2,4,6-Trinitrotoluene
TOAB	tetraoctyl ammonium bromide
TP	thermoplastic polymers
TP	triphosphate
TP	two-photon
Tp	cloud point
TPCA	5-oxo-3,5-dihydro-2*H*-thiazolo [3,2-*α*] pyridine-7-carboxylic acid
TPD	temperature programmed desorption
TPDCA	5-oxo-3,5-dihydro-2*H*-thiazolo [3,2-*α*] pyridine-3,7-dicarboxylic acid
TP-DMT	thermoplasmonic-assisted dual-mode transducing biosensing system
TPEF	two-photon excitation fluorescence
TPGS	D-α-tocopheryl polyethylene glycol succinate
TPP	tetraphenylporphyrin
TPP	triphenylphosphine
TPrA	tripropylamine
TPs	thermoplastic polymers
T-PSA	total prostate-specific antigen
TR	rotational correlation time
TRFN	time-resolved fluorescence nanobeads
TRG	thermally reduced graphene oxide
TRIS–HCl	trihydroxymethyl aminomethane hydrochloride buffer
TRL	technology readiness level

TRY trypsin
TS thermal spraying
TSAs tumor-specific antigens
TSTU N,N,N',N'-tetramethyl(succinimido) uronium tetrafluoroborate
TTA1 trauma team activation
TTCE tetrachloroethane
TTDDA 4,7,10-trioxa-1,13-tridecanediamine
TTHA triethylenetetranitrilohexaacetic acid
TTR transthyretin
TvL Trametes versicolor laccase
TYR tyrosinase
(U)
UCNPs upconversion nanoparticles
UCNs upconverting nanomaterials
UCPL up-conversion photoluminescence
UCST upper critical solution temperature
UGAs unidirectional graphene aerogels
UiO Zr-based metal–organic framework
ULN upper limit normal
(UO)-SWCNTs ultra-oxide single-walled carbon nanotubes
(US)-SWCNTs ultrashort single-walled carbon nanotubes
UV ultraviolet
UVA ultraviolet A radiation between the wavelengths of 315 and 400 nm
UVB ultraviolet B radiation between the wavelengths of 280 and 315 nm
UVC ultraviolet C radiation between the wavelengths of 100 and 280 nm
UV-vis ultraviolet-visible
UV-Vis-NIR ultraviolet-visible near-infrared
(V)
VA Veterans Health Administration
VACNT vertically aligned carbon nanotube
VANTAs vertically aligned carbon nanotube arrays
VB valence band
VC vitamin C
VCD vibration circular spectroscopy
VDC volts of direct current
Vds fixed bias voltage
vdW van der Waals
VEGF vascular endothelial growth factor
V–FITC annexin V binding to apoptotic cells
VGS source gate voltage
Vis visible spectroscopy
VLB vinblastine
VLPs virus-like particles
Vm membrane potential
VMD visual molecular dynamics
VN @C vanadium nitride–coated CNT
VPBA 4-vinylphenylboronic acid
VPc vanadium-phthalocyanine
VPE vapor-phase epitaxy
VRH variable-range hopping model
VSFG vibrational sum-frequency generation spectroscopy
V_T threshold voltage
V_{th} threshold voltage
(W)
WAXD wide-angle X-ray diffraction
WBCs white blood cells
WCA water contact angle
WCDs white fluorescent carbon dots
WCl_6 tungsten hexachloride
WHO World Health Organization
WKY Wistar-Kyoto
WLED white light–emitting diode
WNV West Nile virus
WO_3/g-C_3N_4 tungsten trioxide and graphitic carbon nitride composite materials
WPU water polyurethane
WS_2 tungsten disulfide
wsCNO water-soluble carbon nano-onion
WSe2 tungsten diselenide
(X)
XANES X-ray absorption near-edge structure
XAS X-ray absorption spectroscopy
XeF2 xenon difluoride
XGO xanthogranulomatous orchiepididymitis
XPS X-ray photoelectron spectroscopy
XRD X-ray diffraction
XRF X-ray fluorescence analysis
(Y)
90Y yttrium-90
YAG neodymium-doped yttrium aluminum garnet
YFV yellow fever virus
(Y)-GQDs yellow GQDs
(Z)
ZE Zinnia elegans plants
ZET zebrafish embryo toxicity
ZnCDs zinc-coadsorbed CD nanocomposite
ZGNRs zigzag graphene nanoribbons
ZIF zeolitic imidazolate framework
ZIF-8 zeolitic imidazolate framework-8
ZIKV Zika virus
Zn zinc
ZnO zinc oxide
ZnP zinc phthalocyanine
ZnPc zinc phthalocyanine
ZnS zinc sulfide
ZOL zoledronic acid
ZPE zero-point energy
ZPVE zero-point vibrational energy

Bibliography

Bellet, P., M. Gasparotto, S. Pressi, A. Fortunato, G. Scapin, M. Mba, E. Menna, F. Filippini, Graphene-based scaffolds for regenerative medicine, *Nanomaterials* 11 (2021) 404.

Bhol, P., S. Yadav, A. Altaee, M. Saxena, P.K. Misra, A.K. Samal, Graphene-based membranes for water and wastewater treatment: A review, *ACS Appl. Nano Mater.* 4 (2021) 3274–3293.

Camisasca, A., S. Giordani, Carbon nano-onions in biomedical applications: Promising theranostic agents, *Inorg. Chim. Acta.* 468 (2017) 67–76.

Cui, H., Y. Guo, Z. Zhou, Three-dimensional graphene-based macrostructures for electrocatalysis, *Small* 17 (2021) 2005255.

De Maio, Flavio, Enrico Rosa, et al., 3D-printed graphene polylactic acid devices resistant to SARS-CoV-2: Sunlight-mediated sterilization of additive manufactured objects, *Carbon* 194 (July 2022) 34–41, https://doi.org/10.1016/j.carbon.2022.03.036

Han, J., H. Li, Q.-H. Yang, Compact energy storage enabled by graphenes: Challenges, strategies and progress, *Mater. Today* 51 (2021) 552–565.

Hibino, H., H. Kageshima, M.J.N.T.R. Nagase, Graphene growth on silicon carbide, 8 (8) (2010).

Jampilek, Josef, Katarina Kralova, Advances in drug delivery nanosystems using graphene-based materials and carbon nanotubes, *Materials* 14 (2021) 1059, https://doi.org/10.3390/ma14051059

Katuwavila, N.P., Y. Amarasekara, V. Jayaweera, C. Rajaphaksha, C. Gunasekara, I.C. Perera, G.A.J. Amaratunga, L. Weerasinghe, Graphene oxide-based nanocomposite for sustained release of cephalexin, *J. Pharm. Sci.* 109 (2020) 1130–1135.

Keshwani, Gaurav, Jiten Chandra Dutta, CNT based high-κ dielectric ion sensitive field effect transistor based cholesterol biosensor, *Curr. Trends Biotechnol. Pharm.* 15 (2) (April 2021) 182–188, ISSN:0973-8916 (Print), 2230–7303.

Kim, S.D., A. Sarkar, J.-H. Ahn, Graphene-based nanomaterials for flexible and stretchable batteries, *Small* 17 (2021) 2006262.

Lehto, M., Karilainen, T., Roìg, T., Cramariuc, O., Vanhala, E., Tornaeus, J., et al. (2014). Co-exposure with fullerene may strengthen health effects of organic industrial chemicals. *PLoS One* 9:e114490. doi:10.1371/journal.pone.0114490

Liu et al., Water-soluble supramolecular fullerene assembly mediated by metallobridged β-cyclodextrins, *Angew. Chem. Int. Ed.* 43 (2004) 2690–2694.

Lu, H., J. Tournet, K. Dastafkan, Y. Liu, Y.H. Ng, S.K. Karuturi, C. Zhao, Z. Yin, Noble-metal-free multicomponent nanointegration for sustainable energy conversion, *Chem. Rev.* 121 (2021) 10271–10366.

Madkour, Loutfy H., *Nanoelectronic Materials: Fundamentals and Applications* (2019), Springer Nature, Softcover ISBN: 978-3-030-21623-8, Hardcover ISBN: 978-3-030-21620-7, eBook ISBN: 978-3-030-21621-4, https://doi.org/10.1007/978-3-030-21621-4

Madkour, Loutfy H., *Nucleic Acids as Gene Anticancer Drug Delivery Therapy* (2019), Academic Press, Copyright © 2019 Elsevier Inc., ISBN: 978-0-12-819777-6, https://doi.org/10.1016/C2019-0-00456-6

Madkour, Loutfy H., *Reactive Oxygen Species (ROS), Nanoparticles, and Endoplasmic Reticulum (ER) Stress-Induced Cell Death Mechanisms* (2020), Academic Press, Copyright © 2020, Elsevier Inc., ISBN: 978-0-12-822481-6, https://doi.org/10.1016/C2019-0-04102-7

Madkour, Loutfy H., *Nanoparticles-Based Drug Delivery in Cancer Treatment* (2022), CRC Press, ISBN: 9781003229674, https://doi.org/10.1201/9781003229674

Madkour, Loutfy H., *RNA Delivery Function for Anticancer Therapeutics* (2022), CRC Press, ISBN: 9781003229650, https://doi.org/10.1201/9781003229650

Madkour, Loutfy H., Anticorrosive carbon-based polymer and epoxy nanocomposite coatings, *Handbook of Research on Corrosion Sciences and Engineering*, edited by Younes El Kacimi, Lei Guo (2023), IGI Global, pp. 86–134, https://doi.org/10.4018/978-1-6684-7689-5.ch005

Madkour, Loutfy H., Carbon nanotubes—based intelligent platform for cancer vaccine co-delivery nanocarriers immunotherapy achievements: Challenges in vitro and in vivo, *Int. J. Nurs. Care Res.* 1 (2) (2023) 1–55.

Madkour, Loutfy H., Corrosion resistance potential of metal-matrix composites reinforced with carbon nanofibers and carbon nanotubes, *Handbook of Research on Corrosion Sciences and Engineering*, edited by Younes El Kacimi, Lei Guo (2023), IGI Global, pp. 135–188, Book chapter. https://doi.org/10.4018/978-1-6684-7689-5.ch006. ISBN13: 9781668476895| ISBN10: 1668476894| EISBN13: 9781668476901

Madkour, Loutfy H., Eco-friendly green biosynthesized metallic nanoparticles and biotechnological applications in pharmaceuticals sciences, *J. Mater. Sci. Eng. B.* 13 (1–3) (2023) 1–69, https://doi.org/10.17265/2161-6221/2023.1-3.001; https://www.davidpublisher.com/Public/uploads/Contribute/64866c1700971.pdf

Madkour, Loutfy H., Graphitic carbon nitride quantum dots (g-C3N4): Fundamentals and applications, *Int. Res. J. Basic Clinical Stud.* 8 (4) (August 2023) 1–14, https://doi.org/10.14303/irjbcs.2023.48

Malik, S., S. Marchesan, Growth, properties, and applications of branched carbon nanostructures, *Nanomaterials* 11 (2021) 2728.

Mamidi, N., J. Villela Castrejón, A. González-Ortiz, Rational design and engineering of carbon nano-onions reinforced natural protein nanocomposite hydrogels for biomedical applications, *J. Mech. Behav. Biomed. Mater.* 104 (2020) 103696.

McDonald, A.G., K.F. Tipton, Enzyme nomenclature and classification: The state of the art. *FEBS J.* 290 (9) (2023) 2214–2231, 2021 Federation of European Biochemical Societies, https://doi.org/10.1111/febs.16274

Onyancha, R.B., U.O. Aigbe, K.E. Ukhurebor, P.W. Muchiri, A facile review on the synthesis and applications of carbon nanotubes in heavy-metal remediation and biomedical fields, *J. Mol. Struct.* 1238 (2021) 130462.

Poojari, C., Wilkosz, N., Lira, R. B., Dimova, R., Jurkiewicz, P., Petka, R., et al. (2019). Behavior of the DPH fluorescence probe in membranes perturbed by drugs. *Chem. Phys. Lipids* 223:104784. doi: 10.1016/j.chemphyslip.2019.104784

Rahamathulla, M., R.R. Bhosale, R.A.M. Osmani, et al. Carbon nanotubes: Current perspectives on diverse applications in targeted drug delivery and therapies, *Materials* 14 (2021) 6707.

Reina, G., D. Iglesias, P. Samori, A. Bianco, Graphene: A disruptive opportunity for COVID-19 and future pandemics? *Adv. Mater.* 33 (2021) 2007847.

Rowley-Neale, S.J., E.P. Randviir, A.S. Abo Dena, C.E. Banks, An overview of recent applications of reduced graphene oxide as a basis of electroanalytical sensing platforms, *Appl. Mater. Today* 10 (2018) 218–226.

Salah, Lakhdar Sidi, Nassira Ouslimani, Dalila Bousba, Isabelle Huynen, Yann Danlée, Hammouche Aksas, Carbon nanotubes (CNTs) from synthesis to functionalized (CNTs) using conventional and new chemical approaches, *J. Nanomaterials* (2021) Article ID 4972770, 31 pages, https://doi.org/10.1155/2021/4972770

Saleemi, M.A., M.H. Fouladi, P.V.C. Yong, K. Chinna, N.K. Palanisamy, E.H. Wong, Toxicity of carbon nanotubes: Molecular mechanisms, signaling cascades, and remedies in biomedical applications, *Chem. Res. Toxicol.* 34 (2021) 24–46.

Sepideh, Ketabi, Leila Rahmani, Carbon nanotube as a carrier in drug delivery system for carnosine dipeptide: A computer simulation study, *Mater. Sci. Eng. C.* 73 (2017) 173–181, http://dx.doi.org/10.1016/j.msec.2016.12.058

Shanmugam, Kalaiselvan, J. Manivannan, M. Manjuladevi, *Stupendous Nanomaterials: Carbon Nanotubes Synthesis, Characterization, and Applications*, edited by Simona Clichici (2020), IntechOpen Book Series, ISBN: 978-1-78984-617-1, https://doi.org/10.5772/intechopen.90318; https://www.intechopen.com/chapters/70356

Sidi Salah, L., N. Ouslimani, M. Chouai, Y. Danlée, I. Huynen, H. Aksas, Predictive optimization of electrical conductivity of polycarbonate composites at different concentrations of carbon nanotubes: A valorization of conductive nanocomposite theoretical models, *Materials* 14 (7) (2021) 1687.

Tang, Lu, Qiaqia Xiao, Yijun Mei, Shun He, Ziyao Zhang, Ruotong Wang, Wei Wang, Insights on functionalized carbon nanotubes for cancer theranostics, *J. Nanobiotechnology* 19 (423) (2021) 1–28.

von Ranke, Natalia L., Helena Carla Castro, Carlos R. Rodrigues, Molecular modelling and dynamics simulations of single-wall carbon nanotube as a drug carrier: New insights into the drug-loading process, *J. Mol. Graph. Model.* 113 (June 2022) 108145, https://doi.org/10.1016/j.jmgm.2022.108145

Wang, C., M. Muni, V. Strauss, A. Borenstein, X. Chang, A. Huang, S. Qu, K. Sung, T. Gilham, R.B. Kaner, Graphene's role in emerging trends of capacitive energy storage, *Small* 17 (2021) 2006875.

Winkler, K., A.L. Balch, Electrochemically formed two-component films comprised of fullerene and transition-metal components, *C. R. Chim.* 9 (2006) 928–943.

Zhao, Q., Miriyala, N., Su, Y., Chen, W., Gao, X., Shao, L., et al. (2018). Computer-aided formulation design for a highly soluble lutein-cyclodextrin multiple-component delivery system. *Mol. Pharm.* 15, 1664–1674. doi: 10.1021/acs.molpharmaceut.8b00056

Index

Note: Page numbers in *italic* indicate figures and schemes, and those in **bold** indicate tables.

C

D

N

For Product Safety Concerns and Information please contact our EU
representative GPSR@taylorandfrancis.com
Taylor & Francis Verlag GmbH, Kaufingerstraße 24, 80331 München, Germany

www.ingramcontent.com/pod-product-compliance
Lightning Source LLC
LaVergne TN
LVHW080120011026
849160LV00013B/1140
* 9 7 8 1 0 3 2 6 3 5 9 6 5 *